Student Resources

Online Student Resources are **included** with this textbook.
Visit **http://nursing.pearsonhighered.com** for the following assets and activities:

- Learning Outcomes
- Chapter Review Questions
- Case Studies

- Nursing Process Applications
- Application Activities
- Content Updates

- Weblinks
- Links to additional nursing resources

Additional resources available. For more information and purchasing options visit **nursing.pearsonhighered.com**

CLASSROOM

mynursinglab

- MyNursingLab provides you with a one-of-a-kind *guided learning path*. Its proven personalized study plan helps you to *synthesize vast amounts of information* with an engaging **REVIEW**, **REMEMBER**, and **APPLY** approach. Move *from memorization to true understanding* through application with:
  - Even more alternate-item format questions
  - More analysis and application level questions that gauge true understanding
  - An interactive eText (also available via iPad®) with multimedia resources built right in

CLINICAL

Pearson's Nurse's Drug Guide

- Published annually to be your current, comprehensive, and clinically relevant source for drug information

- Your complete mobile solution!

Real Nursing Skills

- Video demonstrations of over 200 clinical nursing skills
- Each skill includes Purpose, Preparation, Procedure, Post-Procedure, Expected and Unexpected Outcomes, Documentation and References and Resources

NCLEX®

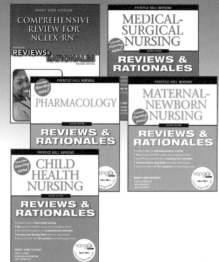

- Concentrated review of core content
- Thousands of practice questions with comprehensive rationales

---

PEARSON

ALWAYS LEARNING

PEARSON NURSING CLASS PREPARATION RESOURCES

New and Unique!

- Use this preparation tool to find animations, videos, images, and other media resources that cross the nursing curriculum! Organized by topic and fully searchable by resource type and key word, this easy-to-use platform allows you to:
  - Search through the media library of assets
  - Upload your own resources
  - Export to PowerPoint™ or HTML pages

Use this tool to find and review other unique instructor resources:

Correlation Guide to Nursing Standards

- Links learning outcomes of core textbooks to nursing standards such as the 2010 ANA Scope and Standards of Practice, QSEN Competencies, National Patient Safety Goals, AACN, Essentials of Baccalaureate Education and more!

Pearson Nursing Lecture Series

- Highly visual, fully narrated and animated, these short lectures focus on topics that are traditionally difficult to teach and difficult for students to grasp
- All lectures accompanied by case studies and classroom response questions for greater interactivity within even the largest classroom
- Use as lecture tools, remediation material, homework assignments and more!

MYTEST AND ONLINE TESTING

- Test questions even **more accessible** now with both pencil and paper (MyTest) and online delivery options (Online Testing)
- **NCLEX®-style** questions
- **All New!** Approximately 30% of all questions are in alternative-item format
- **Complete rationales** for correct and incorrect answers mapped to learning outcomes

BOOK-SPECIFIC RESOURCES
Also available to instructors:

- **Instructor's Manual and Resource Guide** organized by learning outcome
- Comprehensive **PowerPoint™** presentations integrating lecture notes and images
- **Image library**
- **Classroom Response Questions**
- **Online course management systems** complete with instructor tools and student activities

mynursinglab

- **Proven Results:** Pearson's MyLab/Mastering platform has helped millions of students
- Provide your students with a one-of-a-kind guided learning path and personalized study plan! An engaging **REVIEW**, **REMEMBER**, and **APPLY** approach moves students from memorization to true understanding through application with:
  - Even more alternate-item format questions
  - More analysis and application level questions
  - An interactive eText (also available via iPad®) with multimedia resources built right in
- **Trusted Partner:** A network of customer experience managers and faculty advocates are available to help instructors maximize learning gains with MyNursingLab.

REAL NURSING SIMULATIONS

- 25 simulation scenarios that span the nursing curriculum
- Consistent format includes learning objectives, case flow, set-up instructions, debriefing questions and more!
- Companion online course cartridge with student pre-and post-simulation activities, videos, skill checklists and reflective discussion questions

Real Nursing SIMULATIONS *Facilitator's Guide* Institutional Edition

Partnering With Clients and Families

Rx Communication

What Every Nurse Should Know

Why I Became a Psychiatric–Mental Health Nurse

Why I Plan to Become a Psychiatric–Mental Health Nurse

Your Assessment Approach

Contemporary Psychiatric–Mental Health Nursing

Third Edition

Carol Ren Kneisl
Eileen Trigoboff

PEARSON

Boston   Columbus   Indianapolis   New York   San Francisco   Upper Saddle River
Amsterdam   Cape Town   Dubai   London   Madrid   Milan   Munich   Paris   Montreal   Toronto
Delhi   Mexico City   São Paulo   Sydney   Hong Kong   Seoul   Singapore   Taipei   Tokyo

This book is dedicated to Daniel H. Trigoboff, PhD.
Because of you I have seen a better world,
with you I experience the magnificence of life,
and from you I feel the energy to evolve and grow forever.

Publisher: Julie Levin Alexander
Publisher's Assistant: Regina Bruno
Senior Acquisitions Editor: Kim Norbuta
Development Editor: Michael Giacobbe
Editorial Assistant: Marion Gottlieb
Supplement Editor: Molly Ward
Managing Production Editor: Patrick Walsh
Production Liaison: Cathy O'Connell
Production Editor: Lynn Steines, S4Carlisle
   Publishing Services
Manufacturing Manager: Ilene Sanford
Art Director: Christopher Weigand
Interior and Cover Designer: Marta Samsel

Art Editor: Patricia Gutierrez
Director of Marketing: David Gesell
Senior Marketing Manager: Phoenix Harvey
Marketing Specialist: Michael Sirinides
Media Product Manager: Travis Moses-Westphal
Assistant Editor for Media: Sarah Wrocklage
Media Project Managers: Rachel Collett
   and Leslie Brado
Composition: S4Carlisle Publishing Services
Printer/Binder: Courier/Kendallville
Cover Printer: LeHigh Phoenix Color/Hagerstown
Cover Image: shutterstock/fotoecho
Text Font: Times LT Std Roman

Credits and acknowledgments for content borrowed from other sources and reproduced, with permission, in this textbook appear on appropriate page within text or on copyright page.

Photo credits: Unit Openers 1 and 5: Stanislaw Tokarski/Shutterstock; Unit Opener 2: Muellek Josef/Shutterstock; Unit Opener 3: Howard Sandler/Shutterstock; Unit Opener 4: Adam Michal Ziaga/Shutterstock; Unit Opener 6: Lizette Potgieter/Shutterstock

Notice: Care has been taken to confirm the accuracy of information presented in this book. The authors, editors, and the publisher, however, cannot accept any responsibility for errors or omissions or for consequences from application of the information in this book and make no warranty, express or implied, with respect to its contents.

The authors and publisher have exerted every effort to ensure that drug selections and dosages set forth in this text are in accord with current recommendations and practice at time of publication. However, in view of ongoing research, changes in government regulations, and the constant flow of information relating to drug therapy and drug reactions, the reader is urged to check the package inserts of all drugs for any change in indications of dosage and for added warnings and precautions. This is particularly important when the recommended agent is a new and/or infrequently employed drug.

Library of Congress Cataloging-in-Publication Data
Kneisl, Carol Ren.
   Contemporary psychiatric-mental health nursing / Carol Ren Kneisl, Eileen Trigoboff. — 3rd ed.
      p. ; cm.
   Includes bibliographical references and index.
   ISBN-13: 978-0-13-255777-1
   ISBN-10: 0-13-255777-0
   I. Trigoboff, Eileen.   II. Title.
   [DNLM: 1. Mental Disorders—nursing.   2. Psychiatric Nursing—methods. WY 160]
   616.89'0231—dc23

                                                                2011040215

10 9 8 7 6 5 4 3

PEARSON

ISBN-10:   0-13-255777-0
ISBN-13: 978-0-13-255777-1

CAROL REN KNEISL, RN, MS, APRN, DABFN, has had a variety of psychiatric–mental health nursing experiences. She has taught psychiatric–mental health nursing in diploma, baccalaureate, and master's programs that prepared clinical specialists in psychiatric–mental health nursing. She has been a staff nurse, a nurse manager, a nursing supervisor, a clinical nurse specialist, and has supervised the group therapy of clinical nurse specialists and psychiatry medical residents. She is currently an adjunct professor of psychiatric–mental health nursing at William Carey University in New Orleans, Louisiana.

Carol is also a nurse entrepreneur. She founded Nursing Transitions, a corporation that provided continuing education for psychiatric–mental health and corrections/forensic nurses. Her company sponsored the first national nursing conference focused on AIDS. She is a national and international speaker and consults with nurses and mental health and forensic agencies on topics such as group therapy, stress management, self-awareness issues and strategies, implementation of client rights, legal aspects, and creative clinical teaching in psychiatric–mental health nursing.

Carol has authored or contributed to 28 nursing textbooks and several nursing journals. She has been an associate editor of a psychiatric nursing review journal and has served on several editorial boards.

Carol was among the first nurses in the country to develop clinical specialist certification in conjunction with nurses from New York and New Jersey. Their work formed the basis for the national certification granted through the American Nurses Credentialing Center of the American Nurses Association.

She is a graduate of a diploma school, the Millard Fillmore Hospital School of Nursing in Buffalo, New York, from which she received the Alumna of the Century award on the occasion of the school's 100-year anniversary. Carol has a BS in nursing from the University of Buffalo, an MS in nursing as a clinical nurse specialist in adult psychiatric–mental health nursing from the University of California at San Francisco, and has pursued graduate education in community mental health administration and interpersonal communication from the State University of New York at Buffalo.

Carol is the mother of two adult children—a daughter who is a right-brained special effects artist and a son who is a left-brained mathematician and the father of her two grandchildren. When she is not commuting to New Orleans she writes and consults from her home on a Gulf of Mexico beach in Orange Beach, Alabama.

EILEEN TRIGOBOFF, RN, PMHCNS-BC, DNS, DABFN, CIP, is a Clinical Nurse Specialist with a specialty in Adult Psychiatry–Mental Health in a private psychotherapy practice in western New York. An important part of her practice is the national and international interdisciplinary supervision of, and consultation with, other mental health and health care professionals. Dr. Trigoboff is the Director of Program Evaluation at the Buffalo Psychiatric Center in Buffalo, New York and is the Liaison for the Office of Mental Health's Institutional Review Board. She has taught associate degree, bachelor's degree, and graduate-level nursing students on all aspects of the nursing process, research methodologies, statistics, psychiatric nursing, and pharmacology. Dr. Trigoboff is also the Research Preceptor for the Psychiatric Residency program at the State University of New York at Buffalo School of Pharmacy Doctoral Residency Program.

Dr. Trigoboff earned her BSN, her MS as a Clinical Nurse Specialist in psychiatric nursing, and her Doctorate in Nursing Science (DNS) in psychiatric nursing from the State University of New York at Buffalo. She received a National Institutes of Mental Health Individual National Research Service Award Pre-Doctoral Research Fellowship for her dissertation research on medication teaching and psychopharmacology. Dr. Trigoboff's research interests include cognitive–behavioral nursing interventions with seriously and persistently mentally ill clients and the safety and efficacy of neuroleptics. She is a Diplomate and Fellow in the American College of Forensic Examiners Board of Forensic Nurse Examiners, and is board certified as an Institutional Review Board Professional (CIP) and in hospital and program accreditation.

Eileen is author, coauthor, and contributor to 14 books and numerous journal articles. She presents internationally on a wide variety of clinical, research, and professional topics to health care, governmental, and corporate organizations. She continues to be an international speaker and consultant on topics including professional issues, assessment, psychopathologies, and interventions. She also serves on the editorial boards of several professional journals and is on the editorial panel for a magazine on anxiety and depression. She is active in community service venues, including clinical settings and family support groups. She also serves as a computer systems and statistical consultant and belongs to numerous professional nursing organizations.

Eileen enjoys her clinical psychologist husband, her Congo African Grey parrot, a large and loving family, good friends, international travel, and reading.

THANK YOU!

CONTRIBUTORS

We extend a heartfelt thanks to our contributors, who gave their time, effort, and expertise so tirelessly to the development and writing of chapters and resources.

TEXTBOOK CONTRIBUTORS

Carol Bradley-Corpuel, APRN, BC
Psychiatric Clinical Nurse Specialist
Saint Mary's Regional Medical Center
Reno, Nevada
Adjunct Clinical Faculty, Orvis School of Nursing
University of Nevada, Reno
Chapter 26: Adolescents

Sue C. DeLaune, MN, RN
Assistant Professor and Undergraduate Program Coordinator
William Carey University, School of Nursing
New Orleans, Louisiana
President and Education Director
S. DeLaune Consulting
Mandeville, Louisiana
Chapter 18: Anxiety Disorders
Chapter 19: Dissociative, Somatoform, and Factitious Disorders
Chapter 22: Personality Disorders
Chapter 35: Anger Management and Intervention in Psychiatric–Mental Health Settings

Karen Lee Fontaine, RN, MSN, AASECT
Professor
Purdue University Calumet
Hammond, Indiana
Chapter 20: Gender Identity and Sexual Disorders
Chapter 24: Intrafamily Violence: Physical and Sexual Abuse

STUDENT AND INSTRUCTOR RESOURCE CONTRIBUTORS

Melissa Black, MSN, RN, FNP, PhDc
Breckinridge School of Nursing, Greenville, South Carolina

Jane E. Bostick, RN, PhD, PMHCNS-BC
University of Missouri-Columbia, Columbia, Missouri

Amy Mitchell Corbitt, RN, MSN
ECPI University, Newport News, Virginia

Rose M. Kutlenios, RN, MN, MSN, PhD
Wheeling Jesuit University, Wheeling, West Virginia

Susan C. Maloney
Edinboro University of Pennsylvania, Edinboro, Pennsylvania

Cleo Newton-Watkins, RN, MS, PMHCNS-BC
D'Youville College, Buffalo, New York

REVIEWERS

The authors and publisher are grateful for the expertise provided by nursing faculty and clinicians who gave of their time to review chapters for this book and the material that accompanies it. Thank you for your generosity in sharing your insightful comments with us.

Virginia Byer RN, MSN
Community College of Baltimore, Catonsville, Maryland

Nancy Craig-Williams MS, RN, PhD
Greenfield Community College, Longmeadow, Massachusetts

Marianne Eichenberger RN, PhD
Community College of Baltimore, Baltimore, Maryland

Ginette Ferszt PhD, RN, PMHCNS-BC
University of Rhode Island, Kingston, Rhode Island

Norma Katz RN, PMHNP, BC, MS
Westchester Community College, Valhalla, New York

Ann Keeley RN, APRN-BC, PMH/CNS
Georgia Baptist College of Nursing, Atlanta, Georgia

Mary Leveillee PhD, RN, PCNS
University of Rhode Island, Kingston, Rhode Island

Doris Lippman APRN, EdD
Fairfield University, Fairfield, Connecticut

Gloria Mejia RN, BSN
Kenner, Louisiana

Marita Terese Peppard RN, ND, NS
Austin Community College, Leander, Texas

Leah Rowbotham MS, APRN, BC
Seton Hall University, Montclair, New Jersey

Helen Trotter APRN-NP
Southeast Community College, Lincoln, Nebraska

Alexandra Winter RN, MSN
Metropolitan Community College, Omaha, Nebraska

Millions of people around the world face the challenges that mental health disorders bring. In fact, new studies by World Health Organization (WHO) international researchers document that five of the ten leading causes of disability in the world today are psychiatric in nature. Worldwide, depression is the number-one health problem, followed by alcohol and drug abuse disorders and dementia of the Alzheimer's type, schizophrenia, and bipolar depression. At least 15% of persons with a medical illness have a co-occurring psychiatric illness, and almost half of all health-related disability in the United States and Canada can be directly attributed to psychiatric disorders. The prediction of the WHO investigators is that the burden of mental disorders will increase even more by the year 2020 because global mental health resources remain low and improvements in this past decade were minimal at best.

Adding to the challenges that mental health disorders bring is the stigma of mental illness. The stigma of mental illness is based on a societal perception that mental illness is a blemish of individual character. Stigmatizing mental illness is a worldwide problem experienced in all segments of society but is especially prevalent in deprived, marginalized, and minority communities. Stigma hurts, punishes, and diminishes people. Despite advances in psychiatric treatment, stigma continues to grow around the globe and is the main obstacle to better mental health care and quality of life for clients, families, communities, and staff members who deal with mental health disorders.

Our goal for this textbook, *Contemporary Psychiatric–Mental Health Nursing,* and its companion supplements is to provide students and practicing psychiatric–mental health nurses with the most up-to-date, evidence-based, culturally competent, authoritative, and comprehensive resource available and to present it in an accessible, clinically relevant, and professional format. The strategies we present in this book are designed to help you become a therapeutic, comfortable, successful, and safe psychiatric–mental health nurse. We encourage you to think seriously about what constitutes mental health and mental disorder, to appreciate the humanity of people who experience mental disorder, and to approach your psychiatric–mental health experience with confidence.

UNDERLYING THEMES

Throughout this edition, we remain true to the values of clinical competence, cultural competence in an increasingly diverse society, client-centered care, the relevance of meaning to shaping behavior and treatment choices, and the need to improve quality and access to mental health care. We believe that psychiatric–mental health nursing is concerned with the quality of human life and its relationship to optimal psychobiologic health, feelings of self-worth, personal integrity, self-fulfillment, spirituality, and creative expression. Thus, we emphasize the importance of empathy and empowerment in the nurse–client relationship.

Understanding people who are searching for meaning through interaction in complex times demands the most authoritative and contemporary knowledge and clinical competence. It is through the power of knowledge and clinical competence that psychiatric–mental health nurses can help clients from diverse cultures to live with uncertainty, unfamiliarity, and unpredictability and to pursue creative healing on psychobiologic and spiritual levels. The psychiatric–mental health nurse's scope of practice is broad enough to include issues such as alienation, identity crises, sudden life changes, and troubled family relationships. It may involve issues of poverty and affluence, cross-cultural disparities in access to health care, and the human experiences of birth, death, and loss. Psychiatric–mental health nursing is concerned with sustaining and enhancing the mental health of both the individual and the group, while its practice locale is often found in the community.

In exploring the theme of global mental health, each unit of this book opens with compelling photographs and stories of individuals from around the world who face stigmatization because of mental health issues. In presenting this global perspective and exploring science, art, and spirituality as a path toward our shared vision of global mental health, we hope to promote awareness of the relevance of those same global issues in our own culturally diverse society.

The themes, ideas, knowledge, tools, and organization of this textbook were expressly designed for psychiatric–mental health nursing students and clinicians who are committed to developing the habits of mind, responsibility, and practice that will make a difference in view of contemporary trends. Specifically, this text prepares students to tailor and humanize interventions for traditional as well as "new" psychiatric–mental health clients often encountered in forensic settings, homeless shelters, and in other community-based and rehabilitation-oriented settings. Furthermore, because advances in neuroscience and the study of the human genome are redefining our conception of the basis for mental disorders, a solid grounding in psychobiology is threaded throughout the book. Brain imaging assessment and concise yet comprehensive information on the expanding array of psychopharmacologic treatment is yet another strong emphasis. *Contemporary Psychiatric–Mental Health Nursing* is explicitly linked to contemporary trends in our field.

ORGANIZATION

The book is divided into six units. Unit One introduces you to the clients you will encounter, what it means to be a psychiatric–mental health nurse, the professional and personal attributes that enable artful therapeutic practice, and the importance of basing the therapeutic nurse–client relationship on theoretical understandings and appropriate clinical techniques. Unit Two clusters five chapters that provide comprehensive coverage of interdisciplinary psychiatric theories, the biologic basis of mental disorders, the science of psychophar-macology, the methods by which people attempt to handle stress, and the importance of developing cultural competence. In Unit Three, we address topics traditionally associated with psychiatric–mental health nursing, such as therapeutic communication, assessment, ethics, advocacy, clients' rights, legal and forensic issues, and therapeutic environments for care. Unit Four focuses on caring for clients with specific DSM mental disorders. In it, we first outline the defining characteristics of each disorder, then cover the biopsychoso-cial theories necessary to understand them, and finally apply the nursing process to caring for clients with these disorders. Unit Five shifts the focus to vulnerable populations that re-quire comfort and care from psychiatric–mental health nurses. These populations include people at risk for self-destructive behavior, sexual abuse and family violence, and specific age groups. Unit Six provides authoritative coverage of nursing intervention strategies and desired outcomes including a wide range of modalities from therapeutic groups to family-focused strategies, crisis intervention, and cognitive–behavioral inter-ventions; to psychopharmacology, recovery and psychiatric rehabilitation, and complementary, alternative, and integra-tive healing practices; and anger management and violence in psychiatric settings.

NEW TO THIS EDITION

A new chapter, Chapter 32, Recovery and Psychiatric Re-habilitation Strategies, focuses on what it means to recover from a debilitating mental disorder and the proven strategies we can use to help clients achieve recovery. Other chapters have been reorganized for ease of understanding—the ele-ments essential to developing a therapeutic alliance with cli-ents have been brought together in Chapter 4, The Therapeutic Nurse–Client Relationship; knowledge and skills essential for partnering with clients' families have been synthesized in Chapter 29, Family-Focused Interventions; and anger manage-ment has been added to the content on violence in psychiatric settings in Chapter 35, Anger Management and Intervention in Psychiatric–Mental Health Settings.

In this edition we introduce several new and exciting features. "Mental Health in the Movies" boxes reveal how the depiction of mental illness in cinema affects our attitudes and behaviors toward persons with mental disorders. "Men-tal Health in the News" boxes highlight the successes and difficulties faced by others who reveal their own struggles and seek help or fail to seek help. "Developing Cultural Compe-tence" boxes are an important link to the cultural forces that influence the experience and expression of mental disorders and pose critical thinking questions. "Why I Plan to Become a Psychiatric–Mental Health Nurse" boxes present the per-sonal stories of students in psychiatric–mental health nursing courses who chose this nursing specialty over all others.

We strongly believe that it is our responsibility as authors to present all material in clear and understandable language and formats that appeal to a range of learning styles, and many of the changes in this edition promote that purpose.

THE TEXTBOOK AS A MAP, A COMPASS, AND AN INSPIRATION

Psychiatric–mental health nursing is poised at a crossroads. We are challenged to bring complex thinking to a complex world if we are to reduce stigma and actualize our contribu-tion to global mental health—the vision to which this text is dedicated. This book has been crafted to provide you with the best possible evidence generated in research to help you achieve your goal of excellence in practice. It offers a fully integrated biopsychosocial perspective rather than relying on any single theory or ideology. It encourages you to become personally, professionally, and spiritually willing to muster the courage and hope necessary to forge proactive steps in our future and to make a commitment to work globally in a contemporary landscape and mindscape.

We have the opportunity to forge a new synthesis of professional wisdom in the face of tough mind–body–spirit problems and needs and the stigmatization of mental illness. We need to face critical transitions with intelligence, stam-ina, wit, creativity, skill, and moral courage. Global mental health can become a shared emergent vision constructed in a way that is respectful of the rich diversity of the citizens of our contemporary world. We created this book to provide you with a map, a compass, and the inspiration to succeed in your current work. We hope that it encourages you to become a participant and leader in facing the broader chal-lenges ahead of us.

Carol Ren Kneisl
Eileen Trigoboff

ACKNOWLEDGMENTS

Producing a book isn't anything like singing a solo—it rather resembles singing in a choir. We wish to thank the many people in our choir who helped us create this textbook.

First, heartfelt thanks to Michael Giacobbe, our Developmental Editor. Mike patiently answered our questions, fulfilled our requests, and shepherded this textbook through its progress from manuscript to finished product. What patience he has with last-minute changes and additions! Kim Mortimer, Acquisitions Editor, is gracious and accommodating and a friend of nursing as is her editorial assistant, Marion Gottlieb.

The talented professionals at Pearson are an incredibly savvy publishing team. We appreciate Julie Alexander, Publisher, who continues to support us and our work. Many thanks to the production team of Patrick Walsh, Production Manager and Cathy O'Connell, Production Liaison for overseeing the process. Special thanks to Lynn Steines, Production Editor at S4Carlisle for her expertise and knowledge. The beautiful, elegant, and inviting design of the book results from the energy provided by Maria Guglielmo and Chris Weigand.

The excellent media supplements were coordinated by Leslie Brado and Rachel Collett. Molly Ward provided superb leadership in heading the team responsible for the Online Student Resources as well as the instructor supplements.

Our professional colleagues and friends, Carol Bradley-Corpuel, Sue C. DeLaune, and Karen Fontaine, generously shared the power of their collective wisdom and clinical expertise in many chapters.

We also wish to acknowledge the efforts of the writers listed on page iv who developed content for the Online Student Resources and the instructor supplements.

Our thanks go to the many reviewers of the manuscript and the supplements for helping us to prepare a book that is useful for students and faculty alike, accurate in content, and relevant to every specialty area. We always welcome the thoughtful comments of nursing faculty, nursing students, and practicing psychiatric–mental health nurses. We have tried to make this book a reflection of what they want in a psychiatric–mental health nursing text.

A GUIDE TO CONTEMPORARY PSYCHIATRIC–MENTAL HEALTH NURSING

KEY TERMS alert you to the vocabulary used in the chapter. The page numbers indicate where the term is defined.

LEARNING OUTCOMES indicate what important information or skills you will have after studying the chapter.

CRITICAL THINKING CHALLENGE at the beginning of each chapter presents a brief, care-based scenario that asks you to analyze an issue or an assertion related to the chapter topic. The questions that follow stimulate critical thinking.

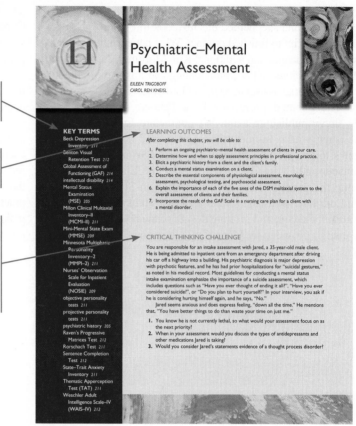

11

Psychiatric–Mental Health Assessment

EILEEN TRIGOBOFF
CAROL REN KNEISL

KEY TERMS
Beck Depression Inventory *211*
Benton Visual Retention Test *212*
Global Assessment of Functioning (GAF) *214*
intellectual disability *214*
Mental Status Examination (MSE) *205*
Millon Clinical Multiaxial Inventory–II (MCMI-II) *211*
Mini-Mental State Exam (MMSE) *209*
Minnesota Multiphasic Personality Inventory–2 (MMPI-2) *211*
Nurses' Observation Scale for Inpatient Evaluation (NOSIE) *209*
objective personality tests *211*
projective personality tests *211*
psychiatric history *205*
Raven's Progressive Matrices Test *212*
Rorschach Test *211*
Sentence Completion Test *212*
State–Trait Anxiety Inventory *211*
Thematic Apperception Test (TAT) *211*
Weschler Adult Intelligence Scale–IV (WAIS–IV) *212*

LEARNING OUTCOMES
After completing this chapter, you will be able to:

1. Perform an ongoing psychiatric–mental health assessment of clients in your care.
2. Determine how and when to apply assessment principles in professional practice.
3. Elicit a psychiatric history from a client and the client's family.
4. Conduct a mental status examination on a client.
5. Describe the essential components of physiological assessment, neurologic assessment, psychological testing, and psychosocial assessment.
6. Explain the importance of each of the five axes of the DSM multiaxial system to the overall assessment of clients and their families.
7. Incorporate the result of the GAF Scale in a nursing care plan for a client with a mental disorder.

CRITICAL THINKING CHALLENGE

You are responsible for an intake assessment with Jared, a 35-year-old male client. He is being admitted to inpatient care from an emergency department after driving his car off a highway into a building. His psychiatric diagnosis is major depression with psychotic features, and he has had prior hospitalizations for "suicidal gestures," as noted in his medical record. Most guidelines for conducting a mental status intake examination emphasize the importance of a suicide assessment, which includes questions such as "Have you ever thought of ending it all?", "Have you ever considered suicide?", or "Do you plan to hurt yourself?" In your interview, you ask if he is considering hurting himself again, and he says, "No."

Jared seems anxious and does express feeling, "down all the time." He mentions that, "You have better things to do than waste your time on just me."

1. You know he is not currently lethal, so what would your assessment focus on as the next priority?
2. When in your assessment would you discuss the types of antidepressants and other medications Jared is taking?
3. Would you consider Jared's statements evidence of a thought process disorder?

DEVELOPING CULTURAL COMPETENCE boxes are an important link to the cultural forces that influence the experience and expression of mental disorders and pose critical thinking questions.

DEVELOPING CULTURAL COMPETENCE

Symptoms of Depression in Various Cultures

Depression may be experienced in somatic terms, rather than with sadness or guilt, in some cultures. People of Latino and Mediterranean cultures may tell you about having headaches and "nerves." People of Chinese and Asian cultures may emphasize weakness and tiredness. Middle Easterners may refer to problems of the "heart." The Hopi may express the depressive experience by being "heartbroken." Cultures may differ regarding the seriousness placed on symptoms and share distinctive culture-specific experiences (such as the feeling of being hexed). It is essential to identify those cultural factors that may facilitate, or deter, desired health-related behaviors.

CRITICAL THINKING QUESTIONS

1. How might your own knowledge about physical illnesses as well as your perceptions and stereotypes interfere with understanding the emphasis on somatic symptoms in some depressed persons from other cultures?
2. What are some essential elements to incorporate in a psychoeducation program on depression for Asian clients being treated for depression in a community setting?
3. If someone believes that her depression is the result of a hex, what adaptations might be necessary in a plan for care for the client?

EVIDENCE-BASED PRACTICE boxes show how research evidence shapes the plan of care for a particular client. Critical thinking questions follow each vignette.

EVIDENCE-BASED PRACTICE

Strategy of Protective Empowering

Lorelei is the nurse manager on an alcohol detoxification unit. James, a 55-year-old man with a 30-year history of alcohol abuse and cigarette smoking, is admitted for alcohol detoxification. Because he had pulled out his IV fluids on the preceding shift, managed to obtain a cigarette lighter in order to smoke, and fallen out of bed, the night shift put him in soft restraints. Every time one of the night shift nurses came into his room, James cursed at them.

Lorelei assigned Kevin, who was newly hired and still in the process of orientation, to James's care. Lorelei and Kevin's joint assessment of James's current mental status, background history, and mental status examination results convinced them that he is at risk for harming himself. Although hospital policy justifies the use of soft restraints, Lorelei felt strongly that James could be kept safe

with one-to-one supervision rather than with soft restraints and that the presence of a staff member would be more comforting and less anxiety provoking for him. Lorelei cautioned Kevin not to take James's cursing personally.

Among the goals that Lorelei and Kevin formulated cooperatively were relating to John in a respectful way, keeping him safe, and encouraging him to regain greater self-control. Although action should be based on more than one study, their strategy of protective empowering was based on the following grounded theory research:

Chiovitti, R. F. (2011). Theory of protective empowering for balancing patient safety and choices. *Nursing Ethics, 18*(1), 88–101.

CRITICAL THINKING QUESTIONS

1. How does protective empowerment fit with the basic premises of humanistic interactionism?
2. How does protective empowerment fit with the basic premises of psychobiologic theory?
3. How does protective empowerment fit with the basic premises of cognitive–behavioral theory?

WHAT EVERY NURSE SHOULD KNOW

provides examples to illustrate that regardless of the specialty, psychiatric–mental health practices are a part of it. These boxes emphasize the importance of recognizing mental health problems and applying these practices in all nursing situations.

PARTNERING WITH CLIENTS AND FAMILIES

emphasizes the value of including the family in psychiatric–mental health care. Families play an important role in the treatment of a family member. Understanding the characteristics of the disorder and how it may arise during family interactions improves the client's ability to function and make family life more comfortable. This feature provides key topics to discuss with families.

WHAT EVERY NURSE SHOULD KNOW

An Agitated Client

Imagine that you are the psychiatric nurse on a crisis response team. The team receives a call about a very agitated man who has a history of paranoid delusions and hallucinations. You and the other team members approach the man, who is on his porch mumbling agitatedly to himself.

Your knowledge of the psychobiology of schizophrenia supports the strategy of having only one person speak clearly and simply to this man so as not to overwhelm him. His executive functioning, and therefore his ability to process incoming information, is challenged when symptoms are acute. You interact with him in a calm, straightforward manner, asking what the problem could be. When he answers you in a loud, menacing tone that he must "strike before the irons have cooled beyond their coloration," you ask him to tell you what he wants you to do. In the conversation that follows, you discover that he has not been eating or sleeping, that he becomes very upset when people interrupt him (to ask him to eat or try to get some sleep), and that he is exhausted from days of trying to accomplish a delusional task.

When it is apparent that an individual such as this man is experiencing severe symptoms, stabilization is needed to protect him and others. Stabilization can be achieved through a combination of a safe environment, psychopharmacology to balance neurotransmitter functions, and compassionate care to help him through this trauma.

PARTNERING WITH CLIENTS AND FAMILIES

Teaching About Genetic Testing for Schizophrenia

At present there is no definitive test for schizophrenia—no blood test or biopsy result that would render a diagnosis—so genetic testing for schizophrenia takes place in research settings. A reliable test using blood and other body cells is sure to be developed in the not-too-distant future. Talking about genetics with clients and families will familiarize them with the potentials for diagnosis, treatment, and risk reduction.

If your clients and their family members have the opportunity to be involved in genetic research, informed consent documents

for participation in these studies explain in detail what is being tested, how the sample will be used, and how long the sample will be kept following the research. Clients and their family members should know that research does not necessarily help study subjects who have the illness. After hundreds of genetic samples have been examined, however, a clearer picture of the genetics of schizophrenia can be developed. Helping clients and families understand the benefits of genetic research now will shape what happens for future generations of people with schizophrenia.

CARING FOR THE SPIRIT

boxes reinforce the belief in the interconnection of mind, body, and spirit. They appear throughout the book and are designed to promote the understanding of the client's essence, meaning, and purpose in life, as well as the nurse's role in supporting spirituality.

CARING FOR THE SPIRIT

Basic Biologic, Safety, and Belonging Needs

Spirituality may be an important connection between mental health and mental illness. In mental illness, most clients describe feeling "disconnected" from their families, their friends, the universe itself, and from their "faith." For example, clients describe depression as similar to being in a gray or black tunnel with a profound sense of disconnectedness.

Imagine what it would be like to go for 24 hours or longer without sleep. How would you look? Would you feel

disconnected or disoriented? Ask someone with mania what that's like. Have you ever awakened suddenly and not known where you are? How would it be to feel like that for an hour, a whole day, or a month? Ask someone with schizophrenia what that's like. Perhaps you've driven down the road and realized that you're confused about where you are and how you got there. And what if you had voices inside your head at the same time? Would this be frightening? Would you feel disconnected?

WHY I BECAME A PSYCHIATRIC–MENTAL HEALTH NURSE boxes share the reasons and events that led the authors and contributing authors of this text to enter the field of psychiatric–mental health nursing.

WHY I PLAN TO BECOME A PSYCHIATRIC–MENTAL HEALTH NURSE boxes present the personal stories of students in psychiatric-mental health nursing courses who chose this nursing specialty over all others.

YOUR SELF-AWARENESS engages the reader in a process of introspection and self-questioning that is essential to the therapeutic use of self.

DSM ESSENTIAL FEATURES provide the most current diagnostic criteria from the APA 2000 *Diagnostic and Statistical Manual of Mental Disorders* in each of the disorders chapters.

RX COMMUNICATION boxes offer sample dialogues between nurses and clients. In addition, they provide the rationale for at least two different but helpful alternatives. This feature is designed to provide students with a beginning repertoire of communication interventions useful when interacting with psychiatric–mental health clients.

R̞X COMMUNICATION

Assessing Your Client

CLIENT: "They're all out to get me. I can't get a day without being interfered with and manipulated. I hear them talking about me even now."

NURSE RESPONSE #1: "You think that others have it in for you?"	NURSE RESPONSE #2: "Tell me the ways you've been coping so we can figure out what would be best for you."
RATIONALE: Focus on process, ventilation/catharsis of feelings.	*RATIONALE:* Focus on emotional process, seeking details of client's behaviors and planned actions.

NURSING CARE PLANS are included in the chapters dealing with specific disorders. They represent a different way to view care for clients diagnosed with specific mental disorders according to the DSM-IV.

NURSING CARE PLAN: CLIENT WITH DELIRIUM

Identifying Information

Mr. Hennessey is a 50-year-old married man who entered the hospital to have colon surgery. He is a physically fit man in a physically demanding job, typically jogging several miles a week for exercise. This is his first serious physical problem. His wife of 25 years is extremely devoted and stayed with him following his surgery. While still in the ICU, Mr. Hennessey became disoriented. Staff members were careful to check his electrolyte balances, which were within normal limits. Within 2 days he began hallucinating. He cried out that the hovering bats he saw in the corners of the room were trying to kill him. He has had other hallucinations and believes that his life is at great risk. When his wife offered him a newspaper, he whispered that she should give him the bucket of pills he'd been hiding under his bed. He lashed out at his wife following this exchange and ripped out his IV and nasogastric tube.

History

Mr. Hennessey has no prior psychiatric history, nor are there any family members with major psychiatric problems. His wife and two grown children, who live nearby, are concerned about his well-being. All are attentive to Mr. Hennessey, love him, and are willing to help with his care.

Mr. Hennessey is a contractor and owns his own business. He and his wife have many friends and activities. He was diagnosed with a colon tumor 1 month ago and had a colon resection. The pathology report was positive for cancer. Mr. Hennessey had been healthy all his life until he noticed rectal bleeding a month ago. He has had regular physicals and responded immediately when symptoms of a problem arose.

Current Mental Status

Mr. Hennessey is disoriented the majority of time, and he is often aggressive. He has been having frightening visual hallucinations, especially at night. He is delusional that people are trying to hurt him.

Other Clinical Data

Mr. Hennessey is on morphine for pain management.

Nursing Diagnosis: High Risk for Violence related to confusion and fear inherent in delirium

Expected Outcome: Mr. Hennessey does not attempt to harm self or others.

Short-Term Goals	Interventions	Rationales
Mr. Hennessey will have decreased symptoms of persecutory delusions.	■ Directly address the fear he is feeling (i.e., "I understand how frightening this all is, and we will make sure you are safe"). ■ Prevent overstimulation and understimulation.	Talking about the feelings is more reassuring and shifts interactions from argumentation. ICUs can be overwhelming in certain sensory areas while not providing enough cues to the outside world (such as windows).
Mr. Hennessey displays considerably less agitation and fear.	■ Orient Mr. Hennessey whenever he is confused. ■ Promote relaxation in both active and soothing modes. ■ Move slowly, speak clearly, and explain all procedures. ■ Make sure only one person is speaking to Mr. Hennessy at a time. ■ Following clearance on neurologic examination, medicate Mr. Hennessey with a low-dose antipsychotic. ■ Explain to family about ICU psychosis and the temporary nature of it.	Decrease the stimuli that can exacerbate symptoms or confusion.

YOUR ASSESSMENT APPROACH and **YOUR INTERVENTION STRATEGIES** present clinically relevant strategies in a succinct, user-friendly format. Your Assessment Approach contains lists of assessment points. Your Intervention Strategies list specific nursing intervention strategies along with their rationales.

YOUR INTERVENTION STRATEGIES
Lessons on Collaboration

1. First, as we often remind you in this text, know your own reality. Determine your values, biases, and goals.
2. Value diversity and turn differences into assets.
3. Acknowledge that conflict is natural and develop constructive conflict resolution skills.
4. Recognize your own power base and share it with others (colleagues and clients and their families).
5. Master interpersonal communication skills and processing skills.
6. Approach collaboration as lifelong learning. The more you collaborate with others, the better you get at it.
7. Place yourself in interdisciplinary situations whenever possible—be present, both physically and mentally, at team forums.
8. Appreciate that collaboration is often spontaneous and you must be ready to seize the moment.
9. Balance unity with autonomy. That is, work neither exclusively as a member of a team (collaboration is not required for all decisions) nor in isolation.

YOUR ASSESSMENT APPROACH Basic Sleep Pattern Assessment

Sample questions for assessing a client's basic sleep patterns are as follows.

Sleep–Wake Schedule

What time do you usually go to bed?
How long does it usually take you to fall asleep after you have turned off the light?
What time do you usually wake up?
What is different about your sleep–wake schedule on the weekend/days off?
How often do you take naps? (Be alert here for cultural influence, such as taking siestas, or occupational influence.) Under what circumstances?

Getting to Sleep

What helps you get to sleep?
What makes it difficult for you to get to sleep?

Staying Asleep

On average, how many times do you wake up during the night?
What seems to waken you?
How long does it usually take to get back to sleep?
What do you do if you are having trouble getting back to sleep?

Waking Up

How difficult is it for you to wake up?
How soon after waking up do you usually get up?
How do you feel when you first get up?

Daytime Functioning

At what time of day do you usually feel most energetic?
At what time of day do you feel most sleepy?
Would you call yourself a "morning person" or an "evening person"?

Satisfaction With Sleep; Potential Problems

How satisfied are you with the sleep you usually get?
Do you think you get enough sleep on average? How do you know?
How has your sleep been during the past 2 weeks in comparison to what is normal for you?
Are you concerned about any of the following things?

- Getting to sleep
- Waking up too many times during the night
- Waking up too early
- Having to fight sleepiness during the day
- Snoring, restlessness, talking or walking in your sleep
- Bad dreams
- Drinking too much coffee (or other caffeine/nicotine sources)

When do you enjoy sleep the most?

MENTAL HEALTH IN THE NEWS

boxes highlight the successes and difficulties faced by others who reveal their own struggles and seek help or fail to seek help.

MENTAL HEALTH IN THE NEWS
The Psychoanalysis of Marilyn Monroe

It is surprising to most people to think of Marilyn Monroe, a film "sex goddess," as a woman with a sexual dysfunction. She engaged in numerous affairs throughout her life from an early age, apparently participated in a stag film and in multiple sex parties at a hotel in New York City (according to a government report), posed nude for a calendar, engaged in sexual activity with women as well as men, had nearly a dozen abortions and multiple miscarriages, but had never had an orgasm until much later after seeking therapy. Marilyn's orgasmic difficulties were the focus of her relationship with a renowned psychoanalyst popular among the Hollywood elite.

She saw her psychoanalyst virtually every day, and in the beginning several times a day. Although she was helped to experience an orgasm for the first time, Marilyn remained in the grips of a severe addiction which continued to be fueled by the routine prescriptions she received from her psychoanalyst for tranquilizers and barbiturates. This relationship lasted for years until her death from an overdose of the barbiturate pentobarbital (Nembutal). Renowned Los Angeles medical examiner, Thomas Noguchi, listed the cause of her death as a "probable" suicide after taking into account several curious facts about her death (among the curious facts is the possibility that the overdose was by rectum, not by mouth, since pentobarbital was not present in her stomach in an amount that would cause death).

Photo courtesy of Superstock.

MENTAL HEALTH IN THE MOVIES

boxes reveal how the depiction of mental illness in cinema affects our attitudes and behaviors toward persons with mental disorders.

MENTAL HEALTH IN THE MOVIES
Rainman

The dichotomy between the deficits of autism and the skills called *savant skills* were displayed in the film *Rainman*. The inspiration for the autistic brother depicted in the movie was Kim Peek, an autistic man (who recently died). Mr. Peek had limited social skills and was taken care of by his father for his day-to-day needs. When Mr. Peek and his father educate people on autism he demonstrated one of his many extraordinary skills at the beginning of every conference. Typically, he was introduced to each person in the audience as they entered the auditorium or conference center. During the talk Mr. Peek demonstrated that he remembered not only the name of every person at the conference, but every person he ever met—over one million people.

The neuroanatomic and biologic difference between Mr. Peek and most other people is that he did not have a corpus callosum. Because he had access to his entire brain without the mediating influence of the corpus callosum, Mr. Peek could think and remember very quickly and completely. This contributed to his great memory in that not only could he remember people, but he could also quote dialogue from any movie, and tell you the day of the week for any date you selected. Despite these unique abilities, problem-solving was always a challenge for him.

Photo courtesy of Alamy.

EXPLORE THE ONLINE STUDENT RESOURCES

Easy access to the online student resources for NCLEX® review, animations, case studies, care plans, and more!

Pearson Nursing Student Resources
Find additional review materials at
nursing.pearsonhighered.com
Prepare for success with additional NCLEX®-style practice questions, interactive assignments and activities, Web links, animations and videos, and more!

OTHER FEATURES

CLINICAL EXAMPLES provide real-life scenarios that students may encounter and point out the challenges involved.

CROSS REFERENCES pinpoint specific content linked to supporting chapters when more depth is required. The icon ∞ refers the reader to content in other sections of the book.

SPECIAL FEATURES

Mental Health in the Movies

Mental Health in the News

Your Intervention Strategies

Your Self-Awareness

DETAILED CONTENTS

UNIT 3 • Psychiatric–Mental Health Nursing Processes 183

UNIT 4 • Clients With Mental Disorders   267

UNIT 5 • VULNERABLE POPULATIONS 507

UNIT 6 • Intervention Strategies 623

1
UNIT

FOUNDATIONS FOR PSYCHIATRIC–MENTAL HEALTH NURSING PRACTICE

SAMUEL looks like any other 35-year-old Ugandan man, standing at the entrance to his home in Agora village with the rest of his family. Samuel is *ebangi* (mad); when his medication runs out and there is no money to buy more medication, Samuel becomes aggressive, threatens people in the village, and is often beaten up when his threats frighten others.

Samuel is not alone—35% of Ugandans, about 11.5 million people, have some form of mental disorder, with depression being the most common. Barely half seek treatment because the people believe that mental illness comes from witchcraft or a supernatural force and, therefore, cannot be cured by modern medicine. Mental illness is believed to run in families—therefore, his family members are shamed and stigmatized because they are also considered mentally ill.

Uganda has only 28 psychiatrists for 33 million people. Medical students believe that if they become psychiatrists they will, in time, develop mental health problems themselves. Many nurses share these beliefs. They keep their work secret because of fear of stigmatization by others, often leaving mental health work for another specialty such as midwifery.

Despite the Ugandan government's newer and more progressive mental health policy, mental health has taken a back seat to communicable diseases such as malaria, tuberculosis, and AIDS. Underfunding, understaffing, and underprioritizing have undercut implementation.

1

Mental Health, Mental Disorder, and Psychiatric–Mental Health Clients: Who Are They?

CAROL REN KNEISL

LEARNING OUTCOMES

After completing this chapter, you will be able to:

1. Analyze why the term *deviant behavior* lacks a definition that covers all situations.
2. Define and explain *mental disorder*.
3. Compare and contrast the essential characteristics of mental health with mental disorder.
4. Name the five mental disorders that rank among the top ten causes of disability worldwide.
5. Explain how societal attitudes, philosophical viewpoints, and definitions of *mental disorder* have shifted throughout history.
6. Explore the meaning of stigma for clients, families, friends, communities, and mental health caregivers and agencies.

CRITICAL THINKING CHALLENGE

Your Aunt Lisa and Uncle Bob are worried about your upcoming mental health clinical experiences. Frightened by the many television programs and movies that portray violent acts committed by supposedly mentally deranged people, they point to dramas whose protagonists are forensic scientists or criminal profilers who solve gory cases based on bizarre circumstances. They worry that the mental health settings for your clinical experiences are full of the sorts of characters they have seen on television and in the movies.

1. Do Aunt Lisa and Uncle Bob have realistic concerns?
2. How will you deal with Aunt Lisa's and Uncle Bob's concerns?
3. What information would be helpful to them?
4. If you have similar concerns, what can you do to attain a sense of comfort in this clinical experience?

Y ou are about to enter upon a journey unlike any other you have had to date in your nursing program. Facing the unknown in a psychiatric–mental health setting invites a variety of feelings and may prompt you to ask yourself several questions:

- What kinds of people will I encounter in the mental health settings I will visit?
- Will they be hard to talk to?
- What do I have in common with them?
- What if they can't, or won't, control themselves?
- How do I know that what I say won't harm them?
- What are they all about and how can I ever figure them out?

This chapter discusses some of these questions. Others that are common concerns of beginning psychiatric–mental health nursing students are fully addressed in Chapters 4 and 10 (see especially Your Self-Awareness on page 48).

What do you have in common with psychiatric–mental health clients? How can you ever hope to understand them? There are many approaches to understanding people—history, sociology, anthropology, philosophy, anatomy, physiology, and psychology, among others. Each is like a searchlight, illuminating some facts while leaving others in shadow. One of the challenges you will face in your clinical experiences, in your classroom lectures and discussions, and in the reading of this textbook is answering these questions by judiciously and appropriately blending knowledge from these diverse areas.

The strategies we present in this book are designed to help you become a therapeutic, comfortable, successful, and safe psychiatric–mental health nurse. In this chapter we discuss what it means to be mentally ill, that is, to have a mental disorder. We review the attitudes and philosophic viewpoints that have influenced our understanding and approach to "madness" throughout history and the stigma connected with mental illness. We also identify the global burden of mental disorder in our country, around the world, in our neighbors and friends, and in prominent people in the news. Our goals in this text are to encourage you to think seriously about what constitutes mental health and mental disorder, to appreciate the humanity of people who experience mental disorder, and to approach your psychiatric–mental health experience with confidence.

In addition to any anxiety, trepidation, or self-doubt you have, we encourage you to approach this experience as we do, with energetic enthusiasm and an eagerness to relate to people whose behavior may be unusual, offensive, socially inappropriate, or even frightening. In doing so, you will find the humanity, creativity, caring, and joy inherent in your clients.

THE CONCEPTS OF DEVIANCE, MENTAL HEALTH, AND MENTAL DISORDER

Defining what is normal AND what is abnormal is not as simple as it might seem. We believe that concepts such as *deviance, mental health,* and *mental disorder* derive their meaning not only from changes in brain structure and biochemistry but also from how we define certain behavior by certain people. Therefore, we also advocate taking a critical look at the social

conditions (Hewitt & Shulman, 2011) under which someone is called "mentally ill."

Deviance

You will undoubtedly hear about, and see, deviant behavior. We use the sociologic definition of **deviance**—behavior outside or away from the social norm of a specific group—in this text. Think back to your sociology courses and recall that in its social context, *deviant* does not mean "bad" or abnormal (Cockerham, 2011). Behavior that is considered bizarre or unreasonable in one cultural context or in one particular time span may be considered desirable in another. Twenty or thirty years ago, the tattoos and piercings of the young people in FIGURE 1-1 ■ would have been thought to be extremely deviant. Today, tattoos and piercings are no longer unique. Not only are they commonplace, they are also considered fashion statements.

Further, your ideas about deviant behavior are likely to be influenced by your upbringing, what you have seen and heard in your own communities and neighborhoods (as illustrated in the clinical example that follows), what you have read about in newspapers or magazines, or what you have seen and read about on the Internet. All of these events influence your attitudes toward, and beliefs about, deviance, mental health, and mental disorder.

Clinical Example

A psychiatric–mental health nurse, recalling her childhood experiences with community deviants, commented on the intense and sometimes morbid excitement that she and her friends found in taunting "Crazy Helen" to run out on her porch and shout incoherently at them, or in telling stories about "Lester the Molester" who hung around the school, the playground, and the community pool and occasionally exposed himself to the children.

The interest these characters held for the children, along with "Vince the Window Peeper," "Eddie the Drunk," and other community deviants, was reawakened in her as she approached her first psychiatric–mental health nursing experience. It was all very frightening, yet intriguing at the same time.

FIGURE 1-1 ■ Nonconforming behavior or appearance that flouts social norms is an example of social deviance—not evidence of psychopathology or abnormal behavior.
Photo courtesy of Michael Newman/PhotoEdit.

You will also find that, unlike the bizarre characters described in the clinical example, most psychiatric–mental health clients are everyday, ordinary people. They are your neighbors, your friends, your family members; your teacher, pharmacist, or physician; or even yourself. It is highly likely that you know someone who has been diagnosed with a mental disorder or has sought mental health counseling to deal with problems in living.

Clients, Not Patients

You cannot help but notice that throughout this text we use the term **client**, not patient, to refer to persons who seek or receive mental health services. We prefer the term *client* over *patient* because of its association with empowerment and self-responsibility, respect, and an optimistic belief that people are capable of change. The term *patient* is associated with the traditional sick role in which people relinquish responsibility to health care experts who have decision-making authority. We believe that in the traditional sick role, people are vulnerable and disempowered.

More people than ever before engage in partnerships with their health care providers and act on their own behalf (or, an advocate does, if the person is unable). Not all people are capable of participating in their own health care—in some emergency situations, when comatose, or when a mental or physical condition prevents it. However, they are more likely to do so when they are informed consumers of mental health care and know that options exist, and when they are encouraged, and even expected, to do so. The term is a reminder—to us and to our clients—that people with mental disorders and their families partner with us (see the Partnering With Clients and Families feature throughout this text) in order to improve their lives.

In health care today, the power balance has shifted. The same principles apply to the use of the terms *adherence* and *compliance*. We prefer encouraging clients to adhere to a treatment protocol; that is, clients are active participants in the treatment regimen. However, when treatment is involuntary (see Chapter 12∞), the achievable goal may be compliance.

Mental Health

There is no one overall accepted definition of **mental health**. In general, however, we consider an individual to be mentally healthy when what that person does (the person's behavior), how that person relates to others (the person's **interpersonal** relationships between oneself and others), and how that person relates to him- or herself (the person's **intrapersonal** relationships within the mind or the self) give evidence of psychological, emotional, and social health. It is a lifelong process of growing toward one's potential. In other words, mental health is more than the mere absence of mental illness.

Mentally healthy people are independent and autonomous. They think well of themselves and others, but are also realistic about their own and others' abilities and shortcomings. They can accept the ups and downs of life and often come out even stronger than before. They have a wide range of behaviors, emotions, and values that are usually consistent

---

> **Box 1-1 Characteristics of Mentally Healthy Individuals**
>
> What are the characteristics of mentally healthy individuals? People who are mentally healthy:
>
> - **Function independently and autonomously.** Mentally healthy individuals respect and seek out the opinions of others but assume responsibility for solving their own problems. They can plan ahead and formulate realistic goals.
> - **Hold a positive attitude toward themselves.** However, their positive self-esteem is combined with a realistic estimate of their abilities and their limitations.
> - **Take life's disappointments in stride.** Mentally healthy people have a variety of coping mechanisms that help them to deal with the ups and downs of everyday life.
> - **Remain healthy even under high levels of stress or in the face of loss or trauma.** This characteristic is called **hardiness**.
> - **Adapt successfully to even very difficult experiences.** This characteristic of being able to bounce back to normal functioning or an even higher level of functioning is called **resilience**.
> - **Integrate their emotions, behaviors, and values into a coherent whole.** Their emotions, behaviors, and values are consistent and fit together.
> - **Experience a wide range of emotions.** The emotions they experience run the gamut—sadness, hopefulness, anger, joy, anxiety, disgust, fear, surprise, elation, and happiness, among others.
> - **Master their environment.** Mastering the environment includes being able to capably deal with what goes on around them, thus achieving a sense of connectedness, harmony, and balance among themselves, their families, their friends, and the community.
> - **Perceive reality clearly.** The mentally healthy person can distinguish between fact and fantasy and lives in the real world.

with one another. These and other characteristics of mentally healthy people are discussed in Box 1-1.

Mental Disorder

Mental illness and mental health, we believe, are outgrowths of both intrapersonal and interpersonal processes. Determining that someone has a mental disorder is often a matter of judgment, even when brain chemicals are altered. The appropriateness of behavior depends on whether it is judged plausible or not (e.g., deviant) according to a set of social, ethical, and legal rules that define the limits of appropriate behavior and reality. For example, if a man on a street corner says he is Napoleon, people will not believe him and will consider him deviant and his statement symptomatic or disturbed. If a man at a masquerade party says he is Napoleon, people reach a different conclusion because in that social setting his behavior fits the norm. We would not label deviant political, religious, or sexual behavior, or conflicts primarily between an individual and society, as a mental disorder unless the deviance or conflict is a symptom of dysfunction in the individual.

With the preceding as philosophic background, we support the concept of **mental disorder**, or **mental illness**, as a psychological group of symptoms, such as a pattern or a syndrome, in which the individual experiences significant **distress** (the person suffers psychologically) and **disability** (impairment in one or more important areas of functioning in daily life), or causes them to harm themselves or others.

The signs and symptoms of mental disorder are known as **psychopathology** (literally, pathology of the mind). Mental health professionals refer to mental disorders as psychopathologic conditions. Mental disorders are identified, standardized, and categorized in the *Diagnostic and Statistical Manual of Mental Disorders* of the American Psychiatric Association (2000), currently being revised but probably not available until 2014 or later. Later in this textbook you will learn about major mental disorders, some of which are as follows:

- Disorders of mood such as depression and bipolar disorder that can significantly interfere with a person's thoughts, behavior, mood, activity, and physical health
- Schizophrenia, a disorder of thinking characterized by social withdrawal, distortions of thinking and perception, and bizarre behavior, that first develops in the later teenage and early adult years
- Anxiety disorders, with the common theme of excessive, irrational fear and dread
- Personality disorders, persistent and rigid behavior patterns that can significantly affect the person's ability to reasonably function in society
- Cognitive disorders or disorders of thinking that usually develop in the later adult years
- Substance-related disorders that include addictions to alcohol, drugs, and other substances
- Dissociative disorders, complex disorders in which a cluster of events is beyond the person's ability to recall
- Somatoform disorders in which symptoms suggest physical disorders for which there is no evidence, and factitious disorder in which a person intentionally produces or feigns physical or psychological symptoms

- Gender identity disorder that affects a person's sense of self as male or female and sexual disorders that affect one's sexual and interpersonal relationships
- Eating disorders in which disturbed eating patterns develop as a way of coping with stress
- Disorders such as autism and disruptive behavior disorders specific to children

Given the right circumstances, anyone can have a mental health problem or disorder, ranging from a mild, temporary increase in anxiety to the most severe of mental disorders. Fame, status, and money do not ensure mental health or happiness, at least not according to the celebrities we hear about—actors, sports stars, authors, musicians, singers, movie directors, and scientists. Many celebrities are speaking out about their experiences with mental illness, such as those in the following list:

- Paula Abdul speaks about her experience with the eating disorder, bulimia.
- Alan Alda speaks about having to come to terms with his mother's schizophrenia.
- Drew Carey and Mike Wallace speak about bouts of depression and suicide attempts.
- Brooke Shields speaks about her postpartum depression.
- David Hyde Pierce speaks about having two family members with Alzheimer's disease, his father and grandfather.

People who openly discuss their mental health problems or write books about their experiences increase public awareness. They make it easier for others to reveal their own struggles and seek help. The Mental Health in the News feature highlights Carrie Fisher's success in coping with problems with drugs and alcohol, addiction to prescription medications, and bipolar disorder.

Like many concepts in the human sciences, the concept of mental disorder lacks a definition that covers all situations. In addition, definitions of mental disorder have shifted throughout history. The historical shifts in attitude and philosophic viewpoints from preliterate cultures to the present day are reviewed later in this chapter. The history of psychiatric–mental health nursing is reviewed in Chapter 2 and the history of psychiatric treatment in Chapter 5∞.

MENTAL HEALTH IN THE NEWS

Carrie Fisher

As the daughter of Debbie Reynolds and Eddie Fisher, Carrie Fisher was a real-life Hollywood princess before she became Princess Leia of the blockbuster Star Wars movie trilogy in the 1970s. A best-selling author, Fisher wrote *Postcards From the Edge (1987)*, a semi-autobiographical novel that discussed her addiction to cocaine and other drugs. *Postcards From the Edge* became a movie, for which she also wrote the screenplay. She became a top Hollywood script doctor, working on and refining the screenplays of other authors, writing other novels and screenplays, and acting in movies, television, and stage plays. Her memoir published in 2008—*Wishful Drinking*—had been a one-woman play and an HBO documentary.

Carrie Fisher has publicly discussed her problems with drugs and alcohol, addiction to prescription medications, and bipolar disorder (for which she receives electroshock treatments every 6 weeks). An extremely productive person, Carrie Fisher's successes provide hope to others in coping with and managing comorbid mental disorders. *Photo courtesy © Allstar Picture Library/Alamy.*

MENTAL DISORDER AS A GLOBAL PROBLEM

How many people worldwide have diagnosable mental disorders? Answers to this important question, most of which are derived from epidemiologic studies, help us to plan and implement mental health services. Psychiatric **epidemiology** is the study of the distribution and determinants of mental disorders in human populations and is used to do the following:

- Determine causative factors for specific disorders
- Identify groups of people at high risk of developing specific disorders
- Recognize changes in health problems, especially the emergence of new problems
- Plan for current health needs and predict future needs
- Evaluate preventive and therapeutic measures

Psychiatric epidemiology is particularly useful to the psychiatric–mental health nurse as the basic discipline for preventive and community psychiatry. The next section presents material from several epidemiologic studies. Additional information about psychiatric epidemiologic studies is available through the National Institute for Mental Health (NIMH) and can be accessed through the online student resources website for this book.

Mental Disorders in the United States

Researchers have found a surprisingly high incidence of mental disorder—ranging from 25% to 64%—in people treated for physical illnesses in primary health care settings in the United States. In fact, most clients with anxiety disorders receive their care from a primary care practitioner (Stein et al., 2011), not from a mental health care practitioner. In addition to anxiety disorders, mood and somatoform disorders are prominent in primary care (Sansone & Sansone, 2010). In fact, mood disorders ranked second after chronic pain as a reason for seeking care (Fernandez et al., 2010). This does not mean that there is equal access for all in primary care. Lamb, Bower, Rogers, Dowrick, and Gask (2011) found exceptional problems in access to mental health treatment in primary care in population groups such as the homeless, adolescents with eating disorders, and depressed elderly people.

The World Health Organization (WHO) estimates that neuropsychiatric disorders are the leading contributor to the total burden of disability in the United States and Canada. Neuropsychiatric disorders contribute almost twice as much as cardiovascular diseases and almost twice as much as cancers (National Institute of Mental Health [NIMH], 2011). Thus, the principles of psychiatric–mental health nursing that you will learn in this textbook have major implications for your work in nursing, regardless of your area of specialization.

In any one 12-month period, 26.2% of all U.S. adults experience a mental disorder (this is called the *prevalence* of active cases of specific mental disorders in a population) and 5.8% of all U.S. adults have a mental disorder classified as severe, that is, illness that results in functional impairment which substantially interferes with or limits one or more major life activities (NIMH, 2011). Further, the *lifetime prevalence* for a mental disorder in the U.S. is 46.4%. This means that at some point in their lives, almost one half of the population of the United States will have had a mental disorder. The most recent 12-month and lifetime prevalence rates and demographics (race, age, and sex) for adults in the United States are illustrated in FIGURE 1-2 ■. Relevant information for children is in Chapter 26∞. Statistics that relate to specific disorders are in the disorders chapters in Unit IV∞.

Comorbidity of Mental Disorders

We are increasingly aware that many people with mental disorders have two or more psychiatric disorders—particularly depression, anxiety, and alcohol and other substance abuse—at any one given time or during their lifetime. This is referred to as **comorbidity** or co-occurring disorder. Issues related to co-occurring disorders are receiving significant attention in psychiatric research.

In 2005, Kessler et al. replicated an earlier congressionally mandated national comorbidity study to examine what changes, if any, had occurred in the prevalence of mental disorders over the previous decade since the original study. The comorbidity replication study is the most extensive research regarding psychiatric disorders to date. Kessler et al. found that the prevalence of mental disorders had not changed during the decade. Their findings are summarized in the following list and were consistent with previous research:

- Women had higher rates of affective and anxiety disorders.
- Men had higher rates of substance abuse disorders and antisocial personality disorder.
- Most disorders declined with age and with higher socioeconomic status.
- Fewer than 40% of those with a lifetime disorder had ever received professional treatment.

A most striking finding is that mental disorders are more highly concentrated than previously recognized in approximately 1/6 (14%) of the population who have had a history of three or more comorbid disorders. When severity is considered, this group also includes the great majority of those with severe disorders. Less than 50% of this highly comorbid group ever obtained specialty mental health treatment, despite the number and severity of their disorders. Findings point to the need for community-based preventive programs aimed at more outreach. There is also a need for more research on barriers, including cultural barriers, to mental health services.

Care-Seeking Patterns in Mental Health Care

The research on care-seeking patterns may be summarized as follows:

- Most people with mental disorders do not seek professional treatment.
- Comorbidity increases the likelihood that a person will seek treatment. Still less than half of the highly comorbid group identified by Kessler et al. ever obtained specialty mental health treatment, despite the number and severity of their disorders.

**Demographics
(for lifetime prevalence)**

- **Sex:** Women are no more or less likely than men to experience any disorder over their lifetime
- **Race:** Non-Hispanic blacks are 30% less likely than non-Hispanic whites to experience any disorder during their lifetime
- **Age:** 18–60+ years

Prevalence

- **12-month Prevalence:** 26.2% of U.S. adult population
- **Severe:** 22.3% of these cases (e.g., 5.8% U.S. adult population) are classified as "severe"

FIGURE 1-2 ■ Prevalence rates and demographics of mental illness in adults (United States).
Source: National Institute of Mental Health. Retrieved 4/17/11 from http://www.nimh.nih.gov

- When seeking treatment, most people with mental disorders seek treatment from primary care physicians, who prescribe the majority of psychotropic medications. Yet, there is a current decrease in primary care physicians, especially in impoverished and rural areas.
- Individuals with chronic mental disorders comprise the majority of those who seek treatment.
- Psychiatrists are the mental health professionals who are most likely to treat individuals with severe disorders, yet there is a current undersupply of psychiatrists in the United States.

Awareness of these care-seeking patterns is essential in order to address the problems of nonuse or misuse of mental health services. Pivotal issues are the availability, accessibility, cost, and quality of mental health services, especially because prognosis is affected by the duration of any mental disorder.

Cost of Mental Health Care

Cost is the most frequently addressed mental health topic in current literature on medical care organizations. Insurance coverage for mental health care appears to lag behind that for other medical care. Only a few states have legislated parity for mental health care—insurance coverage at the same rate as for physical illnesses. Severely underserved groups in relation to mental health services include the following:

- Substance abusers
- Older adults (especially if minority)
- Uninsured persons
- Homeless persons

Unfortunately, mental health policy continues to be reactive rather than proactive, situational rather than long term and strategic, and rehabilitative rather than preventive.

Adequacy of Mental Health Care Services

The National Alliance for Mental Illness (NAMI) is a proactive consumer organization that provides help to clients, families, and mental health professionals. Because the demand for mental health services is increasing at the same time that our nation confronts economic problems, state budget cuts are adversely affecting the nation's mental health care system. NAMI has graded individual states in relation to their provision of mental health services (see FIGURE 1-3 ■). Each state was scored on 39 specific criteria. Note that the national average is D. None received an A and eight received an F.

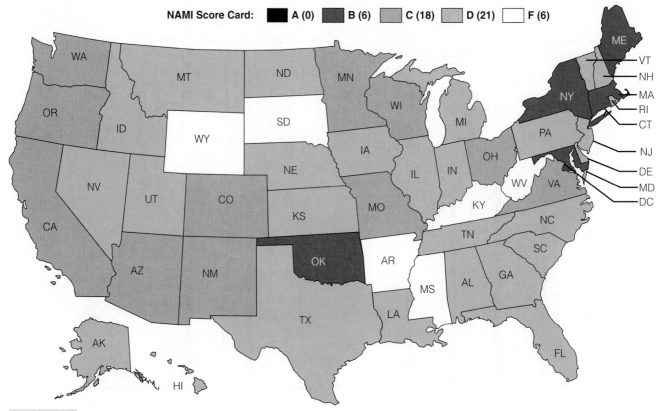

FIGURE 1-3 ■ NAMI's report: Grading the states on mental health services.
Source: www.nami.org/gtsTemplate09.cfm?Section=Grading_the_States_2009.

Mental Disorders Around the Globe

A classic and still relevant major study by WHO has shown that we have underestimated the incidence of mental disorder worldwide. The *Global Burden of Disease* study demonstrated that five of the top ten causes of disability worldwide were psychiatric disorders—depression (ranked number one), schizophrenia, bipolar disorder, alcohol abuse, and obsessive–compulsive disorder (Murray & Lopez, 1996). In fact, although mental disorders are responsible for only 1% of all deaths, they account for a staggering 47% of all disability in economically developed countries such as the United States and Canada (and are the second leading source of disease burden), and 28% of all disability worldwide. These data are illustrated in TABLE 1-1 ■.

A more recent WHO study on the global burden of disease also ranked depression as the leading cause of disability in people ages 15 and older (Moussavi et al., 2007). These researchers also determined that depression is the factor that produced the greatest decrement in health when compared with the chronic physical diseases of angina, arthritis, asthma, and diabetes. The burden of mental disorders is likely to have been underestimated because of inadequate appreciation of the connection between mental illness and other health conditions (Prince et al., 2007). As these researchers say, there is no health without mental health.

Many collaborators from around the world worked intensively to update and provide a more precise, comprehensive

	Women		Men	
TABLE 1-1 ■ Prevalence Rates for Various Mental Disorders	1-year	Lifetime	1-year	Lifetime
Phobic disorder	12.9	17.8	6.3	10.4
Alcohol abuse/dependence	2.2	4.6	11.9	23.8
Major depression	4.0	7.0	1.4	2.6
Antisocial personality	0.4	0.8	2.1	4.5
Obsessive–compulsive disorder	1.9	3.2	1.4	2.0
Panic disorder	1.2	2.1	0.6	1.0
Schizophrenia	1.1	1.7	0.9	1.2
Bipolar mood disorder	0.8	0.9	0.6	0.7

assessment of the global burden of disease and its causes. (The latest text, *Global Burden of Disease and Risk Factors* by Lopez, 2006, is available for download at http://www.dcp2.org. WHO yearly reports are available at http://www.who.int/whr/en) For example, Prince et al. (2007) observed that about 14% of the global burden of disease is attributed to neuropsychiatric disorders, particularly due to the chronic disabling nature of depression, substance use disorders, and psychoses. They suggest that the burden of mental disorders is likely to be underestimated because of a lack of awareness of the connection between mental disorders and other health conditions. Mental disorders may interact to increase risk for communicable diseases (e.g., alcohol and drugs for HIV/AIDS), noncommunicable diseases (e.g., depression and coronary heart disease), and intentional and unintentional injuries (e.g., alcohol as a risk factor in traffic accidents). Conversely, many health conditions may increase the risk of mental disorder (e.g., depression subsequent to debilitating chronic illness).

The prediction of the WHO investigators is that the burden of mental disorders will increase even more by the year 2020 because global mental health resources remain low and improvements in this past decade were minimal at best. Clearly, mental disorders are one of global health's greatest challenges (Patel & Prince, 2011). The website of the WHO has extensive documentation of recent programs and resources related to the global burden of disease and can be accessed through the Online Student Resources for this book.

Throughout this text, we will continue to remind you of these serious concerns. We will remind you of the humanity of those diagnosed with a mental disorder—of the family and friends we love, the neighbors we know, and celebrities we hear about. We will also continue to remind you that the experience of mental disorder not only has devastating effects on the lives of those affected, but also can encourage extraordinary clarity, insight, and creative potential.

HISTORICAL PERSPECTIVES

People who have been called "mentally ill" have been with us throughout history—to be feared, marveled at, ignored, banished, laughed at, pitied, or tortured. A historical review of the place of the "mentally ill," however they have been defined in societies during different periods, brings up the following central points:

- Dominant social attitudes and philosophic viewpoints have influenced the understanding of, and approach to, "madness" throughout recorded history, and probably before.
- Ideas that may be considered contemporary at one time often have roots in earlier centuries.
- The modern medical concept of "madness" as an illness is open to the same scrutiny as interpretations of the past, such as beliefs about witchcraft or mysticism.

The timeline in FIGURE 1-4 ■ illustrates the shifting approaches to mental disorder throughout history.

Era of Magico–Religious Explanations

In preliterate cultures, the causes of mental and physical suffering were not differentiated. Both were attributed to forces acting outside the body. Consequently, no distinctions were made between magic, medicine, and religion. Magic, medicine, and religion were all variously directed against some mortal or superhuman force that had cruelly inflicted suffering on another (Wallace & Gach, 2011). Primitive healers quite logically dealt with the spirits of torment with appeal, reverence, prayer, bribery, intimidation, appeasement, confession, punishment, exorcism, magical ritual, and incantation.

Behavior considered to be a mental disorder by modern Western cultures was attributed in preliterate cultures to the violation of taboos, the neglect of ritual obligations, the loss of a vital substance from the body (such as the soul), the introduction of a foreign and harmful substance into the body (such as evil spirits), or witchcraft.

Era of Organic Explanations

In the 4th century BCE, Hippocrates proposed a medical concept to explain mental suffering. He rejected demonology and proposed that psychiatric illnesses were caused mainly by imbalances in body humors: blood, black bile, yellow bile, and phlegm. For example, an excess of black bile was thought to cause melancholy (Wallace & Gach, 2011).

One important consequence of these beliefs was that psychiatric suffering came within the realm of medical practice to include words (interpretation of dreams and talking) and medical treatments (purging, bloodletting, and ritual purification).

Era of Alienation

At the height of their civilization, the citizens of ancient Greece found their inner security in knowledge and reason. The Romans adopted the intellectual heritage of Greece but placed greater reliance on their social institutions and the rational organization of society supported by law and military might. When these institutions disintegrated and the Roman Empire went into a decline, fear tore apart the fabric of society.

The collapse of Rome signaled a general return to the magic, mysticism, and demonology from which people had retreated during the age of Greek rationality. During the Middle Ages, the period between approximately 400 CE and the Renaissance (1300–1600 CE), madness was seen as a dramatic encounter with secret powers. Troubled minds were thought to be influenced by the moon (see FIGURE 1-5 ■). *Lunacy* literally means a disorder caused by the moon.

In the Arab world, the insane were believed to be divinely inspired and not victims of demons. An asylum for the mentally ill was built in Fez, Morocco, early in the 8th century. Other asylums were soon established in Baghdad, Cairo, and Damascus. The care in these asylums was usually benevolent and kindly.

The first European hospital devoted entirely to mental patients was built in 1409 in Valencia, Spain. The problems of the mind, however, remained the domain of theologians. A book called *Malleus Maleficarum* (*The Witches' Hammer*, 1487) became the basis for witch hunts. The *Malleus* details the destruction of dissenters, heretics, and the "mentally ill," most of whom were women and all of whom were labeled *witches*. Theologic rationalizations and magical explanations were used to justify burning witches at the stake.

The violent insane were shackled in prisons. Others were sent on voyages of symbolic importance. Boatloads of mad people were sent out to sea to search for their reason on "ships of fools." In essence, this opportunity for mental reintegration was really abandonment by society.

Important Dates in the Shifting Approaches to Mental Disorder

- Mental and physical suffering not differentiated.

- "Spirits of torment" acting outside the body are responsible for ills.

- No distinctions made between medicine, magic, and religion.

- Primitive healers address spirits by appeal, prayer, bribery, intimidation, appeasement, punishment.

- Healing methods include exorcism, magical ritual, incantation.

Era of Magico-Religious Explanations

Preliterate Times

- Hippocrates (460-370) rejects demonology and proposes that psychiatric illnesses are caused by imbalances in "body humors": blood, black bile, yellow bile, and phlegm.

- Psychiatric suffering comes within the realm of medical practice.

- Imbalances in body humors often corrected by bloodletting.

Era of Organic Explanations

Early Civilization

- Return to the magic, mysticism, and demonology of preliterate times.

- Madness viewed as dramatic encounter with secret powers and influenced by the moon (lunacy).

- *Malleus Maleficarum* (The Witches' Hammer) by Dominican monks Johann Sprenger and Heinrich Kraemer published in 1487 rationalized mental illness in terms of magical explanation.

- Violent insane shackled in prisons or sent to sea "in search of reason."

Era of Alienation

The Medieval Period

Early 20th Century

Mid 20th Century

Late 20th Century

Era of Psychoanalysis

- Emil Kraepelin (1856-1926) creates system of distinct disease entities and differentiates biopolar disorder from schizophrenia.

- Sigmund Freud (1856-1939) explains human behavior in psychological terms and demonstrates that behavior can be changed through psychoanalysis.

- Pavlov's discovery of the conditioned response forms the basis for modern-day cognitive-behavioral therapy.

Era of Ideologic Expansion

- From the mid-1940s to mid-1950s, a strong rift between biologic orientation and dynamic orientation develops.

- By the early 1950s, several drugs for the treatment of mental disorder were in common use.

- Harry Stack Sullivan developed the interpersonal theory of psychiatry, Erik Erikson formulated his psychosocial theory of development, and Abraham Maslow proposed an order, or hierarchy of basic human needs leading to self-actualization.

- Group therapy, family therapy, and short-term therapy recognized as options to costly long-term therapy.

- Milieu therapy developed by Maxwell Jones in England.

Deinstitutionalization and the Community Mental Health Movement

- By the early 1960s, a shift from institutional to community-based care and toward preventive services, consumer participation, and the development of community mental health centers began.

- Between 1955 and 1975, the number of resident clients in state mental hospitals decreased nearly 66% as the community mental health movement reached its apex.

- By the 1960s, family therapy had become both a diagnostic tool and a mode of treatment.

- Politicians and the public become more aware of the difficulties the mentally ill face.

FIGURE 1-4 ■ *Photo source top to bottom by column:* SZ Photo/Scheri/Alamy; Photo Researchers, Inc.; Maslow, Abraham H./ Frager, Robert D./Fadiman, James, *Motivation and Personality*, 3rd Ed., ©1987. Reprinted and electronically reproduced by permission of Pearson Education, Inc., Upper Saddle River, New Jersey; Philosophical Library; Photo Researchers, Inc.; Photo Researchers, Inc.; Philosophical Library; Philosophical Library; ajt/Shutterstock.

• Physicians classify symptoms of mental disorders without understanding the sources of mental suffering.

• In 1794 Philippe Pinel (1745-1826) treated inmates in the French institutions Bicetre and Salpetriere with humanity and was thus considered mad.

• In 1656, Hópital Générale in Paris founded to confine the mad, poor, and various deviants.

• The "insane" have no recourse to appeal.

• Madness not linked to medicine; could only be mastered by discipline and brutality.

• Radical physicians like Johann Weyer (1515-1588) believed that "those illnesses whose origins are attributed to witches come from natural causes."

• In England, William Tuke (1732-1822) focused on "moral treatment" in a humane milieu called the York Retreat to counter conditions in settings such as "Bedlam."

• In America, Benjamin Rush (1746-1813) focused on moral treatment and humanitarianism at the Pennsylvania Hospital.

• Dorothea L. Dix (1802-1887) founds or enlarges over 30 mental hospitals.

• Moral treatment replaced by custodial care.

• Clifford Beers (1876-1943) published his book describing his own intense suffering and mental anguish, leading to the development of preventive psychiatry and the formation of child guidance clinics.

Era of Confinement

Era of Moral Treatment

Era of Public Mental Hospitals

The Renaissance

The 18th and Early 19th Centuries

Late 19th and Early 20th Centuries

The 1990s

The New Millennium

The Decade of the Brain

Era of Health Care Reform

• The primary innovation of the 1990s is the "biologic revolution": collaboration of science and technology to expand concepts of mental disorder proposed by psychological, behavioral, and psychoanalytic theories.

• The gains made in research-based knowledge about the epidemiology, diagnosis, treatment, and prevention of major mental illnesses constitute a quantum leap in understanding the brain.

• Client advocacy groups welcome psychiatry's shift toward psychosocial rehabilitation for client self-care.

• The National Alliance on Mental Illness (NAMI) established a separate research foundation to study the biologic basis of major mental illness.

• Reform of psychiatric care has decereased length of hospital stays and increased client acuity.

• The advancing explosion in neuroscience has reshaped our conception of the bases of mental disorders.

• Innovations in technology have informed diagnostic practices such as brain imaging.

• The array of available psychopharmacologic treatments continues to expand.

• Populations of psychiatric clients include growing numbers of mentally ill elders, more people with coexisting substance use disorders, more comorbidities with chronic illnesses, and expanding racial and cultural diversity.

• A yearning for spirituality has been reawakened in clients as well as health care providers.

• The study of genomes and the biology of the brain touch ethical, moral, and political nerves.

FIGURE 1-6 ■ A ward in Bethlehem Hospital about 1745. A patient is being chained in the foreground, and in the background are two Sunday visitors on an entertainment outing.
Photo courtesy of Philosophical Library.

FIGURE 1-5 ■ Moonstruck women dancing in a 17th-century square. This activity is the source for the word *lunatic*.
Photo courtesy of Philosophical Library.

Era of Confinement

Unlike the Middle Ages, when the insane were generally driven out of, or excluded from, community life, during the Renaissance they were confined. Tamed, retained, and maintained, madness was reduced to silence through a system of mutual obligation between the afflicted and society. Mad persons had the right to be fed but were morally constrained and physically confined.

Seventeenth-century society created enormous houses of confinement. In these asylums were gathered the mad, the poor, and various deviants. A landmark date is 1656, when by decree the Hôpital Général in Paris was founded. It was not a medical establishment, but rather a threatening institution complete with stakes, irons, and dungeons. The "insane" were completely under the jurisdiction of the institution and had no recourse to appeal their incarceration. The Hôpital Général and other, similar institutions were established to maintain social order. In London, the hospital of St. Mary of Bethlehem became famous as *Bedlam,* illustrated in FIGURE 1-6 ■, where, for the entertainment of onlookers on a Sunday afternoon outing, mad persons were publicly beaten and tortured.

Those chained to cell walls were no longer considered people who had lost their reason or sick persons, but rather beasts seized by frenzy. During this period, it was believed that madness could be overcome only by discipline and brutality.

Era of Moral Treatment

The 18th and early 19th centuries were an era characterized by internal contradictions. Although the insane were unchained, the medical treatment they received consisted of what amounted to torture with special paraphernalia. To grasp the incredible inhumanity with which the mentally disordered were treated in what became known as "the era of enlightenment," consider the following:

- The nature of mental disorders could not be explained by any of the prevailing concepts—black humors could not be seen, demons or animal spirits could not be observed, and knowledge of anatomy could not be applied to the workings of the mind.
- Because mental disorders could not be satisfactorily explained, the deeply felt dread of the insane could not be dispelled.
- Mental disorders were believed to be incurable, and mad persons were thought to be dangerous.

Even the most sensitive physicians did not try to understand the sources of mental suffering. Because they had no way to explain or understand mental disorders, they developed and focused on elaborate and detailed systems of classification (see Chapter 5∞).

At the same time, a general spirit of reform and humanitarianism swept western Europe and the United States (Wallace & Gach, 2011). Physicians developed a zeal for social reform and moral enrichment and began to release inmates from their chains, abolish systematized brutality with chains and whips, feed them nourishing foods, and treat them with kindness. This movement was first led by Philippe Pinel (1745–1826) (see FIGURE 1-7 ■) in France and the Quakers in England under William Tuke (1732–1822).

Moral treatment in the United States—led by Benjamin Franklin, Benjamin Rush (called "the father of American psychiatry," 1745–1813), and others—was an alternative to mere confinement. Despite his association with humanitarianism and moral treatment, Rush was a major follower of

FIGURE 1-7 ■ A landmark event—Philippe Pinel unchaining the insane in the Bicêtre Hospital in Paris.
Photo courtesy of Charles Ciccione/Photo Researchers, Inc.

the ideas of Scotland's William Cullen (1710–1790). Cullen believed that mental disorder was due to decay, either of the intellect or of the involuntary nervous system, that is, a matter of disordered physiology. Rush advocated bloodletting, the restraining chair illustrated in FIGURE 1-8 ■, the gyrating chair, and other devices that we now consider inhumane.

FIGURE 1-8 ■ Benjamin Rush, the "father of American psychiatry" and an idealist and humanitarian, nevertheless favored physical theories such as "excitement of the brain" to explain mental illness. He was preoccupied with somatic treatments such as bleeding and purging and developed the tranquilizing chair to quiet the insane.
Photo courtesy of Philosophical Library.

Era of Psychoanalysis

During the late 19th and early 20th centuries, the number of mental hospitals, both private and government run, grew. Beliefs about mental disorder began to change again. Insanity was linked to faulty life habits and treated with new forms of physical or somatic therapies. Other clinicians were inclined toward an organic, neurophysiologic explanation of mental disorders. The emphasis on the classification of distinct disease entities continued.

These developments formed the background for the work of one of the most influential figures in the history of psychiatry, Sigmund Freud (1856–1939). He succeeded in explaining human behavior in psychologic terms. Freud's contributions to psychiatry are discussed in greater detail in Chapter 5∞.

Contemporary Developments

By the mid-20th century, psychiatric thinking was expanding and moving toward an emphasis on the importance of the social dimension. Dissatisfaction with psychoanalytic explanations for mental disorder became more common, and drug treatment for mental illness was being developed in the early 1950s. Research into chemotherapy and the etiology of mental illness increased.

The primary innovation of the 1990s—known as The Decade of the Brain—was the so-called biologic revolution: the collaboration of science and technology to expand concepts of mental disorder proposed by psychologic and behavioral theories. During this period, a quantum leap was made in understanding the brain. For example, research on brain dysfunction in mental disorders has resulted in a major reconceptualization of the diagnosis and treatment of several mental disorders. Researchers have discovered a variety of brain dysfunctions, including ventricular enlargement, cerebral atrophy, and disturbances in neurotransmitters (discussed in Chapter 6∞).

This up-to-date, research-based knowledge is reflected in contemporary psychiatric and psychiatric–mental health nursing literature, including this text. Research in the 21st century is focused on such areas as:

- The bases of mental disorders
- The continuing development of newer generations of medications with fewer side effects to treat mental disorders
- The effects of various medications on neurotransmitters in the brains of clients with psychiatric disorders
- The role of nutrients in modifying brain function
- The influence on mood and behavior of disruptions of biologic rhythms
- The role of viruses in mental disorders
- The influence of the endocrine system on the brain and behavior
- The role of the brain in producing physical illnesses
- The identification of biologic markers that might alert clients and clinicians to the onset of a mental disorder
- The interrelationship between genetics and mental disorder
- The prevention of major mental disorders

We can expect that, as the result of contemporary research, our conceptualizations of mental disorder will continue to shift.

THE STIGMA OF MENTAL ILLNESS

One of the negative consequences of being diagnosed with a mental disorder is stigmatization. The **stigma** of mental illness is based on a societal perception that mental illness is a blemish of individual character (Cockerham, 2011). Stigmatization of mental illness is a world-wide problem experienced in all segments of society but is especially prevalent in deprived, marginalized, and minority communities (Lamb et al., 2011). A national anti-stigma campaign has been created by the actress Glenn Close, whose sister is coping with bipolar disorder. Called *Bring Change 2 Mind,* Close's efforts are endorsed by NIMH, the Substance Abuse and Mental Health Systems Administration (SAMHSA), and several mental health organizations. You can access this not-for-profit organization through the online student resources for this text. *The Snake Pit,* the film discussed in the movie feature about the treatment of mental illness, has served to both increase stigma as well as decrease it.

Stigma is about disrespect:

- It hurts, punishes, and diminishes people.
- It harms and undermines interpersonal relationships.
- It appears in behavior, language, attitude, and tone of voice.
- It causes others to keep their distance from someone who is "not right" and results in social isolation for the stigmatized person.

Stigma is an attitude that leads to prejudice and discrimination. It affects the judgments of family, friends, coworkers, health care providers, and others about the person labeled mentally ill. Research carried out by the Programme Against Stigma and Discrimination of the World Psychiatric Association (WPA) indicates that approximately 2/3 of people with schizophrenia reported moderate or high perceived discrimination (Brohan, Elgie, Sartorius, Thornicroft; GAMAIN-Europe Study Group, 2011). Almost 3/4 of people with bipolar disorder or depression reported moderate or high perceived discrimination (Brohan, Gauci, Sartorius, Thornicroft; GAMAIN-Europe Study Group, 2011). Examples of inaccurate beliefs about mental illness that lead to or perpetuate stigma and discrimination of people with mental disorders are in Box 1-2.

In his early classic work on stigma, the sociologist Erving Goffman (1963) equated stigma with having a *spoiled identity*. The person incorporates societal perceptions of not being normal, or right, or worthwhile, and comes to believe that he or she does indeed fall short of what he or she should be. This internalization, or self-stigma, leads to feeling unworthy, having low self-esteem, and losing hope, all characteristics that work against coping with, or recovering from, mental illness. This process is illustrated in FIGURE 1-9 ■.

Despite advances, stigma continues to grow around the globe and is the main obstacle to better mental health care and quality of life for clients, families, communities, and staff members who deal with mental health disorders.

Clinical Example

In the United States and Canada, job-seekers who tell a prospective employer about their mental disorder risk not being hired. On the other hand, if they do not tell or have a relapse, they risk being fired. In India, people are reluctant to tell their neighbors about a mental disorder because it might hurt a child's or sibling's chances of being married. In Japan, mentally disordered persons are kept at home to do domestic chores and out of the public eye. In China, mental illness is seen as a family problem that is hidden and the responsibility for managing it is kept within the family. In all these countries, stigmatization is the motivating force.

According to the Programme against Stigma and Discrimination of the WPA, stigma extends to not only clients and their families, but also to the medications used for treatment, the agencies that provide mental health treatment, staff members in those agencies (Sartorius, Gaebel, Cleveland, Stuart, Akiyama et al., 2010), and even the sites on which they are located. Stigma affects everyone in the global mental health community.

Language Matters

Although aberrant behavior is a source of stigma, labels reinforce stigma (Green, 2009). It would be nice if the old saying, "Sticks and stones can break my bones, but words can never hurt me" was true. As it relates to stigma in mental health, words are

MENTAL HEALTH IN THE MOVIES
The Snake Pit

In this 1948 classic film and exposé of the dire conditions at many state hospitals, Virginia Cunningham, played by Olivia de Haviland, is an inpatient in a state insane asylum (as psychiatric hospitals were known then). *The Snake Pit* was an adaptation of a best-selling novel by Mary Jane Ward who had been a patient in a mental hospital for more than 8 months. Many of the characters were composites of the nurses, doctors, and patients she met during her hospitalization.

Prior to *The Snake Pit,* mental illness in the movies was either the butt of jokes in comedies or romanticized as a byproduct of tragic love. The film authentically portrayed the dehumanizing conditions

that existed at the time in large mental institutions—a fearful and insensitive staff focused on regimentation to control and manage the asylum's inmates, overcrowding, facilities designed like prisons, and typical treatments such as electroshock therapy and cold water hydrotherapy. The portrayals of psychoanalysis, hypnosis, and the reasons behind the main character's mental disorder were too simplistic to do justice to the complexities involved in being mentally ill.

The film had a significant impact on the conditions in mental institutions in the United States. By 1949, journalists were keeping track of the number of states to institute reforms and 20th Century Fox claimed that 26 of the 48 states had enacted reform legislation as a result of *The Snake Pit.*

Photo courtesy of Everett Collection.

Box 1-2   Stigmatizing Beliefs About Mental Illness

- **MYTH: Mentally ill people are dangerous and violent.** *FACT: People with mental illness are not more violent than other people when they are on medication. They are more frequently the victims of violence than the perpetrators.*
- **MYTH: Mentally ill people have a low IQ.** *FACT: People with mental illness are not developmentally disabled, that is, they do not have diminished intellectual capacity that is usually present since birth. They may have difficulty performing at a normal level, but this is due to their illness, not their intellectual capacity. However, people who have a developmental disability may also have a mental illness.*
- **MYTH: Mentally ill people cannot hold a job.** *FACT: People with mental illness whose symptoms are under control not only hold jobs, despite an employer's reluctance to hire them, but may excel at their jobs.*
- **MYTH: Mentally ill people have nothing to contribute to society.** *FACT: People with mental illness are contributing members of society. They are scientists, musicians, astronauts, sports stars, singers, actors and contribute to society in a wide range of areas. (See the Mental Health in the News feature on page 5.)*
- **MYTH: Mentally ill people lack willpower.** *FACT: People with mental illness whose symptoms are under control can, and do, exert willpower and control in their daily lives. Any difficulties are due to their illness, not to a lack of willpower.*
- **MYTH: Mentally ill people come from low-income families.** *FACT: People with mental illness come from any income bracket, race, religion, age, and educational background. Mental illness is an equal opportunity disorder.*
- **MYTH: Mentally ill people are lazy.** *FACT: People with mental illness are not inherently lazy. Their symptoms may make it difficult for them to be productive.*
- **MYTH: Mentally ill people cause their own problems.** *FACT: People with mental illness have a neurobiologic brain disorder that disrupts their thinking, feeling, mood, daily functioning, and ability to relate to others.*
- **MYTH: Mentally ill people should just "shape up."** *FACT: People with mental illness cannot just "shape up" just as a person with cancer cannot just "shape up." Mental illness, like physical illness, requires intervention for symptoms.*
- **MYTH: Mental illness does not exist.** *FACT: People with mental illness have an actual neurobiologic brain disorder that is every bit as factual as a physical illness.*

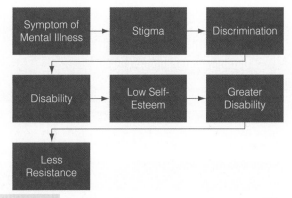

FIGURE 1-9 ■ The effect of stigma on recovery from mental illness. The person's symptom is the marker that leads to stigmatization by society. Eventually, the effects of stigmatization negatively influence the person's ability to recover from mental illness.

it unfounded and negative implications. People probably described "Crazy Helen" as having had a **nervous breakdown**—a general, nonspecific term for an incapacitating but otherwise unspecified type of mental disorder. Other stigmatizing and denigrating terms are *wacko, looney, psycho, lunatic, maniac, bananas, cuckoo, head case,* and *nuts.*

Many of the terms that society uses to describe aberrant behavior have a convoluted history and have traveled over time and between languages, as you will see in the historical perspectives section of this chapter. It is important that you not only educate those who use stigmatizing language and advocate for others to treat clients respectfully and ethically, but also that you serve as a role model. The Code of Ethics for Nurses (Fowler, 2010) identifies respect for persons as a core ethical principal integral to professional nursing. Respectful language is discussed in the Your Self-Awareness feature. We also discuss the ethics of stigmatizing labels in Chapter 13∞.

YOUR SELF-AWARENESS
Respectful Language to Combat Stigma

You can help to combat stigma by using respectful language when you refer to mental disorders or to clients with mental illness. This requires that you become aware of the language you use and modify it, if necessary. The suggestions below are designed for your use. However, they can also be implemented in a psychoeducation teaching plan for clients, family members, mental health staff, and others in the community.

- Say *mental disorder, mental illness,* or *psychiatric disability* (terms that show respect). *Avoid saying* crazy, cuckoo, wacko, nuts, psycho, lunatic, bananas, *or* head case *(terms that disrespect and stigmatize).*
- Say *person with bipolar disorder, person who has schizophrenia, person who has cognitive difficulties* (terms that put people first, not their disabilities). *Avoid saying* manic, bipolar, schizophrenic, *or* demented *(terms that emphasize limitations and depersonalize).*
- Say *person coping with, managing,* or *recovering from depression* (terms that focus on positive abilities). *Avoid saying* afflicted with, suffering from, victim of *(terms that sensationalize a disability).*

powerful. Stigmatizing language builds barriers to the understanding and treatment of persons with mental disorders.

Many terms have been used to describe aberrant behavior or mental disorder. You may have used some or all of these terms yourself, and you may hear them used in mental health settings and in the community at large. As you learn more about mental disorders and the effects of stigma, you will gain a greater appreciation of the humanity of clients with mental disorder and find that you have edited demeaning, denigrating, and stigmatizing labels from your vocabulary.

In the earlier clinical example on page 3, the neighbor was known as "Crazy Helen." **Crazy** is an informal, denigrating, and stigmatizing term for "mentally ill" that carries with

Pearson Nursing Student Resources

Find additional review materials at
nursing.pearsonhighered.com

Prepare for success with NCLEX®-style practice questions,
interactive assignments and activities, web links, animations
and videos, and more!

REFERENCES

American Psychiatric Association. (2000). *Diagnostic and statistical manual of mental disorders* (4th ed., Text Revision) (DSM-IV-TR). Washington, DC: Author.

Brohan, E., Elgie, R., Sartorius, N., Thornicroft, G.; GAMAIN-Europe Study Group. (2011). Self-stigma, empowerment and perceived discrimination among people with schizophrenia in 14 European countries: The GAMAIN-Europe Study Group. *Schizophrenia Research, 122*(1–3), 232–238.

Brohan, E., Gauci, D., Sartorius, N., Thornicroft, G.; GAMAIN-Europe Study Group. (2011). Self-stigma, empowerment and perceived discrimination among people with bipolar disorder or depression in 13 European countries: The GAMAIN-Europe Study. *Journal of Affective Disorders, 129*(1–3), 56–63.

Cockerham, W. C. (2011). *Sociology of mental disorder* (8th ed.). Upper Saddle River, NJ: Prentice Hall.

Fernandez, A., Saameno, J. A., Pinto-Meza, A., Luciano, J. V., Autonell, J., Palao, D., . . . Serrano, A. (2010). Burden of chronic physical conditions and mental disorders in primary care, *British Journal of Psychiatry, 196,* 302–309.

Fowler, M. D. M. (2010). *Guide to the code of ethics for nurses: Interpretation and application.* Silver Spring, MD: American Nurses Association.

Goffman, E. (1963). *Stigma: Notes on the management of spoiled identity.* Englewood Cliffs, NJ: Prentice Hall.

Green, G. (2009). *The end of stigma? Changes in the social experience of long-term illness.* New York, NY: Routledge.

Hewitt, J. P., & Shulman, D. (2011). *Self and society: A symbolic interactionist social psychology* (11th ed.). Upper Saddle River, NJ: Prentice Hall.

Kessler, R.C., Demler, O., Frank, R.G., Olfson, M., Pincus, H.A., Walters, E.E., . . . Zaslavsky, A.M. (2005). Prevalence and treatment of mental disorders, 1990 to 2003. *New England Journal of Medicine, 352*(24), 2515–2523.

Lamb, J. D., Bower, P., Rogers, A., Dowrick, C., & Gask, L. (2011). Access to mental health in primary care: A qualitative meta-synthesis of evidence from the experience of people from "hard to reach groups." *Health.* Advance online publication.

Lopez, A. D., Mathers, C. D., Ezzati, M., Jamison, D. T., & Murray, C. J. L. (2006). *Global burden of disease and risk factors.* Washington, DC: World Bank.

Moussavi, S., Chatterji, S., Verdes, E., Tandon, A., Patel, V., & Ustun, B. (2007). Depression, chronic diseases, and decrements in health: Results from the World Health Surveys. *Lancet, 370*(9590), 851–858.

Murray, C. J., & Lopez, A. D. (1996). Evidence-based health policy: Lessons from the global burden of disease study. *Science, 274,* 740–761.

National Alliance for Mental Illness. *Rating the states.* Retrieved from http://www.nami.org/gtsTemplate09.cfm?Section=Grading_the_States_2009

National Institute of Mental Health. *Leading categories of diseases/disorders.* Retrieved from http://www.nimh.gov

Patel, V., & Prince, M. (2011). Global mental health. *Journal of the American Medical Association, 303*(19), 1976–1977.

Prince, M., Patel, V., Saxena, S., Maj, M., Maselko, J., Phillips, M. R., & Rahman, A. (2007). No health without mental health. *Lancet, 370*(9590), 859–877.

Sansone, R. A., & Sansone, L. H. (2010). Psychiatric disorders: A global look at facts and figures. *Psychiatry, 7*(12), 16–19.

Sartorius, N., Gaebel, W., Cleveland, H. R., Stuart, H., Akiyama, T., et al. (2010). WPA guidance on how to combat stigma of psychiatry and psychiatrists. *World Psychiatry, 9*(3), 131–144.

Stein, M. B., Roy-Byrne, P. P., Craske, M. G., Campbell-Sills, L., Lang, A. J., Golinelli, D., . . . Sullivan, G. (2011). Quality of and patient satisfaction with primary health care for anxiety disorders. *Journal of Clinical Psychiatry.* Advance online publication.

Wallace, E. R., & Gach, I. (2011). *History of psychiatry and medical psychology.* New York: Springer-Verlag.

Psychiatric–Mental Health Nurses: Who Are They?

CAROL REN KNEISL

LEARNING OUTCOMES

After completing this chapter, you will be able to:

1. Apply knowledge of current practice and professional performance standards to the delivery of contemporary psychiatric–mental health nursing.
2. Compare and contrast the differences and similarities among the roles of the psychiatric–mental health nurse and other members of the mental health team.
3. Analyze the factors that influence the success with which the mental health team achieves collaboration among its members and with clients and their significant others.
4. Describe how the role of the psychiatric–mental health nurse changed over the years from that of custodian to a multifaceted role.
5. Discuss the nursing theory concepts and principles that have shaped psychiatric–mental health nursing most directly.
6. Explain why you should be capable of functioning in all theories of care.

CRITICAL THINKING CHALLENGE

You find your psychiatric–mental health nursing clinical experience professionally challenging, intellectually stimulating, and personally rewarding. You are considering becoming a psychiatric nurse upon graduation and have discussed your feelings with a classmate, a neighbor, and your primary care physician.

Your classmate says you won't be a real nurse and that you'll forget all the skills you learned in school. Your neighbor, a critical care nurse, thinks you'll be bored as a psychiatric–mental health nurse. The critical care unit, with its high drama, split-second decisions, and high-tech atmosphere, she says, is the setting where a good student like you would be happiest and make the greatest contribution. Your physician suggests that you be cautious. With the explosion in psychobiologic research and the discovery of more effective psychopharmacologic agents, she thinks that in a few years there may be no need for psychiatric–mental health nurses and you'll be out of a job.

1. What do you think about what they have said? Are they right?
2. What elements of psychiatric–mental health nursing provide excitement, challenge, art, and science?
3. In what ways are psychiatric–mental health nurses valuable to their clients?

What does it mean to be a psychiatric–mental health nurse? According to a coalition of professional groups (American Nurses Association [ANA], American Psychiatric Nurses Association [APNA], & International Society of Psychiatric–Mental Health Nurses [ISPN], 2007), **psychiatric–mental health nursing** is committed to promoting mental health through the assessment, diagnosis, and treatment of human responses to mental health problems and psychiatric disorders. It is a specialized area of nursing practice and a core mental health discipline that employs explanatory theories of, and research on, human behavior as its science and the purposeful use of self as its art. Essential components of the specialty practice of psychiatric–mental health nursing include the following:

- Health and wellness promotion through identification of mental health issues
- Prevention of mental health problems
- Care of persons with mental health problems
- Treatment of persons with psychiatric disorders (ANA, APNA, & ISPN, 2007)

This coalition of professional groups identified standards for professional psychiatric–mental health nursing practice. These standards are discussed later in this chapter. On a more personal level, this specialty is the only one in which your voice, face, body language, and what cannot be seen—the mind, neurotransmitters, self-esteem, your attitude, and the like—shape your work.

The authors and contributors to this textbook, other seasoned psychiatric–mental health nurses and nursing students share their personal reasons for choosing psychiatric–mental health nursing in the Why I Became a Psychiatric–Mental Health Nurse and Why I Plan to Become a Psychiatric–Mental Health Nurse features sprinkled throughout this book. We hope that you will join us in rehumanizing mental health care in a technologic society.

EMERGENCE OF THE DISCIPLINE

The role of the psychiatric–mental health nurse has changed over the years from that of custodian to a multifaceted role, and the settings in which psychiatric–mental health nurses practice have expanded from inside the hospital to all of the communities in which people live.

Although nursing functions have existed since ancient times, the profession of nursing, particularly psychiatric–mental health nursing, is a product of the late 19th and 20th centuries. Theodor and Friedericke Fliedner founded the first systematic school of nursing in Germany in 1836. It was this school at Kaiserwerth that Florence Nightingale (see FIGURE 2-1 ■) visited in 1851 before organizing a school to educate nurses in England after the Crimean War. Her school, Saint Thomas Hospital in London, stressed the importance of providing an optimum environment for clients. Although it is true that in the context of her time she emphasized the physical environment, Nightingale was among the first to note that the influence of nurses on their clients goes beyond physical care and has psychological and

WHY I BECAME A PSYCHIATRIC–MENTAL HEALTH NURSE

Carol Ren Kneisl, RN, MS
Textbook Author

I love challenges. As a beginning nursing student, I thought the excitement and high-tech atmosphere of a large general hospital was the best and most challenging of all worlds. It was in this setting that I discovered that although I could perform the technical skills without a problem, physical care was not enough for many of the clients I saw.

In this medical–surgical setting, I learned that an effective personal coping style, emotional stability, family support, and resilience and hardiness on the client's part; and the comfort, concern, and commitment provided by caring nurses helped people get well or overcome their circumstances. This is most likely when I realized that through artful therapeutic practice, I could create a common ground with my clients and provide a nurturing, healing milieu. What could be more challenging than that?

The practice of psychiatric–mental health nursing has brought me the excitement and the challenge I crave. I know, as an optimistic person, that all people, no matter their circumstances, have the capacity for personal responsibility, growth, and change. It is personally satisfying to know that as a psychiatric–mental health nurse, I have the opportunity to help them in their search for happier and mentally healthier lives.

FIGURE 2-1 ■ Florence Nightingale.
Photo courtesy of Photos.com/Jupiterimages.

social components. This section discusses the history of psychiatric–mental health nursing, which is summarized in the timeline in FIGURE 2-2 ■.

Early Psychiatric Nursing Education

In the early 1870s, the first three American nursing schools, organized in the pattern of Nightingale's school at Saint Thomas Hospital, were opened in New York, Boston, and New Haven. Linda Richards—sometimes called "the first American psychiatric nurse"—spent a significant part of her career developing better nursing care in psychiatric hospitals (see FIGURE 2-3 ■ on page 22). She opened the first American school for psychiatric nurses at the McLean Psychiatric Asylum in Waverly, Massachusetts, in 1880. By 1890, there were 35 such schools in asylums. Unlike graduates of general hospital schools of nursing, these nurses could find employment only in asylums.

By the end of the 19th century, psychiatric nurses attended mainly to the physical needs of clients and did not pursue systematic interpersonal work with them. Psychiatric theory in this period emphasized providing a physical environment that would promote recovery. Thus, nurses administered medications such as chloral hydrate and paraldehyde, supervised the use of hydrotherapy, and oversaw the nutrition and physical care of clients. Much of psychiatric nursing practice was custodial, mechanistic, and directed by psychiatrists. A ratio of 1 trained nurse to 140 clients was not unusual, and some large mental hospitals hired no registered nurses at all.

The notion that nurses caring for clients with physical disorders should be trained in general hospitals, and those caring for clients with mental disorders should be trained in psychiatric hospitals, dominated nursing education for over half a century. In 1913, the school of nursing at Johns Hopkins Hospital in Baltimore included a psychiatric nursing component in its curriculum, heralding the beginning of a slow, but important, change in the structure of nursing programs.

The first psychiatric nursing text, *Nursing Mental Diseases,* was written in 1920 by Harriet Bailey, the Assistant Superintendent of Nurses at the psychiatric service at Johns Hopkins Hospital. It was, for 20 years, the standard textbook in psychiatric nursing. Prior to this time, psychiatric textbooks were written by psychiatrists who devoted only a few pages to the instruction of nurses in procedures such as tube feeding and preparing treatment trays.

In the years between the two world wars, mental hospitals were seriously understaffed. In an effort to cope with understaffing, mental hospitals opened schools of nursing at an incredible rate—67 in 1936 alone.

Moving into the Mainstream

In 1937, the National League for Nursing Education (now the National League for Nursing [NLN]) recommended, but did not require, that psychiatric nursing content and clinical experience be a part of the curriculum in all basic nursing programs. The NLN also took over from psychiatrists the tasks of standardizing and accrediting psychiatric nursing education in single-focus schools for psychiatric nurses.

Psychiatric nursing moved into the mainstream of nursing in the 1940s, and nurses began to assume increasing responsibility for educating their own. However, the focus of psychiatric nursing activities continued to be providing kind, but custodial, nursing care. Nurses supervised or were responsible for providing housekeeping tasks such as scrubbing floors and counting mops and sheets; feeding, clothing, and bathing clients; assisting physicians with treatments; and keeping the keys to locked wards, locked cabinets, even locked toilet tissue containers.

The specialty grew slowly during the 1940s. In the meantime, psychiatric theory expanded to encompass the interpersonal and emotional dimensions of mental illness. During these years, Sigmund Freud published his works on psychoanalysis, Adolph Meyer's *commonsense psychiatry* had great impact in the United States and Great Britain, and Harry Stack Sullivan introduced the concept of *milieu therapy* as a new approach to treating hospitalized psychiatric patients. These ideologic changes in psychiatry, discussed further in Chapter 5∞, did not have a noticeable influence on psychiatric nursing care until the early 1950s.

Although the somatic treatments in use at the time controlled some dramatically bizarre client behavior and made some clients more available for interpersonal interactions, it was not until 1946, with passage of the National Mental Health Act (the government's response to growing recognition of mental illness as a national health problem), that any systematic development of psychotherapeutic roles for nurses began. Most psychiatric clients were being cared for in large state mental hospitals where small numbers of staff were expected to manage large numbers of clients living in crowded conditions. Somatic treatments, rather than talk therapies (or psychotherapy), were more practical in these settings. Talk therapies were often reserved for the private clients of psychiatrists in private psychiatric hospitals or in private practice settings.

Psychiatric Nursing as a Specialty

During World War II, 43% of all people discharged from the army were classified as having a psychiatric disability, creating a sharp increase in the demand for psychiatric services. The National Mental Health Act, enacted in 1946 to cope with the surge in the need for psychiatric services, established the National Institute for Mental Health (NIMH) to be added to the National Institutes of Health in Bethesda, Maryland.

With the establishment of the NIMH, psychiatric nursing was finally added to psychiatry, psychology, and social work as a field in which the highest priority became the preparation of clinically capable persons for positions of leadership. Before this time, fewer than a dozen psychiatric nurses held master's degrees in the United States. The psychiatric nursing education given most students consisted of a few weeks of observation on a psychiatric ward.

Because of new funding, the number of graduate programs increased gradually and steadily and prepared many of the nursing leaders who later developed theoretical frameworks for one-to-one relationship work. Because of its wide-ranging effects, the National Mental Health Act of 1946 is probably the

Important Dates in the History of Psychiatric-Mental Health Nursing

• Florence Nightingale founds school at Saint Thomas Hospital in London. Nightingale among the first to note that the influence of nurses on their clients transcends physical care.

• Linda Richards directs the first American school for psychiatric nurses at the McLean Psychiatric Asylum in Waverly, Massachusetts.

• Trained nurses attend to the physical needs of clients and do not pursue systematic interpersonal work.

• Psychiatric nursing practice is primarily custodial, mechanistic, and directed by psychiatrists.

• A ratio of 1 trained nurse to 140 clients is not unusual.

• *Nursing Mental Diseases*, the first psychiatric nursing text, is written by Harriet Bailey and remains the standard textbook in psychiatric nursing for 20 years.

• Most textbooks are written by psychiatrists; only a few pages address psychiatric nurses in such procedures as tube and rectal feeding and preparing treatment trays.

Emergence of the Discipline of Psychiatric Nursing

1860s	1890s	1920s
1960s	1970s	1980s

Confirmation of Specialist Roles

Period of Decline and Retrenchment

• The Community Mental Health Centers Act pushes trend in psychiatric nursing toward expanded and specialized roles in a variety of community settings.

• First textbook to address group therapy techniques in nursing practice written by Shirley Armstrong and Sheila Rouslin.

• Shirley Burd and Margaret Marshall write and edit the first compilation of papers suitable for graduate students in psychiatric nursing.

• First psychiatric nursing journals *Perspectives in Psychiatric Care* and *Journal of Psychiatric Nursing and Mental Health Services* published.

• The first certification programs for advanced psychiatric nursing practice are developed by the New Jersey and New York State Nurses Associations.

• The psychiatric nurses who developed and implemented the early certification programs (Marian Pettingill, Sheila Rouslin Welt, and Carol Ren Kneisl) recognized the need to acknowledge expertise, distinguish generalist from specialist roles, and safeguard the public.

• Certification in psychiatric nursing becomes the responsibility of the ANA.

• *Standards of Psychiatric-Mental Health Nursing* published by ANA.

• *Issues in Mental Health Nursing* published.

•ANA Council of Specialists in Psychiatric and Mental Health Nursing develops a classification system for Psychiatric Nursing Diagnosis.

• *Standards of Child and Adolescent Psychiatric and Mental Health Nursing* and *Standards of Addictions Nursing Practice* published by ANA.

• American Psychiatric Nurses Association formed.

• *Archives of Psychiatric Nursing* and *Journal of Child and Adolescent Psychiatric and Mental Health Nursing* published.

• Psychiatric nursing leaders recommend incorporating new psychobiologic knowledge into clinical practice.

FIGURE 2-2 ■ *Photo source top to bottom by column:* Photos.com/Jupiterimages; Superstock; Eileen Trigoboff; Carol Ren Kneisl; Eileen Trigoboff; Viktoriya/Shutterstock; Shutterstock; Photo Researchers, Inc.; Letitia Anne Peplau; Photo Researchers, Inc.; Benjamin Albiach Galan/Shutterstock.

• New medical surgical procedures (deep sleep therapy, insulin shock therapy, psychosurgery, and electroshock therapy) promote the role of psychiatric nurses as participants in psychiatric treatment.

• Nursing leaders recommend elimination of single-focus schools marking the beginning of the mainstreaming of psychiatric nursing.

• National Institute of Mental Health (NIMH) established; National Mental Health Act helps develop psychotherapeutic roles for nurses.

• Hildegard Peplau emphasizes psychodynamic concepts and counseling techniques and develops first master's program to prepare clinical specialists in psychiatric nursing.

• Gwen Tudor Will demonstrates nursing interventions with a sociopsychiatric base.

• National League for Nursing introduces the concept of psychiatric nurse specialists; first NIMH grants to integrate mental health concepts into nursing curriculum.

• National League for Nursing Education recommends that psychiatric nursing content and clinical experience be part of the curriculum in all basic nursing programs.

• Psychiatric nursing activities contiue to be custodial nursing care, including housekeeping tasks and keeping the keys to locked wards, cabinets, and even toilet tissue containers.

Movement of Psychiatric Nursing into the Mainstream of Nursing

Confirmation of Psychiatric Nursing as a Specialty

1930s **1940s** **1950s**

The 1990s **2000**

Decade of the Brain

• Several psychiatric nurses appointed to President Clinton's task force on health care reform.

• *Standards of Psychiatric Consultation Liaison Nursing* published by ANA.

• Revised *Standards of Psychiatric-Mental Health Clinical Nursing Practice* published by ANA.

• *Psychopharmacology Guidelines for Psychiatric-Mental Health Nurses,* intended to increase knowledge of psychopharmacology and improve patient care, published by ANA.

• *Journal of the American Psychiatric Nurses Association* published.

• Psychiatric nursing leaders urge nurses to use the challenging circumstances posed by burgeoning information, reduced funding, and health care reform to clarify nursing's unique contribution to mental health care.

Beginning of a New Millennium

• American Nurses Association, in collaboration with the American Psychiatric Nurses Association and the International Society of Psychiatric-Mental Health Nurses, publishes (2000) and revises (2007) the *Scope and Standards of Psychiatric-Mental Health Nursing Practice.*

• An increase in the numbers and types of alternative and nontraditional treatment settings provide new opportunities for psychiatric-mental health nurses to provide mental health care in primary care environments as well as in psychiatric settings.

• As knowledge continues to explode in psychobiology, genetics, and human behavior, psychiatric nursing leaders focus on the need to integrate the biological, psychological, social, spiritual, and environmental realms of the human experience into mental health services while remaining centered in the nursing domain with its focus on caring.

• Primary care becomes a significant point of entry for psychiatric care.

• Nurse practitioner and clinical nurse specialist titles for APRNs.

FIGURE 2-3 ■ Linda Richards, known as the first American psychiatric nurse.
Photo courtesy of Superstock.

most significant piece of legislation affecting the development of psychiatric–mental health nursing.

Nursing leaders began to question the wisdom of single-focus schools of psychiatric nursing. In 1948, a report entitled *Nursing for the Future* (Brown, 1948) recommended their elimination. The needs of nursing could best be served, the report indicated, if the psychiatric hospitals conducting schools of nursing made their facilities widely available instead to students in basic schools of nursing. Shortly thereafter, in 1955, the NLN made the provision of a clinical experience in psychiatric nursing a requirement for the accreditation of nursing schools. Requiring both coursework and hands-on clinical experience further cemented the mainstreaming of psychiatric nursing.

Until the early 1950s, psychiatric nurses formulated only vague concepts about how nurses might participate in one–to–one relationships with clients. Ambiguity about professional psychiatric nursing roles characterized this period.

Role Clarification

The 1950s and early 1960s were a period of role clarification. Three important milestones in psychiatric nursing occurred in 1952.

First, Hildegard Peplau published *Interpersonal Relations in Nursing,* the first systematic theoretic framework in psychiatric nursing, a milestone in the development of psychiatric nursing theory and practice (1952). She delineated several skills, activities, and roles for psychiatric nurses and emphasized the interpersonal nature of nursing and the need for nurses to understand and use psychodynamic concepts and counseling techniques in their practice. Under Peplau's leadership, the first graduate degree in psychiatric–mental health nursing was awarded in 1954 by Rutgers University. Peplau's theoretical contributions are discussed in greater detail later in this chapter.

Second, Gwen Tudor Will published an article in the journal *Psychiatry*. This was a major feat in itself because the journal for psychiatrists had never published an article by a nurse and no psychiatric nursing journals existed at the time. She used sociopsychiatric theory to explain a mutual pattern of avoidance that emerged among the nursing staff, physicians, and one particular female client (Tudor, 1952) and designed and tested a nursing intervention to disrupt the pattern of avoidance. Tudor's unique contribution demonstrated that:

- Psychiatric nurses can have a profoundly positive or a profoundly negative effect on the client
- The social milieu of the psychiatric ward can maintain deviant patterns of behavior
- The psychotherapeutic nursing role can be taught to others
- Nurses can carry out scholarly research

Hers is the classic scholarly psychiatric nursing research study, significant for its dramatic impact on nursing and its contribution to an understanding of the effects of the milieu.

Third, Frances Sleeper, in an address to the American Psychiatric Association, advocated the use of psychiatric nurses as psychotherapists. Her advocacy ushered in a heated, 10-year controversy over caretaker versus psychotherapist roles for psychiatric nurses.

Clinical Nurse Specialist Role

The Community Mental Health Centers Act in 1963, which encouraged the closing of large mental hospitals in favor of treatment in the community, further encouraged the trend in psychiatric nursing toward expanded and specialized roles. The **clinical nurse specialist (CNS)**, prepared at the graduate level in psychiatric–mental health nursing, began providing individual, group, and family psychotherapy in a wide variety of settings and obtaining third-party reimbursement in some states. They broadened their practice to include schools, outreach clinics, transitional services, jails, alternative treatment settings, and private practice as well as the traditional mental hospital.

The launching in 1963 of *Perspectives in Psychiatric Care*—the first psychiatric nursing journal, was edited and published by Alice Clarke, a psychiatric nurse—provided a forum for airing issues and sharing psychiatric nursing knowledge. A second journal, the *Journal of Psychiatric Nursing and Mental Health Services,* began later that same year and changed its name in 1981 to the *Journal of Psychosocial Nursing and Mental Health Services.* Clinical and research papers by psychiatric nursing leaders in these journals and in the *American Journal of Nursing* further established the counseling role as the basis of psychiatric nursing, whether it was defined as psychotherapy or not.

Shortly thereafter, the first textbook to address group therapy techniques in nursing practice was written by Shirley

Armstrong and Sheila Rouslin (1963). Shirley Byrd and Margaret Marshall (1963) wrote and edited the first compilation of psychiatric nursing papers suitable for graduate students in psychiatric nursing.

A 1967 ANA position paper on psychiatric nursing endorsed clinical specialists as therapists in individual, group, family, and milieu work. By 1969, a psychiatric nurse had, as Peplau predicted a few years before, moved into private practice.

The first master's level certification program for advanced psychiatric nursing practice was developed by the New Jersey Nurses Association in 1971, followed in 2 years by the New York State Nurses Association. The psychiatric nurses who developed and implemented these early certification programs—Sheila Rouslin Welt, Carol Ren Kneisl, Marian Pettingill, Marian Krizinofski, and others—recognized the need to acknowledge expertise, distinguish generalist from specialist roles, and safeguard the public. By the mid-1970s, certification at both the generalist and the specialist levels in psychiatric nursing became the responsibility of the ANA.

In 1973, the ANA published the first standards of psychiatric–mental health nursing practice to serve as guidelines for providing quality care. These standards of practice, revised several times since then, delineate psychiatric–mental health nursing roles and functions and are the focus of the next section of this chapter.

President Jimmy Carter's 1977 Commission on Mental Health, unlike earlier commissions on mental health and mental illness that were dominated by physicians, included a nurse (Martha Mitchell, the chairperson of the ANA Division on Psychiatric and Mental Health Nursing Practice), and three other professional nurses who served on adjunct committees. This was the first official high-level document to give visibility to the professional competence of nurses in mental health care.

According to Osborne (1984), the publication in 1979 of *Psychiatric Nursing* by Holly Skodol Wilson and Carol Ren Kneisl (the original edition of this textbook) signaled a significant change in psychiatric nursing textbooks and psychiatric nursing thinking. This was the first in a new era of psychiatric nursing textbooks to provide and consistently use a major conceptual theme based on humanistic interactionism and advocating negotiated goals between nurse and client, client advocacy, and political sensitivity, as well as caring and compassion in a biopsychosocial model. Since that time, other psychiatric nursing textbooks have followed in the tradition of Wilson and Kneisl. Another psychiatric nursing journal, *Issues in Mental Health Nursing,* also began in 1979.

Fiscal Decline and Retrenchment

After two decades of apparently unlimited support from the NIMH in the form of money for educational programs and traineeships for psychiatric nurses at the graduate level, funding for psychiatric nursing education was cut. A major concern for psychiatric nurses in the 1980s was the decrease in the number of nurses selecting psychiatric nursing as a specialty and a shortage of clinical training funding. Psychiatric nursing found itself on the verge of a period of retrenchment that remains to this day.

In 1984, recognizing the need for a set of psychiatric nursing diagnoses to supplement those identified by the North American Nursing Diagnoses Association (NANDA), the ANA Council of Specialists in Psychiatric and Mental Health Nursing developed a classification system for psychiatric nursing. The panel identified relevant and useful categories for psychiatric nursing diagnosis and synthesized its findings with those of NANDA. Psychiatric nursing diagnoses are now an integral part of the NANDA classification system.

In early 1987, another new psychiatric nursing journal, *Archives of Psychiatric Nursing,* made its debut. The purpose of the journal was to provide a forum in which psychiatric nursing clinician–scholars can suggest theoretic linkages between diverse areas of practice and shape public policy for the delivery of psychiatric and mental health nursing services.

Decade of the Brain

The 1990s were designated the "Decade of the Brain" by Congress and the NIMH. During this period, psychiatry underwent a paradigm shift to include the neurobiologic domains. Research studies that focused on psychobiology provided new biologic strategies for assessments and interventions.

Psychiatric nursing leaders urged the inclusion of biologic therapies along with the use of more traditional psychotherapy, psychosocial therapies, and combination therapies. McBride cautioned psychiatric–mental health nurses to stop devaluing biologic knowledge and to become fundamentally reassociated with care and caring (1990). Peplau (1989) made additional recommendations to:

- Promote political savvy in advocating psychiatric–mental health care resources
- Continue developing out-of-hospital services, including those offered on a private practice basis
- Pursue evaluation and outcome clinical studies
- Inform the public and others of the work we do
- Keep emphasizing the human aspects of mental health work even as psychiatry moves in the direction of psychobiologic practice

The specialty needed to create a new image for psychiatric–mental health nurses, foster cultural diversity among psychiatric–mental health nurses, and integrate philosophic and theoretic perspectives in both practice and research.

Health care reform was a political concern during the 1990s, and nursing organizations (Krauss, 1993) figured prominently in advocating for reform and equitable access to basic mental health care, a goal that has yet to be met.

During this period, there was tremendous growth in the development of new psychopharmacologic treatments for mental disorder. The ANA named a task force, the Psychiatric–Mental Health Nursing Psychopharmacology Project, to study the issues and strategies associated with the administration of psychopharmacologic agents. The task force published a set of psychopharmacology guidelines for psychiatric–mental health nurses in 1994 (American Nurses Association Task Force on Psychopharmacology, 1994). The guidelines recommended integrating current data from the neurosciences, demonstrating

Case Study: The Multifaceted Role

knowledge of psychopharmacologic principles, and providing safe and effective clinical management of clients taking these medications (see Chapters 7 and 32∞).

A specialty organization for psychiatric–mental health nurses, the American Psychiatric Nurses Association (APNA), was established in the 1990s and began publication of a new psychiatric nursing journal, the *Journal of the American Psychiatric Nurses Association.*

The New Millennium

Early in the new millennium, the ANA collaborated with the APNA and the International Society of Psychiatric–Mental Health Nurses to revise the standards for the practice of psychiatric–mental health nursing. In 2007, these guidelines were revised into the most forward-looking set of standards developed to date (ANA, APNA, & ISPN, 2007). They are discussed later in this chapter.

The knowledge explosion in psychobiology continues, characterized by a broader understanding of the biology of the mind and the biologic foundations of behavior and temperament. Significant knowledge about the genetic basis of inherited mental disorders has resulted from the genetic research undertaken at the NIMH. A growing arsenal of psychopharmacologic agents with fewer side effects helps clients enjoy a higher quality of life. The greatest challenge that psychiatric–mental health nursing faces is integrating psychobiologic knowledge into clinical practice while maintaining a focus on the caring dimension.

Other trends, early in this new millenium, have sparked several significant changes in the delivery of mental health services and provide new challenges for the practice of psychiatric–mental health nursing:

- Concern with the physical health problems of psychiatric clients, a sometimes overlooked dimension of care. In particular, Chafetz and her associates (Chafetz, White, Collins-Bride, & Nickens, 2008), concerned about the physical health of severely and persistently mentally ill clients who live in community settings, have developed wellness clinics especially for them.
- The shift to primary care as a point of entry for psychiatric care (Jackson, Passamonti, & Kroenke, 2007; Kroenke, Spitzer, Williams, Monahan, & Lowe, 2007).
- A curriculum shift in graduate programs in psychiatric–mental health nursing that encompasses an increased emphasis on comprehensive health assessment, management of common physical health problems, and a focus on meeting the requirements for prescriptive authority for advanced practice nurses.
- A shift at the advanced level of practice toward the use of psychiatric–mental health nurse practitioner as a title. The role competencies for psychiatric–mental health nurse practitioners have been clearly delineated (National Panel for Psychiatric–Mental Health NP Competencies, 2003). Advanced-practice psychiatric–mental health nurses now practice under the clinical nurse specialist or nurse practitioner titles, but share the same core competencies.

- An expansion of the settings for psychiatric–mental health nursing practice from hospitals and traditional psychiatric settings to alternative and nontraditional settings.

At the same time, in most schools, nursing students receive only brief and limited exposure to mental health clients and mental health settings. It is difficult to appreciate a specialty when you do not experience its many facets. This textbook will, we hope, enhance those limited clinical experiences. We hope not only to challenge you but also to awaken in you a sense of excitement about the possibilities for professional fulfillment that psychiatric–mental health nursing holds.

STANDARDS AND LEVELS OF PRACTICE

Two sets of standards guide professional psychiatric–mental health nursing practice. The Standards of Practice are reproduced in Box 2-1. Note that Standard 5 specifically discusses the unique role functions of the psychiatric–mental health nurse. The Standards of Professional Performance are reproduced in Box 2-2. The chapters in this textbook are firmly guided by the Standards of Practice and the Standards of Professional Performance and demonstrate client-centered care in this specialty area. The chapters identify how you would assess, diagnose, identify outcomes, plan, implement, and evaluate the care of clients with mental health disorders in nonpsychiatric as well psychiatric settings.

Basic Level of Practice

There are two levels of professional practice in psychiatric–mental health nursing. The *basic level psychiatric–mental health nurse* (PMH) may have received basic nursing preparation in a diploma, associate degree, or baccalaureate program. Essentially a generalist who works in a specialized setting, this nurse provides the bulk of the nursing care to clients. Registered nurses offer direct and indirect care through the nurse–client relationship. They have major responsibility for the milieu and have contact with clients at all stages of daily life. Nurses at this level may seek **certification** as generalists through the ANA's American Nurses Credentialing Center (ANCC). Certification by a professional nursing organization recognizes competence and also protects the consumer of mental health services. Credentialing information can be found on ANCC's website and accessed through the online student resources for this book.

Advanced Level of Practice

According to the ANA, APNA, and ISPN (2007), the **advanced practice registered nurse (APRN)** in psychiatric–mental health (APRN-PMH) is a licensed registered nurse who is educationally prepared as a clinical nurse specialist or a nurse practitioner at the master's or doctorate degree level in the specialty of psychiatric–mental health nursing. Advanced practice psychiatric–mental health nurses may also seek certification at the advanced level through ANCC. They may use the initials CS (certified specialist). The advanced-level certification is a means of protecting consumers. In addition to the basic-level role functions, several advanced-level role functions are listed in Box 2-2 (see Standards 5E, 5F, and 5G).

Box 2-1 Psychiatric–Mental Health Nursing Standards of Practice

The six standards of practice describe a competent level of nursing care organized around the nursing process. Note that Standards 5E, 5F, and 5G apply to advanced practice only.

Standard 1. Assessment The Psychiatric–Mental Health Registered Nurse collects comprehensive health data that is pertinent to the patient's health or situation.

Standard 2. Diagnosis The Psychiatric–Mental Health Registered Nurse analyzes the assessment data to determine diagnoses or problems, including level of risk.

Standard 3. Outcomes Identification The Psychiatric–Mental Health Registered Nurse identifies expected outcomes for a plan individualized to the patient or to the situation.

Standard 4. Planning The Psychiatric–Mental Health Registered Nurse develops a plan that prescribes strategies and alternatives to attain expected outcomes.

Standard 5. Implementation The Psychiatric–Mental Health Registered Nurse implements the identified plan.

Standard 5 A. Coordination of Care The Psychiatric–Mental Health Registered Nurse coordinates care delivery.

Standard 5 B. Health Teaching and Health Promotion The Psychiatric–Mental Health Registered Nurse employs strategies to promote health and a safe environment.

Standard 5 C. Milieu Therapy The Psychiatric–Mental Health Registered Nurse provides, structures, and maintains a safe and therapeutic environment in collaboration with patients, families, and other health care clinicians.

Standard 5 D. Pharmacological, Biological, and Integrative Therapies The Psychiatric–Mental Health Registered Nurse incorporates knowledge of pharmacological, biological, and complementary interventions with applied clinical skills to restore the patient's health and prevent further disability.

Standard 5 E. Prescriptive Authority and Treatment (APRN only) The Psychiatric–Mental Health Advanced Practice Registered Nurse uses prescriptive authority, procedures, referrals, treatments, and therapies in accordance with state and federal laws and regulations.

Standard 5 F. Psychotherapy (APRN only) The Psychiatric–Mental Health Advanced Practice Registered Nurse conducts individual, couples, group, and family psychotherapy using evidence-based psychotherapeutic frameworks and nurse–patient therapeutic relationships.

Standard 5 G. Consultation (APRN only) The Psychiatric–Mental Health Advanced Practice Registered Nurse provides consultation to influence the identified plan, enhance the abilities of other clinicians to provide services for patients, and effect change.

Standard 6. Evaluation The Psychiatric–Mental Health Registered Nurse evaluates progress toward attainment of expected outcomes.

Source: Reprinted with permission from American Nurses Association, American Psychiatric–Mental Health Nurses Association, & International Society of Psychiatric–Mental Health Nurses. *Psychiatric–mental health nursing: Scope and standards of practice,* © 2007. Silver Spring, MD: Nursesbooks.org

---

Box 2-2 Psychiatric–Mental Health Nursing Standards of Professional Performance

The nine standards of professional performance describe a competent level of behavior in professional role activities.

Standard 7. Quality of Practice The Psychiatric–Mental Health Registered Nurse systematically enhances the quality and effectiveness of nursing practice.

Standard 8. Education The Psychiatric–Mental Health Registered Nurse attains knowledge and competency that reflect current nursing practice.

Standard 9. Professional Practice Evaluation The Psychiatric–Mental Health Registered Nurse evaluates one's own practice in relation to the professional practice standards and guidelines, relevant statutes, rules, and regulations.

Standard 10. Collegiality The Psychiatric–Mental Health Registered Nurse interacts with and contributes to the professional development of peers and colleagues.

Standard 11. Collaboration The Psychiatric–Mental Health Registered Nurse collaborates with patients, family, and others in the conduct of nursing practice.

Standard 12. Ethics The Psychiatric–Mental Health Registered Nurse integrates ethical provisions in all areas of practice.

Standard 13. Research The Psychiatric–Mental Health Registered Nurse integrates research findings into practice.

Standard 14. Resource Utilization The Psychiatric–Mental Health Registered Nurse considers factors related to safety, effectiveness, cost, and impact on practice in the planning and delivery of nursing services.

Standard 15. Leadership The Psychiatric–Mental Health Registered Nurse provides leadership in the professional practice setting and the profession.

Source: Reprinted with permission from American Nurses Association, American Psychiatric–Mental Health Nurses Association, & International Society of Psychiatric–Mental Health Nurses. *Psychiatric–mental health nursing: Scope and standards of practice,* © 2007. Silver Spring, MD: Nursesbooks.org

American Nurses Credentialing Center

PARTNERSHIP AND COLLABORATION

As a psychiatric–mental health nurse, you will collaborate with other members of the mental health team and with the client's family and significant others. Psychiatric–mental health nurses, wherever they practice, must plan and share with others to deliver maximum mental health services to clients and their families. The purpose of partnering and collaborating with others is to make the best use of the different abilities of mental health team members so that the client and the family receive the most effective service available.

The Mental Health Team

The psychiatric–mental health nurse is an integral and important part of the mental health team. Of all the disciplines involved in mental health care, nursing is the one most likely to have an overall view of the client's situation.

Mental health services are provided by a variety of professionals—psychiatric–mental health nurses, psychiatrists, clinical psychologists, psychiatric social workers, marriage and family therapists, occupational therapists, recreational therapists, and creative arts therapists—who have received many forms of specialized training. These professions require formal academic instruction, often at the graduate level, and extensive clinical experience. Psychosocial rehabilitation workers and psychiatric attendants also provide mental health services and may have formal or on-the-job training.

In general, the number of professionals who supply mental health services has expanded dramatically since the 1990s, while the number of psychiatric–mental health nurses has declined. Most of the growth has occurred among non-physicians. The descriptions in TABLE 2-1 ■ of the education and functions of mental health team members reflect more traditional distinctions. Role definitions that were traditionally assigned to specific disciplines have become increasingly blurred. Many of the functions are now shared across disciplines when the team member has been appropriately educated for the task and when laws and regulations permit the sharing of functions. Psychiatric–mental health nurses, social workers, and psychologists, among others, have more direct influence than ever before. Roles are less specifically defined, and in many community settings, mental health professionals take on whichever functions they do best. However, these roles involve more than the transfer of skills—they also involve a reconfiguration of power relationships from one professional group to another (Rana, Bradley, & Nolan, 2009). This is the subject of the next section.

TABLE 2-1 ■ The Mental Health Team

Team Member	Education/Preparation	Role
Psychiatric–mental health nurse	A registered nurse with specialized preparation in psychiatric–mental health nursing; level of expertise depends on education, which may include up to the doctoral level	Responsible for the nursing care of mental health clients; has major responsibility for the milieu
Clinical specialist	A registered nurse with specialized preparation in psychiatric–mental health nursing at the graduate level	Provides a complete spectrum of services for individuals, groups, and families in inpatient, outpatient, and private practice settings to assess, manage, and treat mental health problems
Nurse practitioner	A registered nurse with specialized preparation in psychiatric–mental health nursing at the graduate level	Similar core competencies as the clinical specialist
Psychiatrist	A medical physician whose specialty is mental disorders; has completed an approved psychiatric residency	Responsible for diagnosis and treatment of persons with mental disorders
Clinical psychologist	A psychologist specially educated and trained in mental health; certification requires completion of an approved doctoral program and a clinical internship	Performs psychotherapy; plans and implements programs of behavior modification; selects, administers, and interprets psychological tests
Psychiatric social worker	A graduate of a master's program in social work with an emphasis in mental health; may have a doctoral degree	Helps clients and their families cope more effectively; identifies appropriate community resources; may perform counseling and psychotherapy
Marriage and family therapist	May be a member of any mental health discipline, usually prepared at the master's or doctoral level	Provides psychotherapy usually focusing on couples or families
Occupational therapist	Prepared in occupational therapy at the baccalaureate or master's level with a specialty in mental health care	Uses manual and creative techniques to elicit desired interpersonal and intrapsychic responses; teaches self-help activities; helps clients prepare to seek employment
Recreational therapist	May be prepared at informal or formal levels in university physical education and health education programs	Plans and guides recreational activities to provide socialization, healthful recreation, and desirable interpersonal and intrapsychic experiences
Creative arts therapist	May be prepared at informal or formal levels in colleges and universities	Uses art, music, dance, and literature to facilitate interpersonal experiences and increase social responses and self-esteem
Psychosocial rehabilitation worker/psychiatric attendant	Most have either a high school education or a bachelor's degree	Teaches clients practical, day-to-day skills for living in the community and provides case management services

Cooperation Versus Competition

Relationship problems among mental health team members must be resolved to avoid distorting the team's efforts. The key to working together on a problem with a common purpose is cooperation rather than competition. Working together in cooperation ensures movement toward the common goal, whereas inappropriate competition hinders goal achievement and may be destructive to the competing individuals.

Much of our present understanding of cooperative and competitive behavior has come from the efforts of game theorists, who have researched player behavior. According to game theorists, players can be identified and placed in categories as follows:

- *Maximizers*—those interested only in their own gain
- *Rivalists*—those interested only in defeating their partners
- *Cooperators*—those interested in helping both themselves and their partners

Mental health providers who are maximizers jeopardize the client's welfare because they put themselves first and the client last. Rivalists direct their energies toward being "one up" through put-downs of others. They also are concerned not with the client but with the process of winning. Cooperators are interested in helping both themselves and their colleagues to aid the client. Participants who actively recognize the importance of each individual member of the mental health team can influence maximizers and rivalists to become cooperators.

Effective collaboration is based on respect for the position from which another participant acts. Our values and our culture direct our beliefs and the climate in which we operate. Knowing this, we can become aware of the values and culture of others and, in turn, respect them. For a full discussion of culture and what it means to be culturally competent, refer to Chapter 9∞.

Unfortunately, the process of socialization into a profession may make it difficult for a person to respect, accept, and trust the position of another. As students become committed to a profession through the process of socialization, they tend to view members of other disciplines with suspicion. Review the lessons on collaboration in Your Intervention Strategies.

Administrative and peer support creates an atmosphere in which nurses are free to share their knowledge, skills, and evolving ideas. Such support increases creativity, depth, and perspective in nursing. Self-exploration and self-assessment, through reading and dialogue with other nurses and mental health team members, can help nurses embrace a spirit of cooperation.

Clients and Families

Family members, friends, and members of the mental health team are a central influence in each client's life. Partnership includes clients and their significant others in the collaborative process of the mental health team whenever possible. Clients' participation in their own health care assures nurses that their clients are informed consumers of mental health services. To help you develop partnerships with your clients and their families and friends, we have provided a special feature entitled

---

YOUR INTERVENTION STRATEGIES
Lessons on Collaboration

1. First, as we often remind you in this text, know your own reality. Determine your values, biases, and goals.
2. Value diversity and turn differences into assets.
3. Acknowledge that conflict is natural and develop constructive conflict resolution skills.
4. Recognize your own power base and share it with others (colleagues and clients and their families).
5. Master interpersonal communication skills and processing skills.
6. Approach collaboration as lifelong learning. The more you collaborate with others, the better you get at it.
7. Place yourself in interdisciplinary situations whenever possible—be present, both physically and mentally, at team forums.
8. Appreciate that collaboration is often spontaneous and you must be ready to seize the moment.
9. Balance unity with autonomy. That is, work neither exclusively as a member of a team (collaboration is not required for all decisions) nor in isolation.

"Partnering With Clients and Families," which you will find throughout this textbook and a separate chapter that features family-focused interventions (Chapter 29∞).

Clients and family members can also be invited to participate in case conferences. These conferences often have an important place in the functioning of mental health agencies and may have a number of purposes. Encourage clients to participate in case conferences involving collaboration among several agencies or several mental health care workers who are moving toward similar goals.

Consult the client about the information to be shared with family members and other members of the mental health team. It is not always easy for the nurse to determine exactly how much to share and with whom. When the boundaries of confidentiality are not clear, confer with your nursing instructor or a supervisor to determine what should be shared. Decisions should take safety measures into consideration as well as what agreement exists between nurse and client about sharing information and how the person or agency receiving information will use that information in the client's best interest. Refer to Chapter 12∞ for a thorough discussion of client rights and your professional responsibilities as they relate to confidentiality.

NURSING'S THEORETIC HERITAGE

The concept of nursing as primarily technologic has been replaced by the idea that nursing is theory based. We use theories to organize assessment data, identify problems, plan interventions, generate goals and nursing actions, and determine and evaluate outcomes.

A few of the best-known nursing theorists and the concepts and principles of their theories or models most relevant to psychiatric–mental health nursing are examined in this section. Each of the early nursing theorists has revisited her original formulation to move closer to psychiatric–mental health nursing values of humanism, interactionism, cultural competence, the relevance of meaning, and the importance of empathy and empowerment in the nurse–client relationship. Hildegard Peplau, Joyce Travelbee, Josephine Paterson, Loretta Zderad, Jean Watson, and Patricia Benner are theorists whose existential and interactional origins and subsequent conceptualizations are particularly congruent with the philosophy of psychiatric–mental health nursing advocated in this text.

Peplau

Hildegard Peplau (see FIGURE 2-4 ■) has had greater impact on psychiatric–mental health nursing than any other nursing theorist to date. Peplau published her groundbreaking nursing theory in the classic book *Interpersonal Relations in Nursing* (1952). She defined nursing as a significant therapeutic interpersonal process. Peplau was strongly influenced by the psychiatrist Harry Stack Sullivan and other theorists of the interpersonal school (see Chapter 5∞).

Peplau conceptualized the one–to–one nurse–client relationship as the situation in which clients can accomplish developmental tasks such as learning to trust or learning to collaborate and practice healthy communication and behaviors. The core concepts of Peplau's theory of interpersonal relations (1997) were the three phases of what she identified as the nurse–client relationship, as follows:

1. *Orientation Phase:* defining the problem mutually with the client

FIGURE 2-4 ■ Hildegard Peplau. Peplau's theory continues to guide the heart of psychiatric–mental health nursing practice.
Photo courtesy of Letitia Anne Peplau.

2. *Working Phase:* assisting the client with problem-solving alternatives
3. *Termination Phase:* dissolving the links between nurse and client

There are several similarities between Peplau's stages and the nursing process. Some say that Peplau's stages are the ancestor of the phases of the nursing process.

One of Peplau's many major contributions was the development of a step-by-step nursing intervention into anxiety. To this day this classic nursing intervention remains an important strategy not only for psychiatric–mental health nurses, but also for any nurse who works with an anxious client in any setting (George, 2011). Peplau's step-by-step nursing intervention into anxiety is discussed in detail in Chapter 18∞. This nursing intervention into anxiety demonstrated how nurses could implement the nursing roles she wrote about (1978) that were central in the creation of a therapeutic relationship, as follows:

- *Teacher:* imparting knowledge that sheds light on a need or interest
- *Resource:* providing specific information that aids in understanding a problem or a new situation
- *Counselor:* using specific skills and attitudes to help another to identify, cope with, and resolve problems that interfere with well-being
- *Leader:* carrying out and maintaining the therapeutic relationship through interacting with the client in specific phases
- *Technical expert:* using clinical skills in giving physical care
- *Surrogate:* taking the role of another (as in providing a corrective emotional experience; see Chapter 4∞)

Memorial tributes to Peplau upon her death in 1999 by nurses around the world recognized her as the "mother of psychiatric nursing" (Barker, 1999; Haber, 1999). She developed the first master's level clinical specialist program in psychiatric–mental health nursing at Rutgers University in 1954 and also practiced what she preached in a private practice in psychiatric nursing, with the World Health Organization and the NIMH, the Nurse Corps, and in other schools of nursing in North America and abroad. Psychiatric–mental health nurses continue to use Peplau's teachings to understand and guide decisions in the one–to–one therapeutic relationship. Chapter 4∞ details the one–to–one therapeutic relationship between client and nurse.

Travelbee

Joyce Travelbee is another nurse theorist who focuses on the meaning in nurse–client interactions. Travelbee (1966) explained in detail the concepts of sympathy, rapport, and suffering and emphasized the importance of communication and stages of nurse–client relationships. She emphasized the importance of being motivated by compassion—of "walking the walk with you" (George, 2011). Her view of humanity, uniqueness, existential encounters, and nursing is highly congruent with values in psychiatric–mental health nursing.

Paterson and Zderad

Paterson and Zderad's 1976 book, republished in 1988, and again in 2008, reflected the contemporary nature of their original ideas. They were a decade ahead of their time in rejecting a mechanistic cause-and-effect view of nursing science and urged instead that observations of the experience of nurses in practice should be the basis of any useful nursing theory.

Their theory portrays nursing as a live dialogue in which both nurse and client are present in the experience in an existential way that includes mutuality and intimacy. Their theory relies heavily on existential philosophers and emphasizes humanism—the freedom of human choice and responsibility for one's actions (George, 2011). It is a highly abstract theory with a major focus on the process of interaction (or dialogue) between nurse and client.

Watson

Jean Watson's theory of human caring was influenced by Jungian psychology, feminist theory, and Maslow's concept of self-actualization (Watson, 1988). She credits much of her thinking on therapeutic relationships and communication to the work of Carl Rogers, identifying congruency, empathy, and warmth as foundational to a caring relationship that conveys authenticity and genuineness and facilitates the client's expression of emotions.

According to George (2011), the elements of Watson's theory are reminiscent of Nightingale's concept of nursing as a calling. Caring–healing within Watson's framework is based on values such as kindness, concern, love of self and others, and the ecology of the earth and involves what she originally called *carative* factors: a humanistic–altruistic value system, faith–hope, and sensitivity of self and others (Watson, 1999). Watson now uses the term *clinical caritas processes; caritas* meaning "to cherish, to give special and/or loving attention." This shift in terminology demonstrates Watson's emphasis on the spiritual dimensions of the human experience. In fact, she likens caring science to sacred science (2008). Watson's 10 clinical caritas concepts are described in Box 2-3.

Her theory emphasizes sensitivity to self and values clarification regarding personal and cultural beliefs that might pose barriers to transpersonal caring. Establishing a helping–trusting human care relationship is pivotal to Watson's theory.

Watson (2008) also develops the notion of spiritual environment and the interconnectedness of all things, including the connection between natural healing approaches, self-knowledge, self-control, self-caring, self-healing potential, and caring, healing relationships with self and others. Watson's theory is philosophically congruent with contemporary global approaches to health and health promotion (Pilkington, 2007) and with the philosophical approach of this textbook.

Benner

Patricia Benner (1983, 1996, 1999), part philosopher, part theorist, has added to nursing's understanding of the language of caring. Her ideas have been generated by observing and interviewing expert nurses engaged in clinical practice. Her goal has been to disclose the nature of clinical wisdom,

---

Box 2-3   Watson's Clinical Caritas Processes

1. Embrace altruistic values and practice loving kindness with others.
2. Instill faith and hope and honor others.
3. Be sensitive to self and others by nurturing individual beliefs and practices.
4. Develop helping–trusting–caring relationships.
5. Promote and accept positive and negative feelings as you authentically listen to another's story.
6. Use creative scientific problem-solving methods for caring decision making.
7. Share teaching and learning that addresses the individual needs and comprehension styles.
8. Create a healing environment for the physical and spiritual self that respects human dignity.
9. Assist with basic physical, emotional, and spiritual human needs.
10. Open to mystery and allow miracles to enter.

Source: Dr. Jean Watson's human caring theory: Ten caritas processes. Retrieved from http://watsoncaringscience.org/caring_science/10caritas.html

---

particularly around caring and comforting practices. She argues for the importance of forming nurse–client relationships, teaching and coaching, and bearing witness to the illness experience.

Implications for Psychiatric–Mental Health Nursing Practice

The interpersonal theory of psychiatric–mental health nursing originated by Hildegard Peplau remains the nursing theory that has shaped psychiatric–mental health nursing most directly. More contemporary nurse theorists, however, have also laid the foundation for concepts that are central to psychiatric–mental

---

WHY I PLAN TO BECOME A PSYCHIATRIC–MENTAL HEALTH NURSE

Kirstie's Story: Actually, my first career goal was to become an elementary school teacher. If you had told me that one day I'd be telling my story about choosing psychiatric nursing as my future career, I would have told you that you are dead wrong. I never, ever, considered being a psychiatric nurse. I always thought that I would work in some sort of high-tech environment—emergency room or a trauma unit, even a flight nurse. But, once I had my first clinical experience, I just knew this was the place for me. On that first day, there was a client who became increasingly agitated until he finally exploded and threw a chair at another client. In our postconference we discussed how to observe for instances of increasing anger and how to assess for and recognize these symptoms before they become out of control and before it becomes necessary to administer an IM PRN medication for agitation. Another client was experiencing several side effects from his medication so we developed a psychoeducation teaching plan for him and the next week did a group on side effects for all the clients on the unit. I could actually see that the things I was doing were making a difference in their lives.

health nursing practice. The nursing theorists discussed here have had the following effects on psychiatric–mental health nursing:

- Differentiated nursing from medicine with emphases on caring and comforting rather than curing
- Placed the importance of interpreting meaning at the center of their theories
- Focused on interaction between the nurse and the client
- Advocated humanistic and existential values of client dignity, freedom, and responsibility and nurse authenticity and caring as crucial to quality of care

These theories provide the beginnings for directing practice, focusing nursing research, and developing a framework of concepts integral to the preparation of professional nurses.

Approaches associated with two or more different nursing theories or the psychiatric theories discussed in Chapter 5∞ are often used in combination. For example, bizarre, self-destructive behavior may be controlled with medications so that the client is more available for a caring, healing relationship with a psychiatric–mental health nurse. Such a combined or eclectic approach demands that you be capable of functioning according to all theories of care, depending on which is best for the client and best fits the resources and limitations of the situation. If you give adequate consideration to the theoretic framework of your psychiatric–mental health nursing, you will foster practice-oriented research and clinical judgments that you can articulate and teach to others. Research is a tool for developing psychiatric–mental health nursing theory that synthesizes the most useful elements of these theories.

Pearson Nursing Student Resources
Find additional review materials at
nursing.pearsonhighered.com
Prepare for success with NCLEX®-style practice questions, interactive assignments and activities, web links, animations and videos, and more!

REFERENCES

American Nurses Association, American Psychiatric Nurses Association, and International Society of Psychiatric–Mental Health Nurses. (2007). *Psychiatric–mental health nursing: Scope and standards of practice.* Silver Spring, MD: Nursesbooks.org

American Nurses Association Task Force on Psychopharmacology. (1994). *Psychiatric–mental health nursing psychopharmacology project.* Washington DC: Author.

Armstrong, S. W., & Rouslin, S. (1963). *Group psychotherapy in nursing practice.* New York, NY: Macmillan.

Barker, P. (1999). Hildegard E. Peplau: The mother of psychiatric nursing. *Journal of Psychiatric and Mental Health Nursing, 6*(3), 175–176.

Benner, P. (1983). Uncovering the knowledge embedded in clinical practice. *Image: Journal of Nursing Scholarship, 15*(2), 36–41.

Benner, P. (1996). *Expertise in nursing practice: Caring, clinical judgment and ethics.* New York, NY: Springer.

Benner, P. (1999). *Clinical wisdom and interventions in critical care: A thinking-in-action approach.* Philadelphia, PA: Saunders.

Brown, E. L. (1948). *Nursing for the future.* New York, NY: Russell Sage Foundation.

Byrd, S., & Marshall, M. (1963). *Clinical approaches to psychiatric nursing.* New York, NY: Macmillan.

Chafetz, L., White, M., Collins-Bride, G., & Nickens, J. (2008). Clinical trial of wellness training: Health promotion for severely mentally ill adults. *Journal of Nervous and Mental Diseases, 196*(6), 475–483.

George, G. B. (2011). *Nursing theories: The base for professional nursing practice* (6th ed.). Upper Saddle River, NJ: Pearson.

Haber, J. (1999). Hildegard Peplau. The mother of psychiatric nursing. *Nursing and Health Care Perspectives, 20*(4), 228.

Jackson, J. L., Passamonti, M., & Kroenke, K. (2007). Outcome and impact of mental disorders in primary care at 5 years. *Psychosomatic Medicine, 69*(2), 217–229.

Krauss, J. B. (1993). *Health care reform: Essential mental health services.* Washington, DC: American Nurses Publishing.

Kroenke, K., Spitzer, R. L., Williams, J. B., Monahan, P. O., & Lowe, B. (2007). Anxiety disorders in primary care: Prevalence, impairment, comorbidity, and detection. *Annals of Internal Medicine, 146*(5), 317.

McBride, A. B. (1990). Psychiatric nursing in the 1990s. *Archives of Psychiatric Nursing, 4*(1), 21–27.

National Panel for Psychiatric–Mental Health NP Competencies. (2003). *Psychiatric–mental health nurse practitioner competencies.* Washington, DC: National Organization of Nurse Practitioner Faculties.

Osborne, O. H. (1984). Intellectual traditions in psychiatric–mental health nursing: A review of selected textbooks. *Journal of Psychosocial Nursing and Mental Health Nursing, 22*(11), 27–32.

Paterson, J. G., & Zderad, L. T. (2008). *Humanistic nursing.* Retrieved from http://www.paterson-zderad-humanistic-nursing.com. Previously published 1988 (Publication No. 41–2218). New York, NY: National League for Nursing.

Peplau, H. E. (1952). *Interpersonal relations in nursing.* New York, NY: Putnam.

Peplau, H. E. (1978). Psychiatric nursing: Role of nurses and psychiatric nurses. *Journal of Psychosocial Nursing and Mental Health Services* (16), 17–24.

Peplau, H. E. (1989). Future directions in psychiatric nursing from the perspective of history. *Journal of Psychosocial Nursing, 27*(2), 18–27.

Peplau, H. E. (1997). Peplau's theory of interpersonal relations. *Nursing Science Quarterly, 10*(4), 162–167.

Pilkington, F. B. (2007). Envisioning nursing in 2050 through the eyes of nurse theorists: Leininger and Watson. *Nursing Science Quarterly, 20*(1), 8.

Rana, T., Bradley, E., & Nolan, P. (2009). Survey of psychiatrists' views of nurse prescribing. *Journal of Psychiatric and Mental Health Nursing, 16*(3), 257–262.

Travelbee, J. (1966). *Interpersonal aspects of nursing.* Philadelphia, PA: Davis.

Tudor, G. (1952). A sociopsychiatric nursing approach to intervention in a problem of mutual withdrawal on a mental hospital ward. *Psychiatry, 15,* 174+.

Watson, J. (1988). New dimensions in human caring theory. *Nursing Science Quarterly, 1*(4), 175–181.

Watson, J. (1999). *Postmodern nursing and beyond.* New York, NY: Churchill Livingstone.

Watson, J. (2008). Nursing: *The philosophy and science of caring* (Rev. ed.). Denver, CO: University of Colorado Press.

Wilson, H. S., & Kneisl, C. R. (1979). *Psychiatric nursing.* Menlo Park, CA: Addison-Wesley.

Self-Awareness and the Psychiatric–Mental Health Nurse

CAROL REN KNEISL

LEARNING OUTCOMES

After completing this chapter, you will be able to:

1. Explain how self-knowledge and self-reflection are important to psychiatric–mental health nurses.
2. Discuss the concept of personal integration and how it relates to psychiatric–mental health nursing practice.
3. Describe the qualities that enable psychiatric–mental health nurses to practice the use of self artfully in therapeutic relationships.
4. Provide examples of how the concepts of blame and control affect artful therapeutic practice.
5. Foster culturally competent care for clients with psychiatric–mental health disorders by understanding the influence of your own sociocultural background on your nursing practice.
6. Demonstrate empathy in psychiatric–mental health clinical practice.
7. Maintain a respectful attitude toward clients, their families, and colleagues.
8. Demonstrate a commitment to practicing self-care and connecting with self and others.

CRITICAL THINKING CHALLENGE

Ruby Ann is a 19-year-old African-American mother of three small children. She lives with her boyfriend in a one-bedroom mobile home in a crime-ridden area of a major Southern city. Ruby Ann has been treated several times in the city hospital's emergency department for bruises, lacerations, and broken bones. She has called 911 four times in the past year because her boyfriend was threatening to kill her and her children. Your assessment interview upon her arrival at the battered women's shelter reveals that Ruby Ann is anxious and depressed and has experienced frequent, severe verbal and physical abuse. She reports that she is unable to sleep, has no appetite, and has lost 20 pounds over the past 9 months. Ruby Ann also confides that her spiritual beliefs have sustained her in her suffering and distress. She says, "If God wasn't with me, I wouldn't have got out of there, but I'm starting to doubt Him because how could He let all this happen to my babies?"

1. Based on this data, what specific type of spiritual assistance would you offer Ruby Ann?
2. Does it matter if you and Ruby Ann are of different faiths?
3. What feelings do you think Ruby Ann might be experiencing?
4. How would spiritual support help to reduce untoward feelings?

The value of self-knowledge is a recurring theme in both popular and professional literature. Libraries are stocked with volumes dealing with the undiscovered self, the expansion of human awareness, spirituality and the care of the soul, strategies for self-realization, and the like. A common thread in all these is the idea that the quality and nature of a person's relationships with others are strongly influenced by the person's self-view. Consider the comments made by students in their psychiatric nursing clinical experience in the following clinical example.

Clinical Example

Laurie: "I just can't take it. I feel myself getting confused about who is the crazy one. There's such a fine line. Sometimes I think I'll be a patient here."

Eric: "I hated psych—it just didn't seem like nursing to me. I really like to keep busy. When you change someone's dressing, you really feel like you've helped them. Here it's all so uncertain."

Makayla: "All I kept thinking about was that a lot of the patients had done really weird things. This one guy had lived in an apartment with his dead mother's body for 3 months before they brought him in. Another had tried to shoot the governor. I never felt safe turning my back on them."

Throughout this text, you will be encouraged to attend to the mind–body–spirit of your clients. This chapter explores some dimensions of self-awareness and self-knowledge through the examination of personal integration and recurring problems that pertain to the nurse's identity, the personal qualities on which the artful use of self in therapeutic relationships is based, and strategies for taking care of your mind–body–spirit. In this text, we pay significant attention to the stresses psychiatric nurses experience in attempting to relate fully to clients while maintaining their own personal integration.

PERSONAL INTEGRATION

Many students and practitioners faced with relating to people whose behavior they view as offensive, frightening, curious, or socially inappropriate find that their personal attitudes, expectations, myths, and values make it difficult for them to fulfill their professional roles. This was the case in the following clinical example.

Clinical Example

Penny, a baccalaureate nursing student, had selected a clinical placement at a substance abuse clinic in the community. Despite her initial interest, she developed a pattern of absences from the clinic. When her faculty adviser discussed this observation with her, Penny blurted out that, much to her surprise, she was unable to assist with the group meetings for pregnant heroin addicts. The thought of addicting babies before they were born—babies who would ultimately suffer because of their mothers' self-indulgence—horrified Penny. She found herself judging their choices constantly and avoiding interaction with them. "I feel like they should be shot instead of given all this support and sympathy."

For many nurses, confrontation with deviance (defined in Chapter 1 as behavior outside the social norm of a specific group that should not be construed to mean negative behavior) reinforces a personal sense of stability. Others are threatened by such confrontation.

Recall the clinical example of "Crazy Helen," "Vince the Window Peeper," "Eddie the Drunk," and "Lester the Molester" on page 3 in Chapter 1∞. Dealing with people whose personal integration is fragmented, dissolving, divided, or alienated puts the nurse's own identity on the line as well. To respond with both compassion and the critical distance necessary to be effective (a personal quality we call detached concern), psychiatric professionals must confront their own identity; separate it from the client's identity, which may indeed be dissolving; and finally integrate different values and behaviors comfortably in the therapeutic relationships they develop with clients.

This personal quality is called **detached concern**—the ability to distance oneself in order to help others. It is an essential quality not only in avoiding *burnout,* a problem discussed later in this chapter, but also in using appropriate *assertiveness* when collaborating with colleagues, and in maintaining *empathic abilities* in highly stressful situations.

Creating a Common Ground

Because people are constantly building and protecting their own self-images, they try to get others to see their image of themselves. However, it is impossible to see another's self-image or worldview exactly as that person experiences it. Despite this fact, psychiatry has traditionally attempted to have certain people, labeled *crazy,* assume the perspective of certain other people, called *mental health professionals.*

A more acceptable alternative seems to lie in the creation of some common ground, a mutually understood, negotiated reality or shared perspective (Hewitt and Shulman, 2011). Even to this common ground the nurse and the client bring their own conceptions, feelings, and attitudes toward and images of each other and themselves. In many instances, our image of the client—how we expect the client to act or feel— is not the same as the client's self-image. This is confusing to both client and nurse and hinders our attempts to establish therapeutic relationships and communicate effectively.

Searching for Meaning

Psychiatric–mental health nurses work with clients in a search for meaning in clients' lives. It is essential that we establish our own personal meaning and integration of self, for these are key resources in treatment. In order to be effective, we must already possess the personal skills to deal with the client's symptoms. And, we must have personally worked through any problems that resemble those of the client. For example, if your goal is to be liked and admired by everyone you meet, you are likely to find it difficult to set reasonable and rational limits.

Feelings: The Affective Self

The ultimate effectiveness of efforts to relate to and communicate with others depends on how well people know themselves (**self-awareness**) and develop the ability to be sensitive to and care about others. In the following clinical example, Josh's limited self-awareness hampers him in his clinical work.

Clinical Example

Josh is a middle-aged man who sought out nursing as a career. Although he is highly proficient in technical skills and charming and engaging in relationships with most clients, he has discovered a surprising intolerance for some of the tears, complaints, and self-preoccupation of depressed clients. He finds himself responding with admonitions to stop it, to bite the bullet, to grow up. He personally has seldom allowed himself to experience his own sadnesses and jokingly characterizes himself as a firm believer in repression and denial. The need to empathize with severely depressed people unable to control their feelings evokes discomfort, and he is unable to work with such clients.

Self-awareness and caring seem to go hand in hand. At the root of social interaction is people's ability to understand and care about each other's attitudes and feelings. Because each human being is unique, this ability, called *empathizing,* is a difficult and challenging task. (Empathy is discussed in greater detail later in this chapter, and empathy as a communication skill is discussed in Chapter 10∞.) One way to develop this ability is to practice it. Learning to be aware of your responses to the expression of feelings from another person is a starting point. The film, *Harry Potter and the Deathly Hallows,* illustrates the importance of self-awareness.

Self-Awareness of Feelings

Feelings are like icebergs: Only the tips stick up into consciousness, and the deeper parts are submerged. One such feeling, illustrated in Figure 3-1 ■, is fear. The conscious part may be experienced as dislike, avoidance, or reluctance. At a deeper level, the feeling is reported as anxiety. Even deeper,

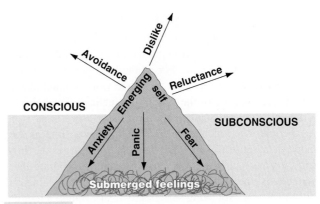

FIGURE 3-1 ■ Self-awareness of feelings. Superficial feelings are visible; deeper feelings are submerged.

the person may acknowledge, "I feel scared." Deeper yet, the person may experience genuine panic. Such an iceberg may well explain Josh's attitude toward tearful, depressed clients. His annoyance, irritation, sarcasm, and disdain may represent the tip of the iceberg of Josh's fear of depression. The iceberg comparison also applies to other feelings, such as love, hurt, and guilt.

Nurses may also erect rigid defenses aimed at denying their personal feelings because of the emotional demands of nursing. For example, some procedures actually require the nurse to violate a client's emotional or physical state (injections, dressings). Defending against feelings becomes one way for the nurse to cope with inflicting pain on another person. You can deal effectively with the feelings of clients only to the extent that you explore your own personal feelings.

MENTAL HEALTH IN THE MOVIES
Harry Potter and the Deathly Hallows

For the main characters in the Harry Potter film series, the battles never seem to end. In this film, Harry, Ron, and Hermione battle Voldemort, Dementors, and other various villains. But, how about their own internal battles? From the first film in 2001, *Harry Potter and the Sorcerer's Stone,* the personality traits with the potential to hinder Harry, Ron, and Hermione were evident.

The circumstances of Harry's early life were not the best. His mother and father were killed while he was still an infant. Brought up by his aunt and uncle in an abusive household, Harry was forced to live in a small closet beneath the stairs, he carried out the household chores, and he was treated either as if he did not exist or as if he was an immense bother. And, not only that, there is a powerful villain with many disciples bent on killing Harry. Yet, despite these events and the anxiety and depression they engender, Harry is remarkably self-confident and balanced. Kind teachers, hard work, and steadfast friends help him to face fearsome challenges.

Ron was born into a household in which he was the last in a long line of boys and could be easily overlooked or overshadowed by his successful older brothers and his cute and perky little sister. Ron's insecurities and low self-esteem are often dealt with by joking behavior—perhaps fearing that his opinions are unimportant or will be disregarded—and continually plague Ron in all the films. His reluctance to talk about his feelings distances himself from others. Yet, Ron always overcomes his doubts and fears. He seems to hold it together well enough to save both Harry and Hermione on a number of occasions.

Hermione is fastidious, a workaholic, and often at the head of her class in the school of wizardry. Hermione sets such high standards for herself that she often feels unfulfilled and unsuccessful. She sometimes seems unable to recognize the effect of workaholism on her health and continues to try to please her friends as well as her teachers. Her stubbornness and need to control cause interpersonal difficulties. But, because she is steadfast in her determination, smart, skillful, brave, and willing to use her talents to benefit others, Hermione helps Harry and Ron overcome obstacles.

The Harry Potter films help to educate others about hardiness and resilience in the face of untoward circumstances. A common thread is the value of self-awareness and the means by which self-knowledge can enhance the quality and nature of one's relationships with others.
Photo courtesy of Newscom.

Problems With Submerged Feelings

One characteristic of icebergs of feeling is that at the tip of the iceberg, feelings lose their experiential quality and are translated into impulses to act. For example, a person with submerged guilt may express it by frequent worrying and may be completely unaware of the underlying feelings. The behavior is the only outward manifestation.

People lose touch with their feelings over time as they shape their sense of self. They hear such messages as "boys don't cry" or "girls are too sensitive" and incorporate these injunctions into their emerging self-system (explained in Chapter 5∞). Not being sufficiently aware of one's feelings has several disadvantages:

- What people don't know *can* hurt them. Repressed feelings may reappear in behaviors that are difficult to alter. For example, hidden anger may emerge in migraine headaches or the use of sarcasm.
- People who are not aware of their feelings find it difficult to make decisions. It is hard to tell a "should" from a wish. Without some awareness of their real wants, they may have trouble saying no or requesting something they need. They are more likely to rely on others—experts, authorities, rules and regulations, and so forth—for guidance.
- People who, like Josh, are "out of touch with" or unaware of their feelings may find it difficult to be really close to and empathic toward others. Intimacy and empathy demand the expression of here-and-now feelings, whether positive or negative.

As a professional, you realize the value of thinking clearly. You understand that it is a learned ability and takes practice. Feeling clearly (authentically) is just as important as thinking clearly. It too can be practiced and learned.

Dominant Emotional Themes

In order to be effective, we need to explore the dominant emotional themes in our personalities. If you find that you respond to many situations with the same feelings, you are probably narrowing your range of potential feelings, much as Marge, Joan, and Ed in the following clinical example.

Clinical Example

Whatever the occasion, Marge was tired or bored. Fatigue and chronically depressed states were routine for her. Holidays, vacations, dinner engagements all evoked the same predictable response.

Joan was afraid of everything. When she met her brother at the plane, her first question was, "Aren't you afraid of flying?" She was afraid driving home from the airport. The prospect of starting back to school also frightened her.

Regardless of the circumstances, Ed always questioned the intentions of his wife, his children, his coworkers, and his friends. According to Ed, the motives for their behavior were always up for debate.

People who feel the same way in a variety of situations may be missing a lot of what is happening in those situations. They perceive only what will fit a narrowed range of feelings.

Becoming aware of limited emotional themes is a way to begin to widen one's range of feelings.

Acceptance of Disapproved Feelings

Most people have been taught to block off awareness and expression of certain feelings. Children are taught that being rude or ungrateful or cranky is rarely acceptable. To retain love and approval, they usually comply, not by stopping the feelings but by acting as if they didn't have them. Nursing students often get similar messages from their teachers. That is, it is not acceptable to find a client repulsive, to dislike someone who is sick and dependent, or to express anger at or criticism of the teacher. Positive feelings of attraction and love may also seem unacceptable. Failure to recognize these feelings can interfere with interactions.

Recognizing and accepting our own feelings make us less vulnerable to other people's ideas about how we should feel. Nurses often feel guilty when they don't feel what others imply they should feel. Nurses who can allow themselves the right to their own feelings can also allow clients the right to have and express theirs.

Beliefs and Values

Our personal values are the "shoulds" that direct our behavior. Beliefs and values take three major forms:

1. Rational beliefs are beliefs that are supported by available evidence.
2. Blind belief is belief in the absence of evidence.
3. Irrational belief is belief held despite available evidence to the contrary.

Blind and irrational beliefs will cause problems in our relationships with others, including our relationships with clients.

Dogmatic Belief

Dogmatic belief (opinions or beliefs held as if they were based on the highest authority) includes both blind belief and irrational belief. Dogmatically held beliefs are not based on personal experience. Operating on the basis of dogmatically held beliefs often causes us to distort our personal experiences of the world to fit our preconceptions. Box 3-1 has examples of some strongly held beliefs about behaviors that are labeled "mental illness."

Issues of Blame and Control

Inherent in these strongly held beliefs about mental illness are the issues of *blame* and *control*. Believing that people cause their own problems involves the issue of blame. Believing that people are responsible for solutions to their problems involves the issue of control. Your assumptions about personal responsibility affect the way you go about your clinical work. For artful therapeutic practice, you need to be aware of your beliefs about blame and control as well as your client's orientation. The help you offer may not be effective if the person desiring help and the person offering help have different views on personal responsibility.

Box 3-1 Blind and Irrational Beliefs
About Mental Illness

- Most clients in mental hospitals are dangerous.
- People who seek counseling are mentally disordered.
- If parents loved their children more, there would be fewer mental disorders.
- When a person has a worry, it is best not to think about it.
- Many people become mentally disordered just to avoid the problems of life.
- People would not become mentally disordered if they avoided bad thoughts.
- Anyone who is in a hospital for a mental disorder should not be allowed to vote.
- To become a psychiatric client is to become a failure in life.
- One of the main causes of mental disorders is a lack of moral strength.

Most research on strongly held beliefs indicates that people usually know more about the things they believe than about those they don't believe. By staying ignorant about anything they don't already agree with, they can avoid changing. This posture cuts off personal growth and learning that could be derived from the unknown. Obviously, clients are better served by nurses who are aware of their own dogmatically held beliefs and then challenge those beliefs.

Attitudes and Opinions

A feeling is a transitory experience. A feeling held over a period of time is called an *attitude*. An attitude linked to an idea or belief becomes an *opinion*. An opinion, then, involves both thinking and feeling. Research in this area has shown that people are more comfortable when their beliefs are consistent with their attitudes. People do several things to keep their attitudes and beliefs consistent:

- They repress any belief or attitude that seems inconsistent
- They distract their awareness from conflict either physically (such as by leaving the room) or psychologically (such as by daydreaming)
- They distort their perceptions to fit an existing attitude or belief

These maneuvers take place in an attempt to keep actions consistent with attitudes or beliefs.

Arriving at Values

Every day, each person meets life situations that call for thought, opinion forming, decision making, and action. At every turn in our personal and professional lives, we are faced with choices. Our choices are based on the values we hold, but often those values are not really clear. People actively value something to the degree that they are willing to put energy into doing something about it. Their values are demonstrated in their interests, preferences, decisions, and actions, as in the following clinical example.

Clinical Example

In talking with colleagues, Susan, a psychiatric–mental health nurse, claims to value interacting with clients more than doing paperwork. Yet a quick assessment of how she spends her time—sitting at the nurse's station talking with colleagues, filling out forms, making her grocery list—reveals that she acts on other values.

Mel, a nurse working in a state hospital unit for profoundly developmentally disabled children, says that he believes these clients are human beings, despite their uncommunicative, immobile forms. He demonstrates this value in the hours he spends trying to communicate his presence and concern for them, using acupressure and touch performed slowly and with genuine feeling.

The distinction in the above examples is between *cognitive* and *active values.* Susan verbally subscribes to values but fails to act on them. These are cognitive values. Mel's actions demonstrate that he gives more than lip service to the idea of the dignity of all living beings. He follows active values.

Culture and Social Class

Cultural and social class differences between you and the client may impede your best intentions. Gaining awareness of sociocultural differences requires that you first come to understand your own background and the influence of that background on your practice. Nurses are better able to meet the sociocultural needs of a client when they acknowledge that a culture and a society influence their beliefs, values, attitudes, and behavior. Quality nursing care is culturally sensitive; that is, aware of cultural issues that are important to the client and may affect the client's response to treatment.

In planning nursing interventions, do not follow a predetermined plan, but plan care that is culturally competent for each person. For example, if a Latina teenage girl is obese and wants to lose weight, you would not hand her a printed 1,000-calorie diet plan but would work with her and a nutritionist to plan a diet based on the foods she prefers. If an Asian client who is a Buddhist wants time each day to meditate, you would allow for that time in the care plan. It is not easy to take a client's culture into consideration when planning care. It takes time and requires patience, insight, and creativity.

Sociocultural Heritage

The questions in the Your Self-Awareness feature are designed to facilitate acknowledgment of your own sociocultural heritage. Answering these questions honestly and completely will help you to understand which sociocultural factors impact your ability to communicate in a culturally sensitive way.

Avoiding Misdiagnosis

Clients from different cultures may be misdiagnosed by Western health care providers. Culturally competent nurses can play a role in assessing clients' social, psychological, and behavioral symptoms in light of clients' own cultural norms. For example, a psychiatrist may diagnose a man who talks to the dead as *schizophrenic,* but for someone from Puerto Rico who believes in *espiritismo,* talking to the dead is a common practice. A

> ## YOUR SELF-AWARENESS
> ### Influence of Sociocultural Heritage
>
> Ask yourself the following questions:
>
> - What ethnic group, socioeconomic class, religion, age group, and community do you belong to?
> - What experiences have you had with people from ethnic groups, socioeconomic classes, religions, age groups, or communities different from your own?
> - What were those experiences like? How did you feel about them?
> - When you were growing up, what did your parents and significant others say about people who were different from your family?
> - What about your ethnic group, socioeconomic class, religion, age, or community do you find embarrassing or wish you could change? Why?
> - What sociocultural factors in your background might contribute to your being rejected by members of other cultures?
> - What personal qualities do you have that will help you establish interpersonal relationships with persons from other cultural groups?
> - What personal qualities do you have that may be detrimental?
> - What cultural assumptions do you hold about the people who populate our world?

client who is a charismatic Christian may lapse into an altered state of consciousness and speak in tongues. To interpret these behaviors as evidence of schizophrenia is inappropriate. Obtaining a cultural profile helps to prevent misdiagnosis. Culturally competent psychiatric–mental health nursing practice is more thoroughly discussed in Chapter 9∞.

TAKING CARE OF THE SELF

Knowing who you are is just a beginning. Taking care of others requires that nurses respect and care for themselves. Those who have the quality of hardiness (see Chapter 1∞), that is, they rise to meet challenges, pace themselves in order to sustain the effort needed to deal with stress and strain (Phillips, 2011). This section on assertiveness, the need for solitude, maintaining physical health, attending to cues of personal stress, and avoiding burnout will help you to pace yourself and preserve your personal integration.

Solitude

Most people need time alone to assimilate what has happened in time spent with other people. They also need it for relief from responding to the demands of others. Aloneness need not mean physical distance. People can be alone in a crowded library. The crucial factors are that they are making no demands on others and that no one is making demands on them.

After a sanctioned time away, most people return refreshed to their relationships, work, and usual circumstances. Planning for time alone is highly preferable to reaching a breaking point and then aggressively and irresponsibly running away from others.

Physical Health

An important way of taking care of oneself is to provide for the physical health of the body. A proper diet, adequate rest, and exercise, rejuvenate and restore the body. All these activities potentially make nurses more alive and better able to share themselves with their clients. As students, you are coping with pressures to study, to prepare for clinical experiences, and to complete assignments, as well as performing other roles that are important to you.

Sleep Deprivation and Shift Work Disorder

Sometimes we manage these pressures by sleeping less. However, being chronically sleep deprived works against maintaining physical health. Sleep debt accumulation results in chronic fatigue (Niu et al., 2011). Take the quiz in the Your Self-Awareness feature to see whether you are getting enough sleep to meet your needs.

> ## YOUR SELF-AWARENESS
> ### Are You Sleep Deprived?
>
> Ask yourself the following questions:
>
> - Do you usually fall asleep within 5 minutes after you turn off the lights?
> - Do you struggle to stay awake in lectures?
> - Do you "get by" all week and then try to catch up by sleeping in on the weekend?
> - Do you do shift work?
> - Do you often wake up with a headache?
> - Do you have trouble getting going in the morning?
> - Do you push yourself to keep going?
>
> If you answered "yes" to more than two of these questions, you may not be getting as much sleep as you need.

More than 14 million Americans—such as nurses, bakers, pilots, train conductors, truck drivers, police officers, firefighters, factory workers, gambling casino employees—work evening, night, or rotating shifts. This number accounts for 15% of all full-time workers in the United States, 10% of whom have shift work disorder (Krystal, 2011). As you might expect, shift work—in which the 24-hour sleep–wake schedule is disturbed—is a major source of circadian rhythm disruption for nurses (O'Malley, 2011) and other shift workers, as demonstrated in the clinical example that follows.

Clinical Example

Years after he had retired from his bakery business, Yürgen continued to awaken very early in the morning. This pattern further complicated a sleep disorder related to his medical condition of Parkinson's disease.

Jane was working rotating shifts in an intensive care unit. She noted that she had worsening insomnia and feared that her judgment would be affected by increasing sleep deprivation.

There are several behavioral and physical effects of shift work circadian rhythm disruption and sleep deprivation. The behavioral effects are: decreased vigilance, general malaise, decreased mental efficiency, impaired ability to function at work and at home, depression, increased auto accidents from the impaired ability to drive safely, and increased stress on personal relationships. Some physical effects are gastrointestinal disturbances (ulcers and functional bowel disorders) and hypertension (Krystal, 2011; Niu et al., 2011). The impact of shift work and sleep deprivation on sleep patterns and sleep disturbance often extends beyond the period of shift work.

Specific suggestions for obtaining a good sleep despite an evening, night, or rotating shift work schedule can be found on http://www.goodsleep.com. Although studies in sleep labs indicate that light exposure, melatonin, hypnotic agents, caffeine, and central nervous system stimulants are helpful, these measures have not yet been evaluated in persons with shift work disorder. Another circadian rhythm sleep disorder, jet lag, is discussed in Chapter 6∞.

Attending to Internal Stress Signals

Nursing students who read about mental disorders in their textbooks or encounter emotionally disturbed clients commonly begin seeing in themselves all the "symptoms" about which they are learning. This perception is probably due more to the heightened awareness of, and attention to, the emotional aspects of their lives than to anything else. However, it is important for us to learn to recognize and respond to our own genuine stress signals. Difficulty in admitting the inability to cope was acknowledged by all nursing student subjects in a study that looked at nursing students' experience of stress (Freeburn & Sinclair, 2009). Be aware that all people have times in their lives when they may become very upset at small disturbances or see things out of proportion to their ultimate importance. These feelings are significant warning signals that one is not coping adequately with stress.

Times of stress can be important turning points in people's lives. They are strong messages that change is needed. It is foolish to ignore these messages. In their daily lives, nurses are often tempted to handle their own symptoms of stress by suppressing them with tranquilizers or other drugs. They could serve themselves better by really experiencing their feelings and attending to what the signals are saying. Help in managing stress creatively is the subject of Chapters 8 and 33∞. As Montes-Berges & Augusto put it: "It is better to prevent stress than to suffer from it" (2007, p. 169). Using the strategies and therapies recommended in these chapters will help you prevent stress, ease tension before it becomes unmanageable, and gain control of your life.

Pain and suffering are sources of some of the most intensely experienced stresses in life. Events such as the death of loved ones, divorce, illness, separation from loved ones, and failure are all part of the cycle of life's experience. Being told that they deserve it, or that they really don't have it so bad and therefore have no right to feel the way they feel, does not help people cope with pain and suffering. People want to continue what *was* instead of living with what *is*. They need to find ways of handling suffering without being destroyed by it. Some people need to replace what they have lost with something similar. Others need to explore a new dimension in their lives. Classmates, friends, and family members can be great sources of support. Being able to both give and receive support strengthens the individual.

Realizing that pain and hardship are part of what it is to be a human being makes the pain a bit gentler. It is important to attend to genuine feelings about loss or prospective loss. The alternative to experiencing pain is to live on the surface, out of touch with the joyful experiences in life as well as the painful ones. A more life-enhancing approach is to experience all aspects of life.

Burnout

The nurse in the following clinical example verbalizes one of the possible consequences of working intensely with troubled people.

Clinical Example

"After hours, days, and months of listening to other people's problems, something inside you can go dead and you don't care anymore. That's when you'd rather sit at the desk and do the paperwork than be out talking to clients on the floor."

Burnout is the name given to this phenomenon, a condition in which health care professionals lose their concern and feeling for their clients and come to treat them in detached or even dehumanized ways. Burnout happens to some, but not all, mental health professionals, poverty lawyers, social workers, clinical psychologists, childcare workers, prison personnel, and others who struggle to retain both their objectivity and their concern for the people with whom they work. Burnout involves physical, mental, and emotional exhaustion that is attributed to long-term involvement in emotionally demanding situations. Burnout is a less healthy and problematic attempt to cope—by distancing oneself—with the stresses of intense interpersonal work. It hurts not only clients but also mental health professionals, in that they become ineffective and dissatisfied.

In many cases, burning out involves not only thinking in derogatory terms about clients but also believing that somehow clients deserve any problem they have. Benner and Wrubel, nurse theorists discussed in Chapter 2∞ who have studied both caring and burnout, caution us to avoid making the mistake of thinking that caring is the cause of burnout and thus trying to prevent the "disease" of burnout by protecting ourselves from caring (1989). According to them, the sickness is the loss of caring, and the return of caring is the recovery.

There is little doubt that burnout plays a major role in the poor delivery of psychiatric care. It is also a key factor in low staff morale, absenteeism, and high job turnover.

Cues to Burnout

Cues to burnout can be found in the language used to describe clients. Burnout victims may refer to their clients as "crocks," "vegetables," "wackos," and so forth, or they may become highly analytic and abstract: "That's just a manifestation of his primary process thinking." Another cue is lack of involvement with clients. Some nurses "hide" in the nurses' station or staff conference room to avoid interacting. Some openly reject bids for human contact. "Going by the book" rather than considering the unique factors in a situation is a way of minimizing personal involvement with the client. By rigidly applying the rules, one can avoid thinking about the client's specific problems. Be careful: Burnout can transform an original and creative nurse into a mechanical bureaucrat.

Another cue to burnout is joking put-downs, such as those in the following clinical example, which make mental health work seem less frightening and overwhelming.

Clinical Example

When the nurse is asked where Mr. Grant is, she laughingly reports that he's taking a shower in preparation for his MMPI test. Everyone in the nurses' station breaks up in gales of laughter.

In a discharge conference, the psychiatrist says he'd like to discharge Earl, a young male client with a history of violent outbursts. The nurse replies, "With or without a baseball bat?" and everyone chuckles.

Reducing Burnout

Most research, such as that referenced in the Evidence-Based Practice feature, indicates that the causes of professional burnout are rooted not in the permanent psychological characteristics of individuals but rather in the social context of their work; specifically, lack of resources and workload pressures. Most nurses usually expect the presence of negative conditions: large client loads, time pressures, and daily confrontation with suffering, pain, and death. It is the absence of

positive factors—a sense of significance, rewarding interpersonal relationships, the appreciation of others, challenge, and variety—that is most distressing (Onyett, 2011). The strategies listed in the Your Intervention Strategies feature can be used to reduce and modify the occurrence of burnout.

> ## YOUR INTERVENTION STRATEGIES
> ### Reducing and Modifying the Occurrence of Burnout
>
> - Request a lower staff–client ratio. You can then give more attention to each client and have time to focus on the positive, nonproblematic aspects of the client's life.
> - Recognize that no one is perfect. Your clients deserve the best care you can provide; it may not always be perfect care, and it isn't 24-hours-a-day, 7-days-a-week care.
> - Take all sanctioned breaks rather than guilt-provoking escapes from the work situation.
> - Talk over your problems to get advice and support when you need it.
> - Express, analyze, and share your feelings about burning out. This lets you get things off your chest and gives you the chance to get constructive feedback from others and perhaps a new perspective as well.
> - Understand your own motivations in pursuing a psychiatric–mental health nursing career and recognize your expectations for work with clients. Deal with your clients' problems, not your own.
> - Attend to your own internal stress signals.
> - Pursue happiness and satisfaction in your personal life through family, friends, social or spiritual organizations, and hobbies and recreational interests.

(margin) Care Plan: Managing Burnout on the Unit

> ## EVIDENCE-BASED PRACTICE
>
> ### Improving Practice and Avoiding Burnout
>
> You and a colleague work in the medication clinic of a community mental health center. Both of you have talked about your increasing dissatisfaction with your job. You feel burdened. There are too many clients and too little time. You feel that you don't get enough feedback on your performance from the more experienced nurses. The improvements you would like to make—medication education groups for family members, for example—are impossible to implement given the workload. Neither you nor your colleague feels that you are doing the best you can for your clients and their families. You decide to approach the administration to ask for the following:
>
> 1. Hiring another nurse to decrease the workload
> 2. Regularly scheduled time for clinical supervision by the more experienced nurses
> 3. Adding a weekly medication education group for family members
>
> Your requests are based on the following nursing research:
>
> Hameideh, S. H. (2011). Burnout, social support and job satisfaction among Jordanian mental health nurses. *Issues in Mental Health Nursing, 32*(4), 234–242.
>
> Hooper, C., Craig, J., Janvrin, D. R., Wetsel, M. A., & Reimeis, E. (2010). Compassion satisfaction, burnout, and compassion fatigue among emergency nurses compared with nurses in other selected inpatient specialties. *Journal of Emergency Nursing, 36*(5), 420–427.
>
> Yoder, E. A. (2010). Compassion fatigue in nurses. *Applied Nursing Research, 23*(4), 191–197.
>
> *CRITICAL THINKING QUESTIONS*
>
> 1. What relationship do you see between your experience at the medication clinic and the issue of burnout?
> 2. How do you deal with feeling that you are not doing the best you can for your clients and their families?
> 3. What are the essential elements to keep in mind when approaching the administration to make your request?

QUALITIES THAT ENHANCE THERAPEUTIC RELATIONSHIPS

Self-awareness, empathy, and moral integrity all enable psychiatric nurses to practice the use of self artfully in therapeutic relationships. Some characteristics of artful therapeutic practice are respect for the client, availability, spontaneity, hope, acceptance, sensitivity, vision, accountability, advocacy, spirituality, empathy, critical thinking, and self-disclosure. These personal characteristics will enhance your therapeutic relationships. The therapeutic relationship with individual clients is the subject of Chapter 4 ∞.

Respect for the Client

Respect emerges from the belief that human beings have inherent worth and dignity. The behavior of many mental health clients demonstrates their loss of self-respect. Some may appear dirty and disheveled. Others may plead, beg, or cry. Still others may try to do physical harm to themselves or others. A relationship in which they experience a sense of dignity and receive messages of respect from you is of inestimable value. Suggestions for how you can convey respect in relationships with clients are in Your Intervention Strategies. Expressions of joy and assessments of client abilities, talents, and capabilities are often neglected, but are an essential and respectful element of artful therapeutic practice.

YOUR INTERVENTION STRATEGIES
Conveying Respect for the Client

Keeping the following principles in mind will help you to convey respect for clients:

- Hold personal judgments in check.
- Take the time and energy to listen.
- Take care not to invalidate clients' experience of their world with comments such as "It's not so bad," "Don't be that way," "Time heals all wounds," or "Keep a stiff upper lip."
- Give clients as much privacy as possible during examinations and treatments or when they are upset.
- Minimize experiences that humiliate clients and strip them of identity, thus allowing them to make as many of their own choices and be in control of as much of their own lives as possible.
- Be honest with clients about medicines, treatments, privileges, length of stay, and so on, even when the truth may be difficult to handle.
- Create an atmosphere that conveys permission for the client to express pain as well as joy and pleasure.
- Hold an inherent but realistic belief in the client's abilities and talents.

Availability

Of all the members of the mental health team, the nurse has the richest opportunity to be available to clients when needed.

Because we are with clients on a relatively constant basis, nurses have the responsibility for the following:

- Creating a nurturing, healing milieu
- Assisting suffering clients to meet their basic human needs
- Collecting and conveying crucial data about clients that will influence decisions around them

Spontaneity

Many nurses have come to believe that therapeutic relationships with psychiatric clients require them to be stiff, stilted robots uttering clichés from a list of unnatural-sounding communication "techniques." Nurses who are comfortable with themselves, aware of therapeutic goals, and flexible about using a repertoire of possible interventions find that being natural and spontaneous, while keeping therapeutic goals uppermost in their minds, is their most effective "technique." Clients experience such nurses as authentic, that is, showing their real selves, rather than hiding behind the role of nurse. You are unique and necessarily bring your own personal style to practice. We have different ways of putting the words together to convey to clients that we accept and care about them. Sometimes we say it with nonverbal behavior: keeping promises, being on time, touching, and staying with a client who needs someone. We need to trust our own natural styles, combined with sound communication principles such as those discussed in Chapter 10 ∞, in working toward therapeutic goals.

Hope

Effective mental health–psychiatric nursing practice is characterized by hope and optimism that all clients, no matter how debilitated, have the capacity for growth and change. Even clients whose most marked attributes are chronicity and deterioration can be helped to some optimal level of well-being by a nurse, such as the one in the clinical example that follows, who believes in their possibilities and is willing to search for some strengths on which to build.

Clinical Example

Jamal, a creative nurse in a day treatment center, encouraged David, a client, to partner with him to assist less-able clients toward self-care. Jamal believed that this strategy—increasing the connectedness between himself and David and between David and other clients—would decrease David's feeling of aloneness while emphasizing David's ability to manage his illness.

A key role in psychiatric–mental health nursing is helping clients to maintain and engender hope in mastering the challenges and complexities of mental health problems (Clarke, 2009).

The primary obstacle to instilling hope is stigma (discussed in Chapter 1 ∞). Keep in mind that many people lead fulfilling lives despite fairly disabling mental illness. You can have a negative impact on clients if you fail to believe in the client's eventual recovery; if you fail to see the client as a person; if you fail to lobby to reduce stigma in both the public and the health care communities; or if you fail to persevere with clients in their journey of recovery.

Case Study: Therapeutic Alliance

Acceptance

There is a distinction between acceptance and approval. Acceptance means refraining from judging and rejecting a client who you personally dislike or who behaves in a way that makes you uncomfortable, as in the clinical example that follows.

Clinical Example

Joan, a staff nurse on an inpatient unit for severely and persistently mentally ill clients, considered herself a faithful Christian who followed the teachings of the bible. Two clients often provided challenges to Joan's ability to accept them. Mary frequently cursed and used vulgarities. Sinesha bragged about her sexual prowess and her sexual encounters. Joan overcame these challenges by reminding herself that their behavior was often influenced by their psychiatric symptoms.

Clients may feel offended and demeaned if they perceive the nurse as rejecting them. Therapeutic work requires that clients be able to examine, explore, and understand their coping mechanisms without feeling the need to cover up or disguise them to avoid negative judgments or punishments. Nurses who tell clients what they should say, or do, or feel, deny these clients the acceptance they need to explore their problems.

Sensitivity

Genuine interest and concern provide the basis for a therapeutic nurse–client relationship. Clients recognize the falseness of memorized phrases and assumed postures. You convey general interest and concern by trying to understand the client's perspective, working with the client on mutually formulated goals, and persisting even when breakthroughs and improvements are subtle and slow instead of dramatic and quick. A study by Shattell, McAllister, Hogan, and Thomas (2006) determined that understanding the client's perceptions and concerns helps us to connect with our clients, acknowledges their importance, and facilitates the relationship between nurse and client.

Assertiveness

Assertiveness is the ability to express one's feelings, thoughts, and beliefs openly even if doing so is emotionally difficult or personal risk is involved. Assertiveness is a style of interacting with others that protects your rights without depriving others of theirs. It involves standing up for yourself in a nondestructive manner even if your stance is unpopular.

Being assertive in a therapeutic context with clients means that you are able to take advantage of opportunities to make interpersonal contact with clients. Confident nurses are assertive nurses. They recognize that assertiveness and caring are compatible (McCartan & Hargie, 2007).

Often, people are either so timid that they do not get what they want or so aggressive and belligerent that they offend and alienate others. Being assertive in one's professional life builds upon being assertive in one's personal life. **Assertive behavior** is asking for what one wants or acting to get it in a way that respects other people. It is midway between **passive behavior** (timid holding back) and **aggressive behavior** (inconsiderate, offensive aggression).

Compare the passive, aggressive, and assertive behaviors listed in the Your Self-Awareness feature to see which descriptions best characterize your behavior with others. Fortunately, old behaviors can be unlearned, and new behaviors can be learned.

Passive Behavior

Fear tends to be the major feeling in passive responses—fear of being embarrassed, of disappointing someone, or making someone angry. Because of fear, passive people frequently say "yes" at the expense of their own happiness or well-being, even when they want to say "no." To these individuals, everyone else's feelings and needs are more important than their own. Imagine what could happen if four passive individuals arrive at a four-way traffic stop at approximately the same time. Believing that the others have more important things to

---

YOUR SELF-AWARENESS
Comparing Your Own Passive, Aggressive, and Assertive Behaviors

Determine which of the following descriptions most closely match your behavior. Once you have finished, develop a personal plan for adopting a wider range of assertive behaviors in both your personal and professional life.

Passive	Aggressive	Assertive
"I'm not angry (but I am scared)!"	"I'm not scared (but I am angry)!"	"I'm both angry and scared!"
"I always do everything wrong."	"They always do everything wrong."	"Neither one of us is perfect, and there's nothing wrong with that."
"I'll try to make it (but I don't intend to because I'm resentful of your demands)."	"You must be crazy if you think I'll be there. Who do you think you are?"	"We should spend some time together and talk about our relationship."
"I never achieve my goals."	"The only way I can achieve my goals is by forcing others to agree with my way of thinking."	"I almost always achieve the goals I set for myself."
"I wish someone else would speak up."	"Be quiet and let me speak. You always monopolize the conversation."	"We can both have a chance to speak."

do and places to be, no one takes the initiative. All are fearful of angering or insulting the others. They sit there, waving one another on. People who consistently give up control are often left with resentment in their interpersonal relationships.

Aggressive Behavior

Aggressive responses are at the other end of the continuum of interaction. The three hallmarks of aggressive behavior are as follows:

1. The major feeling is anger.
2. The person says "no" even when "yes" could, or should, be said.
3. The aggressive person believes that his or her feelings are more important than the feelings of others.

Generally speaking, people who feel in the least control can be the most aggressive (Dupre & Barling, 2007). Some examples are: a bully, a subordinate at work with little control over others, or someone who shouts angrily, talks over others, and insists there is only one way to do something. Imagine what could happen if four aggressive individuals arrive at a four-way stop at the same time. Each believes that he or she has the most important thing to do or place to be. Each is angry with the others and attempts to be the first to cross the intersection. Perhaps all four crash in the middle of the intersection.

Assertive Behavior

People who focus on neither anger nor fear, respect their own and others' feelings, and say "yes" and "no" appropriately, behave assertively. Imagine what could happen if four assertive individuals arrive at a four-way stop at the same time. Recognizing traffic rules and the rights of others, each allows the person on the right the opportunity to proceed first.

Everyone has assertiveness potential, but not everyone has learned how to be assertive. You can teach clients and families how to behave assertively by incorporating the guidelines in the Partnering With Clients and Families features on page 376 in Chapter 17 and page 766 in Chapter 35∞.

Vision

Because psychiatric–mental health nurses focus their work on enhancing the quality of life for all human beings, you must come to terms with a personal and professional vision of what quality of life means. Some conditions of life associated with high quality are influence or power, freedom, accountability, self-determinism, openness to gratifying experience, action, mastery, a sense of purpose or meaning, privacy, hope, stability, nonviolence, and intimacy. The nurse with vision enhances clients' quality of life by providing opportunities for these life conditions.

Accountability

According to Peplau (1980), the need for personal accountability—professional integrity—is greater in psychiatric practice than in any other type of health care. Clients in mental health settings are usually more vulnerable and defenseless than are clients in other health care settings, particularly because their conditions hinder their thinking processes and their relationships with others.

You are accountable for the nature of the effort you make on behalf of clients and answerable to clients for the quality of your efforts. As Peplau put it, "Personal accountability is an attitude—a quality of the heart and mind of those professionals who are competent and determined that every psychiatric patient will have the best problem-resolving assistance possible" (1980, p. 133).

Psychiatric–mental health nurses are accountable to themselves, their peers, their profession, and the public in the following ways:

- Accountability to self involves bringing personal behavior under conscious control so that the nurse becomes the person-as-nurse she or he wants to be.
- Accountability to peers involves engaging in peer review with nurse colleagues to give and receive feedback intended to improve the quality of care.
- Accountability to the profession involves clarifying the role of the psychiatric–mental health nurse, keeping current with changes in the field, and encouraging self-regulation to protect the public and enhance the quality of care.
- Accountability to the public requires keeping abreast of knowledge in the field, becoming credentialed according to level of competence, applying the ANA standards of psychiatric–mental health nursing practice (discussed in Chapter 2∞), and protecting the rights of clients and their families (discussed in Chapter 13∞).

The personally accountable psychiatric–mental health nurse will insist on clinical supervision. Supervision provides novice as well as experienced nurses with the opportunity to learn therapeutic techniques and attitudes. It enables them to receive validation, insight, and support during the difficult times that may accompany a therapeutic relationship and enables them to analyze how they affect the outcome of the relationship.

Advocacy

Throughout history, psychiatric–mental health nurses have been ardent supporters of a neglected, ignored, and forgotten population—the mentally ill. In the 21st century, there is a need for new energy and political activism. In this era of health care reform, there is an especially important concern—ensuring that the needs and the rights of mentally disordered people are not overlooked or ignored while the explosion of knowledge in science and technology revolutionizes how nurses practice mental health care.

Nurses are more politically aware than ever before. A newly energized political activism calls for you to speak out publicly for the health, welfare, and safety of your clients; to take steps to protect client rights; to write articles for the popular press; to lobby your congressional representatives on behalf of better mental health for all people; and to run for political office. The power that such a large group of citizen nurses could wield on behalf of their clients would be awesome. As Brian, a psychiatric–mental health nursing student

CARING FOR THE SPIRIT

Spirituality: Helping Clients Rediscover Their Spiritual Path

Spirituality is the third part of the triad known as mind–body–spirit in the holistic practice of nursing. In ancient times, spirit meant breath—as essential to life as air. Spirituality is that part of every person that yearns to share the beauty, love, and joyfulness of the universe.

We take our spirituality from many sources: Nature, God, Buddha, Higher Power, Goddess, Krishna, B'ahaullah, Mohammed, Yahweh, and a connection to other people. Although many of these sources are incorporated into organized religions, spirituality is not religion, nor is religion spirituality. Religion is the organization of a set of beliefs, practices, and rituals, whereas spirituality is a reflection of one's "spirit" and its relationship to the rest of the universe. Some people develop their spirituality throughout life with prayer, meditation, and reflection. Others may leave the spiritual path because of conflicts with religious beliefs, values, and practices; because of toxic family relationships; or because they are too busy trying to survive physically and mentally.

Helping clients rediscover their spiritual path is a fulfilling role for psychiatric–mental health nurses. You can help clients find out who they really are, beyond, for example, simply husband, father, lover, police officer. Help them identify the source of their inner energy and how to get in touch with their "center" or their "soul." Keep in mind that spirituality is a deeply personal inner experience as opposed to a set of behaviors tied to an externally imposed doctrine or ritual. By offering a simple spirituality inventory, such as that in the Caring for the Spirit: Spiritual Health Assessment box in Chapter 11∞ on page 215, you encourage clients to look at the strength of their faith, which will help them with their recovery. Faith is a way of being—being open to possibilities, and to healing.

---

at William Carey University in New Orleans, put it: "The moment that we stop fighting for one another is the moment we lose our own humanity."

Successful advocacy is a positive experience for nurses as well as for clients. Clients derive a benefit, and we feel good about our ability to be agents of change. Be aware, however, that not all advocating will be successful. Sometimes, despite our most earnest and well-intentioned efforts, we fail in our attempt to advocate for positive change for our clients.

Spirituality

Spirituality, the search for meaning and purpose in life through a connection with others, nature, and/or a belief in a higher power, is at the core of each person's existence. Spirituality varies in strength from person to person. Some people already have a meaningful philosophy of life. Others, on a spiritual journey, search for life's meaning and purpose. Still others experience hopelessness, despair, and spiritual distress. Helping clients find meaning and purpose in their lives empowers them.

For some clients, their spirituality becomes a central focus in their treatment. They may attempt to resolve internal conflicts or conflicts with others through religious rituals or practices. Other clients will have maladaptive behavior that involves religiosity rather than spirituality (Sessanna, Finnell, Underhill, Change, & Peng, 2011). To differentiate between religiosity and spirituality, see the Caring for the Spirit feature.

Recent research indicates that the connection between mind, body, and spirit is complex and that spirituality is influenced by culture. You need to be aware of the client's source of hope and strength; the significance or insignificance of religious practice and rituals in the client's life; the client's thinking about the relationship between spiritual beliefs and mental health; the client's fear of alienation, loneliness, or solitude; and the client's concept of God (Wilkinson, 2012).

Helping clients in their search for meaning and purpose is possible when nurses have beliefs that sustain them rather than beliefs that are sources of conflict. You must meet your own spiritual needs satisfactorily before you can have a meaningful relationship with your clients. Take the time to carefully consider the questions in Caring for the Spirit: Your Personal Journey of Spiritual Growth to determine whether you meet your own spiritual needs satisfactorily.

CARING FOR THE SPIRIT

Your Personal Journey of Spiritual Growth

To help you on your personal journey of spiritual growth, contemplate these questions:

1. What gives the greatest meaning or purpose to your life?
2. How do you express your spirituality or your philosophy of life?
3. How does God/Higher Power/Ultimate Other/The Transcendent function in your personal life?
4. What kinds of confusion or doubt do you have about your religious beliefs?
5. What do you do to show love for yourself?
6. What brings you joy and peace in your life?
7. How do you heal your spirit?
8. What art, music, or literature nurtures your spirit?
9. How does your spirituality affect your experience as a nurse?

Answering these questions, in part or in whole (with the goal of eventually fully answering them), and asking yourself how you can change your situation will make you a spiritual activist for yourself and for your clients.

Empathy

Comprehension of, and ability to use, the process of empathy is one strategy for responding to the feelings of aloneness often experienced by people who are psychiatric clients. Perhaps the most important function of empathic understanding is to give the client the very precious feeling of being understood and cared about.

Empathy is a pervasive phenomenon in the life experience of all people. **Empathy** can be defined as the ability to feel what others feel and respond to and understand the experience of others on their terms. A nurse who empathizes with a client momentarily abandons the personal self and relives the emotions and responses of someone else. People in everyday life tend to empathize most with those to whom they feel closest. In mental health work, we must seek to empathize with those from whom we feel most separate or whose closeness threatens our own sense of integration.

The capacity for empathy relies on personal integration. A firm sense of self is necessary for a person to be a good empathizer. As we continue to interact with others, we learn to be sensitive to others without losing our own integration. The role of empathy in facilitating communication is discussed in Chapter 10∞.

Critical Thinking

Critical thinking is the means by which we transfer nursing knowledge into clinical practice (Wilkinson, 2012). It is a purposeful mental activity in which ideas are produced and evaluated and judgments are made. A critical thinker analyzes information before drawing conclusions about it. **Critical thinking** can be defined as purposeful, reasonable, reflective thinking that drives problem solving and decision making and aims to make judgments based on evidence.

The ability to think critically is crucial for psychiatric–mental health nurses because the complexity of care makes critical thinking skills urgent. Critical thinking mobilizes intrapersonal, interpersonal, perceptual, moral/ethical, experiential, practical, scientific, and contextual knowledge (Lechasseur, Lazere, & Guilbert, 2011) all of which are elemental in providing safe and effective care.

To encourage you to think critically, we have provided critical thinking challenges at the beginning of every chapter and critical thinking questions at the end of every Evidence-Based Practice feature and every Developing Cultural Competence feature. To develop effective, critical thinking habits, implement the strategies suggested in Your Intervention Strategies.

YOUR INTERVENTION STRATEGIES   Promoting Critical Thinking

Strategy	Rationale
Anticipate questions others might ask, such as "What will my supervisor or instructor want to know?"	This helps identify a wider scope of questions that must be answered to gain relevant information.
Ask "What if" questions like "What if something goes wrong?" or "What if we try?"	This helps you be proactive and creative.
Look for flaws in your thinking. Ask questions like, "What is missing?" "Have I recognized my biases?" "How could this be made better?"	Such questions help you evaluate your thinking and make improvements.
Ask someone else to look for flaws in your thinking.	You are usually too close to your own work to be objective; others bring a fresh eye and possibly new ideas and perspectives.
Develop "good habits of inquiry" (habits that aid in the search for the truth, such as always keeping an open mind, verifying information, and taking enough time).	These habits can make critical thinking more automatic.
Develop interpersonal skills, such as conflict resolution and getting along with those who have different communication styles.	If you do not have good interpersonal skills, you are unlikely to get the help or information you need to think critically.
Replace "I do not know" and "I am not sure" with "I will try."	This demonstrates you have the ability to find answers and mobilizes you to locate resources.
Turn errors into learning opportunities.	We all make mistakes; they are stepping stones to maturity and new ideas. If you are not making mistakes, maybe you are not trying hard enough.

Pearson Nursing Student Resources

Find additional review materials at
nursing.pearsonhighered.com

Prepare for success with NCLEX®-style practice questions,
interactive assignments and activities, web links, animations
and videos, and more!

REFERENCES

Benner, P., & Wrubel, J. (1989). Coping with caregiving. In *The primacy of caring: Stress and coping in health and illness* (pp. 365–406). Menlo Park, CA: Addison-Wesley.

Clarke, L. (2009). Hope: The eternal paradigm for psychiatric/mental health nursing. *Journal of Psychiatric and Mental Health Nursing, 16*(9), 843–847.

Dupre, K. E., & Barling, J. (2007). Predicting and preventing supervisory workplace aggression. *Journal of Occupational Health, 11*(1), 13–26.

Freeburn, M., & Sinclair, M. (2009). Mental health nursing students' experience of stress: Burdened by a heavy load. *Journal of Psychiatric and Mental Health Nursing, 16*(4), 335–342.

Hameideh, S. H. (2011). Burnout, social support and job satisfaction among Jordanian mental health nurses. *Issues in Mental Health Nursing, 32*(4), 234–242.

Hewitt, J. P., & Shulman, D. (2011). *Self and society: A symbolic interactionist social psychology* (11th ed.). Upper Saddle River, NJ: Allyn & Bacon.

Hooper, C., Craig, J., Janvrin, D. R., Wetsel, M. A., & Reimeis, E. (2010). Compassion satisfaction, burnout, and compassion fatigue among emergency nurses compared with nurses in other selected inpatient specialties. *Journal of Emergency Nursing, 36*(5), 420–427.

Krystal, A. D. (2011). Recognition and assessment of shift work disorder. *Journal of Clinical Psychiatry, 72*(2), 248–257.

Lechasseur, K., Lazere, G., & Guilbert, L. (2011). Knowledge mobilized by a critical thinking process deployed by nursing students in practical situations: A qualitative study. *Journal of Advanced Nursing.* Advance online publication.

McCartan, P. J., & Hargie, O. D. W. (2007). Assertiveness and caring: Are they compatible? *Journal of Advanced Nursing, 13*, 707–713.

Montes-Berges, B., & Augusto, J. M. (2007). Exploring the relationship between perceived emotional intelligence, coping, social support and mental health in nursing students. *Journal of Psychiatric and Mental Health Nursing, 14*(2), 163–171.

Niu, S. F., Chung, M. H., Chen, C. H., Hegney, D., O'Brien, A., & Chow, K. R. (2011). The effect of shift rotation on employee cortisol profile, sleep quality, fatigue, and attention level: A systematic review. *Journal of Nursing Research, 19*(1), 68–81.

O'Malley, P. (2011). Staying awake and asleep: The challenge of working nights and rotating shifts: Managing shift work disorder for the clinical nurse specialist. *Clinical Nurse Specialist, 25*(1), 15–17.

Onyett, S. (2011). Revisiting job satisfaction and burnout in community mental health teams. *Journal of Mental Health, 20*(2), 198–209.

Peplau, H. E. (1980). The psychiatric nurse—accountable? To whom? For what? *Perspectives in Psychiatric Care, 18*(3), 128–134.

Phillips, J. (2011). Hardiness as a defense against compassion fatigue and burnout. *Journal of Emergency Nursing, 37*(2), 125.

Sessanna, L., Finnell, D. S., Underhill, M., Chang, Y. P., & Peng, H. L. (2011). Measures assessing spirituality as more than religiosity: A methodological review of nursing and health-related literature. *Journal of Advanced Nursing.* Advance online publication.

Shattell, M. M., McAllister, S., Hogan, B., & Thomas, S. P. (2006). "She took the time to make sure she understood": Mental health patients' experiences of being understood. *Archives of Psychiatric Nursing, 20*(5), 234–241.

Wilkinson, J.M. (2012). *Nursing process and critical thinking* (5th ed.). Upper Saddle River, NJ: Prentice Hall.

Yoder, E. A. (2010). Compassion fatigue in nurses. *Applied Nursing Research, 23*(4), 191–197.

The Therapeutic Nurse–Client Relationship

CAROL REN KNEISL

LEARNING OUTCOMES

After completing this chapter, you will be able to:

1. Explain the common shared characteristics of one–to–one relationships.
2. Encourage the client's systematic use of abilities and behaviors most often associated with growth-producing outcomes.
3. Analyze how phenomena such as resistance, transference, countertransference, critical distance, gift giving, the use of touch, and the values held by both client and nurse affect the therapeutic relationship.
4. Incorporate an understanding of the three phases of the therapeutic nurse–client relationship and the main objectives and therapeutic tasks of each phase into one–to–one work with clients.
5. Apply the nursing process to the three phases of the nurse–client relationship.
6. Establish and maintain one–to–one relationships within the context of the client's cultural background.

CRITICAL THINKING CHALLENGE

Your worst fear has just been realized. You have just met with your first psychiatric–mental health client to develop a therapeutic nurse–client relationship. Despite your best efforts, your client, Sammy, gave you "a hard time." There were long periods of silence broken by angry and explosive statements about your abilities and the fact that you are "only a student." You are uncertain whether Sammy will meet with you again.

1. What are your ideas about why Sammy behaved the way he did?
2. How might your feelings about Sammy's behavior influence your performance as a student of psychiatric–mental health nursing?
3. What steps can you take to deal with this first contact and the uncertainty of subsequent contacts with this client?

In the 21st century, psychiatric–mental health nursing continues to expand its neuropsychiatric focus. There has been an explosion of knowledge concerning the neurobiologic basis of mental illness in diagnostic technology and in the discovery of newer and better psychopharmacologic approaches (see Chapters 7 and 31∞) that has moved us toward a neuropsychiatric paradigm of care. At the same time that clients may have their needs for safety, structure, and medication met, they may also express their longing for a deeper connection to mental health staff and more insight-oriented treatment. The challenge for us is to integrate both biologic and psychosocial concepts while maintaining our nursing focus on caring. The therapeutic nurse–client relationship provides the opportunity to meet this challenge.

The **therapeutic nurse–client relationship**, also called the *one–to–one relationship,* is one in which you use theoretical understandings, personal attributes, and appropriate clinical techniques such as those in FIGURE 4-1 ▪ to provide the opportunity for a corrective emotional experience for clients. The therapeutic relationship has evolved as the cornerstone of psychiatric–mental health nursing theory and practice, largely based on nearly five decades of work by Hildegard Peplau. Her theory of interpersonal relations in nursing, discussed earlier in Chapter 2∞, was the basis for psychotherapeutic nursing (Peplau, 1952, 1997).

We are challenged to creatively adapt the time-honored principles of Peplau's work under changing conditions such as briefer psychiatric hospitalizations and the increase in outpatient and community treatment. The current health care economic climate has changed the face of the traditional therapeutic nurse–client relationship advocated by Peplau. Nevertheless, we incorporate the principles in our everyday work—brief encounters as well as consistent long-term relationships.

This chapter demystifies the characteristics, processes, phases, and problems of one–to–one relationships so that beginning psychiatric–mental health nurses can approach them with increased awareness of their own interpersonal effectiveness. Practical guidelines on how to facilitate interpersonal effectiveness with clients are included. The principles, processes, and phases discussed in this chapter also apply to family, group, and community interventions or therapies.

THE ONE–TO–ONE RELATIONSHIP

The one–to–one relationship between psychiatric–mental health nurse and client is a mutually defined, collaborative, and goal-oriented professional relationship. It may be viewed as a series of sequential nurse–client interactions with the following additional elements:

- The interactions occur over a designated period of time (daily, weekly, monthly).
- The interactions take place in a unique nurse–client structure, characterized by specific phases, processes, and problems.
- The interactions occur in a designated setting (home, private practice office, mental health clinic, inpatient psychiatric unit, medical unit).

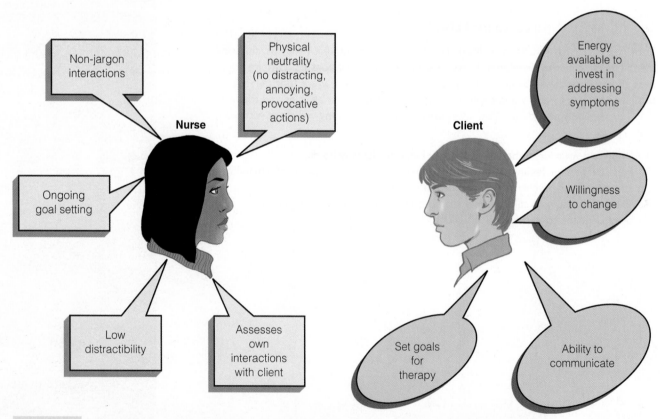

FIGURE 4-1 ▪ Nurse and client characteristics that enhance the one–to–one therapeutic relationship.

In addition, a one–to–one relationship has three distinct phases, as follows:

1. The orientation (beginning) phase, characterized by the establishment of contact with the client
2. The working (middle) phase, characterized by the maintenance and analysis of contact
3. The termination (end) phase, characterized by the termination of contact with the client

Each phase of a one–to–one relationship is distinguished by important goals and therapeutic tasks. These phases are discussed in detail later in the nursing process section of this chapter.

The time required for each phase ideally depends on the severity of client dysfunction, the number and types of problems that surface, and the type of therapeutic contract. Although these phases are presented in this chapter in their entirety in order to develop a comprehensive theoretic framework, nurses rarely experience them in such detail and sequence. You are more likely to experience the development of several short-term goals and to experiment with several subsequent interventions in any phase of relationship work. Nevertheless, an exploration of each phase will increase your familiarity with the flow—that is, "what comes next"—and may also provide a framework in which you can see client and nurse behaviors as partial expressions of a specific phase.

The amount of time a client may have available to establish a one–to–one relationship can be contingent on a variety of circumstances. The client's health care insurance resources may restrict access to mental health care services either by limiting the length of a hospital stay or by limiting the number of allowable outpatient sessions. A reality of health care, particularly mental health care, is the timeframe imposed from without, often without a surplus of options.

Characteristics of Therapeutic Nurse–Client Relationships

In addition to having three distinct phases, the therapeutic nurse–client relationship has several specific, inherent characteristics.

Although the components themselves do not change, the schedule will.

Therapeutic Alliance

The one–to–one relationship begins with the creation of a therapeutic alliance between nurse and client. A **therapeutic alliance** is a conscious, growth-facilitating relationship between a helping person (the psychiatric–mental health nurse) and the client. It is fundamental to the process of making adaptive change (Horvath, Del Re, Fluckiger, & Symonds, 2011). Beginning psychiatric–mental health nursing students have several common anxiety-provoking concerns about the process of creating a therapeutic alliance. The questions and answers in Your Self-Awareness address those concerns.

The goal in the therapeutic alliance is to facilitate the client's growth by helping the client address personal problems and concerns in order to handle unresolved problems constructively. More specifically, the nurse identifies and provides feedback regarding the client's patterns of reaction, abilities, and potentials using therapeutic communication skills (discussed in Chapter 10 ∞). The client can use these assets to handle unresolved problems constructively.

Establishing a therapeutic alliance is essential in one–to–one relationships. Such a binding alliance between you and the client allows the one–to–one relationship to continue, especially when the client experiences increased anxiety and resistance to change. Investing time, persistence, and patience in the therapeutic relationship promotes the long-term goal of helping the client change established response patterns. Forming a strong therapeutic alliance may enhance recovery and rehabilitation among persons with major mental illnesses (Priebe, Richardson, Cooney, Adedejo, & McCabe, 2011). The personal qualities of the nurse that enhance the ability to forge a therapeutic alliance are discussed in Chapter 3 ∞. One version of forming a therapeutic alliance is critiqued in Mental Health in the Movies.

Professional

One–to–one relationships reflect a professional, rather than a social, relationship. We use our personalities, interpersonal skills and techniques, and theoretic knowledge of psychiatric–mental

---

MENTAL HEALTH IN THE MOVIES
Analyze This

Analyze This is the story of a calm, cool, and collected psychiatrist (Dr. Ben Sobel, played by Billy Crystal) and his new client, the most powerful mobster in New York City (Paul Vitti, played by Robert DeNiro), an emotionally vulnerable man who has begun to experience incapacitating panic attacks. The odd-couple chemistry between the two men is engaging as the psychiatrist is forced to help the mobster get in touch with his feelings. The sessions between psychiatrist and client are witty—as Dr. Ben Sobel puts it,

"What is my goal here, to make you a happy, well-adjusted gangster?" Later in the movie, Vitti tries out some of what he has learned in therapy, attempting to talk about his feelings to a rival mobster with whom he is angry.

The movie is not all slapstick comedy. It treats Vitti's emotional problems seriously. We come to understand the mob boss's feelings of stress, anxiety, and depression, as well as the psychiatrist's complicated family situation that brings him stresses of his own. In *Analyze That*, the sequel to the film, Sobel and Vitti continue to deal with the nuances of their therapeutic relationship in a variety of unusual situations.

Photo courtesy of Alamy A.F. Archive.

YOUR SELF-AWARENESS
Common Concerns of Beginning Psychiatric–Mental Health Nursing Students

Review these common concerns and the suggestions that relate to them before your first psychiatric nursing clinical experience.

- **The client won't talk to me.** It is true that at times clients may not want to talk, or their symptoms may make it difficult for them to interact with you. You can offer to remain with the client (if that is acceptable to the client) without an expectation that the client talks to you. Demonstrate your genuine interest in the client by offering to return at another time and offering the client the opportunity to seek you out or let you know when he or she wishes to talk.

- **The client tells me to go away or seems angry when I approach him or her.** Refrain from imposing your goals on the client and tell the client that you respect the client's wishes. Let the client know that you will try again at another time. Recognize that the rejection or anger is not likely to have anything to do with you, but is probably a reflection of the client's emotional distress.

- **Being afraid of hurting the client by saying the wrong thing.** There is no one wrong thing that will make things worse for the client. If you show genuine interest, respect the client's dignity, and truly care about the client, these qualities will be apparent in your nonverbal behavior. If you say something that you think is wrong or came out in a way you did not intend, let the client know. You can always say something like: "That didn't sound right. What I really meant to say is . . .".

- **The fear that mentally ill people can be dangerous.** If this is your first experience in a psychiatric setting, much of what you think you know about mentally ill people comes from movies and television. Actually, few mentally ill clients are dangerous to others. Of course, you must keep safety factors in mind—note which clients the staff say are aggressive, be with the client in an open area rather than a closed room, provide space between yourself and the client, seek the assistance or presence of your instructor or a staff person.

- **Feeling sorry for clients who do not have money for cigarettes or treats.** Giving clients money or cigarettes is a form of gift giving (see the section on gift giving in the nursing process section) that may impair the therapeutic relationship. In addition, money or cigarettes may be part of a token economy plan of care in some agencies—there are specific purposes and times for the giving of money and cigarettes. Instead, help clients to look at what they themselves can do to get money or cigarettes.

- **Being asked to give personal information—home address, telephone number, or being asked to see the client socially outside of the psychiatric setting.** Realize that some clients have difficulty recognizing interpersonal boundaries. Explain to the client the difference between a social and a professional relationship and tell the client that yours is a professional relationship. Giving personal information or seeing the client socially would be a professional boundary violation.

- **The client is sexually inappropriate.** Recognize that sexually inappropriate behavior is a boundary violation on the client's part. You can use the same strategies described earlier. Let the client know that the behavior is inappropriate but do so in a way that protects the client's dignity.

- **Seeing someone you know being treated in the mental health facility.** Take your cue from the client—the client may not wish to acknowledge your previous relationship. Let your instructor know so you will not be assigned to the client. Respect the client's privacy and do not read the client's record.

- **Running into a client at a restaurant, grocery store, or other public place.** Again, take your cue from the client. The client may not wish others to know that the client receives, or has received, mental health treatment. Do not acknowledge the client unless the client acknowledges you first. Monitor what you say in order to keep the client's confidentiality.

- **Being fearful of admitting anxiety about the clinical experience.** Most beginning students are anxious about the clinical experience connected with the psychiatric–mental health nursing course, and instructors recognize that. Your instructor can be a source of help to you to overcome or reduce your anxiety, but not if you do not share these concerns in the spirit of learning and growing.

health nursing practice in a purposeful, goal-directed manner to facilitate a useful change in the client's life. This professional relationship differs from a social relationship in several significant ways that are summarized in Table 4-1 ■.

A professional one–to–one relationship can be either informal or formal. Spontaneous, informal nurse–client relationships are at one end of the continuum, and formal individual counseling or psychotherapy (by advanced practice psychiatric–mental health nurses) is at the other end.

Informal Relationships Informal nurse–client relationships may be prearranged and planned, but more often they occur spontaneously—between a nurse and a client with leukemia, between a nurse and an offender in jail, between a nurse and a high-risk pregnant woman, between a home care nurse and a client with emphysema, or between a nurse and a psychiatric client. An example of an informal one–to–one relationship is described in What Every Nurse Should Know.

These relationships consist of a set of interactions limited in time. There is minimum structure and a sense of immediacy. They occur in numerous medical and nonmedical settings and are particularly common in psychiatric institutions and community mental health settings.

Formal Relationships The more formal one–to–one relationship is used in crisis intervention, counseling, or individual psychotherapy. It requires more planning, structure, consistency, nursing expertise, and time. The formal one–to–one relationship occurs in various psychiatric settings,

Characteristic	Professional Relationship	Social Relationship
Purpose	Systematic working-through of troublesome thoughts, feelings, and behaviors Planned evaluation (through stages)	Companionship, pleasure, sharing of interests Evolves spontaneously
Role delineation	Specific roles for nurse and client with explicit use of psychiatric nursing skills and interventions	Generally not present, except for broad social norms governing the particular type of relationship (friend versus lover)
Satisfaction of needs	Client is encouraged to identify, develop, and assess ways to meet own needs more effectively Does not address personal needs of the nurse	Mutual sharing and satisfaction of personal and interpersonal needs
Timeframe	Usually time-limited interactions with an expected termination	Usually not time limited, in either duration or frequency of contact No planned termination

TABLE 4-1 ■ Differences Between Professional and Social Relationships

WHAT EVERY NURSE SHOULD KNOW

The Therapeutic Relationship With Parents of a Premature Infant

Imagine that you are a neonatal intensive care nurse. When an infant has been born prematurely or has physical problems upon birth (such as low birth weight), the infant may be placed in a neonatal intensive care nursery (NICU). Emotions can run high in the NICU as the infant's health fluctuates.

Your ability to act as a liaison between the medical system and the parents throughout the infant's tenure in the NICU will likely take place within a one–to–one relationship. You will incorporate a number of one–to–one strategies when you work with parents: recognizing and respecting the boundaries of the therapeutic relationship, acknowledging how the parents' anxiety affects communication with their infant as well as the NICU staff, adjusting the speed and volume of your information sharing so as not to overwhelm the stressed adults, and discussing the emotional tone the parents have while interacting with their infant.

You can use the information in this chapter, specifically information about the therapeutic alliance, cultural context, and goal-directed behaviors, to shape how you proceed.

including psychiatric institutions, community mental health centers, and private practice.

High levels of symptoms can compromise the client's level of functioning, and thus the ability to establish a formal relationship. If a one–to–one relationship already exists when symptoms exacerbate, that is, they worsen, your therapeutic interactions must be skilled and flexible enough to change your pace and expectations. When the goal of the therapeutic relationship is to promote major changes in emotional states, the client must be able to participate in a focused and abstract effort (Smith & Greenberg, 2007). The nurse must be an expert partner in achieving that goal.

TABLE 4-2 ■ highlights the similarities and differences of informal and formal relationship work. The differences are also discussed throughout this chapter.

Mutually Defined

A one–to–one relationship is mutually defined by the two participants. That is, both you and the client voluntarily enter the relationship and specify the conditions under which it is to evolve (Spiers & Wood, 2010). For example, the client may seek immediate relief from symptoms rather than long-term individual psychotherapy. You and the client identify together where and when you will meet and other conditions of your participation. This is a part of the contract that is explored further in the discussion of the beginning (orientation) phase of therapy later in the chapter. Once the one–to–one relationship is established, maintaining it depends on the commitment of both participants.

Collaborative

Both you and the client enter a relationship in which goals, strategies, and outcomes evolve within the context of the therapeutic work together. Mutual collaboration implies that each of you brings personal abilities, capabilities, and power to the relationship. You have an impact on the client, and the client has a personal impact on you as well. However, it is important to not assume responsibility for client behaviors but to actively work with the client to assess the self-defeating and growth-promoting aspects of specific behaviors. Recognizing, supporting, and emphasizing clients' capacity to have control over their own health and life (Hudson, St. Cyr-Tribble, Bravo, & Poitras, 2011) is a growth-producing opportunity for clients.

The client is in charge of change following a joint assessment of problematic behaviors and emotional states (Hudson et al., 2011). Working in concert with a nursing professional in a therapeutic alliance has the added effect of supporting psychological well-being by crafting healthy interdependence (Steelman, 2007). Mutual collaboration also means that we assess and are accountable for our own behavior with clients. Ongoing supervision often helps us to meet these particular goals.

TABLE 4-2 ■ Similarities and Differences in Informal and Formal One–to–One Relationships

Characteristic	Informal Relationship	Formal Relationship
Setting	Varied	Generally psychiatric settings
Frequency and duration of contact	Flexible, depending on client need or tolerance; example: short, frequent intervals daily	Structured; example: once weekly, with possible crisis sessions; duration usually set at 30 minutes or 1 hour
Duration of relationship	May or may not involve time commitment Generally a few days to a few weeks	Involves time commitment: weeks to months, for short-term work; months to years, for long-term work
Type of dysfunction	In general, more effective with severe dysfunction	In severe dysfunction, may be useful after client is stabilized on medication
Use of therapeutic contract	May involve simple therapeutic contract	Utilizes therapeutic contract; the more specific, the better
Fees	Usually not relevant	May be relevant; may be part of therapeutic contract
Degree of skill required	Nursing student or psychiatric nurse	Advanced degree beneficial but not essential
Degree of supervision	Some degree and type of supervision always necessary	Consistent supervision or consultation usually necessary
Degree of effectiveness	Depends on client's level of functioning, skills of the psychiatric–mental health nurse, and time allotment	Depends on client's level of functioning, skills of the psychiatric–mental health nurse, and time allotment

Goal Directed

A therapeutic nurse–client relationship is always goal directed. The client is expected to identify and achieve specific physical, emotional, and social goals within the context of the relationship. Client goals vary widely in type and depth. For example, in informal relationship work a client's goal may be to initiate one peer relationship within an inpatient psychiatric unit. Other examples include resolution of a divorce involving children and shared personal possessions, or coming to terms with the client's impending death. Often, the client's initial goal is to solve an immediate problem, and this serves as a basis for establishing more extensive psychosocial goals.

The psychiatric–mental health nurse also formulates therapeutic goals to enhance the growth-producing elements of the relationship. Inpatient clients with serious symptomatology may have difficulty in connecting behaviors and modifying them in the time allotted. Goals that can be worked on in the future and in various settings are more likely to be achieved.

Open

The one–to–one relationship between nurse and client may be viewed as an experience in *shared dignity*. The psychiatric–mental health nurse adapts to allow clients to reveal their humanness freely and openly. Each aspect of your verbal and nonverbal behavior either encourages or inhibits clients from being open themselves. Evidence-Based Practice shows how one nurse demonstrated openness using several interventions to encourage a client to discuss a difficult topic.

Negotiated

In the one–to–one relationship, the client is an active decision maker and is personally accountable for the work. The atmosphere of give-and-take within the relationship emphasizes mutuality, reciprocity, and interpersonal fairness.

Establishing a clearly defined, mutually agreed-upon therapeutic contract represents a prime example of negotiation in one–to–one work. (The therapeutic contract is covered later in the chapter.)

Committed

Commitment is based on the therapeutic contract between nurse and client. The contract establishes the limits of the relationship as well as the time and energy allotted to it. At some point in the relationship, you will be confronted by the reality of the client's dysfunction. Because of personal discomfort, some beginning psychiatric–mental health nurses may respond by actively colluding with the client to deny or ignore the dysfunction and remain on a superficial, social level of communication. This collusion protects the nurse from having to address the client's helplessness, desperation, hostility, or raw grief. Not allowing the client to express these feelings signals that you are not sufficiently committed to the client.

The opposite is also nontherapeutic. Assuming an omnipotent or rescuer role to "cure" the client signals your overcommitment. This role robs the client of active decision-making power and accountability.

Be aware that the client will test your commitment in some phase of the relationship. Both you and the client need to deal with this test explicitly on verbal and nonverbal levels. A sense of positive connectedness with the client strengthens the sense of commitment.

Culturally Sensitive

Because cultural context influences nursing care, a sensitive and systematic consideration of the client's cultural and ethnic background is an essential part of the psychiatric nursing process in one–to–one relationship work. Cultural forces shape the expression of distress and the formation of symptoms.

Pregnancy and Antidepressants

Sharon is a 25-year-old with a history of depression. She is currently pregnant and is wondering if she should continue taking antidepressant medications during her pregnancy or stop and risk having her symptoms return. Sharon has been discussing her concerns with you and the rest of the team during her prenatal care appointments. She has not discussed them with anyone other than her health care providers, because she is afraid of what they might say.

During your one–to–one interactions with Sharon, you state your concern for her welfare and assure her that her concerns will be discussed on a regular basis. You tell her that you and she will work on a solution together as you have in the past with other problems.

The one–to–one relationship maintained in this situation has a positive effect on Sharon's ability to discuss a difficult topic. You remain available, without withdrawing, despite Sharon's distress, fears, or silence. You promote trust by stating your concern for Sharon's welfare and offering to discuss the issue together. Your nursing intervention should be based on more than one study, but the following research would be helpful in this case.

Gawley, L., Einarson, A., & Bowen, A. (2011). Stigma and attitudes toward antenatal depression and antidepressant use during pregnancy in healthcare students. *Advances in Health Science Education, Theory, and Practice.* Advance online publication.

Gentile, S. (2011). Drug treatment for mood disorders in pregnancy. *Current Opinion in Psychiatry, 24*(1), 34–40.

Petersen, I., Gilbert, R. E., Evans, S. K., Man, S. L., & Nazareth, I. (2011). Pregnancy as a major determinant for discontinuance of antidepressants: An analysis of data from The Health Improvement Network. *Journal of Clinical Psychiatry.* Advance online publication.

CRITICAL THINKING QUESTIONS

1. If antidepressants have even an unlikely potential to affect the baby, should Sharon stop taking them?
2. Should women who take psychotropic medications avoid pregnancy?
3. Why is it important that Sharon's symptoms of depression symptoms do not return?

Culture also influences the client's expectations of the nurse–client relationship and the client's interpretations of the events that take place within it. It is important to consistently evaluate the influence of culture within the one–to–one relationship as well as the effects of the therapeutic relationship on the client's values and life experiences. A sensitive and systematic consideration of the client's cultural and ethnic background is important at each phase of the one–to–one relationship. How to keep culture in mind is interwoven throughout this and other chapters and is further described in Chapter 9∞.

PHENOMENA OCCURRING IN ONE–TO–ONE RELATIONSHIPS

Sometimes you may initially feel a sense of unease or confusion about what is happening in the nurse–client therapeutic relationship. This uneasiness may be difficult to identify, describe, and explore. Remember to keep the following phenomena in mind when you are attempting to "make sense" of a one–to–one relationship.

Resistance

Resistance refers to all the phenomena that interfere with and disrupt the smooth flow of feelings, memories, and thoughts. It inevitably surfaces in the course of any informal or formal psychotherapeutic work and most often occurs as the client begins to address self-defeating thoughts, feelings, and behaviors.

Resistance is often mistakenly seen as the client's struggle against the nurse. Instead, the client is struggling against the anxiety associated with change, against self-awareness, and against responsibility for actions (Smith & Greenberg, 2007). Thus, resistance in therapeutic one–to–one relationships is best understood as the client's struggle against change. The client's behavior patterns may have self-defeating aspects, but at the same time they have also provided some satisfaction or prevented some discomfort. In other words, they have "worked" in the past.

Evaluating Behavior as Resistive

In general, you may suspect resistance when the client's behavior appears to block the progress of the relationship. However, exercise caution in evaluating a client's behavior as resistive. There may be other explanations for the emotional atmosphere in the one–to–one interaction. For example, a client's silence may indicate pensiveness, a pause before emotive expression, or a sense of completion. The client who is habitually late may have real difficulties adjusting a full personal schedule to accommodate the sessions. The client who resists discussing specific topics or concerns may not be ready for investigative work. Likewise, a client may resist giving up a defense mechanism such as rationalization or projection (see Chapter 8∞) because it is desperately needed to keep anxiety about unbearable thoughts and impulses, or anxiety about a present situation, at manageable levels.

Remember that the client has a right to resist any aspect of, or the entire, therapeutic process as a matter of choice. However, the client's resistive behavior should be openly discussed, rather than ignored.

General Intervention Strategies With Resistance

Several consecutive approaches are used as general nursing intervention strategies for resistance. They begin with the nurse's awareness of the resistance. Helpful intervention strategies include the following:

- Label the resistant behavior with the client. You may allow the resistance to occur several times to demonstrate its presence to the client. It is as if you were holding up a mirror for the client, reflecting and clarifying the specific resistant behavior.
- Explore the accompanying emotion and the history of its development.
- Explore what function the resistance may serve, especially any self-defeating aspects.
- Facilitate working through the resistance by fully understanding and appreciating its implications in the client's life.

This sequence may occur repeatedly before a resistant behavior is resolved.

Acting Out as Resistance

Acting out is a particularly destructive form of resistance in which the client puts into action (that is, "acts out") emotional conflicts. It is important to recognize that the client is externalizing an inner conflict to people in the immediate environment. Rather than verbalizing conflicts or feelings, the client displays inappropriate behaviors. Some examples of acting out include forcefully slamming a door, dressing provocatively, or slapping someone.

In acting out, the client acts toward a mate, friend, relative, or other person those feelings and attitudes that the client does not express toward the nurse. An example of acting out is developing third-person relationships to absorb the emotions and fantasies that belong in the therapeutic relationship. Exaggerated feelings of intense hostility toward the nurse may lead to violence or physical harm to the client, nurse, or the third person. Intense feelings of love for the nurse or therapist may precipitate an affair or marriage with the third person.

Intervention Strategies With Acting Out Acting out contains a vital seed for change. That is, it can form the basis for the client's understanding of, and eventual giving up of, destructive and inappropriate behaviors. The one–to–one therapeutic relationship can transform a client's acting out (for example, rageful behaviors) into adaptive emotions and behaviors by facilitating change (Smith & Greenberg, 2007). Acting out is difficult to deal with because the client does not talk about the feelings that precipitate the behavior and later tends to conceal or rationalize the behavior. Acting out can abruptly disrupt the relationship or psychiatric treatment, unless it is identified and dealt with explicitly.

Specific nursing interventions relating to acting out include the following:

- Bring the acting out behavior to the client's attention.
- Encourage the client to *talk about* impulses rather than to act them out.

- Encourage identification of feelings *before* putting them into action.
- Increase frequency of contact.
- Look for evidence of transference phenomena toward the nurse (discussed in the next section).

With repeated dangerous acting out behaviors, consider withdrawing from the relationship unless the client sets limits on these behaviors.

Transference

Transference is a normal phenomenon that may surface and inhibit effectiveness in any phase of one–to–one relationship work and in any setting, including nonpsychiatric settings. **Transference** is a set of feelings and thoughts about significant others in the client's past and current life that is transferred to the caregiver. It can be considered a lens through which the client sees his or her relationships. Transference typically happens quickly, and generally unconsciously, in the therapeutic relationship (Boag, 2007). Therapeutic effectiveness requires working with transference issues within the client's cultural framework and developing options for the client to emote and behave adaptively in interpersonal relationships.

A study of early transference reactions (Beretta et al, 2007) noted that people tend to have a limited number of types of relationship patterns (parents, romantic, family, friendship, colleague, and impersonal). It is likely that clients will repeat their particular patterns with you and re-enact the patterns they use outside the therapeutic relationship. The following clinical example illustrates how transference may surface in a clinical setting.

Clinical Example

Conrad, hospitalized for depression, was assigned to a primary counselor, a male psychiatric–mental health nurse. Over the course of several meetings with his counselor, Conrad assumed a cowering, ingratiating manner. He seemed to resemble a little boy awaiting punishment from an intimidating, punitive father. This interpersonal orientation was observed by other male staff members in their informal interactions with Conrad. Conrad was eventually able to discuss his views of older men based on his relationship with a stern, demanding father.

The recognition of transference signals that it is time to explore this interaction in order to reduce interpersonal problems in the one–to–one relationship (Ryum, Stile, Svartberg, & McCullough, 2010). Expect that clients will have transference issues. Work collaboratively with clients, using the transference as a therapeutic tool, to foster adaptive and positive changes in their relationships.

Explore the meaning of individual words, gestures, events, and situations in the current one–to–one relationship to determine how these reflect or replay distortions in other past or current relationships. The therapeutic task is to separate feelings, thoughts, and behaviors that belong to the current one–to–one relationship from those that represent unresolved conflicts in other relationships.

Increasing awareness of the transference process often frees the client to work through conflicts and explore the more creative, self-actualizing aspects of personal identity as they evolve. You must not interact as the client's parent or any other transference figure. Rather, help the client bring an unconscious event into consciousness, to examine its cause and meaning. Remember to seek supervision from your instructor when you suspect a transference reaction.

Positive Transference

Transference may be positive or negative. *Positive transference*—that is, positive feelings for the therapist—occurs when the client generally has had satisfying past relationships with significant others during childhood. The therapeutic relationship is usually able to progress in this instance.

Negative Transference

In *negative transference*, the client shows a number of reactions based on forms of hate (hostility, loathing, bitterness, contempt, annoyance). Although there are both positive and negative aspects to every transference, a predominantly negative transference is uncomfortable for both you and the client. The client does not like to be aware of and express this hate, and you will not like being the target of it. When negative transference appears unresolvable, seek clinical supervision with a knowledgeable colleague. It may be advisable to terminate the relationship work rather than run the risk of further client dysfunction.

Countertransference

While transference involves the client's reactions to the psychiatric nurse, **countertransference** involves the nurse's reactions to the client. You may develop powerful counterproductive fantasies, feelings, and attitudes in response to the client's transference or personality. Countertransference is thought by some to be almost inevitable in psychotherapeutic situations (Ellis, 2001).

Countertransference is suspected when the nurse repeatedly assigns meaning to the nurse–client relationship that belongs to the nurse's other relationships. In countertransference, the psychiatric–mental health nurse's ability to assess nurse–client interactions becomes confused or thwarted by unresolved conflicts. This conflict may be expressed in acts of omission or commission that may be covert or overt. That is, you may unconsciously use behaviors (as parent, sibling, lover, or friend) that attempt to replay some conflict with significant others. Some examples are as follows:

- Placing hands on the hips or pointing a finger while setting limits on a client's behavior (parental)
- Patting a client on the shoulder and offering reassurance (parental)
- Dressing suggestively (erotic)
- Blushing and giggling when a client makes a sexual remark (sexual)
- Being sarcastic in response to a client's concern (hostile)

Parental or caretaker behaviors that express the need to nurture the client are the most common among beginning psychiatric–mental health nurses. These behaviors may discount the client's ability to ensure his or her own well-being and encourage acting out by the client. Be alert for actions with clients that are out of line with standard expectations for professional psychiatric–mental health nursing care. Look for cues to the presence of countertransference such as those discussed in Your Self-Awareness.

Countertransference is a normal occurrence, requiring clinical supervision or consultation to prevent degeneration of the one–to–one relationship. Clinical supervision may enable you to separate feelings, thoughts, and behaviors that belong to the current relationship from those that represent unfinished conflicts in other relationships. It is reassuring that most countertransference problems can be resolved by self-assessment with professional supervision. Once the countertransference process is identified, you can consciously develop therapeutic, goal-directed responses. Avoid self-disclosure of countertransference to clients. Sharing these feelings may overwhelm clients and burden them in a destructive way (Beretta et al., 2007). In the rare instance that controlling these disturbed attitudes and emotions requires extended work, referring the client to another nurse or mental health professional is appropriate.

Conflict Between Caretaker and Therapist Roles

A one–to–one relationship requires that you help the client actively explore the meaning underlying the client's personal pain, distress, or discomfort. Avoid the caretaker role in which you alleviate pain. Rather, encourage clients to develop ways to do so for themselves. Similarly, the caretaker role requires nurses to make decisions for clients. It does not encourage clients to be accountable for their own decisions.

Assuming the caretaker role also undermines your therapeutic effectiveness. The caretaker role tends to involve sympathy rather than empathy. The difference between these two responses (discussed in Chapter 10∞) is significant

---

YOUR SELF-AWARENESS
Countertransference

Look for the following cues in your own behavior that signal the presence of countertransference:

- Irrational friendliness toward the client
- Irrational concern about the client
- Reacting with annoyance or irrational hostility toward the client
- Feeling uneasy during or after meeting with the client
- Dreaming or fantasizing about the client
- Being preoccupied with thoughts of the client during leisure time
- Any actions that are out of line with standard expectations for professional and therapeutic behaviors

to therapeutic outcomes. How effective you are when you interact with a client in a one–to–one relationship is based on your intentions and emotions. The path of the relationship depends on your self-knowledge of these factors discussed in Chapter 3∞.

Critical Distance

It is important to observe how the client uses physical space. Individual preferences as well as culture will dictate the specific distance between individuals, depending on the relationship between them. Allow physical distance between yourself and clients, especially early in a relationship. This distance promotes verbal communication and minimizes any existing anxiety and hostility the client may have. Moving rapidly toward closeness, especially in establishing the nurse–client relationship, may overwhelm the client and increase anxiety.

The physical distance between you and the client can be indicative of other therapeutic processes. For example, a client may sit in a chair at a great distance from you during initial meetings but move closer and closer as the working relationship is established. Assess the possible interpersonal implications of proximity (nearness) for each client. As the relationship progresses, assess whether physical distance or proximity reduces client anxiety. The client's need for critical distance during the therapeutic process usually increases as the client experiences panic or near-panic levels of anxiety. See Chapter 10 and Figure 10-3∞.

Gift Giving

The giving of gifts may be a special concern in therapeutic relationships (Forrester, 2010). Gift giving may take various forms: a fleeting social amenity (the purchase of a cup of coffee), a gesture (the loan of a favorite book), or the presentation of a valued object (the giving of an original painting). Like self-disclosure (discussed later in this chapter), gift giving in any instance must be met with ongoing assessment and evaluation to determine its form, intent, appropriateness, and meaning in the context of the therapeutic relationship. Nurses from specialty areas other than psychiatry may have more leeway in this regard (Weeks, Cowell, Scullion, & Tanton, 2007). However, professional ethics and therapeutic integrity bar many but the most token of gifts. No rule covers all instances of gift giving. Several broad guidelines to help you evaluate particular situations are discussed in each phase of the one–to–one relationship in the nursing process section of this chapter.

Use of Touch

Physical contact is used cautiously in therapeutic work. It is best to avoid unplanned physical contact without therapeutic rationale. Some clients with poor ego boundaries may become intensely threatened and feel overwhelmed by physical contact. For example, a client may lose the ability to distinguish self from the nurse during simple hand contact. Such contact may be perceived as a hostile or sexual gesture, although you

do not intend it that way. In contrast, an acutely grief-stricken client, too distraught to focus on words, might receive needed support from being held. When considering any use of touch, ask yourself:

1. Does touch meet the client's therapeutic goals, or does it meet my needs?
2. Does touch foster a more productive therapeutic relationship?
3. Will touch honor this client's personal space?
4. How does touch fit with the client's cultural background?

Evaluate the use of touch, like self-disclosure, in the context of the therapeutic relationship, paying attention to its timing, appropriateness, and type. For example, a client is thrilled to achieve an on-the-job goal that has taken much personal time and effort. You determine that a firm handshake and a statement of congratulations are facilitative in this instance and at this working phase of the relationship. If you are unsure of the effect of such a gesture, a frank inquiry may be in order: "How did you feel when I shook your hand a few moments ago?" Again, the client's reaction and subsequent exploration can be a gauge for measuring how the client perceives and responds to the use of touch.

Self-Disclosure

Self-disclosure means being open to personal feelings and experiences, being "real" as opposed to hiding behind a facade. This is an expectation we have of our clients—we encourage them to be real, to self-disclose as a necessary step in their move toward mental health. But what about self-disclosure on our part? While being "real" is a quality of authenticity (see Chapter 3∞), it is important to also recognize that self-disclosure is a complex phenomenon.

How much should you share with a client? Under what circumstances is it appropriate? The wisdom of disclosing personal information to clients has been the subject of much debate. Some argue that self-disclosure impedes therapeutic work and undermines the relationship because it violates boundaries between professional and social roles (Pope & Keith-Spiegel, 2008). Others argue just the opposite—that self-disclosure can facilitate therapeutic work depending on the circumstances—in cognitive–behavioral therapy, with children, with persons with diminished capacity, in social skills training, and in psychopharmacologic and supportive treatments (Psychopathology Committee of the Group for the Advancement of Psychiatry, 2001). A recent review of the literature on self-disclosure found divergent results from one study to the next, indicating that the implications of self-disclosure on the mental health professional's part are unclear (Henretty & Levitt, 2010). How much to share, and under what circumstances, remains an area for further research. Beginning psychiatric–mental health nursing students should be cautious about personal self-disclosure to clients and should always discuss self-disclosure with an instructor first.

Pay attention to the timing, appropriateness, and degree of self-disclosure. For example, use self-disclosure cautiously with a severely dysfunctional client with poor ego boundaries. This client may not be able to separate thoughts and feelings that belong to the self from those that belong to you. The client might misinterpret your self-disclosure or might not be able to make sense of the disclosure. The client may also fear engulfment; that is, your feelings might be perceived as threatening or overwhelming. Self-disclosure should foster the development of the therapeutic relationship rather than threaten its continuance. The right time and reason for self-disclosure become clearer after answering the questions in Your Self-Awareness.

Personal self-disclosures require evaluation. Students should seek consultation from a faculty member. Practicing nurses should seek consultation through peer review (Jain & Roberts, 2009).

Culture, Values, and Beliefs

Address client values and beliefs that interfere with adaptive functioning. Some examples of people who hold values and beliefs that may interfere with constructive change are:

- The spouse who believes the partner should be subservient, and, conversely, the partner who defers personal needs to preserve the relationship
- The parent who believes that to "spare the rod" is to "spoil the child"
- The child raised with the family injunction that family problems should not be discussed outside the home and may view your actions as an invasion of privacy
- The woman who believes that because God takes care of His people there is no need to solve personal problems
- The man who believes that divorce and homosexuality are sins that will never be forgiven

Initially, you should become aware of the specific values and beliefs that influence the immediate relationship work. It is often useful to label the value or belief with the client, exploring its history, importance, cultural context, and impact. Nonjudgmental, alternative values may be discussed if the client initiates such an exploration. The humanistic nurse respects the client's values and beliefs and the client's ultimate choices regarding personal value systems. Your earnest

---

YOUR SELF-AWARENESS
Self-Disclosure

Determining whether or not to self-disclose will be made clearer by answering the following questions:

- What is the purpose of the revelation; who is this self-disclosure for?
- Does this self-disclosure meet the client's therapeutic goals, or does it meet my needs?
- Will this self-disclosure take the focus away from the client?
- Does this self-disclosure foster the development of a more productive therapeutic relationship?
  1. Will it encourage the client to disclose what the client has withheld or suppressed?
  2. Will it encourage the client's cooperation?
  3. Will it help the client to consider another point of view?
  4. Will it support the client's positive movement in addressing life problems?
  5. Will it encourage empathic understanding?

---

interest in how the client is coping with emotional stressors provides the encouragement and support that facilitates health-related behavior change (Weiss & Lewis, 2007).

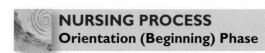

NURSING PROCESS
Orientation (Beginning) Phase

The primary goal of the orientation phase is to establish contact and begin developing a working relationship with the client. Establishing contact includes the initial encounters between nurse and client—how they approach and interact with each other, both verbally and nonverbally. An example of early dialogue in the orientation phase can be found in Rx Communication.

In informal relationships, contact usually begins when the nurse seeks out the client. Establishing contact may involve developing client awareness of your presence, followed by working to communicate with the client verbally. In formal relationships, contact may begin when the client inquires about services or when the psychiatric–mental health nurse contacts the client following referral. In both formal

Case Study: Orientation Phase

R$_X$ COMMUNICATION

The Initial Contract

CLIENT: "What, exactly, are we supposed to be doing together?"

NURSE RESPONSE 1: "I'd like to meet with you every day while you're here. This will give you an opportunity to talk about yourself and the things that are of concern to you."	**NURSE RESPONSE 2:** "That's something that you and I can decide together tomorrow morning when we meet here at 9:30."
RATIONALE: In addition to providing structure about the sessions, the nurse lays the groundwork for the focus on the client.	*RATIONALE:* The nurse reminds the client of the time for their meeting and sets the stage for mutual collaboration and negotiation.

and informal relationships, the sense of working together in a therapeutic alliance enables the client to endure anxiety and deal with resistance to change, which inevitably surface during the course of one–to–one relationships.

This phase of the therapeutic relationship concludes with mutual agreement on a therapeutic contract, which may be verbal and quite simple. The contract spells out the client's goals for treatment and the nurse's professional responsibilities.

Assessment

Client assessment begins at the first moment of contact. Assessment continues throughout the therapeutic relationship but is particularly important during the orientation phase. Remember that shortcuts taken in assessment procedures almost always jeopardize the ultimate quality of care because crucial areas of concern may go unaddressed or be treated superficially.

An important part of client assessment is to determine what the client is likely to accomplish in the time allotted. Consider the extent of the client's responsiveness to you during this early stage of relating, the severity of the client's symptoms, the client's level of resistance, and the priorities for the care of the client. Emphasize the treatment needed to reach the most important and obtainable goals. Together, you and the client take this opportunity to shape the nature of the client's care within the limits of the current health care environment.

Subjective Data

Observation, a process long regarded as essential to clinical nursing practice, is of particular importance in one–to–one relationship work. Note elements in the nurse–client interaction that are missing, distorted, or imbalanced. What the client avoids discussing is often more crucial than what is shared.

An effective one–to–one relationship requires observation of the client's behavior and facial expressions, the content of the client's communication, and other cues about the client's involvement in the process. Keep in mind that you will also be sending the message that you understand, care about, and respect the client. Being aware of and using the cues you observe helps you adjust your interventions as necessary during the session. Your goal is to promote the therapeutic relationship and allow the therapeutic process to continue.

An awareness of changes in the client's nonverbal behavior—such as crossing the arms across the chest, leaning back in the chair, and appearing to withdraw from the interaction with you—is an important component of maintaining a one–to–one relationship. In this instance, an appropriate therapeutic response is, "I'm noticing as we're talking that you've crossed your arms and leaned back in the chair away from me. I wonder how you're feeling right now." This therapeutic response acknowledges the **here-and-now**, that is, the processes and dynamics at that very moment in the interaction. The importance of tuning in to process is emphasized later in this chapter.

Objective Data

Objective data collection ideally includes the following: mental status examination, complete physical examination, nursing history, and psychologic testing, as needed. Which examinations are done and by whom are generally determined by the agency or institution in which the psychiatric–mental health nurse works, and by the psychiatric–mental health nurse's expertise in these specific areas.

The Initial Interview

Interviewing is a process that serves several purposes in the orientation phase of one–to–one relationships. Although a psychiatric–mental health nurse may use a structured initial interview in formal one–to–one work, it is rarely used in informal relationships. In informal relationships, consider using the applicable principles and concepts during your initial meeting with the client.

The initial interview has the following purposes:

- To initiate trust building
- To establish rapport with the client
- To obtain pertinent client data
- To initiate client assessment
- To make practical arrangements for treatment

The initial interview is crucial because it sets the stage for subsequent therapeutic contact. As you begin to work together with the client to identify the issues the client intends to work on, you further the development of the one–to–one relationship. You are more likely to intervene effectively if you understand how a therapeutic relationship will fit into the client's life and consider the direction the client wishes to take (Gary, 2007).

Structure Structure the initial interview to establish rapport, decrease anxiety, and convey willingness to address the client's distress. Begin by introducing yourself, inviting the client to be seated, and making a statement about information thus far known about the client's seeking of services. An open-ended question, such as, "How is it that you are here today?" or "What brought you to the hospital?" provides an opportunity for the client to talk about concerns. Inform the client that the purpose of the initial interview is to obtain an overview of the client's current situation and then determine the availability of appropriate services.

Essential Data One primary purpose of structuring the initial interview is to collect essential data (see Chapter 11 ∞). Address client resistance if it surfaces during the initial interview. This resistance may occur when the client has initiated services at someone else's request or insistence, has fears and misconceptions about therapy, or has had an unsatisfactory therapeutic experience in the past. Explore resistance before collecting further data.

Anxious clients may be confused about or misinterpret information you give during the initial interview. You may need to repeat information several times or in subsequent meetings. You will also need to determine whether the client's confusion or misinterpretation could be a manifestation of resistance instead of anxiety, as in the clinical example that follows.

Clinical Example

Selena, a 35-year-old woman, has been referred to the outpatient mental health clinic following several visits for minor medical problems. You note from the record a pattern of medication refills for antianxiety medication from her primary care provider. You also note that she was referred for mental health care on two other occasions, but failed to keep those appointments.

In thinking about the information Selena presented in the first session, you review her comments on her failures to follow through on the other two referrals. There are many possible reasons a client may miss appointments, some having to do with insufficient motivation for treatment, some having to do with psychiatric symptoms, and others attributable to unavoidable life circumstances. Selena's explanations indicate no external interfering life stressors or difficulties with transportation.

During that first session, Selena was distraught and apologetic for not following through on the referrals, which she attributed to her anxiety symptoms. Specifically, she has been experiencing increasing difficulty leaving her home. The farther she gets from home, the more anxious she becomes. She cannot leave her home, even to run important errands, without taking antianxiety medications. Selena cannot really specify the reason for her anxiety other than a sense of impending catastrophe. Selena's behavior, self-reports, and history are all consistent with what would be expected in an anxiety disorder. You note the lack of defensiveness in her presentation and you conclude that, at this point, there is no avoidance or resistance that would sabotage the initiation of a one–to–one relationship.

Knowing about a client's typical emotions and defenses is valuable because it provides direction for formulating appropriate nursing diagnoses related to both behavior and affect, identifying appropriate outcomes, setting specific client-centered goals, and implementing appropriate interventions.

Nursing Diagnosis: NANDA

Organize all the data collected during the assessment phase and formulate preliminary nursing diagnoses. The word *preliminary* is used to imply the ongoing potential for revision as client behaviors unfold during the course of the nurse–client relationship.

The goal in organizing the data is to understand the data as they reflect the client's unique, private world. Look for dominant themes or central issues in the client's responses.

The dominant themes and central issues will be unique to each individual client. Select NANDA nursing diagnoses that derive from these themes and issues.

Outcome Identification: NOC

The major outcomes of the orientation phase are establishing contact and beginning to form a working relationship between client and nurse. The working relationship in this initial phase is the framework on which the client constructs behavioral change, a challenging task, in the next phase. Your Assessment Approach highlights common signs of a working relationship. Look for these signs to determine whether the one–to–one relationship is moving into the working phase. Other individual outcomes will be determined by the client's specific dominant themes and central issues.

Planning and Implementation: NIC

The following interventions are common elements during the orientation phase. The development of additional interventions is based on assessment and nursing diagnoses for each individual client.

Developing the Therapeutic Contract

A plan for action actually forms the *therapeutic contract* negotiated in a one–to–one relationship. The therapeutic contract is a concrete, detailed, and mutually negotiated acknowledgment of the client's personal goals for treatment plus the nurse's professional responsibilities. Essentially, you and the client discuss how you will work together. Be certain to announce the timeframe for your work together during this phase, and reinforce it during the other phases so that it does not come as a surprise when it is time to terminate the relationship.

The contract may be modified over time but always serves as a tool for evaluating the benefit to the client and the effectiveness of the nurse. In an informal therapeutic relationship, the therapeutic contract may differ from the usual care plan often developed in outpatient and inpatient settings. For example, an initial contract may begin as a very simple agreement concerning the time and place of subsequent meetings together.

The client's personal goals for treatment may be long-term or short-term goals, but they always specify detailed, observable outcomes, as in the following clinical example.

YOUR ASSESSMENT APPROACH   Signs of a Working Relationship

The following criteria may be useful in determining whether a one–to–one relationship is moving into the working, or middle, phase.

For Nurse
- Sense of making contact with the client
- Sense that the client is responding well to the relationship
- Sense that the nurse can facilitate client growth regardless of the severity of client dysfunction
- Sense of commitment to addressing the client's problems

For Client
- Nonverbal and verbal evidence of liking the nurse
- Sense of relaxation with the nurse
- Sense of confidence in the nurse
- Nonsuperficial (in nature and depth) problems addressed

Clinical Example

Nicole is a 30-year-old woman admitted to an inpatient psychiatric unit following an overdose of risperidone (Risperdal). During past hospitalizations, Nicole has been emotionally labile, has had trouble following her treatment schedule, was easily frustrated by the limits and compromises of living in the hospital, demanded medication, and threatened suicide. Nicole's primary nurse proposed that they work together to identify goals and behaviors for improved personal and interpersonal functioning. Nicole identified problems of feeling empty, having poor relationships with others, and being angry; she chose to focus on the overall goal of improved social skills. Nicole agreed to the following expectations:

- I will participate in a one–to–one relationship with my nurse and express my feelings verbally.
- I will identify uncomfortable situations involving other people and discuss the interactions with my nurse at appointed times.
- I will continue my routine treatment activities until the appropriate time to meet with my nurse.

Client goals most often contribute to the establishment of a working relationship when they are specific, address intrapersonal or interpersonal behavior patterns, and specifically delineate the degree of change necessary for client self-satisfaction. Strive for the most concise, detailed, and accurate description of client goals in the beginning phase. Clearly stated goals facilitate subsequent mutual evaluation during the middle and end phases of one–to–one work. Goals may focus on the following:

- Decreasing or eliminating troublesome behaviors
- Increasing socialization
- Increasing living skills

At times, client goals may be long term or even inappropriate. In this situation, help the client define initial steps toward the long-term goal. For example, a readmitted mentally ill client may pinpoint discharge as an important goal. You may then work with this client to identify the steps needed to achieve this goal. One step may be to maintain self-care in the area of bathing/hygiene. When severe dysfunction limits client input into planning, the nursing staff may supplement goals that are determined to be beneficial to the client.

In a formal therapeutic relationship, as in individual psychotherapy, the therapeutic contract is more detailed and generally includes three practical matters:

1. Determining the place, duration, and time of the meetings
2. Establishing fees and payment intervals, if any
3. Considering optional referral sources, should the client be unable to negotiate an agreement on the first two matters

The therapeutic contract does not always reflect client problems and strengths in their entirety. For example, the client may not determine that an area is, in fact, a problem. Thus, the therapeutic contract reflects the *client's* definition of personal goals at one moment in time. In this instance, remain aware of other probable problem areas and engage with the client in reassessing these areas and modifying or deleting goals in subsequent phases.

Regardless of the form that goal identification takes, the therapeutic contract serves the following purposes:

- Facilitating humanistic involvement with the client as an individual
- Involving the client as a full partner in the therapeutic process
- Serving as a basis for communication in the therapeutic process
- Providing continuity for the client and everyone involved with the client

Establishing Trust

Concerns about trust surface in this first phase of the relationship. Trust between nurse and client evolves over time as the client tests the emotional climate of your interactions together, risks self-disclosure, and observes that you are responsible and do what you say you are going to do. You can promote trust by responding to all of the client's feeling states without being judgmental or attempting to control the client's expression of emotions. The process recording in TABLE 4-3 ■ demonstrates how one nurse began to promote trust early in the orientation phase. Note that she was self-assured enough to encourage the client to share his concerns about trust. It is important to be consistent and to be self-aware of the part your feelings play in the interactions.

In addition to being consistent and self-aware of the part your feelings play in interactions with clients, the following positive and helpful behaviors encourage initial trust and help the client to feel safe while disclosing uncomfortable, even forbidden feelings, wishes, or behaviors:

- Listening attentively to client feelings
- Responding to client feelings
- Exhibiting consistency
- Viewing situations from the client's perspective

These behaviors constitute positive, helpful influences in encouraging trust. It is also important to avoid giving premature reassurances about trust, which may inhibit exploration of this vital therapeutic issue and create distance between you and the client.

Keeping Confidentiality

Client concerns about the level of confidentiality also surface in this first phase of the therapeutic relationship. Keeping clients' confidentiality is a legal and ethical responsibility (see pages 224–225 and 237–239 in Chapter 12∞). However, circumstances do exist (for example, intent to commit suicide, intent to harm others) in which it is necessary to disclose a client's information. Be sure to inform clients of the limits of confidentiality. Doing so actively demonstrates caring behavior by protecting the dignity and respecting the autonomy of clients (Fisher & Oransky, 2008).

Be aware of your responsibilities in relation to confidentiality. Explicitly address the issue of confidentiality when the client makes even vague reference to it. Explicitly state which people will have access to client revelations (clinical

TABLE 4-3 ■ Process Recording of an Orientation Phase Session

Verbatim Interaction	Nursing Intervention	Rationale
Client: "It's so difficult for me to talk . . . to let you know about me." (30-second pause)	None	Allows client to proceed at own pace; if silence is uncomfortably long in first few contacts, you may use reflection, e.g., "I sense how difficult talking is for you."
Client: "Every time I start to tell anybody about myself, they usually end up laughing at me."		
Nurse: "Give me an example."	Encourage elaboration.	Explores meaning of this statement to the client.
Client: "Well, just last week I started talking to my neighbor. I told him that I was laid off from work again. Next thing you know, he's laughing, slapping my back, and saying, 'Hey, hard times, eh?'" (Shifts in chair, avoids eye contact.)		
Nurse: "What was this like for you?"	Explore client's personal reaction, especially accompanying feelings.	Further explores meaning of this specific incident as perceived by the client.
Client: "Awful . . . lousy . . . that's all." (Pause.)		
Nurse: "I wonder if you're concerned that the same might happen here—that you'll be laughed at?"	Connect the client's concern regarding this emotionally difficult interaction to the here-and-now, i.e., the one–to–one therapeutic relationship.	Issues concerning client's immediate life situations often reflect parallel issues in nurse–client relationship.
Client: "Well, maybe . . . I don't know you, so how do I know what you might do? You don't look like the type, but then again, how do I know?"		
Nurse: "It sounds like you're wondering if it's safe to trust me."	Identify what appears to be the underlying central concern or theme.	Reflection of what appears to be the central concern (theme) encourages client assessment by validation or correction of your statement.
Client: "Yeah . . . no offense, though."		
Nurse: "Let's talk about how safe you feel today and as we continue to work together."	Focus on trust as an issue for further exploration; acknowledge that there is stress in evolving a working relationship.	Avoid premature reassurances so that trust can evolve and be assessed periodically.

instructor, case supervisor, consultant, colleague), and explore how the client feels in response to this information.

Tuning In to Process

The beginning nurse often attends carefully to the *content* of the client sessions—what the client says—and only after considerable experience becomes actively attuned to *process,* the dynamics of the here-and-now situation. Avoid focusing solely on your technique. This produces mechanical, unfeeling responses and interferes with your ability to be aware of process. *Process* as used here (and discussed in Chapter 10 ∞) does not mean nursing process. Processing is a complex communication skill that enables the nurse to focus on several aspects of the nurse–client relationship at the same time. Process involves attending to all nonverbal and verbal client behaviors. It involves responding to client themes, such as anger, hopelessness, and powerlessness.

The experienced nurse is simultaneously aware of both content and process, interweaving both for maximum therapeutic effectiveness. The challenge is to become savvy enough to learn what to ignore and sensitive enough to know what to emphasize (Guy & Brady, 2001).

Addressing the Client's Suffering

Directly address the client's suffering within the context of the client's cultural and ethnic background. This intervention allows clients to share how they perceive, experience, and manifest the problem. The following clinical example illustrates how a nurse encouraged a depressed client to "move outside himself."

Clinical Example

Client: "This depression is like a big log weighing on my chest."

Nurse: "How would I know that you are suffering in this way? What would I see and hear?"

Client: "Well . . . I sigh a lot . . . I don't move a lot, only when I have to . . . I wouldn't look at you, or bother to talk to you. I guess when I feel like this, I close people out. Yeah, I close everyone out, even my wife."

Nurse: "So when you suffer in this way, you close people out. And what is this like for you?"

Client: "I'm alone and lonely. Not a soul on earth cares for me."

YOUR INTERVENTION STRATEGIES   Goals, Tasks, and Interventions of the Orientation Phase

Goal: Establish contact and begin to form a working relationship with the client

Therapeutic Tasks	Nursing Interventions
Clarify the purpose of relationship work, the role of the nurse, and responsibilities of the client.	Provide information regarding purpose, roles, and responsibilities in relationship work to alleviate initial client anxiety.
	Immediately and explicitly address any misconceptions, fantasies, and fears regarding relationship work and/or the nurse.
Address client suffering directly, offering to work with the client toward its alleviation.	Use therapeutic communication techniques, especially empathic understanding, discussed in Chapter 10∞.
	Avoid premature reassurance (allow trust to evolve).
Address issues of confidentiality.	Be explicit about the degree of confidentiality and who has access to client's revelations.
Negotiate a therapeutic contract (client's definition of personal goals for treatment and the nurse's professional responsibilities).	Whenever possible, encourage delineation of goals that are specific, address intrapersonal and interpersonal behavioral patterns, and designate the degree of change necessary for client self-satisfaction.

Addressing the client's suffering is not easy at first. Avoid the temptation to offer reassurance or sympathy, or change the topic, in the hope that you will ease the client's burden. Doing so will only demonstrate to the client that it is not safe to talk about painful topics.

Clarifying Purpose, Roles, and Responsibilities

An additional therapeutic task in this beginning phase is to intervene directly in clarifying the purpose of the relationship work, the role of the nurse, and the responsibilities of the client. When this preliminary exploration of purpose, roles, and responsibilities is explicit and detailed, each participant better understands how to move within the relationship. It also decreases anxiety and the chance that a client may use the relationship to obtain special privileges. From the first meeting, you have the opportunity to reinforce effective coping skills and increase client self-esteem. Your Intervention Strategies summarizes the goals, tasks, and subsequent nursing interventions of the orientation phase of one–to–one relationships.

Gift Giving During the Orientation Phase

During the orientation phase of a therapeutic relationship, the client may overtly offer or ask for a gift. This gesture may be as incidental as offering you a cigarette or asking you for one. Examine this overture, keeping in mind several possible motivations:

- The client may seek to bribe or manipulate you, thereby seeking to control the direction of the therapeutic relationship. (Chapter 22∞ deals with manipulation.)
- The client may seek to "buy" your time and attention.
- The client may ask for small gifts to reinforce a helpless, "take-care-of-me" interpersonal stance.
- Of course, the client may have no covert intent and may simply need a cigarette.

In the orientation phase, it may be helpful not to accept or give any gift you feel uncomfortable about or that may signal a boundary violation (Forrester, 2010). Explore the client's intent. Often, this mutual exploration not only clarifies the client's intent but also helps define the parameters of the evolving relationship and models the exploratory process for the client.

Evaluation

In the orientation phase, evaluation includes your initial comprehensive evaluation of client behaviors, any initial steps toward the development of client self-evaluation, and your ongoing self-evaluation. The more specific and goal-oriented the therapeutic contract, the easier it is for the client and nurse to evaluate the effectiveness of the therapeutic relationship.

In addition to evaluating the effectiveness of each therapeutic task, you must evaluate the important goal of the orientation phase: Has a working relationship evolved between the client and yourself, and, if so, to what degree? Review Your Assessment Approach: Signs of a Working Relationship on page 57 to assess readiness to move into the working phase.

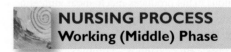

NURSING PROCESS
Working (Middle) Phase

Once contact is established, attention turns to maintenance and analysis of contact in the working phase. *Analysis of contact* refers to an in-depth exploration of how the client relates to others as manifested in the nurse–client relationship. In this working phase, the client may address developmental and situational problems, as well as interpersonal problems. It is called the *working phase* because during this phase, you and the client actively and systematically identify, explore, link, modify, and evaluate specific behaviors, especially those determined to be dysfunctional for the client.

The client's clearly stated goals in the therapeutic contract are now explored. The nurse has the following two therapeutic goals:

■ *Behavioral analysis.* The nurse and client determine the dynamics of the client's response patterns, especially those considered to be dysfunctional. Such analysis also addresses dysfunctional thought and emotive patterns, because these inevitably alter the client's behavior.
■ *Constructive change in behavior.* This applies particularly to dysfunctional response patterns.

Thus, you and the client work together to analyze behavior and institute behavioral change.

Assessment

Assessment is continued, detailed, and expanded upon. Your observations of nonverbal, verbal, and environmental responses continue to have vital importance as the client begins to address personal response patterns. In addition, you continue to assess emotive, cognitive, cultural, and behavioral aspects.

By filling in gaps of information not obtained in the orientation phase, you may now acquire a detailed assessment about a subject the client was unable to share or ignored earlier. The following clinical example illustrates that what is not said (that is, what is avoided, blocked, rejected) by the client may have more significance than what the client shares.

Clinical Example

During initial sessions, 18-year-old Maureen avoided any inquiries about her parents, other than to say that she lived alone. After several sessions, the nurse again asked about the parents. Maureen replied softly, with tears welling in her eyes, "They're dead. They died in a car crash 2 years ago." She slowly related how, since their deaths, she had spent so much energy trying to survive that she barely felt much of anything. Subsequent sessions dealt with her apparent delayed grief reaction.

The new data caused the nurse to revise and update the tentative nursing diagnoses and initiate a marked change in the direction of the sessions. Such shifting is not uncommon in one–to–one relationships. When a change in direction occurs, assess if the sudden change indicates either the need to avoid a certain topic or a move toward a deeper level of emotive expression.

In the working phase, you facilitate many aspects of assessment with the client. First, collaborate with the client in identifying important behavioral trends and patterns. Knowing the issues that promote or inhibit therapeutic progress is essential to success (Balkin, Leicht, Sartos, & Powell, 2011). Once you identify a pattern, explore it in elaborate detail to determine its origin, causes, operation, and effects on the client and the people in the client's world. Environmental factors (familial, political, economic, or cultural) are separated from intrapersonal factors (depression or anxiety) contributing to the pattern. The client figuratively holds the pattern to the light to examine and make sense of its every aspect. The

elements of one pattern will inevitably link with others, so that the major life patterns gradually unfold. The first part of Your Intervention Strategies summarizes the therapeutic tasks undertaken to achieve the objective of behavioral analysis and offers specific nursing approaches to helping the client.

There are two noteworthy considerations regarding therapeutic tasks of the first goal, behavioral analysis:

1. As clients begin to describe and re-experience conflict, they consciously or unconsciously use defenses to ward off the anxiety this awakens. The development of a good working relationship enables clients to tolerate increased anxiety in the working phase.
2. As clients become familiar with self-assessment, they may modify original personal goals, or develop additional goals, in keeping with what they have learned.

It is important during the working phase to encourage the client's self-assessment of growth-facilitating and growth-inhibiting behaviors. After assessing one specific response, the client is often able to transfer this skill to begin assessing other aspects of life as well. A realistic self-assessment process is perhaps the most valuable skill that the client can "take home." It is often thrilling to experience the client "taking over" and further applying realistic assessment skills developed in one–to–one work.

Nursing Diagnosis: NANDA

In the working phase, nursing diagnoses may be revised, expanded, or deleted to more accurately reflect a central pattern of concern in the evolving one–to–one relationship. As the working phase proceeds, the priority assigned to a nursing diagnosis may change—for example, when the client is able to implement positive change in some areas. Those nursing diagnoses designated as "risk for" may move up or down on the priority list, depending on what interventions, if any, have been effective. A potential diagnosis may decrease in priority after preventive health education, if both the client and the nurse decide that this intervention is beneficial.

Outcome Identification: NOC

The initial goal of behavioral analysis of the client's response patterns continues throughout the working phase. The major identified client outcomes are as follows:

■ Develops an awareness of current behavioral patterns
■ Understands how and when those patterns manifest themselves
■ May gain insight into the potential causes of those patterns
■ Assesses which behavioral patterns are ineffective and self-defeating
■ Attempts to change ineffective behavioral patterns and develop new, more effective behaviors

Be aware that the quality of the therapeutic relationship predicts outcomes—the better the relationship, the better the client outcomes (Priebe et al., 2011).

YOUR INTERVENTION STRATEGIES   Goals, Tasks, and Interventions of the Working Phase

Goal: Behavioral analysis (mutual determination of dynamics of response patterns identified by client, especially those considered dysfunctional)

Therapeutic Tasks	Nursing Interventions
Identify and explore important response patterns in detail.	Explore the origin, causes, operation, and effect of response pattern (intrapersonally and interpersonally). Separate environmental factors (familial, political, economic, cultural) from intrapersonal factors. Link elements of one response pattern to other patterns as appropriate for a gradual unfolding of central life patterns.
Analyze, with the client, the client's mode of conflict resolution.	Encourage detailed exploration of how the client reacts to reduce anxiety associated with conflict. Increase awareness of defenses employed to ward off anxiety awakened by such exploration.
Facilitate client self-assessment of growth-producing and growth-inhibiting response patterns.	Encourage client to evaluate each response pattern to determine which are self-defeating and/or thwart gratification of basic needs.

Goal: Constructive change in behavior, especially in dysfunctional response patterns identified by the client

Therapeutic Tasks	Nursing Interventions
Address forces that inhibit desired change (troublesome thoughts, feelings, and behaviors).	Help the client challenge personal resistance to change. Use problem-solving strategies, active decision making, and personal accountability. Help the client learn and apply problem-solving strategies. Encourage the client to assert own needs when external environmental conditions (group, agency, institution) are an inhibiting force.
Create an atmosphere offering permission for active experimentation to test and assess the effectiveness of new behaviors.	Allow freedom to make and assess mistakes and blunders. Avoid parental judgment of any behavioral experimentation; encourage client self-assessment instead.
Facilitate development of coping skills to deal with anxiety associated with constructive changes in behavior.	Address, rather than avoid, anxiety and its manifestations. Strengthen existing growth-promoting coping skills, especially regarding unalterable conditions (terminal illness, physical deformity, loss of significant other by death). Encourage development of new coping skills and their application to actual life experiences.

Planning and Implementation: NIC

In the working phase, planning is ideally done collaboratively between client and nurse. When planning has been systematic and thorough, there is hardly a moment to worry about "what to do." The short-term and long-term treatment goals in the form of the therapeutic contract comprise a map indicating the direction, momentum, and the steps that are needed to reach a designated point.

There is, however, a potential danger in the implementation of the planning component: moving too quickly and incompletely through an exploration of the client's feelings and thoughts in an attempt to reach a designated goal. *Slowness* and *thoroughness* are all-important here. Change needs to take place in the client's feelings, thoughts, and behaviors. If change does not occur in all aspects, then it is destined to be short-lived and ineffectual in the long run and may cause the client to feel discouraged.

When the client is working on an issue that is unresolved at the end of a meeting, it is often helpful to summarize the unfinished work for the next meeting. This technique may help the client anticipate, plan, or prepare to tackle this area of concern again. Personal experiments, such as trying out new behaviors in real situations, may be encouraged between sessions. Some clients may be able to continue working through a problem on their own between meetings.

Active intervention is especially important to achieve the second goal of the working phase, constructive changes in behavior, particularly in self-defeating, growth-inhibiting behavior patterns. Behavioral change flows from the first goal of behavioral analysis. The objectives are interrelated and essential for successful therapeutic work. Understanding and insight need to be complemented by behavioral implementation. The client's failure to make adaptive behavioral changes stymies progress and sabotages the therapeutic experience (Martin & Pear, 2007). Clients may consistently generate and thrive on sophisticated insights while continuing to assume a powerless stance about implementing constructive change in their condition. Your Intervention Strategies on page 62 highlights therapeutic tasks and specific nursing interventions for both goals of the working phase, behavioral analysis, and constructive change in behavior.

Testing the Effect of New Behaviors

You can also use active experimentation to test the effect of new behaviors. The introverted male client who resolved to establish relationships with women may try out various postures (cavalier, paternal, seductive) with a female nurse to determine the appropriateness of these behaviors. Permission to "try on" or role-play new behaviors must also include the freedom to make mistakes. Errors and blunders are rich sources of additional learning and occasional fun. Clients who can see humor in errors in a nondefeatist manner have acquired a new skill. Encourage them to apply this skill, and any other coping skills learned in relationship work, to normal maturational and situational crises encountered throughout life.

In inpatient settings, communicate with other staff members to make the whole team aware when the client is trying out new behaviors that may be exaggerated at first. For example, a depressed client may be encouraged to verbalize anger and begin by shouting. If there is no staff collaboration, the client may receive negative feedback such as room restrictions or a loss of certain privileges for testing out new coping skills.

Implementing Problem-Solving Strategies

Problem-solving strategies, as a mode of intervention, are particularly important in the working phase. Problem-solving strategies are essential after the client has identified, explored, and assessed important behavioral patterns. Encourage clients to use the sequential problem-solving strategies discussed in Your Intervention Strategies below. Reminding clients to be patient is supportive and reassuring. Problem-solving abilities improve with time and experience.

Challenging the Client's Resistance to Change

Challenging the client's resistance to change is an appropriate intervention in the working phase. There are two major categories of forces that inhibit desired change, as follows:

1. *Intrapersonal forces,* which may arise from troublesome thoughts, feelings, or behaviors; thoughts that hamper the client's sense of worth, the client's inability to control and express emotion appropriately, or the client's inability to relate to others in a meaningful manner.
2. The client's personal *resistance to change,* which is the greatest inhibiting force. In fact, the client's challenge to this resistance constitutes the major work in one–to–one relationships.

Problems of resistance and general intervention strategies were discussed earlier in the chapter. Of equal significance is the previous discussion of transference and countertransference phenomena, since these may require careful, planned nursing interventions. Sometimes transference and countertransference are so intense that they become a problem for the beginning psychiatric–mental health nurse.

Gift Giving During the Working Phase

During the working phase, particularly after the client has shown positive growth, the client may offer a gift in the form of a craft or skill. As in the orientation phase, the intent of the gift needs to be made explicit. Most ethics and professional conduct boards set overall limits on the monetary value of gifts and agree that professionals must consider the symbolic meaning of the gift. Encourage this exploration by

---

YOUR INTERVENTION STRATEGIES   Problem-Solving Strategies

- **Observation.** Observation as a problem-solving strategy involves gathering and analyzing facts about a potential problem area. It eliminates opinions and impressions and emphasizes facts. Observation as an aspect of assessment is discussed in the section on subjective assessment.
- **Definition.** Definition is perhaps the most significant and far-reaching problem-solving strategy. It involves an initial specification of a problem, followed by a question. Starting a problem-solving exploration with the word "How" ("How is it?" "How does it manifest itself?" "How has this come about?") puts the focus on the process of a specific problem. It is generally more useful than asking "Why?" which emphasizes rationale. Questioning as a communication technique is explored in Chapter 10 ⚭.
- **Preparation.** Preparation involves collecting additional pertinent data related to the basic problem that may prove useful in later stages of problem-solving strategies. This

enables the nurse and client to anticipate which data might be most useful.
- **Analysis.** As a problem-solving strategy, analysis involves breaking down the relevant material into subproblems so that each subproblem may be assessed separately.
- **Ideation.** Ideation involves accumulating alternative ideas on how to resolve the basic problem.
- **Incubation.** Incubation involves setting aside the problem-solving process or one aspect of it for a period of time to allow for illumination.
- **Synthesis.** Synthesis involves putting together all elements of the basic problem, subproblems, and possible alternatives.
- **Evaluation.** Evaluation consists of making judgments about the ideas that result.
- **Development.** As a final problem-solving strategy, development involves planning the implementation of these ideas.

asking questions such as, "How is it that you're sharing this gift with me?" or "What feelings might you want to share with this gift?" Be careful to establish and maintain professional boundaries in relation to client gifts (Forrester, 2010).

A client might give a gift during the working phase for several reasons:

- The client may wish to acknowledge the mutual work that has taken place.
- The client may wish to show appreciation for being allowed to share concerns with another person.
- The gift may be a smoke screen to block further exploration of a major dynamic.
- The gift may outwardly cover up anger or frustration felt inwardly.
- Finally, the gift may indicate the client's perception that the therapeutic work is finished.

In every instance, assess the intent of the gift, as well as its timing and appropriateness, in the context of the therapeutic relationship. Beginning psychiatric–mental health nurses should always discuss gifts with their clinical instructor.

Evaluation

Several levels of evaluation occur simultaneously in the working phase. First, do an ongoing evaluation of the client's various levels of intrapersonal and interpersonal functioning. Feedback from family, community agencies, or the client's employer may enhance any current comprehensive evaluation. For example, does the client seem to be facing an impending crisis? If so, you may choose to switch from intrapersonal exploration to a crisis intervention strategy. Second, encourage client self-evaluation, as explored in previous discussion. Finally, constantly perform self-evaluation as a helping person growing in skill and experience. Nursing self-evaluation is done by informal discussions with staff and other mental health care personnel and by formal clinical supervision.

On-the-spot evaluations of relevant short-term and long-term goals can occur during any meeting with the client. For example, as the client talks about increasing socialization skills, you may reflect: "Let's look at our contract together. You originally wanted to date a woman of your choice for 2 hours during an evening without having to leave. How do you think this compares with what you're now saying has happened?" Support any effort at evaluation on the part of the client and explore what else needs to happen for the client to achieve the short-term goal. An additional area of evaluation involves the client's "trying on" alternative behaviors to determine whether these new behaviors may work.

The client and nurse should mutually evaluate the appropriateness of goals in any one of the following areas in light of the client's current functioning:

- Degree of the client's success in achieving specific goals
- The client's growth-producing and growth-inhibiting behavior patterns
- Unfinished business that must be resolved to achieve a desired goal

The working phase may also involve ongoing evaluations of the status, characteristics, and depth of the nurse–client relationship. The client may view you in different ways (parent, sibling, friend) at various times. It is only when the client makes these views explicit that you may intervene to clarify roles and responsibilities in a facilitative manner.

The psychiatric–mental health nurse and the client have moved through the first two phases of therapeutic relationships when the following occurs:

- They have established a working relationship.
- They have analyzed the dynamics of the client's behavioral patterns.
- The client has effectively instituted behavioral changes in keeping with the therapeutic contract.

In informal relationship work, you may touch on only one or two aspects of the working phase. Even the advanced psychiatric–mental health nurse rarely addresses all therapeutic tasks in this phase of relationship work.

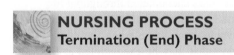

NURSING PROCESS
Termination (End) Phase

During the termination or resolution phase of one–to–one relationships, the psychiatric–mental health nurse works toward discontinuing contact. This phase is as important as the previous two phases, although both the nurse and the client frequently avoid it because of past difficulties with separation.

The goal of the end phase is termination of the one–to–one relationship in a mutually planned, satisfying manner. Remind the client that termination was first addressed in the orientation phase, when the duration of the relationship was discussed. Also emphasize the client's growth and the positive aspects of the relationship, rather than focusing exclusively on separation.

A smooth and complete termination sometimes occurs in actual practice. In informal relationship work in inpatient settings, termination more often occurs with the client's abrupt departure or planned medical discharge. Even in formal relationship work in community settings, contact often ceases without explanation after a series of missed appointments, or with a phone call in which the client voices the decision to terminate, or with the client abruptly leaving a session and failing to resume subsequent contact. If this happens, you can call or write the client and suggest an additional session to deal with either the therapeutic good-bye or continue the relationship work. Termination requires careful preparation, adequate time for the client to work through the feelings about ending, and an opportunity for you to explore your personal reactions with a clinical instructor, colleague, supervisor, or consultant.

Assessment

Assessment as a component of the nursing process in the resolution phase deals primarily with determining when the client may be ready to terminate, how the client deals with termination, and how the nurse deals with termination. Criteria that

Care Plan: Termination Phase

indicate a client's readiness for termination are presented in Your Assessment Approach.

Many factors influence how the client reacts to termination. These factors include the following:

- *Degree of client involvement.* The greater the degree of client involvement, the more intense the client's reaction to termination.
- *Length of treatment.* In general, the longer the nurse–client relationship lasts, the more time should be spent in exploring all aspects of termination.
- *Client's past history of significant losses.* A client who has lost significant others may re-experience past conflicts and emotional responses.
- *Ability to separate from others.* The reaction to termination is influenced by how well the client has mastered the early separation–individuation phase of development (see Erikson's eight developmental stages in Chapter 5∞).
- *Degree of success achieved.* Reaction to termination depends on how successful and satisfying the relationship has been for the client.
- *Degree of transference in the relationship.* The greater the transference in the nurse–client relationship, the more intense the client's reaction to termination.

Be alert to client responses during termination. Any number of responses—repression, regression, anger, denial, sadness, withdrawal, avoidance, acceptance, joy—may surface, and it is not unusual for several to surface at once. When repressing, the client shows no emotional response. Regression on the part of the client is an extremely common response to termination. Regressive behavior may range from statements of abandonment and hopelessness to an inability to tend to personal hygiene. The central message conveyed is: "See? I can't make it without you!"

Nurse's Self-Awareness

Finally, assessment involves how you personally manage separation in the one–to–one relationship. Like the client, you can have any number of responses. Some common responses are as follows:

- Regret that the client did not achieve more than the client actually did
- Being dependent upon and hesitant to give up the relationship
- Colluding with the client to prolong sessions to avoid the inevitability of separation

Nursing Diagnosis: NANDA

Nursing diagnoses during termination should reflect the termination behaviors the client manifests. A wide variety of nursing diagnoses may be relevant. Potential nursing diagnoses that stem from regression during the termination phase may be: Self-Care Deficit, Hopelessness, Powerlessness, and Ineffective Coping. Modify nursing diagnoses as necessary, as the client moves through the termination experience.

Outcome Identification: NOC

The ideal outcome occurs when the nurse–client relationship terminates after achieving all identified and measurable personal behavioral changes. Such resolution seldom occurs in acute care inpatient settings, especially since brief hospital stays are now the rule rather than the exception. Often, the client achieves more limited behavioral changes and agrees to return for future work or referral as necessary. At other times, the client achieves symptom relief only.

Outcomes are compromised when the client is unable to make progress due to lack of insight or mental capacity. Chronic catastrophic life circumstances (such as severe medical illness, life-threatening poverty, prison, and so on) may interfere with growth-producing behaviors. On rare occasions, the client's condition deteriorates and the client is unable to benefit from the nurse–client relationship.

Planning and Implementation: NIC

Planning involves preparing for the final good-bye and for where and under what circumstances the client may seek future help if the need arises.

Intervening in Specific Client Termination Behaviors

Intervention strategies vary according to the client's behaviors. You may respond to the client who is repressing the reality of termination by repeatedly observing that he or she is not addressing the issue of the impending separation. You may then attempt to explore this avoidance with the client.

YOUR ASSESSMENT APPROACH
Termination Readiness

The following criteria may be useful to determine whether the client is ready to terminate:

- **The client has experienced relief from the presenting problem.** Symptoms no longer interfere with the client's comfort.
- **The client's treatment goals have been achieved.** These ideally are planned goals included in the therapeutic contract between the nurse and client.
- **The client's social functioning has improved.** The client experiences increased satisfaction in interpersonal relationships.
- **The client has acquired adaptive coping strategies.** Ideally, these strategies include the client's use of effective problem-solving strategies on a daily basis.
- **The client has acquired more effective defense mechanisms.** A client who cannot achieve adaptive coping strategies should develop more effective defense mechanisms to ensure stabilization.
- **The client has increased self-dependence.** The client experiences self-satisfaction and no longer needs to depend on the nurse for a sense of well-being.
- **There has been a major impasse in the one–to–one relationship.** Stubborn resistances may surface and persist on the client's part. Uncontrollable countertransference may develop on the nurse's part.

YOUR INTERVENTION STRATEGIES   Goals, Tasks, and Interventions of the Termination Phase

Goal: Terminate contact in a mutually planned, satisfying manner

Therapeutic Tasks	Nursing Interventions
Help the client evaluate the therapeutic contract and the therapeutic experience in general.	Encourage the client's realistic appraisal of personal therapeutic goals (motivation, effort, progress, outcome) as these evolved in treatment.
	Provide appropriate feedback regarding the appraisal of goals.
	Review the client's assets and therapeutic gains.
	Review areas for further therapeutic work.
Encourage the transference of dependence to other support systems.	Encourage the client to develop reliance on others in client's immediate environment (spouse, relative, employer, neighbor, friend) for empathic, emotional support.
Participate in explicit, therapeutic good-bye with the client.	Be alert to the surfacing of any behavior arising on termination (repression, regression, acting out, anger, withdrawal, acceptance).
	Help the client work through feelings associated with these behaviors.
	Anticipate your own reaction to separation and share in a manner that does not burden the client.
	Allow time and space for termination; the longer the duration of the one–to–one relationship, the more time is needed for the termination phase.

Useful interventions for clients who are regressing in response to termination include the following:

- Addressing the possible underlying fears of abandonment
- Emphasizing the growth achieved by the client
- Continuing to focus on the realities of separation

The client who acts out may protest termination in numerous ways before the termination date, such as attempting suicide, requiring psychiatric hospitalization, quitting a job, or rejecting the nurse.

In general, underlying feelings, fears, and fantasies need ventilation, exploration, and working through, as do reactions of anger, depression, and grief. An exception to this general guideline is the client who uses distraction maneuvers to prevent termination, such as introducing explosive new material in final sessions. In this situation, you may use limit setting rather than exploration because of time constraints. In other words, there may be "unfinished business" despite appropriate planning and effort.

Providing for an Explicit and Therapeutic Good-Bye

You have the final task of participating in an *explicit and therapeutic good-bye* with the client. Nursing responsibilities in this final phase include anticipating your own personal reaction to separation and, optionally, expressing this reaction in a manner that does not burden the client. In addition, you may share a special wish for the client, based on the client's particular assets within the therapeutic relationship.

A therapeutic good-bye gives the client a sense of freedom to move on to other relationships. The end phase may take from one meeting to several months of meetings, depending on the duration of the one–to–one relationship. In general, the longer the duration of the relationship, the longer the time needed to

deal explicitly with the termination of contact. Your Intervention Strategies summarizes the goal, therapeutic tasks, and specific nursing interventions of the termination phase.

Ideally, the client can completely work through feelings regarding separation so that there is no unfinished business between nurse and client. The nurse–client relationship has given the client the opportunity to depend on another in a realistic and mature manner. The direct, explicit good-bye is frequently the first such experience for the client. It is usually a moment of unique humanness for both the nurse and the client.

Gift Giving During the Termination Phase

Gifts are most often given during the termination phase of one–to–one relationships. In this phase, a gift may have several overt and covert meanings, as follows:

- The client may wish to give a token of appreciation for positive personal growth that has taken place.
- The client may desire to change the therapeutic relationship into a social one.
- The client may wish to prolong sessions to avoid the final good-bye.

Some nurses accept a small gift from a client at the time of termination if feelings regarding the gift have been explored and clarified. (The gift may be an appropriate remembrance of a mutual and positive growth experience.) Exploring the significance of a termination gift will ensure the maximum therapeutic benefit for the client. A nurse's refusal to accept a gift of any type may prevent the client from learning the important skill of being able to accept gifts from others (Duffin, 2007). The nurse, as role model, has an opportunity to model appropriate gift giving and gift receiving. You may find receiving a gift at times awkward and "artificial."

Yet, such a situation gives you the opportunity to help the client toward further self-expression and self-knowledge.

Referring the Client for Follow-Up

When a referral is made to another psychiatric–mental health nurse or therapist, a home care nurse, a self-help group, a community agency, or a job training program, it is often wise to arrange for an initial contact with the referred person or agency before the nurse–client relationship terminates. This is a way to identify and deal with any initial misconceptions about what will take place after discharge and to ensure follow-up. The shift to dependence on other support systems (family, friends, referrals) is a therapeutic task that should be jointly managed, at least initially, by the nurse and the case manager.

Evaluation

Evaluation is a vital component of the nursing process during the termination phase. You have the task of helping the client evaluate the therapeutic contract. The criteria for evaluation are the goals formulated in the orientation and working phases of the one–to–one relationship. Each goal is evaluated in terms of measurable, observable behavior. Were the goals appropriate, practical, and specific to the client? What are the therapeutic gains? What are the areas for possible further therapeutic work? How does the client evaluate motivation, effort, progress, and outcome? Has the client worked through most feelings about separation from the nurse?

You will also help the client evaluate the therapeutic experience in general, which may set the stage for future psychotherapeutic work. Would the client seek a similar experience in the future if deemed necessary? Having the opportunity to discuss the work and the outcome is an empowering exercise for clients.

The nurse's own personal, ongoing self-evaluation also warrants emphasis here. It is essential to continuously evaluate which of your own behaviors consciously or unconsciously promote, inhibit, or actively block growth-producing client abilities.

Clinical Supervision

Clinical supervision is essential if the one–to–one relationship is to be effective. Professional supervision helps you use transference effectively and recognize countertransference phenomena. The supportive function of supervision may be used to monitor your own needs, thereby minimizing the likelihood of severe clinical stress and burnout. There are various methods of evaluation: process recordings, videotapes, client evaluations, audiotapes, didactic instruction, and referral to specific clinical readings. There are several kinds of supervision available, such as intradisciplinary supervision with a psychiatric–mental health clinical nurse specialist or with a faculty member if a student, or interdisciplinary supervision by another mental health care professional (psychologist, psychiatrist, psychiatric social worker). Supervision helps the psychiatric–mental health nurse effectively define, initiate, use, and evaluate client and self in any therapeutic relationship.

CASE MANAGEMENT

The likely possibility that not all client goals would be achieved during typical brief hospitalizations makes case management and community-based care more important than ever. Performing case management functions involves assisting the client on an almost daily basis in managing frequent challenges or problems associated with dysfunction. You will need to work at promoting the client's confidence in your skills during the therapeutic relationship to ensure the client makes the effort to seek help to manage problems. The client's confidence in your knowledge promotes improved health maintenance behaviors so that he or she does not sabotage the treatment or recovery process.

Guiding or accompanying clients through the mental health care system is another facet of the case manager role. Each geographic area differs in the kind of services that are available. In order to obtain treatment, the psychiatric client has to know how to work the system. Case management services assist clients in this process. Working the system may involve making appointments for clients, accompanying clients to disability interviews, and explaining forms and paperwork required by agencies or providers. Maneuvering around barriers or obstacles is a special skill of the nurse case manager.

The clinical example that follows illustrates how a primary nurse in an inpatient setting can continue the therapeutic nurse–client relationship after discharge and can also function as a case manager.

WHY I PLAN TO BECOME A PSYCHIATRIC–MENTAL HEALTH NURSE

Jonathan's Story: No matter what happens, there will always be a place for psychiatric–mental health nurses. If mental disorders could be totally treated with medications alone, then it would be a different story. However, mental disorders are so very complex. Besides being an actual disorder of neurons or chemicals within the brain, they are disorders of interpersonal functioning. That's where we come in as psychiatric nurses. I've always been pretty good with people, so I see psychiatric nursing as a perfect fit for me. It will give me a chance to use my people skills as well as my technical skills.

Clinical Example

You have worked with Francisco, a 65-year-old male, during his brief 5-day stay on your unit. The treatment team's goal was to stabilize his mood and begin antidepressant medication. You have spent 45 minutes each day developing a therapeutic nurse–client relationship with Francisco.

Following his discharge, you function as his case manager, connecting him with a job training program, a social club for mental health clients, and a medication psychoeducation group. You also meet with Francisco in the outpatient clinic weekly for 4 weeks, then every 2 weeks for the next 2 months, and finally, monthly for the next 4 months.

COMMUNITY-BASED CARE

Community-based care is a commonly used forum for treating people who have psychiatric problems. It is much more cost effective to treat clients on an outpatient than an inpatient basis. The nurse working in a community care setting will likely see particular outpatients repeatedly in that setting. Even though considerable time may elapse between sessions, you should help the client develop a strong, ongoing relationship with the provider, thus encouraging the client to seek needed help and to disclose important information. Information about symptoms, side effects, and recovery throughout the client's care in the community is essential to determining appropriate and effective interventions.

HOME CARE

Acceptance of home care and other services by the client and the client's significant others involves a variety of cultural, demographic, and personal preferences. In one study, there was resistance to several types of home care services. However, ethnic and racial minority clients accepted services from psychiatric nurses (Joosten, 2007), demonstrating that the decision to accept counseling at home can be positively influenced by the interaction between nurse and client. Counseling an individual in his or her home requires sensitivity—about both the therapeutic process and the therapeutic content.

A major consideration in psychiatric–mental health nursing is continuity of care. An important feature of effective care is making sure the same nurse who had a one–to–one relationship with the client sees the client afterward during home care when possible. Organizations could create new positions or expand duties within existing positions to achieve this continuity. Sometimes, to maximize available services and budgets, mental health systems combine the duties of nurses providing care to clients. This leads to multitasking, not an unusual feature of many nursing positions.

Pearson Nursing Student Resources
Find additional review materials at
nursing.pearsonhighered.com
Prepare for success with NCLEX®-style practice questions, interactive assignments and activities, web links, animations and videos, and more!

REFERENCES

Balkin, R. S., Leicht, D. J., Sartos, T., & Powell, J. (2011). Assessing the relationship between therapeutic goal attainment and psychosocial characteristics for adolescents in crisis residence. *Journal of Mental Health, 20*(1), 32–42.

Beretta, V., Despland, J. N., Drapeau, M., Michel, L., Kramer, U., Stigler, M., & de Roten, Y. (2007). Are relationship patterns with significant others reenacted with the therapist? A study of early transference reactions. *Journal of Nervous & Mental Disease, 195*(5), 443–450.

Boag, S. (2007). *Decoding the meaning of transference and countertransference: An integrative perspective.* Washington, DC: American Psychological Association.

Duffin, C. (2007). NMC proposal to ban gifts "could harm staff–patient relationships." *Nursing Standard, 21*(32), 10.

Ellis, A. (2001). Rational and irrational aspects of countertransference. *Journal of Clinical Psychology, 57*(8), 999–1004.

Fisher, C. B., & Oransky, M. (2008). Informed consent to psychotherapy: Protecting the dignity and respecting the autonomy of patients. *Journal of Clinical Psychology, 64*(5), 576–588.

Forrester, K. (2010). What you see may not be what you get: Beware of patients bearing gifts. *Journal of Law and Medicine, 18*(2), 268–274.

Gary, J. M. (2007). Counseling adult learners: Individual interventions, group interventions, and campus resources. In J. A. Lippincott & R. B. Lippincott (Eds.), *Special populations in college counseling: A handbook for mental health professionals* (pp. 99–113). Alexandria, VA: American Counseling Association.

Gawley, L., Einarson, A., & Bowen, A. (2011). Stigma and attitudes toward antenatal depression and antidepressant use during pregnancy in healthcare students. *Advances in Health Science Education, Theory, and Practice.* Advance online publication.

Gentile, S. (2011). Drug treatment for mood disorders in pregnancy. *Current Opinion in Psychiatry, 24*(1), 34–40.

Guy, J. D., & Brady, J. L. (2001). Identifying the faces in the mirror: Untangling transference and countertransference in self psychology. *Journal of Clinical Psychology, 57*(8), 993–997.

Henretty, J. R., & Levitt, H. M. (2010). The role of therapist self-disclosure in psychotherapy: A qualitative review. *Clinical Psychology Review, 30*(1), 63–77.

Horvath, A. O., Del Re, A. C., Fluckiger, C., & Symonds, D. (2011). Alliance in individual psychotherapy. *Psychotherapy, 48*(1), 9–16.

Hudson, C., St. Cyr-Tribble, D., Bravo, G., & Poitras, M. E. (2011). Enablement in health care context: A concept analysis. *Journal of Evaluation in Clinical Practice, 17*(1), 143–149.

Jain, S., & Roberts, L. W. (2009). Ethics in psychotherapy: A focus on professional boundaries and confidentiality practices. *Psychiatric Clinics of North America, 32*(2), 299–314.

Joosten, D. (2007). Preferences for accepting prescribed community-based, psychosocial, and in-home services by older adults. *Home Health Care Services Quarterly, 26*(1), 1–18.

Martin, G., & Pear, J. (2007). *Behavioral modification: What it is and how to do it* (8th ed.). Upper Saddle River, NJ: Pearson Education.

Peplau, H. E. (1952). *Interpersonal relations in nursing.* New York, NY: Putnam.

Peplau, H. E. (1997). Peplau's theory of interpersonal relations. *Nursing Science Quarterly, 10*(4), 162–167.

Petersen, I., Gilbert, R. E., Evans, S. K., Man, S. L., & Nazareth, I. (2011). Pregnancy as a major determinant for discontinuance of antidepressants: An analysis of data from The Health Improvement Network. *Journal of Clinical Psychiatry.* Advance online publication.

Pope, K. S., & Keith-Spiegel, P. (2008). A practical approach to boundaries in psychotherapy: Making decisions, bypassing blunders, and mending fences. *Journal of Clinical Psychology, 64*(5), 638–652.

Priebe, S., Richardson, M., Cooney, M., Adedejo, O., & McCabe, R. (2011). Does the therapeutic relationship predict outcomes of psychiatric treatment in patients with psychosis? A systematic review. *Psychotherapy and Psychosomatics, 80*(2), 70–77.

Psychopathology Committee of the Group for the Advancement of Psychiatry. (2001). Reexamination of therapist self-disclosure. *Psychiatric Services, 52*(11), 1489–1493.

Ryum, T., Stile, T. C., Svartberg, M., & McCullough, L. (2010). The role of transference work, the therapeutic alliance, and their interaction in reducing interpersonal problems among psychotherapy patients with Cluster C personality disorders. *Psychotherapy, 47*(4), 442–453.

Smith, K. W., & Greenberg, L. S. (2007). Internal multiplicity in emotion-focused psychotherapy. *Journal of Clinical Psychology, 63*(2), 175–186.

Spiers, J. A., & Wood, A. (2010). Building a therapeutic alliance in brief therapy: The experience of community mental health nurses. *Archives of Psychiatric Nursing, 24*(6), 373–386.

Steelman, J. R. (2007). Relationship dynamics: Understanding married women's mental health. *Advances in Nursing Science. Women and Aging, 30*(2), 151–158.

Weeks, S., Cowell, R., Scullion, J., & Tanton, E. (2007). Readers panel. Refusing gifts. *Nursing Standard, 21*(39), 26–27.

Weiss, M. A., & Lewis, L. (2007). Respect for the patient. *American Journal of Nursing, 107*(Supp.), 12.

2
UNIT

THEORETICAL BASIS FOR PSYCHIATRIC–MENTAL HEALTH NURSING PRACTICE

MAI LEE, seen here in traditional dress, is a member of the Hmong (pronounced "mung"), an ethnic and cultural group from the mountainous regions of Vietnam, Laos, Thailand, and China. Many Hmong in Laos, including Mai Lee's family, became refugees because they fought with United States soldiers against the Communist regime, settled in Minnesota, and are among the more than 250,000 Hmong from Laos who have migrated to the United States.

In this culture, mental illness is not accepted as a group of diseases of the mind; thus, people are not aware of the signs and symptoms of mental illness and psychological and emotional pain may be expressed through physical symptoms. Illness is believed to stem from a combination of natural causes, and supernatural causes (such as spells, curses, violation of taboos, and fright in which the soul is believed to leave the body).

Hallucinations and delusions are often seen as a form of spiritual unrest meted out to the individual by a vengeful spirit. Because a *dab*, or bad spirit, can cause illness when offended, many Hmong hesitate to discuss their symptoms and risk offending a dab even more. From this standpoint, symptoms (punishment for transgressions) are stigmatized and it is shameful to talk about emotional problems with people outside the family. Young people such as Mai Lee often experience frustration, stress, and depression as they feel caught in the middle of two often conflicting worlds—traditional Hmong culture and contemporary American society.

5

Theories for Interdisciplinary Care in Psychiatry

CAROL REN KNEISL

LEARNING OUTCOMES

After completing this chapter, you will be able to:

1. Discuss the major ideas of interactionism.
2. Discuss the major principles of humanism.
3. Describe the influence of the knowledge explosion in psychobiology.
4. Explain how the premises of human interactionism and psychobiology relate to psychiatric–mental health nursing.
5. Compare and contrast the assumptions and key ideas of medical–psychobiologic, psychoanalytic, cognitive–behavioral, and social–interpersonal theories.
6. Discuss the implications of each theory for the practice of psychiatric–mental health nursing.

CRITICAL THINKING CHALLENGE

Sonia Jones, a 38-year-old musician, came to the mental health clinic complaining of depression, anxiety, and fear about her increasing use of methamphetamines (speed) and alcohol. Sonia's reason for seeking help to is get clean and sober. Some members of the treatment team, however, cite a randomized clinical trial and a psychobiologic theory that support treating the depression prior to addressing Sonia's coexisting addictive disease. Your own clinical wisdom and past experience convince you that both conditions must be addressed simultaneously.

1. When you do not have established theory or clear research findings to guide your clinical decisions, how important are clinical preferences and clinical wisdom?
2. Do you think they constitute evidence on which to base practice?

To practice psychiatric–mental health nursing humanistically, you must devote yourself to understanding what makes people human, how they express their joy of living, their sadness, their desire to love, their hopes for growth. Understanding these phenomena becomes even more crucial when trying to explain how the joy of living suddenly turns to the desire to die, how love of self and others turns to violence and hate, how the hope for growth turns to withdrawal and despair, and how alterations in the brain relate to these human experiences.

This chapter introduces you to a holistic philosophy that includes humanism, interactionism, and the knowledge explosion in psychobiology. In this chapter, we also compare the basic assumptions and implications for practice in the dominant theories for interdisciplinary psychiatric care. These are as follows:

- Medical–psychobiologic theory
- Psychoanalytic theory
- Cognitive–behavioral theory
- Social–interpersonal theories

Clinicians often say they are *eclectic,* that is, they choose one or a combination of these theories in determining what information to assess about clients, what intervention outcomes and approaches to recommend, and what ultimate evaluation criteria to set. We believe that clinicians *should* be eclectic, choosing strategies based on scientific evidence about their effectiveness for any given client. The best strategies based on the best available evidence are reviewed in every chapter of this book.

Your approach to understanding psychiatric–mental health clients is influenced by your philosophy. We believe, further, that humanistic interactionism is the philosophy that fits best with psychiatric–mental health nursing goals. Theories such as those discussed in this chapter provide the conceptual tools to formulate that understanding and to interpret clinical data. Blend an understanding of these theories with the nursing theories discussed in Chapter 2∞, especially the psychiatric–mental health nursing theory of Hildegard Peplau.

SCOPE OF PSYCHIATRIC–MENTAL HEALTH NURSING PRACTICE

All nurses are concerned with the quality of human life and its relationship to health. The psychiatric–mental health nurse is especially concerned with the relationship between the individual's optimal psychobiologic health and feelings of self-worth, personal integrity, self-fulfillment, and creative expression. Just as important are the satisfying of basic living needs, comfortable relationships with others, and the recognition of human rights. These elements, as you read in Chapter 1∞, collectively define mental health.

Our scope of practice is broad enough to include issues such as alienation, identity crises, sudden life changes, and troubled family interactions. It may deal with poverty and affluence, the experiences of birth and death, the loss of significant others, or the loss of body parts. It is concerned with sustaining and enhancing the individual and the group.

Yet it also must address basic life issues shared by psychiatric clients—eating, sleeping, grooming, and hygiene. This broad-ranging, humanistic, interactional, and psychobiologic view of the scope of psychiatric–mental health nursing is dramatically different from the exclusively medical or behavioral science orientations of the last 50 years.

Psychiatric–mental health nurses are concerned with the care of clients who have identified mental disorders. However, our concerns extend to the wide range of human responses to mental distress, disability, and disorder. For example, an addicted parent may not only suffer from shame, unemployment, and abusive outbursts of anger but may also lose a sense of purpose and meaning and experience a disturbed self-concept and spiritual distress. These responses have detrimental effects on the health of children, partners, and other significant people in the person's life.

Like many concepts in the human sciences, the concept of mental disorder lacks a definition that covers all situations. Faced with such a diverse array of human problems, the psychiatric–mental health nurse is challenged to synthesize a holistic philosophy for practice that can be the basis for care.

HUMANISTIC INTERACTIONISM AND PSYCHOBIOLOGY: THE MIND–BODY–SPIRIT CONNECTION

The classic psychiatric and psychological approaches have described and classified signs and symptoms of *illness,* then accounted for it by individual psychological dynamics such as character disorder, weak ego, or failed defense mechanisms. The basis for this text is a synthesis of psychosocial and psychobiologic knowledge required for practice in the 21st century.

Basic Premises of Interactionism

One central idea in the approach we advocate has come to be known as **symbolic interactionism** (Hewitt & Shulman, 2011), a term that describes an approach to the study of human conduct. It is based on the philosophic premises identified in Box 5-1 on page 74.

Implications for Psychiatric–Mental Health Nursing Practice

Interactionism offers psychiatric–mental health nursing a perspective of human beings as having purpose and control over their lives, even if they have altered brain structure and chemistry and stressful environments. Interactionism as interpreted here provides the premise for a philosophy of caring with a strong humanistic cast, such as that described in Evidence-Based Practice. Interactionism acknowledges the interaction of psychology, psychobiology, and sociocultural contexts.

The First Premise: Behavior Is Purposeful We believe that people act with plans and purposes in mind. That is, human conduct is directed toward some goal or purpose. However, once people set their conduct in motion they may be deflected from their intended paths by obstacles or more appealing objects. Goals and purposes are not fixed and final—they

---

Box 5-1   Symbolic Interactionism: Philosophic Premises

1. People act with plans and purposes in mind and have the capacity to think of new ways to act by finding alternative goals and alternative methods.
2. Human beings act toward things (other people, events) on the basis of the meaning that the things have for them, that is, meaning is a basis for behavior. Life experiences may have different meanings for different people.
3. The meaning of things in a person's life arises from, and is transformed by, the social interactions that person has with others. We learn meanings during our experiences with others.
4. People handle and modify the meanings of the things they encounter through an interpretive process. They come to their own conclusions.
5. People want to regard themselves favorably and to maintain and enhance their self-esteem.
6. When human beings encounter situations they have not faced before, they must find new meanings, new purposes, and new methods to deal with novel situations.
7. As human beings, we inherit a society and a culture within which we live; however, we do not have to reproduce it.

---

emerge and change as we go about our lives. Behavior arises from, and is affected by, our interactions with others.

The Second Premise: Different Meanings for Different People We believe that all behavior has meaning. To understand clients' actions, you must identify the meanings those actions have for them. Be wary of interventions that ignore, discount, or discredit the meaning an experience has for the client in favor of your own definition of the situation. Thus, you must develop skill in observing, interpreting, and responding to the client's lived experiences in the hope of arriving at a common ground of negotiated meanings and authentic communication.

The Third Premise: Meanings Arise in One's Social World We believe meanings arise in the *process* of interaction with others. It is essential, therefore, that psychiatric–mental health nurses take into account the social and cultural environment of each client. A holistic assessment of a client accounts for the interaction patterns in that person's social world. A shaved head, tattoos, baggy denim pants worn low on the hips, and a woolen cap, which appear deviant in a milieu of business suit-wearing bankers and executives, may represent a close adherence to the dress and demeanor codes of some street gang subcultures.

The Fourth Premise: Meaning Is Individually Interpreted We believe that people come to their own conclusions. You need to keep this premise in mind when responding to an expression of human distress. People handle situations in terms of what they consider vitally important about the situation. Avoid saying, "I wouldn't worry about it," or "Don't feel that way," "You are reacting inappropriately," or "It's not so bad." Such clichés are not usually helpful, not because they are inherently nontherapeutic but because voicing them invalidates the basic premise that people interpret the world in their own way.

The Fifth Premise: Self as a Valued Object We believe that human beings want to regard themselves favorably and to attach a positive value to the self. Human beings desire to act in ways that will develop and sustain coherent images of themselves. They also wish to find a sense of security and place—a sense of social identity—by integrating themselves into group life. They take themselves—their feelings, their interests, and their images of self—into account as they act.

EVIDENCE-BASED PRACTICE

Strategy of Protective Empowering

Lorelei is the nurse manager on an alcohol detoxification unit. James, a 55-year-old man with a 30-year history of alcohol abuse and cigarette smoking, is admitted for alcohol detoxification. Because he had pulled out his IV fluids on the preceding shift, managed to obtain a cigarette lighter in order to smoke, and fallen out of bed, the night shift put him in soft restraints. Every time one of the night shift nurses came into his room, James cursed at them.

Lorelei assigned Kevin, who was newly hired and still in the process of orientation, to James's care. Lorelei and Kevin's joint assessment of James's current mental status, background history, and mental status examination results convinced them that he is at risk for harming himself. Although hospital policy justifies the use of soft restraints, Lorelei felt strongly that James could be kept safe with one-to-one supervision rather than with soft restraints and that the presence of a staff member would be more comforting and less anxiety provoking for him. Lorelei cautioned Kevin not to take James's cursing personally.

Among the goals that Lorelei and Kevin formulated cooperatively were relating to John in a respectful way, keeping him safe, and encouraging him to regain greater self-control. Although action should be based on more than one study, their strategy of protective empowering was based on the following grounded theory research:

Chiovitti, R. F. (2011). Theory of protective empowering for balancing patient safety and choices. *Nursing Ethics, 18*(1), 88–101.

CRITICAL THINKING QUESTIONS

1. How does protective empowerment fit with the basic premises of humanistic interactionism?
2. How does protective empowerment fit with the basic premises of psychobiologic theory?
3. How does protective empowerment fit with the basic premises of cognitive–behavioral theory?

The Sixth Premise: New Ways of Being We believe that it is within interpersonal interaction that clients can learn new definitions for life situations and new repertoires for action. This is the heart of the psychiatric–mental health nurse's therapeutic and caring role. The sensitive, intelligent, and humanistic use of self within interpersonal relationships is a key part of the psychiatric–mental health nurse's skill. You have the potential for helping clients redefine their experiences in more satisfying ways, learn new patterns of coping with stress, and generally enhance the quality of their lives and social worlds. Such is the essence of psychiatric–mental health nursing.

The Seventh Premise: Culture Shapes Conduct We believe that people are born into an already existing society and culture and are surrounded by others who define reality for us. Human beings are not required to keep cultural definitions set by others. Culture is an environment in which we all live. However, we do not have to reproduce the society and culture that we inherit. In many instances, our survival depends upon coming to terms with the culture we have inherited.

Basic Premises of Humanism

One of the purposes of this chapter is to specify a philosophic basis for subsequent chapters. The seven premises of interactionism provide us with a basic orientation. A theory of life centered on human beings, called **humanism**, adds to the philosophic perspective. The humanistic perspective views human nature as basically "good," emphasizes present conscious processes, and places strong emphasis on people's inherent capacity for self-direction (Butcher, Mineka, & Hooley, 2010). It pays less attention to the unconscious processes and past causes emphasized by some of the theories (see, for example, psychoanalytic theory) discussed later in this chapter. It first arose as a reaction against the psychoanalytic and behaviorist perspectives (Cicarelli & White, 2009).

The central concept of humanism is that the chief end of human life is to work for well-being within the limitations of life in today's world. Humanism is a philosophy of service to benefit humanity through reason, science, and democracy. The humanistic perspective has seven central propositions (Lamont, 1967) identified in Box 5-2.

Implications for Psychiatric–Mental Health Nursing Practice

As a philosophy underlying psychiatric–mental health nursing practice, having a humanistic perspective means devotion to the interests of human beings wherever they live and whatever their status or culture. It reaffirms the spirit of compassion and caring toward others. It is a constructive philosophy that wholeheartedly affirms the joys, beauty, and values of human living.

The subsequent chapters in this text show how these basic premises can be put to use in psychiatric–mental health nursing practice. Some fundamental concepts are described briefly in the following sections.

A Holistic View of the Mind–Body Relationship Our humanistic interactional view is that physical and mental factors are interrelated and that a change in one may result

---

Box 5-2 Humanistic Perspective: Philosophic Premises

1. The human being's mind is indivisibly connected with the body.
2. Human beings have the power or potential to solve their own problems.
3. Human beings, while influenced by the past, possess freedom of creative choice and action and are, within certain limits, masters of their own destinies.
4. Human values are grounded in life experiences and relationships, and our highest goal must be the happiness, freedom, and growth of all people.
5. Individuals attain well-being and a high quality of life by harmoniously combining personal satisfactions with activities that contribute to the welfare of the community.
6. We should apply reason, science, and democratic procedures in all areas of life.
7. We must continually examine our basic convictions, including those of humanism.

---

in a change in another. For example, anger may result in increased blood pressure. An invading organism, a decrease in a neurotransmitter, or a structural change in the body can alter thought processes. Low self-esteem can result in hunched shoulders and skeletal muscle contractures.

The implications for psychiatric–mental health nursing are clear. Healing and caring must be approached in a **holistic** manner, recognizing physical and psychosocial needs. That is, the psychiatric–mental health nurse deals with the biologic aspects of a primarily psychological or emotional pattern and the psychological or emotional aspects of biologic experiences, as in the following clinical example.

Clinical Example

Kate, a prominent television personality who wants to remain anonymous, is hospitalized for a severe eating disorder on an integrated behavioral unit, and you are assigned to provide her care. She weighs under 90 pounds, which is extremely thin for her 5'7" frame and is dehydrated, malnourished, and obsessed with getting back to work and looking good in an industry that expects bone-thin women anchors for the news.

As a nurse educated to recognize both her physical and psychosocial needs, you are challenged to formulate a holistic, integrated care plan.

What you will learn in this text is relevant not only in mental health care settings. You can use the philosophies, theories, concepts, and principles in the care of any client, no matter the setting, even if their immediate problems are primarily physical.

An Expanded Role for Nurses The humanistic interactional perspective on mental disorders implies an expanded role for psychiatric–mental health nurses. We believe that psychiatric nurses should be prepared to work for change within social and political systems. Psychiatric–mental health nursing must not be limited to client-oriented activities designed exclusively to control symptoms and increase the

Care Plan: Humanism: A Basis for Care

capability of individuals to adjust satisfactorily to the existing social condition. Instead, psychiatric–mental health nursing must be involved in social goals that advance health holistically. Because psychiatric–mental health nursing has political consequences, it is essential that you begin to develop a philosophic and ethical framework to guide and evaluate the political outcome of therapeutic intervention.

Negotiation and Advocacy In this book, the model for intervention and change is one of negotiation and advocacy. The responsibility for change remains with the person who seeks psychiatric help or consultation. Clients are held accountable for their own behavior. They are not the passive recipients of care given by psychiatric professionals. Instead, they are empowered in the process of developing new perspectives and encouraged to weigh alternatives and make self-directed choices. They and their families are educated about their disorder and its treatment.

Basic Premises of Psychobiology

The last decades have seen major breakthroughs in knowledge about the brain, the mind, the spirit, and behavior. This knowledge explosion has taken place in a field of study called **psychobiology**. Research has generated new understandings of how genetics, immunology, biorhythms, brain structure, and brain biochemistry influence mental disorders (discussed in Chapter 6∞).

New imaging techniques make it possible to view what has never been seen before. Neuroscientists have found that our thoughts, sensations, joys, and aches consist of physiological activity in the 100 billion neurons in the tissues of the brain. They can almost read people's thoughts from the blood flow in their brains. They can tell whether a person is thinking about a face or a place, or whether the person is looking at a bottle or a shoe.

New medications to correct biochemical imbalances in the brain are being prescribed. Psychobiologic interventions such as exposure to bright light and white noise, and the restriction of nutrients and nonnutrients believed to affect behavior, have become commonplace.

Implications for Psychiatric–Mental Health Nursing Practice

Some authorities argue that psychiatric–mental health nurses should continue to focus on the human aspects of care as psychiatry moves toward "remedicalization." They fear that by embracing the biologic sciences we will diminish the art of psychiatric–mental health nursing. Others, ourselves included, contend that, to bring a contemporary holistic perspective to psychiatric–mental health nursing care, we must integrate the rapidly accumulating knowledge in psychobiology. We do not give up our humanistic, psychosocial, and interactional premises simply because we recognize the value of the breakthroughs being made in psychobiology. Instead, as we redefine the traditional art of psychiatric–mental health nursing care and caring in contemporary society, our practice and research must integrate "high tech" and "high touch," nature and nurture, the biologic sciences and the behavioral sciences.

THEORIES FOR INTERDISCIPLINARY PSYCHIATRIC CARE

Dominant social attitudes and philosophic viewpoints have influenced the understanding of and approaches to mental disorder throughout history. Concepts and theories that we consider modern may have roots in earlier eras (see Chapter 1∞ for a thorough discussion of the history of social attitudes toward mental illness and Figure 1-4 on pages 10–11 for a timeline illustrating these shifts in viewpoints).

TABLE 5-1 ■ compares the major features of the medical–psychobiologic, psychoanalytic, cognitive–behavioral, and social–interpersonal theories discussed next. While the approaches suggested by these theories appear to be very different, it is up to the individual psychiatric–mental health nurse to use the best aspects of each approach in clinical practice. For example, a biologically oriented clinician can see the value of psychotherapy or cognitive–behavioral therapy, as well as medication, for a man who has a fear of flying, and a cognitive–behavioral therapist can appreciate the anxiety-reducing effects of medication for the client.

Medical–Psychobiologic Theory

The medical–psychobiologic model in psychiatry originated in the era of classification. The classification of mental disturbances brought the emotional and behavioral aspects of people into the domain of the medical doctor during a period when the systematic observation, naming, and classification of symptoms were emphasized.

Emil Kraepelin's monumental descriptive diagnostic classification system of mental disorders is acknowledged as the first comprehensive medical model (Wallace & Gach, 2011).

TABLE 5-1 ■ Comparison of Major Features of Traditional Psychiatric Theories

Theory	Assessment Base	Problem Statement	Goal	Dominant Interventions
Medical–psychobiologic	Individual client symptoms	Disease	Symptom management; cure	Psychopharmacology and other biologic therapies
Psychoanalytic	Intrapsychic; unconscious	Conflict	Insight	Psychoanalysis
Cognitive–behavioral	Behavior	Learning deficit	Behavior change	Behavior modification or conditioning
Social–interpersonal	Interactions between individual and social contexts	Interpersonal dysfunction	Enhanced awareness and quality of interpersonal interactions	Group, family, and milieu therapies

He noted that certain patterns of symptoms occurred with enough frequency to be considered as specific types of mental disorders. Kraepelin described these types of mental disorders and worked out a classification scheme that is the basis of our present system, the *Diagnostic and Statistical Manual of Mental Disorders (DSM)* published by the American Psychiatric Association (2000). The DSM classification system is reproduced in Appendix A and discussed in Chapter 11∞ and throughout the text.

Kraepelin also formulated the notions that the cause of mental illness was organic, that it was located in the central nervous system, that the disease followed a predictable course, and that treatment should be based on accurate diagnosis. Contemporary research findings in the field of psychobiology lend support to some of these early ideas but advance them and make them specific in important ways.

Assumptions and Key Ideas

Medical–psychobiologic theories view emotional and behavioral disturbances like any physical disease. Thus, abnormal behavior is directly attributable to a disease process, a lesion, a neuropathologic condition, a toxin introduced from outside the body, or (most recently) a biochemical abnormality of neurotransmitters and enzymes or a genetic predisposition. The medical–psychobiologic position is summarized in Box 5-3.

Implications for Psychiatric–Mental Health Nursing Practice

Nurses who were first involved in the care of psychiatric clients were primarily responsible for the client's physical well-being. Their responsibilities included administering medications prescribed by the physician and caring for clients undergoing treatments such as insulin shock therapy, electroshock therapy, hydrotherapy, or psychosurgery (see Chapter 12∞).

Psychobiologic theories are the conceptual basis for the continued use of biologic therapies in the care of mental health clients, the hospital as the setting for care, research into the genetic transmission of mental illness, research on biochemical and metabolic variables among diagnosed psychiatric clients, and dominance of the medical doctor—the psychiatrist—in the mental health team. As long as psychiatric clients are admitted to, and reimbursed for, care according to medical diagnoses, knowledge of this framework is crucial. Furthermore, as long as psychobiologic knowledge expands, psychiatric–mental health nurses are responsible for translating that knowledge into care practices that recognize the biologic factors related to mental disorders. Chapter 6∞ of this text provides an authoritative source of such contemporary psychobiologic knowledge. Advances in psychobiologic theory and research are also integrated throughout specific disorders and interventions chapters.

Psychoanalytic Theory

Psychoanalytic theory is usually credited to the Viennese physician Sigmund Freud (FIGURE 5-1 ■). Freud believed that all psychological and emotional events, however obscure, were understandable. For the meanings behind behavior, he looked to childhood experiences that he believed caused adult neuroses that interfered with productive and satisfying living. Freud's work shifted the focus of psychiatry from classification to a dynamic view of mental phenomena.

Assumptions and Key Ideas

There are several basic principles that are central to psychoanalytic theory.

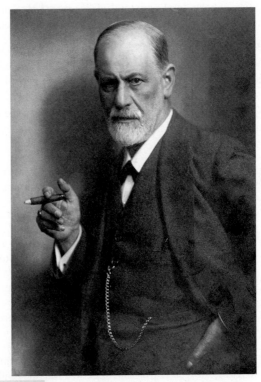

FIGURE 5-1 ■ Sigmund Freud, founder of psychoanalysis.
Photo courtesy of Alamy SZ Photo/Scherl.

Box 5-3 Medical–Psychobiologic Views

- The individual suffering from emotional disturbances is sick and has an illness or defect.
- The illness can, at least presumably, be located in some part of the body (usually the brain's limbic system and the central nervous system's synapse receptor sites). Factors related to mental disorders include, but are not limited to, excesses or deficiencies of certain brain neurotransmitters; alterations in the body's biologic rhythms, including the sleep–wake cycle; and genetic predispositions.
- The illness has characteristic structural, biochemical, and mental symptoms that can be diagnosed, classified, and labeled.
- Mental diseases run a characteristic course and have a particular prognosis for recovery.
- Mental disorders respond to physical or somatic treatments, including drugs, chemicals, hormones, diet, or surgery.
- Psychobiologic explanations of mental disorders can reduce the stigma often associated with them, and can discourage claims that mental disorders result from a lack of willpower or moral character.

Psychic Determinism Psychic determinism states that no human behavior is accidental. Each psychic event is determined by the ones that preceded it. Events in people's mental lives that seem random or unrelated to what went before are only apparently so. Thus, psychoanalysts never dismiss any mental phenomenon as meaningless or accidental. They always search for what caused it, why it happened. For example, people commonly forget or misplace things. They usually view this as simply an accident. Psychoanalysts seek to demonstrate that the accident was caused by a wish or intent of the person involved. Psychoanalysts also view dreams as subject to the principle of psychic determinism, each dream and each image in each dream bearing some relationship to the rest of the dreamer's life.

Role of the Unconscious The distinction between conscious and unconscious thought was made famous by Freud. Some kinds of information in the brain—your plans for the day, the faces of the people near you, your pleasures and your pains—are **conscious**. You think about them, discuss them, and let them guide your behavior. Others—the control of your heart rate and the sequence of muscle contractions that allow you to turn the pages of this book—are **unconscious**. They are in your brain someplace, but are sealed off from your planning and reasoning circuits. Likewise, any mental event that occurs outside of conscious awareness represents the unconscious region.

Significant unconscious mental processes occur frequently in normal as well as abnormal mental functioning. Much of what goes on in people's minds is unknown to them, and this accounts for the apparent discontinuities in their mental life. According to psychoanalytic theory, if the unconscious motivation of behavioral symptoms is discovered, the apparent discontinuities disappear, and the connection becomes clear.

Psychoanalysis The most powerful method for studying the unconscious is the technique that Freud evolved over several years called **psychoanalysis**. The basic logic behind psychoanalysis is discussed in Box 5-4.

Strategies used in psychoanalysis are hypnosis, the interpretation of dreams, and *free association,* in which the client is

encouraged to express every idea that comes to mind—no matter how insignificant, irrelevant, shameful, or embarrassing—ignoring all self-censorship and suspending all judgment.

Structure of the Mind With the publication of *The Ego and the Id* in 1923, Freud introduced the *structural model* of the mind (1962a). The structural model of the mind contends that there are three distinct entities: the id, the ego, and the superego. The **id** is a completely unorganized reservoir of energy derived from drives and instincts. The **ego** controls action and perception, controls contact with reality, and, through defense mechanisms, inhibits primary instinctual drives. One of its fundamental functions is also the capacity for developing mutually satisfying relationships with others. The **superego** is concerned with moral behavior. Frequently, the superego allies itself with the ego against the id, imposing demands in the form of conscience or guilt feelings. The relationship between Freud's levels of conscious and unconscious awareness and his concepts of id, superego, and ego is often depicted as an iceberg (see FIGURE 5-2 ■).

The id operates according to what Freud called the *pleasure principle:* the tendency to seek pleasure and avoid pain. This is not always possible, so the demands of the pleasure principle have to be modified by the *reality principle.* The reality principle is a learned ego function by which people develop the capacity to delay the immediate release of tension or achievement of pleasure.

Instinctual Drives Freud believed that psychic energy was derived from drives. He used the word *cathexis* to refer to the attachment of psychic energy to a person or a thing. The greater the cathexis, the greater the psychological importance of the person or object.

Freud accounted for the instinctual aspects of a person's mental life by assuming the existence of two drives, the *sexual*

Box 5-4   The Basic Logic Behind Psychoanalysis

1. The client underwent a *traumatic experience* that stirred up intense and painful emotion.
2. The traumatic experience represented to the client some ideas that were incompatible with the dominant ideas constituting the ego. Thus, the client experienced a *neurotic conflict.*
3. The incompatible idea and the neurotic conflict associated with it force the ego to bring into action *defense mechanisms.* (Chapter 8◗◗ describes in detail common defense mechanisms.)
4. Therapy is directed toward resolving the conflict by uncovering its roots in the unconscious. If the client is able to release the repressed feelings associated with the conflict, the symptoms disappear.

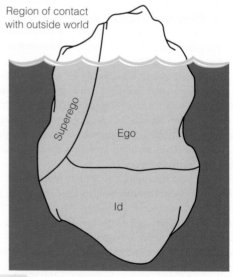

FIGURE 5-2 ■ Levels of awareness in relation to id, ego, and superego. In this image, the id is completely below the water's surface and the superego is partially below and partially above the surface. In comparison to the superego, the ego is more fully above the surface in the realm of conscious awareness.

TABLE 5-2 ■ Freud's Psychosexual Stages

Stage	Age Span	Task	Key Concept
Oral	0–18 months	Satisfaction and anxiety management from oral activity	Oral activity gives pleasure and is a source for learning
Anal	18 months–3 years	Learning muscle control for toilet training	Delayed gratification and rule internalization
Phallic	3–6 years	Gender identification and genital awareness	Repression of attraction to the opposite-sex parent (Oedipus and Electra complexes), leading to same-sex identification
Latency	6–12 years	Repression of sexuality	Oedipal conflict resolved with a shift to other interests and friends
Genital	12 years–young adult	Channeling sexuality into relationships with members of the opposite sex	Re-emerging sexuality to motivate behavior

drive and the *aggressive drive*. The former gives rise to the erotic component of mental activity, and the latter gives rise to the destructive component. The sexual drive came to be known as the *libido*. According to Freud, we all pass through five stages of psychosexual development from infancy through puberty (see TABLE 5-2 ■). Each stage is characterized by a dominant mode of achieving libidinal (sexual) pleasure.

The Oedipus Complex and the Electra Complex Freud believed that each person must resolve the conflicts that arise in each psychosexual stage of development in order to avoid later fixations. He termed one of the most important conflicts the **Oedipus complex**. Freud believed that each young boy symbolically relives the Greek myth, in which Oedipus unknowingly kills his father and marries his mother, in the phallic stage of psychosexual development. However, the young boy, although longing for his mother sexually, fears that his father will cut off his penis as punishment. This fear, termed **castration anxiety**, forces the young boy to repress his hostility toward his father and his sexual desire for his mother. In successful resolution, the young boy has affection for his mother (but not sexual desire) and is able to channel his sexual impulses into relationships with other potential partners.

The **Electra complex** is the female counterpart, and is also drawn from Greek mythology. Freud believed that young girls

desire to replace their mothers in order to possess their fathers. It is at this stage that young girls experience what Freud termed **penis envy**, the wish to be more like one's father or brothers.

Decline of Freudian Psychoanalysis

We have seen a steady decline in the reliance on psychoanalytic theory and psychoanalysis as a treatment measure. The most frequent cited criticisms are that psychoanalytic theory is based on inferences (not proof) from clinical experiences, no single verifiable cure exists, and psychoanalysis is the costliest and most time-consuming treatment, often requiring expensive weekly meetings between client and psychoanalyst for years (Crews, 1998; Webster, 1995). The Mental Health in the News feature discusses Marilyn Monroe's psychoanalysis to treat sexual dysfunction.

In addition, because it requires a person to be relatively well functioning, introspective, and financially secure, psychoanalysis is not accessible to many mental health clients. People with psychotic disorders or personality disorders are especially unlikely to benefit. However, as you will see later in this chapter, variations on Freudian theory led to the development of various insight-oriented therapies such as those described in the section on social–interpersonal theories. Most psychiatric-mental health clinicians continue to use

MENTAL HEALTH IN THE NEWS

The Psychoanalysis of Marilyn Monroe

It is surprising to most people to think of Marilyn Monroe, a film "sex goddess," as a woman with a sexual dysfunction. She engaged in numerous affairs throughout her life from an early age, apparently participated in a stag film and in multiple sex parties at a hotel in New York City (according to a government report), posed nude for a calendar, engaged in sexual activity with women as well as men, had nearly a dozen abortions and multiple miscarriages, but had never had an orgasm until much later after seeking therapy. Marilyn's orgasmic difficulties were the focus of her relationship with a renowned psychoanalyst popular among the Hollywood elite.

She saw her psychoanalyst virtually every day, and in the beginning several times a day. Although she was helped to experience

an orgasm for the first time, Marilyn remained in the grips of a severe addiction which continued to be fueled by the routine prescriptions she received from her psychoanalyst for tranquilizers and barbiturates. This relationship lasted for years until her death from an overdose of the barbiturate pentobarbital (Nembutal). Renowned Los Angeles medical examiner, Thomas Noguchi, listed the cause of her death as a "probable" suicide after taking into account several curious facts about her death (among the curious facts is the possibility that the overdose was by rectum, not by mouth, since pentobarbital was not present in her stomach in an amount that would cause death).

Photo courtesy of Superstock.

several relevant psychoanalytic concepts—the structure of the mind, the role of the unconscious, defense mechanisms (discussed in Chapter 8∞), dream interpretation, and the three concepts of resistance, transference, and countertransference (discussed in Chapter 4∞)—to understand mental processes and the process of the therapeutic relationship.

Implications for Psychiatric–Mental Health Nursing Practice

Psychoanalytic theory has historically provided an extremely limited treatment role for the nurse. Psychoanalytic clients are usually seen in the analyst's office as private clients. With the emergence of psychoanalytically oriented private hospital treatment settings, nurses became somewhat more involved. In these settings, nurses shared at least in the psychoanalytic language, concepts, and speculations about client dynamics and personality development, but usually not in the psychotherapeutic treatment role, unless they chose to train and function as psychoanalysts.

Cognitive–Behavioral Theory

Cognitive–behavioral theory focuses on the present rather than the past. Behaviorist theory in psychiatry has its roots in psychology and neurophysiology. The term *behavior therapy* has largely been replaced by the term *cognitive–behavior therapy,* although they may be used interchangeably throughout this text. The specifics of cognitive–behavioral therapy are thoroughly discussed in Chapter 30∞.

To the behaviorist, symptoms associated with neuroses and psychoses are clusters of learned behaviors that persist because they are somehow rewarding to the individual. One of the most important contributions to this framework was made by Ivan Pavlov (1849–1936), who in 1902 discovered a phenomenon he called the **conditioned response** in a famous experiment with a dog and a bell (FIGURE 5-3 ■). The basic principle of the conditioned response is described as follows:

1. A response is a reaction to a stimulus.
2. If a new and different stimulus is presented with, or just before, the original stimulating event, the same response reaction can be obtained.

FIGURE 5-3 ■ Pavlov's famous experiment demonstrated the part conditioning plays in behavior. Pavlov is shown here with the staff and some of the apparatus used to condition reflexes in dogs.
Photo courtesy of Photo Researchers, Inc.

3. Eventually the new stimulus can replace the original one, so that the response occurs in reaction to the new stimulus alone.

The conditioned or learned response is viewed as the basic unit of all learning, the unit on which more complex behavioral patterns are constructed. Such construction occurs through a process called **reinforcement**, in which behaviors are rewarded and persist. Pavlov's theories have influenced contemporary cognitive–behavioral therapists and are valued for their simplicity, concreteness, and objectivity. Some behaviorists see them as the key to understanding and controlling the whole range of undesirable human behavior.

Assumptions and Key Ideas

The fundamental premises of cognitive–behavioral theory are presented in Box 5-5. Both Joseph Wolpe (1956) and B. F. Skinner (1971) are associated with psychiatric treatment approaches that represent one form of **conditioning** (using a specific stimulus to elicit a specific response) and reflect the assumptions in Box 5-5.

Wolpe defined *neurotic behavior* as unadaptive behavior acquired in anxiety-generating situations. He based his therapeutic method on the introduction of a response that inhibits anxiety when situations occur that ordinarily evoke anxiety. Relaxation, for example, was considered incompatible with anxiety and, therefore, effective in inhibiting it. Thus, Wolpe would direct his intervention to a counterconditioning technique, usually putting the client under hypnosis and using various techniques for gradual *desensitization*. For example, a man afraid of dying might gradually attempt to overcome his

---

Box 5-5 Fundamental Principles of Cognitive–Behavioral Therapy

- The self in humans is the sum or repository of past conditionings or simply the behavioral repertoire. Therapists can know clients only by the clients' behavior.
- Behavior is the way in which a person acts. It can be observed, described, and recorded.
- There is no autonomous person. People are what they do and what they are reinforced for doing by conditions in their environment.
- The self is a structure of stimulus–response chains or hierarchies of habit. It is possible to know and predict conditions under which behavior will occur.
- The symptoms of a mental disorder are, in fact, the substance of that person's troubles. There is no hidden motive, no underlying cause, no internal pathogenic process. There is only the symptom or the behavior, and the aim of cognitive–behavioral therapy is to change the behavior.
- The therapist determines what behavior should be changed and what plan should be followed. Change comes about by identifying events in the client's life that have been critical stimuli for the behavior and then arranging interventions for *extinguishing* those behaviors. A changed way of acting precedes a changed way of thinking, according to behaviorist theory.

anxiety at seeing a coffin, attending a funeral, and so on, by trying to relax in these situations.

Skinner's approach, called **operant conditioning**, emphasizes discovering why the behavioral response was elicited in the first place and what actively reinforces it. The key concept in operant conditioning is reinforcement. Skinner originally used the term **positive reinforcement** to describe an event that increases the probability that the response will recur—a reward for behavior. A **negative reinforcement** was defined as an event likely to decrease the possibility of recurrence because it penalizes the behavior.

The term for an intervention designed to change a person's behavior is **shaping**. It is a procedure of manipulating reinforcement to bring the person closer to the desired behavior. According to Skinner, there are times in a client's life when responses are accidentally reinforced by a coincidental pairing of response and reinforcement. This accidental pairing may play a role in the development of phobias (irrational fears) and other distressing and/or dysfunctional behaviors.

In addition to these classics, contemporary cognitive–behavioral therapists use a vast array of techniques based on basic psychological science and developed out of psychological research and validated in thousands of treatment outcome studies.

Implications for Psychiatric–Mental Health Nursing Practice

In many institutional environments, clients follow prescribed schedules for daily living that include a **token economy**. Clients are rewarded for desired behavior by token reinforcers, such as food, candy, verbal approval, and even money. The use of this approach raises issues of control, responsibility for behavior, and the morality of using negative or punitive stimuli in a therapeutic context, to name only a few. Mental health professionals who successfully resolve such basic philosophic issues have designed and implemented successful behavior modification plans with disturbed, overtly aggressive children, developmentally disabled clients, violently self-destructive people and people who are severely and persistently mentally ill.

The movement toward community-based psychiatric treatment has made plain some of the shortcomings and economic realities of therapies aimed toward resolving everyone's intrapsychic conflicts. The movement has instead attempted to replace maladaptive behavior with behavior that allows people to function effectively within their natural environment. When parents or others in the client's environment are taught to implement behavior change procedures, therapy moves away from the artificial situation of the therapist's office into the client's total environment. It no longer requires the presence of highly trained, often expensive experts and thus makes treatment more affordable.

Psychiatric–mental health nurses have had a special role in teaching behaviorist principles to people with little training so that they can act as change agents. Nonprofessional staff can be taught the effective use of behaviorist principles to eliminate chronic, maladaptive behavior. Hyperactive children or children with borderline intelligence can be treated in the home by their parents when nurses teach the parents to use approaches such as frequency counts on specific behaviors to be modified, time-outs (short periods of isolation) for undesired behavior, and the bestowal of attention, praise, and affectionate physical contact as rewards.

Cognitive–behavioral interventions focus on the individual—what that person feels, thinks, and assigns meanings to—and empowers clients to learn new skills. How psychiatric–mental health nurses can use cognitive–behavioral strategies, such as behavioral contracting, in their clinical practice is the subject of Chapter 30∞.

Social–Interpersonal Theories

Social–interpersonal theories of psychiatry grew out of a general dissatisfaction with approaches that account for mental illness in terms of either intrapersonal mechanisms (the symptoms of a disease) or individual personality dynamics such as anxiety, ego strength, and libido. Advocates of this perspective assert that other theories neglect the crucial social processes and cultural variation involved in the development, identification, and resolution of disturbed human responses.

Assumptions and Key Ideas

Two separate but philosophically congruent schools of thought contribute to social–interpersonal theories. These are the interpersonal–psychiatric (Harry Stack Sullivan, Abraham Maslow, Carl Rogers, and Erik Erikson) and the general systems approaches (von Bertalanffy, Menninger). The assumptions and key ideas of each are discussed next.

Interpersonal–Psychiatric Theory: Harry Stack Sullivan Psychiatrist Harry Stack Sullivan (1953) made significant contributions to social–interpersonal theory in the first half of the 20th century and greatly influenced the work of Hildegard Peplau (see Chapter 2∞). He is viewed as the least reductionist of psychiatric theorists and emphasizes **interpersonal theory** (the client's past and present relationships with others and modes of interaction) as the real focus of psychiatric inquiry. Sullivan's views were influenced by his teacher, Alfred Adler (1971), who defected in 1911 from the dominant psychoanalytic viewpoint of his teacher, Sigmund Freud. Sullivan became the theoretic and ideologic leader of the interpersonal school of psychiatry.

One concept that plays a crucial role in the organization of behavior, according to Sullivan, is **self-system** or *self-dynamism.* The self-system enables people to deal with the tasks of avoiding anxiety and establishing security. The self is a construct built from the child's experience and initially develops in the process of seeking satisfaction of bodily needs and safety. To feel secure, the self essentially requires feelings of approval and prestige as protection against anxiety.

The self-system is comprised of **reflected appraisals**—that is, the view of ourselves that we learn in interactions with significant others. Rewarding appraisals from others yield what Sullivan calls the *good-me* aspect of the self. Anxiety-producing appraisals result in the *bad-me* aspect. The *not-me*

TABLE 5-3 ■ Sullivan's Stages of Interpersonal Development

Age	Stage	Task/Key Concept
Birth–18 months (to appearance of speech)	Infancy	Experiences anxiety in interaction with mother figure; learns to use maternal tenderness to gain security and avoid anxiety
18 months–6 years (from first speech to need for playmates)	Childhood	Learns to delay gratification in response to interpersonal demands; uses language and action to avoid anxiety
6–9 years	Juvenile	Develops peer relationships and uses environment outside the family to shape self
9–12 years	Preadolescence	Develops a caring relationship with same-sex peer, chum relationship
12–14 years	Early adolescence	Develops interest in opposite-sex relationships
14–21 years	Late adolescence	Has satisfying relationships; directs sexual impulses
21 years +	Adulthood	Establishes a love relationship

aspect exists normally in dreams and in aspects of experience that are poorly understood and later experienced as dread, horror, and loathing among mentally disordered people.

In summary, Sullivan emphasizes the pervasive interaction between the organism and the environment as well as the developmental tasks of the personality (TABLE 5-3 ■). Nonetheless, Sullivan has little to say about the impact on behavior of specific variations in the social or cultural scene.

Like Sullivan, other advocates of the interpersonal school of psychiatry, such as Karen Horney (1950) and Erich Fromm (1941), stress the general climate in the immediate family. The interpersonal school of psychiatry in general takes a developmental–interpersonal view of the self.

Hierarchy of Basic Human Needs: Abraham Maslow

The *self-actualization* and hierarchy-of-needs theories of Abraham Maslow (1962) belong squarely in this school (FIGURE 5-4 ■). Maslow was one of the early humanistic psychologists who rejected the dominant views of psychoanalysis and behaviorism in favor of a more positive view of human behavior.

Maslow proposed an order, or hierarchy, of basic human needs. According to Maslow, there are eight categories of needs (Maslow & Lowery, 1998). First, we must meet elemental and basic physiological needs for food and water. Once these needs have been met, second-tier or safety needs come next. After safety needs are belongingness and love needs, needs for friends and companions. See Caring for the Spirit for a discussion of what a client might experience when there are problems meeting these first three levels.

The self-esteem need is the need to feel that one has accomplished something good and earned the esteem of others. Next come the cognitive needs—the need to gather knowledge so that one can know and understand the world. Aesthetic needs have to do with appreciating beauty and expressing oneself artistically. It is not until all these needs have been met that one can concern oneself with **self-actualization** or reaching full human potential. The times that we achieve self-actualization are called *peak experiences*. The highest need, transcendence, involves helping others achieve their full potential.

Moving up and down the pyramid, and then back up, is quite common. A shift in life circumstances, such as that described in the clinical example, may require a shift to a lower need.

Clinical Example

Donna had been retired for 4 years from her job as a consulting engineer. When she was actively employed, Donna was held in high esteem by her colleagues. She often travelled internationally as a "trouble-shooter" to Thailand, Indonesia, France, Germany, and the Czech Republic. When Donna's husband, Jim, died after a long battle with cancer, Donna found herself in some financial difficulty. There were many bills and a mortgage and car to pay for. Jim's retirement income ended upon his death, and the economy took a nose-dive. Currently, Donna works as a cashier at the local supermarket in her community in order to ease her financial problems. While Jim was alive, he and Donna spent lots of time together. Now that Jim is dead, Donna has increased the time she spends with people from her church and friends from the senior center in her community.

CARING FOR THE SPIRIT

Basic Biologic, Safety, and Belonging Needs

Spirituality may be an important connection between mental health and mental illness. In mental illness, most clients describe feeling "disconnected" from their families, their friends, the universe itself, and from their "faith." For example, clients describe depression as similar to being in a gray or black tunnel with a profound sense of disconnectedness.

Imagine what it would be like to go for 24 hours or longer without sleep. How would you look? Would you feel disconnected or disoriented? Ask someone with mania what that's like. Have you ever awakened suddenly and not known where you are? How would it be to feel like that for an hour, a whole day, or a month? Ask someone with schizophrenia what that's like. Perhaps you've driven down the road and realized that you're confused about where you are and how you got there. And what if you had voices inside your head at the same time? Would this be frightening? Would you feel disconnected?

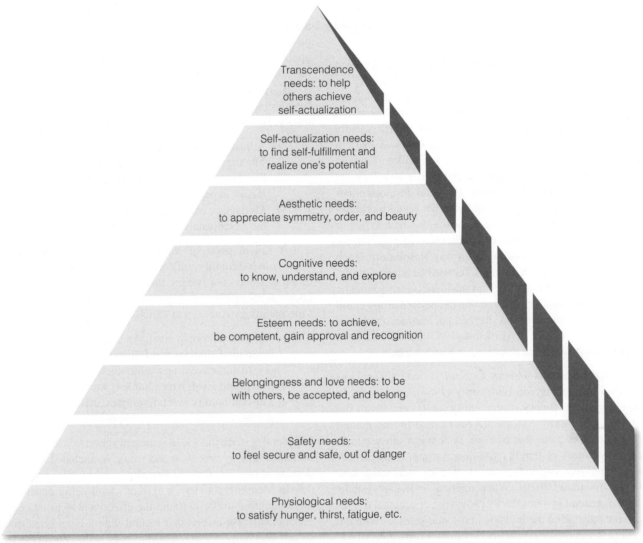

FIGURE 5-4 ■ Maslow's hierarchy of needs. The most basic needs for survival that must be met first are at the bottom and the highest needs are at the top.
Source: Ciccarelli, S. K., & White, J. N. (2009). *Psychology.* Upper Saddle River, NJ: Pearson, p. 367.

Client-Centered Therapy: Carl Rogers Like Maslow, Carl Rogers was an early humanistic psychologist who emphasized human potential, the ability of each person to become the best he or she could be. Rogers is probably the first to use the term *client,* rather than patient, for the person seeking counseling or mental health services. **Client-centered therapy** focuses on the client as the healer, rather than the therapist.

Rogers identified four elements as key in successful therapeutic relationships:

1. *Reflection.* Rogers believed that it was important to allow the ideas coming from the client to flow freely in order to attain insight. To this end he believed that therapists should not interfere with their own interpretations and biases. Reflection is literally a mirroring of the client's statements. Reflection as a therapeutic communication technique is discussed in Chapter 10∞.

2. *Unconditional positive regard.* Therapists should be warm and accepting and provide an uncritical atmosphere for clients. Having **unconditional positive regard** means that therapists respect clients and their feelings, values, and goals, even if they differ from those of the therapist.

3. *Empathy.* Empathy is the ability to understand clients by acknowledging what they are feeling and experiencing. Empathic therapists listen closely to what their clients are saying and try to feel what their clients feel without getting their own feelings mixed up with the client's feelings.

4. *Authenticity.* Authenticity is the ability to be open, genuine, and honest in response to the client. Being authentic means not hiding behind the role of therapist. It does mean that the therapist treats the client as a partner in the counseling process.

Like Maslow, Rogers believed in helping clients move toward self-actualization. Rogers was also an influence on Hildegard Peplau and her work.

Developmental Theory of Personality: Erik Erikson

Erik Erikson also formulated a developmental theory of personality that took much more into account than just biologic instincts. He elaborated and broadened Freud's psychosexual stages into more socially, culturally, and interpersonally oriented concepts. For example, Erikson believed that, in what Freud described as the "oral stage" in which the child is focused on oral gratification, the child's real development centers around issues of basic trust. The child develops either "basic trust" or "basic mistrust" of his or her social world.

Erikson described eight stages of life in which crises or conflicts develop. Each crisis or conflict has the potential for being resolved in a healthy or unhealthy way. Resolution of each stage is required in order to move forward developmentally. Erikson's developmental theory is considered more optimistic than Freud's because he believed that clients in therapy could return to a developmental task that had not been accomplished previously and relearn it (Erikson, 1963). Erikson's eight developmental stages are discussed in TABLE 5-4 ■.

General Systems Theory

General systems theory was pioneered by Ludwig von Bertalanffy (1968), a biologist. In **general systems theory**, every entity, or system, from the atom to rapid transit systems are maintained by the mutual interaction of its parts, that is, every system is a subsystem of larger systems. A system is more than the sum of its parts—when things are organized into a system, something new emerges (Nichols, 2010). When applied to living systems (people), general systems theory provides a conceptual framework for integrating the biologic and social sciences with the physical sciences. In psychiatry, it offers a resolution of the mind–body dichotomy, an integration of biologic and social approaches to the nature of human beings, and an approach to psychopathology, diagnosis, and therapy. The most common application of general systems theory today is in understanding how families function (see Chapter 29∞).

Karl Menninger (1963) views normal personality functioning and psychopathology in terms of general systems theory. His work addresses four major issues, as follows:

1. Adjustment or individual–environment interaction
2. The organization of living systems
3. Psychological regulation and control, known as *ego theory* in psychoanalysis
4. Motivation, which is often called *instinct* or *drive* in the psychoanalytic framework

A salient point of Menninger's theory is the idea of *homeostasis* (equilibrium). He asserts that the greater the threat or stress on a system, the greater the number of system components involved in coping with or adapting to it. Therefore, pathology can exist at various levels, as follows:

- The cell and organ level: An example might be the behavioral changes that follow cellular alterations due to addictive drugs, a blood clot, or a tumor.
- The group level: An example is family violence.
- The community level: Examples are overpopulation, pollution, homelessness, and poverty.

In general systems theory, all represent abnormalities or stresses on matter–energy processes and would be included within the domain of psychiatric professionals.

In Menninger's view, a system's well-being depends on the amount of stress on it and the effectiveness of its coping mechanisms. He asserts that mental illness is an impairment of self-regulation in which comfort, growth, and production

TABLE 5-4 ■ Erikson's Eight Developmental Stages

Age	Stage of Development	Task/Area of Resolution	Concepts/Basic Attitudes
Birth–18 months	Infancy	Trust versus mistrust	Ability to trust others and a sense of one's own trustworthiness; a sense of hope; withdrawal and estrangement
18 months–3 years	Early childhood	Autonomy versus shame and doubt	Self-control without loss of self-esteem; ability to cooperate and to express oneself; compulsive self-restraint or compliance; defiance, willfulness
3–5 years	Late childhood	Initiative versus guilt	Realistic sense of purpose; some ability to evaluate one's own behavior; self-denial and self-restriction
6–12 years	School age	Industry versus inferiority	Realization of competence, perseverance; feeling that one will never be "any good," withdrawal from school and peers
12–20 years	Adolescence	Identity versus role diffusion	Coherent sense of self; plans to actualize one's abilities; feelings of confusion, indecisiveness, possibly antisocial behavior
18–25 years	Young adulthood	Intimacy versus isolation	Capacity for love as mutual devotion; commitment to work and relationships; impersonal relationships, prejudice
25–65 years	Adulthood	Generativity versus stagnation	Creativity, productivity, concern for others; self-indulgence, impoverishment of self
65 years to death	Old age	Integrity versus despair	Acceptance of the worth and uniqueness of one's life; sense of loss, contempt for others

are surrendered for the sake of survival at the best level possible but at the sacrifice of emergency coping devices. Therapists using the general systems approach emphasize current conflicts, restoration of impaired systems of functioning, and subsequent reintegration of the restored function into future coping strategies.

Implications for Psychiatric–Mental Health Nursing Practice

Social–interpersonal theories give independent and collaborative psychiatric–mental health nursing clear theoretic direction and support. Nursing roles are associated with shifts in the delivery of psychiatric services variously termed *case management*, *social psychiatry*, *community psychiatry*, *psychoeducation*, and *milieu therapy*. According to these orientations, all social, psychologic, and biologic activity (including research developments in psychobiology) that affect the mental health of the population is important to professionals in community psychiatry. Therapeutic interventions may include programs for social change, political involvement, community organization, social planning, family support groups, and education about medications, symptom management, genetic risk, and family environment. Many implications for practice can be derived from this theoretic model, which are reflected in the following examples:

- Clients are approached in a holistic way, reflecting the interrelationship and interaction between the biophysical, psychologic, and socioeconomic–cultural dimensions of human life.
- Definitions of the client must include the concept of the client system. A family, a couple, an aggregate, or even a community may collectively constitute the client.
- Intervention strategies include primary prevention achieved through psychoeducation, social change, and research.
- Therapy focuses on helping troubled people gain a useful perspective on their lifestyle and social environment.
- Therapy also focuses on helping trouble people develop coping skills and resources rather repressing and controlling their symptoms.
- Psychiatric–mental health nurses must synthesize psychobiologic knowledge with psychosocial rehabilitations skills (see Chapter 32∞) and psychoeducation.
- Psychiatric–mental health nurses must be prepared to function as autonomous members of the mental health team and to assume more responsibilities in the shift away from the dominance of the physician in decision making and toward diffusion of roles.

Once clients are viewed as becoming dysfunctional in the context of unhealthy or problem-filled interpersonal relationships, establishing healthy, constructive interpersonal relationships becomes important in their care. Psychiatric–mental

health nurses can apply concepts of milieu therapy, primary prevention, social psychiatry, community psychiatry, and psychobiologic interventions to implement this fundamental idea. The following clinical example and discussion that follows demonstrate how these concepts can be applied in clinical practice.

Clinical Example

Mrs. Seminara is a 67-year-old woman in good physical health. She has become increasingly untidy, forgetful, reclusive, sad, and suspicious since the death of her aggressive, bank-president husband from a heart attack 6 months ago. She recently sold the large house where she had lived for the past 45 years and moved into a two-bedroom apartment in a nearby town. Because of apartment rules, she was unable to take her 12-year-old cat. She sold the house because her husband had told his lawyers that she should do so. (He made all the family decisions while he lived.) Mrs. Seminara has taken to skipping meals except for candy bars because she must rely on a friend to drive her to the grocery store. (Her husband believed she did not need to learn to drive.) Her younger sister (age 59), seeking advice about Mrs. Seminara's behavior, phoned the community mental health center at the suggestion of the family physician.

The social–interpersonal psychiatric–mental health nurse assessing this situation would tend not to view Mrs. Seminara's symptoms as psychological conflicts reflecting her ambivalence toward her dead husband or as manifestations of a mental disorder, such as major, single-episode depression. Instead, the nurse would focus on the way Mrs. Seminara is functioning in her current interpersonal situation and her holistic human responses to it. In this analysis, the nurse does not view Mrs. Seminara as "diseased" and therefore in exclusive need of a somatic treatment such as medication.

Instead, treatment consists of helping Mrs. Seminara develop strategies for coping with her new situation and satisfying her needs. The nurse would seek out the younger sister and other family members in an attempt to enhance Mrs. Seminara's social support network. Efforts may be directed toward mobilizing other environmental forces (including the nurse) to provide company, stimulation, and proper nutrition for Mrs. Seminara, since the absence of all three contributes to her symptoms and discomfort. The clinical situation would undoubtedly reinforce the psychiatric nurse's political efforts to point out the potential consequences of lifelong passive dependence for some adult women. The nurse may also become involved in community organizations working for better services for older clients.

The shifts in the delivery of psychiatric services toward a social psychiatry or community psychiatry view are associated with efforts to provide psychiatric services more efficiently to large groups of people (particularly those previously neglected), and attempts to counteract the debilitating effects of long-term institutionalization. Social psychiatry or community psychiatry are associated with a movement to address the client's social context in providing psychiatric care.

Pearson Nursing Student Resources
Find additional review materials at
nursing.pearsonhighered.com
Prepare for success with NCLEX®-style practice questions,
interactive assignments and activities, web links, animations
and videos, and more!

REFERENCES

Adler, A. (1971). *The practice and theory of individual psychology.* New York, NY: Humanities Press.

American Psychiatric Association. (2000). *Diagnostic and statistical manual of mental disorders* (4th ed., Text Revision) (DSM-IV-TR). Washington, DC: Author.

Butcher, J. N., Mineka, S., & Hooley, J. M. (2010). *Abnormal psychology* (14th ed.). Boston, MA: Allyn & Bacon.

Chiovitti, R. F. (2011). Theory of protective empowering for balancing patient safety and choices. *Nursing Ethics, 18*(1), 88–101.

Ciccarelli, S. K., & White, J. N. (2009). *Psychology* (2nd ed.). Upper Saddle River, NJ: Pearson.

Crews, F. C. (1998). *Unauthorized Freud: Doubters confront a legend.* New York, NY: Viking Press.

Erikson, E. (1963). *Childhood and society* (2nd ed.). New York, NY: Norton.

Freud, S. (1962). *The ego and the id.* New York, NY: Norton.

Fromm, E. (1941). *Escape from freedom.* New York, NY: Irvington.

Hewitt, J. P., & Shulman, D. (2011). *Self and society: A symbolic interactionist social psychology* (11th ed.). Boston, MA: Allyn & Bacon.

Horney, K. (1950). *Neurosis and human growth.* New York, NY: Norton.

Lamont, C. (1967). *The philosophy of humanism.* New York, NY: Frederick Ungar.

Maslow, A. (1962). *Toward a psychology of being.* New York, NY: Van Nostrand.

Maslow, A., & Lowery, R. (1998). *Toward a psychology of being* (3rd ed.). New York: Wiley & Sons.

Menninger, K. (1963). *The vital balance.* New York, NY: Viking Press.

Nichols, M. P. (2010). *Family therapy.* Boston, MA: Allyn & Bacon.

Skinner, B. F. (1971). *Beyond freedom and dignity.* New York, NY: Prentice Hall.

Sullivan, H. S. (1953). *The interpersonal theory of psychiatry.* New York, NY: W. W. Norton.

von Bertalanffy, L. (1968). *General systems theory.* New York, NY: Braziller.

Wallace, E. R., & Gach, J. (2011). *History of psychiatry and medical psychology.* New York, NY: Springer-Verlag.

Webster, R. (1995). *Why Freud was wrong: Sin, science, and psychoanalysis.* New York, NY: Basic Books.

Wolpe, J. (1956). Learning versus lesions as the basis of neurotic behavior. *American Journal of Psychiatry, 112,* 923–931.

The Biologic Basis of Behavioral and Mental Disorders

EILEEN TRIGOBOFF

LEARNING OUTCOMES

After completing this chapter, you will be able to:

1. Describe five neuroanatomic structures that affect thought, behavior, memory, understanding of consequences, and emotions.
2. Systematically compare and contrast alterations of the neuromessengers that occur in schizophrenia, bipolar disorder, and major depression.
3. Provide three examples of genetic contributions to mental disorder.
4. Identify two ways in which communication between the endocrine and immune systems affects a person's mood and behavior.
5. Explain how understanding the biologic contribution to emotional problems contributes to your nursing practice.
6. Partner with clients and families to teach the biologic implications of psychiatric illnesses.
7. Analyze how your own personal feelings, opinions, or beliefs about psychobiology can enhance or diminish your ability to be a support person and advocate for clients and their families.

CRITICAL THINKING CHALLENGE

Imagine you are the nurse at a family care clinic, and Kay, a 30-year-old woman with mood swings, is being assessed. During your clinical interview you discover she is currently a caretaker for several family members: her father, who has dementia of the Alzheimer's type; her mother, who is depressed and unable to function; and her 38-year-old brother, who has severe symptoms of paranoid schizophrenia. Major psychiatric illnesses are now understood as brain diseases that affect behavior, cognition, learning, and emotion. This knowledge has ramifications as it relates to your role, because the interventions that are aimed at improving overall functioning must consider Kay's unique biologic, environmental, and psychosocial strengths and weaknesses.

1. How can you integrate the understanding of the biologic components of Kay's functioning when providing comprehensive care?
2. Do you have a responsibility to integrate the biologic information with the behavioral and affective components of Kay's life? Why, or why not?

Psychobiology is neither a new concept nor a recent discovery. It has existed since the birth of humankind and has been a subject of discussion for at least the last 2,000 years. What *is* new in psychobiology is a broader understanding of the biologic basis of the mind and behavior. This understanding lowers the likelihood that people with psychiatric disorders will experience stigma. Current knowledge about the biologic components of behavior is revolutionizing not only psychiatry but also our view of behavior, temperament, and psychiatric disorders and their treatment.

Psychobiology encompasses an enormous amount of information and current research contributes to its growth. The study of the brain structures, biochemical foundations, molecular and genetic influences on cognition, mood, emotion, affect, and behavior and the interactions among them make up the realm of psychobiology. This comprehensive view takes into consideration both internal and external influences across a person's life span, including genetics, the effects of other body systems such as the endocrine and immune systems, temperament, resilience in the face of stress, and the environment.

A major barrier to seeking care for psychiatric symptoms can be stigma. Stigma results from lack of knowledge, misunderstanding how a severe mental disorder comes about, and not a small contribution from media sources that sensationalize events, issue misinformed and ill-conceived explanations, and demonize those who are ill. In addition, there are a great many sites on the Internet that do not offer entirely accurate information. Every instance of erroneousness and distortion can fuel someone's frightened or angry interaction. Stigma is often the result (see Chapter 1∞).

Science has provided more relevant explanations for psychiatric symptomatology than the long-held myth that parenting styles and lack of character are, in and of themselves, responsible. Understanding the working hypotheses of psychobiology is important for removing the guilt and stigma associated with psychiatric disorders. Teaching clients and families about the biologic aspects of the disorder increases their understanding of the illness and its treatment, and can increase the client's motivation to continue to seek appropriate treatment.

The standards of practice for psychiatric–mental health nursing (American Nurses Association, American Psychiatric Nurses Association, & International Society of Psychiatric–Mental Health Nurses, 2007) urge the inclusion of biologic therapies along with the use of the more traditional psychotherapy, psychosocial therapies, and combination therapies in the ongoing shift to a community-based care system. Excellence-based psychiatric–mental health nursing integrates psychobiologic concepts with our traditional practice to provide holistic caring for both clients and their families. Our understanding of the role biologic factors play in the client's illness and recovery can assist the client in adhering to medication regimens and other therapeutic interventions through psychoeducation and partnerships.

In this chapter we highlight the psychobiologic principles that can be used in the nursing care of a client. The scope of this chapter curtails how much psychobiology we can explore, therefore we crafted this chapter to help you apply basic psychobiologic principles to your professional work. To help integrate these psychobiologic principles into your clinical practice, this chapter will focus on structure and function and how they both play key roles in behavior and emotional communication.

BRAIN, MIND, AND BEHAVIOR

Communication is a vital aspect of psychiatric–mental health nursing. Through neurobiologic discoveries we now know that communication, behaviors, and thought patterns have a molecular, anatomic, and chemical basis. Who we are originates from order or disorder at any of these levels.

The brain encodes or decodes information through complex interactions of neuromessengers, chemical processes, and anatomic systems. When clients ask about their symptoms you can provide useful information using current neurobiologic knowledge. For example, a client who has panic attacks certainly feels like they are real, but may not know why they occur. You can bring an understandable scientific explanation of how panic attacks result from the triggering of an over-reactive alarm center in the brain. This trigger sends a message of fear via the release of a neurotransmitter, causing a racing heart and shortness of breath.

Certain portions of the brain function in concert with other parts to create a system with a specific action; the limbic system is a good example. Other systems that are of special interest to psychiatric–mental health nurses include the reticular activating system and the extrapyramidal system, which are discussed later in this chapter.

Neuroanatomy

Volumes have been written about the anatomy of the brain and the other components of the nervous system. The definition that best suits the perspective of this chapter is that the brain is a part of the central nervous system (CNS; that also includes the spinal cord) encapsulated by the skull. The brain is the core of our humanity. Intercommunication among different parts of the brain yields the experiences of love, hate, joy, fear, silliness, and sadness. The brain provides the underlying biology for will, determination, hopes, and dreams as well as the ability to problem solve, to establish memory, and to learn and use acquired knowledge productively. The major features of the brain discussed here are the cerebrum, diencephalon, mesencephalon, pons, medulla oblongata, and cerebellum.

Cerebrum

The cerebrum includes the following structures and functions:

- Cerebral hemispheres
- Conscious thought processes and intellectual functions
- Memory storage and processing
- Conscious and subconscious regulation of skeletal muscle contractions

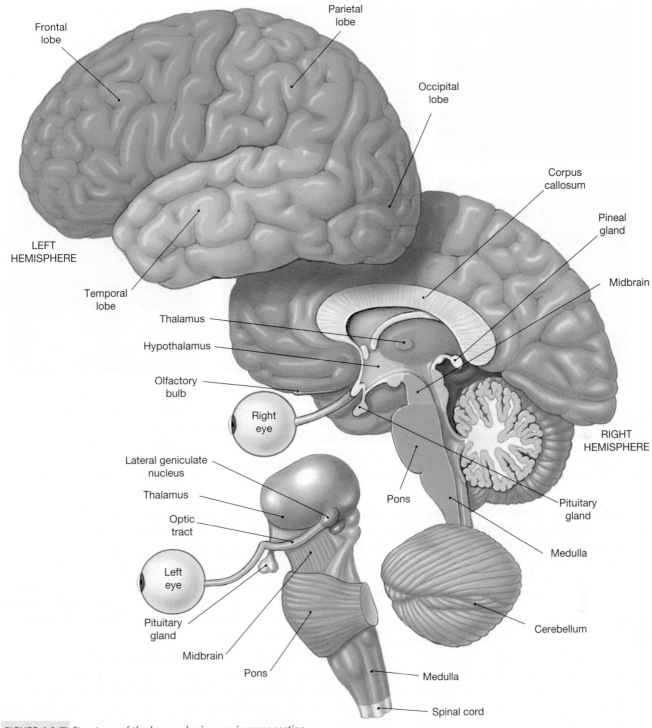

FIGURE 6-1 ■ Structures of the human brain seen in cross-section.
Source: Smock, T. K. (1999). *Physiological psychology: A neuroscience approach.* Upper Saddle River, NJ: Prentice Hall.

If you were to dissect the brain, you would see only indistinguishable gray matter, layer after layer. It is remarkable that such homogenous-looking tissue can be fundamentally varied. See FIGURE 6-1 ■, a cross-sectional view of the structures of the brain. Advantages of technological advances such as brain imaging allow us to study the brain in a number of ways. Electroencephalograms (EEGs), computerized tomography

(CT) scans, magnetic resonance imaging (MRI), and positron emission tomography (PET) scans all give us a glimpse of how the brain works. FIGURE 6-2 ■ shows these techniques.

The **cerebrum** comprises the largest part of the human brain. It is divided into two components, the *cerebral hemispheres*. The deep furrow that divides the hemispheres is the *longitudinal sulcus*. A small but important piece of tissue,

FIGURE 6-2 ■ Studying the brain. These are four methods researchers use to study the brain: EEGs, CT scans, MRIs, and PET scans. (a) An example of an EEG readout. (b) A CT scan (colored by a computer) showing the detail of a center cross-section of the brain. (c) An MRI (colored by a computer) showing enhanced detail of the same view of the brain as in the CT scan. (d) A PET scan showing activity of the brain, using colors to indicate different levels of activity; areas that are very active are white, whereas areas that are inactive are dark blue. (e) An fMRI tracking the oxygen levels in the brain shows the difference between brain activity when preparing to make a gesture and brain activity when actually making the gesture.
Source: Ciccarelli, S. K., & White, J. M. (2009). *Psychology* (2nd ed.). Upper Saddle River, NJ: Pearson Education, p. 66.
Photo courtesy of (a) SPL/Photo Researchers, Inc.; (b) Alfred Pasieka/Photo Researchers, Inc.; (c) © Pete Saloutos/Corbis; (d) Tim Beddow/Photo Researchers, Inc.; (e) Corbis.

the *corpus callosum,* connects the two hemispheres medially and allows communication between them through networks of neurologic fibers. In the past, scientists believed that each hemisphere had separate functions, such as logic or creativity and spatial accommodation. With technologies such as positron-emission tomography (PET) it is now possible to assess metabolic activity in the brain as it occurs (see Box 6-1). Scientists are now able to observe brain activity and have concluded that creative as well as logical activities require input from both cerebral hemispheres.

The cerebral hemispheres are divided into four lobes, named after the parts of the skull under which they lie: frontal, parietal, temporal, and occipital (see Box 6-2). The lobes have pairs on each side of the corpus callosum, which splits the brain in half. These lobes comprise the *neocortex.* The neocortex is involved in the subjective experience of emotion, motivation, learning, memory, and gross motor skills. Each lobe has unique functions that contribute to a person's ability to move, process information, and have thoughts and feelings.

Frontal Lobe The frontal lobe has functional responsibilities for muscular movement and *vegetative effects* (slowing effects) on respiration and circulation. After receiving information from the limbic system, the frontal lobe affects motivation, thinking, and how one understands consequences to behavior. You may have already seen during clinical rotations how lesions in the

frontal lobe lead to a host of problems. See Box 6-3 for information on the practical impacts of frontal lobe damage or a lesion.

Temporal Lobe The temporal lobe is the emotional center and is involved with memory and cognition. This lobe helps us understand the acoustic aspects of language. It is the primary auditory cortex. The limbic system, which is involved in emotions, memory, and thought patterns, will be covered later in this chapter.

Parietal Lobe The parietal lobe facilitates complex motor and cognitive skills, such as a mastery of visual and spatial balance, math abilities, and spelling. The parietal lobe is also the primary somatosensory area receiving input from the thalamus—you know what your body is trying to tell you because the parietal lobe is working.

Occipital Lobe The occipital lobe is involved in visual perception and recognition (Ankney & Colbert, 2011). All the lobes contain many gyri (ridges), fissures, and sulci (grooves) that serve to maximize the surface area of the brain.

The brain in general, and the cerebral hemispheres in particular, are well protected not only by the skull but also by a protective fluid, called *cerebrospinal fluid (CSF),* that circulates around and within the brain. Deep within the brain are three spaces, or ventricles, that aid in the circulation of CSF. Normal CSF volume is about 125 mL in an average adult and

---

Box 6-1 Tools of Psychobiology

Brain Imaging

- *Computed tomography (CT).* An X-ray beam (radiation exposure) is passed through serial sections of the brain to look at structural images.
- *Magnetic resonance imaging (MRI).* Reconstructs detailed images of cerebral anatomy from multiple perspectives, including subcortical structures, using radio frequency signals emitted by relaxing hydrogen atoms. It delineates gray and white matter. New instruments image elements other than hydrogen, allowing an MRI to be used for structural imaging. An fMRI (functional MRI) is used to detect the functional and metabolic processes under review. Contraindicated for clients with any metal objects in their bodies such as pacemakers, due to the presence of a magnetic field.
- *Positron emission tomography (PET).* Imaging of active neurochemical substrates and physiological processes; regional localization of metabolic functions through the measurement of radioactive labels or tags attached to molecules as glucose; density of neuroreceptors; regional cerebral blood flow (rCBF) of the brain. Operates on the principle that blood rushes to the busiest area of the brain to deliver oxygen and nutrients to the active neurons.
- *Single photon-emission computed tomography (SPECT).* Measures rCBF; visualizes and measures the density of neuroreceptors, using tracer isotopes such as xenon, a gas; iodine 123; or technetium.

Neurophysiological Techniques

- *Electroencephalogram (EEG).* Measures electrical activity patterns of the brain from leads connected to surface electrodes placed on the scalp and nasopharyngeal area.
- *Polysomnography (sleep EEG).* Measures electrical brain activity data during all-night sleep.

- *Brain electroactivity mapping (BEAM).* Extends the EEG by generating computerized maps of brain electrical activity to produce images; permits visualization of the brain performing tasks or specific functions. Useful with children.
- *Event-related potential (ERP).* Repeated auditory or visual stimuli associated with tiny electrical events in the cerebral cortex or subcortical structures, measured by surface electrodes.

Pharmacologic Challenge

A pharmacologic challenge involves the use of a medication to provoke (challenge) a neuronal system to better understand its physiological effects and changes. Examples are the dexamethasone suppression test (DST), thyrotropin-releasing hormone (TRH) challenge, or giving a medication known to have specific receptor affinity such as clonidine to examine the alpha-2-adrenergic system in panic disorder.

Molecular Genetics

- *Linkage map.* A genetic map that represents the relationship between two genes, often revealed by the inheritance of traits in families, to determine the relative position of genes on a given chromosome.
- *Restriction fragment length polymorphisms (RFLPs).* Method of molecular genetics using restriction enzymes, which cuts a DNA strand at sites where the enzyme recognizes a sequence between coding information. Differences in the lengths of these restriction fragments are believed to be inherited. The transmission can be mapped within families and a genetic pattern of transmission identified.
- *Candidate genes.* Identification of a specific gene thought to have pathophysiological relevance to the illness being studied.

Box 6-2 Functions of the Cerebral Lobes

Frontal Lobes

- Responsible for movement; the right frontal lobe controls the left side of the body's movements, the left controls the right-sided movements
- Contain the premotor cortex, which organizes complicated movement
- Contain prefrontal fibers with capacities for planning and problem solving; also responsible for social judgment, volition, attention, learning, spontaneity, thinking, and affect
- Responsible for executive functioning, which determines how information is interpreted; starting and stopping certain functions (such as verbal exchanges); and filtering and screening out extraneous information

Parietal Lobes

- Contain the sensory cortex, which interprets contact sensations such as touch and pressure
- Facilitate spatial orientation

Temporal Lobes

- Involved in hearing, memory, language comprehension, and emotions
- Connect with the limbic system (the "emotional brain") to allow for the expression of emotions such as rage, fear, sexual and aggressive behavior, and possibly love; damage to temporal lobes is sometimes seen as extreme and inappropriate expressions of these feelings

Occipital Lobes

- Facilitate the interpretation of visual images and visual memory
- Involved in language formation
- Collaborate with many other brain structures in the formation of memory

---

Box 6-3   Practical Impacts of Frontal Lobe Damage or Lesion

The frontal lobe organizes various aspects of everyday interactions and functioning. Examples of the effects of damage to this lobe are as follows:

Speech

- In a slow-moving supermarket line, someone with frontal-lobe damage might curse and shout at others in line in a way not typical of that person prior to the injury.
- The capacity to restrain or inhibit expressions of strong emotion may be impaired, regardless of the circumstances. The person will make inappropriate sexual comments, ask rude questions, or say things that others may think but do not say, such as "You're not too bright, are you?" or "Your breath really stinks."
- The person may have difficulty comprehending a moderately abstract idea, such as an assignment to oversee an area or a process and would not be likely to tell you when he was feeling overwhelmed.

Motor and Voluntary Movement

- There will be considerable trouble using a straw, groping for objects, and gripping objects (objects are often dropped).

Drive and Motivation

- There will be a noticeable loss of energy to participate in activities.
- Hygiene activities are neglected or not completed.

Thinking

- Reactions occur without trying to think it through because it is too demanding.

Planning

- The person has difficulty developing and keeping to a schedule.
- Arranging any type of transportation (bus schedules, calling for a ride) is challenging.

Concentration

- The person will have regular and remarkable forgetfulness.
- Someone with a frontal lobe problem will not be able to track events that occur in the environment.

Ability to Sort Out What Is Happening in the Environment

- Stimuli, both internal and external, are disorganized and affect the ability to react.
- The person is easily overwhelmed.

Shifting from One Mental Activity to Another

- The person will have difficulty making the shift from, for example, watching TV to talking to another person.

Behavior

- The person demonstrates an easy loss of self-control and has temper tantrums.
- Mood changes are common.
- The person is apathetic (not caring about events or ideas).

---

is replaced approximately four times in 24 hours. The CSF reflects neurochemical activity of the brain and is one method for studying in vivo (within the living organism) communication. The purposes of spinal taps are to measure the volume and pressure of the CSF; to look for trauma, blood, or infection; and to measure metabolites, which are the products or substances produced from the breakdown of metabolic processes of the brain's neuromessengers.

The cerebral hemispheres consist of both white and gray matter. Gray matter consists of fibers called *nerves;* bundles of nerves are called *tracts.* The cerebral cortex consists solely of gray matter with underlying white matter. The white matter is an indication of myelination. The white matter increases with age, while gray matter decreases with age. The corpus callosum, a white matter structure, grows in size about 1.8% each year between the ages of 3 and 18 years. This structure

MENTAL HEALTH IN THE MOVIES
Rainman

The dichotomy between the deficits of autism and the skills called *savant skills* were displayed in the film *Rainman.* The inspiration for the autistic brother depicted in the movie was Kim Peek, an autistic man (who recently died). Mr. Peek had limited social skills and was taken care of by his father for his day-to-day needs. When Mr. Peek and his father educate people on autism he demonstrated one of his many extraordinary skills at the beginning of every conference. Typically, he was introduced to each person in the audience as they entered the auditorium or conference center. During the talk Mr. Peek demonstrated that he remembered not only the name of every person at the conference, but every person he ever met—over one million people.

The neuroanatomic and biologic difference between Mr. Peek and most other people is that he did not have a corpus callosum. Because he had access to his entire brain without the mediating influence of the corpus callosum, Mr. Peek could think and remember very quickly and completely. This contributed to his great memory in that not only could he remember people, but he could also quote dialogue from any movie, and tell you the day of the week for any date you selected. Despite these unique abiities, problem-solving was always a challenge for him.
Photo courtesy of Alamy.

Seizure Videos and Animations

integrates the activity between the left and right cerebral hemispheres. The increase in corpus callosum may be a sign of an increased ability for problem solving (Boyd & Bee, 2012). See Mental Health in the Movies for an excellent example of what happens when a person does not have a corpus callosum.

The cerebral cortex produces results much like those produced by the central processing unit (CPU) of a computer. The cortex is the part of the brain that makes sense out of volumes of input. It processes and synthesizes information, thought, reasoning, will, and choice. Our dreams come from the cortex.

Limbic System

The **limbic system**, often called the *emotional brain,* the *primitive brain,* or the *reptilian brain,* is believed to be responsible for the experience and expression of emotion, as well as memory and some aspects of attention. It is involved in the creation of our emotional states, drives, and behaviors associated with feelings and motivations. The limbic system is not a cohesive structure located in one place in the brain; it is a functional grouping rather than an anatomic one. The limbic system consists of structures from the cerebral hemispheres and the *diencephalon,* a part of the brain located between the cerebrum and midbrain (see Box 6-4).

The following two limbic structures play an especially important role in how emotions and memories are generated:

1. Amygdala
2. Hippocampus

Learning and memory are two aspects of the interaction between the amygdala and the hippocampus.

The limbic structures also include the olfactory area. If the olfactory sensors determine a scent, the memory of the event will include this cue. For example, does the smell of baking cookies trigger a pleasant memory of being in a kitchen when cookies are being baked? This is the combined effect of amygdalar and hippocampal functions using the cue of the aroma of cookies as the stimulus for the memory.

Amygdala The **amygdala** gauges certain emotional reactions and plays a role in social behavior. It serves as the behavioral awareness center and helps pattern appropriate emotional and behavioral responses such as fear, sexual desire, rage, and appetite. It is hypothesized that the amygdala is also important in seeking love and sustaining long-term emotional memories.

Hippocampus The **hippocampus** is also involved in emotional reactions and in learning. It helps process, store, and retrieve information in our memory. It provides new information for permanent storage. Hallucinations may, in part, originate from hyperexcitability of psychomotor effects of olfactory, visual, auditory, and tactile stimulation in this region (Brown, 2010). Weak stimuli in the hippocampus can cause epileptic seizures.

The limbic system has numerous functions beyond those addressed here, and the neuronal connections are so widespread and intricate within the brain that their complex interactions involve many different areas. Other neuronal groups that participate with the limbic system are the thalamus, hypothalamus, and pituitary gland.

Reticular Activating System The reticular activating system (RAS) consists of nerve pathways that originate in the spinal cord and connect in the reticular formation, a system of neurons that modulates awareness and states of consciousness. By screening stimulation from the environment and helping us filter out what we don't need at the moment, the RAS enables us to concentrate. The RAS also permits us to not pay attention for a period of time, allowing us to sleep. During sleep, excitatory neurons of the RAS gradually become more and more excitable because of prolonged rest, while inhibitory neurons of sleep centers become less excitable because of overactivity, leading to a new cycle of wakefulness. This helps explain the rapid transitions between sleep and wakefulness. Arousal, as experienced by people with psychiatric conditions, can be the insomnia that occurs when a person's mind becomes preoccupied with a thought. In states of mental disorder, there is obviously some biologic disequilibrium of the RAS because it involves motivation and levels of arousal. However, the details of this imbalance are not yet well understood.

Extrapyramidal System The extrapyramidal system (so labeled because it lies alongside the outer aspects of the pyramidal system) consists of tracts of motor neurons from the brain to parts of the spinal cord. This system has complex relays and connections to areas of the cortex, cerebellum, brain stem, and thalamus. The tracts play an important role in gross movements and responses of emotional tone, such as smiling and frowning. Antipsychotic medications create side effects that affect the extrapyramidal system and are called *extrapyramidal side effects (EPSE).* A complete discussion of EPSE is in Chapters 7 and 31∞.

Diencephalon

The diencephalon is composed of the thalamus and the hypothalamus. The thalamus functions as a relay and processing center for sensory information. The hypothalamus controls emotions, autonomic functions, and hormone production.

Box 6-4 Structures of the Limbic System

Cerebral Components

Cortical areas: Limbic lobe (cingulate gyrus, dentate gyrus, and parahippocampal gyrus)
Nuclei: Hippocampus, amygdaloid body
Tracts: Fornix

Diencephalic Components

Thalamus: Forward (anterior) nuclear group
Hypothalamus: Center for emotions, appetites (thirst, hunger), and related behaviors

Other Components

Reticular formation: Network of nuclei throughout the brain stem

Thalamus The thalamus receives impulses from the spinal cord, brain stem, and cerebellum. With the aid of numerous connections in the cerebral hemispheres and cortex, the thalamus regulates activity and movement, sensory experience (except smell), and emotional expression.

Hypothalamus The **hypothalamus** is a "hub" between the mind and body, giving physical form to thoughts and emotions. It weighs approximately 4 grams and accounts for less than 1% of the total volume of the brain. Its size, however, is not a good indication of its importance. The hypothalamus regulates many of the body's critical activities, including hormone levels, appetite (hunger), body temperature (thermoreceptors), sex drive (libido), water balance (thirst), circadian rhythms, pleasure, and pain. See FIGURE 6-3 ■ for a graphic representation of the hypothalamus as a hub.

The hypothalamus is the critical link between the cerebral cortex, the limbic system, and the endocrine system. It serves as a pipeline to the brain stem and acts as a conduit for control of the autonomic nervous system. The mammillary bodies, located at the back of the hypothalamus, help transfer information about the activities of the hypothalamus to other parts of the brain. The amygdala controls hypothalamic impulses due to the direct neurologic connection. This control is important in the regulation of hunger, thirst, sexual behavior, rage, and/or pleasure.

The infundibulum, a narrow stalk, connects the hypothalamus to the pituitary gland, a part of the endocrine system. The hypothalamus is involved in hormonal balance along with the pituitary gland, which is crucial when the individual experiences a stress response (Ankney & Colbert, 2011). The thalamus and hypothalamus, as well as the pituitary gland, are illustrated in Figure 6-1.

Pituitary Gland

The pituitary gland, under the direction of the hypothalamus, secretes hormones. These hormones are carried through the bloodstream and trigger the activities of other endocrine glands. The pituitary also receives input from the fornix and includes connections to the thalamus, which in turn communicates to and from the frontal cortex. The pituitary gland is the primary link between the nervous and endocrine systems.

Basal Ganglia

The basal ganglia are collectively a set of structures that include the caudate nucleus, putamen, globus pallidus, and substantia nigra. Their functions include starting and stopping movements, planning motor activities, mediating hallucinations and delusions, and processing emotions and memories. The basal ganglia have a high concentration of dopamine receptors, acetylcholine, gamma-aminobutyric acid (GABA), and peptides. A deficit of dopamine in this area is associated with Parkinson's disease. Parkinson's disease is characterized by rhythmic tremors of the extremities, slurred speech, and an unchanging facial expression. Former boxer Muhammad Ali, who demonstrates all these symptoms, sustained numerous blows to his head that resulted in damage to the basal ganglia.

Cerebellum

The **cerebellum** lies below the posterior section of the cerebrum. It is our second largest brain structure. Like the cerebral hemispheres, the cerebellum has an outer layer of gray matter and is mainly composed of underlying white matter. The main function of this highly specialized part of the brain is movement, posture, balance, and sensory–motor coordination. The hand–eye coordination of a diamond cutter, the fluid movements of a ballerina, and the success of a quarterback's moves all depend on cerebellar functions. The cerebellum also coordinates complex somatic motor patterns and adjusts the output of other somatic motor centers in the brain and spinal cord.

Brain Stem

Beneath the structures in the limbic system is the **brain stem**. The brain stem consists of three smaller structures: the medulla oblongata, the pons, and the midbrain.

Medulla Oblongata The medulla oblongata (Latin for "oblong marrow," or the inner, oblong portion of the organ) relays sensory information to the thalamus and other portions of the brain stem. As the connecting piece of tissue between the brain stem and the spinal cord, it functions as the autonomic center for the regulation of visceral function (cardiovascular, respiratory, and digestive system activities). It is less than 5 cm long but is responsible for controlling many vital functions, including respiration, regulation of blood pressure, and partial regulation of heart rate. It also controls vomiting, swallowing, some aspects of talking, and the perception of pain. Incoming fibers from the spinal cord cross over in the medulla; thus, the left cerebral hemisphere controls the right side of the body, and vice versa.

Pons The pons (Latin for "bridge") contains conduction paths between the spinal cord and the brain, relaying sensory information to the cerebellum and thalamus and serving as a visceral and motor center. It is truly a bridge. It also contains reflex centers that mediate sensations of the face, chewing,

FIGURE 6-3 ■ The hypothalamus hub.

Control of autonomic nervous system

Cerebral cortex

Endocrine system

Hypothalamus

Limbic system

Brain stem

Hormone balance in partnership with pituitary gland

abduction of the eyes, facial expressions, balance, and the regulation of respiration. Located within the pons is the locus ceruleus, a tiny oval structure that contains 70% of the neurons (nerve cells) that release norepinephrine, a neurotransmitter affecting the entire brain. One projection of the pons is to the amygdala, resulting in emotional and cardiovascular control. Activation of the locus ceruleus is associated with fear, pain, and alarm.

Midbrain The midbrain, also called the *mesencephalon,* is located above the pons and below the cerebral hemispheres. The midbrain processes visual and auditory data and is a reflex center for the regulation of eye movement, visual accommodation, and regulation of pupil size. The midbrain is also essential for relaying impulses to the cerebral cortex, generating reflexive somatic motor responses (sending behavior-producing messages back to the rest of the body), and maintaining consciousness.

Autonomic Nervous System Within the brain stem is an area of the autonomic nervous system (ANS) known as the parasympathetic division. In stressful emotional circumstances, the sympathetic division of the ANS (also called the sympathetic nervous system), located in the spinal cord, prepares for fight or flight; the parasympathetic initiates the relaxation response with the aid of the endocrine system. Prolonged stress can weaken the immune system (Miodrag & Hodapp, 2010). Long-term effects may trigger mood disorders. Chapter 8∞ includes a complete review of stress reactions. The goal of meditation and other forms of stress management is to inhibit the sympathetic response and strengthen the parasympathetic response. Chapter 8 includes a complete review of stress reactions and Chapter 34∞ discusses stress management.

Genetics

Clients may tell you that others in their family experience "moodiness," "crazy thoughts," or that they "worry constantly for no reason." These are important clues to how major psychiatric disorders tend to run in families. A new area of research, genomics, explores genetic material for clues to a possible heritable basis of behavior in order to answer the question: What are the molecular consequences of abnormal genes? Applying genetic strategies to clinical practice will bring many new challenges and ethical dilemmas (some of these ethical dilemmas are discussed in Chapter 12∞). Alterations in genetic coding, or designer genes, are currently being used with diseases such as cancer and cystic fibrosis to supply healthy genes or block a defective gene. In the future, perhaps the following questions will be answered for us:

- How can understanding the biologic markers determine what medications may help an individual?
- What specific steps can a family take to decrease the incidence of a severe mental disorder if there is a high genetic loading based on history?
- How can nurses help clients understand the role genetics may play in emotional illness?
- Do the same genes, but a different environment, result in depression or an anxiety disorder?
- Does a stressful life event trigger genetically vulnerable neurons to promote rapid-cycling mood disorder or panic disorder?

To begin to answer these questions, a review of the chemical composition of genes and certain aspects of cell structure and function is necessary.

Gene Structure

In 1990, the Human Genome Project was established to discover gene structure, provide a map of how genes work, and locate the chemical base pairs that comprise DNA and the spaces between the chemical pairs, to determine abnormal or disease-linked genes.

The gene is the functional unit of information within the chromosome. The human genome consists of 23 pairs of chromosomes, one from each parent; 22 pairs are the somatic chromosomes, and one pair is the sex chromosome (XX female, XY male). Genes are segments of *DNA* (deoxyribonucleic acid), the complex molecule that comprises chromosomes, and are found in all the body's cell nuclei. Each cell uses its complement of genes in a specific way. The genes make proteins that are necessary for the cell to do its assigned task. For example, a bone cell gene differs from a brain cell gene in structure and function. Our *genotype,* or our genetic makeup, differs from our *phenotype,* how our genes are actually expressed.

RNA (ribonucleic acid) is another complex molecule that plays a role in translating DNA's coding instructions for making protein. Each strand of the complex molecule of DNA is compactly formed into a double helix. The strand of DNA is composed of chemical nucleotides consisting of one sugar

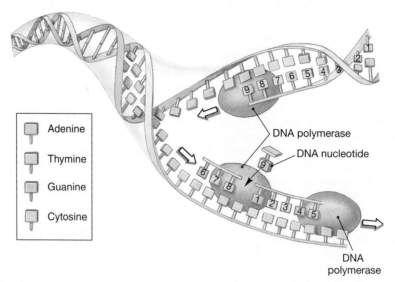

Adenine

Thymine

Guanine

Cytosine

DNA polymerase

DNA nucleotide

DNA polymerase

FIGURE 6-4 ■ The structure of DNA shows how each strand of the complex molecule is compactly formed into a double helix and the strand of DNA is composed of the chemical nucleotides adenine (A), thymine (T), guanine (G), and cytosine (C), which fit together like the teeth of a zipper.
Source: Martini, F. H. (2001). *Fundamentals of anatomy and physiology.* Upper Saddle River, NJ: Prentice Hall.

molecule (DNA or RNA), one phosphate group, and one of four nitrogen bases. The nucleotides are as follows:

■ Adenine (A)
■ Thymine (T)
■ Guanine (G)
■ Cytosine (C)

The nucleotides line up next to each other like two sides of a zipper, with the phosphate and sugar forming the outer strand; the bases (A, T, G, and C) act like interlocking teeth (see FIGURE 6-4 ■). The sequence of amino acids, which are proteins, is coded by genes. The sequence or code is like a language and is not arbitrary. The nucleotides, or two sides of the zipper, can fit together in only one way: A pairs with T, and G pairs with C. This base pairing allows for the known sequence of one strand to predict the partner strand. Each strand of the double helix thus specifies its complement and allows for the duplication of genetic information in dividing cells.

Gene Function

Variations in the chemical composition of the genes can produce abnormal structural proteins or enzymes, altering how signals are sent or received and resulting in dysfunction or disease. The main component of all living matter is protein, which consists of large molecules or long chains of amino acids linked together. The sequence of amino acids along the chain determines each protein's physical and biologic properties, acting as information molecules.

The transfer of DNA from the nucleus requires messenger RNA (mRNA), which serves as the instructor for making proteins outside the nucleus. Ribosomes, which float in the cytoplasm or sit on the rough endoplasmic reticulum, translate the mRNA into proteins. Also in the cytoplasm are the mitochondria, which generate energy, via ions and adenosine

triphosphate (ATP), from the oxidation of fats and sugars, and also contain RNA and DNA.

Instructions for synthesizing and metabolizing molecular messengers of the brain are coded in the DNA. A typical protein has a useful life of about 2 days, so new protein molecules are constantly being synthesized. Genes can be mutated by a single mismatch of the wrong base in the DNA, or a piece of the DNA can be mistakenly repeated, deleted, or altered. This error could cause the cell to function in a changed manner. This may help explain how a client's symptoms or behavioral expression can change over time. New messages among the complex combinations of proteins change the code in the physical environment, resulting in different expressions of temperament, behavior, and individuality.

New technologies enable researchers to modify DNA and RNA so that both the messages and the expression of the messages can be manipulated experimentally. DNA markers, from fragments of DNA (restriction fragment length polymorphisms, or RFLPs), are making it possible to identify and localize the genes involved in a disease process. RFLPs represent a direct reflection of the DNA sequence and can be used to determine accuracy on kinship and group relationships. RFLP separation has led to a large library of DNA sequence markers and a human mutation database. This information has assisted researchers in determining the probability that a mutation can take place at any specific area of the genome and can affect functioning and symptoms (Kareken et al., 2010). The data gathered in the mutation database help us to understand the pathophysiology of a disease and its treatment and possibly, in the future, its prevention.

The polymerase chain reaction (PCR) is another technology used with DNA. Even a single cell would be enough to start the process of analyzing a DNA fragment with PCR, because the amounts needed for analysis can be generated from that cell. This process reproduces individual fragments of DNA and is used in genetic engineering efforts and research investigations (Morgan, Dudley, & Rosenberg, 2010). PCR was used to develop a number of diagnostic tests to detect disease-causing agents, and it is used in determining paternity. Also, in forensic medicine, PCR has proved indispensable for criminal investigations.

Genetic Research

Psychiatric-focused genetic studies are conducted by examining the blood of family members who have mental disorders. Linkage studies are a type of genetic blood study used to locate genes that are thought to be involved in susceptibility to emotional illness. These studies examine the inheritance patterns of known DNA markers. This research assists in understanding the possible location of a suspect gene for an identified disorder, although the results thus far have not shown one particular gene as the culprit for any major mental disorder (Avramopoulos, 2010).

The National Human Genome Research Institute (NHGRI), part of the National Institutes of Health (NIH), is encouraging research that would lower the cost of sequencing a mammalian-sized genome. Lower costs would enable researchers to sequence the genomes of hundreds or even thousands of people to identify genes that contribute to common, complex diseases. If the cost of whole-genome sequencing is cut to a manageable level, sequencing individual genomes may become part of routine medical care and would allow us to tailor diagnosis, treatment, and prevention to each person's unique genetic profile.

Ethics in Genetic Research

When a genetic loading component has the potential to create a mental disorder, the ethical implications can be controversial:

- How should a mental health professional proceed in discussions about heritability of the illness?

- What treatments are offered if, in the future, a gene is identified as causing a mental disorder and a child with no symptoms has that gene?

The ethical dilemmas include waiting until the child experiences symptoms and treating at that point, or treating before any symptoms appear. These are not clear choices. But overall, nurses need to be familiar with the biologic mechanism of the illness to help clients make decisions about their care, their choices about childbearing, and to avoid the potential stigma associated with the genetics of mental disorders. See the Evidence-Based Practice feature for a perspective on this issue.

The ethics of genetic research is another area under examination. Consent for study participation includes being given information about the study and understanding the risks and benefits of the research, what is involved in study participation, and what will be done with the genetic information obtained during the course of the study. Researchers must define how the information that is gathered during the study is secured, how the client's identity will be protected, and what will be reported. Confidentiality in keeping the genetics of the study sample anonymous is an essential consideration for the participants. Study participants have the right in every study to ask questions of the principal investigator (Sterling, 2011).

Questions might include, among others:

1. What do the individual results mean?
2. What implications might genetic results have for children?
3. What implications could genetic results have for developing physical illnesses?

More on this topic is included in Chapter 12∞.

The Genetic Basis of Psychiatric Illness

The field of genetics maps the genetics of psychiatry more completely each year. Research on the genetic basis of inherited

---

EVIDENCE-BASED PRACTICE

Genetic Counseling

Your work as a nurse involves contacts with those in rural areas or low–population density sectors. Access to genetics specialists can be limited, or nonexistent, in these areas. With all the advances being made in genetic determinations and the potential, as well as the reality, of genetic treatments, it is important for you to keep your knowledge base about genetics current.

Evidence is strong that developing strategies for translating research discoveries and pilot project findings into realities will be essential to improving health care for the whole community. Some strategies that will improve fairness and create a more equitable distribution of genetic services for society as a whole, not just those fortunate enough to live close to a major genetic center, are as follows:

- Enabling genetic technologies, with proven utility, to be implemented in a timely and effective manner
- Providing educated professionals who can discuss and counsel regarding genetics

Hawkins, A. K., & Hayden, M. R. (2011). A grand challenge: Providing benefits of clinical genetics to those in need. *Genetic Medicine, 13*(3), 197–200.

CRITICAL THINKING QUESTIONS

1. What ethical questions do genetic testing and the subsequent counseling raise?
2. What legal questions does genetic counseling raise?
3. Why should the ethical and legal issues raised by genetics be of concern to psychiatric–mental health nurses?

psychiatric illnesses has been a focus of the Office of Human Genetics and Genomic Resources in the National Institute of Mental Health (NIMH). This group supports research on the identification, localization, function, and expression patterns of genes that produce susceptibility to mental disorders.

Research findings will set the stage for our understanding of the complexity of the genetic and environmental influences on mental disorders. All the genetic models must consider the roles of environmental influences, perinatal events, trauma, infections, and stress. When evaluating clients and families for possible genetic links to an emotional disorder, it is important to consider the interaction between the genetic factors and the environment (Miodrag & Hodapp, 2010).

Nurse scientists and those from other disciplines have discovered the following:

- There is no single gene responsible for a mental disorder.
- There may be several susceptibility genes that interact with one another.
- Environmental influences interact with genes to increase the risk of developing a mental disorder.

Current research is developing in two directions. The Human Genome Project and genetic mapping have enabled researchers to look for chromosomes that may be implicated in a disease. For example, researchers identified molecular approaches to the genetics of psychiatric disorders (Avramopoulos, 2010; Stewart & Pauls, 2010). Another area of study you will see often in the literature involves examining the altered genetic material of mouse brains. This type of research is vital in helping us understand the structure and behavior patterns demonstrated in these altered animals. This body of research is useful in testing hypotheses about the nature of mental disorders in humans as well as in testing new medications.

Neurons, Synapses, and Neurotransmission

The brain's structural complexity increases as one considers the biochemical processes that occur with every thought, emotion, memory, dream, or hope. Thoughts and feelings are made possible by the complex interplay and communication between cells in the central nervous system (CNS) in response to stimuli in the environment.

The specialized cells of the nervous system are called **neurons**. Like other cells in the body, each neuron has a cell body that contains cytoplasm and a nucleus. Unlike other cells, a neuron has at least two other extensions: an axon and one or more dendrites. An axon is the portion of a neuron that conveys electric impulses from the cell body to other neurons. Axons are covered with a white myelin sheath and are the white matter in the brain and spinal cord. Dendrites are unmyelinated and conduct electrical messages to the cell body. There are approximately 100 billion neurons in the brain and nearly an equal number of supporting (glia) cells.

Neurons are classified according to the direction in which they conduct impulses. Sensory neurons, also known as *afferent neurons,* send messages from the peripheral body parts to the brain. For example, if you place your foot into a tub of scalding water, the message that the water is too hot is sent to your brain via sensory neuron pathways. Motor neurons, or efferent neurons, carry messages that originate in the brain and yield a behavioral change in the peripheral body parts. When your foot is in the hot water, the message from your brain is to remove the foot quickly; this message travels via motor neuron pathways, causing your foot to jerk out of the water.

Communication among and between neurons is complex and specific and is believed to be the basis of behavior. Each neuron forms anywhere from 1,000 to 10,000 synaptic connections. The synapse is a gap in the synaptic cleft between neurons. See FIGURE 6-5 ■ for a structural view of how a neuron conveys its messages. These reciprocal synapses form positive and negative feedback loops. Neurons are arranged in networks or pathways where neuronal communication is facilitated by repetition. Interneuron communication is electrical and chemical and occurs at synapses, or points of contact between neurons, as well as along the neuron itself.

Synaptic Transmission

Neuromessenger is a collective, generic term for neurotransmitters, neuromodulators, and neurohormones. **Neurotransmitters (NTs)** are neuromessengers that are rapidly released at the presynaptic neuron on stimulation, diffuse across the synapse between two neurons, and have either an excitatory or inhibitory effect on the postsynaptic neuron. The membrane of the axon terminal of a neuron contains many saclike projections called *synaptic vesicles,* which contain the NT molecules that transmit messages across the synapse.

Neurons are encased in cell membranes that function as a complex regulation site. The membranes contain proteins, some of which are phospholipids, enzymes, and ion channels. Ion channels are water-filled molecular tunnels that pass through the cell membrane and allow electrically charged atoms (ions) or small molecules to enter or leave the cell. The neuron exists in a state of tension because of the various ions in its membrane. Changes in ion concentrations cause the nerve impulse, or *action potential,* which transmits information between the neurons. The four major ions are sodium, potassium, calcium, and chloride. Each ion passes in or out of the neuron via its own channel. Nerve impulses involve the opening or closing of the ion channels by gates.

Once the action potential reaches the end of the axon, the electrical transfer of the information ends, and messages are then conveyed by chemicals, the NT molecules. The signal is mediated by binding to specific receptors on the cell surface (Ciccarelli & White, 2009). Depending on the type of channel, the action potential can be one of the following:

- Excitatory, influencing the neuron to fire
- Inhibitory, preventing it from firing

Presynaptic axon terminals contain large numbers of calcium channels, which determine the quantity of NT that is released into the synaptic cleft.

At the synapse, the membrane of the postsynaptic neuron contains receptor proteins. Receptors are highly specialized proteins embedded in the membrane of the neuron that are

Neurological Synapse Animation

FIGURE 6-5 ■ Synaptic contacts. A neuron is capable of making many different types of synaptic contacts. Shown here are:
(a) a synapse contact on a dendrite, called *axodendritic contact*;
(b) a contact on the soma, called *axosomatic contact*; (c) a synapse contact on another axon, called *axoaxonic contact*; and (d) an area where signals are sent and received, called *axosynaptic contact*.
Source: Smock, T. K. (1999). *Physiological psychology: A neuroscience approach*, p. 23. Upper Saddle River, NJ: Prentice Hall.

in part exposed to the extracellular fluid and recognize the neuromessenger. Receptors are located on the axon (presynaptic) or on the dendrite (postsynaptic). Neurotransmitters and receptors vary in their affinity for each other, depending on the NT involved. They may bind like a lock and key, or the outcome may depend on what is available. Every neuron is more or less sensitive to a constant amount of neuromessenger, and this is an important principle in pharmacology. The NT that remains in the synapse after the postsynaptic response is either dissolved by synaptic enzymes or reabsorbed for recycling by the presynaptic neuron, a process known as *reuptake*.

FIGURE 6-6 ■ Common neurotransmitter pathways. Purple = DA, black = NE, dashed line = 5-HT. The dotted line indicates the pons.

Neurotransmitters

Neurotransmitters include three classes—biogenic amines (monoamines), amino acids, and peptides—as well as dissolved gases and a number of other compounds. Neurotransmitters are discussed in TABLE 6-1 ■. Biogenic amines are synthesized in the axon terminals and released into the synapse. The era of neuropsychopharmacology began with the identification of these neurotransmitters.

Functional imaging techniques now enable researchers and clinicians to visualize the pathways of neuron clusters at work and better understand their functional association with behavior. The original belief that a neuron contained only one NT is no longer valid. FIGURE 6-6 ■ illustrates the basic pathways of three of the major biogenic amines.

Dopamine Dopamine (DA) is released in many areas in the brain, where it influences how we interact in the world. One example of the excitatory effects of DA is when cocaine inhibits the removal of DA from the neuronal synapse. This causes a rise in the concentration of DA at those synapses, the excitatory impact takes effect, and the "high" associated with cocaine use is created.

Because of the presence of DA pathways in all of these areas of the brain, DA disturbance is involved in psychosis. See TABLE 6-2 ■ for specific DA areas and functions.

Norepinephrine Norepinephrine (NE) is also called *noradrenalin*, and synapses that release NE are adrenergic synapses. Receptors for the neurotransmitter norepinephrine are widespread in the brain. Locations of the receptors for NE are listed in TABLE 6-3 ■. NE plays a major role in mediating mood and anxiety. Normally NE is considered to have an excitatory impact. Regulation of norepinephrine has been examined

TABLE 6-1 ■ The Major Known Neurotransmitters

Neurotransmitter	Function
Biogenic Amines (Monoamines)	
Acetylcholine (Ach) Precursor: choline	Attention; memory; promotes preparation for action; conserves energy; thirst; defense and/or aggression; sexual behavior; regulates mood; REM sleep; voluntary movement of the muscles; stimulates parasympathetic division of the ANS; controls muscle tone in balance with DA in the basal ganglia
Dopamine (DA) Precursor: tyrosine	Integrates thoughts and emotions; regulates pleasure and reward-seeking stimuli; controls complex movements; motivation; cognition; stimulates hypothalamus to release hormones affecting adrenal, thyroid, and sex hormones
Histamine (H) Precursor: histidine	Mediates allergic and inflammatory responses; smooth muscle constriction; stimulates gastric acid secretion; role in biorhythms and thermoregulation; role in second messenger transmission
Norepinephrine (NE) or noradrenalin Precursor: Tyrosine	Stimulates sympathetic division of the ANS; role in stress response; fluctuates with sleep and wakefulness; role in attention and vigilance, arousal, ability to focus or learn, feeling of reward, and regulation of mood and anxiety
Serotonin (5-HT) Precursor: Tryptophan	Inhibits activity and behavior; role in level of arousal; increases sleep time; reduces aggression, play, sexual, and eating activity; regulates temperature; controls pain; controls mood states; role in circadian rhythms; regulates senses; helps focus the brain; regulates pituitary
Amino Acids	
Aspartate	Excitatory
Gamma-aminobutyric acid (GABA), also written as γ-aminobutyric acid Precursor: Glutamic acid	Reduces aroused aggression, anxiety, and excitation; sedation; motor behavior; anticonvulsant and muscle-relaxant properties
Glutamate	Excitatory; role in learning and memory; neural degeneration
Glycine Precursor: serine	Inhibitory; spinal reflexes; motor behavior
Peptides (Neuromodulators)	
Cholecystokinin (CCK)	Role in schizophrenia; eating and movement disorders; panic disorder
Corticotropin-releasing hormone (CRH)	Stress, mood, memory, and anxiety
Neurotensin	Role in schizophrenia
Opioids: endorphins and enkephalins	Alter emotional behavior; pain control; hallucinations; pleasure; motor coordination; water balance
Somatostatin	Mood disorders; Alzheimer's disease; negative feedback control of thyrotropin secretion; role in positive symptoms of schizophrenia; excites limbic neurons
Substance P	Excitatory; role in pain syndromes, mood, and movement disorders
Vasopressin	Role in mood disorders

TABLE 6-2 ■ Dopamine Location and Function

Area/Location	Dopamine Is Associated With	
Basal ganglia area	The control of complex movement	
Limbic system	Memory Mood Reward	Pleasure Motivation
Hypothalamic tract	Endocrine functions Circadian rhythms	Food and water intake Temperature
Frontal cortex pathway	Insight Judgment Problem solving	Inhibition Social awareness

TABLE 6-3 ■ Norepinephrine Location and Function

Area/Location	Norepinephrine Is Associated With	
Pons, specifically locus ceruleus	Stress response Arousal	Alertness
Cerebral cortex	Cognitive functioning	
Limbic system	Emotional responses Ability to focus or learn Reward	Regulation of mood Pleasure
Hypothalamus	Endocrine functions Temperature	Appetite Biologic rhythms

closely in the treatment of mood and anxiety disorders and contributes to current psychopharmacologic interventions.

Serotonin The **serotonin** (referred to as 5-HT) neurons arise in the raphe nuclei and project to the same areas as the NE pathways. A raphe, anatomically, refers to a seam in the tissue. A raphe nucleus is a moderate-sized cluster of nuclei found in the brain stem. This cluster releases serotonin to the rest of the brain. Selective serotonin reuptake inhibitor (SSRI) antidepressants are believed to act on these nuclei. Serotonin appears to be a modulator. Its effects influence the temperature, sensory, sleep, and assertiveness areas of the brain. Serotonin serves as a chemical mediator in pain perception, normal and abnormal behaviors, moods, drives, the regulation of food intake, and neuroendocrine functions. Receptor subtypes decrease cerebral blood flow during a migraine episode and increase the response to pain.

Acetylcholine The first chemical to be identified as a true neurotransmitter, acetylcholine (ACh), is the "grandparent" of neurotransmitters. Dopamine and ACh share a concentration of activity within the basal ganglia, and medications used to block EPSE are cholinergic stimulants, suggesting a reciprocal relationship between these two neurotransmitters in the modulation of movement and possibly the development of psychosis. ACh plays a major role in the encoding of memory and in cognition. It also plays a mediation role in mood disorders, stress, and sleep regulation. It is considered to be highly significant in neuromuscular transmission.

Histamine The role of histamine (H) in psychiatric illness is less understood. It is a chemical messenger that mediates a wide range of cellular responses, including allergic and inflammatory reactions, gastric acid secretions, and neurotransmission. Some psychiatric medicines block H receptors, resulting in the side effects of sedation, weight gain, and drowsiness (Preskorn, 2011).

Amino Acids These neurotransmitters are natural substances found throughout the brain and body and in the proteins of the food we eat. The amino acid GABA is the most prevalent inhibitory NT. GABA neurons are widely distributed in the CNS. Glycine, also an inhibitory NT, exists primarily in the brain stem, spinal cord, and cerebellum. GABA has a prominent role in arousal; when the neuron is stimulated, GABA acts as a brake, decreasing neuronal excitability.

Glutamate and aspartate are the two primary excitatory amino acid neurotransmitters. Glutamate is primarily located in the cerebral cortex and hippocampus and has a role in long-term memory and learning. Too much glutamate can be a neurotoxin, as seen in Huntington's chorea and phencyclidine (PCP) psychosis.

Psychoendocrinology and Psychoneuroimmunology

This section examines the interaction of the brain with two body subsystems: the endocrine and immune systems. The interaction of the brain with the endocrine system is known as *psychoendocrinology*. The interaction of the brain with the immune system is known as *psychoneuroimmunology*.

The immune and endocrine systems are integrated through a shared set of hormone receptors.

Endocrine System

The endocrine system functions through neurochemical messengers in the bloodstream called *hormones.* The rise or fall in the blood level of one hormone can cause an increase or decrease in the level of another hormone. Hormones have a broader range of responses than nerve impulses and require seconds to days to cause a response that may last from weeks to months.

Irregularities of Neuroendocrine Function Neuroendocrine function irregularities have been linked to depression, postpartum psychosis, schizophrenia, polydipsia in clients with psychosis, panic disorder, obsessive–compulsive disorder, anorexia nervosa, dementia of the Alzheimer's type (DAT), and circadian rhythms.

Psychopharmacologic challenge tests, described in Box 6-1 earlier in this chapter, enhance our understanding of the pathophysiology of these conditions. One such test is the **dexamethasone suppression test (DST)**, which attempts to assess the hypothalamic–pituitary–adrenal (HPA) axis and neuroendocrine feedback (FIGURE 6-7 ■). Dexamethasone, a

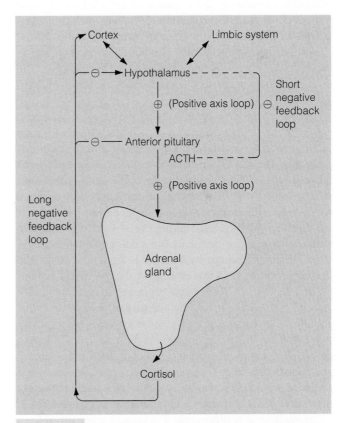

FIGURE 6-7 ■ Example of neuroendocrine feedback. The positive loop in the axis is depicted by the hypothalamus. Upon stimulation from the cortex or limbic system, the release of trophic peptide CRH (corticotropin-releasing hormone) tells the pituitary gland to signal the adrenal cortex, via ACTH (adrenocorticotropic hormone), to release the glucocorticoid cortisol. Cortisol released into the bloodstream provides negative feedback to the hypothalamus or anterior pituitary. Additionally, ACTH can provide negative feedback to the hypothalamus.

synthetic glucocorticoid, is given by mouth at 11:00 p.m. to "challenge" the axis. By measuring blood samples of the hormone cortisol drawn at 4:00 p.m. the day before the pill is taken, and at 8:00 a.m. (highest level of normal rhythm), 4:00 p.m. (lowest level of rhythm), and 11:00 p.m. the day after the pill is taken, one can assess the relationship between the pituitary and the hypothalamus.

Dexamethasone "turns off" adrenocorticotropic hormone (ACTH) secretion at the pituitary, which in turn suppresses cortisol secretion from the adrenals. In a normally functioning axis, cortisol is reduced for the next 24 hours. However, in many psychiatric conditions, nonsuppression, or "escape," is observed by a rise in the 4:00 p.m. level, when it should be low. There are no side effects or long-lasting changes as a result of taking dexamethasone. The results are not diagnostic of the illness, but suggest some pathology in the HPA axis function.

Neuropeptides Hormones secreted by the hypothalamus and pituitary are neuropeptides, which are large, complex chains of amino acids linked together and synthesized by ribosomes in the neuronal cell body through the transcription of DNA. Their physiology is complex; they bind to specific receptors, modulating the response of the postsynaptic cell to the NT. These effects are slow, involving such prolonged actions as changes in the number of receptors, synapses, and closures of ion channels. They also have an important role in the memory process (Adams, Holland, & Urban, 2011). The most commonly understood neuropeptides are summarized in Table 6-1.

Researchers have been studying the effect substance P has on human beings. Substance P is a prototype neuropeptide that is thought to cotransmit with serotonin in the neuronal pathways. The role of substance P has been studied in altered mice (discussed later in this chapter). The synthesis of substance P along with other neuropeptides is necessary during a neurogenic inflammatory response in mice.

Substance P is released during stress—both physiological stress, such as pinching the mouse's tail, and environmental stress. In human beings, substance P is thought to contribute to changes in the CNS that predispose the individual to anxiety and depression. We are now beginning to understand substance P's role in signaling the intensity of pain and aversive stimuli and substance P's involvement with depression and psychological stress. The direction of this research will lead to the development of medication compounds that are substance P antagonists that may treat diseases that have an emotional response to aversive stimuli, such as post-traumatic stress disorder (PTSD). Antagonists of the neuropeptide substance P, vasopressin, and neuropeptide Y represent a departure from traditional monoamine receptor–based mechanisms (Pongor, Altdorfer, & Feher, 2011).

Immune System

Psychoneuroimmunology (PNI) is the study of the links between thoughts, emotions, the nervous system, and the immune system. The relationships between these systems have been known

to clinicians for a long time. New research is being dedicated to further the *why* of the interactions. The National Institutes of Health (NIH) National Center for Complementary and Alternative Medicine (NCCAM) investigates methods and techniques of complementary and alternative treatments. The goal for most practitioners is to combine effective treatments from complementary and alternative options with commonly understood mainstream medicine to provide the best care. This combination is referred to as an *integrative approach.* An enormous reservoir of choice for promoting health for an individual can be opened up by determining how complementary and alternative techniques, discussed in Chapter 33∞, can influence healing. This field holds great potential for nurses and clinicians in all specialties including psychiatry as we strive to understand the influence stress has on mental disorders (Miodrag & Hodapp, 2010).

Our understanding of chemical communication between the brain and immune system comes from the study of receptors. Cells in the limbic system have many receptors for neuropeptides such as endorphins, and immune system cells contain receptors for endorphins and other peptides such as corticotropin-releasing hormone (CRH). The brain can directly influence the immune system by sending messages along nerve cells. This series of communications affects the cell nucleus, producing changes in the DNA and RNA that alter the shape of the neuron or even cause cell death. In the fight-or-flight response, immune system function is slowed, and energy is directed toward helping the body meet the immediate challenge.

Kindling and Behavioral Sensitization

Kindling is the repeated administration of a subconvulsant stimulus, such as repeated stress, to the neuron. The stimulus can come from a variety of sources and may be a chemical cascade from stress. When stress occurs over and over, it can sensitize the neuron rather than creating a tolerance to the stimulus. The theory about kindling includes the idea that stress induces symptomatic episodes and, as the illness progresses, the individual becomes more and more vulnerable to stress and further episodes. Soon only a slight stressor tips the person into a symptomatic episode (Kanner, 2011; Wilhelm et al., 2011).

Behavioral sensitization is a chemical phenomenon in which changes occur in the person's behavior. Short-term and long-term memory are affected. Following a series of these "behavioral seizures," the neuron requires less stimulus to produce the seizure-like response. Kindling appears to be a kind of learning, independent of cognition, and it can set off an autonomous process.

Alcohol withdrawal, PTSD, panic disorder, and rapid-cycling mood disorders are all similar in that stress or a chemical substrate produces kindled seizures in the amygdala region of the brain, which, over time, produces behavior changes (Stroud, Davila, Hammen, & Vrshek-Schallhorn, 2011; Claycomb, Hewett, & Hewett, 2011).

Carbamazepine, an anticonvulsant, and the benzodiazepines act on kindled episodes. Some anticonvulsant medications are also mood stabilizers for those with bipolar disorder and raise the question about the relationship between mood instability and kindling. The current working hypothesis is examining the correlation of the first episode of bipolar disorder with a stressful life event. The thinking is that repetitions of illness (episode sensitization) may trigger further psychopathology and also provide some explanation for why people with rapid-cycling mood disorders become refractory to medications over time. The neuron actually goes through changes, so different medications or combinations of medications are required to stabilize the progressive course.

Circadian Rhythms

Circadian rhythm (biologic rhythms or biorhythms) program our 24-hour day–night cycles. Chronobiology is the relationship between time and biologic rhythms and their effect on living systems. There are rhythms in endocrine secretion, NT synthesis, receptor number, enzyme levels and affinities, brain electrical activity, duration of cell cycle times, and the transcription regulation of DNA. Rhythms can have different cycle lengths, as follows:

- Ultradian: less than 24 hours
- Circadian: 24 hours
- Infradian: more than 24 hours

Plasma cortisol, core body temperature, and growth hormones are all paced in a particular manner. *Zeitgebers* are time cues or synchronizers, environmental cues about timing, and they set the biologic rhythms. See Box 6-5 for examples of zeitgebers. When there is a problem with someone's cycle length, you can assess the typical cues that may contribute to the cycle distortion. Assess the environment including social, occupational, and contributions from the surroundings. Family patterns of activities influence biologic rhythms and cycles, and disturbances of body rhythms impacting psychological functioning are well substantiated in the literature (Tsai, Barnard, Lentz, & Thomas, 2011; Quera-Salva, Hartley, Claustrat, & Brugiéres, 2011).

One of the major functions of circadian timing is organizing and prioritizing metabolic and physiological events. The suprachiasmatic nucleus (SCN), a cluster of neurons in the hypothalamus, is the body's own internal synchronizer for temperature and sleep. External influences work as cues to your body and include the light–dark cycle, mealtime patterns, and work schedules.

One theory of depression is that it represents a phase advance disorder (as evidenced by early morning awakening), decreased onset of rapid eye movement (REM) sleep, and neuroendocrine changes. Research into the question of whether estrogen shortens the circadian period, lengthening the sleep phase, advancing sleep onset, and consolidating sleep, would help our understanding of the phenomenology of depression and menopause related to changes in the sleep–activity cycle for women. Symptoms of people with seasonal affective disorder (SAD) vary, but common symptoms are increased sleep and appetite, decreased energy, weight gain, low self-esteem, and negativism. A common treatment for this desynchronization is exposure to broad-spectrum light. Melatonin, synthesized from tryptophan in the pineal gland, allows the individual to become drowsy and promotes sleep. Light suppresses melatonin production. Therefore, broad-spectrum light can decrease the physiological source of increased sleep.

You can teach clients who have a recurrent pattern of winter depression (seasonal affective disorder; see Chapter 17∞) to begin preparing for their symptoms by seeking light treatment in the early fall. Usually, early morning exposure to pale blue bright light treatment (BLT) of approximately 7,500 lux may be sufficient to promote a change (Lieverse et al., 2011). Additional strategies include the following:

- Cautioning individuals with bipolar disorder not to stay up all night studying or partying, as that disrupts the sleep–wake cycle
- Helping postpartum mothers with a history of mood disorders prepare for night feedings to avoid becoming sleep deprived
- Advocating that people with mood disorders not work irregular shift patterns

The Americans with Disabilities Act (ADA) supports the idea that people with psychiatric disabilities should have a "reasonable" work schedule. This could include stable shift assignments.

Circadian Sleep Rhythm Disorders

Shift work disorders and sleep deprivation in nurses is discussed in Chapter 3∞. The **circadian rhythm sleep disorders** are those disorders in which the 24-hour sleep–wake schedule is disturbed through internal cues (e.g., phase delay is more common in teenagers and young adults; phase advance is more common in young children and older adults) or external cues (e.g., shift work, travel across time zones). The cycle of human biologic rhythms (as seen in FIGURE 6-8 ■) determines much of our mammalian activity level. Three circadian rhythm sleep disorders are discussed here—jet lag type, delayed sleep phase type, and advanced sleep phase type.

Chronobiology (the scientific study of the impact of time on the body) is rapidly expanding and has implications for

---

Box 6-5   Zeitgebers

Zeitgebers are the external environmental synchronizers that help us adjust to a 24-hour day and include the following:

- Light
- Eating schedules
- Work
- Sounds (birds chirping, clocks chiming)
- Dark
- Social activities
- Smells (coffee brewing)
- Other time-enforced activities

The solar light–dark cycle is considered the most important environmental cue.

FIGURE 6-8 ■ Continuum of human biologic rhythms.

coping with shift work. Inquiries about shift work should be a routine part of a sleep assessment because the impact on sleep patterns and sleep disturbance often extends beyond the period of shift work. Specific suggestions for obtaining good sleep despite a night-shift work schedule can be developed. Although studies in sleep labs indicate that light exposure, melatonin, hypnotic agents, caffeine, and central nervous system stimulants are helpful, clock entrainment is also studied as a helpful tactic (Alvarez-Saavedra et al., 2011).

Jet Lag Type Jet lag was unknown until the middle of the 20th century when large numbers of people began flying long distances in high-speed aircraft. Many noticed their body clocks become disoriented and confused after crossing several time zones. The impact on a passenger depends on the direction flown (east or west) and the number of time zones crossed. The impact on a passenger of flying east is illustrated in FIGURE 6-9 ■, and the impact of flying west in FIGURE 6-10 ■.

Sleeping pills are not recommended for trips of 8 hours or less. The medication may still have an effect if one has slept for only 4 or 5 hours, and disorientation, memory problems, or amnesia is possible for several hours following the flight. For long-haul flights, a sleeping pill may help you fall asleep and keep airplane distractions from waking you up.

In a client with bipolar disorder, jet lag and the associated sleep deprivation may further exacerbate a manic phase.

Clinical Example

Mr. Bernstein traveled from the United States to the Middle East on business. Upon his return to the United States, he made a series of irrational business decisions that he blamed on the stress of jet lag. However, it was subsequently determined that Mr. Bernstein had bipolar disorder.

Jet lag, a known stressor, may have precipitated Mr. Bernstein's first manic episode. The stressor may have also contributed

From New York

When you leave
New York, it is
9:30 p.m., and your
body thinks it
is 9:30 p.m.

7-hour flight

To Paris

When you arrive in
Paris, it is 10:30 a.m.
(Paris time) but
your body thinks
it is 4:30 a.m.

FIGURE 6-9 ■ Flying east.

To Tokyo

When you arrive in
Tokyo 12 hours later,
it is 4 p.m. (Tokyo time),
but your body thinks
it is midnight.

12-hour flight

From Los Angeles, California

When you leave
Los Angeles at
12 noon, your body
thinks it is 12 noon.

FIGURE 6-10 ■ Flying west.

to sleep deprivation experienced by travelers flying across several time zones. However, the body clock can be adjusted by both pharmacologic and behavioral interventions (Alvarez-Saavedra et al., 2011). Two Internet resources that provide information on preventing or reducing jet lag are http://www.circadian.com and http://www.goodsleep.com.

Delayed Sleep Phase Type An abnormality in sleep phase can contribute to what may appear to be socially inappropriate or uncooperative behavior. Clients with the circadian rhythm disorder known as *delayed sleep phase type* seem programmed to stay up late and sleep in late. This syndrome should not be confused with normal tendencies to be either a "night owl" or "morning lark." Delayed sleep phase syndrome is a persistent problem that is resistant to standard attempts to get up earlier.

Treatment measures include chronotherapies to change the delayed sleep circadian rhythm, such as morning bright light exposure, the administration of melatonin, and behavioral strategies (Mottram, Middleton, Williams, & Arendt, 2011). However, most people with delayed sleep phase type do not seek treatment. Many will say, "That's just how I'm programmed." It is not unusual to encounter people with this disorder who have adapted by seeking types of employment and entertainment that are conducive to late nights and late rising. The disorder can also contribute to social isolation.

Advanced Sleep Phase Type *Advanced sleep phase type* is the reverse of delayed sleep phase type in that early evening sleepiness regularly accompanies early wakening. A mildly advanced sleep phase is common among older adults and should not be confused with the early wakening associated with depression. With depression, other symptoms and sleep changes are evident.

The main consequences of delayed or advanced sleep phase syndrome are the disruption of family, work, and/or social activities. If the circadian pattern is problematic, phase shifting can be modified through *chronotherapy* or light therapy. Chronotherapy consists of systematically delaying

bedtime, usually in 3-hour increments, over a period of several weeks until the client reaches the desired bedtime hour, after which the new schedule is carefully maintained. Light therapy is timed to coincide with the time of day that sleepiness should be reduced. For people with advanced sleep phase syndrome, light therapy may be administered in the early evening.

As our understanding of biorhythms grows, we can expect that certain clinical decisions, such as the optimal time to administer medications or perform surgery, will change. Knowing a client's circadian patterns will help you administer appropriate medication dosages, resulting in greater efficacy and minimal side effects.

PSYCHOBIOLOGY AND MENTAL DISORDERS

This section examines current hypotheses about the psychobiologic basis of schizophrenia, mood disorders (major depression and bipolar disorder), anxiety disorders (panic disorder and OCD), dementia of the Alzheimer's type (DAT) personality disorders, and substance-related disorders. Research is continuing to examine most major psychiatric problems for issues related to biologic changes. The disorders described in this section are examples of how biologic research helps us understand and treat these disorders.

Schizophrenia

The evolution of the diagnosis of schizophrenia has been dramatic, shifting from a narrowly focused definition of the illness to one with specific criteria that acknowledge the many ways this illness is manifested. No single neurobiologic hypothesis as the source of schizophrenia exists. The variability of the psychopathology requires the implementation of multifaceted, or multifocal, treatments.

Neuron Loss

Researchers are trying to determine why there is a neuronal degeneration in the brain tissue of people with schizophrenia (Monji, Kato, & Kanba, 2009). While there are fewer nerve cells overall, there are more pyramidal cells (containing DA, ACh, and glutamate) that are excitatory in nature, bringing sensory inputs (sights, sounds, thoughts) to the cerebral cortex. This suggests that the illness may result from an increased flow of activity up to the cortex and may explain why people with schizophrenia become overwhelmed by stimuli such as hallucinations and misperceptions (Vyas, Patel, & Puri, 2011).

Cognitive Abnormalities

Changes in electroencephalograms (EEGs) may indicate a deficit in the processing of data in individuals with schizophrenia. Abnormalities in the GABA minergic system can result in cognitive abnormalities such as hallucinations, and association problems in the thought pattern. Studies of DA receptors, especially DA type II (D_2) receptors, provide clues to the neuropathology of schizophrenia. Most D_2 receptors are in the basal ganglia, as observed with neuroimaging studies. The presence of D_2 receptors in structures with receptors having connections to the limbic and cortical pathways helps link the functions or behaviors of the cognitive and emotional aspects of schizophrenia. Postmortem studies are looking at serotonin receptors to clarify the relationship of the central neurocognitive deficits and the pathophysiology of the disease syndrome (Rasmussen et al., 2010).

Molecular Genetics

The conventional and less frequently used antipsychotic medications, haloperidol and fluphenazine, bind to block D_2 receptors in the basal ganglia and target the symptoms of hallucinations, delusions, and loose associations (also called *positive symptoms*). From the application of molecular genetics techniques, the cloning of other DA receptors (D_3, D_4, and D_5) has led to the development of more specific psychotropic medications. The newer antipsychotics, sometimes called *atypical antipsychotics,* are discussed in Chapter 7∞.

Structural Brain Abnormalities

A second major hypothesis about schizophrenia is that structural brain abnormalities are associated with being schizophrenic. Brain computed tomography (CT) scans show enlarged ventricles and widened sulci and fissures that appear to have been present from the onset of symptoms, so are not a result of treatment. When a twin has schizophrenia, the nonaffected twin's ventricles appear normal in size; the ventricles of the twin with schizophrenia are larger. A prenatal injury, postnatal maturational change in brain cells, or delayed myelination of nerve cells may explain the delay of the syndrome until adolescence. Myelin forms the insulating lining of axons and is associated with the maturation of behavior during normal development. Myelination is thought to assist with the emotional component of cognition and behavior. The ability to think abstractly is related to myelination in the limbic system and is thought to be established by midadolescence, with full maturity taking place during adulthood. A decrease in myelination would cause an increase in anxiety, difficulty socializing, abrupt or muted styles of interacting, and difficulty in modulating affect. Think about the medical syndromes that involve a decrease in myelination (such as multiple sclerosis) and how that affects emotions and interactions.

Genetic Alterations

Genetic polymorphisms—many genetic alterations as opposed to a single gene mutation—are now generally thought to be responsible for the development of schizophrenia. Recent research has concentrated on determining the specific chromosomal locations of those genes. For example, genes 1q22–q24 and 1q42 demonstrate that genetic changes in the brain increase the likelihood of developing schizophrenia or bipolar disorder. Research on genetic location may assist in determining genetic counseling and treatment, and true genotype variants for schizophrenia could be discovered in the near future. Such a discovery would allow us to predict who will get the illness and who will respond to which specific medication. The variable expression of the illness likely occurs through epigenetic modification of gene activation (Liao et al., 2009). We see this variability in monozygotic twins when only one twin has schizophrenia even though they have the same genes; in the difference in the risk for schizophrenia between dizygotic twins and siblings, when both share about the same percentage of parental genes; in the considerable drop in elevated risk for schizophrenia from first-degree to second-degree relatives; as well as in multiple documented environmental factors of modest but elevated risk. See the Partnering With Clients and Families feature.

The CATIE study (Clinical Antipsychotic Trials of Intervention Effectiveness) selected subjects (N=738) with

PARTNERING WITH CLIENTS AND FAMILIES

Teaching About Genetic Testing for Schizophrenia

At present there is no definitive test for schizophrenia—no blood test or biopsy result that would render a diagnosis—so genetic testing for schizophrenia takes place in research settings. A reliable test using blood and other body cells is sure to be developed in the not-too-distant future. Talking about genetics with clients and families will familiarize them with the potentials for diagnosis, treatment, and risk reduction.

If your clients and their family members have the opportunity to be involved in genetic research, informed consent documents for participation in these studies explain in detail what is being tested, how the sample will be used, and how long the sample will be kept following the research. Clients and their family members should know that research does not necessarily help study subjects who have the illness. After hundreds of genetic samples have been examined, however, a clearer picture of the genetics of schizophrenia can be developed. Helping clients and families understand the benefits of genetic research now will shape what happens for future generations of people with schizophrenia.

schizophrenia who were then genotyped (Lieberman et al., 2005). The genome-wide approach seeks to detect genetic variation underlying individual differences in response to treatment with the antipsychotics olanzapine, quetiapine, risperidone, ziprasidone, and perphenazine. This effort, which is ongoing at this printing, demonstrates the potential of genome-wide association studies to discover novel genes that will mediate the effects of antipsychotics for people who have schizophrenia. Ultimately, this research could help tailor drug treatment to clients who have schizophrenia.

Stress–Diathesis Model

Contemporary treatment of schizophrenia is influenced by a stress–diathesis model (a biologic predisposition to a disease that is activated by stress). We know that merely having a predisposition for the illness does not necessarily mean the individual will develop the illness. Resilience in response to stress can make the difference between developing the illness or not. These interactions between psychobiologic vulnerability and environmental events can stress the person's adaptive abilities and precipitate the onset of the syndrome or the recurrence of symptoms. Nurses can target interventions that alter the neurochemical systems with pharmacotherapy and psychosocial treatments (such as social skills, case management, client and family education). Chapter 16∞ includes a thorough discussion of nursing interventions for clients with schizophrenia.

Mood Disorders

Because of the variability in both the genetics and the symptoms of major depression and bipolar disorder, the psychobiologic basis of mood disorders can be difficult to determine. Research has focused on 5-HT and NE receptors. Brain stem nuclei that project to the amygdala, hippocampus, mammillary bodies, and cerebral cortex help account for the symptoms of appetite change, insomnia, depressed affect, loss of interest and pleasure (anhedonia), decreased problem-solving skills, and thoughts of self-harm. The association of decreased 5-HT with aggression may account for the suicide potential of this population. Postmortem findings show reduced 5-HT reuptake sites in the hypothalamus and hippocampus. Much further investigation is needed to determine whether more severe functional deficits are related to the neurotoxic effects of severe manic episodes on medial temporal structures, or to the neurobiologic differences that occur over time (Bora, Yucel, Pantelis, & Berk, 2011).

Neuroendocrine challenge tests report increased cortisol, blunted ACTH response, hypothalamic–pituitary–thyroid axis alterations, and a higher-than-expected rate of autoimmune thyroiditis. When clients ask you, as their nurse, what these results indicate, you can emphasize they are state-dependent findings, that is, these are markers that occur while the person is in a depressed mood (state), and do not demonstrate a genetic characteristic of the illness.

Recent NT studies suggest that complex interactions among NE, 5-HT, DA, ACh, GABA, peptides, and second messengers contribute to bipolar disorder. There may be as many as six different types of bipolar disorders; further research to distinguish among them will refine our assessments and clinical treatments. Bipolar disorder tends to accelerate over time if left untreated. Early episodes tend to be precipitated by stress, either positive or negative stress. But once recurrent episodes have occurred, the illness accelerates independently of external causes. Even with a genetic predisposition, there can also be changes in gene expression based on life experiences. Cognitive alterations may reflect genetic influences as well as mood, medication, and thyroid function (Arts, Jabben, Krabbendam, & van Os, 2011). The skill of resilience—knowing how to manage and cope with negative events—can mitigate a major portion of a person's genetics. In other words, even if you had a very strong genetic loading for a major mental illness, if you were able to show resilience in the face of stress, there would be less likelihood you would develop a major mental illness.

Because of the various clinical symptoms associated with mood disorders, you have an excellent opportunity to assess clients for their unique psychobiologic profile. The outcome of this specific assessment with each client over time will promote improved efficacy of treatment for the target symptoms and potentially prevent future disruptive episodes. Promoting client self-care, which involves the client's becoming aware of his or her symptoms in order to report clinical changes early in a recurrence of the depression, will assist in limiting the severity of the mood disorder (see Chapter 17∞).

Anxiety Disorders

Anxiety disorders have many subtypes, which are discussed in detail in Chapter 18∞. Therefore, this chapter will not provide a complete review. As you know from an earlier discussion in this chapter, the question of whether anxiety disorders are a separate type of disorder or a variant of a depressive spectrum is still unanswered. MRI and PET scans reveal right hippocampal changes, high brain metabolism, and an abnormal sensitivity to hyperventilation in people with panic disorder.

Anxiety is a psychobiologic condition that responds to both behavioral and pharmacologic interventions and is recognized as amenable to our nursing care. Through the use of nursing science, you conduct a thorough assessment of a client's symptoms of anxiety, using various assessment tools. Cognitive–behavioral and supportive approaches have been effective interventions for anxious clients. Clients with any of the anxiety disorders benefit from being taught about the use of medications to decrease anxiety symptoms. How is your approach with mildly anxious clients different from your approach with clients who have moderate, high, or crisis levels of anxiety? Provided that you assess the client's anxiety accurately, how prescriptive are your interventions, and what objective evaluative measures of anxiety control do you use? See What Every Nurse Should Know for an example. Refer to Chapters 8 and 18∞ for further information about caring for an individual with an anxiety disorder.

WHAT EVERY NURSE SHOULD KNOW

An Agitated Client

Imagine that you are the psychiatric nurse on a crisis response team. The team receives a call about a very agitated man who has a history of paranoid delusions and hallucinations. You and the other team members approach the man, who is on his porch mumbling agitatedly to himself.

Your knowledge of the psychobiology of schizophrenia supports the strategy of having only one person speak clearly and simply to this man so as not to overwhelm him. His executive functioning, and therefore his ability to process incoming information, is challenged when symptoms are acute. You interact with him in a calm, straightforward manner, asking what the problem could be. When he answers you in a loud, menacing tone that he must "strike before the irons have cooled beyond their coloration," you ask him to tell you what he wants you to do. In the conversation that follows, you discover that he has not been eating or sleeping, that he becomes very upset when people interrupt him (to ask him to eat or try to get some sleep), and that he is exhausted from days of trying to accomplish a delusional task.

When it is apparent that an individual such as this man is experiencing severe symptoms, stabilization is needed to protect him and others. Stabilization can be achieved through a combination of a safe environment, psychopharmacology to balance neurotransmitter functions, and compassionate care to help him through this trauma.

Panic Disorder

Neurochemical changes are associated with NE, 5-HT, GABA, and peptides in panic disorder. The discharge of NE in the brain stem, chemoreceptors in the medulla, and 5-HT sets off a series of communications that extend through the limbic system, rich in benzodiazepine receptors, to the prefrontal cortex. This pathway may explain why the cortex interprets the rapid pulse from the NE discharge as a life-threatening heart attack. These neural connections allow for a hypervigilant cognitive appraisal or an inability to integrate the sensory information with any biologic sensation. The inappropriate behavioral outcome is anticipatory anxiety and avoiding stimuli that might be the associated precipitant of the arousal.

Obsessive–Compulsive Disorder (OCD)

PET scans show higher metabolic rates in the left prefrontal cortex and caudate nuclei in people with OCD. The caudate or "gating station" dysfunction may lead to overactive circuits that fail to properly integrate cognitive, emotional, and motor responses to sensory inputs. The prefrontal hyperactivity in the brain's error-detection circuits give messages something is deadly wrong and may give rise to the tendency to ruminate and plan excessively, as well as to think in an abstract way (Meyer, Chapman, & Weaver, 2009). Increased frontal lobe activity manifests as a heightened sense of judgment (guilt and worry), intense affect (depression), and hyperjudgmental rigidity.

Abnormal regulation of the 5-HT subsystem has a role in the pathophysiology of OCD. This possibility is supported by improvement in response to treatment with SSRIs. In addition, increased levels of arginine, vasopressin, somatostatin, and CRH are found in the CSF of people with OCD. These neuropeptides promote grooming activity and perseverative (repetitive) motor behaviors and increase arousal (anxiety), which are part of the OCD symptomatology.

Voyiaziakis et al. (2011) describe the genetics of OCD as equivocal (not definitive in one direction or another). OCD is a complex illness with a variety of presentations. In a family with a high rate of OCD, the illness will look different clinically as well as genetically among affected family members. A further complication arises with nonfamilial cases of OCD. A reasonable question would be, "Where does OCD come from?" It appears to arise from genetic, neurochemical, neuroanatomical, and environmental influences that are being thoroughly explored. The existence of a possible gender effect is being explored. Indications that people who have OCD show differences in their serotonin transporter gene as well as abnormalities in the brain's white matter is also of interest; however, there does not seem to be an OCD syndrome gene.

Dementia of the Alzheimer's Type (DAT)

Working with clients suffering from DAT and their family caregivers calls for creativity based on knowledge of the structure and function of the brain. In assessing and intervening with the DAT client, be aware that disorientation results in fear and agitation. Thus any change, such as bed reassignment or facility transfer, is a significant stressor. For those with parietal involvement, walking down a hall with a patterned carpet, stepping up on a weight scale, or managing steps is difficult because they cannot orient themselves in relation to the space around them. Chapter 14∞ includes a thorough discussion of the nursing care of individuals with DAT.

Neurobiology

People with DAT have decreased cerebral blood flow or metabolic function in the posterior temporoparietal regions. DAT is the only major mental disorder to show this characteristic pattern of hypometabolic function. Thus, PET and SPECT studies may be useful in differentiating DAT from other disorders that include confusion and intellectual deterioration as symptoms. Structural neuronal degeneration occurs, producing neurofibrillary tangles and amyloid deposits, or plaques. Nerve receptor density and distribution studies promise improved diagnostic accuracy.

Decreases in cholinergic neurons in a region of the basal ganglia that connect to the amygdala, hippocampus, and cortex are seen in DAT. Functionally, these decreases result in the short-term memory loss characteristic of the disease. While the deficits are considered central, other NT systems are involved in the pathology, including NE, 5-HT, DA, peptides, and nerve growth factor. If receptors in the limbic structures are affected, depression or labile mood results; a decrease in social skills, inhibition, and impaired judgment can also be a part of the behavioral pattern.

Genetics

DAT research investigates chromosomal abnormalities. Understanding the causal factors in early onset DAT has led to assessing for mutation in presenilin-1. This research used altered mice that lacked the gene for presenilin-1. The mice demonstrated that the presenilin-1 did not cleave in the usual way and the beta-amyloid plaques that are present in DAT did not occur. The research concluded that when the gene for presenilin-1 is present and overactive, there is excessive cleaving of the amyloid precursor protein that forms the plaques. Further genetic research in DAT is focusing on the effect amyloid-beta-derived diffusible ligands (ADDLs) have on the nerve cells. ADDLs disrupt the neurons responsible for learning and memory, then cause neuronal death. Understanding the changes in the genetic composition of the nerve cells can lead to new medications that block ADDLs or decrease the excessive cleaving of the amyloid precursor protein. Compounds called [gamma]-secretase modulators (GSMs) inhibit the generation of amyloidogenic A[beta]42 peptides and are proving to be promising agents for treatment or prevention of Alzheimer's disease through breaking the attenuating effects of presenilin mutations (Hahn et al., 2011). Research will contribute to the information needed to develop effective treatments for this complex disease.

Where does DAT come from? Inheritance is well documented and accounts for approximately one third of all cases of DAT. Evidence of mutations in at least four genes that can cause DAT has now been documented: mutations in the amyloid precursor gene; mutation in a chromosome 14 gene encoding presenilin-1; mutation in a gene on chromosome 1 that encodes presenilin-2; and association with the APOE-4 allele on chromosome 19. Each mutation depicts different aspects of the disease (e.g., early onset, cardiovascular disease). APOE 4-allele confers a risk for both sporadic and familial DAT and may be better labeled a risk gene, although there are no widely accepted definitions of risk versus cause. Keep in mind that more factors than simply the presence of the APOE-4 allele are necessary for the expression of DAT; other yet-to-be-identified environmental or genetic factors may contribute to the development of DAT.

Personality Disorders

Personality disorders, by definition, cause distress and impairment severe enough to lead clients to seek help. You are sure to come in contact with someone with a personality disorder at some point in your practice.

Neurobiology

Recent neurobiologic evidence indicates that the origin of personality disorders rests in biology as well as psychology. Antisocial personality disorder, three to six times more prevalent in men, is evident when someone who is literally against society is caught and their story publicized in the media (Ciccarelli & White, 2009). Narcissistic personality disorder is also inordinately represented by men. One of the largest groups of personality disorders, borderline personality disorder (BPD), remains a rich area of study. Women are more likely than men

to be diagnosed with this disorder. Legitimate gender differences in the prevalence of a diagnosis has been found in other mental health disorders as well (i.e., depression in women and OCD in men) and you will likely become aware of other possible genetic and sociocultural factors that influence the development and course of a disorder. Chapter 22∞ explores the underlying features of personality disorders in greater detail.

Neurochemistry

The neurochemistry of personality disorders, especially catecholamine activity, differs, depending on the mental health diagnosis. An individual with more than one personality disorder—also called *heterogeneity of diagnosis*—will demonstrate a wide variety of clinical symptoms. For example, catecholamine regulates and modulates visual, visiospatial, and verbal working memory tasks. The result of catecholamine activity would likely be different with each individual where mood and stress, and a sense of well-being, are impacted by catecholamine activity (Rief et al., 2010).

Genetics

Both quantitative and molecular approaches are important in understanding the genetics of personality disorders. A comingling of mental disorders, or heterogeneous diagnoses, blurs the picture. High comorbidity rates in this group make genetic testing for personality disorders difficult. Hypotheses are being tested for commonalities between mood, behavioral, and personality disorders on a neurobiologic substrate. The frequent combination of fear and anger traits among persons with personality disorders suggests a direction for research.

The same factors that help create healthy personalities—genetics, social relationships, and parenting—also create disordered personalities (Ciccarelli & White, 2009). Understanding the underlying features of personality disorders contributes to effective goal setting and treatment.

Substance-Related Disorders

The psychobiology of substance abuse is a rich field of study. So many substances are destructive not only to the users' health but also to the integrity of families and communities. Exploring this area to its greatest extent is necessary to promote public health. Research moves us toward that goal.

Because 4% to 5% of people in Western societies have difficulty with alcohol dependence and the relapse rate is 50% to 80% in a year, understanding its origins and having a reliable genetic analysis are vital. We know from decades of studies that there is heritability and predisposition to alcohol dependence as well as complex environmental influences. The latest research indicates an association of alcohol dependence with single-nucleotide polymorphism in a GABA receptor gene, especially in those with a presumed genetic predisposition (Kareken et al., 2010). Identifying the genetic components of the disease helps identify high-risk individuals. Once someone is identified as being at high risk, you can intervene as a nurse on an interpersonal basis. Interventions include defining weaknesses in stress responses, improving resilience to adversity, and teaching the person how to increase support

Care Plan: Genetic Implications

PARTNERING WITH CLIENTS AND FAMILIES

Teaching About the Genetic Basis of Substance-Related Disorders

When someone is diagnosed with a substance-related disorder such as alcoholism, your involvement with that client and the family will revolve around teaching. The genetic basis for alcohol dependence includes heritability and a predisposition for offspring to be alcohol dependent as well. While the immediate concern is for the client, a future concern will be the life-impacting ramifications that a substance-related disorder will have for the client's children.

Whether the client's children are biologically related or adopted, there are also complex contributions from environmental conditions. Once a blood relative has been identified as alcohol dependent, there is a presumed genetic predisposition to alcoholism. You may introduce the topic and explain how genetics can serve as advance notice for people to take action. A proactive environment helps the at-risk individual maximize coping skills without turning to substances to cope and begins the process of prevention for future generations.

Your role can include mapping out how an at-risk person reacts when exposed to a stressor. Is the reaction adaptive? The following are all healthy responses:

- Learning
- Exploring options

- Thinking about consequences
- Reviewing how well one's coping skills worked in a situation
- Making changes when things didn't turn out well
- Adjusting and fine-tuning the changes made

If you detect less-than-ample adaptive coping skills in an at-risk individual, you would proceed with shoring up the weaker areas to prevent (or at least minimize the possibility of) maladaptive coping such as substance abuse. These are some client-centered strategies to promote better coping:

- Become actively involved in shaping a personal support system.
- Identify stressors such as the following:
  - Timing—time of year, holidays, anniversaries, schedule disruptions, varying work shifts
  - Interpersonal issues—arguments, intimacy, loneliness, crowding, demands from others, financial problems
  - Intrapersonal issues—feelings of anger, incompetence, fatigue, frustration, fear
- Rehearse and practice healthy responses to difficult situations.
- Develop an array of activities or behaviors that minimize or reduce stressful times and situations.

---

systems. Genetic research has helped to develop meaningful and effective pharmacologic treatments. See Partnering With Clients and Families for an example of counseling clients and families about the genetic basis of substance-related disorders.

The combination of substance abuse or dependence and another identified psychiatric problem is common and complicates the picture. The characteristics of one illness meld with the features of another, resulting in a deepening and difficult situation from which few effectively extricate themselves. Psychiatric care settings that address this problem are better equipped to improve outcomes for these clients. See Chapter 15∞ for detailed discussions of substance-related disorders and their genetics and heritability.

PSYCHOBIOLOGY AND NURSING

We remind you frequently in this text that linking body, mind, brain, and behavior is the essence of a holistic psychiatric–mental health nursing practice. Integrating psychobiologic principles enhances that goal. To function as a professional nurse, it is important to be aware of any personal feelings, opinions, or beliefs that you have that may diminish your ability to be an advocate for and support person to clients and their families.

Your attitude about the underlying neurobiology of behavior can influence therapeutic outcomes. It is important to consider how treatment outcomes are potently influenced by both the style and the knowledge incorporated into nursing interventions. If the comprehensive nursing assessment, interpretation of the assessment, client teaching, and evaluation

of the intervention are based on knowledge of the biologic, cognitive, and behavioral factors that affect the client, the client has a greater opportunity for successful reduction of symptoms. If, however, you are ambivalent about the value of biologic or somatic therapies, you will inevitably communicate this attitude to the client and the family, and your interventions may not be as effective as they could be. Remember, you integrate your own viewpoint into client teaching, and its expression can hinder or help your clients and their families.

Integrating psychobiology into nursing care involves our skills as nurses throughout our assessment, integration of assessment information into a cogent plan of action, and interventions with psychological and biologic foci (medications and physiological-based strategies). It enables the nurse to fine-tune assessments, diagnoses, interventions, and evaluations of clients' response patterns. The synthesis of this critical thinking provides clients and families with quality, cost-effective care. The Evidence-Based Practice feature on genetic profiles is an example of how relevant psychobiologic research can contribute to our nursing practice.

Being a nurse is an opportunity for you to be flexible, creative, and a visionary. Keep a diary of how you made a difference for a client. Was a biologic variable involved? Articulate how you made that difference, and link it with cost-effective care. The care of people who have psychiatric disorders uses technology to address the neuropathology. Technology assists you in determining diagnostic impacts and targeting symptoms in order to effectively intervene as a psychiatric–mental health nurse. Your psychobiologic nurse–client relationship remains the core of your nursing practice.

EVIDENCE-BASED PRACTICE

The Role of Genetic Profiles in Treatment

Exciting advances are being made in psychobiology as a result of research evidence. One example is a study on the neuropeptide Y (NPY). This particular neuropeptide helps restore calm after experiencing stress. People whose genes predispose them to produce lower levels of NPY are more responsive to negative stimuli in key psychobiologic circuits related to emotion and are therefore less resilient when faced with stress. As you have seen in other discussions, less resilience may put people at higher risk for developing a major depressive disorder.

NPY is a genetic feature that can be measured in anyone to determine what the overall impact might be on how one responds to stress. Individuals with the genotype that produced lower amounts of NPY had measurably stronger brain responses to negative stimuli and psychological responses to physical pain. This is called a *low-expression NPY genotype*. These individuals were also over-represented in a population diagnosed with a major depressive disorder.

Examining this genetic feature can guide us toward assessing someone's risk for developing depression and anxiety. Recognition of this link between a genetic predisposition and an emotional outcome will help in early diagnosis and early intervention for depression.

Other psychiatric illnesses eventually will be the target in developing tailored therapies based on genetic profiles. This is the personalized medicine we have been striving toward in psychobiologic research. Valid, reliable, and clinically applicable psychobiologic research evidence such as this is of the highest standard. This expansion of our understanding of the physiology of depression has the potential to change how we treat psychiatric disorders with medications.

Mickey, B. J., Zhou, Z., Heitzeg, M. M., Heinz, E., Hodgkinson, C. A., Hsu, D. T., . . . Zubieta, J. K. (2011). Emotion processing, major depression, and functional genetic variation of neuropeptide. *Archives of General Psychiatry, 68*(2),158–166.

CRITICAL THINKING QUESTIONS

1. How can this test be used to individualize treatment selection?
2. How can this test be used to individualize medication dosing?
3. How do clients benefit when nurses are knowledgeable about genetic testing?

The exact biologic determinants for psychiatric disorders and behaviors are yet to be discovered. To date, there is no definitive biologic test to identify a psychiatric disorder. We still rely on expert nursing observations and assessment.

However, multifocal and multidisciplinary care that incorporates psychobiologic dimensions advances our ability to offer new, more effective assessments and interventions for our clients.

Pearson Nursing Student Resources
Find additional review materials at
nursing.pearsonhighered.com
Prepare for success with NCLEX®-style practice questions, interactive assignments and activities, web links, animations and videos, and more!

REFERENCES

Adams, M. P., Holland, L. N., & Urban, C. Q. (2011). *Pharmacology for nurses: A Pathophysiologic approach* (3rd ed.). Upper Saddle River, NJ: Prentice Hall.

Alvarez-Saavedra, M., Antoun, G., Yanagiya, A., Oliva-Hernandez, R., Cornejo-Palma, D., Perez-Iratxeta, C., . . . Cheng, H. M. (2011). miRNA-132 orchestrates chromatin remodeling and translational control of the circadian clock. *Human Molecular Genetics, 20*(4), 731–751.

American Nurses Association, American Psychiatric Nurses Association, & International Society of Psychiatric–Mental Health Nurses. (2007). *Psychiatric–mental health nursing: Scope and standards of practice.* Silver Spring, MD: Nursesbooks.org

Ankney, J. J., & Colbert, B. J. (2011). *Anatomy & physiology for health professions: An interactive journey* (2nd ed.). Upper Saddle River, NJ: Prentice Hall.

Arts, B., Jabben, N., Krabbendam, L., & van Os, J. (2011). A 2-year naturalistic study on cognitive functioning in bipolar disorder. *Acta Psychiatrica Scandinavica, 123*(3), 190–205.

Avramopoulos, D. (2010). Genetics of psychiatric disorders methods: Molecular approaches. *Clinics in Laboratory Medicine, 30*(4), 815–827.

Bora, E., Yucel, M., Pantelis, C., & Berk, M. (2011). Meta-analytic review of neurocognition in bipolar II disorder. *Acta Psychiatrica Scandinavica, 123*(3), 165–174.

Boyd, D. A., & Bee, H. L. (2012). *Lifespan development* (6th ed.). Upper Saddle River, NJ: Pearson.

Brown, S. A. (2010). Implementing a brief hallucination simulation as a mental illness stigma reduction strategy. *Community Mental Health Journal, 46*(5), 500–504.

Ciccarelli, S. K., & White, J. N. (2009). *Psychology* (2nd ed.). Upper Saddle River, NJ: Pearson Education.

Claycomb, R. J., Hewett, S. J., & Hewett, J. A. (2011). Prophylactic, prandial rofecoxib treatment lacks efficacy against acute PTZ-induced seizure generation and kindling acquisition. *Epilepsia, 52*(2), 273–283.

Hahn, S., Bruning, T., Ness, J., Czirr, E., Baches, S., Gijsen, H., Korth, C., . . . Weggen, S. (2011). Presenilin-1 but not amyloid precursor protein mutations present in mouse models of Alzheimer's disease attenuate the response of cultured cells to [gamma]-secretase modulators regardless of their potency and structure. *Journal of Neurochemistry, 116*(3), 385–395.

Hawkins, A. K., & Hayden, M. R. (2011). A grand challenge: Providing benefits of clinical genetics to those in need. *Genetic Medicine, 13*(3), 197–200.

Kanner, A. M. (2011). Depression and epilepsy: A bidirectional relation? *Epilepsia, 52* Suppl. 1, 21–27.

Kareken, D. A., Liang, T., Wetherill, L., Dzemidzic, M., Bragulat, V., Cox, C., . . . Foroud, T. (2010). A polymorphism in *GABRA2* is associated with the medial frontal response to alcohol cues in an fMRI study. *Alcoholism: Clinical and Experimental Research, 34*(12), 2169–2178.

Liao, S. Y., Lin, S. H., Liu, C. M., Hsieh, M. H., Hwang, T. J., Liu, S. K., . . . Chen, W. J. (2009). Genetic variants in COMT and neurocognitive impairment in families of patients with schizophrenia. *Genes, Brain, & Behavior, 8*(2), 228–237.

Lieberman J. A., Stroup T. S., McEvoy J. P., Swartz M. S., Rosenheck R. A., Perkins D. O., & Hsiao J. K. (Clinical Antipsychotic Trials of Intervention Effectiveness [CATIE] Investigators). (2005) Effectiveness of antipsychotic drugs in patients with chronic schizophrenia. *N Engl J Med* 353:1209–1223.

Lieverse, R., Van Someren, E. J., Nielen, M. M., Uitdehaag, B. M., Smit, J. H., & Hoogendijk, W. J. (2011). Bright light treatment in elderly patients with nonseasonal major depressive disorder: A randomized placebo-controlled trial. *Archives of General Psychiatry, 68*(1), 61–70.

Meyer, R. G., Chapman, L. K., & Weaver, C. M. (2009). *Case studies in abnormal behavior* (8th ed.). Upper Saddle River, NJ: Prentice Hall.

Mickey, B. J., Zhou, Z., Heitzeg, M. M., Heinz, E., Hodgkinson, C. A., Hsu, D. T., . . . Zubieta, J. K. (2011). Emotion processing, major depression, and functional genetic variation of neuropeptide. *Archives of General Psychiatry, 68*(2), 158–166.

Miodrag, N., & Hodapp, R. M. (2010). Chronic stress and health among parents of children with intellectual and developmental disabilities. *Current Opinion in Psychiatry, 23*(5), 407–411.

Monji, A., Kato, T., & Kanba, S. (2009). Cytokines and schizophrenia: Microglia hypothesis of schizophrenia. *Psychiatry & Clinical Neurosciences, 63*(3), 257–265.

Morgan, R. A., Dudley, M. E., & Rosenberg, S. A. (2010). Adoptive cell therapy: Genetic modification to redirect effector cell specificity. *Cancer Journal, 16*(4), 336–341.

Mottram, V., Middleton, B., Williams, P., & Arendt, J. (2011). The impact of bright artificial white and 'blue-enriched' light on sleep and circadian phase during the polar winter. *Journal of Sleep Research, 20*(1pt2), 154–161.

Pongor, E., Altdorfer, K., & Feher, E. (2011). Colocalization of substance P with tumor necrosis factor-[alpha] in the lymphocytes and mast cells in gastritis in experimental rats. *Inflammation Research, 60*(2), 163–168.

Preskorn, S. H. (2011). CNS Drug Development: Part III: Future Directions. *Journal of Psychiatric Practice, 17*(1), 49–52.

Quera-Salva, M. A., Hartley, S., Claustrat, B., & Brugiéres, L. (2011). Circadian rhythm disturbances associated with psychiatric symptoms in a patient with a pineal region tumor. *American Journal of Psychiatry, 168*(1), 99–100.

Rasmussen, H., Erritzoe, D., Andersen, R., Ebdrup, B. H., Aggernaes, B., Oranje, B., . . . Glenthoj, B. (2010). Decreased frontal serotonin2A receptor binding in antipsychotic-naive patients with first-episode schizophrenia. *Archives of General Psychiatry, 67*(1), 9–16.

Rief, W., Mills, P. J., Ancoli-Israel, S., Ziegler, M. G., Pung, M. A., & Dimsdale, J. E. (2010). Overnight changes of immune parameters and catecholemines are associated with mood and stress. *Psychosomatic Medicine, 72*(8), 755–762.

Sterling, R. L. (2011). Genetic research among the Havasupai: A cautionary tale. *American Medical Association Journal of Ethics, 13*(2), 113–117.

Stewart, S. E., & Pauls, D. L. (2010). The genetics of obsessive-compulsive disorder. *Focus, 8*, 350–357.

Stroud, C. B., Davila, J., Hammen, C., & Vrshek-Schallhorn, S. (2011). Severe and nonsevere events in first onsets versus recurrences of depression: Evidence for stress sensitization. *Journal of Abnormal Psychology, 120*(1), 142–154.

Tsai, S., Barnard, K. E., Lentz, M. J., & Thomas, K. A. (2011). Mother-infant activity synchrony as a correlate of the emergence of circadian rhythm. *Biological Research for Nursing, 13*(1), 80–88.

Voyiaziakis, E., Evgrafov, O., Li, D., Yoon, H. J., Tabares, P., Samuels, J., . . . Knowles, J. A. (2011). Association of SLC6A4 variants with obsessive-compulsive disorder in a large multicenter US family study. *Molecular Psychiatry, 16*(1), 108–120.

Vyas, N. S., Patel, N. H., & Puri, B. K. (2011). Neurobiology and phenotypic expression in early onset schizophrenia. *Early Intervention in Psychiatry, 5*(1), 3–14.

Wilhelm, J., Heberlein, A., Karagulle, D., Groschl, M., Kornhuber, J., Riera, R., . . . Hillemacher, T. (2011). Prolactin serum levels during alcohol withdrawal are associated with the severity of alcohol dependence and withdrawal symptoms. *Alcoholism: Clinical & Experimental Research, 35*(2), 235–239.

The Science of Psychopharmacology

EILEEN TRIGOBOFF

7

LEARNING OUTCOMES

After completing this chapter, you will be able to:

1. Explore how psychopharmacology has changed psychiatric–mental health nursing since 1958.
2. Incorporate psychiatric medications into treatment for two diagnostic groups.
3. Apply biologic impacts of medications to the care of clients from three ethnically distinct groups.
4. Identify two manifestations that require you to differentiate psychiatric symptomatology from medication side effects.
5. Describe how you would document the positive and negative impacts of psychiatric medications on behavior.
6. Compare and contrast the general classifications of medications used for particular psychiatric symptoms.
7. Explain the psychobiologic mechanisms important in psychopharmacology.
8. Teach clients and their families about the effects and uses of psychotropic medications.

CRITICAL THINKING CHALLENGE

Psychiatric medications could address the clinical problems of psychiatric symptoms a client is having, but they are capable of creating additional clinical problems because of side effects. Unpleasant side effects may cancel out whatever relief is felt. Consider the following situation with a client with schizophrenia.

Roberta has symptoms that cause severe difficulties in her thinking, information processing, communication, and relationships. The discomfort she experiences from these symptoms is exceeded only by a sense of demoralization as she realizes she has a chronic and debilitating disease for which there is no cure and the medication she takes causes the chronic side effects of stiffness and dry mouth. Rehabilitating Roberta to a lifestyle with psychotic symptoms, or with fewer or no psychotic symptoms, requires a realistic view of her needs and abilities and specific training to cope with the mental illness and its impact on her life.

1. What solutions would medications provide and what problems could be created for Roberta?
2. Under what conditions might there be unethical use of medications for psychiatric treatment?
3. What steps could you take to reduce the sense of demoralization Roberta feels?

This chapter explores the science of the psychopharmacologic agents used to treat symptoms of mental disorders and disabilities. The categories and main effects of these medications are detailed here, as well as some rationales for certain medication choices. Ways to help clients manage their medications and the side effects they may experience are discussed in Chapter 31∞. The science and management of psychopharmacology are intertwined; however, this chapter's discussion of the basics of major medication groups used in psychiatric–mental health nursing can help you create a useful platform on which to build your therapeutic interactions.

Psychopharmacologic nursing interventions deal with the side effects, drug interactions, psychosocial implications, and education activities among you, your clients, and their families. Psychiatric–mental health nursing demands both areas of expertise, but it may be easier to understand psychopharmacology—one of the major tools of your work—in the way we have structured it in this book in two separate chapters.

Psychiatric medications form the primary treatment for many psychiatric diagnoses. As you can see in the psychopharmacologic timeline in FIGURE 7-1 ■ on pages 116–117, in the years prior to the 1950s (when psychopharmacology became available and widely used), the focus was on behavioral interventions and sedative substances. The past six decades have shown us the beginning use, then enormous leaps of generations of compounds with major impacts, and even success, in treating many of the serious symptoms of mental illness. FIGURE 7-2 ■ on page 118 illustrates the drop in numbers of inpatients as a result of biologic and pharmacologic interventions. Just as the symptoms of an endocrine disorder such as diabetes respond to treatment with insulin, mental illness is an imbalance of brain chemicals that can be addressed or corrected with medications.

Psychopharmacology is a primary treatment mode of psychiatric–mental health nursing care and requires nurses to monitor client response as well as identify problems or side effects. Ours is a holistic function, incorporating the client's life, likes and dislikes, and activities along with symptomatology into a comprehensive view of treatment. One of the aims of psychopharmacologic nursing interventions is to teach clients about their medications, including over-the-counter medications and supplements, and their likely impact.

PSYCHOPHARMACOLOGY AND NURSING

The knowledge base of psychopharmacology continues to grow as a result of research and clinical expertise. Psychiatric–mental health nursing has similarly grown, and our responsibilities to recipients of mental health care services involve, to a large degree, psychopharmacologic expertise. Once we integrate current data from the neurosciences about psychopharmacologic compounds, we can provide safe and effective clinical management of clients taking these medications.

Every nurse is responsible for maintaining an updated knowledge base in psychobiology and pharmacology to intervene during clinical work. Our national professional organization, the American Nurses Association (ANA), examined this issue, and the ANA's Task Force on Psychopharmacology set forth guidelines for this aspect of nursing practice (ANA, 1994). The guidelines remain current and delineate three areas that unite the practice of psychiatric–mental health nursing with expertise in psychopharmacology. The goal of psychopharmacologic interventions is to promote clients' physiologic stability so they can achieve psychologic, social, and spiritual growth.

The word *drugs* conjures up a variety of powerful positive and negative images. Media messages depict the devastating negative effects of IV drug use, alcoholism, and methamphetamine use. They also give a picture of people leading productive lives, professionals demonstrating relief of symptoms, and schoolchildren being inoculated against diphtheria, polio, and pertussis. All these images are powerful, and each is backed by truth. But every media representation, positive or negative, must be viewed critically, because misunderstanding and outright ignorance about psychiatric disabilities can lead to inaccurate portrayals of symptoms and treatments. Powerful media messages can influence and interfere with proper care.

Examine your attitudes about medications, in particular psychiatric medications, by looking at the Your Self-Awareness box. Exploring your personal feelings will be a healthy challenge throughout your psychiatric–mental health nursing practice, and psychopharmacology could evoke very strong feelings in either direction for you. Make sure you are aware of your biases and that you have well-informed opinions so that you give your clients the best possible care.

Neuroleptics and Psychotropics

The complexities of psychiatric disorders and the desire to address the difficulties that face people who have these symptoms have resulted in a number of innovative medication regimens. Research has further expanded our knowledge, and a clearer vision of the capabilities of these compounds is emerging. Now many medications have multiple indications beyond their original ones, which have necessitated more global terms to describe the medication. We still use classification names such as "antipsychotic" and "antidepressant"; however, this is changing and some medications are labeled "neuroleptic" or "psychotropic" with the understanding that they can be used across some diagnostic groups. See TABLE 7-1 ■ on page 118 for some examples of the changing psychopharmacologic landscape.

One example of this phenomenon is fluoxetine (Prozac), used originally as an antidepressant, indicated as an antiobsessional medication and for the treatment of premenstrual dysphoric disorder (PMDD; a proposed category under study but not yet included in the DSM [Diagnostic and Statistical Manual of Mental Disorders]). A second example is risperidone (Risperdal), an atypical or newer antipsychotic, indicated for use in stabilizing the manic phase of bipolar disorder but also used in dementia. There are clinical applications of

YOUR SELF-AWARENESS
Your Views on Psychopharmacology

Your cultural inclinations have an influence on your attitudes toward medications. These attitudes have an impact on one of the major interventions in psychiatry—psychopharmacology. Which of these views do you hold about medications? How will they affect the care you give clients?

- They will make me healthier.
- This stuff will kill me.
- It is only for a short time.
- They are addictive.
- I will take medications only if my life depends on it.
- Isn't modern pharmacology a wonderful thing?
- I take the right medication for the problem.
- Taking the medications will mean I am a bad/weak person because I couldn't battle my disorder on my own.
- Medicine is made from herbs—it is the same thing, so I would rather take the herbs.
- Medications are too strong for me, so they are too strong for everybody.
- I cannot contaminate myself with these chemicals.
- If I take psychiatric medications, people will think I am crazy.
- What if the people at work find out I am taking these pills? They will think I cannot do my job.
- I am flawed because I need medication.
- People are more sophisticated these days. They would understand that I am taking the exact same medications as a well-known public figure.

multicultural environment such as mental health care, these are important considerations in assessing responses to psychopharmacologic treatments.

Important factors are the variation in genetics and in metabolic rates among ethnic groups (an important point in evaluating the effectiveness of a medication). McClay et al. (2011) examined genetic variations and their impact on response rates for those with schizophrenia. Metabolizing a medication more quickly or more slowly than expected changes what we observe during our clinical assessments. A high metabolic rate may produce effects below the optimal level, resulting in ineffective treatment. A low metabolic rate increases side effects. Because people of Asian descent have low metabolic rates, almost all Asians (95%) experience extrapyramidal side effects (EPSE) as compared to European- and African-Americans, two thirds of whom experience EPSE (defined and discussed in Chapter 31 ∞). Also because of metabolic differences, the therapeutic range for lithium differs among Asian, African-American, and Caucasian groups. The determination of effective lithium levels must take ethnicity into account.

Recognizing how ethnicity determines the way in which people respond to medications promotes the provision of culturally competent care. How ethnicity affects the expression of abnormal biologic processes is a growing field of study as is recognizing how to involve cultural competence in organizational functioning (Purnell et al., 2011; Mallinger & Lamberti, 2010). Exploring the related literature will help you to incorporate this expanding knowledge base into your psychiatric–mental health nursing practice and promote your cultural competence.

psychiatric medications to a different diagnostic group, or for a different set of psychiatric symptoms, than originally intended. There may not be a Food and Drug Administration (FDA) indication for the medication in those circumstances; however, clinical appropriateness has established the use pattern. This holds true for risperidone as a treatment for dementia with agitation.

Clinical application of nonpsychiatric medications to treat a psychiatric diagnostic group or a set of psychiatric symptoms also occurs. The complexity of the brain's involvements in physical and emotional problems indicates the need for overlapping and interwoven treatments. One of the most apparent examples is the anticonvulsant class. Valproic acid (Depakote), carbamazepine (Tegretol), and lamotrigine (Lamictal) are all used as mood stabilizers as well as for their original indications.

Biologic Impact on Ethnically Distinct Groups

You may notice in your psychiatric–mental health practice that the effects of medications may differ in ethnically distinct groups. Factors such as medication toxicity levels and autonomic nervous system (ANS) responses are not the same for all groups of individuals (Seripa et al., 2011). In a

ANTIPSYCHOTIC MEDICATIONS

Antipsychotic medications are those used to treat hallucinations, delusions, disorganized thinking, and other psychiatric and nonpsychiatric conditions and symptoms). The discovery of the first antipsychotic medications, such as chlorpromazine (Thorazine), is a prime example of the role of chance in the history of psychopharmacology. Chlorpromazine was initially synthesized as an antihistamine to facilitate operative procedures and was not tried as a tranquilizer for clients with schizophrenia until 1952. Its effects on the behavior, thinking, affect, and perception of clients with schizophrenia were so profound that information about its properties was rapidly disseminated, and it became widely used within 3 to 4 years.

Chlorpromazine's effects on the hospital practice of psychiatry were staggering. Its use contributed to reversing a steady rise in the population in U.S. mental institutions, and that population has progressively decreased ever since. It is not hard to imagine that chlorpromazine gave birth to the modern notions of psychiatric treatment—unlocked wards, milieu treatment, occupational and recreational therapy, psychiatric rehabilitation, and supervised living environments. The entire field of community mental health is ultimately linked to its

Important Dates in the Treatment of Mental Disorder with Psychopharmacology

• Quite by chance, chlorpromazine was first used to treat schizophrenia in 1952 after it was observed that its use as an antihistamine also calmed preoperative clients. It changed

forever the face of psychiatry, dramatically decreasing the number of inpatients and gave birth to modern notions of psychiatric treatment.

• In this decade, other antipsychotics, trifluoperazine, perphenazine and thioridazine were developed.

• Olive oil infused with narcotics, opium, morphine, or other sedatives was used to medicate "insane" and "deranged" people.

Before Psychopharmaceuticals

164 BCE to 1951 CE

Conventional Antipsychotics

1950s

2000s

Psychopharmaceuticals for the New Millenium

• Nonbenzodiazepine anxiolytic, ramelteon, used to treat anxiety.

• The first sedative–hypnotic for long-term treatment of insomnia, eszopiclone, is released.

• Synaptic action developments lead to antidepressant SSRI medications sertraline, paroxetine, and citalopram.

• Antidepressants called serotonin and norepinephrine reuptake inhibitors desvenlafaxine and duloxetine— which treat depression and pain—are developed and released or newly indicated for depression.

• The first antidepressant medication in a patch, seligiline, is made available.

• Atypical antipsychotics ziprasidone, aripiprazole, paliperidone, asenapine, and iloperidone add to treatment options.

• The first long-acting atypical antipsychotic, Risperdal Consta, provides long-acting antipsychotic without the side effects of the conventional antipsychotic. This leap forward in treating psychosis was followed by other long-acting atypical antipsychotics Zyprexa Relprevv and Invega Sustenna.

• Mood stabilizer medication, Symbyax, is a combination of olanzapine and fluoxetine for the treatment of acute mania and depression in bipolar disorder and as maintenance treatment in bipolar disorder and psychotic depression.

• Acetylcholinesterase inhibitor medication, galantamine, is developed and released.

• The first medication for dementia modifying the brain's glutamate pathway, memantine, pioneers alternative modes of dementia treatment.

FIGURE 7-1 ■ *Photo source top to bottom by column:* Philosophical Library; Smock, Timothy K., *Physiological Psychology: A Neuroscience Approach,* 1st Ed., ©1999. Reprinted and electronically reproduced by permission of Pearson Education, Inc., Upper Saddle River, New Jersey; Everett Collection; Shutterstock; Eileen Trigoboff; Shutterstock; Eileen Trigoboff; Pearson; Pearson; Pearson; Pearson; suravid/Shutterstock.

- Other antipsychotics such as haloperidol and thiothixene are made available.

- During this period, antianxiety agents were developed to relieve anxiety and induce sleep. Meprobamate was the first antianxiety agent in common use.

- Medications help people move out of institutions into less restrictive settings and homes.

- The antipsychotics mesoridazine and loxapine were developed.

- Long acting injections of haloperidol and fluphenazine allow clients to maintain steady levels of antipsychotic without depending on oral formulations. Injections can be given every 2, 3, or 4 weeks.

First Generation Antipsychotics and Anxiolytics

1960s - 1970s

2010s

- Atypical antipsychotic clozapine is re-released after extensive research to establish safety and use in North America. Becomes the "gold standard" in managing a treatment-resistant or treatment-refractory psychosis. Different dopamine action has decided impact on both negative and positive symptoms of schizophrenia.

- Atypical antipsychotics risperidone, olanzapine, and quetiapine are developed and released and have the advantage of being easier on the body, have fewer side effects due to advances in neurotransmitter effects, and do not require blood monitoring.

- Antidepressant SSRIs sertraline, paroxetine, and citalopram are made available.

- The first acetylcholinesterase inhibitor for memory enhancement in dementia, tacrine, is a new approach to treat the most problematic symptom.

- Acetylcholinesterase inhibitors donepezil and rivastigmine are developed and released.

- The first nonbenzodiazepine anxiolytic, zolpidem, is made available to treat anxiety, followed by zaleplon.

Advances in the Decade of the Brain

1990s

Contemporary Developments

- Psychiatric drug manuals (such as that written by psychiatric nurse Eileen Trigoboff) demonstrate nursing involvement in psychopharmacology.

- Atypical antipsychotic lurasidone is synthesized, adding yet another compound to treat psychosis.

- New research in seratonin reuptake leads to latest SSRI antidepressant vilazodone.

- Genetic phenotypes and variations, as well as the effects of ethnicity on psychiatric pharmacology (ethnopharmacology), are being explored so that someday soon we may be able to have exactly the right medication to help a client reach stability and recovery.

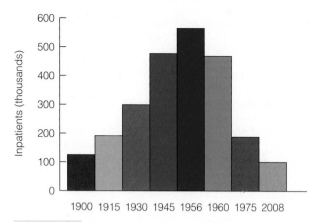

FIGURE 7-2 ■ The great success of biologic psychiatry. This graph illustrates the dramatic decrease in psychiatric inpatient numbers since the inception of psychopharmacology.

discovery because it enabled clients to return to their lives outside an inpatient facility.

In the decades since that discovery we learned a great deal about which medications generally work under which circumstances. Studies demonstrated that taking antipsychotic medication is far more effective than taking no medicine, and that taking it regularly is essential to the long-term treatment of schizophrenia. We know that medications alone are not sufficient to cure the disease, but they are necessary to manage it. These medications make psychosocial interventions

possible. Decades of experience demonstrate how psychopharmacology assists clients in managing anxiety, stress, and other symptoms so nurses can intervene with education about coping strategies and developing or strengthening support systems.

The National Institute of Mental Health funded a landmark study, the Clinical Antipsychotic Trials of Intervention Effectiveness (CATIE) study (Lieberman et al., 2005), that looked at treatment outcomes. This major study was designed to learn whether there were differences among the newer medications and whether they had significant advantages over older medications. It is still an important study although even newer medications exist. The results of the CATIE study are summarized in Box 7-1.

Understanding the psychobiology of antipsychotic medications requires a basic knowledge of the functions of the central nervous system. Chapter 6 ∞ provides an inside look at the psychobiologic mechanisms that are important in psychopharmacology. Illustrations and animations are also available through the Online Student Resources website. Here is an overview of the basic mechanisms of action.

Basic Mechanisms of Action

Generally, neuroleptics (medications that work on the central nervous system) work by blocking a variety of central nervous system (CNS) receptors. Most medications work on more than one neurotransmitter system. Therefore, it is likely that several types of neurotransmitters and

TABLE 7-1 ■ Medications and Their Cross-Diagnostic Uses														
	Psychosis	Dementia	Depression	Obsessions/ Compulsions	Mood Instability	PTSD	PMDD	Panic Disorder	Social Phobia	Autism	Convulsions	Cigarette Smoking	Migraine	Pain
Aripiprazole (Abilify)	✓		✓		✓									
Bupropion (Wellbutrin, Zyban)			✓									✓		
Carbamazepine (Tegretol)					✓						✓			
Divalproex (Depakote)		✓			✓						✓		✓	
Duloxetine (Cymbalta)			✓											✓
Fluvoxamine (Luvox)			✓	✓				✓						
Fluoxetine (Prozac, Sarafem)			✓	✓			✓	✓						
Olanzapine (Zyprexa)	✓				✓									
Paroxetine (Paxil)			✓					✓	✓					
Quetiapine (Seroquel)	✓	✓			✓									
Risperidone (Risperdal)	✓	✓			✓					✓				
Sertraline (Zoloft)			✓	✓		✓		✓						
SSRIs			✓					✓						
Tricyclic antidepressants			✓					✓						✓
Ziprasidone (Geodon)	✓		✓		✓									

Box 7-1 CATIE Study Summary

The 18-month Clinical Antipsychotic Trials of Intervention Effectiveness (CATIE) study, whose results were published in 2005, involved more than 1,400 participants at 57 sites around the United States. Its findings, based on a wide range of clients in a variety of treatment settings, are considered reliable and relevant to the 3.2 million Americans with schizophrenia. CATIE directly compared an older medication (perphenazine), available since the 1950s, to four atypical antipsychotics (olanzapine, quetiapine, risperidone, and ziprasidone) introduced in the 1990s. The goal of the study was to learn whether there are differences among the newer medications and whether the newer medications hold significant advantages over the older medications. The study was conceptualized before the newer antipsychotics such as aripiprazole (Abilify) and lurasidone (Latuda) were available in the United States.

These were the results:

- Several factors, such as adequacy of symptom relief, tolerability of side effects, and treatment cost, influence a person's willingness and ability to adhere to a medication regimen.
- Three fourths of the participants discontinued their antipsychotic medication and changed to another because of intolerable side effects or inadequately controlled symptoms.

- Olanzapine performed slightly better than the other medications but also was associated with significant weight gain and metabolic changes.
- Clients taking olanzapine were less likely to be hospitalized for a psychotic relapse and tended to stay on the medication longer than those taking other medications.
- Quetiapine, risperidone, ziprasidone, and olanzapine had a modest advantage over the older generic medication perphenazine.
- The study's highest olanzapine dose exceeded current label recommendations. Prescribers use higher doses of the other antipsychotics clinically than the study did.
- People taking ziprasidone, on average, experienced no weight gain and fewer of the neurologic tremors that can be a serious problem for people with schizophrenia.
- An important issue still to be considered is individual differences in response to these medications.
- Each medication has tradeoffs that must be considered for each client.

Source: Lieberman, J. A., Stroup, T. S., McEvoy, J. P., Swartz, M. S., Rosenheck, R. A., Perkins, D. O., . . . Hsiao, J. K. (Clinical Antipsychotic Trials of Intervention Effectiveness [CATIE] Investigators). (2005). Effectiveness of antipsychotic drugs in patients with chronic schizophrenia. *New England Journal of Medicine, 353,* 1209–1223.

neuromodulators are affected by the administration of a single medication. While most neuroleptics have an affinity for several types of neurotransmitters, others are more specific and work more selectively. These differences account for the effects of the various neuroleptic medications. Blockade of postsynaptic dopaminergic receptors (in other words, receptors that are designed specifically for dopamine are prevented from receiving dopamine) is one way these medications can have their main effect. Other pathways and mechanisms may also contribute. The side effects that result from this mechanism are consistently dry mouth, blurred vision, constipation, urinary retention, and parkinsonian side effects.

Major Effects

The beneficial effects of antipsychotic medications in all psychotic states have been demonstrated beyond question. Multiple and varied criteria have been used to measure improvement. These medications have been used successfully in clients with delusional thinking, hallucinations, confusion, motor agitation, and motor retardation. Antipsychotic medication treatment also decreases thought disorder, blunted affect, bizarre behavior, social withdrawal, belligerence, and uncooperativeness.

The most common disintegrative condition treated with antipsychotic medication is the group of symptoms traditionally labeled *schizophrenia* (see Chapter 16∞). The problem of assessment is complicated by the fact that many diseases can cause syndromes with features like those of schizophrenia. For example, delusions may indicate a variety of DSM conditions, including schizophrenia, bipolar mania, and dementia of the Alzheimer's type. All clients manifesting psychotic symptoms should have a thorough review of their medical history and a physical examination to rule out treatable medical illnesses, many of which are accompanied by behaviors considered psychotic or psychobiologic. Consider this: Would it be unjust to treat someone's symptoms with neuroleptic medications when a basic physical would have determined that the problem was a result of infection or a tumor?

The Choice of a Specific Medication

There are currently many older antipsychotic medications and several newer antipsychotic medications on the market in the United States. Two of the newer antipsychotics come in a long-acting injectable form. Medications have varying success rates because individual responses frequently dictate use. The choice of a particular medication, then, depends on its pharmacologic properties and likely side effects, the client's or a family member's history of response to that medication, and the prescriber's experience with various compounds. Important client variables are past successes with specific medications, a history of allergies, a history of serious or intolerable side effects, and current ability to manage a medication schedule. Some medications may have side effects such as sedation, which, while not necessarily desired by the prescriber, may nevertheless prove helpful in treatment. Expect a certain amount of trial and error with each clinical application.

TABLE 7-2 ■ lists the major antipsychotic medications. The list is extensive and growing, and it makes sense for each member of the treatment team to become familiar with just a few representative medications, their predictable effects, and their common side effects. As the nurse, you will likely be a resource for the other non–medically trained team members in this regard (that is, social workers, rehabilitation counselors, and psychologists). Some characteristics of these medications are discussed in the sections that follow.

More than seven distinct chemical classes of antipsychotic medications are now commonly used in the United States. (One class, the phenothiazines, is subdivided into three different types of medications.) As a result, there are choices in terms of side effects and potential client responsiveness. A client who is unresponsive to one class may respond to another that circumvents a problem in absorption, accumulation at neurotransmitter receptor sites, or metabolism. However, there are many people for whom the available medications are not especially helpful, or, if major symptoms are addressed, the side effects reduce the overall benefit of the medication.

You will see in the course of your career, whether it is as a psychiatric–mental health nurse or in any other specialty practice, that more choices are still needed.

Table 7-2 also shows the wide range among antipsychotic medications in milligram-per-milligram potency. This fact is most relevant when treating clients who require large doses. In such cases, a potent medication is best. Consumer issues and clinician concerns are addressed at http://www.FDA.gov, the website for the U.S. Food and Drug Administration. You can access the FDA through the Online Student Resources.

Newer Antipsychotics

The newer antipsychotics (also called *atypical antipsychotics*) have a drastically different physiologic action than do the traditional or conventional antipsychotics. Conventional antipsychotics primarily affect the positive symptoms of psychotic disorders, with little or no effect on the negative or cognitive symptoms. Their mechanism of action is thought to occur through nonselectively blocking the neurotransmitter dopamine D_2 receptors in the brain. To be clinically effective,

TABLE 7-2 ■ Antipsychotic Medications*

Class	Generic Name	Trade Name	Usual Dosage Range (mg/day)
Atypical/SGA			
Benzoisothiazol derivative	Lurasidone	Latuda	40–80
Benzisothiazolyl piperazine derivative	Ziprasidone	Geodon	40–200
Benzisoxazole derivative	Risperidone	Risperdal	4–6
	Paliperidone	Invega	3–12
Dibenzodiazepines	Clozapine	Clozaril	12.5–900
Dibenzo-oxepino pyrrole	Asenapine	Saphris	10–20
Dibenzothiazepine derivative	Quetiapine	Seroquel	300–400
Dichlorophenyl piperazinyl butoxydihydroquinolin	Aripiprazole	Abilify	10–30
Piperidinyl-benzisoxazole derivative	Iloperidone	Fanapt	12–24
Thieno-benzodiazepine	Olanzapine	Zyprexa	10–20
Conventional/Typical			
Butyrophenones	Haloperidol	Haldol	2–40
Dibenzoxazepines	Loxapine	Loxitane	10–100
Dihydroindolones	Molindone	Moban	15–225
Phenothiazines			
Aliphatic	Chlorpromazine	Thorazine	150–1500
Piperazine	Trifluoperazine	Stelazine	10–60
	Fluphenazine	Prolixin	3–45
	Perphenazine	Trilafon	12–60
Piperidine	Thioridazine	Mellaril	150–800
Thioxanthenes	Thiothixene	Navane	10–60
	Chlorprothixene	Taractan	40–600

*Atypical antipsychotics currently not available in the United States: sulpiride, amisulpiride, melperone, sertindole.

these medications occupy between 70% and 90% of the D_2 receptors, while the advent of EPSEs occurs at above 80% occupancy (Veselinovi et al., 2011; Muller et al., 2010). The newer antipsychotics have a much reduced affinity, or attraction, for D_2 receptors, and they all have an affinity for the serotonin receptors, a profile that appears to lessen EPSEs and can improve the negative symptoms of psychotic disorders.

The newer antipsychotics offer a wider range of options for the care and treatment of clients experiencing psychotic conditions. The search continues for more psychopharmacologic treatments for psychoses. Medications are being researched and tested every day, and if they provide relief from symptoms without undue side effects, clients will be more likely to continue taking them, and will therefore have fewer symptoms of their illness and stay healthier longer.

Uncomfortable side effects are reasons many people do not continue taking any prescription medication. If someone with a major mental illness such as schizophrenia stops taking an antipsychotic, becoming very sick and losing the ability to function well is likely. Mental Health in the Movies provides one such example.

There is a variety of atypical antipsychotics including clozapine (Clozaril), risperidone (Risperdal, Risperdal Consta), paliperidone (Invega, Invega Sustenna), olanzapine (Zyprexa, Zyprexa Relprevv), asenapine (Saphris), iloperidone (Fanapt), and lurasidone (Latuda). An overall look at two examples follows.

Clozapine (Clozaril)

The first atypical antipsychotic on the market in the United States was clozapine (Clozaril). Clozapine is an antipsychotic medication with an unusual pharmacologic and clinical profile. It was used in Europe for several years and is now generally used in the United States with clients who cannot tolerate the EPSEs of other antipsychotics, or who have a treatment-resistant or treatment-refractory psychosis, as is the case with certain clients with schizophrenia. Reviews of studies regarding the effectiveness of clozapine have demonstrated its

decided impact on both negative and positive symptoms, with improvement evident on follow-up as well.

Serious Side Effects Despite its remarkable capacity to ameliorate some very recalcitrant symptoms for people, clozapine has some serious side effects. The most serious is **agranulocytosis** (a marked decrease in granulated white blood cells), which occurs in less than 1% of clients taking this medication. It is essential to monitor the white blood cell count (WBC) and absolute neutrophil count (ANC) of clients taking clozapine. Immediately discontinuing the medication when agranulocytosis is detected and before signs of an infection develop will usually resolve the episode. There are specific guidelines for treating a client who experiences agranulocytosis as a result of using clozapine. Clozapine can be reinstituted (called *re-challenging*) under certain circumstances but not others.

There is a risk for agranulocytosis with a variety of other psychotropic medications (conventional antipsychotics, benzodiazepines, anticonvulsants); however, there is a higher risk with clozapine. There have been reported rates of agranulocytosis at significantly lower levels than the currently estimated 1% (that is, 0.25%, according to Snowdon & Halliday, 2011). One of the important questions for clozapine treatment remains, "Is there a specific risk period for agranulocytosis, and if there is, when does it occur?" The risk period establishes the frequency of blood monitoring, which can be an impediment to clients' initial and continued use of the antipsychotic.

Currently, it is estimated that this rare side effect of agranulocytosis may occur up to a year following initial treatment with clozapine, although the vast majority of cases appear within 5 months. As a result of these data, blood monitoring for agranulocytosis is completed weekly for the first 6 months of therapy. If WBC levels remain normal and regular use is not interrupted throughout those 6 months, then blood monitoring can be reduced to biweekly frequencies. After another 6 months of regular use and normal blood results, monitoring can be done monthly. Because the medication stays in the

Teva Clozapine Patient Registry

MENTAL HEALTH IN THE MOVIES
The Soloist

The movie *The Soloist* is based on the true story of a homeless musician with schizophrenia, Nathaniel Ayers (played by Jamie Foxx), befriended by a Los Angeles Times correspondent, Steve Lopez (played by Robert Downey, Jr.), who wrote a series of articles that brought the plight of the homeless and the seriously mentally ill to attention. Nathaniel, a cello prodigy at Juilliard, dropped out of the prestigious music school and ended up on the streets when he was no longer able to handle the voices in his head. An accomplished musician, Nathaniel also plays the violin, French horn, clarinet, and oboe. The movie shows Nathaniel sleeping each night on one of skid row's filthy,

rat-infested streets in which thousands of homeless, mostly mentally ill, people sleep. *The Soloist* is essentially the story of the ups and downs, and bumps in the road, in a friendship between a person with schizophrenia who has the right to refuse treatment such as medications and a person who tries to help from his own frame of reference. The movie does not end with Ayers magically getting better and rejoining mainstream society. In 2009, Ayers was honored by the National Association on Mental Illness for decreasing the stigma associated with being mentally ill. Their friendship continues to this day.

Photo courtesy of Alamy.

system for some time after discontinuation, remember that blood monitoring must continue for 4 weeks following the discontinuation of clozapine regardless of where your client is in this schedule.

Another serious side effect is the potential for seizure, which seems to be dose related at over 600 mg/day. Less acute, but nonetheless important, side effects include sedation, tachycardia, sialorrhea (drooling), weight gain, and hypotension. Balancing positive symptom control and negative symptom relief with these side effects—a consideration with all antipsychotic medications—is explored in Chapter 31 ∞.

Risperidone (Risperdal)

Risperidone was introduced in the United States in 1994. It was the first of a new class of antipsychotics, benzisoxazole derivatives, that does not clinically relate to any existing antipsychotic medication. Its unique feature is the relative absence of EPSE at the therapeutic dosing level. It addresses the positive, negative, and affective symptoms of schizophrenia and may also alleviate depression and anxiety. Side effects similar to those experienced with haloperidol (Haldol) are seen in doses above 10 mg per day.

Dosage for risperidone has been described as "the 1-2-3" regimen, in which the client receives 1 mg bid, the next increase (slowly titrated according to the client's tolerability and response) is to 2 mg bid, and the next increase after that is to 3 mg bid. This places the client at 6 mg/day, which is in the currently recommended therapeutic window of 4 to 8 mg/day. Doses less than 3 mg/day have been linked with a better outcome than higher doses (Gafoor et al., 2010). Risperidone can be administered up to 16 mg/day, but the absence of EPSEs fades at doses over 10 mg/day. Response within 1 to 10 weeks gives the medication a fair trial. Dosage for older clients is lower; the initial dosage is generally cut in half (0.5 mg bid, 1 mg bid, and 1.5 mg bid) and there is at least 1 full week between dosage changes.

Risperidone has been very useful in the treatment of psychotic symptoms, and the clinical knowledge gained from using it regularly has been valuable. Risperidone is now available in depot injection form. (**Depot injection** is a term used to describe the slow release of a long-term medication given by intramuscular or subcutaneous injection using the body as a temporary storage device for the entire dose.) This compound, called Consta, is injected every 2 weeks. This additional administration mode for risperidone offers another choice in the array of treatments for psychotic symptoms. (See Unique Routes of Administration.)

Other uses for risperidone include its 2003 indication for treating extreme mood swings in bipolar disorder in addition to its antipsychotic features. In 2006, the orally disintegrating tablets of risperidone, M-tab, received an indication to treat symptoms of irritability in autistic children and adolescents. Aggressiveness, deliberate self-injury, and the temper tantrums associated with autism are also addressed by this medication.

Dosage

Dosage ranges for antipsychotic medications vary widely among clients. Medications must be titrated against the psychotic target symptoms and the appearance of side effects. Most clients are initially given a relatively low dose of an antipsychotic to test for adverse effects for 1 to 2 hours. Consider chlorpromazine, with an initial dose of 20 to 50 mg orally (PO) or 25 mg intramuscularly (IM). Later the medication is typically given in doses of 300 to 400 mg (or IM equivalent) per day, and gradually increased by 25% to 50% each day until maximum improvement is noted or intolerable side effects are encountered. This type of progression is common with the various antipsychotic medications.

Treatment settings frequently influence the medication regimen. In a crowded hospital emergency room, for example, hourly doses of medication may be given until a client is sedated. In more completely staffed, private inpatient units, a client may be observed for several days before medication is given. Symptoms and behavioral problems are addressed by the antipsychotic medication, but cognitive functioning studies have been inconclusive. When looking at long-term outcome and length of time until eventual remission, neither approach has been found to be superior to the other (Preskorn, 2011).

Clients who are extremely agitated, violent, severely withdrawn, or catatonic require significant doses during the first few days of treatment, delivered by injection to ensure rapid relief. Chlorpromazine, 50 to 100 mg IM, may be used, particularly if sedation is required. Be aware that this is an irritating medication; injections must be deeply intramuscular in either the buttocks or upper arms, and sites must be rotated. Substantial IM doses of the more potent antipsychotics, such as haloperidol 10 mg or trifluoperazine 10 mg, may be given to agitated clients.

There are options for short-term injections, such as ziprasidone (Geodon), aripiprazole (Abilify), and olanzapine (Zyprexa), that replace the use of older, conventional antipsychotic medications. This approach frequently avoids some of the more troublesome side effects while ameliorating behavioral and cognitive symptoms. Use of an atypical antipsychotic reduces side effects and therefore has a positive impact on a client's perceptions of psychiatric medications. The role atypical antipsychotics play in helping clients remain on their medications and experience fewer troublesome side effects is discussed more fully in Chapter 31 ∞.

After maximum clinical improvement has been obtained, antipsychotic medications are generally reduced in a gradual manner. Continuing to give a client modest doses of an antipsychotic following a psychotic episode lowers the chances of relapse and rehospitalization. Rehabilitation and recovery interventions (Chapter 32 ∞) are especially helpful for individuals who have psychiatric symptomatology. Psychotherapy with clients who have schizophrenia may not be particularly effective without maintenance medications in conventional treatment settings, but it does improve psychosocial functioning in clients who are also taking maintenance medications. It is generally believed that clients should be kept on doses of antipsychotics sufficient to suppress symptoms for 3 months to 1 year following an acute episode. After that interval, the client's course and life situation must be considered and treatment individualized. Some clients recover from a psychotic episode completely within 6 months. Clients with schizophreniform disorder should not receive long-term maintenance medication treatment. For individuals who have already experienced recurrent episodes of psychosis and demonstrate a deteriorating course, it is clearly advantageous to prevent relapses with medications if possible.

The Decision to Use a Medication

Today, the following general principles govern antipsychotic medication use:

- Medications are given to treat target symptoms of schizophrenia or other psychotic disorders.
- Initial treatment may require parenteral doses or rapidly dissolving forms. These are changed to oral forms such as pills or liquid concentrate as the behavior disturbance subsides.
- Total dosages are tailored to individual needs; wide variations exist among clients.
- For medications with sedating side effects, divided doses are changed as soon as is practical to a single dose, given at bedtime to maximize the medication's sedative properties.
- Most clients with a chronic course require maintenance doses for sustained improvement and to minimize the number of relapses.

Other considerations for using a particular medication include the use of adjunctive therapies. Adjunctive treatment may be necessary when an available compound has a necessary, but insufficient, impact on symptoms and another medication using different pathways or different mechanisms is able to provide an additional and sufficient impact. This package of two or three medications can work in concert for the client. The ever-present danger with this practice is called *polypharmacy* where too many medications are used without careful consideration of when medications can and should be discontinued from the mix (Mojtabai & Olfson, 2010).

Do the medications needed to treat one problem blend well with any or all of the other medications the client may need? Clients often have more than a single mental disorder. Multiple diagnoses require a more complex palette of biologic therapies. See Your Assessment Approach for antipsychotic medication interactions with other medications and substances to which your client may be exposed.

Special Considerations

The following special considerations apply to the use of antipsychotic medication.

Unique Routes of Administration

The phenothiazines, fluphenazine (Prolixin) and haloperidol, are available in long-acting intramuscular injectable forms that behave like time-release capsules. These medications are gradually released over a long period of time, 2 to 4 weeks. Long-acting fluphenazine and haloperidol are available in decanoate, long-acting depot injection preparations that are oil based. The long-acting parenteral form of risperidone (Risperdal Consta) is also a depot medication available for injection every 2 weeks but instead of being oil based, the microspheres containing the medication are suspended in water. This injection is easier to tolerate and, because it is an atypical antipsychotic, has fewer side effects and can address the negative symptoms of schizophrenia. Olanzapine has a long-acting injectable atypical antipsychotic—Zyprexa Relprevv. The standard of care is to observe the client for 4 hours following the injection. Research is nearing completion for the depot route of administration for aripiprazole (Abilify).

As with any depot medication, the oral form of the same medication must be administered before the depot is used to ensure the client tolerates the medication. The main advantages

---

YOUR ASSESSMENT APPROACH   Antipsychotic Medication Interactions

Combining One of These	With One of These Antipsychotics	Can Lead to These Problems
Antacids	Phenothiazine antipsychotic	Decreased phenothiazine effect
Anticholinergics	Clozapine	Potentiated anticholinergic effect of clozapine
	Antipsychotic	Increased level of neuroleptic in the system, with extrapyramidal side effects
Benzodiazepines	Clozapine	Respiratory arrest, circulatory difficulties
Carbamazepine	Haloperidol	Decreased effect of either medication
	Clozapine	Additive bone marrow suppression
CNS depressants such as: narcotics, anxiolytics, alcohol, barbiturates, or antihistamines	Antipsychotic	Additive CNS depression
Coffee, tea, milk, or fruit juices	Phenothiazine antipsychotic	Decreased phenothiazine effect

of depot forms are that they reduce clients' ambivalence about taking medication, eliminate the need for constant pill taking, and can help clients who have illness-related cognitive impairments. Memory and concentration difficulties are typical among those with executive functioning deficits, one of the major impairments that must be overcome by people who have schizophrenia. (Chapter 6∞ discusses executive functioning.) Making sure clients have a steady level of medication in their system minimizes the fluctuations in blood level seen in nonparenteral forms of medication administration. A fluctuating blood level leads to more difficulty managing symptoms, especially if the client is sensitive to minor fluctuations. A depot antipsychotic with considerably fewer side effects than haloperidol and fluphenazine, such as Risperdal Consta, has the potential to prolong antipsychotic medication use and minimize dissatisfaction with, and discontinuation of, treatment.

The psychiatric–mental health nurse in a community setting may frequently have occasion to administer long-acting fluphenazine, haloperidol, Risperdal Consta, or Zyprexa Relprevv. With a client whose treatment will include a long-acting medication, a dose of the oral form is taken first to rule out the possibility of allergic reactions. Such reactions can be devastating if discovered after a 2- or 3-week supply of medicine has been given as a depot treatment. If no adverse reactions are noted, the long-acting form is injected, usually in a large muscle mass. Ongoing research and clinical experience provides us with options for muscles such as the deltoid to use for these injection sites (Saxena et al., 2008).

Various pharmaceutical companies have explored better routes for medication administration for years. As a result, there is yet another way to give a number of antipsychotic preparations. Clozapine, risperidone, olanzapine, and aripiprazole are all available in orally disintegrating tablet formulations. The clozapine version is called FazaClo, risperidone's oral formulation is called M-tab, the olanzapine version is called Zyprexa Zydis, and aripiprazole has a Discmelt product. (You may see the Zydis form used with a variety of compounds in medical–surgical settings.) These tablets begin disintegrating in the mouth within seconds, so they can be swallowed with or without liquid, thus reducing problems with swallowing and cheeking (hiding) behaviors and offering a more discreet option for taking medication during activities. This vehicle for administering full doses of medication promotes adherence.

In the future we will see a variety of innovative and effective technologies for enhancing the administration and absorption of psychiatric medications. Currently, research is investigating the following:

- Multiphase, multicompartment capsules using gelatin, natural hydroxypropyl methylcellulose, and alternative capsule materials
- Quick-dissolving strips and films
- Inhalers
- Implanted pumps

The first patch for transdermal delivery of an antidepressant is selegiline (Emsam). More are being developed. These opportunities for medication delivery platforms, coupled with research for new compounds to treat disorders, help normalize psychiatric disorders—that is, they are treated just as all other physical disorders are treated—and provide more options. Over the course of your career in nursing, you will see innovative and effective absorption-enhancing delivery systems and routes for administration of medications to treat and improve the quality of life for your clients.

Potential Side Effects of Antipsychotic Medications

Continuous contact with clients gives nurses an advantage over other professionals who may see a client only every other day or, at best, once a day. Both the dangerous and the more uncomfortable side effects frequently have a rapid onset and need prompt attention.

The side effects of antipsychotic medications that nurses must recognize can be divided into the following classes:

- Autonomic nervous system
- Extrapyramidal
- Other central nervous system
- Allergic
- Blood
- Skin
- Eye
- Endocrine
- Weight gain

See Chapter 31∞ for details about these side effects and how to help clients manage the side effects they experience.

Metabolizing Psychiatric Medications

A liver enzyme called cytochrome P_{450} (abbreviated as CYP) is responsible for metabolizing psychiatric medication out of the client's system. The two main directions that can influence how your clients metabolize psychiatric medications are called *inhibition* and *activation* (or *induction*). Inhibition of the enzyme allows the medication and its metabolites to remain in the system longer than usual, accumulating and causing higher blood levels, enhanced effects of the medication, and greater side effects. Imagine a jammed parking lot or gridlock on a city street as the medication is unable to flow out of the system easily.

Induction (or activation) of the enzyme speeds the medication and its metabolites out of the system faster than usual. When a medication does not have enough time to take full effect, it may appear that symptoms are not being competently addressed. The medication is considerably less effective in this case than if it had the time to be fully utilized by the body. Picture the medication being washed out of the system faster than intended.

Other coadministered medications, your client's genetics, foods eaten, and cigarettes smoked are some of the factors that can induce or inhibit cytochrome P_{450}. The entire field of study on CYPs is an extensive one, covering the intricacies of medication interactions, metabolism, and coadministration cautions.

Liver Enzyme Cytochrome P450 Animation

ANTIDEPRESSANT MEDICATIONS

Classes of **antidepressant medications** (pharmaceutical compounds used to treat the symptoms of depression) that currently exist include: **tricyclic antidepressants (TCAs)**, **monoamine oxidase inhibitors (MAOIs)**, **selective serotonin reuptake inhibitors (SSRIs)**, phenethylamine antidepressants (also known as **serotonin and norepinephrine reuptake inhibitors [SNRIs]**), and atypical antidepressants (so called because of their variety of formulation and actions). For a look at some of the variety of antidepressant medications currently available from different classes with differing actions, see TABLE 7-3 ■.

Like antipsychotic medications, the original antidepressant medications were discovered accidentally. In the case of imipramine (Tofranil), the first of the tricyclic antidepressants, investigators were actually searching for effective antipsychotics similar to chlorpromazine. The "tri-" in *tricyclic antidepressants* refers to the triple chemical rings at the center of each of the medications. Iproniazid, a MAOI, was discovered when people with tuberculosis who were regularly treated with a similar medication, isoniazid, became less depressed. Antidepressants have shed considerable light on the biochemical mechanisms of the brain in both normal and abnormal emotional expression. See the Evidence-Based Practice feature regarding psychopharmacology in the treatment of depression.

Psychobiologic Considerations

Knowledge about the pharmacology of antidepressant medications has led to a theory of the biochemistry of depression. Basically, all the true antidepressants make the neurotransmitters norepinephrine (NE) and serotonin (5-HT) more available to the synaptic receptors in the central nervous system. Tricyclics block the reuptake of these substances into the neuron after their release, thereby postponing their degradation. MAOIs interfere with the enzymes responsible for the actual breakdown of the neurotransmitter molecules. Because both are antidepressants, these observations have led to the theory that NE and 5-HT shortages in the brain cause depression, at least the type of depression that responds to medication therapy.

The initial distinction to be understood in the psychopharmacology of depression is between true antidepressants and stimulants or euphoriants. TCAs and MAOIs are not stimulants and do not induce euphoria in healthy people. In a single dose they have a sedative effect. Amphetamines and methylphenidate (Ritalin), on the other hand, are stimulants but not antidepressants in the pharmacologic sense. They can induce an increased sense of well-being in certain individuals, but do nothing to combat depression on a lasting basis.

Tricyclic antidepressants are the "first generation" of antidepressant medications, that is, they were among the first medications identified as effective in the treatment of depression. New developments and ideas in chemical motivations to help treat symptoms of depression are labeled as subsequent generations.

Since the introduction of the first antidepressants, a number of medications have been developed to treat the symptoms of major depression and the depressive features of schizoaffective disorder. Among these medications are the MAOIs, the SSRIs, the SNRIs, and a number of atypical antidepressants with a variety of neurotransmitter actions.

Bupropion (Wellbutrin) is an oral antidepressant medication that is not a TCA and is unrelated to other known antidepressants. Bupropion has been well tolerated in people who experience orthostatic hypotension when taking TCAs. This medication has the potential to cause seizures to a greater extent than other antidepressants depending on the dose. It has few anticholinergic side effects and essentially no important cardiovascular effects. Bupropion is also indicated for use as an aid to smoking cessation. Sustained-release formulations of this medication are available under two trade names, Wellbutrin SR and Zyban. For smoking cessation, the medication is used for up to 14 weeks.

As each new group of medications became available, practitioners initially used the new medications to the partial exclusion of the old. When a client is not responding to a medication, it is helpful to have an array of choices from which to select further treatment. The side effect profiles of antidepressants remain one of the linchpins of successful care. If sedation is a side effect and the client is sleeping at a higher-than-preferred level, then a class of medications with less sedating side effects may be a better choice. Experience reinforces the truth that a number of treatment and medication options are necessary to effectively treat

Methylphenidate Drug Mechanism in Action Animation

TABLE 7-3 ■ Antidepressant Medications				
TCA	**Other Antidepressants**	**SSRI**	**MAOI**	**SNRI**
Amitriptyline (Elavil)	Amoxapine (Asendin)	Sertraline (Zoloft)	Phenelzine sulfate (Nardil)	Venlafaxine (Effexor)
Desipramine (Norpramin)	Trazodone (Desyrel)	Paroxetine (Paxil)	Tranylcypromine sulfate (Parnate)	Duloxetine (Cymbalta)
Imipramine (Tofranil)	Maprotiline (Ludiomil)	Fluoxetine (Prozac)	Isocarboxazid (Marplan)	Desvenlafaxine (Pristiq)
Nortriptyline (Aventyl)	Bupropion (Wellbutrin)	Citalopram (Celexa)	Selegiline (Emsam)	
Protriptyline (Vivactil)	Mirtazapine (Remeron)	Escitalopram (Lexapro)		
		Vilazodone (Viibryd)		

EVIDENCE-BASED PRACTICE

Depression and Antidepressant Medications

You are working in an acute psychiatric setting with an individual who is severely depressed and is receiving a tricyclic antidepressant. This African-American client, Ryan, told you he feels so much better after only a few doses of medication, although his mouth is uncomfortably dry. You ask a number of questions about his latest symptoms, and he reports significantly less depression. You have a few theories about why this is happening. One is the "flight into health" people sometimes demonstrate, especially those with depressive symptoms. The diagnosis of depression and the need for therapeutic interventions may frighten or disrupt them to the point where they downplay symptoms or actually feel less depressed temporarily and declare themselves much better.

Another theory is that the energizing impact of the antidepressant is taking place before a significant difference has been made in depressive thinking, including lethality. This energy can be mobilized into suicide attempts. The third theory for Ryan's improvement is the faster therapeutic response and higher serum concentrations of tricyclics in African-Americans. His dry mouth is evidence that the higher serum concentration is causing more adverse effects than are experienced by other groups.

Your discussion with Ryan focuses on his treatment, side effects, and a lethality assessment. You have seen journal articles regarding these issues and are able to assess a depressed individual at this stage of treatment, keeping the possible explanations in mind. Findings from ethnopharmacology research, such as the following reference citations, support the differences seen with extensive metabolizers (EM) and poor metabolizers (PM) in genetic phenotypes. (Remember that action should be based on more than one study.)

Lea, D. H., Skirton, H., Read, C. Y., & Williams, J. K. (2011). Implications for educating the next generation of nurses on genetics and genomics in the 21st century. *Journal of Nursing Scholarship, 43*(1), 3–12.

Nichols, A. I., Focht, K., Jiang, Q., Preskorn, S. H., & Kane, C. P. (2011). Pharmacokinetics of venlafaxine extended release 75 mg and desvenlafaxine 50 mg in healthy CYP2D6 extensive and poor metabolizers: A randomized, open-label, two-period, parallel-group, crossover study. *Clinical Drug Investigations, 31*(3), 155–167.

CRITICAL THINKING QUESTIONS

1. How would you go about determining whether Ryan is downplaying his symptoms?
2. How would knowing the racial and cultural differences in main effects and side effects of medications help you assess a depressed client?
3. Why would Ryan's energy level be a helpful indicator of medication effectiveness?
4. How would you go about determining Ryan's suicide risk?
5. Of what value are Ryan's responses to your therapeutic interventions in interpreting whether his depressive thoughts have been disrupted?

psychiatric disorders; therefore, all categories of antidepressants remain useful.

Tricyclic Antidepressants (TCAs)

One of the commonly used classes of antidepressant medications is tricyclic antidepressants (TCAs), named for their consistent triple-ringed chemical structure. These compounds are close in chemical structure to phenothiazines and have many similar side effects, but they have profoundly different effects on mood, behavior, and cognition. TCAs are not antipsychotic agents when given to clients with schizophrenia and may in fact aggravate a disintegrative pattern or precipitate overt symptoms in a client with latent disintegrative behavior. Imipramine (Tofranil) and amitriptyline (Elavil) are the two prime representative TCAs. Desipramine (Norpramin, Pertofrane), nortriptyline (Pamelor), and protriptyline (Vivactil) are reported to reduce the incidence of side effects.

Monoamine Oxidase Inhibitors (MAOIs)

Clients who do not respond to TCAs may respond to another major class, monoamine oxidase inhibitors (MAOIs). These medications inhibit the enzyme monoamine oxidase from breaking down the neurotransmitter. Generally, MAOIs are not as effective as tricyclics and are somewhat slower to act, sometimes requiring a month of treatment before improvement shows. Isocarboxazid (Marplan) is considered the most effective, with phenelzine (Nardil) and tranylcypromine (Parnate) slightly behind. Complicating the decision to use MAOIs is their association with several very severe side effects. Hepatic necrosis, commonly fatal, and **hypertensive crisis** (severe elevation in diastolic blood pressure above 120 to 130 mmHg) leading to intracranial bleeding are among the most threatening. The latter reaction, heralded by severe headache, stiff neck, nausea, vomiting, and sharply increased blood pressure follows the ingestion of foods that contain the amino acid tyramine and the ingestion of sympathomimetic medications. The potential to have an antidepressant interact with other medications is explored in Your Assessment Approach: Antidepressant Medication Interactions.

Introduction of a patch system for treatment with a MAOI, selegiline (Emsam), does not require the dietary restrictions at the lower dose (Gillman, 2011). This transdermal method of delivering an antidepressant dose is also less stigmatizing. See

YOUR ASSESSMENT APPROACH   Antidepressant Medication Interactions

Combining One of These	With One of These Antidepressants	Can Lead to These Problems
Antiarrhythmic	TCA	Additive antiarrhythmic effect, myocardial depression
Anticholinergic	TCA	Additive anticholinergic effect
Anticonvulsant	TCA	Decreased TCA effect, lower seizure threshold
Antihypertensive	TCA	Hypertensive crisis
Antipsychotic	TCA	Increased TCA effect, confusion, delirium, ileus
CNS depressants such as: Alcohol Antihistamines Anxiolytics Barbiturates Narcotics	TCA	Decreased TCA effect, additive CNS depression
Foods or medications containing tyramine	MAOI	Hypertensive crisis
Levodopa	MAOI	Hypertensive crisis
MAOI	SSRI	Serotonin syndrome, serious adverse reactions
MAOI	TCA	Hyperpyrexia, severe excitation
Nicotine	TCA	Decreased TCA serum level
St. John's wort (herb)	SSRI	Sedative–hypnotic intoxication
SSRI	TCA	Increased TCA serum levels, elevated nortriptyline serum levels with adverse effects

the feature Partnering With Clients and Families: Teaching About a Low-Tyramine Diet in Chapter 31∞.

Further development of antidepressants has been the result of a scientific search for medications with fewer toxic side effects and greater biologic predictability in the treatment of depression. Newer antidepressants are believed to be more neurotransmitter specific and better able to treat conditions related to dopamine, serotonin, or norepinephrine dysfunctions.

The earlier antidepressants have certain disadvantages. Uncomfortable and sometimes intolerable side effects and a number of use restrictions with certain populations, combined with the dietary restrictions of the MAOIs, make these medications inappropriate for many people.

Selective Serotonin Reuptake Inhibitors (SSRIs)

The next class of antidepressant medications developed was the selective serotonin reuptake inhibitors (SSRIs). While chemically different, SSRIs inhibit the reuptake (and thus the deactivation) of the neurotransmitter serotonin, allowing for the increased availability of serotonin at synapses. The first SSRI developed was fluoxetine. There are now a number of potent and highly specific medications with this action including the latest vilazodone (Viibryd). A profound difference with this group of medications is their much safer and more tolerable side effects.

The SSRIs shed light on the workings of synapses. For the first time, psychiatric–mental health nurses were able to

see the direct impact of changing neurotransmitter concentrations. FIGURE 7-3 ■ shows the structure of the synapse. To see an animation of the synaptic action of these medications, see the Online Student Resources accompanying this text.

An important consideration for clients taking SSRIs is the proximity of the administration of MAOIs. Fluoxetine and a MAOI together may cause serious and fatal interactions. The half-life of fluoxetine is such that there must be a 5-week gap between taking fluoxetine and taking a MAOI, and vice versa. Sertraline (Zoloft), paroxetine (Paxil), citalopram (Celexa), and escitalopram (Lexapro) have shorter half-lives, and there must be a 1- or 2-week gap (both directions) between taking these medications and taking MAOIs. Keep in mind that St. John's wort is a naturally occurring MAOI and, although as a botanical it is much less potent than a pharmaceutical-grade compound, can also interact with an SSRI and cause a negative episode for your client. FIGURE 7-4 ■ illustrates the process of serotonin neurotransmission, which is so important to the effectiveness of SSRIs. Imagine the movement of neurotransmitters back and forth across the synapse—this is the movement that SSRIs affect.

Of note is the cross-diagnostic use of medications initially indicated for other conditions (discussed earlier in this chapter and referred to in Table 7-1). Fluoxetine (Prozac) is an antidepressant and was the first SSRI developed. This compound has an indication for another treatment regimen. Under the trade name Sarafem, fluoxetine is used to treat the mood and physical symptoms of premenstrual dysphoric disorder (PMDD), which is differentiated from depression and

Neurological Synapse Animation

Fluoxetine Drug Mechanism in Action Animation

(a)

(b)

FIGURE 7-3 ■ Structure of the synapse. The synapse at the top has many specialized characteristics. The electron micrograph shows the vesicles containing the synaptic transmitter, the abundance of mitochondria necessary for energy production, and the abundance of protein in the presynaptic and postsynaptic densities. Above are incoming axons (purple) contacting dendrites (yellow) with nonneural cells nearby (green).
Photo courtesy of (top) Photo Researchers, Inc., Don W. Fawcett; (bottom) Photo Researchers, Inc.

(c)

FIGURE 7-4 ■ Serotonin neurotransmission. (a) A highly schematic model of normal serotonin (5-HT) neurotransmission.
(b) In depression, there may be a shortage of 5-HT in the synapse.
(c) The action of an antidepressant medication blocking 5-HT reabsorption (reuptake).

other mental disorders. The dosing is flexible and is usually 20 mg/day.

Serotonin and Norepinephrine Reuptake Inhibitors (SNRIs)

Venlafaxine (Effexor) is the first in a class of new-generation antidepressants called *phenethylamine antidepressants,* also called serotonin and norepinephrine reuptake inhibitors (SNRIs). They have two mechanisms of action: inhibiting the reuptake of both serotonin and norepinephrine. Anticholinergic-like side effects may occur. The newest compound in this class is desvenlafaxine (Pristiq). A time buffer is also necessary when a SNRI is used in conjunction with MAOIs: a 14-day gap after discontinuing a MAOI before starting the SNRI, and at least a 7-day gap after discontinuing SNRI and before starting a MAOI.

Another SNRI is duloxetine (Cymbalta). The starting dose is 30 mg/day, usually given for 1 week, with the target therapeutic dose of 60 mg/day. Higher doses have occasionally been used for treatment-resistant neuropathic pain and treatment-resistant depression. Like venlafaxine, duloxetine can occasionally disturb sodium metabolism and disrupt lab values. Notable is that duloxetine may enhance the effects of benzodiazepines, but does not enhance the effects of alcohol (Knadler, Lobo, Chappell, & Bergstrom, 2011).

Other Medications Used for Depression

Stimulants, such as amphetamines and methylphenidate (Ritalin), and the phenothiazines are less commonly used antidepressants. Stimulants are not a proven treatment. Phenothiazines may be particularly useful in the presence of agitation. Some clinicians and researchers believe that major depressive episodes with psychotic features (delusional depressions) respond better to a combination of an antidepressant and an antipsychotic agent or to electroconvulsive therapy (ECT) than to antidepressants alone. Others simply recommend higher-than-usual doses of antidepressants.

Age-Related Considerations

Antidepressant use raised the concern that children, adolescents, and adults might, as a result of certain medications, demonstrate an increased risk of suicidal behavior. This has not been fully supported by the data; however, following an FDA Public Health Advisory in 2005, all antidepressants now have specific labeling. This labeling reinforces what clinicians have always been vigilant of—that children, adolescents, and adults who are being treated for depression with antidepressants, and therefore experiencing an increase in energy prior to resolution of depressive and suicidal thinking, can have an increase in suicidal ideation and behavior during the first few months of treatment. Clients who are new to therapy with these compounds should be assessed for clinical worsening, changes in behavior, or suicidality. See Chapters 23 and 31 ∞ for more information on this topic.

MOOD STABILIZERS

The earliest discovery of a mood-stabilizing medication was made in 1948 by Australian physician John Cade. Cade found that lithium worked to subdue wild behavior in animals. To the astonishment of his colleagues, he went one step further and gave lithium to humans.

The psychopharmacologic treatment of conditions collectively labeled *mania* used to be virtually synonymous with lithium carbonate therapy in the United States. Many well-controlled clinical studies indicated unequivocally that lithium was initially the most effective agent for treating the vast majority of acute manic and hypomanic episodes. In addition, because of the absence of sedative side effects, clients felt much more connected to their environment and able to function normally while under the influence of lithium.

In the last few years, several medications have been added to the list of pharmacologic treatments for bipolar disorder. The first was carbamazepine, used to control bipolar symptoms in people who either could not take lithium or did not respond therapeutically to it. Recognizing the potential effectiveness of carbamazepine in certain mood disorders, another seizure medication, divalproex (Depakote), was prescribed for clients with diagnoses of bipolar mood disorder or schizoaffective disorder.

Pharmacologic treatments for bipolar disorder have expanded and are a substantial improvement over the clinically efficacious choices available even a decade ago. New guidelines for bipolar treatment have been created and have thus expanded our abilities to care for clients with bipolar disorders. (See Chapter 17 ∞ for more information on treating mood disorders.) Current treatment guidelines for bipolar disorders emphasize the following key recommendations:

- A mood stabilizer is used in all phases of treatment.
- Atypical, or newer, antipsychotics are preferable to conventional antipsychotic medications (first-line use only when mania is accompanied by psychosis).
- Mild depression is treated initially with a mood stabilizer. Severe depression is treated from the beginning with an antidepressant plus a mood stabilizer.
- Rapid cycling (mania or depression) is treated from the beginning with a mood stabilizer alone, preferably divalproex.

Divalproex or lithium is the foundation of acute-phase and preventive treatment for mania. An additional treatment feature is the use of atypical antipsychotic medications in the acute manic phase of the disorder. The Clinical Example provides a description of a manic episode with psychotic features. The medications that are effective during the acute manic phase are also used for long-term prevention of mania. Bipolar depression usually necessitates lithium to stabilize clients in monotherapy for depression. If, for some reason, lithium is not used, divalproex or even lamotrigine can be used.

The various treatments for bipolar disorder necessitate an in-depth view of medication interactions. See Your Assessment Approach for examples of potential problems.

YOUR ASSESSMENT APPROACH   Mood Stabilizer Medication Interactions

Combining One of These	With One of These Mood Stabilizers	Can Lead to These Problems
Aminophylline	Lithium	Increased lithium secretion
Benzodiazepines	Valproic acid	Excessive CNS depression
Carbamazepine	Lithium	Increased effect of lithium, lithium toxicity
Carbamazepine	Topiramate	Decreased topiramate level
Chlorpromazine	Valproic acid	Valproic acid toxicity
Clozapine	Carbamazepine	Additive bone marrow suppression
CNS depressants	Topiramate	Possible topiramate-induced CNS depression as well as other adverse cognitive and neuropsychiatric effects
Diuretics	Lithium	Increased lithium levels and potential lithium toxicity (monitor electrolytes, especially sodium)
Haloperidol	Carbamazepine	Decreased effectiveness of either compound
Lamotrigine	Valproic acid	Increased lamotrigine levels, decreased valproic levels
MAOI	Lithium	Increased depressant and anticholinergic effects
Marijuana	Lithium	Increased lithium levels and potential lithium toxicity
Neuroleptics	Lithium	Encephalopathy
NSAIDs	Lithium	Increased effect of lithium, lithium toxicity
SSRI	Lithium	Increased effect of lithium, lithium toxicity
Tetracyclines	Lithium	Lithium toxicity
Thyroid hormones	Lithium	May induce hypothyroidism

Dosage

The management of an acute manic episode involves rapid initiation of the selected mood stabilizer, increased to substantial doses during the first week of treatment. Lithium is available only in oral form in capsules and time-release tablets or as a liquid known as lithium citrate. Because lithium is an ion, its concentration can be measured in the blood. In the acute phase, the blood level must usually attain a concentration of 1 to 1.5 mEq/L. After 1 week to 10 days, as the bipolar symptoms subside, the dosage of lithium can be decreased to 900 to 1,200 mg/day, with the blood level maintained in the range of 0.6 to 1.2 mEq/L for continuing control of symptoms.

The basic principles for lithium medication therapy are as follows:

- Blood levels must be monitored after each dosage increase.
- Blood levels are checked every 2 to 3 months, or sooner if there is evidence of mood instability.

For symptoms of breakthrough depression seen with bipolar depression, the dosing of divalproex or lithium must be maximized before other stabilizing or antidepressant agents are added to the regimen. After that episode resolves, the doses of the antidepressant medication are tapered slowly over the following 2 to 6 months. Special assessment skills are called into service during the tapering process to detect any resurgence of depressive symptoms.

Length of treatment with medication for bipolar disorder is a debated issue. Clinical practice suggests prophylactic use of a mood stabilizer, preferably the compound effective during the acute phase of treatment, for at least 2 years. If the client has no intention of taking the medication for that long a period of time, there may be a premature recurrence of the mania. The following Clinical Example illustrates the appropriate use of medication in the case of a client with bipolar disorder.

Clinical Example

Chris, a 32-year-old legal aide, was brought to the clinic by her sister after she was fired from her position at a law firm. She had been arguing constantly with the lawyers and legal secretaries and stood on the conference room table, loudly telling people how to do their jobs. She had not slept in 3 days and was so irritable that she shoved a court clerk when approached about seeking care. Her sister stated that Chris was grandiose; spoke very quickly, moved from topic to topic in a rapid-fire style; and belittled everyone around her. The family was very concerned. She had not taken any prescription or recreational compounds as far as the family knew. In the past 5 years she had been prescribed lithium, which seemed to help; however, Chris refuses to take it now because it leaves a metallic taste in her mouth.

On interview, Chris spoke about having special powers such as bringing people back from the dead because she was a "sanctioned deity." Her episodes in the past did not include delusional thinking, and this was the first time her family could not contain her. Chris had some awareness that her behavior had frightened her family. She was told she had bipolar disorder with delusions. She was given divalproex sodium 250 mg tid and risperidone 1 mg bid initially to control the mania and the psychosis. Chris was not hospitalized because her family agreed to supervise her care. After 1 week, the divalproex dosage was increased to 250 mg qid and Chris's behavior was under considerably better control.

The use of anticonvulsants as mood stabilizers has its own unique set of effects and termination-of-treatment issues. Divalproex, carbamazepine, topiramate, and lamotrigine all have sedation, gastrointestinal (GI) disturbances, and dizziness as side effects, along with others more specific to each compound. The body needs time to adapt to the medication; therefore, some side effects are temporary. However, dosage adjustments can minimize the impact of these side effects so that the quality of life is not shifted downward.

Important client teaching points when using anticonvulsants as mood stabilizers are twofold. When using an anticonvulsant as a mood stabilizer, especially for example the medication topiramate, the dose is initially going to be too low to address symptoms and must be gradually increased to prevent negative cognitive impacts. The result is less-than-optimal symptom control until a therapeutic dose is reached. Clients and significant others need to be prepared for this stage. The other relevant and vital issue is the body's inability to handle the abrupt discontinuation of these medications. Frank discussions must highlight the increased chance of having a seizure, even if the client has never had one, if the dose is not tapered slowly to discontinuation.

Remaining on a mood stabilizer can be a challenge for those with bipolar disorder, but effective nursing interventions and medication teaching can promote adherence. The success seen with maintenance medication for someone with bipolar disorder is described in Mental Health in the News. Even the stressors and pressures of a life in the Arts can be managed with the help of psychopharmacology.

Psychobiology of Lithium

The psychobiology of bipolar disorder has not yet been mapped, but much can be said about the psychobiology of lithium. Lithium is a salt that occurs naturally in our bodies. People who have bipolar disorder and respond to lithium do not have a deficit of lithium in their systems. Lithium, not unlike the antidepressants, affects neurotransmitters, especially norepinephrine and serotonin. In short, lithium aids in the reduction of neurotransmitter release into the synapse and enhances its return, yielding a lower overall amount of the neurotransmitter in the synapse. Behaviorally, these biologic changes can be observed as an absence of mania or depression. What is unclear is why lithium takes up to a few weeks to be fully effective, when its effects can be observed on synaptic activity almost immediately. Also, why do some people with bipolar disorder *not* respond at all to lithium therapy? Many psychobiologists believe that lithium's effects are likely to be based on neurocellular changes that occur over weeks or months after a client begins lithium therapy. A similar explanation may hold true concerning the effectiveness of other mood stabilizers.

ANXIOLYTIC MEDICATIONS

Medications in this class are used to treat a variety of problems from high levels of anxiety and panic to insomnia.

Effects

Anxiolytic medications, or antianxiety agents—sedatives and hypnotics—have very similar pharmacologic attributes. All can be used in small or moderate doses to relieve anxiety and in larger doses to induce sleep. Although they share the major clinical effect of tranquilization or **disinhibition** (loss or reduction of an inhibition) of fear-induced behavior, their side effects, including their addictive potential and overdose sequelae, make certain medications in this category more suitable for routine use and others better reserved for limited, special circumstances.

Antianxiety medications are sometimes called *minor tranquilizers,* but this is a misleading term. Their effects on anxiety have qualities that are different from those of the "major tranquilizers" or antipsychotic medications, but the quantity of the impact is the same.

Meprobamate

Meprobamate (Miltown, Equanil) was the first antianxiety agent to gain popularity in the 1960s. The results of controlled studies of the effects of meprobamate compared to placebos are generally favorable but not overwhelmingly convincing. This, and the addictive and fatal overdose potentials of the medication, prompted investigators to develop more effective and safer medications that have made meprobamate all but obsolete. You will seldom see the use of this medication in clinical settings.

MENTAL HEALTH IN THE NEWS

Patty Duke Aston

Patty Duke Aston is an actress who shares her story of bipolar disorder and how she struggled, and succeeded, over the years. An actress with her own show, The Patty Duke Show, Patty Duke had pressures and responsibilities at a very young age. She also had remarkable symptoms of bipolar disorder that few recognized and some took advantage of for the benefit of the fast-paced world of entertainment. Once Patty Duke finally received treatment after years of bizarre behavior and outrageous stunts, she was able to reach stability and share her story. She speaks at professional conferences, does public speaking to explain mental illness, and established The Patty Duke Online Center for Mental Wellness. She is an example of how stability, recovery, and rehabilitation are not only possible, but highly probable with proper treatment.

Photo courtesy of Alamy.

Benzodiazepines and Nonbenzodiazepines

The major class of medications used today in the management of anxiety is benzodiazepines and nonbenzodiazepines. This group, represented by alprazolam (Xanax), lorazepam (Ativan), and others, accounts for a very high percentage of all the psychoactive medications prescribed in the United States. This fact usually evokes a mixed response in professional circles. The easy distribution of medications for such a ubiquitous human phenomenon as anxiety fosters the development of a pill-oriented and pill-dependent society, say critics. If someone's anxiety level is low to moderate and they are not interested in learning how to effectively cope with anxiety, or the person is unaware they could develop the skills in therapy, then taking a pill seems like the only logical course of action. Using a medication instead of a skill leaves the individual vulnerable to distress when the medication is not available or is no longer effective. Sympathizers focus on the proven effectiveness of the medications, which help people achieve higher levels of functioning, more pleasurable experiences, and even more productive psychotherapies in some instances.

The dosing and timing of an antianxiety medication determine whether the treatment of anxiety is effective or interferes with a client's ability to learn how to cope. These are two entirely different pathways in the treatment of anxiety. Anxiety is a normal human response to threats of varying intensities and is not necessarily an experience to be avoided at all costs. At low to moderate levels, anxiety can be motivating and instructive and helps one to be more aware of one's environment. Treatment is not needed for this entirely healthy human reaction. But when anxiety passes these stages and becomes excessive, high anxiety and panic can occur. Extreme feelings of anxiety and panic are not motivating—in fact, they are immobilizing and make learning impossible (see Chapter 8 ∞). Treatment with psychotherapy and possibly also medication would be introduced at that point, because anxiety has surpassed a normal level reaction and become a symptom.

The clinical application and purpose of antianxiety medications is primarily to support clients through episodes of stress and anxiety at moderate to high levels. Medicating so that higher levels of anxiety are prevented allows the individual to have a lower level of anxiety that can be managed with the coping skills taught by nurses, and to gauge the effectiveness of his or her coping skills. If antianxiety medications are given without regard for the actual anxiety level and the individual's need to learn coping skills, it is possible to obliterate the need to learn to cope. Instead, the client learns to rely on the medication to become less anxious. Having taken the medication and experienced no level of anxiety whatsoever, the client would not be motivated to do anything. The lesson the client will have learned is: When anxious, take pills. For a list of currently available benzodiazepines and nonbenzodiazepines, see TABLE 7-4 ■.

New Medications

In recent years, anxiety-related research has expanded tremendously, and several new anxiolytic medications have been introduced. The newer benzodiazepines give prescribers a wider range of therapies to target the often idiosyncratic

TABLE 7-4 ■ Generic and Trade Names of Benzodiazepines and Nonbenzodiazepines

Generic Name	Trade Names
Benzodiazepines	
Adinazolam	Deracyn
Alprazolam	Xanax
Bromazepam	Lexotan, Lexotanil, Lexomil
Brotizolam	Lendormin
Camazepam	Albego
Chlordiazepoxide	Librium, Libritabs, Elenium
Clobazam	Frisium
Clonazepam	Klonopin
Clorazepate	Tranxene
Clotiazepam	Clozan, Trecalmo
Cloxazolam	Enadel
Diazepam	Valium
Estazolam	ProSom, Nuctalm
Ethyl loflazepate	Meilax, Victan
Etizolam	Depas
Flunitrazepam	Rohypnol
Flurazepam	Dalmane, Dalmadorm
Halazepam	Paxipam
Ketazolam	Anxon, Unakalm
Loprazolam	Dormonoct
Lorazepam	Ativan
Lormetazepam	Loramet
Medazepam	Nobrium
Midazolam	Versed, Dormicum
Nitrazepam	Mogadon
Oxazepam	Serax
Oxazolam	Tranquit
Pinazepam	Domar
Prazepam	Centrax
Quazepam	Doral, Oniria, Dormalin, Quazium
Temazepam	Restoril
Tetrazepam	Musaril, Myolastan
Tofizopam (tofisopam)	Grandaxin, Seriel, Tavor
Triazolam	Halcion
Nonbenzodiazepines	
Buspirone	BuSpar
Eszopiclone	Lunesta
Meprobamate	Miltown, Equanil
Ramelteon	Rozerem
Zaleplon	Sonata
Zolpidem	Ambien
Zopiclone	Imovane

manifestations of anxiety. Some of the new medications have more rapid onsets and shorter half-lives (triazolam, quazepam [Doral]), while others have the usual benzodiazepine onset time and an extended half-life (clonazepam [Klonopin]).

With what we know now about psychobiology, a great variety of benzodiazepine medications can be used more effectively in the treatment of a number of disorders. Benzodiazepines are used for the following:

- Anxiety disorders
- Sleep disorders
- Mood disorders
- Anxiety associated with medical illness
- Psychotic symptoms and disorders
- Convulsive disorders
- Involuntary movement disorders
- Spastic disorders and acute muscle spasms
- Intoxication and withdrawal from alcohol and other substances
- Preanesthesia
- Nausea and vomiting associated with chemotherapy
- Anxiolytic, sedative, and amnestic effects in a wide range of stressful diagnostic procedures

Uses for Anxiolytics

There is no question that benzodiazepines offer a rapid, effective, and safe treatment for the emotional state commonly known as anxiety. Caffeine interferes with the effectiveness of these medications, both pharmacologically and as an irritant to the client's mood and systems.

These medications are absorbed much more rapidly and completely from the gastrointestinal tract than from intramuscular injection and are almost always administered orally. Exceptions are the intramuscular injections of lorazepam (Ativan) for extreme agitation and the use of intravenous diazepam (Valium) to induce sleep before anesthesia or to manage status epilepticus. Peak levels of chlordiazepoxide (Librium) are reached in the bloodstream 2 to 4 hours after oral ingestion, and peak levels of diazepam are reached in 1 to 2 hours.

The major side effects of benzodiazepines are related to their sedative qualities. Clients may complain of excessive drowsiness and must be cautioned against driving a car or operating other machinery.

Other medications used to treat anxiety, generally less effectively, include the antihistamines diphenhydramine (Benadryl) and hydroxyzine (Vistaril, Atarax), the beta blocker propranolol (Inderal), and methaqualone (Quaalude), which is a synthetic nonbarbiturate sedative. Methaqualone has been a much-abused medication, probably because of the intense euphoria associated with peak blood levels. See Chapter 15∞ for discussions of substances of abuse.

Another common use of benzodiazepines, especially diazepam and chlordiazepoxide, is in the detoxification of individuals who are alcohol dependent. Given adequate doses of benzodiazepines to induce sedation (usually starting at 30 to 40 mg/day of diazepam or 150 to 350 mg/day of chlordiazepoxide), alcoholic clients can be smoothly withdrawn by stepwise reductions in chlordiazepoxide dose over a 1- to 2-week period, without encountering alcohol withdrawal delirium or generalized seizures.

Psychobiology of Anxiolytic Medications

Antianxiety medications probably work through a process of synaptic activity involving the neurotransmitter gamma-aminobutyric acid (GABA) in the brain and spinal cord. Benzodiazepines most likely potentiate GABA, producing muscle relaxation. This mechanism involves a complex process of presynaptic and postsynaptic receptor activity. The antianxiety effectiveness seen with these medications is related to their impacts on GABA receptors. Recent research has yielded information about the presence of a postsynaptic receptor called the *benzodiazepine receptor*. As the term implies, benzodiazepines bind perfectly and with great specificity to these receptors, allowing for the sensation of relaxation. Two types of benzodiazepine receptors have been identified in the CNS. Type 1 receptors are located in parts of the brain responsible for sedation, and nonbenzodiazepines bind exclusively to the Type 1 receptors. This makes nonbenzodiazepines an excellent choice for the treatment of sleep disturbances. Type 2 receptors are positioned in parts of the brain responsible for cognition, memory, and psychomotor functioning. Benzodiazepines bind with either Type 1 or Type 2 receptors.

Researchers continually work to develop next-generation benzodiazepines by adjusting the chemical design to deliver a more selective main effect that avoids the many unwanted side effects. Alternatives such as an anxiolytic fatty acid isolated from the plant *Aethusa cynapium* and an omega-3 fatty acid containing eicosapentaenoic acid (EPA) are also being explored. Some advances have been made but are still in clinical trials at this writing. Your Assessment Approach points out potential medication interactions between existing anxiolytics and other medications and substances.

YOUR ASSESSMENT APPROACH   Anxiolytic Medication Interactions

Combining One of These	With One of These Anxiolytics	Can Lead to These Problems
Cimetidine	Alprazolam	Decreased alprazolam clearance
CNS depressants	Anxiolytics	Increased CNS depression, increased risk of apnea
Digoxin	Clorazepate, lorazepam, oxazepam	May increase serum digoxin level, digoxin toxicity
Kava (herb)	Alprazolam	May cause coma
MAOIs	Buspirone	Elevated blood pressure
TCA	Alprazolam	Increased TCA plasma level

TREATMENT FOR INSOMNIA

The pharmacologic management of insomnia presents an interesting and challenging clinical problem. Many of the truly hypnotic medications tend to have undesirable effects, including physiologic dependence, fatal overdose potential, and dangerous interactions with other medications because of liver enzyme induction. The first principle of treatment is to assess whether the insomnia is related to one of the major mental disorders, such as schizophrenia or major depression. If so, the insomnia can and should be treated as part of the larger problem, and sedative antipsychotics or antidepressants may be given at bedtime for this purpose.

In the management of simple insomnia without an associated major mental disorder, sedative–hypnotics are indicated for short-term treatment. Overall, the available sedative–hypnotics include certain antidepressants, benzodiazepines, nonbenzodiazepines, over-the-counter (OTC) medications, barbiturates, and some miscellaneous substances such as chloral hydrate and alcohol (Adams, Holland, & Urban, 2011; Samuel, Zimovetz, Gabriel, & Beard, 2011). Prescription medications are more effective than OTCs, while barbiturates are rarely, if ever, prescribed due to safety and substance dependence problems. The benzodiazepine compound flurazepam (Dalmane), 15 to 30 mg at bedtime, is an example of

WHAT EVERY NURSE SHOULD KNOW

Medications That Affect Sleep

Type	Examples	Comments
Antidepressants	Tricyclic antidepressants such as amitriptyline (Elavil)	Induce drowsiness to varying degrees; effect on insomnia associated with depression usually occurs earlier than antidepressant effect. Suppress REM.
	Selective serotonin reuptake inhibitors such as fluoxetine (Prozac)	Generally decrease total sleep time, increase wakefulness, may induce vivid dreaming.
Antiepileptics	Phenytoin (Dilantin) and phenobarbital	Sedation common, less so with newer seizure control medications.
Antihistamines	Chlorpheniramine (Chlor-Trimeton) and pseudoephedrine compounds (Benylin cold capsules)	Induce drowsiness to varying degrees. Sometimes used as sleep-promoting agents because of their availability over the counter.
Antimanic medications	Lithium (Lithane)	Improves sleep but may cause daytime sleepiness initially.
Antiparkinson medications	Levodopa–carbidopa combinations (Sinemet)	Low doses may improve sleep, but generally persons on medication for Parkinson's have poor sleep with insomnia, vivid dreaming.
Antipsychotics	Traditional antipsychotics such as chlorpromazine (Thorazine) and haloperidol (Haldol)	Chlorpromazine very sedating, haloperidol less so.
	Atypical antipsychotics such as clozapine (Clozaril), risperidone (Risperdal)	High incidence of sedation with clozapine, less so with risperidone.
Anxiolytics	Benzodiazepines such as temazepam (Restoril)	May be used as hypnotics to induce and sustain sleep (note differences between short- and long-acting types).
	Buspirone (BuSpar)	Little effect on sleep and alertness.
Caffeine	Additive to some pain and headache remedies, coffee, tea, colas	Increases wakefulness, effects may last 8–14 hours.
Cardiovascular medications	Antihypertensives such as propranolol (Inderal), clonidine (Catapres), captopril (Capoten)	Insomnia, sedation, and nightmares, less so with captopril and other angiotensin-converting enzyme inhibitors.
Corticosteroids	Prednisone	Generally disturb sleep, especially if taken late in the day; suppress REM sleep.
Hypnotics	Zopiclone (Imovane)	Effective for sleep-onset insomnia because of rapid absorption.
	Zolpidem (Ambien), zaleplon (Sonata), eszopiclone (Lunesta)	Indicated for treatment of insomnia by U.S. Food and Drug Administration.
	Flurazepam (Dalmane)	Longer half-life, useful for sleep onset and maintenance insomnia.

a commonly used historical insomnia treatment. This medication can be used on consecutive nights for about 1 month. Other benzodiazepine compounds that are used for their hypnotic qualities include triazolam and lorazepam.

The rapid absorption of nonbenzodiazepines, within 30 minutes, along with efficient elimination and the minimal hangover effects of sedation the following day, make them the treatment of choice for insomnia. Zolpidem (Ambien), zaleplon (Sonata), and eszopiclone (Lunesta) are nonbenzodiazepines structurally very different from each other but equally effective in the treatment of insomnia. Fast-acting, competent sleep-inducing, and quickly eliminated medications such as these can be used without the difficulties associated with other commonly used compounds. Clinical reports of unusual side effects from the nonbenzodiazepines include sleep walking, sleep eating, and other behaviors that the individual does not remember. Inform your clients about these and other side effects of treatment with these compounds. Eszopiclone is the first sedative–hypnotic medication approved by the FDA for long-term treatment of insomnia. Clients using zolpidem may find it a little more difficult to fall asleep the first night without the medication, but zaleplon only has minimal withdrawal or rebound effects.

Sleep hygiene is an important topic for nurses to discuss with clients who are being treated for sleep problems. Behavioral and pharmacologic circumstances can affect sleep as well as interfere with effective treatment. See What Every Nurse Should Know about relevant information for medications that affect sleep.

TREATMENT OF DAT

A group of medications that is used to treat some of the behavioral symptoms of dementias, including DAT, are atypical antipsychotics. They are common choices for treating the delusions, hallucinations, aggression, and agitation seen with clients who have dementia. Lower doses of these medications than would be used in the treatment of younger clients with psychotic disorders are usual.

There is ongoing debate about whether the adverse effects of atypical antipsychotics offset the advantages. As these concerns are explored, atypical antipsychotics offer good symptom control with far fewer side effects than haloperidol, the antipsychotic previously used to treat the symptoms of dementia.

ACETYLCHOLINESTERASE INHIBITORS

The class of medications with specific abilities for dementia treatment is **acetylcholinesterase inhibitors**, also called *cholinesterase inhibitors*. The title of this class describes how these compounds affect the CNS. The enzyme responsible for the breakdown of a particular neurotransmitter is inhibited from acting by the medication. The enzyme is acetylcholinesterase, and the neurotransmitter it specifically works on is acetylcholine. The cholinergic system is involved in memory, the ability to logically progress from one step to the next in problem solving, and the identification of objects and people in the environment, among other skills. Clients with dementia

of the Alzheimer's type (DAT) have acetylcholine neurotransmitter deficits at the root of some of their problems. When the breakdown of acetylcholine is slowed, it allows more of the neurotransmitter to remain in the synapse, thus promoting acetylcholine's function—transmitting information from one cell to another. In mild to moderately affected individuals, when there is more acetylcholine in the CNS, cognitive functioning and memory improve. This is essentially the path by which these medications slow the progression of the memory deficits in clients with early stage DAT.

Acetylcholinesterase inhibitors are best utilized early in the dementing process when deficits are still mild to moderate in scope. But the best timing and the most effective use of the compounds are frequently thwarted by the realities of human nature. Instituting treatment at early stages may be difficult because many people are not aware they are in the early stages of dementia. Frequently they are unable to grasp their own level of symptomatology and lack information on the early signs, symptoms, or issues of dementia. Confabulation or denial prevents a client or loved ones from noting deficits or recognizing the implications of low-level difficulties. For example, a woman who is unable to tie her shoes may ask her husband to do that for her; both of them attribute her difficulty to arthritis, musculoskeletal problems, or side effects of medications. Another example is the man who stops balancing his checkbook, ostensibly because the bank has always been correct when in reality he has lost the basic math skills required.

Think of this medication class as a treatment for specific symptoms, not a cure. Acetylcholinesterase inhibitors do not alter the course of the underlying disease process or have an impact on the progressive nature of the disease. They are a way to temporarily improve neurotransmission and thus ameliorate memory deficits. The first of the acetylcholinesterase inhibitors was tacrine (Cognex). Although it did not help all clients with DAT, it was the first step in the direction of active treatment for a major portion of people with dementing processes. Problems with this medication included liver toxicity, which could be controlled, and several common side effects including GI disturbances and headache. From this beginning, other compounds were developed. Donepezil (Aricept) and rivastigmine (Exelon) are acetylcholinesterase inhibitors with improved impacts and fewer difficulties from side effects. Donepezil (Aricept) is approved for the treatment of all degrees of severity of DAT. GI disturbances occur at a much lower level than with the original compound, and headaches are reported at only a slightly higher level than with clients taking a placebo. There is even hope that these medications can play a role in preventing individuals with cognitive deficits from converting to DAT. See Chapter 14 ∞ for a discussion of DAT and its progression.

GLUTAMATE PATHWAY MODIFIER

Another approach to address the memory difficulties in the pathologic process of DAT involves looking at glutamate. Glutamate is a primary excitatory neurotransmitter in the brain and glutamate receptor activity is associated with information processing, storage, and retrieval. Glutamate triggers

N-methyl-D-aspartate (NMDA) receptors to allow calcium to flow into a nerve cell, creating the chemical environment required for information storage. Too much glutamate overstimulates NMDA receptors to allow too much calcium into nerve cells, leading to disruption and death of cells. It may be that overexcitation of these receptors contribute to the impaired cognition and memory in DAT.

The medication memantine (Namenda) is the first glutamate pathway modifier and is used to mitigate the impacts of DAT on functioning. Its job is to moderate the glutamate such that it does not overexcite the NMDA receptors. As a result, nerve cells are not negatively impacted or destroyed and degradation is minimized over time. While the mechanism of action of memantine in DAT is not known, the principal pharmacologic actions at a therapeutic dose are inhibition of NMDA receptors. Memantine can reverse the decreased metabolic activity associated with DAT, possibly accounting for its beneficial effects on cognition and global functioning. Memantine also has neuroprotective properties and can inhibit amyloid-beta-induced toxicity and neurodegeneration.

MEDICATION COUNTERFEITING

Medications available through prescription can be, and are, counterfeited and sold through nonprescription means. Counterfeit medications are illegal and inherently unsafe and are a growing public health problem. A counterfeit medication is a fake medication. It may be contaminated or contain the wrong—or no—active ingredient, be made with the wrong amount of ingredients, or be packaged in phony packaging. Typically, a person who cannot afford a particular medication may purchase it over the Internet and unknowingly receive a counterfeit medication instead, with unintended and possibly serious consequences.

The World Health Organization (WHO) has the International Medical Products Anti-Counterfeiting Taskforce, or IMPACT, to protect people from counterfeit medicines. Regulation and technology are being employed to try to minimize this public health problem. To ensure your clients are receiving safe medications, advocate that they obtain medications only from a licensed pharmacy. Legitimate Internet pharmacies carry accreditation (the Verified Internet Pharmacy Practice Sites Accreditation Program, or VIPPS) to show they are a reputable source. The FDA is preparing requirements to track the pedigree of prescription medications from the manufacturer, through the medication distribution chain, to the end retailer. For up-to-date information on this subject, visit the FDA website at http://www.fda.gov/counterfeit.

HERBAL MEDICINES

Herbal medicines are widely used as an alternative or complementary therapy. (See Chapter 34 ∞ for another discussion of these interventions.) One quarter of prescription medications and hundreds of OTC medications are derived from plants. Herbs and plants generally take longer to act than pharmaceuticals, and few have the potency of a prescription. However, many herbal agents have powerful medicine-like actions and side effects.

One of the vital features of safe and effective nursing care is communication about complementary and alternative treatments. Keep in mind the variety of terms used to describe these treatments: complementary, alternative, botanical, nutriceutical, herbal medicine; home remedy, natural remedy, homeopathic remedy; health food, vitamin therapy, dietary supplement, phytomedicine, supplements, herbal tea; and others.

The concomitant use of herbal medicines with psychiatric pharmaceuticals can be accomplished safely only when health providers know that their clients use them and the safety and effectiveness for the client's specific condition have been thoroughly appraised. Be sure to assess your clients for the use of herbal medicines.

There are many benefits to using alternative substances. For example:

- Self-treatment can be empowering.
- The very low concentrations of these substances could be helpful and might not be harmful for those who are sensitive to even low doses of pharmaceutical compounds.
- Some people feel safer using "natural" products and distrust chemical formulations.
- Standard labeling and dosing are possible.

However, there are potential problems with the use of alternative substances in psychiatry even though these substances have lower potencies. Psychiatric indications for alternative substances currently exist only for St. John's wort for depression and ginkgo biloba for dementia, although alternative substances are frequently used for several other psychiatric symptoms and disorders. You may encounter clients using ma huang (ephedra) for general malaise, kava for anxiety and stress (see the FDA caution in Table 33-2 on page 732), and ginseng and SAMe for depression. Competent assessment and evaluation requires our awareness of the potential for difficulties with alternative substances. Problems with using herbs may include:

- Contamination of the product
- Dosing inconsistencies
- Delayed absorption of other coadministered medications
- Worsening of high blood pressure, potassium imbalance, and coagulation problems
- Side effects such as nerve damage, kidney damage, and liver damage
- Advertising of unproven claims
- Aggravation of allergic reactions
- Interference with breastfeeding
- Believing that one is treating the problem, when in reality the symptoms could continue to worsen, making effective treatment much more difficult

Assessing Herb Consumption

Many clients do not tell health care providers about their herbal use for fear of being ridiculed or criticized. How do you find out what alternative therapies your clients are taking? Good interviewing skills—tolerance, a nonjudgmental stance,

FDA: Counterfeit Drugs

℞ COMMUNICATION

Communicating With Your Client About Herbal Medicines

CLIENT: "I do not like taking all these chemicals. It is not natural."

NURSE RESPONSE 1: "Are you more comfortable taking medicine to help you when you know it is natural?" *RATIONALE:* This question gathers more data about what the client needs in order to feel better and raises the possibility of alternative substance use.	**NURSE RESPONSE 2:** "Have you had bad experiences with anything in particular?" *RATIONALE:* This response makes the connection for the client between the idea and a possible result. It may also encourage discussion of recreational substance use.

and some expressive questions—will bring much of your client's life into the light. Questions such as "Do you do anything to improve your health?" or "What do you buy at the grocery store or health food store besides food?" can open the subject. See Rx Communication for examples of a conversation about this topic.

Be aware of the client's need to talk to a knowledgeable professional. The client may tell you about someone else who is taking alternatives while watching for your reaction. A nonjudgmental response would include questions about what the client thinks about it, whether it has helped the individual, or whether the client would consider using this particular treatment. Not knowing about your client's use of botanicals risks dangerous medication interactions or costly and painful tests or treatments when an herb causes an unrecognized side effect.

Psychopharmacology is an important aspect of the treatment of people who have mental health issues. When you understand the science of pharmacology, you can more easily perform some of the main tasks of psychiatric–mental health nursing—educating clients about medications as a vital part of psychiatric treatment, promoting self-care, and advocating for the best possible outcomes.

Pearson Nursing Student Resources
Find additional review materials at
nursing.pearsonhighered.com
Prepare for success with NCLEX®-style practice questions, interactive assignments and activities, web links, animations and videos, and more!

REFERENCES

Adams, M. P., Holland, L. N., & Urban, C. Q. (2011). *Pharmacology for nurses: A pathophysiologic approach* (3rd ed.). Upper Saddle River, NJ: Prentice Hall.

American Nurses Association Task Force on Psychopharmacology. (1994). *Psychiatric–mental health nursing psychopharmacology project.* Washington, DC: American Nurses Association.

Gafoor, R., Landau, S., Craig, T. K. J., Elanjithara, T., Power, P., & McGuire, P. (2010). Esquire trial: Efficacy and adverse effects of quetiapine versus risperidone in first-episode schizophrenia. *Journal of Clinical Psychopharmacology, 30*(5), 600–606.

Gillman, P. K. (2011). Advances pertaining to the pharmacology and interactions of irreversible nonselective monoamine oxidase inhibitors. *Journal of Clinical Psychopharmacology, 31*(1), 66–74.

Knadler, M. P., Lobo, E., Chappell, J., & Bergstrom, R. (2011). Duloxetine: Clinical pharmacokinetics and drug interactions. *Clinical Pharmacokinetics, 50*(5), 281–294.

Lea, D. H., Skirton, H., Read, C. Y., & Williams, J. K. (2011). Implications for educating the next generation of nurses on genetics and genomics in the 21st century. *Journal of Nursing Scholarship, 43*(1), 3–12.

Lieberman, J. A., Stroup, T. S., McEvoy, J. P., Swartz, M. S., Rosenheck, R. A., Perkins, D. O., ... Hsiao, J. K. (Clinical Antipsychotic Trials of Intervention Effectiveness [CATIE] Investigators). (2005). Effectiveness of antipsychotic drugs in patients with chronic schizophrenia. *New England Journal of Medicine, 353*, 1209–1223.

Mallinger, J. B., & Lamberti, J. S. (2010). Psychiatrists' attitudes toward and awareness about racial disparities in mental health care. *Psychiatric Services, 61*(2), 173–179.

Masi, G., & Liboni, F. (2011). Management of schizophrenia in children and adolescents: Focus on pharmacotherapy. *Drugs, 71*(2), 179–208.

McClay, J. L., Adkins, D. E., Aberg, K., Stroup, S., Perkins, D. O., Vladimirov, V. I., ... van den Oord, E. J. C. G. (2011). Genome-wide pharmacogenomic analysis of response to treatment with antipsychotics. *Molecular Psychiatry, 16*(1), 76–85.

Mojtabai, R., & Olfson, M. (2010). National trends in psychotropic medication polypharmacy in office-based psychiatry. *Archives of General Psychiatry, 67*(1), 26–36.

Muller, D. J., Zai, C. C., Sicard, M., Remington, E., Souza, R. P., Tiwari, A. K., ... Kennedy, J. L. (2010). Systematic analysis of dopamine receptor genes (DRD1-DRD5) in antipsychotic-induced weight gain. *Pharmacogenomics Journal.* Advance online publication. doi:10.1038/tpj.2010.65

Nichols, A. I., Focht, K., Jiang, Q., Preskorn, S. H., & Kane, C. P. (2011). Pharmacokinetics of venlafaxine extended release 75 mg and desvenlafaxine 50 mg in healthy CYP2D6 extensive and poor metabolizers: A randomized, open-label, two-period, parallel-group, crossover study. *Clinical Drug Investigations, 31*(3), 155–167.

Preskorn, S. H. (2011). CNS drug development: Part III: Future directions. *Journal of Psychiatric Practice, 17*(1), 49–52.

Purnell, L., Davidhizar, R. E., Giger, J. N., Strickland, O. L., Fishman, D., & Allison, D. M. (2011). A guide to developing a culturally competent organization. *Journal of Transcultural Nursing, 22*(1), 7–14.

Rosner, F. (1978). *Julius Preuss' biblical and Talmudic medicine.* New York: Sanhedrin Press.

Samuel, S., Zimovetz, E. A., Gabriel, Z., & Beard, S. M. (2011). Efficacy and safety of treatments for refractory generalized anxiety disorder: A systematic review. *International Clinical Psychopharmacology, 26*, 63–68.

Saxena, A., Grace, J., Olympia, J. L., Trigoboff, E., Watson, T., Cushman, S., & Newcomer, D. (2008). Risperidone long-acting injections: Successful alternative deltoid muscle injections for refractory schizophrenia. *Psychiatry, 5*(9), 40–46.

Seripa, D., Bizzarro, A., Pilotto, A., D'Onofrio, G., Vecchione, G., Gallo, A. P., ... Pilotto, A. (2011). Role of cytochrome P4502D6 functional polymorphisms in the efficacy of donepezil in patients with Alzheimer's disease. *Pharmacogenetics and Genomics, 21*(4), 225–230.

Snowdon, J., & Halliday, G. (2011). A study of the use of clozapine in old age psychiatry. *International Clinical Psychopharmacology, 26*(4), 232–235.

Trigoboff, E., Wilson, B. A., Shannon, M. T., & Stang, C. L. (2005). *Psychiatric drug handbook* (1st ed.). Upper Saddle River, NJ: Prentice Hall.

Veselinovi, T., Schorn, H., Vernaleken, I. B., Schiffl, K., Klomp, M., & Gerhard Grunder, G. (2011). Impact of different antidopaminergic mechanisms on the dopaminergic control of prolactin secretion. *Journal of Clinical Psychopharmacology, 31*(2), 214–220.

Stress, Anxiety, and Coping

CAROL REN KNEISL

8

LEARNING OUTCOMES

After completing this chapter, you will be able to:

1. Explain how stress affects an individual.
2. Identify the sources of anxiety.
3. Describe the everyday methods people use to cope with stress and anxiety.
4. Compare and contrast the common defense-oriented behaviors (defense mechanisms) people use to cope with stress and anxiety.
5. Implement nursing intervention strategies specific to each defense-oriented behavior listed.
6. Discuss common medical conditions with an onset or a course influenced by psychological and behavioral factors.

CRITICAL THINKING CHALLENGE

At the scene of an auto accident in which a couple in their eighties lost control of the RV trailer they were towing, the husband remained immobile in the driver's seat, hands firmly fixed to the steering wheel, eyes focused on some distant spot despite the threat of explosion from the smoking car. The wife ran around in circles. She had lost her shoes in the accident, but despite numerous bleeding cuts, she was unaware she was running barefoot through broken glass from the windshield.

Two nurses who were the first drivers on the scene had differing opinions about which person displayed the healthier response. One said the gentleman's "control" was positive, but the wife's "hysteria" was negative.

1. What is your opinion?
2. Does everyone react in the same way to stress? Anxiety?
3. Are some strategies for handling stress and anxiety better than others? In what ways?

How do we handle the ups and downs of life? Our brains have built-in chemical circuit breakers that shut off stress hormones and networks of nerves whose job it is to calm us down. The circuit breakers and the nerves require us to take regular breaks from our everyday routines—that is, we have a biologic need to periodically disengage. Consider how advances in technology have affected our lives: cell phones, text messaging, tweeting, handheld computers for e-mails—with instant messaging we are on call 24/7/365. In a survey of over 1,000 people, 40% of 18- to 25-year-old students said they couldn't cope without their cell phones. Yet, when they do, the students reported feeling less stressed and had lower heart rates and blood pressure (Gallegos, 2011). Instant communication technology makes it harder, not easier, to get away, to decompress, or to disengage.

In addition, personal and professional expectations have risen exponentially in a culture that favors constant, measurable productivity. At work and at school we feel that we must hit the benchmarks that are set for us. Then there is the driver who cut you off this morning, the argument with the person you are dating, and the newest tuition increase at school. The global condition keeps us on edge everyday—terrorist attacks, wars in Iran and Afghanistan, threats of bird and swine flu, medication-resistant strains of staphylococcus, oil spills in the Gulf of Mexico. Insurance claims for stress, job burnout, and depression are among the fastest-growing disability categories in the United States. Are our nervous systems designed to take this kind of beating?

The study of stress raises other questions:

- Why is the same event stressful for one person but not another?
- Is change always stressful?
- How do people typically cope with stress?
- How does stress affect psychological and physical health?

In this chapter, we show how the traditional view of stress as a purely biologic phenomenon has given way to a biopsychosocial model. That is, stress is caused by a complex interaction of biologic, psychological, and sociocultural factors.

STRESS

Stress is part of being alive. Standing erect stresses the muscles and bones that must work together to keep the body erect; eating stresses the digestive system, which must produce enzymes and absorb nutrients; and breathing stresses the respiratory system, which must exchange carbon dioxide and oxygen. Facing a demanding situation is stressful. We define stress more broadly and holistically as an interaction. **Stress** is what happens when threats such as demanding situations or daily challenges are greater than our coping abilities or resources and upset our balance. The threats may be to physical safety, long-range security, self-esteem, reputation, peace of mind, or other things that one values.

This broader definition fits more closely with the humanistic perspective of this textbook. In this view, stress is a person–environment interaction. That is, our interpretation or perception of what is happening to us. The source of the stress, the demanding situation, is known as a **stressor**. The internal state the stress produces is one of tension, anxiety, or strain. See FIGURE 8-1 ■ for an example of stress as a person–environment situation.

There is no one universally accepted definition of stress among stress theorists and researchers. An interactional view of stress, such as the one given earlier, is consistent with how nurses view human experiences. The theories of stress that follow in this chapter are those in common use. Although they do tell us a great deal about responses to stressful situations, these explanations are not necessarily consistent with nursing's orientation. The causes, the situational context in which the stressful event occurs, and the psychological interpretation of the demanding situation must be considered in a holistic, humanistic approach to the client. These and other important factors related to stress are illustrated in FIGURE 8-2 ■. The DSM-IV-TR (American Psychiatric Association [APA], 2000) offers some general parameters for assessing the severity of stress. The DSM-IV-TR is discussed in Chapter 11∞.

Conflict as a Stressor

The concept of conflict is useful in identifying the stresses that help cause disturbed coping patterns. Conflict often explains such behaviors as hesitation, vacillation, blocking, and fatigue. **Conflict**—having opposing desires, feelings, or goals—is frequently seen in the behavior of psychotic clients, who may have difficulty making even the simplest decisions.

The following conflicts are the most likely to cause stress:

- Conflicts that involve social relations with significant people
- Conflicts that involve ethical standards

FIGURE 8-1 ■ A family is shocked at the devastation caused by the powerful March 11, 2011 earthquake in their hometown in Fukushima Prefecture, Japan. The stressed and anxious family has an additional worry—the state of emergency at the nearby Fukushima nuclear power plant damaged by the earthquake and its strong aftershocks. *Photo courtesy of* Photoshot Holdings.

FIGURE 8-2 ■ Factors involved in stress. Several important factors are involved in understanding stress. They include personality factors (such as how we handle anger), cognitive factors (such as whether we perceive an event as a challenge or threat), physical factors (such as how the body responds to stress), environmental factors (such as fog, fire, or snow), cultural factors (such as our learned beliefs about religion, health, and family), and coping strategies (such as what we do to manage stress).

■ Conflicts that involve meeting unconscious needs
■ Conflicts that involve the problems of everyday family living

A conflict proceeds according to the following four steps:

1. The person holds two goals simultaneously.
2. The person moves in relation to both of the goals, using approach–avoidance, avoidance–avoidance, or approach–approach movements.
3. The person shows hesitation, vacillation, blocking, or fatigue.
4. Resolution occurs either temporarily or permanently.

Approach–Avoidance Conflict

When a person is faced with a single goal that has both attractive and unattractive aspects the person is in an either–or situation. If the person chooses one goal, the other goal is rejected or abolished automatically. The following is an example.

Clinical Example

Mrs. Reynolds wants to talk with the nurse about her fears of going back to work. At the same time, she wants not to be perceived as weak or "a bother." Mrs. Reynolds makes a movement in relation to her goal—talking to the nurse—by walking up to her. When the nurse stops and turns toward her, Mrs. Reynolds asks some superficial question about the time of the next group meeting. In this way, she avoids discussing her real concerns. When the nurse offers an opening to talk further, Mrs. Reynolds avoids the conversation she needs by saying she wants to rest. An hour later, she approaches the nurse with an apologetic but vague question about her medication.

Vacillation (moving first one way, toward a desirable goal, that is, talking to the nurse, then moving another way to avoid what is undesirable, that is, being perceived as weak or as a bother) describes Mrs. Reynolds' behavior.

Avoidance–Avoidance Conflict

In avoidance–avoidance conflict, a person is faced with two undesirable or unattractive goals at the same time. This is the sort of situation we find ourselves in when we say we are "between a rock and a hard place." The person attempts to avoid the nearer of these two goals, but with the retreat from the nearer goal, the tendency to avoid the second goal increases. Unless the tendency to avoid one of the goals overpowers the tendency to avoid the other goal, or unless there is a third way out of the conflict, the person feels trapped by the conflict. Obviously, avoidance–avoidance conflicts are most unpleasant and highly stressful.

Clinical Example

Robert, the 35-year-old son of wealthy parents, was strongly attracted to "the good life." He wanted to live in a creative, esthetic environment, read good books, attend the opera, and drink quality wine. Simultaneously, he wanted both to avoid working to earn the money for the lifestyle he desired and to not depend on his parents for support. His lifestyle became one of waiting to find a resolution to his conflict. He neither worked nor accepted "handouts" from his family, but his preferred lifestyle became one that he talked about rather than lived.

Using avoidance-oriented strategies can also pose both behavioral and physical risks (Wong & Moulds, 2011).

Approach–Approach Conflict

In an approach–approach conflict a person must make a choice between two desirable goals. The old saying "six on one hand, half a dozen on the other" describes this conflict nicely.

Clinical Example

Niesha is shopping at the mall for a dress to wear to the prom. She has narrowed her choices down to two dresses that she really likes—an indigo blue chiffon dress with a bouffant skirt and spaghetti string straps and a slinky red dress with one shoulder strap. She cannot afford both and must decide which one to buy.

Among the three types of conflict, approach–approach conflict tends to be the least stressful. Deciding which of two equally beautiful prom dresses to buy is not usually exhausting. However, approach–approach conflicts may sometimes be troublesome especially if the alternative not chosen represents a loss of sorts.

BIOPSYCHOSOCIAL THEORIES OF STRESS

Each of the theories discussed in this section contributes to our understanding of stress and coping. However, none is complete in and of itself. Psychoneuroimmunology, the final theory discussed in this section, offers a comprehensive framework for understanding stress–disease relationships by taking the best of what the other theories offer and integrating them with the increasing body of evidence on how stress can alter immunologic functioning and, consequently, disease susceptibility and pathology.

The Fight-or-Flight Response to Stress

Beyond the routine and essential stress of everyday life, humans risk encountering undesirable or excess stress that threatens well-being and may even be life threatening. They cope with such threats through either a fight (aggression) or flight (withdrawal) response. The **fight-or-flight response** was first discussed by the physician Walter Cannon in 1932, when he identified stress as an actual cause of disease. The fight-or-flight response is mediated by the sympathetic division of the autonomic nervous system which controls blood vessels, smooth muscles, and glands.

Consider the following situation of extreme stress: A woman is walking down a dark, deserted street when a man with a knife emerges from the shadows just in front of her. Does she try to defend herself? Does she run away? Whichever action she takes is a result of a variety of physiological responses to extreme danger. The following signs of adrenaline rush are likely to happen when a person faces such a situation:

- The heart beats strong and fast to circulate the blood more quickly.
- Airways in the lungs dilate so that the extra blood becomes oxygenated.
- Glucose is released into the blood by the liver.
- The blood vessels dilate to permit the oxygen-rich blood to get to where it is needed most.
- The pupils of the eyes dilate to let more light through, making vision more acute.
- Peristalsis in the gastrointestinal system is inhibited so that the energy peristalsis would consume becomes available for other purposes.
- Norepinephrine-containing cells in the central nervous system are active.
- The palms become sweaty; the mouth becomes dry.

Although these physiological responses seem appropriate, imagine the wear and tear on the body if humans responded to all stress in all of these ways.

Many specialists in the field of behavioral medicine believe the fight-or-flight response to be maladaptive. For example, some forms of hypertension are caused or made worse by chronic activation of the heart due to either an excessive amount of stress or an excessive response to stress. See the section on Psychological Factors Affecting Medical Conditions later in this chapter for a discussion of the relationship between stress and hypertension, heart disease, and a variety of other medical conditions.

Selye's Stress–Adaptation Theory

Hans Selye, a Canadian endocrinologist and the most well-known and widely recognized stress researcher, developed a response-oriented framework for understanding the effects of stress on the human body (1956). He disputed the idea that only serious disease or injury causes stress. Selye believed that any emotion or activity requires a response or change in the individual. Stressors can be physical, chemical, physiological, developmental, or emotional. Playing a game of tennis, going out in the rain without an umbrella, having an argument, and getting a promotion are all examples of stressful events. Life itself is basically stressful because it involves a process of adaptation to continual change. Though the experience of adaptation is stressful, it is not necessarily harmful. Indeed, it can be exciting and rewarding under certain circumstances; and although we cannot avoid the stress of living, we can learn to minimize its damaging effects.

Selye observed that, regardless of the diagnosis, most physically ill people had certain symptoms in common; they lost their appetite, they lost weight, they felt and looked ill, they were anxious and fatigued, and they had aches and pains in their joints and muscles. A long series of experiments led to more objective evidence of actual body damage: enlargement of the adrenal glands; shrinkage of the thymus, spleen, and lymph nodes; and the appearance of bleeding gastric ulcers. Feelings of anxiety, fatigue, or illness are subjective aspects of stress.

Though stress itself cannot be perceived, Selye found that it can be objectively measured by the structural and chemical changes that it produces in the body. These changes are called the **general adaptation syndrome (GAS)** because when stress affects the whole person, the whole person must adjust to the changes. The GAS occurs in three stages: alarm, resistance, and exhaustion. The three stages of the GAS are illustrated and summarized in FIGURE 8-3 ■.

Selye's theory has stimulated extensive research on the neuroendocrine mechanisms underlying stress. The consequent research into psychoendocrinology brought Selye's model into question. Now classical research has demonstrated that neuroendocrine response differs for different stressors, and that there is individual variance in the sensitivity to psychosocial stimuli (Lazarus & Folkman, 1984; Smith, 1998). In addition, a response-based model of stress such as Selye's is not consistent with our view that each individual is unique and people respond differently to similar situations.

Life Changes as Stressful Events

Most people are accustomed to thinking of untoward events as stressful, but they do not realize that desirable events such as job promotions, vacations, or outstanding personal achievements may also prove stressful. Holmes and Rahe (1967) studied life changes—noticeable alterations in one's living circumstances that require readjustment—as stressful events and devised the Social Readjustment Rating Scale (SSRS)—a way to measure the amount of stress in a person's life. These authors believe that life events that require coping behavior tend to decrease a person's ability to handle illness or subsequent stress. Since Holmes and Rahe began their research, other investigators have raised cautions about applying this stimulus-based explanation indiscriminately. These cautions are discussed later in this section.

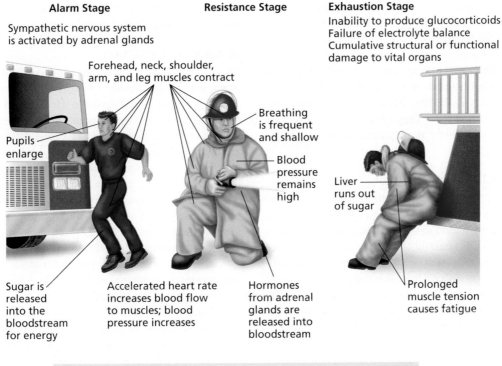

Alarm Stage

Sympathetic nervous system
is activated by adrenal glands

Forehead, neck, shoulder,
arm, and leg muscles contract

Pupils
enlarge

Sugar is
released
into the
bloodstream
for energy

Accelerated heart rate
increases blood flow
to muscles; blood
pressure increases

Resistance Stage

Breathing
is frequent
and shallow

Blood
pressure
remains
high

Hormones
from adrenal
glands are
released into
bloodstream

Exhaustion Stage

Inability to produce glucocorticoids
Failure of electrolyte balance
Cumulative structural or functional
damage to vital organs

Liver
runs out
of sugar

Prolonged
muscle tension
causes fatigue

FIGURE 8-3 ▪ Selye's general adaptation syndrome. The diagram at the top shows some of the physical reactions to stress in each stage. The diagram at the bottom shows the relationships of the stages to the individual's ability to resist a stressor. In the alarm stage, resistance drops at first as the sympathetic nervous system quickly activates. But resistance then rapidly increases as the body mobilizes its defense systems. In the resistance stage, the body is working at a much increased level of resistance, using resources until the stress ends or the resources run out. In the exhaustion stage, the body is no longer able to resist because resources have been depleted. At this point, disease and even death are possible. The third stage of exhaustion may be reversible if the total body is not affected and if the person can eventually eliminate the source of stress. *Source:* Adapted from Ciccarelli, S. K., & White, J. N. (2009). *Psychology* (2nd ed.) Upper Saddle River, NJ: Prentice Hall, p. 445.

Their research assigned ratings to 43 different life changes, called *life change units (LCUs)*. They asked subjects to indicate what life changes had occurred in the past year and then to add up the points assigned to each one (some life changes have higher ratings than others). According to these researchers, a low score indicated that the subject was not likely to have an adverse reaction. A "mild" score meant that there was a 30% chance that the person would manifest the impact of stress through physical symptoms. People in the "moderate" category had a 50% chance of a change in health status, and a "high" score meant an 80% chance of major illness in the next 2 years. High LCU scores also correlated with an increased probability of accidental injury. The following clinical example demonstrates the LCU model.

Clinical Example

Marcia Montes, a 22-year-old woman, had recently been divorced from her husband (LCU 73) after attempting to achieve a marital reconciliation (LCU 45). Marcia's pregnancy (LCU 40) earlier in the year was uneventful, and the couple's healthy son was born on June 2 (LCU 39). At 6 weeks of age, the child suddenly and unexpectedly died in his crib (LCU 63). The couple began to argue frequently (LCU 35) before they made the decision to divorce. After the divorce, Marcia found herself short of funds (LCU 38) and went to work as a waitress in a pizza restaurant (LCU 36). She found it necessary to move to a less expensive apartment (LCU 20). In the period of 1 year, Marcia accumulated an LCU score of 390 and was in the high-risk group.

The SSRS was subsequently revised (Miller & Rahe, 1997) to reflect a 45% increase in the ratings found in the 1967 studies.

A review of the findings of recent research supports classic observations of a close link between stressful life events and physical health related to binge eating (Woods, Racine, & Klump, 2010), skin disorders such as psoriasis (Manolache, Petrriescu-Seceleanu, & Bevea, 2010), and maternal well-being (Ngai & Chan, 2010). They also stress the need for early recognition and timely management of stress-induced illnesses.

Application to Clinical Practice

This model is based on several assumptions that depict a person as a passive recipient of stress caused by life changes. At present, there is little reason to believe that change in itself is inherently or inevitably stressful. To understand the effects of life changes on health, you need to identify what each individual perceives as stressful. Only then can you help people become aware of the stress they face in their lives and plan for the future. In the clinical example that follows, we return to the example of Marcia Montes, who had accumulated an LCU score of 390.

Clinical Example

During the course of group therapy, Marcia shared her desire to return to college and complete the junior and senior years of a medical technology program in which she had been enrolled before her marriage. To do so, she would have to make a number of changes: move to an apartment close to the college because she could not afford to own a car, change her working hours or job so that she could attend day classes, change her sleeping habits, change her recreational and social activities, and reduce her other expenses to pay school costs. The changes required would add almost 200 LCUs to her score.

In group therapy, Marcia was able to consider this information and re-evaluate her goals. She decided to delay her return to school until she could get on her feet financially. She chose not to make any other changes in her life for the present time.

Clients can identify the life change events in their lives, much as Marcia did, to help decide when it might be advantageous or disadvantageous to engage in a life change. This knowledge helps them make responsible decisions about the directions their lives will take. Partnering With Clients and Families

includes some strategies based on the inter-relationship between life changes and stressful events.

Stress as a Transaction

Richard Lazarus, a pioneering theorist and researcher in stress, coping, and health, is known for his transaction-based approach to understanding stress. He believed that measuring major life events misses the point. Instead, the constant minor irritants or hassles that go on day in and day out in a person's life are more important than large or landmark changes. His view is reflected in the definition of stress given at the beginning of this chapter and his transactional model—stress is a process of complex interplay among the perceived demands of the environment and the perceived resources one has for meeting these demands (Lazarus & Folkman, 1984)—is consistent with nursing's holistic approach.

In the Lazarus model, perceived threat—what the person appraises as taxing or exceeding his or her resources and endangering his or her well-being—is the central characteristic of stressful situations because it threatens a person's most important goals and values (Monat & Lazarus, 1991). Once a person has perceived a threat, the person evaluates it by thinking about it. This process is termed *cognitive appraisal.* According to Lazarus, the process works like this:

1. The person assesses the potential for benefit, harm, loss, threat, or challenge in a situation. This is called *primary appraisal.*
2. The person who has identified a threat or a harmful effect then evaluates his or her coping resources and options in the situation. This is called *secondary appraisal.*
3. The person applies the coping resources and options at his or her disposal. This is called *coping.*
4. The person engages in ongoing reinterpretation of the situation based on new information. This is called *reappraisal.*

Lazarus believes that stress depends not only on external conditions but also on the person's physical vulnerability and the adequacy of that person's coping styles.

Cognitive appraisal and coping style are influenced by the person's culture. Providing culturally competent care requires understanding the client's perspective and recognizing

PARTNERING WITH CLIENTS AND FAMILIES

Teaching About Life Changes

You can assist clients by incorporating the following guidelines:

- Help clients recognize when a life change occurs.
- Encourage clients to think about the meaning of the change and identify some of the feelings associated with the change.
- Discuss with clients the different ways they might best adjust to the event.
- Encourage clients to take time in arriving at decisions.

- If possible, encourage clients to anticipate life changes and plan for them well in advance.
- Encourage clients to pace themselves. It can be done, even if they are in a hurry.
- Encourage clients to consider the accomplishment of a task as a part of daily living and to avoid looking at such an achievement as a stopping point or a time for letting down.

that a client's cognitive appraisal of a situation may, and probably will, differ from your own.

Psychoneuroimmunology Framework

The most comprehensive framework for understanding the relationship between stress and disease and the biopsychosocial nature and complexity of the stress process is the **psychoneuroimmunology (PNI)** framework. As discussed in Chapter 6 ∞, PNI is concerned with interaction among the neurologic, endocrine, and immune systems and takes into account the nature of the influence of psychosocial factors on immune function and health outcomes. In other words, the PNI framework integrates the person–environment transactions of the stress process with the psychological and pathophysiological processes involved in stress. An important key that has surfaced in some of the recent research on stress and first-episode psychosis (Pruessner, Iver, Faridi, & Malla, 2011) is the importance of improving resilience. Resilience is defined and discussed in Chapter 1 ∞.

What is emerging is a complex picture of the body's response to stress that involves several related pathways. Over the past few decades, corticotropin-releasing factor (CRF) signaling pathways have been shown to be the main coordinators of the endocrine, behavioral, and immune responses to stress (Taché & Bonaz, 2007). Cortisol, as well as adrenaline (recall the signs of adrenaline rush described earlier on page 142 ∞ that helps us to either take flight or to fight in the presence of immediate danger), is a stress hormone. Cortisol, however, is produced more slowly, and lingers longer in the bloodstream. Because it is primarily immunosuppressive, cortisol contributes to reductions in lymphocyte numbers and function and NK-cell activity (natural killer lymphocytes that attack infected cells and tumor cells in the body). Neuropeptides, the chemical messengers that are links between the mind and the body, are produced in the brain and in the endocrine and immune systems.

In addition to the physiological research, forty decades of sociologic research tell us that stressors have measurable damaging impacts on physical and mental health (Thoits, 2010). Caring for the Spirit is an example of the multifaceted nature of the psychoneuroimmunology framework.

Self-Healing Personalities

Neuropeptide manufacture is activated by positive mental states and suppressed by negative mental states. Several stress and coping-related studies have suggested that some people have *self-healing personalities,* while others have *disease-prone personalities*. Self-healers are emotionally stable people who bounce back from stressful situations. These are people whom others describe as enthusiastic, joyful, secure, energetic, alert, and content. They are likable and have close, warm relationships with others. The nurse-theorist Jean Watson, whose nursing theory identifies the centrality of caring and is discussed in Chapter 2 ∞, also stresses people's self-healing potential (Pilkington, 2007).

Hardiness, Resilience, and Health

A now-classic study on hardiness and health found that individuals who have strong feelings of confidence in their ability to control circumstances, a willingness to see life events as

---

CARING FOR THE SPIRIT

Long-Term Survivors of HIV

Wars wage within our bodies every minute of every day. Most of the time we are unaware of the battles that go on within us. We have evolved legions of defenders—specialized cells that silently rout the unseen enemy. Their victories go unheralded. When our defenses are penetrated, our defenders are caught unprepared, or our defenders are routed and we've lost the battle. Then we develop a cold, the flu, or something worse. Why did I catch a cold from the sick toddler on the airplane when the woman next to me did not? Why didn't you come down with the flu when your roommate was sick? Why do only some of the people exposed to HIV develop the disease? Why do some people with HIV die within a year or two while others have survived, or even thrived for 10, 20, or more years? We don't, as yet, have all the answers to these questions.

Perhaps the most common characteristics of people with AIDS who live long past the time predicted for them is their refusal to accept the diagnosis of HIV disease as a death sentence. They do not deny the diagnosis, but *they do defy the fatal outcome* that is supposed to be connected to it. Long-term survivors are extremely goal oriented and social. They treat their symptoms as if they were minor impediments in their lives; they are determined to prevail. Their immune systems seem to function better. They have higher T-cell counts and, in many cases, other immune system cells compensate for the ravaged T cells. Emotional distress, on the other hand, has been found to accompany negative immune function factors in HIV-infected individuals.

The highest incidence of illness and death occurs in people who experience stress after infection with HIV. This suggests that HIV-seropositive people should reduce their exposure to stressful events. Assertive coping, less stress, more self-nurturing, regular exercise, and a spiritual outlook have been associated with better immune status, suggesting that stress-reduction behaviors may be helpful in slowing the progression of HIV disease.

While we cannot promote the idea that clients are in total control of the disease process and the state of their health, or that the mind or the spirit can cure AIDS, we can and should teach clients the self-care and self-nurturing behaviors that long-term survivors are using to maintain their health. Assess the level of stress, quality of social support, and mood factors that influence the quality of life of people with HIV disease. Nursing interventions to help clients enhance neurologic, immunologic, and cognitive functioning should focus on improved nutrition, adequate sleep–wake patterns, hygiene, stress reduction, and social and spiritual support.

challenges rather than as obstacles, and a strong commitment to the experiences and demands of daily living have fewer illnesses than those who lack these qualities (Kobasa, 1979). These people have the quality known as hardiness discussed earlier in Chapter 1 ∞. Martin Seligman (2011), the father of positive psychology, has spent 30 years researching failure, helplessness, optimism, and resilience. He has developed a program for teaching resilience that has been used with children and young adults and is currently being tested by the U.S. Army.

Disease-Prone Personalities

Disease-prone personalities, on the other hand, tend to display negative emotions. They are suspicious of others and tend to be chronically anxious, angry, or depressed. These chronic negative emotional patterns are linked with various physiological changes such as activation of the sympathetic nervous system, increase in the level of cortisol, and suppression of the immune system, leading to increased vulnerability to illness.

ANXIETY

Anxiety is a state of varying degrees of uneasiness or discomfort. It is frequently coupled with guilt, doubts, fears, and obsessions. Beyond the mild level, anxiety is often described as a feeling of terror or dread; anxiety is believed to be the most uncomfortable feeling a person can experience. In fact, anxiety is so uncomfortable that most people try to get rid of it as soon as possible.

Anxiety is a potent force because the energy it provides can be converted into destructive or constructive action. When used constructively, anxiety can stimulate the action necessary to alter a stressful situation, fill a painful need, or arrange a compromise. A client who understands the source of anxiety is best able to use it constructively.

Neurobiologic Basis of Anxiety

Contemporary thinking about anxiety includes a neurobiologic component. Anxiety is now thought to result, at least in part, from dysregulation of one or more neurotransmitters and their receptors. Most research has focused on the BZ–GABA–chloride complex, although several other neurotransmitters and their receptors such as serotonin, norepinephrine, and the neuropeptide cholecystokinin may play a role in the development of anxiety. Other research using MRIs and PET scans focuses on brain structure itself. The neurobiologic component of anxiety is more fully discussed in Chapters 6 and 18 ∞.

Sources of Anxiety

Anxiety is an inevitable result of the attempt to maintain equilibrium in a changing world. People experience anxiety in many different situations and interpersonal relationships. However, the general causes of anxiety have been classified into two major kinds of threats, discussed in Box 8-1. It is crucial to understand that *either* actual *or* impending interference may cause anxiety; actual interference with a biologic or psychosocial need is not a necessary condition. All that is necessary is the *anticipation* of one of these major threats.

Box 8-1   General Causes of Anxiety

1. Threats to biologic integrity: actual or impending interference with basic human needs such as the needs for food, drink, or warmth
2. Threats to the security of the self:
   a. Unmet expectations important to self-integrity
   b. Unmet needs for status and prestige
   c. Anticipated disapproval by significant others
   d. Inability to gain or reinforce self-respect or gain recognition from others
   e. Guilt, or discrepancies between self-view and actual behavior

---

Threats to biologic integrity or to the fulfillment of such basic human needs as food, drink, warmth, and shelter are a general cause of anxiety. Threats to the security of self are not as easily categorized. In some instances, they are obvious; in others, they are more obscure because each person's sense of self is unique. To one person, power and prestige may be essential; to another, independence; to a third, being of service to others.

Consider the last category—being of service to others.

Clinical Example

Mrs. C, a nurse, is convinced that a client would feel much better if he expressed his fears to her. But no matter how often she provides the opportunity, he insists, "This is not the time to talk about it," and thwarts her attempt. She is not able to help him in a way that is important to her sense of self. In addition, she believes that the unit's nurse manager (whose skills she admires) expects her to have been successful in this endeavor.

Mrs. C is worried and anxious. When unmet needs or expectations related to essential values (such as being of service to the client) are coupled with the actual or anticipated disapproval of others who are important (the nurse manager), anxiety is generated.

Anxiety as a Continuum

Many theorists conceptualize anxiety as a continuum (FIGURE 8-4 ■). Mild to moderate anxiety can be functionally effective in that it helps us focus our attention and generates energy and motivation. Thus, anxiety is an aspect of problem solving in that it alerts us to the need to concentrate our resources. However, severe anxiety and panic narrow our attention to a crippling degree. Under these conditions alertness is greatly reduced, and learning does not usually take place.

Mild Anxiety

Mild anxiety helps one deal constructively with stress. A mildly anxious person has a broad perceptual field because mild anxiety heightens the ability to take in sensory stimuli. Such a person is more alert to what is going on and can make better sense of what is happening with others and the environment. The senses take in more; the person hears better, sees better, and makes logical connections between events. The person feels relatively

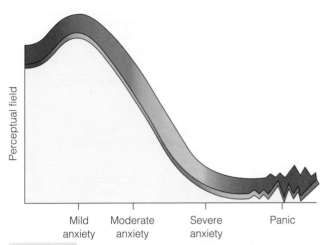

FIGURE 8-4 ■ The effect of anxiety on the perceptual field. Notice that the perceptual field is increased in mild anxiety, becomes increasingly constricted as anxiety increases, and is completely disrupted at the panic level.

safe and comfortable. Because learning is easier when one is mildly anxious, mild anxiety helps clients learn, for instance, how best to administer their own insulin. Mild anxiety can also help a nursing student review psychiatric–mental health nursing before a final examination.

Moderate Anxiety

In moderate anxiety a person remains alert, but the perceptual field narrows. The moderately anxious person shuts out the events on the periphery while focusing on central concerns.

Clinical Example

A nursing student who is moderately anxious about the final examination may be able to focus so intently on studying that she or he is not distracted by an argument between roommates, loud music on the stereo, and a rousing chase scene on television. The student shuts out the chaos in the environment and focuses on what is of central personal importance—preparing for the exam.

This process of taking in some sensory stimuli while excluding others is called **selective inattention**.

People also use selective inattention to cope with anxiety-provoking stimuli. This phenomenon may account for the anxious preoperative client who fails to remember what the nurse said about postoperative pain or about the need to cough and deep breathe after surgery.

Although the perceptual field is narrowed and the person sees, hears, and grasps less, there is an element of voluntary control. Moderately anxious individuals can, with direction, focus on what they have previously shut out.

Severe Anxiety

In severe anxiety, sensory reception is greatly reduced. Severely anxious people focus on small or scattered details of an experience. They have difficulty in problem solving, and their ability to organize is also reduced. They seldom have the

complete picture. Selective inattention may be increased and may be less amenable to voluntary control. The person may be unable to focus on events in the environment. The person may experience new stimuli as overwhelming and may cause the anxiety level to rise even higher.

The sympathetic nervous system is activated in severe anxiety, causing an increase in pulse, blood pressure, and respiration as well as in epinephrine secretion, vasoconstriction, and even body temperature. A multitude of physiological changes may be observed, which are described in the following sections.

Panic

The panic level of anxiety is characterized by a completely disrupted perceptual field. Panic has been described as a disintegration of the personality experienced as intense terror. Details may be enlarged, scattered, or distorted. Logical thinking and effective decision making may be impossible. The person in panic is unable to initiate or maintain goal-directed action. Behavior may appear purposeless, and communication may be unintelligible.

Assessing Anxiety

Anxiety can be assessed in the physiological, cognitive, and emotional/behavioral dimensions. This observation illustrates the relationship between the mind and the body. Anxiety is a multidimensional phenomenon in that the total person is involved in every aspect of it. Objective data, particularly nursing observations, may be critical because of the nature of anxiety. Selective inattention interferes with the client's awareness of anxiety and ability to give accurate reports. Families and friends also can contribute data useful to the assessment of anxiety.

Physiological Dimension

Observations of the client's physiological state are likely to indicate autonomic nervous system responses, particularly sympathetic effects. Sympathetic nervous system dominance is associated with arousal as occurs during anxiety or as the body's response to a physical emergency. The parasympathetic nervous system maintains normal, smooth functioning. Various organs may be affected, such as the adrenal medulla, heart, blood vessels, lungs, stomach, colon, rectum, salivary glands, liver, pupils of the eyes, and sweat glands. FIGURE 8-5 ■ illustrates the sympathetic and parasympathetic nervous systems in detail. Anxious clients may have an increased heart rate, increased blood pressure, difficulty breathing, sweaty palms, trembling, dry mouth, "butterflies in the stomach" or a "lump in the throat," as well as other symptoms.

Laboratory tests are not routinely done to evaluate anxiety because observation is faster and more accurate. However, anxiety affects the results of laboratory tests done for other purposes. Blood studies may show increased adrenal function, elevated levels of glucose and lactic acid, and decreased parathyroid function and oxygen and calcium levels. Urinary studies may indicate increased levels of epinephrine and norepinephrine.

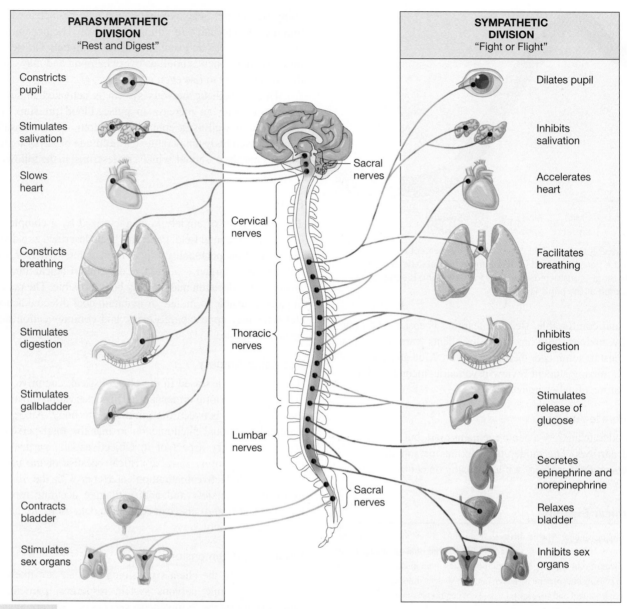

FIGURE 8-5 ■ Involuntary control of bodily functions. The autonomic nervous system has two divisions, the sympathetic and the parasympathetic, which exercise automatic control over the body's organs, generally in opposing ways. The parasympathetic generally has inhibitory or relaxing effects, while the sympathetic has stimulatory effects. Axons of the parasympathetic division emerge not only from the spinal cord, but from the brain as well.
Source: Krogh, D. (2000). *Biology: A guide to the natural world.* Upper Saddle River, NJ: Prentice Hall, p. 515.

Cognitive Dimension

Assessment of cognitive function may indicate difficulty in logical thinking, narrowed or distorted perceptual field, selective inattention or dissociation, lack of attention to details, difficulty concentrating, or difficulty focusing. The level of anxiety determines the extent to which cognitive function is affected. Mild, moderate, severe, or panic-level anxiety is assessed according to the descriptions earlier in this chapter.

Emotional/Behavioral Dimension

In the emotional/behavioral dimension, clients may be irritable, angry, withdrawn, and restless, or they may cry. The affective response can often be assessed through the client's subjective

description. Clients may describe themselves as "on edge," "uptight," "jittery," "nervous," "worried," or "tense." They may feel dizzy or faint and may experience a feeling of impending doom as if something terrible were about to happen.

COPING WITH STRESS AND ANXIETY

Reactions to threatening situations can be divided into two general categories: task-oriented responses and defense-oriented responses.

When we feel competent to deal with stress and the situation is not too threatening to our sense of self, our behavior tends to be *task oriented.* Task-oriented behavior is geared toward problem solving such as occurs in the clinical example.

Clinical Example

Samantha is a psychiatric–mental health nursing student who has been assigned to a psychiatric hospital for her clinical experience. Samantha does her best to avoid interacting with the clients on the unit and busies herself reading charts, chatting with classmates, and running errands for the staff. When clients approach her, Samantha's hands shake, her heart races, and she wishes that she was anyplace else. Once she drives home after the clinical experience she falls into bed exhausted.

After three uncomfortable weeks pass, Samantha decides to discuss her reactions with her clinical instructor.

Because Samantha was not too frightened by the possibility that she may be thought of by the instructor as incompetent or weak, she was able to acknowledge her need for assistance and seek help. This is a task-oriented reaction. It is based on a realistic appraisal or assessment of the situation and involves a series of carefully thought-out judgments about what course of behavior would be most effective. Had Samantha not taken a task-oriented route she would likely inhibit her own growth and development (Freeman & Sinclair, 2009).

When we feel inadequate to cope with stress and the situation is extremely threatening to our sense of self, we tend to engage in *defense-oriented* behavior. Everyone uses defense-oriented behavior from time to time as a protective measure. The diagnosis of a terminal illness, for instance, may be so overwhelming that a person must temporarily defend against acknowledging this reality.

YOUR SELF-AWARENESS
What Coping Strategies Do You Use?

When you are feeling competent to deal with stress and the situation is not too threatening to your sense of self, which task-oriented coping strategies do you use? Review the everyday ways of coping with stress discussed on pages 149–151 and answer the following questions:

- Which everyday ways of coping with stress do you use most often? Be specific.
- Can you identify a pattern or common thread among them? If so, what is it?
- What effects do they have on your sense of comfort or well-being?
- What effects do they have on your interpersonal relationships (include professional relationships)?

When you are feeling inadequate to cope with stress and the situation is extremely threatening to your sense of self, which defense-oriented behaviors do you use? Review the defense-oriented ways of coping (defense mechanisms) discussed on pages 151–158 and answer the following questions:

- Which defense-oriented ways of coping do you use most often? Be specific.
- Can you identify a pattern or common thread among them? If so, what is it?
- What effects do they have on your sense of comfort or well-being?
- What effects do they have on your interpersonal relationships (include professional relationships)?

Such behavior becomes harmful only when it is the predominant means of coping with stress. In such cases, problem-solving and reality-based behaviors are continually avoided. Defense-oriented behavior is discussed later in this chapter.

Coping strategies are a set of behaviors people under stress use in struggling to improve their situations. Once you have finished reading this section, thoughtfully consider how you cope with stress by answering the questions posed in Your Self-Awareness in this section. Coping strategies can be thought of simply as ways of getting along in the world.

Everyday Ways of Coping With Stress

Everyday coping strategies offer an immense repertoire of defenses to maintain control and balance in the face of stress. A person can cope on different levels, including physical, social, cognitive, and emotional levels. However, the devices people choose to cope with stress depend on many factors. Among them are the external circumstances, the suddenness and intensity of the stress, the resources available to the person, and the person's predisposition to certain coping patterns, established over the course of one's development. One man who is late for an appointment because he gets caught in a traffic jam may react with a furious outburst of anger. Another may begin to daydream and forget where he is going. A third may use the time to solve some problem.

Most often, individuals use behaviors that have worked well for them in the past. Sometimes they behave in a certain way because it is the only method they have of coping with stress or because other coping strategies failed to work. Some people learn to turn to others for protection and nurturance; some learn to turn to chemicals or food; some rely on self-discipline and keeping a stiff upper lip; others feel better after the intense expression of feelings; some withdraw physically and/or emotionally; still others exercise or talk the problem out. Common coping methods are discussed in the next section.

Seeking Comfort

The earliest coping strategy is probably the familiar method of turning to a nurturing person for soothing, comfort, and protection. Receiving love is being reassured that one is lovable. Love from supportive others may take the form of physical touching, rocking, patting, or verbal reassurances of various kinds ("Don't be afraid, I'll stay with you"). Sustained touch, such as that in massage, can reduce the stress response (Lindgren et al., 2010). Nurturing may also come about in the form of Bible study or listening to religious tapes, which is comforting to many people.

Some people, like Scott in the clinical example that follows, use less positive behaviors such as alcohol, nicotine, and other chemicals to enhance well-being in the face of stress.

Clinical Example

Scott is a student of economics preparing to apply to law school. He comes to the campus mental health clinic because of difficulty sleeping; a vague, uneasy feeling of dread and apprehension; difficulty working on his final course papers; irritability; and hypervigilance. From time to time, he is sweaty and feels his heart pounding. He describes himself as "stressed out" and smokes pot to calm down almost every day.

This category also includes eating in times of stress and for general support. While comfort foods can soothe in the short term, they can sabotage the long-term stress response by increasing the number of inflammatory proteins in the body. In addition to comfort foods, alcohol, nicotine, and other chemicals are often used to enhance well-being in the face of stress. Many theorists view these alternatives as substitutes for the dependent comfort of being a baby in the care of a nurturing parent.

Relying on Self-Discipline

Wheareas some people under stress tend to turn to the comfort of friendly company, food, or alcohol, all of which are reminiscent of childhood dependence, others rely on self-discipline. Self-control ranks high in the value system of many cultures and subcultures (De Bono, Shmueli, & Mursven, 2011). This coping style involves pride in the ability to laugh off problems, endure frustrations, and discount anxiety. Keep a stiff upper lip, bite the bullet, and get over it are all admonitions that people address to themselves when self-discipline is their patterned response to stress.

Clinical Example

Amanda is under considerable stress. After retiring from her job she was forced to go back to work for financial reasons at age 68. Now at age 74, she is taking care of her younger sister who is incapacitated by rheumatoid arthritis. Amanda becomes annoyed when friends make statements of support or comment on how difficult things must be for her. Her rudeness toward those who attempt to be supportive is driving her friends away.

People such as Amanda are unlikely to want the company of supportive others and may even push them away. They are often unresponsive when others seek comfort from them, for they see such dependent behavior as weak.

Intense Expression of Feeling

Crying, swearing, and laughing all tend to relieve tension. Swearing loses its usefulness as an escape valve if it becomes a habit. This is less true of both crying and laughing. Crying and laughing tend to release energy and exert a soothing effect on a person who is experiencing tension.

Avoidance and Withdrawal

While some people find it hard to sleep when they are under tension, others react to worries, bad news, or an argument with somnolence. Still others respond with a form of waking sleep like apathy or emotional withdrawal, which accomplishes the same thing.

Talking It Out

Many people relieve tension by talking it out. Talking implies establishing and maintaining a contact of sorts with another human being. In addition, it enables new ideas to emerge and new perspectives to be entertained. Obviously, this device is the medium of most therapeutic interventions. This has profound implications for nursing because nurses are the health care providers who spend the most time with clients. It also has profound implications for clients whose communication is dysfunctional or whose ability to communicate freely is restricted. Psychiatric clients generally fall into these categories.

Privately Thinking It Through

Some people believe that the unexamined life is not worth living. When faced with a problem that causes them anxiety, these individuals become introspective about it. The rationalizations that emerge serve as effective tension relievers.

Working It Off

Physical activity to relieve tension may range from simple gestures such as finger tapping, floor pacing, and door slamming to activities purposely designed to alter the tension-producing circumstances, such as aerobic exercise. In addition, some tense individuals feel a lot of aggressive energy. Physical exertion in the form of demanding sports, like jogging or racquetball, or manual labor, like scrubbing the floor, is a way to use this energy constructively. Physical exercise has been found to reduce the symptoms of anxiety and depression. In fact, exercise has been found to compare favorably to antidepressant medication as a first-line treatment for mild to moderate depression (Carek, Laibstain, & Carek, 2011). Even low-impact physical activity can result in improvements in stress, mood, and quality of life.

Engaging in Self-Healing Mind–Body Practices

Increasing numbers of people are integrating self-healing practices such as yoga, meditation, massage, visualization, and relaxation exercises into their everyday lives. While Western medicine continues its explosive growth in psychobiologic knowledge and technology, more of us are finding that these ancient principles and practices have significant therapeutic value.

Clinical Example

Four young mothers who have been friends since the first year of high school get together three mornings a week after their children are picked up by the school bus. On Mondays they meditate using a CD that combines deep breathing, meditation, and imagery. On Wednesdays they take an early morning tai chi class in which the graceful movements help their balance, flexibility, and mindfulness. A Zumba class on Friday gives them energy for the active weekend ahead.

Meditation has been found to significantly reduce chronic insomnia (Gross et al., 2011), and enhance inner strength (Woods-Giscombe & Black, 2010). It has also been associated with enhanced quality of life and decreased depressive symptoms in women with fibromyalgia (Sephton et al., 2007). A thorough discussion of healing practices is in Chapter 33 ∞.

Spirituality and Prayerfulness

We define spirituality as the search for self-transcendence—the search for meaning and purpose through connection with others, nature, and/or a Supreme Being. Spirituality may, but does not always, involve religious structure or traditions. A failure to let the world in, to perceive it and to engage it fully, leads to the emptiness that some people feel in their lives.

Many people's spirituality includes prayerfulness and attendance at religious services. Attending religious services can enhance the recovery process of people with mental illness despite the severity of their symptoms (Fukui, Starmino, & Nelson-Backer, 2011). Prayer can be individual or communal, private or public. People pray for different reasons—to ask for something for themselves, to ask for something for others, to repent of wrongdoing and ask for forgiveness, to give honor and praise to a Higher Power, to offer thanksgiving. Recent research shows that praying can positively affect high blood pressure, the course and extent of heart attacks, migraine headaches, and anxiety. Further, nursing activities that support prayer may be seen by some clients as equally as important as encouraging and reassuring them and speaking up for them (Wilson, 2010).

Using Symbolic Substitutes

Stress may be relieved by ascribing symbolic values to acts or objects. These acts or objects may or may not have other meanings. There are symbolic devices for the management of tension in religious practices such as confession, prayer, or sacrifice. For some people, the automobile has a symbolic significance; others ascribe symbolic significance to their annual

income or their physical appearance. The list is almost endless, but the principle is always the same. Some people attach a meaning beyond the obvious one to objects, experiences, and people, through which they find a means to reduce their tensions.

Somatizing

Many organs of the body have an expression and communication function. This is sometimes known as *somatizing* or *organ language*. Somatizing is not uncommon in people with chronic illnesses such as chronic obstructive pulmonary disease (COPD). Those with somatization tendencies report more severe dyspnea (Albuquerque et al., 2011). Some organs communicate their messages only to their owner. For example, the heart may communicate by means of palpitation. Other demonstrations are public, such as blushing or stuttering. Urination and defecation, increased sweating, and altered sexual activity are other familiar examples of organ language.

Evidence-Based Practice illustrates how nurses can apply everyday ways of coping with stress in helping clients influence the course of their lives.

Defense-Oriented Ways of Coping: Defense Mechanisms

The coping strategies described earlier are considered normal. They are simply ways of getting along. In some people, however, what passes for a normal adjustment is actually a very

---

EVIDENCE-BASED PRACTICE

Psychoeducation for Managing Stress

As the nurse in a day treatment unit located in a suburb of a large city in the southeastern United States, you are especially aware of the difficulty your older clients have in handling stress. Most of your clients are diagnosed with a psychotic disorder or post-traumatic stress disorder and have difficulty maintaining relationships with friends and family and finding or keeping a job. Thus, most have become marginalized, and the day treatment unit has become the core of their daily activities.

You understand that it is important to strengthen life control among those who have become marginalized. People who are in charge of their lives have a sense of coherence. They are more likely to be able to cope with stressful situations in ways that decrease, or even eliminate, their distress. To help your clients develop a sense of coherence and strengthen their resilience to stress, you develop a psychoeducation program for them, focusing on the following:

1. Achieving understanding of the internal environment (what thoughts, feelings, and wishes drive the individual)
2. Achieving understanding of the external environment (what forces affect what an individual is able to accomplish)
3. Exploring human relationships to include client–family, client–friend, client–client, client–employer, client–staff,

client–landlord, and whatever other dyads are active relationships or potential relationships in the clients' lives
4. Exploring the meaning of present events, that is, focusing on the here-and-now, rather than the there-and-then, to gain an understanding of what the stressors are in the lives of the clients
5. Partaking in a program of regular physical activity that includes flexibility training and walking in place

The psychoeducation program you developed is based on the following research citations:

Chan, D., Fan, M. Y., & Unutzer, J. (2011). Long-term effectiveness of collaborative depression care in older primary care patients with and without PTSD symptoms. *International Journal of Geriatric Psychiatry, 26*(7), 758–764.

Chou, K. L., Mackenzie, C. S., Liang, K., & Sareen, J. (2011). Three-year incidence and predictors of first-onset DSM-IV mood, anxiety, and substance use disorders in older adults: Results from wave 2 of the national epidemiologic survey on alcohol and related conditions. *Journal of Clinical Psychiatry, 72*(2), 144–155.

CRITICAL THINKING QUESTIONS

1. What actual activities would help clients to understand their internal environment and explore human relationships?
2. What does it mean to explore the meaning of present events by focusing on the here-and-now?

tenuous one with few outlets for controlled aggression, few love objects, few opportunities for satisfaction and growth. These people find it more and more difficult to cope with additional stress. Ultimately, the external stress the person is trying unsuccessfully to ward off is matched by a mounting internal stress. The person suffers both from increased anxiety and from the strain on overworked stabilizers. And what happens to the person who has no one to talk with, who cannot jog 5 miles, or who cannot laugh off the problem?

When a person is unable to ward off stress or reduce tension in the usual way, anxiety mounts as the person feels increasingly inadequate to cope with the situation. Under these circumstances, the person is more likely to engage in *defense-oriented behavior*. Defense-oriented behavior is not a specific attempt to solve a problem; it consists of using mental mechanisms to lessen uncomfortable feelings of anxiety and to prevent pain regardless of cost. These characteristic mental mechanisms are commonly called **defense mechanisms**. Defense mechanisms are automatic psychological processes that protect the self by allowing the person to deny or distort a stressful event or to restrict awareness and reduce the sense of emotional involvement. Defense mechanisms are mostly unconscious and often inflexible coping patterns that protect a person through intrapsychic (coming from within) distortions that are really self-deceptions. The person usually has little awareness of what is happening or even less control over events.

Although these reactions may help keep the lid on anxiety, they also limit the ability to grow from and savor the experience, they interfere with rational decision making and the ability to work productively, they can easily become a substitute for addressing the underlying cause, and they impair and erode interpersonal relationships. Even adaptive devices can go wrong. Being unable to ward off stress is at the heart of the film discussed in Mental Health in the Movies.

You will notice that definitions of various defense mechanisms overlap, and the same observed behavior may often be explained by more than one type of defense. In addition, people do not use one method of defense at a time; they usually rely on a combination of defenses. For study purposes, the more common defense mechanisms are discussed here: repression, regression, suppression, dissociation, identification, introjection, projection, denial, fantasy, rationalization, reaction formation, displacement, undoing, and intellectualization. They are summarized in Table 8-1 ■.

Repression

Repression, the basis of all defense mechanisms, is the dynamic behind much of "forgetting." When people repress, they unconsciously exclude distressing emotions, thoughts, or experiences from awareness. Repression bars access to conscious awareness of feelings and thoughts that would cause anxiety and disrupt the self-concept. At best, repression protects the individual from overattention to a distressing experience (Scholes & Martin, 2010). It also affords protection from a sudden trauma until the person can deal with the shock. From the individual's point of view, a repressed memory is "forgotten" and cannot be deliberately brought to awareness (see Caring for the Spirit for an example of repression). Although the repressed feelings remain unconscious, they continue to exert pressure for expression. The self tries to maintain the repression, but in people experiencing extreme stress or anxiety, or in febrile (feverish) or toxic states, repression may begin to fail. Clients who are intoxicated by alcohol or drugs or who are emerging from anesthesia may verbalize feelings that they usually repress.

Clinical Example

Susan was raped. She was brought to an outpatient clinic by her roommate. Susan said she felt very anxious and could not recall the circumstances surrounding her rape or what the rapist looked like. Her use of repression protected her from facing her fears and humiliation.

Nursing Intervention Strategies Nursing intervention in such cases should be supportive and protective of the client's defenses. This means that interventions into repression are not called for until after the initial shock has lessened and the client's anxiety level has been reduced. Then, you can help the client examine the traumatic event.

Regression

Regression is falling back to an earlier psychosexual developmental stage (see Freud's psychosexual stages on page 79 in Chapter 5 ∞) involving less mature behavior and

MENTAL HEALTH IN THE MOVIES
Black Swan

Desperately wanting the lead in a production of Swan Lake, Nina is a fragile ballerina in the stressful world of a prestigious New York dance company. Kept in a state of perpetual childhood by a hovering, unfulfilled, and controlling mother, she has dedicated her life to the pursuit of her art, obsesses over being perfect, and lacks the coping resources that help people deal with a stress-laden life. Her journey begins with tension and anxiety and moves rapidly to purging, drugs, and gruesome self-mutilation. Her all-consuming drive to become the best leads to growing paranoia and hallucinations and she becomes increasingly unstable. Nina achieves her goal as the Black Swan, but dies on stage as the result of her self-mutilation. A very dark movie, Black Swan emphasizes Nina's inability to cope that leads to an inevitable tragic ending.

Photo courtesy of Newscom/g90.

TABLE 8-1 ■ Common Defense Mechanisms

Name	Definition	Example
Denial	Blocking out painful or anxiety-inducing events or feelings	A manager tells an employee he may have to fire him. On the way home, the employee shops for a new car.
Displacement	Discharging pent-up feelings on people less dangerous than those who initially aroused the emotion	A student who has received a low grade on a term paper blows up at his girlfriend when she asks about his grade.
Dissociation	Handling emotional conflicts, or internal or external stressors, by a temporary alteration of consciousness or identity	A woman has amnesia for the events surrounding a fatal automobile accident in which she was the speeding driver.
Fantasy	Symbolic satisfaction of wishes through nonrational thought	A student struggling through graduate school thinks about a prestigious, high-paying job she wants.
Identification	Unconscious assumption of similarity between oneself and another	After hospitalization for minor surgery, a girl decides to become a nurse.
Intellectualization	Separating an emotion from an idea or thought because the emotional reaction is too painful to be acknowledged	A man learns from his doctor that he has cancer. He studies the physiology and treatment of cancer without experiencing any emotion.
Introjection	Acceptance of another's values and opinions as one's own	A woman who prefers a simple lifestyle assumes the materialistic, prestige-oriented values of her husband.
Projection	Attributing one's own unacceptable feelings and thoughts to others	A man who is quite critical of others thinks that people are joking about his appearance.
Rationalization	Falsification of experience through the construction of logical or socially approved explanations of behavior	A man cheats on his income tax return and tells himself it's alright because everyone does it.
Reaction formation	Unacceptable feelings disguised by repression of the real feeling and by reinforcement of the opposite feeling	A woman who dislikes her mother-in-law is always very nice to her.
Regression	Reverting to an earlier stage of development	A man exposes his genitalia to women he sees in public places.
Repression	Unconsciously keeping unacceptable feelings out of awareness	A man is jealous of a good friend's success but is unaware of his feelings.
Suppression	Consciously keeping unacceptable feelings and thoughts out of awareness	A student taking an examination is upset about an argument with her boyfriend but deliberately puts it out of her mind so she can finish the test.
Undoing	Attempting to take back an unconscious thought or behavior that is unacceptable or hurtful	A young woman realizes that she has just insulted her boyfriend and spends the rest of the evening complimenting him on his looks and his athletic ability.

responsibility as a way of coping with stressful situations. For example, an individual fixated at the oral stage might eat or smoke excessively or be verbally aggressive. An individual fixated at the anal stage might display excessive messiness or excessive tidiness. Many of the clients in psychiatric inpatient settings demonstrate regressive behavior.

A common example of regression is the young child who reverts to thumb-sucking or bed-wetting upon the birth of a baby brother or sister. It has to do with the young child's fear of change in the parent–child relationship and the fear of losing the parent's love to the newborn sibling. Regressing to an earlier stage of helplessness guarantees the parent's attention and helps the child avoid having to deal with feelings of aggression toward the newcomer. An example of regression in an adult is in the clinical example that follows.

Clinical Example

Marie's husband, Bill, recently passed away. Since his death, Marie remains in her night clothes and stays in bed most of the day. When her daughter comes to check on her, Marie either refuses the meal her daughter has prepared for her, or insists on having it on a tray and being served in bed.

Regression, secondary to illness, is a well-known psychological phenomenon. Illness and hospitalization with its consequences of disability, dependency, unpleasant and restrictive therapeutic regimens, and diminished ability to function in social, familial, and occupational roles often results in regression to more dependent behavior.

Nursing Intervention Strategies Nursing interventions would focus on acknowledging what preceded the regression (illness, death, disability), making supportive statements, and gradually reminding clients of events or situations in which they demonstrated competence before the regression. For a discussion of nursing intervention strategies for regressed behavior see Unit IV, especially Chapters 14–16. ∞

Suppression

Suppression is an intentional (therefore, conscious) act that helps keep thoughts, feelings, wishes, or actions that cause anxiety out of conscious awareness. Suppression is the conscious form of repression.

CARING FOR THE SPIRIT

Repressed Memories or False Memories?

Over 100 years ago, Sigmund Freud proposed that we actively and deliberately bury painful or dangerous memories beyond the reach of consciousness. He called this process *repression*.

According to Freud, repressed memories influence behavior, thinking, and emotions, and produce mental symptoms. Early in his career, Freud wrote that sexual abuse in childhood was common and was the cause of repression. This abuse, and the resulting repression, caused the "hysteria" he diagnosed in his patients. After 1897, Freud abruptly abandoned his theory on repression. Instead, he said, children have fantasies of being seduced. These imagined seductions, according to Freud, cause internal conflict, and repression is a way of coping with this internal conflict.

It is unclear why Freud abandoned his theory. Some of his critics believe that Freud bowed to social pressure and the threat of professional ostracism because the notion of rampant childhood sexual abuse was outrageous. Others of his critics believed that Freud himself distorted his patients' stories because of his own psychological problems.

To understand the concept of repression, we need to understand how memory works. Memories are stored in a portion of each of the millions of neurons in the brain. Each neuron represents a little bit of memory. Because the brain is such a complex organ, it parcels out bits and pieces of an experience to different parts of the brain. For example, memories of sound are parceled out to the auditory cortex, memories of appearance to the visual cortex, memories of sensation to the sensory cortex, memories of smell to the olfactory cortex, and source memory to the frontal cortex. All scattered memory fragments remain physically linked. It is the limbic system that takes on the job of assembling these bits and pieces. The limbic system actually acts as a neural file clerk by pulling memory fragments from various file drawers. Intensely traumatic events produce unusually strong nerve connections.

Memory can go awry if the terror of an experience is so great that the biologic processes underlying information storage are disrupted. However, the right biologic stimulus can set the nerve circuits firing and trigger fear. The source of the fear is *not* remembered. Memory blocks come at great cost. They leave a person without an explanation for bewildering emotional distress that causes turmoil.

Memory can also be confounded; that is, snippets of memory from a real event can be interwoven with snippets of an imagined event. Recent research has demonstrated that the mere suggestion that you could have once been lost in a shopping mall can leave a memory trace in the brain. This memory trace can then become linked to the memory of a friend's or sibling's story of being lost or a fairy tale such as Hansel and Gretel, as well as actual memories of shopping malls. Under stress and over time, the knowledge that being lost in a mall was only a suggestion deteriorates. If you are asked at a later time if you were ever lost in a mall, your brain will activate these assorted images, and eventually you "remember" being lost in a mall as a child.

These findings—that memories are open to faulty recollection or that they can be created through a suggestion from another—have caused great distress for survivors of childhood sexual abuse who experience the phenomenon called **recovered memory**. Recovered memories of childhood sexual abuse are those that emerge into consciousness after being repressed for a period of time, sometimes for years. Imagine what it must be like having recalled long-forgotten memories of painful and humiliating sexual abuse by a trusted or loved adult. Imagine further what it must be like to have your unsettling memories viewed with suspicion. You might feel helpless, hopeless, and lost. Your sense of self would be fragmented, and your self-esteem diminished; your spiritual distress would be heightened.

The recent rise in reported cases of recovered memory has led to a large number of lawsuits against perpetrators accused of having committed acts of abuse years ago. Essentially, people who have recovered repressed memories, often through hypnosis, are pitted against alleged perpetrators who claim these memories are actually manufactured **false memories**. Therapists who work to help people recover repressed memories are pitted against memory researchers who claim that false recovered memories are fabricated in the highly charged atmosphere of mental health therapy.

Psychiatric–mental health nurses need to be aware of both sides of the issue. There are many therapists who are skilled at helping individuals remember events that happened in the past without suggesting possible false memories. At the same time, research has shown that even though hypnosis may make it easier for people to recall real memories, it also makes it easier to create false memories. Be aware that many persons who have experienced sexual abuse have a history of not being believed by parents or others they love or trust. Expressing disbelief will only cause the client further pain. Being compassionate will help clients in the struggle to examine their own lives.

Clinical Example

A woman who is an only child learns that her elderly widowed mother has been diagnosed with cancer. The woman recognizes that she will be the sole support of her mother during this trying time. She also has some professional responsibilities that cannot be put off. The woman decides to put off worrying about what the future may bring or anticipating her mother's death until her mother's diagnostic studies are completed, an accurate staging of the cancer can be performed, the first chemotherapy sequence has been completed, and a realistic prognosis is made of her mother's chances for a remission. As she puts it: "I've got too much to do and can't afford to fall apart right now."

Clients may refuse to consider their difficulties by saying that they "don't want to talk about it" or that they will "think about it some other time." This, too, is suppression.

Nursing Intervention Strategies Suppression can be dealt with in the same way as repression with initial support and protecting the client's need to suppress. Suppression is generally easier to deal with because the material remains conscious. You can be somewhat more directive in assessing why the client avoids talking about a situation. Suggest that the client try to look at the situation because it affects future plans.

Offering information about the situation may help clients look at their situations objectively. As they learn more, they may feel less threatened.

Dissociation

In **dissociation**, the individual handles emotional conflicts, or internal or external stressors, by a temporary alteration of consciousness or identity (see Chapter 19 ∞ for specific mental dysfunctions in which dissociation is the major mental mechanism). Dissociation resembles repression, but it has a different origin. The self is formed through the process of disapproval and approval from significant other people. Therefore, the self *dissociates,* or refuses awareness of, the expression of personal qualities and experiences of which significant others disapprove. These feelings come to exist separately from the person's self-concept. A little girl with artistic abilities that are not validated by her parents will not think of herself as artistic. She may deny her abilities even when other people point them out.

People who dissociate do not "notice" what they are doing. This limitation of awareness is maintained because they experience anxiety whenever permissible levels for the self are trespassed.

Clinical Example

Jennifer consciously believes that sexual overtures are wrong, yet she behaves seductively toward men. She cannot understand why men see her behavior as a sexual invitation. The use of dissociation complicates Jennifer's problems. She needs to ignore or deny aspects of her situation to feel comfortable in it. Other people notice and point out Jennifer's seductive behavior, but she cannot recognize it because it is not a part of her self-concept. If Jennifer admitted her sexual feelings, she would experience severe anxiety and personality disorganization.

Nursing Intervention Strategies To intervene with a dissociated client, nurses would introduce discussions about the client's definition of self-concept. Unrealistic self-concepts, such as Jennifer's, would be addressed over time while helping Jennifer cope with her anxiety. For a discussion of nursing intervention strategies for dissociation, see Chapter 19 ∞.

Identification

Identification is the wish to be like another person and to assume the characteristics of that person's personality. It represents a turning away from our own personality. Identification is unconscious. In this it differs from *imitation,* which is the conscious copying of another person's qualities. Identification with people we admire can serve an important function in maturation by evoking latent qualities. For instance, a little girl who identifies with her mother and sisters learns the behavioral characteristics of womanhood.

The most primitive type of identification is seen in the infant's relationship with the mother. Infants seem to perceive no difference between their mothers and themselves and only gradually become aware that their mothers exist apart from them. Small children deal with people in terms of how these people meet their needs. They do not see them as separate individuals with needs of their own. Such identifications may

persist into adult life in people who have not differentiated themselves psychologically from seemingly powerful parents.

One specific manifestation of identification is passivity in relationships. People who feel they have no resources of their own will overvalue the resources of others and expect to be taken care of. People who are most identified with their parents tend to be people who were not allowed to develop their own individuality. Part of the process of self-realization occurs in adolescence, when we discard, with much anxiety and insecurity, our identification with the parents on whom we have been so dependent. Some clients may not have achieved a degree of self-identity sufficient to do this. Identification can inhibit our usefulness, because it prevents us from focusing on our own capacities.

Identification can be seen in clients who rely heavily on the nurse's advice and support. They expect that all their needs will be met and that nothing will be expected of them.

Clinical Example

Louie has bipolar disorder and is taking lithium. He is not interested in learning about the medication he must take, dietary recommendations, or blood tests he needs. He expects the nurse to take responsibility for seeing that he gets the right medicine and that everything else is in order. Identification prevents him from being self-reliant.

Nursing Intervention Strategies Nurses who work with clients like Louie should clarify what the client's expectations of the nurse are and then correct any misperceptions about the nurse's role. It is important to help the client increase his own skills and take responsibility for his own care. Initially, you can offer the client collaboration and interdependence. The long-term goal in dealing with identification is for the client to formulate a self-care plan independently.

Introjection

Introjection is closely related to identification. It is the process of accepting another's values and opinions as one's own if they contradict the values one previously held.

Clinical Example

Joe Kaufmann, a cabinet maker, has worked for a furniture manufacturing company for 10 years. Joe's employer has asked him to cut some corners to help stem the company's financial losses. Afraid of losing his job, Joe compromises his values by providing shoddy workmanship as his employer requests.

Introjection also occurs in severe depression following the death of a loved one. The depressed person may assume many of the deceased person's characteristics, and in so doing lose some self-awareness.

Nursing Intervention Strategies Treat introjection as you would identification, remembering that introjection is more primitive and more intractable. It originates in our experience of being fed as infants. We incorporate people and objects into ourselves in the same way that we swallowed food. We felt a sense of oneness with everything in the external world and could not differentiate ourselves from others. Because thinking processes are not involved in the first experience of introjection, this defense mechanism tends to be difficult to explore on the verbal level.

Projection

Projection is an unconscious means of dealing with personal difficulties or unacceptable wishes by attributing them to others. We blame other people for our shortcomings or see them as harboring our own unacceptable feelings or thoughts. In the course of development, the child, needing parental approval, will identify with the parents and will also deny what they seem to condemn or fail to acknowledge. For instance, if her parents do not openly express and recognize angry feelings, a little girl will tend to regard anger as dangerous. She will then deny awareness of her own anger. Anger in others will disturb her, and she will tend to condemn in others the anger she cannot accept in herself. It is common knowledge that people often tend to criticize others for their own unacknowledged inferiorities. The person who fears being taken advantage of is often an opportunist.

In adult life, projection can be destructive if it interferes with our ability to acknowledge our own feelings. The tendency to attribute our own undesired feelings to others also blurs the boundaries between ourselves and others. This, in turn, makes it difficult to understand other people's feelings. People who make excessive use of projection tend to attribute to others hostile or seductive motives that do not actually exist. This prevents them from forming trusting and reciprocal relationships.

Clinical Example

Linda is wary and suspicious of every man she meets. Regardless of how they behave toward her, Linda says: "They only want one thing." She interprets their behavior as sexually suggestive but has no awareness of her own sexual interest in them.

A tendency to projection may also interfere with problem solving. A young woman who believes she is failing a course because of her teacher will not focus her energies on her studies.

Nursing Intervention Strategies Clients who must deal with the stress of serious illness may shift the blame for their condition onto you, the nurse. They may complain of poor nursing care to a nurse who is actually very skillful. They may believe that they are being "paid back" for wrongdoing in the past. If such a client is accusing you falsely, do not show anger or retaliate but show, through consistency and attention, that you respect the client and are concerned about his or her welfare.

As clients feel more secure in the nurse–client relationship, encourage them to explore the realistic aspects of their situation. For example, you can help a man who blames his spouse and his job for his alcoholism objectively explore what is known about the etiology of alcoholism. This may help him come to terms with his feelings of guilt and anger. This type of intervention helps the client separate his own feelings from the objective facts of the situation.

Denial

Denial of reality is one of the simplest of the defense mechanisms. In denial, painful or anxiety-producing aspects of awareness are blocked out of consciousness. The reality of a situation is either completely disregarded or transformed so that it is no longer threatening. Denial is one of the most common defenses against the stress of diagnosis and illness and is typically present in the first few minutes of adjustment to the death of a loved one. It may be helpful as a temporary protection against the full impact of a traumatic event.

Clinical Example

A father reacts with denial when he shouts, "No, it can't be true; there must be a mistake," when told his 8-year-old son has just died in the trauma unit of injuries incurred when his bicycle collided with an automobile.

A young woman admitted to a psychiatric hospital because of acute anxiety and frightening hallucinations says she just "needs a rest."

Nursing Intervention Strategies Sometimes denial is the best solution for the client. In such situations, support the denial. A terminally ill client who believes she will soon recover and who cannot think about her illness should be allowed the protection of denial. Not all clients need to face up to reality. You should recognize that the use of denial may be preventing serious personality disorganization.

Sometimes, however, denial is directly harmful to the client, as when a man refuses to take medication that is crucial to his survival or to his mental health. In such cases, you should assess the motivation for the client's behavior. After discovering the protective function the denial is serving, focus on helping the client meet these needs in a way that is not self-destructive. You can also help by not reinforcing patterns of denial but rather focusing on instances when the client seems to be dealing with reality.

Fantasy

Fantasy is a form of nonrational mental activity that enables the individual to temporarily escape the demands of the everyday world. Fantasies are not confined by the reality considerations of cause and effect and time and space. Fantasy normally characterizes the thinking of children before they are able to engage in consensually validated communication. Adults revert to fantasy during times of stress to obtain a symbolic satisfaction of wishes.

Clinical Example

A businesswoman facing financial difficulties temporarily escapes by daydreaming that she is enjoying a luxurious vacation on a Caribbean island.

Another woman with advanced multiple sclerosis imagines herself a famous ballerina with complete control of her body.

A man whose wife has told him she wants a divorce imagines how much his wife will appreciate him now that he has been diagnosed with cancer.

Fantasy may offer temporary relief from pressures, but people who spend too much time in fantasy may be unable to meet the requirements of reality.

Clients who are very ill may fantasize that when they recover, many good things will happen to them. They may imagine that they will receive special recognition in their work or that they will get along better with their families. These fantasies may help such clients deal with the deprivations caused by illness. However, they may also create unrealistic expectations. The fantasies may make one feel good temporarily but interfere with problem solving.

Nursing Intervention Strategies Clients who engage in fantasy related to their illness need gradual help in assessing the responses others are likely to make and the achievements they themselves may realistically expect. Clients who fail to adjust to reality will be disappointed when their expectations are not met.

A helpful approach that will not devastate clients who need to hold on to some fantasy is to ask them to discuss their specific future plans. Examining the details of work and interpersonal adjustment may help a person relinquish unrealistic expectations and make more realistic plans. For example, the man who believes that a diagnosis of cancer will improve his marriage because his wife will appreciate him more fully must recognize that this is improbable. He needs to examine the real effects his illness will have on her. He must plan how to make specific improvements in their communication by anticipating problem areas.

Imagination does have a creative aspect, however. Fantasies have a richness and variety that is lacking in the everyday world. Certain artists, such as Dalí and Picasso, enriched their works of art through fantasy. Evidence also exists that insights leading to scientific discovery do not come about as the result of step-by-step logical thinking. Rather, they are created through fantasy.

Rationalization

Rationalization is the attribution of "good" or plausible reasons for questionable behavior to justify it or to deal with disappointment. Rationalizing helps us avoid social disapproval and bolster flagging self-esteem.

Clinical Example

A nurse fails to return to the bedside of a nursing-home client despite a promise to do so before leaving work. She believes her behavior is justified because the client has problems with recent memory and probably wouldn't remember anyway.

Many people use rationalization because they wish to prove to themselves or others that their actions are governed by reason and common sense, even though they may not fully understand the reasons for their own behavior. Such explanations may be essential to maintaining personal integrity. They are not destructive as long as they do not prevent one from solving everyday problems.

Rationalization becomes more of a hindrance when it prevents us from making necessary changes in our behavior by interfering with our ability to examine that behavior. One sign of rationalization is an active search for reasons to justify our behavior or beliefs. Another is an inability to recognize inconsistencies in our beliefs. A third is being upset when our reasons are questioned, because each questioning threatens our defenses.

Clients may use rationalization to soften the blow of losses caused by illness. For instance, a man who is ill may give up work prematurely after rationalizing that he would not have been successful in that field anyway. Such unnecessary restrictions deprive us of possible achievements.

Nursing Intervention Strategies Nurses must respect their clients' need to rationalize fears and insecurities they cannot face. However, hold out to clients the possibility for change. You can help clients face the reality of their situation by encouraging them to explore ways they can deal with it more effectively. One way is to help them explore past instances in which they did change in order to cope with a stressful situation. Believing and recognizing that we have real strengths helps us face our areas of insecurity.

Reaction Formation

Reaction formation is a defense through which we keep an undesirable impulse out of awareness by emphasizing its opposite. To protect ourselves from recognizing dangerous feelings, we develop conscious attitudes and behavior patterns that are just the opposite of those feelings. For example, the desire to be sexually promiscuous may be concealed behind a moralistic demeanor. Some people who crusade passionately against alcohol or pornography may have an underlying wish to enjoy these things. Hostility may be concealed behind a facade of love and kindness.

Clinical Example

Sue has been married to Colin for 25 years. Sue's friends and family view Colin as a typical chauvinist. Both of them are professional people—Colin is a banker and Sue is a freelance writer. Colin seldom lifts a hand around the house or drives the children to any of their lessons or sporting events. He drops his clothing all over the bedroom floor and expects Sue to clean up after him. One day, while Sue and her colleague were polishing an article for a travel magazine, Colin arrived home after lunch in a restaurant and rushed upstairs to the bathroom. In a few minutes, he rushed out the door, saying, "Sorry, Susie, but there's a bit of a mess in the upstairs bathroom." Colin had been nauseated and vomited and did not clean the toilet or the towels he used. Although Sue's colleague's astonishment at Colin's behavior turned to anger, Sue remained unnaturally sweet and loving and unable to consider the possibility of being angry with him. Sue is probably using this excess sweetness and loving kindness to counteract an unacceptable (to her) degree of anger.

People who use this defense are not conscious of their true feelings. Clues that reaction formation is occurring are an inappropriate intensity of feeling and the inability to consider alternative points of view.

Nursing Intervention Strategies A client manifesting reaction formation requires essentially the same approach as one manifesting repression. Respect and support the client's defenses while providing a secure relationship in which to explore feelings and new behavioral alternatives. Also be aware that it is easy to be annoyed at clients who cannot face their true feelings. The rigid and excessive display of what seems to be an insincere emotion can be frustrating. Remember that these clients are not "lying" or pretending. They are unconsciously protecting themselves against recognizing threatening feelings.

Displacement

Displacement is the discharging of pent-up feelings, generally hostility, on an object less dangerous than the object that aroused the feelings. This defense is used when emotions are aroused in a situation in which it would be dangerous to express them.

Clinical Example

John has just failed an important examination. He believes his failure was the instructor's fault. He cannot express the full extent of his anger, because that would get him into worse trouble with the instructor. John goes quietly back to the dormitory. But when his roommate turns the stereo on too loud, John explodes. He doesn't fear retaliation from his roommate—they are peers and friends.

In some cases, we turn our anger toward another person inward upon ourselves. When this happens, we experience exaggerated self-accusations and guilt.

Nursing Intervention Strategies Clients may express inappropriate anger to the nurse when they are actually angry at someone or something else. The client may feel more secure with the nurse, who offers a safe target for displaced feelings. Displacement differs from projection in that people who use displacement are not distorting their feelings and attributing them to someone else. The feelings are clear, and the person acknowledges them. They are simply being directed at the wrong person. Therefore, it may be easier to help these clients acknowledge the real situation by remaining calm and accepting during an angry outburst. For example, after the outburst is over, say, "You seem so angry; I wonder if you really are angry because your breakfast is cold or if there might be some other reason." Opening up the possibility for a discussion of anger may help these clients to sort out just why and at whom they are angry.

Undoing

Undoing is an attempt to counteract the effects of an earlier behavior or thought that is inappropriate or hurtful in the hope that it will balance out. Undoing is an attempt to take charge—to make things better, and perhaps patch up a relationship. Undoing involves feeling guilty. Because one cannot change the past, however, undoing is essentially symbolic.

Clinical Example

Over a period of several weeks, Elizabeth has failed to return the phone calls and messages that her friend, Lynda, who lives in another city, has left for her. Once she did call Lynda, Lynda told her that she not only had been very worried about Elizabeth, wondering if she was alright, but her feelings were also hurt. Shortly thereafter, Elizabeth sent Lynda a Valentine's Day card.

The symbolic message is: "See, I'm not such a bad person after all." Freud would probably say that Elizabeth's unconscious purpose was to convince *herself* that she was a good person.

Undoing is commonly associated with obsessive–compulsive behaviors. For example, Freud believed that some rituals such as compulsive hand washing were attempts to atone for sexual thoughts, feelings, fantasies, or behaviors.

Nursing Intervention Strategies Clients can be helped to recognize their undoing behaviors as after-the-fact responses to anxiety-provoking situations. You can help clients to rework situations that engendered undoing by avoiding inappropriate or hurtful behaviors. Working with clients with obsessive–compulsive behaviors is discussed in Chapter 22 ∞.

Intellectualization

Intellectualization is the process of separating the emotion aroused by an event from ideas or opinions about the event because the emotion itself is too painful to acknowledge. The painful emotion is avoided by means of a rational explanation that divests the event of any personal significance. Failures are less significant if one believes that the situation could have been worse.

Clinical Example

A woman whose husband recently died deals with her grief by telling her friends in a rational manner that it was better that he died suddenly by heart attack rather than to have died at the end of a long, chronic illness.

A boy who breaks his pelvis while skiing consoles himself after the accident by saying, "I would rather have a broken hip than a broken neck."

Clients may use intellectualization to blunt the emotional impact of their problems. This may be difficult for the nurse to perceive, because such clients often seem to know a great deal about their condition. They may be able to discuss in great detail the metabolic processes in diabetes or the psychodynamics of anxiety. At the same time, they cannot apply these concepts to their own situation in an emotional sense.

Nursing Intervention Strategies Intellectualization resembles rationalization in that it provides a verbal means of dealing with anxiety. Its use closes off the possibility of accepting and working out problems. Clients often use intellectualization at the onset of a crisis, and the need for this defense may decrease in a supportive nurse–client relationship. You can help the client relate emotionally to a problem by not forcing the expression of feeling. This will only frighten the client further. Asking these clients to explain how their knowledge relates to them personally may encourage them to accept and explore their emotional reactions.

PSYCHOLOGICAL FACTORS AFFECTING MEDICAL CONDITIONS

Physical illnesses with a major emotional component are often called *psychophysiologic* or *psychosomatic* disorders. Because these terms are vague and have limited value for diagnosis, treatment, and research, the term **psychological factors affecting medical conditions (PFAMC)** is used in the DSM-IV-TR (APA, 2000) (see the Diagnostic Criteria feature in this section). The essential feature of this category is the presence of one or more specific psychological or behavioral factors that adversely affect a medical condition. These factors may influence the course of a medical condition, interfere with the condition's treatment, or constitute an additional health risk. They may be any one or a combination of the following:

- A mental disorder affecting the course or treatment of a general medical condition, such as bipolar disorder (manic episode) complicating hemodialysis
- A psychological symptom affecting the course or treatment of a general medical condition, such as anxiety complicating the ability to carry out self-care for diabetes mellitus
- A personality trait or coping style affecting the course or treatment of a general medical condition, such as denial interfering with the timely treatment of cancer
- A maladaptive health behavior affecting the course or treatment of a general medical condition, such as a sedentary lifestyle and overeating affecting treatment for coronary artery disease
- A stress-related physiological response affecting the course or treatment of a general medical condition, such as stress-related dysrhythmias in a person recovering from myocardial infarction

The DSM-IV-TR distinguishes PFAMC from several related disorders. A **mental disorder due to a general medical condition** can be defined as the presence of mental symptoms that are judged to be the direct physiological consequence of a general medical condition. In mental disorder due to a general medical condition, the presumed causality is in the opposite direction. For example, an individual may have catatonic disorder due to a neurologic condition such as a neoplasm, encephalitis, or cerebrovascular disease. Personality change may be due to HIV disease, head trauma, or lupus erythematosus. For situations in which delirium, dementia, amnestic disorder, mood

disorder, psychotic disorder, anxiety disorder, sleep disorder, or sexual dysfunction are factors, see the appropriate chapters related to these diagnoses in this text. While somatoform disorders (discussed in Chapter 19 ∞) are characterized by both psychological and physical symptoms, no medical condition completely accounts for the physical symptoms seen in people with this disorder. Other psychiatric disorders excluded from PFAMC include conversion disorder, hypochondriasis, physical complaints associated with a mental disorder, and substance-related physical complaints.

Holistic Theory of Illness

Because all illnesses may ultimately stem from multiple factors, a holistic theory of illness serves as a basis for understanding all human disorders. As you appreciate the complex, interwoven pattern of emotional and physical elements, you will more fully comprehend the essential unity of the body and the mind. For a partial list of physical conditions having psychological components, see TABLE 8-2 ■.

Clients who come to the attention of health care professionals because of physical complaints frequently have their psychological needs neglected. Those unmet needs may be contributing to the complaint, may be the primary cause of symptom development, or may be the reason for the client's decision to seek help. Even if the most technologically advanced diagnostic and treatment approaches are applied, ignoring the psychological components of illness can be as disastrous as ignoring the biological components. Such psychological components can undermine medically appropriate treatment. The following clinical example illustrates these ideas.

Clinical Example

Peter G., 5 years old, was admitted for the fourth time in 6 months because of an acute asthma attack. While Peter was being treated medically, his parents waited in the family room. Mrs. G. sat crying and wringing her hands while Mr. G. paced the floor with a strained expression on his face. A staff nurse was able to talk to them and trace the sequence of events leading up to Peter's admission to the hospital.

It was a Saturday afternoon, and Mr. and Mrs. G. had been arguing about whether to send Peter to kindergarten in the fall. Two points of view had emerged. Mr. G. was all for it. He wanted Peter to grow up quickly and leave his "babyish ways" behind. Mrs. G. was against it. Peter was the baby of the family, and Mrs. G. felt that her husband was always pushing him to do things too advanced for a 5-year-old child. Peter had awakened from his nap to hear his parents shouting at each other. The quarrel ended abruptly when Peter started to wheeze, and both parents rushed to his bedside, united in their concern for him.

DSM ESSENTIAL FEATURES

Psychological Factors Affecting Medical Condition

- A general medical condition is present.
- The psychological factors and the general medical condition are closely related in time.

- The psychological factors not only interfere with the treatment of the medical condition, they also present additional health risks.
- Stress-related physiological responses either cause the medical symptoms or make them worse.

TABLE 8-2 ■ Examples of Physical Conditions Having Psychological Components

System	Condition
Cardiovascular	Essential hypertension, angina pectoris, tachycardia, arrhythmia, cardiospasm, coronary artery disease, mitral valve prolapse, myocardial infarction, migraine headache
Gastrointestinal	Irritable bowel syndrome, gastric ulcer, duodenal ulcer, pylorospasm, regional enteritis (Crohn's disease), ulcerative colitis, nausea and vomiting, gastritis, chronic diarrhea
Hormonal	Hypoglycemia, diabetes mellitus, hyperthyroidism, hypothyroidism, hyperparathyroidism, hypoparathyroidism, premenstrual syndrome, obesity
Immune	Allergic disorders, cancer, autoimmune disorders (systemic lupus erythematosus, rheumatoid arthritis, Hashimoto's thyroiditis, myasthenia gravis, psoriasis), AIDS
Integumentary	Neurodermatitis (atopic dermatitis), pruritus, psoriasis, hyperhidrosis, urticaria, alopecia, acne, herpes, genital warts
Neuromuscular/skeletal	Chronic pain, headache, sacroiliac pain, temporomandibular joint (TMJ) pain, rheumatoid arthritis, Raynaud's disease
Respiratory	Asthma, hyperventilation syndrome, tuberculosis

What factors brought on Peter's asthma attack at that particular time?

1. The biologic factors include Peter's physiological makeup. His mother had been asthmatic as a child. She and Peter are both allergic to chocolate, eggs, feathers, and dust. Peter inherited certain genetic features that make him susceptible to certain environmental stressors—in this case, the specific allergens.
2. Sociologic components of Peter's illness revolve around his family's functioning. Mr. and Mrs. G. have different viewpoints on what Peter's role in the family should be. Their conflicts create a second source of stress for Peter.
3. A third component is Peter's psychological state. A 5-year-old boy views the integrity of his family as extremely important, and parental conflicts may threaten his sense of security. Peter had discovered that his parents rallied together when he was ill.

In view of these contributing factors, the treatment plan for Peter should not end when Peter stops wheezing. To reduce the number of such emergencies, caregivers need to devise a long-range treatment plan. This plan should encompass the physiological, psychological, and sociologic components of Peter's asthma attacks. Peter's condition further illustrates the importance of examining cultural, environmental, developmental, genetic, constitutional, and historical factors in all disease processes.

Therefore, in all illness, a holistic approach is necessary in order for you to address each facet of the client's overall problem. For each of the disorders, we suggest nonmedical interventions that reduce stress while increasing the client's understanding and control over troublesome symptoms. Promoting a healthy lifestyle and advocating lifestyle modifications are important nursing responsibilities regardless of the clinical area in which you practice.

Selected Conditions Affected by Psychological Factors

The following sections review the characteristics of several conditions often considered to be affected by psychological factors. For most of these conditions, an exact etiology is unknown. Current research focuses on the complicated interrelationships among such factors as stress, genetic susceptibility, personality, environment, and hormones. Treatment is eclectic and holistic, focusing on mind, body, and spirit. Chapter 33 ∞ discusses the complementary and alternative therapies that may be used to help clients with these conditions.

Gastrointestinal Disorders

Gastrointestinal (GI) functional disorders are chronic or recurrent GI symptoms with no identifiable physiological basis. GI symptoms are widespread throughout the population and vary according to such factors as gender and socioeconomic status. Women, for example, tend to more frequently report irritable bowel syndrome or functional constipation, while men more frequently report bloating symptoms. Social, economic, and lifestyle factors all appear to affect susceptibility to GI disorders to varying degrees, although whether such increased susceptibility results from differences in social stress, dietary factors, or other socioeconomic factors is unclear.

Peptic Ulcer Peptic ulcer disease (PUD) has been one of the most thoroughly studied illnesses thought to be influenced by psychological factors. Most peptic ulcer disease has been attributed to the bacterium *Heliobacter pylori*, which can be treated with antimicrobial medication. However, PUD is prevalent among people with stressful lifestyles and is associated with "getting ahead" in Western cultures. PUD appears to run in families and may be brought on or exacerbated by diet, stress, and certain infections. Duodenal ulcers, seen more frequently in men, are associated with hypersecretion of hydrochloric acid, probably stimulated by stress and anxiety.

Emotions such as anxiety and anger are also associated with the secretion of acid and pepsin, predisposing susceptible individuals to duodenal ulcer formation. Personality features of hostility, irritability, hypersensitivity, and impaired coping ability may also contribute to ulcer formation.

While studies of the relationship between psychological factors and ulcer formation and chronicity are somewhat controversial, psychological intervention is often recommended for PUD clients, especially in the absence of *Heliobacter pylori*. Such intervention is often directed toward resolving dependence conflicts and may include biofeedback and relaxation therapy (see Chapter 33 ∞), individual and group educational approaches, and pharmacologic and dietary management.

Inflammatory Bowel Disorders The role of psychological factors in inflammatory bowel disorders is unclear, although studies have demonstrated a relationship between psychological factors and the GI system, particularly such conditions as irritable bowel syndrome and inflammatory bowel disease (Hertzer, Denson, Baldassano, & Hommel, 2011), multifactorial disorders for which stress has been implicated in the pathophysiology. Autoimmune factors and infections, coupled with psychological factors, may contribute to these disorders. Clients with ulcerative colitis tend to have a compulsive personality style with the following features: neatness, orderliness, punctuality, indecisiveness, emotional guardedness, humorlessness, conscientiousness, obstinacy, conformity, moral rigidity, and worry. Recent research, however, raises many questions about the validity of these personality features. Contemporary researchers say that the psychological traits these clients display are similar to those of clients with other chronic illnesses, with dependence being the most common trait. In many cases, onset and flare-ups seem linked to stressful life events, such as separations, failures, and disappointments.

Regardless of the source of the client's illness, treatment should focus on present troublesome areas, particularly concerns about the uncertain nature of the disease. Because of inherent differences between Crohn's disease and ulcerative colitis, the clinician must consider different approaches in planning treatment. The plan may include individual psychotherapy, family therapy, and environmental manipulation along with the medical regimen. These clients do best when they are involved in solid and long-term supportive relationships with nurses and physicians who help them develop coping and self-care skills.

Cardiovascular Disorders

The cardiovascular system is a sensitive indicator of emotional arousal, whether it is fear, anger, or pleasurable excitement. High levels of stress are suspected to have harmful effects on the heart and vascular system, especially if stress is chronic or repeated (Doering & Eastwood, 2011). Experience, learning, and symbolic meaning, along with their emotional content, can influence heart rate, heart rhythm, and blood pressure. These cardiovascular changes can in turn create emotions, mostly unpleasant, that affect perception and ideation. A number of indicators have been identified as high-risk factors for heart disease. They include genetic, physiological,

social, and psychological influences. Stress researchers have found that persons who perceive a lack of control over their work situation, and experience high demands at the same time, may be prone to cardiovascular diseases. Situations such as these, common in nursing, may place nurses at risk for health problems.

A variety of psychosocial factors are believed to contribute to coronary artery disease (CAD). Many of these have been studied extensively, including affective states, personality or coping style, psychological reaction to environmental stimuli, sociocultural factors, and interpersonal factors. Psychological factors that have been linked to CAD, sudden death, and ventricular arrhythmias include anxiety and depression, a behavior pattern involving feelings of hostility and anger, work overload, life stress, and a lack of social support.

The highly competitive, urgent, impatient, hostile, and driving **type A personality** displays the classic constellation of personality characteristics associated with CAD, angina pectoris, and myocardial infarction. Of all these behaviors, anger, in particular, is the best predictor of future heart disease (Haukkala, Kontinnen, Laatikainen, Kawachi, & Uutela, 2010). Adverse conditions in the client's environment, either social or economic, can also create the stress that leads to cardiac dysfunction.

Essential hypertension, cardiac dysrhythmias, and so-called cardiac neurosis are three syndromes of cardiovascular functioning with major psychological inputs. The classical hypothesis in hypertension has been that people have conflict between their dependent and aggressive inclinations. This causes chronic repression of all displays of anger or resentment. The repressed emotions are eventually transformed into disorders of blood pressure regulation. Although this specific hypothesis has been difficult to prove, experiments have shown that fear, anger, frustration, and guilt (along with several medical conditions) all cause rises in diastolic blood pressure in vulnerable individuals. Likewise, anxiety, hostility, depression, interpersonal conflict, and disruptive life events have all been shown to potentially precipitate dysrhythmias, such as sinus tachycardia, paroxysmal atrial tachycardia, and both atrial and ventricular ectopic beats.

Cardiac neurosis is a syndrome consisting of cardiac distress, exercise intolerance, easy fatigability, respiratory discomfort, and dizziness. These features are similar to those found in panic disorder (see Chapter 18 ∞) and mitral valve prolapse.

The treatment of cardiac disease must be multifaceted. In addition to medical or surgical treatment, other approaches involve stress management, relaxation training, biofeedback, weight control through diet and exercise, and behavioral interventions to help people give up smoking. More efforts are being geared toward prevention, including programs by industry and corporations to promote healthy lifestyles among employees.

Endocrine Disorders

A large number of disorders of endocrine functioning are associated with psychological factors. The endocrine system has particular significance for psychiatry, because there is a close relationship between the emotions and a variety of active chemical substances released in tissues by nerve impulses.

Studies on the relationship between emotions and endocrine function have shown the following:

- Various neurotransmitters affect hormone-releasing factors.
- Psychoactive medications whose action is mediated by neurotransmitters also affect the delivery of hormone-releasing factors.
- Stress activates the autonomic nervous system, which can stimulate the adrenal medulla to produce epinephrine or the pancreas to secrete insulin.
- Corticosteroid production of the adrenal cortex increases greatly during some psychotic episodes in clients with schizophrenia.
- Steroid levels also increase in agitated or anxious depressive people.

It seems fair to conclude that the emotional centers of the brain—the cerebral cortex and limbic system—are intimately tied to the endocrine organs, through the axis of the hypothalamus and the anterior pituitary. Their secretions act as communication messengers. It is not surprising, then, to find expressions of emotional arousal through endocrine changes and major effects on emotional states from endocrine diseases. These are both, in fact, common. Endocrine disorders and their physical and mental symptoms are listed in Your Assessment Approach.

Adrenal dysfunction characteristically produces prominent mental as well as distinctive physical symptoms. Thyroid disorders are commonly accompanied by cognitive or emotional changes. Stress has been implicated, though inconclusively, in the precipitation of thyrotoxic crises. Stress may influence the course of diabetes, either directly by promoting a flare-up or indirectly by causing the client to neglect a usually rigid medical regimen. So many mental symptoms are associated with hypoglycemia that many clients are classified and treated as "classic neurotics."

It is evident that numerous problems can be caused by endocrine dysfunction. The treatment approach must be individualized to meet the client's physical and psychological needs. An important role for the nurse is primary prevention. Adequately preparing a person for developmental changes by offering accurate information about likely physical and emotional alterations can help prevent severe psychiatric disturbances during these periods. Reliable support and open channels of communication are necessary. New coping strategies can be successful if their design, timing, and presentation are appropriate.

Asthma

Asthma is among the most widely studied illnesses of the respiratory system. Because breathing is essential to life, there has been much speculation about the emotional and symbolic significance that can become attached to the processes of air exchange.

There are allergic, immunologic, and emotional inputs to asthmatic attacks. The emotional components may lead directly to alterations in bronchus size. Contemporary researchers examine the interplay of both psychological and physiological aspects of asthma such as the relationship between asthma, anger, quality of life, early stress, and maternal stress (Wright, 2011) as well as the neurologic and humoral bases of asthma pathogenesis. However, certain personality types are linked by some researchers and clinicians to asthma susceptibility: those with extreme inhibition, covert aggression, marked dependence needs, a high need for affection, and those prone to depression, anxiety, and disturbances of self-esteem.

Asthmatic people may be extremely frightened by asthmatic attacks, particularly in childhood. This fear may make them feel helpless and vulnerable. In response, they often adopt a clinging style of relating. The emotional and physical aspects of the illness seem to interrelate in a complex system of feedback loops. See the clinical profile of Peter G. (on page 159) for an example.

You must assess each person with asthma individually to determine what factors are contributing to the disease process. In addition to medication, a treatment plan may include family therapy, relaxation training, behavior modification, and hypnosis.

Arthritis

Rheumatoid arthritis (RA) has long been identified as an illness that is strongly influenced by emotional life. Its etiology remains uncertain. Psychological stresses are thought to precipitate attacks and flare-ups.

Early psychological studies of individuals with RA attempted to define the "rheumatic personality." These people were described as self-sacrificing, masochistic, inhibited, perfectionistic, and retiring. While a high percentage of people with RA are depressed, they do not differ from others with chronic illness in this respect; that is, chronic illness increases the risk of depression. Thus, in RA, depression may stem from actual and perceived functional and other losses (such as mobility). The diagnosis cannot be based on personality type, however, because there are many exceptions to the rule. Physical findings, deformities, subcutaneous nodules, and blood studies remain the criteria for identification.

A treatment plan for clients with arthritis may include pain control, surgery, drugs, vocational counseling, occupational therapy, and interventions to alleviate or prevent depression and to deal with depression and anger more directly.

Headache

The experience of headache resulting from emotional tension is common. Headaches account for many physician visits and for job absenteeism. Headaches are also highly associated with depressive and anxiety disorders. Some theorists support the notion that headache sufferers are likely to maintain rigid control over emotions, feel hostility toward others, use introjection as a defense, and be perfectionists.

YOUR ASSESSMENT APPROACH   **Common Features of Endocrine Disorders**

Disease	Physical Symptoms	Mental Symptoms
Addison's disease (adrenal insufficiency)	Weakness, fatigue, anorexia, weight loss, nausea and vomiting, pigmentation of skin, hypotension	Depression, irritability, psychomotor retardation, apathy, memory defect, hallucinations
Cushing's syndrome (adrenal cortex hyperfunction)	Truncal obesity, moon facies, abdominal striae, hirsutism, amenorrhea, hypertension, osteoporosis, weakness	Impotence, decreased libido, anxiety, increased emotional lability, apathy, insomnia, memory deficits, confusion, disorientation
Diabetes mellitus	Polydipsia, polyuria, polyphagia, weight loss, blurred vision, fatigue, impotence, fainting, paresthesia	Stupor, coma, fatigue, impotence
Hyperthyroidism	Exophthalmos, goiter, moist warm skin, weight loss, increased appetite, weakness, tremor, tachycardia, heat intolerance	Anxiety, tension, irritability, hyperexcitability, emotional lability, depression, psychosis, or delirium
Hypoglycemia	Tremor, light-headedness, sweating, hunger, nausea, pallor, tachycardia, hypertension	Anxiety, fugue, unusual behavior, confusion, apathy, psychomotor agitation or retardation, depression, delusions, hallucinations, convulsions, coma
Hypothyroidism	Dull expression, puffy eyelids, swollen tongue, hoarse voice, rough dry skin, cold intolerance	Psychomotor retardation, decreased initiative, slow comprehension, drowsiness, decreased recent memory, delirium, stupor, depression or psychosis
Premenstrual syndrome	Headache, breast engorgement, lower abdominal bloating, GI complaints, increased sweating, craving for sweets, other appetite changes	Irritability, depression, anxiety, emotional lability, fatigue, crying spells

---

Headaches may be divided into the five following types:

1. Vascular headache of migraine type
2. Muscle contraction headache (tension headache)
3. Combined vascular–muscle contraction headache
4. Delusional, depressive, conversion, or hypochondriacal headache
5. Structural or disease-related headache from infections, tumors, hematomas, and eye, ear, nose, throat, sinus, and tooth diseases

Interventions are based on the diagnosis and the contributing factors that have been identified. Possible treatments and approaches include measures that increase circulation, such as massage or heat application; use of medications; alterations in diet, rest, and exercise patterns; psychotherapy; and biofeedback, meditation, hypnosis, relaxation, and other stress-management approaches.

Skin Disorders

Allergic illnesses, particularly those involving the skin, have been shown to have psychological elements in etiology or course (Picardi et al., 2006). The skin, with its critical sensory functions, mediates between the outside world and internal states. Itching (pruritus), excessive sweating (hidrosis), urticaria (hives), and atopic dermatitis are all commonly classified as psychophysiological conditions. Because of the skin–nervous system interactions, there may be a significant psychophysiological or behavioral component to many dermatologic conditions.

A variety of stressful or emotional states are associated with flare-ups of allergic skin disorders. Attempts have been made to correlate specific emotional states or stresses such as aggression, anxiety, anger, and longing for love with specific skin disorders. In truth, these feelings and conflicts are seen in normal, disordered, and other psychophysiological states.

Therefore, you should be cautious about accepting psychopathogenic mechanisms as the only valid explanations.

The location of skin lesions has, historically, had symbolic significance. Thus, conflict over an extramarital affair has been associated with dermatitis in the wedding ring area. Head and face locations have been classically associated with conflict over affective display. Affliction of the hands is associated with practical or professional conflicts. A genital distribution of lesions may be associated with sexual concerns.

Resistance to Psychosocial Intervention

Behavioral therapy, cognitive therapy, biofeedback, hypnotherapy, and psychotherapy have all been used successfully with appropriate clients. However, despite the wealth of psychosocial interventions available to people with psychophysiological disorders, many are resistant to approaches that are not strictly medical. Reasons for this include the following:

- These clients are believed to lack insight because they express conflict through somatic complaints rather than verbalization.
- Conflicts over unresolved dependence and aggressive wishes may make it difficult to relate to these clients interpersonally.
- These clients focus steadfastly on their somatic complaints, apparently indicating that alternative defense mechanisms are unavailable or inadequate.
- They are rarely highly motivated to heighten their self-awareness, which is the goal of many forms of psychotherapy.
- Even when they are somewhat motivated, they may be unable or unwilling to delay gratification and thus are impatient with the slow process of growth usually required in psychotherapeutic work.

For these reasons, traditional psychotherapy is not the most useful intervention. Approaches that enhance medical and surgical intervention and allow the client's primary bond to remain with nonpsychiatric health care providers are more successful. Programs geared toward stress management (such as those discussed in Chapter 33 ∞) are very useful because they present stress as part of the human condition and the participants do not feel labeled as having psychiatric problems. Cognitive and behavioral approaches have also gained increasing favor because they alleviate symptoms over a short period of time and thus prove effective in terms of outcome and cost. Cognitive and behavioral approaches are thoroughly discussed in Chapter 30 ∞.

Pearson Nursing Student Resources
Find additional review materials at
nursing.pearsonhighered.com
Prepare for success with NCLEX®-style practice questions, interactive assignments and activities, web links, animations and videos, and more!

REFERENCES

Albuquerque, S. C., Carvalho, E. R., Lapes, R. S., Marques, H. S., Macedo, D. S., Pereira, E. D., ... Carvalho, A. F. (2011). Ego defense mechanisms in COPD: Impact on health-related quality of life and dyspnea severity. *Quality of Life Research*. Advance online publication. doi: 10.1007/s11136-011-9884-9

American Psychiatric Association, (2000). *Diagnostic and statistical manual of mental disorders* (4th ed., Text Revision) (DSM-IV-TR). Washington, DC: Author.

Carek, P. J., Laibstain, S. E., & Carek, S. M. (2011). Exercise for the treatment of depression and anxiety. *International Journal of Psychiatric Medicine, 41*(1), 15–28.

Chan, D., Fan, M. Y., & Unutzer, J. (2011). Long-term effectiveness of collaborative depression care in older primary care patients with and without PTSD symptoms. *International Journal of Geriatric Psychiatry, 26*(7), 758–764.

Chou, K. L., Mackenzie, C. S., Liang, K., & Sareen, J. (2011). Three-year incidence and predictors of first-onset DSM-IV mood, anxiety, and substance use disorders in older adults: Results from wave 2 of the national epidemiologic survey on alcohol and related conditions. *Journal of Clinical Psychiatry, 72*(2), 144–155.

DeBono, A., Shmueli, D., & Mursven, M. (2011). Rude and inappropriate: The role of self-control in following social norms. *Personality and Social Psychology Bulletin, 37*(1), 136–146.

Doering, L. V., & Eastwood, J. A. (2011). A literature review of depression, anxiety, and cardiovascular disease in women. *Journal of Obstetrical, Gynecological, and Neonatal Nursing, 40*(3): 348–361.

Freeman, M., & Sinclair, M. (2009). Mental health nursing students' experience of stress: Burdened by a heavy load. *Journal of Psychiatric and Mental Health Nursing, 16*(4), 335–342.

Fukui, S., Starmino, V. R., & Nelson-Backer, H. B. (2011). Spiritual well-being of people with psychiatric disabilities: The role of religious attendance, social network size and sense of control. *Community Mental Health Journal*. Advance online publication. doi: 10.1007/s10597-011-9375-z

Gallegos, D. (2011). Americans spend more time with computer than spouse. *The Denver Post*. Retrieved from http://www.denverpost.com/search/ci_5075438

Gross, C. R., Kreitzer, M. J., Reilly-Spong, M., Wall, M., Winbush, N. Y., Patterson, R., ... Cramer-Bornemann, M. (2011). Mindfulness-based stress research versus pharmacotherapy for chronic primary insomnia: A randomized control clinical trial. *Explore, 7*(2), 76–87.

Haukkala, A., Kontinnen, H., Laatikainen, T., Kawachi, I., & Uutela, A. (2010). Hostility, anger control, and anger expression as predictors of cardiovascular disease. *Psychosomatic Medicine, 72*(6), 556–562.

Hertzer, M., Denson, L. A., Baldassano, R. N., & Hommel, K. A. (2011). Patient and parent psychosocial factors associated with health-related quality of life in pediatric inflammatory bowel disease. *Journal of Pediatric Gastroenterology and Nutrition, 52*(3), 95–99.

Holmes, T. H., & Rahe, R. H. (1967). The social readjustment rating scale. *Journal of Psychosomatic Research, 11*, 213–218.

Kobasa, S. C. (1979). Stressful life events, personality, and health: An inquiry into hardiness. *Journal of Personality and Social Psychology, 37*, 1–11.

Lazarus, R. S., & Folkman, S. (1984). *Stress, appraisal, and coping*. New York, NY: Springer.

Lindgren, L., Rundgren, S., Winso, O., Lehtipalo, S., Wiklund, U., Kerbeson, M., ... Brulin, C. (2010). Physiological responses to touch massage in healthy volunteers. *Autonomic Neuroscience, 158*(1–2), 105–110.

Manolache, L., Petrriescu-Seceleanu, D., & Bevea, V. (2010). Life events involvement in psoriasis onset/recurrence. *International Journal of Dermatology, 49*(6), 636–641.

Miller, M., & Rahe, R. H. (1997). Life changes scaling for the 1990s. *Journal of Psychosomatic Research, 43*(3), 279–292.

Monat, A., & Lazarus, R. S. (1991). *Stress and coping* (3rd ed.). New York, NY: Columbia University Press.

Ngai, F. W., & Chan, S. W. (2010). Psychosocial factors and maternal well-being: An exploratory path analysis. *International Journal of Nursing Studies, 48*(6), 725–731.

Picardi, A., Porcelli, P., Pasquini, P., Fassone, G., Mazzatti, E., Lega, I., ... Fava, G. A. (2006). Integration of multiple criteria for psychosomatic assessment of dermatological patients. *Psychosomatics, 47*(2), 122–128.

Pilkington, F. B. (2007). Envisioning nursing in 2050 through the eyes of nurse theorists: Leininger and Watson. *Nursing Science Quarterly, 20*(1), 8.

Pruessner, M., Iver, S. N., Faridi, K., & Malla, A. K., (2011). Stress and protective factors in individuals at high risk for psychosis, first episode psychosis and healthy controls. *Schizophrenia Research, 129*(1), 29–35.

Scholes, B., & Martin, C. R. (2010). Could repressive coping be a mediating factor in the symptom profile of individuals diagnosed with schizophrenia? *Journal of Psychiatric and Mental Health Nursing, 17*(5), 403–410.

Seligman, M. E. (2011). Building resilience. *Harvard Business Review, 89*(4), 100–106, 138.

Selye, H. (1956). *The stress of life*. New York, NY: McGraw-Hill.

Sephton, S. E., Salmon, P., Weissbecker, I., Ulmer, C., Floyd, A., Hoover, K., & Studts, J. L. (2007). Mindfulness meditation alleviates depressive symptoms in women with fibromyalgia: Results of a randomized clinical trial. *Arthritis & Rheumatism, 57*(1), 77–85.

Smith, J. C. (1998). *Understanding stress and coping*. Upper Saddle River, NJ: Prentice Hall.

Taché, Y., & Bonaz, B. (2007). Corticotropin-releasing receptors and stress-related alterations of gut motor function. *Journal of Clinical Investigation, 117*(1), 33–40.

Thoits, P.A. (2010). Stress and health: Major findings and policy implications. *Journal of Health and Human Behavior, 51*(Suppl), S41–53.

Wilson, D. W. (2010). Culturally competent psychiatric nursing care. *Journal of Psychosocial and Mental Health Nursing, 17*(8), 715–724.

Wong, Q. J., & Moulds, M. I. (2011). The relationship between maladaptive self-beliefs characteristic of social anxiety and avoidance. *Journal of Behavior Therapy and Experimental Psychiatry, 42*(2), 171–178.

Woods, A. M., Racine, S. E., & Klump, K. L. (2010). Examining the relationship between dietary restraint and binge eating: Differential effects of major and minor stressors. *Eating Behavior, 11*(4), 276–280.

Woods-Giscombe, C. L., & Black, A. R. (2010). Mind-body interventions to reduce risk for health disparities related to stress and strengths among African American women: The potential of mindfulness-based stress reduction, loving kindness and the NTU therapeutic framework. *Complementary Health Practitioner Review, 15*(3), 115–131.

Wright, R. J. (2011). Epidemiology of stress and asthma: From constricting communities and fragile families to epigenetics. *Immunology and Allergy Clinics of North America, 31*(1), 19–39.

9

Cultural Competence

CAROL REN KNEISL

LEARNING OUTCOMES

After completing this chapter, you will be able to:

1. Explain what it means to be a culturally competent nurse.
2. Describe the role of the psychiatric–mental health nurse as culture broker.
3. Incorporate the strategies discussed here in your work with specific cultural groups.
4. Identify the risk factors associated with mental disorders that affect the experience, expression, reporting, and evaluation of mental disorders among culturally diverse groups.
5. Apply personal strategies for developing knowledge, motivation, and skills that can improve your intercultural competence.

CRITICAL THINKING CHALLENGE

Janiece is a nurse in a psychiatric outpatient clinic in a downtown medical center of a large city near the Gulf of Mexico. Her clients come from a variety of backgrounds. Some are local people who have lived and farmed in the surrounding towns or work in the tourist industry. Others are retirees who have moved from the North. Many are Central American immigrants who originally came to help out in reconstruction after a hurricane but now live and work there. There is also a large Czech community. Janiece meets with clients in one-to-one counseling or with clients and families in therapeutic or psychoeducation groups. Clients may or may not have a cultural background similar to hers. Even more complex relationships exist when groups of clients or family members from varied cultural backgrounds meet together with her in a psychoeducation group.

1. How might the clients' cultural beliefs, values, practices, and healing traditions influence the goals Janiece has set for their treatment in one-to-one counseling?
2. How might the clients' and families' cultural beliefs, values, practices, and healing traditions influence the goals Janiece has set for their treatment in therapeutic or psychoeducation groups?
3. How can you apply principles of cultural competence to your psychiatric–mental health nursing experiences with culturally diverse groups as well as individual clients?

To meet global needs and opportunities in the 21st century, nursing is addressing cultural diversity in a health care system in which multicultural individuals are both recipients of care and care providers. America is continuing to undergo demographic shifts that include increasing numbers of diverse cultural groups. Fifty-year projections (2000 to 2050) from the U.S. Bureau of the Census highlight increases in each of the major cultural groups (African-American, Native American, Eskimo and Aleut, Asian and Pacific Islander, and those with Hispanic origins) other than Caucasian. It is estimated that these diverse cultural groups will comprise almost half (47%) of the population by 2050. Population trends reveal that Hispanics will comprise 25% of the population by 2050. Census information can be found on the Census Bureau website (http://www.census.gov) and accessed through the Online Student Resources for this book.

Culture shapes human behavior and assigns unique meanings to the world around us. Be aware that cultural forces are powerful determinants of health-related behaviors in any population. Thus, culture can influence the experience, expression, reporting, and evaluation of mental disorders. Symptoms related to major depression, such as those discussed in Developing Cultural Competence, illustrate this point.

You are being called upon to participate in a health care system that includes people from differing national, regional, ethnic, generational, socioeconomic, religious, and health status backgrounds. The range and variety of health care beliefs, rituals, traditions, and healing practices across cultures are staggering (see FIGURE 9-1 ■). It is your professional responsibility to understand, respect, and work with these cultural differences.

To be professionally effective in this multicultural health care environment, you must develop certain skills that are essential to an understanding and integration of cultural phenomena in all aspects of your professional nursing care. Developing cultural competence is an important link to the reduction of mental health disparities. Thus, this chapter will emphasize the knowledge you need in order to develop an understanding of cultural competence, especially in relation to nursing practice.

Specific strategies for cultural competence are also integrated elsewhere throughout this text. For example, Chapter 3 ∞ discusses the nurse's own sociocultural background and its influence on nursing practice. The chapters in Unit 4 discuss sociocultural theories that expand our understanding of specific mental disorders. Chapters 7 and 31 ∞ discuss psychotropic medications and how ethnicity or cultural background affect how specific medications work. Chapter 33 ∞ discusses a variety of complementary and alternative treatments that stem from non-Western traditions. Several special features in this chapter and throughout the text such as Developing Cultural Competence, What Every Nurse Should Know, Your Self-Awareness, Your Assessment Approach, Your Intervention Strategies, Rx Communication, and Partnering With Clients and Families also provide specific strategies for cultural competence.

DEVELOPING CULTURAL COMPETENCE

Symptoms of Depression in Various Cultures

Depression may be experienced in somatic terms, rather than with sadness or guilt, in some cultures. People of Latino and Mediterranean cultures may tell you about having headaches and "nerves." People of Chinese and Asian cultures may emphasize weakness and tiredness. Middle Easterners may refer to problems of the "heart." The Hopi may express the depressive experience by being "heartbroken." Cultures may differ regarding the seriousness placed on symptoms and share distinctive culture-specific experiences (such as the feeling of being hexed). It is essential to identify those cultural factors that may facilitate, or deter, desired health-related behaviors.

CRITICAL THINKING QUESTIONS

1. How might your own knowledge about physical illnesses as well as your perceptions and stereotypes interfere with understanding the emphasis on somatic symptoms in some depressed persons from other cultures?
2. What are some essential elements to incorporate in a psychoeducation program on depression for Asian clients being treated for depression in a community setting?
3. If someone believes that her depression is the result of a hex, what adaptations might be necessary in a plan for care for the client?

FIGURE 9-1 ■ This young American girl and her mother are dressed in traditional costumes at a Cambodian New Year celebration in Long Beach, California. The mother is helping her daughter to understand and appreciate the customs and traditions associated with her heritage.
Photo courtesy © Kayte Deioma/PhotoEdit.

DEVELOPING AN UNDERSTANDING OF CULTURAL COMPETENCE

In the Western biomedical model, illness is often reduced to a particular disease, there is an emphasis on pathophysiology, and the focus is most often on the client's body rather than on the whole individual. To understand the client's experience of illness, you must attempt to enter the client's world, understand the client's beliefs about what is wrong, what happened, and what should be done to achieve well-being. Thus, the client's perceptions, understandings, and approaches to health and disease are an integral part of any nursing care plan activities.

Cultural Competence

Cultural competence refers to the capacity of nurses or health service delivery systems to effectively understand and plan for the needs of a culturally diverse client or group. Spector (2009) views cultural competence as a complex combination of knowledge, attitudes, and skills used by the health care provider to deliver services that attend to the total context of the client's situation across cultural boundaries. With cultural competence, you are able to move beyond a superficial analysis of cultural differences, having the capacity to understand and work with cultural nuances.

The concept of cultural competence may be applied to health service delivery systems as well. It embraces the notion that health care systems should be able to understand and plan for the health needs of a specific cultural group. Thus, agencies that acknowledge, accept, and work with cultural differences may be viewed as "culturally competent," whereas those agencies that ignore culture when delivering services are viewed as "culturally blind." Developing a culturally competent organization depends upon input from people at all levels in every department (Purnell et al., 2011).

The National Center for Cultural Competence assists health care and mental health organizations in promoting culturally competent values, policy, structures, and practices. The center's mission is to design, implement, and evaluate culturally and linguistically competent service delivery systems. Its website (http://www11.georgetown.edu/research/gucchd/nccc) can be accessed through the Online Student Resources for this book.

Worldview

Simply put, cultural competence incorporates the client's worldview. A *worldview* is the way a group of people (culture or subculture) see their social world, symbolic system, and physical environment and their own place in each. Worldview is revealed in people's religion, art, language, values, and health care beliefs and practices. A people's worldview provides a sense of identity as a Native American, a Puerto Rican, or a Masai tribesman. It promotes a group's survival and gives members a generally useful picture of the universe.

Ethnicity and Ethnocentrism

Ethnicity refers to one's sense of identity, providing social belonging and loyalty to a particular reference group within society. This sense of identity may be based on common

ancestry and religious, national, language, tribal, or cultural origins. In contrast, **ethnocentrism** is the belief that one's own cultural values and behaviors are superior and preferable to those of any other cultural group. The nurse may be unaware of personal ethnocentric behavior that can undermine establishment of a balanced and respectful partnership with a multicultural client or group.

The terms *culturally diverse, multicultural,* and *ethnic* are used throughout this chapter. Likewise, the terms *cross-cultural* and *transcultural* are used interchangeably.

Cultural Sensitivity

Related to cultural competence is the concept of **cultural sensitivity,** the process of increasing professional effectiveness through understanding, respecting, and appreciating the importance of cultural factors in the delivery of health services. These cultural factors may include health beliefs, values, practices, and healing traditions of a client or group from another culture. Refer to What Every Nurse Should Know to expand your knowledge as you develop cultural sensitivity.

It is also important to appreciate the subculture, or culture within a culture. Researchers have referred to the "culture" of the hospital, the operating room, or the nursing school and the "subculture" of the mentally ill, the physically handicapped, or the elderly. Anthropologists point out that simply sharing some common characteristics does not make people members of a culture or subculture. There must be considerably more homogeneity in the group for it to be considered a culture or a subculture. For example, the Choctaw Indians living on a reservation in Philadelphia, Mississippi, are a subculture because they share a language, values and beliefs, and behavioral

WHAT EVERY NURSE SHOULD KNOW

The "Hot and Cold" Healing Practice

Many cultures believe that health is the result of equilibrium between the vital elements of hot and cold—an imbalance between hot and cold causes illness. To cure the illness, the opposite element is given to restore balance in the body. For example, among Afghans and Afghan-Americans, a "hot" illness (such as a fever or infection) may be treated with a diet emphasizing cold foods and medicines. In contrast, a "cold illness" (such as arthritis) may be treated with hot foods and herbs.

Cultures, in addition to Afghan, that tend to embrace this hot and cold healing practice include Puerto Rican, Mexican, Chinese, Filipino, Korean, and Vietnamese. Illnesses and treatments (foods, medications, and/or herbs) are all classified according to their hot or cold properties and vary from culture to culture. Chinese, Vietnamese, and Korean people may connect a person's internal balance to harmony with nature. Note that Koreans may believe that certain mental states are related to excessive cold (depressive and hypoactive) or excessive hot (hyperactive and irritable) imbalances.

patterns. They are part of the larger Native American culture. In contrast, the physically handicapped are not a subculture because they have various disabilities, come from different socioeconomic levels, and may only rarely come into contact with other physically handicapped people.

A case can be made for viewing a hospital or part of it as a culture or subculture. The transient inhabitants of the hospital share a language, standards of acceptable behavior, and a similar worldview. This can be seen even more clearly in specialty units, such as intensive care or psychiatric units. People can be viewed as working within a hospital culture while living within the American culture. Applying the term *culture* or *subculture* to these environments may help us understand a hospital, an emergency room, a school, or a church. Some nurse anthropologists view nursing as a subculture (the health care provider subculture) and document its definite set of beliefs, practices, habits, rituals, and values, often stemming from dominant American cultural values.

Cultural Values

Be aware that perceptions of health, disease, prevention, and treatment may differ among multicultural groups and that many interpretations of reality exist in the world. Acknowledging divergent values can be a significant first step toward improving one's cultural competence and sensitivity to differences, especially when the nurse is from the dominant culture (i.e., of white Anglo-American origin). Table 9-1 highlights

TABLE 9-1 ■ Common Values That may Differ Between Dominant and Nondominant Cultural Groups

Anglo-American (Dominant)	Other Cultural Groups (Nondominant)
Competition	Cooperation
Control over environment	Fate
Directness/honesty	Indirectness/"saving face"
Doing	Being
Efficiency	Idealism
Future orientation	Past or present orientation
Human equality	Hierarchy/ranking
Individualism	Group welfare
Informality	Formality
Mastery over nature	Harmony with nature
Materialism	Spiritualism
Self-help	Birthright inheritance
Time dominates	Personal interaction dominates
Youth	Elders

Sources: Ember, C. R., & Ember, M. R. (2010). *Cultural anthropology* (13th ed.). Upper Saddle River, NJ: Prentice Hall; Ferraro, G., & Andreatta, S. (2011). *Cultural anthropology: An applied perspective* (9th ed.). Albany, NY: Cengage Learning; Gezon, L., & Kottak, C. (2011). *Culture.* New York, NY: McGraw-Hill; Miller, B. (2010). *Cultural anthropology* (6th ed.). Upper Saddle River, NJ: Prentice Hall.

common values that may differ between dominant Anglo-American and nondominant cultural groups.

Cross-Cultural Communication

Consider the challenge of learning to communicate across cultures. The need to increase awareness of your own communication style is important in becoming competent and sensitive to cultural differences. For example, you may carefully choose a rate of speaking that promotes understanding and respect of the client. Other helpful techniques may be to speak in simple sentences and avoid use of slang, jargon, or technical words. Practical suggestions to improve cross-cultural communication skills may include the following:

- Attending multicultural events
- Reading about different cultural groups
- Talking to members of the cultural group
- Spending time in a particular ethnic community
- Learning another language

In everyday practice, you may find yourself working with a client from a cultural background that is unfamiliar to you. Mirroring the client's communication style is one technique for effective cross-cultural communication. Mirroring is more fully discussed in Chapter 10 ∞.

Language and Dialect

You may need to determine the client's level of fluency in English and assess the degree to which another language is used as the primary language. Such language use may vary by generational level as well as by age and gender. In a given setting, language differences represent a serious barrier to all aspects of health care delivery. When you are unfamiliar with the client's language, you must take great care to pay attention to nonverbal communication. The linguistically isolated client may look to your nonverbal behavior in an attempt to understand what is expected in an unfamiliar situation. The nuances of nonverbal communication are discussed in Chapter 10 ∞.

The use of a well-trained, effective interpreter is essential if the client does not speak the language or dialect of the dominant culture. An interpreter can also help you to determine whether the words you hear are actually the language of another culture or an example of *neologistic behavior* (private meanings such as those discussed in Chapter 10 ∞).

Clinical Example

The staff of an inpatient unit enlisted the help of an interpreter from the anthropology department of a local university. Nikolai, a recently admitted client, was an immigrant from Russia and spoke a language that sounded Russian or Eastern European to their ears, and none of the staff were able to understand him. However, the interpreter discovered that not only was Nikolai not speaking Russian, but that he was not speaking any recognizable language at all. The staff was then able to move further in the direction of confirming a diagnosis of schizophrenia and determined that Nikolai was speaking in neologisms.

Examples of people who may assist you in the delivery of linguistically appropriate services may include other health care workers familiar with the culture, a professional interpreter, a cultural consultant, multicultural community resources, or an anthropologist. Family members may be helpful if their presence would not violate the client's confidentiality. In these instances, allow extra time for careful translation and back-translation.

Working With an Interpreter

When you must give a client information through an interpreter, avoid using medical euphemisms and Anglocentric health concepts. Be clear and descriptive. When giving feedback, regardless of the cultural orientation, it is best to focus your input on the client's behavior and not on who the client is personally or spiritually. Information about behavior can cut across cultural differences and be useful input. Even when language is not an issue and interpreters are not involved, it has been argued that it is difficult to incorporate non-Western sensibilities into our present psychiatric classification system which is described for you in Chapter 11 ∞. Your recognition of the validity of cultural backgrounds other than Western will promote client rights and afford clients legitimate entry into health care delivery systems. Remember that the information you share will be shaped by your own culture and beliefs.

Degree of Literacy

Determine the client's reading ability in English or other languages before using written materials related to health care. If the client cannot read English, then determine how best to provide appropriate translated materials that are culturally relevant in the particular setting.

Other Cultural Phenomena Affecting Health and Health Care

In addition to cross-cultural communication, pay attention to the following five cultural phenomena that also affect health and health care among diverse cultural groups: environmental control, biologic variations, social organization, space, and time orientation (Giger & Davidhizar, 2008). Attend to these factors during any cultural assessment, because each may influence health perceptions, beliefs, practices, and healing traditions.

Control Over One's Environment

Environmental control refers to the ability to organize activities that attempt to control nature or environmental factors. Thus, a multicultural group may embrace specific health and illness beliefs, practices, use of folk healers, and healing traditions in attempts to intervene with the complex environment.

Biologic Variations

There may be distinct genetic and physical differences from one multicultural group to another. Examples of such differences include: nutritional habits and preferences, skin color, body build and structure, selective susceptibility to certain diseases, and variation in the metabolism of psychoactive medications (discussed in Chapter 7 ∞).

Social Organization

Social organization describes the type of family unit (e.g., extended, nuclear, or single-parent family) and type of social organizations (e.g., religious or multicultural) that shape the identity of a culturally diverse client or group. Socialization from one's early family life strongly contributes to cultural identification and development.

Space

How a person uses space may be defined and have different meanings based on one's particular culture. There may be different norms for intimacy as well as personal, social, and public distances among various cultural groups (refer to the discussion of space on page 188 and Figure 10-3 in Chapter 10 ∞).

Time Orientation

Emphasis on the past, present, or future varies among culturally diverse groups. Nondominant cultural groups may value the past and present, whereas the dominant Anglo-American culture may emphasize the future.

Cultural Assessment

An appropriate cultural assessment is essential to culturally competent nursing care. You may incorporate cultural assessment into routine assessment procedures as the first step of the nursing process when working with any client or group.

Degree of Acculturation

Assess the degree of acculturation for any client or group in a multicultural setting. **Acculturation** may be defined as the degree to which a particular client or group from another culture has adopted the values, attitudes, and behaviors of mainstream U.S. culture. Acculturation may be one of the most important factors that explain health status and risk behaviors.

One cannot assume that there is acculturation into the mainstream culture because a client or group from another culture is in the United States. There is likely to be a range of acculturation levels from the very traditional to the very acculturated. You will probably find that the more traditional the client or group, the less likely it is for the client or group to be familiar with, understand, or practice Western approaches. It is important to assess the degree of acculturation in a multicultural setting because there may be a natural tendency on the part of many culturally diverse clients to resist acculturation. The measurement of acculturation is an important assessment activity.

Heritage Assessment

The Heritage Assessment Tool for the multicultural client in Your Assessment Approach represents a practical, useful way for you to investigate a client's (or your own) ethnic, cultural, and religious heritage as well as the client's acculturation

YOUR ASSESSMENT APPROACH   Heritage Assessment Tool

An assessment tool like the one that follows will help you structure your assessment to include the salient points that are important to cover. *Note:* The greater the number of positive responses, the greater the degree to which the person may identify with his or her traditional culture. The one exception to positive answers is the question about whether a person's name was changed.

1. Where was your mother born? _____
2. Where was your father born? _____
3. Where were your grandparents born?
   a. Your mother's mother? _____
   b. Your mother's father? _____
   c. Your father's mother? _____
   d. Your father's father? _____
4. How many brothers _____ and sisters _____ do you have?
5. What setting did you grow up in? Urban _____ Rural _____
6. What country did your parents grow up in?
   Father _____
   Mother _____
7. How old were you when you came to the United States? _____
8. How old were your parents when they came to the United States?
   Mother _____
   Father _____
9. When you were growing up, who lived with you? _____
10. Have you maintained contact with the following people?
    a. Aunts, uncles, cousins? (1) Yes _____ (2) No _____
    b. Brothers and sisters? (1) Yes _____ (2) No _____
    c. Parents? (1) Yes _____ (2) No _____
    d. Your own children? (1) Yes _____ (2) No _____
11. Did most of your aunts, uncles, cousins live near your home?
    (1) Yes _____ (2) No _____
12. Approximately how often did you visit your family members who lived outside your home?
    (1) Daily _____ (2) Weekly _____
    (3) Monthly _____ (4) Once a year or less _____
    (5) Never _____
13. Was your original family name changed?
    (1) Yes _____ (2) No _____
14. What is your religious preference?
    (1) Catholic _____ (2) Jewish _____ (3) Protestant _____
    (4) Denomination _____ (5) Other _____ (6) None _____

15. Is your spouse the same religion as you?
    (1) Yes _____ (2) No _____
16. Is your spouse the same ethnic background as you?
    (1) Yes _____ (2) No _____
17. What kind of school did you go to?
    (1) Public _____ (2) Private _____ (3) Parochial _____
18. As an adult, do you live in a neighborhood where the neighbors are the same religion and ethnic background as yourself?
    (1) Yes _____ (2) No _____
19. Do you belong to a religious institution?
    (1) Yes _____ (2) No _____
20. Would you describe yourself as an active member?
    (1) Yes _____ (2) No _____
21. How often do you attend your religious institution?
    (1) More than once a week _____ (2) Weekly _____
    (3) Monthly _____ (4) Special holidays only _____
    (5) Never _____
22. Do you practice your religion at home?
    (1) Yes _____ (If yes, please specify) (2) No _____
    (3) Praying _____ (4) Bible reading _____ (5) Diet _____
    (6) Celebrating religious holidays _____
23. Do you prepare foods of your ethnic background?
    (1) Yes (2) No
24. Do you participate in ethnic activities?
    (1) Yes _____ (If yes, please specify) (2) No _____
    (3) Singing _____ (4) Holiday celebrations _____
    (5) Dancing _____ (6) Festivals _____
    (7) Costumes _____ (8) Other _____
25. Are your friends from the same religious background as you?
    (1) Yes _____ (2) No _____
26. Are your friends from the same ethnic background as you?
    (1) Yes _____ (2) No _____
27. What is your native language other than English? _____
28. Do you speak this language?
    (1) Prefer _____ (2) Occasionally _____ (3) Rarely _____
29. Do you read your native language?
    (1) Yes _____ (2) No _____

Source: Spector, R. E. (2009). *Cultural diversity in health & illness* (7th ed.). Upper Saddle River, NJ: Prentice Hall, pp. 365–367.

level. You may use such assessment to understand a client's health traditions and reveal how deeply a client may identify with any particular tradition. It is important to emphasize that multicultural clients may embrace health beliefs and traditions from more than one culture, based on their unique heritage (Spector, 2009). A heritage assessment will help you to identify positive elements that can be reinforced to facilitate health promotion and disease prevention and anticipate rigid adherence to health beliefs and traditions that may conflict with effective Western practices.

Cultural assessment applies to agencies and health service delivery systems as well as to individuals or groups. Thus, you may have an opportunity to assess where a particular agency stands in terms of cultural competency and sensitivity.

Transcultural Care Planning

Evaluate the information that you have obtained thus far through cultural assessment and think about what additional information (such as in Partnering With Clients and Families on pages 172–173) may be helpful as you prepare or revise the nursing care plan. Include the client's cultural preferences in your

PARTNERING WITH CLIENTS AND FAMILIES

Developing Cultural Competence With Specific Cultural Groups/Nations of Origin

Use the information below to help yourself understand the health beliefs and practices of clients and families from cultural backgrounds that differ from yours. Think about incorporating the suggestions in your plan of care.

Cultural Groups/Nations of Origin	Health Beliefs and Practices	Suggestions to Consider
Hispanic (including Spain, Cuba, Puerto Rico, Mexico, Central and South America)	Belief in folk illnesses may characterize many traditional Hispanic groups. *Curanderismo* is the traditional health care system that may be used first, but not discussed, with a Western health care provider. Traditional folk healers may be the first health practitioners consulted. They are culturally acceptable, much less expensive than Western health care, and are willing to make house calls. *Fatalism* (i.e., the belief that an individual cannot control one's health) may be a common attitude among traditional groups. Health care decisions may involve the head of the household who decides what is best for the family.	Be aware that family and family support are very important core values. Respect is an extremely important factor in all relationships. Avoiding conflict and achieving harmony are strong cultural values.
African-American (including West Indian Islands, Haiti, Dominican Republic, Brazil, England, many West African countries)	Traditional explanations for disease and illness may involve natural causes (e.g., stress, poor eating habits) and unnatural causes from witchcraft practices (e.g., voodoo, bad spirits, other works of the devil). The Western health care system is generally well respected and used for serious illness, although folk healing traditions may also be utilized. Traditional folk healers may be the only health practitioners used by African-Americans of low income.	Be aware that there may be caution about using programs from inside and outside some black communities. Prior programs and services may have lost funding and personnel. African-Americans who have been trained "outside" the community may need to earn trust by demonstrating sincere interest in the community's particular needs and concerns. Churches often have been used as sites for health education and intervention.
Native American and Alaskan Native (including First Nation and indigenous American Indian Nations, Alaskan Aleuts and Eskimos)	Traditional ceremonies may be practiced among tribal groups to promote well-being and balance. Many tribal groups feel distrustful and exploited by Westerners. Medicine men, traditional healers, and herbal treatments are very important to some groups. Taboos and modesty are important in tribal life.	Be aware that every tribal group has its own unique history, traditions, and values. Become familiar with acceptable verbal and nonverbal communications of the group. Respect tribal sovereignty and work within the tribal group. Be aware that "talking circles" together with tribal stories have been useful for culturally appropriate educational interventions.

(Continued)

care plan where possible. Some specific and practical techniques to consider in transcultural care planning are as follows:

- Describe any language barriers. Note what strengths or resources the client might have available to reduce any language barrier.
- When assessing religious beliefs, note any specific religious rituals or religious dietary requirements that the client observes.

- Note any lack of financial resources, including the ability to purchase prescription medicines or food for specific diets. Note whether any local agencies provide financial assistance to the client.
- Identify other barriers to care such as lack of transportation or lack of child care.
- Once barriers are identified, explore alternative resources available to the client's family and community.

PARTNERING WITH CLIENTS AND FAMILIES *(Continued)*

Cultural Groups/Nations of Origin	Health Beliefs and Practices	Suggestions to Consider
Asian-American (including Asian Indians, Chinese, Cambodians, Thais, Vietnamese, Laotians, Filipinos, Hmong, Koreans, Japanese)	A central concept of the traditional health care system is the need to attain a harmonious relationship with nature. This traditional health care system may be the first one used for any illness. There may be a tendency not to discuss this with a Western health care practitioner. Teachings of Buddhism, Confusianism, and Taoism may emphasize upholding a public presentation that avoids admission of physical or mental illness. Many Asians may prefer traditional forms of native medicine, seeking help from Chinatown "masters" who treat with traditional herbs and other methods. Asians may not use the Western health care system because of painful diagnostic tests and lack of information.	Be aware that balance or equilibrium and kinship solidarity are two beliefs that may be prominent among Asians. Kinship solidarity refers to the belief that an individual is subservient to the family or kinship-based group. Thus, separation from family members may be stressful. Respect for elders and male authority may determine decision-making practices regarding health care for recent immigrants. Use "active listening" and watch for nonverbal cues because some Asian groups may not disagree openly with health care providers. Likewise, conflicts are generally handled within the family and may not be shared with a health care provider unless trust is established. It is helpful if outreach workers are perceived as nonthreatening and nonintrusive.
Pacific Islander (including Guamanian, Samoan, Hawaiian, Pacific Islander–American)	Health beliefs and practices among these cultural groups may vary greatly. Thus, knowledge of the geographic location and particular ethnic group is essential. In general, indigenous illnesses may be treated with traditional healing practices, whereas Western illnesses may be treated with Western medical approaches. Taboos, modesty, and traditional healing practices are very important to these cultural groups.	Be aware that health data may not be available for the particular Pacific Islander group of interest. It may be helpful to involve women in all aspects of health care because many island cultures are matriarchal. Emphasize concepts of wholeness and interconnectedness, which are central features of several Pacific Islander groups. Culturally acceptable and appropriate strategies for health promotion may include use of "talk stories," role playing, pictures, and folk media (e.g., song, dance, music).
Anglo-American/European-American (including Germany, Ireland, England, Italy, the former Soviet Union, and all other European countries)	Often the dominant cultural group that influences the determination of health care needs, beliefs, practices, and programs in communities. Primary reliance on a "modern" or "Western" health care system, emphasizing use of technology and diagnostic tests. There may be reliance on traditional health beliefs and practices that may vary greatly, depending on the country of ancestry. There is a recent increased interest in complementary and alternative (CAM) practices, which emphasize holistic, naturalistic healing. Judeo-Christian beliefs may influence health practices.	Individualism, materialism, and emphases on time and youth may be strong cultural values. Directness and efficiency may be factors in relationships with health care providers. Assess the utility of self-help literature and groups when planning health care interventions.

Sources: Huff, R. M., & Kline, M. V. (Eds.). (2008). *Promoting health in multicultural populations: A handbook for practitioners.* Thousand Oaks, CA: Sage Publications; and Spector, R. E. (2009). *Cultural diversity in health & illness* (7th ed.). Upper Saddle River, NJ: Prentice Hall.

- Assess any cultural demands that the client may face at home that may conflict with important health care needs.
- Describe any culturally generated feelings such as shame that may interfere with the client's willingness to embrace a health care plan.
- Note the multicultural client's concerns and address them in the care plan where possible.

Culture Brokering

You are challenged to develop critical skills on behalf of clients, especially when clients and their families do not understand or accept biomedical interventions or treatments. This process, most useful when working with multicultural clients, is called *culture brokering*. **Culture brokering** is defined as the act of bridging, linking, or mediating between groups of people of different cultural systems to reduce conflict or produce change.

Jezewski (1993, 1995) is credited with the development of a culture brokering model evolved from health-related, anthropologic, and business literature sources. This model of conflict resolution is based on several studies of clients displaying vulnerability from extreme circumstances that hindered their autonomous use of the health care system. Jezewski's studies focused on clients who were politically and economically powerless (migrant farmers and homeless people) as well as critical care and oncology nurses working with clients experiencing life-threatening illness who needed to make informed do-not-resuscitate decisions.

The Nurse-as-Culture-Broker

The term *culture broker* is used in many disciplines—nursing, medical anthropology, psychology, and social work in relation to numerous client populations, such as clients in hospitals and community settings, persons with disabilities, prisoners, and immigrants. Within nursing, the effective use of health care services may be thwarted by cultural, social, economic, political, and institutional constraints. Conflict in interactions in health care settings between the client seeking care and the provider giving care is the most important event that signals the need for culture brokering. A conflict may arise when there are differences in values, beliefs, or behaviors between a client and provider concerning the appropriateness and feasibility of a treatment plan.

The **nurse-as-culture-broker** serves as a bridge between the client and the providers in the health care system by "stepping in," or intervening, to facilitate the acquisition of effective heath care. You may act as a broker of information about regulations that control health benefits or facilitate a multicultural client's entry into various hospital departments. A skilled culture broker may develop and maintain working relationships with multicultural and bilingual professionals, staff, and members of the local community. You may act as a culture broker if conflict occurs in a culturally diverse staff. Finally, you may use culture brokering within your own profession to bridge the gap between disparate areas of nursing.

Conditions That Affect Brokering

Several conditions may either enhance or hinder effective health care. Powerlessness of the client is a primary reason for brokering. For example, a disadvantaged client may be in desperate need of intervention but politically, economically, or personally powerless to access health care. Other conditions may include economics (the ability to pay for services), politics, and stigma associated with mental disorder. Two very important conditions in the culture brokering model are cultural background (including ethnicity) and cultural sensitivity. The nurse-as-culture-broker demonstrates cultural sensitivity by being aware of, and sensitive to, the needs of clients from backgrounds other than your own. Note that there may be an increased risk of breakdown or conflict in health care services when providers lack cultural sensitivity.

Stages of Culture Brokering

The resolution of conflict or breakdown in the health care situation occurs in three stages: perception, intervention, and outcome. These stages briefly describe the process of facilitating care by maintaining a client's connectedness to the health care system. Staying connected is the overall dimension that involves linking the client to the health care system, as well as helping the client remain engaged to that health care system in a manner that meets the client's needs.

Stage 1: Perception (perceiving the need for brokering). Assess the impact of conflict or breakdown in health care interaction. Breakdowns in health care interactions are generally less serious than conflict. Assess the conditions that may enhance or hinder the resolution of conflict. Identify barriers to access and health care utilization.

Stage 2: Intervention (strategies to resolve conflict or breakdown). Establish rapport and trust with clients to foster and maintain connections between those clients and their providers. Facilitate links with personnel within and outside the health care setting, using strategies such as networking, negotiating, advocating, and innovating.

Stage 3: Outcome (evaluating strategies to resolve identified conflict or breakdown). Maintain connectedness across various systems. Evaluate connections between the client and the health care system. Evaluate whether conflicts or breakdowns are resolved. If they are not resolved, return to Stage 1 for further assessment or Stage 2 and try different strategies.

Partnering with Clients and Families provides a specific example of how you could apply the key components of culture brokering activities in a health care setting.

DEVELOPING CULTURAL COMPETENCE IN NURSING PRACTICE

Developing an understanding of cultural competence requires paying attention to considerations of global health, cultural values, cultural phenomena affecting health, and the importance of cultural assessment as part of the nursing process. Cultural competence in nursing practice requires practical strategies (general as well as specific to a particular cultural group), considerations of community-based health care promotion and disease prevention programs, and the need to advocate for cultural diversity in nursing practice, research, and education. At the same time, it is important to be aware that there are varying degrees of acculturation and individual differences—assessment of one Chinese person may be dramatically different than another and from one generation to another. In Why I Became a Psychiatric–Mental Health Nurse on page 176, you will read about one psychiatric–mental health nurse whose career focused on cultural phenomena and global health.

The Transcultural Nursing Society (TCNS) promotes knowledgeable culturally based care. You can obtain information about this organization through its website, which can be

PARTNERING WITH CLIENTS AND FAMILIES

Culture Brokering

Imagine that you are a psychiatric consultation–liaison nurse at a local medical center and are contacted by a busy and frustrated family health nurse unable to communicate with an elderly Asian man. The man apparently arrived at the family-practice clinic alone that morning and did not appear to speak English. He would gently shake his head as if to indicate "yes" to any question, repeat the words "Laos" and "Mr. Phet" (pronounced "pet"), but refuse any attempt at physical examination. Drawing on your past experiences in culture-specific clinical nursing care, you recall several Laotian beliefs, values, practices, and healing traditions of which you are aware. You also recall the intervention strategies used in other, similar situations, because past experiences may provide valuable working knowledge to guide your culture brokering activities in the present context. They are as follows:

Laotian Belief, Value, Practice, or Healing Tradition	General Intervention Strategy
"Saving face," i.e., the Laotian tendency to respond in a manner to please the inquirer. Not knowing an answer may be viewed as extremely embarrassing.	Create an environment in which the client is comfortable describing symptoms as well as answering questions. Find ways to help the client to demonstrate that he or she understands what is happening or what needs to be done.
Incomplete use of prescribed medication or unwillingness to refill a prescription.	Give a clear, simple description of how a particular medication works. Explore, if possible, the client's understanding of the illness and your role as provider in relation to the illness.
Possible misunderstanding about the use of vaccines. For example, a yearly flu vaccine may protect against bird flu.	Give a clear, simple description of how each particular vaccine works. Spell out specifically what a vaccine may or may not prevent.
May relate feeling ill to the temperature inside the body. The need to ingest warm food (soups, hot water, etc.) when ill.	Try to incorporate this healing practice into any nursing care plan whenever possible. (Refer back to What Every Nurse Should Know on page 168.)
Belief that the top of the head is sacred but the feet are vulgar.	During physical examination, always ask permission to touch the client's head. When necessary, touch the head first and feet last during any physical assessment. *Never point your feet at someone.*

As a culture broker, your goals are to facilitate care by linking Mr. Phet to the health care system and by helping him "stay connected" to that system. There is a perceived need for brokering because the system has broken down. You quickly recognize Mr. Phet's position of powerlessness because of the language barrier. Based on your perception of Mr. Phet's powerlessness, you immediately implement several intervention strategies to resolve the breakdown.

- You negotiate with a family health nurse interested in developing cultural competence to participate in transcultural care planning and to volunteer as the designated client care coordinator.
- Because a professional medical interpreter is not available, you call on a bilingual Asian staff member to participate in information gathering for transcultural assessment and care planning.
- You identify as assessment priorities other conditions that may affect culture brokering such as the client's ability to pay and stigma associated with illness.
- You attempt to identify family members and community resources that might serve to alleviate the language barrier where possible.
- You network, if necessary, to locate a Laotian consultant in the community who may help to interpret Laotian cultural beliefs, values, practices, and healing traditions.
- You consider a referral to the local home health service to further assess Mr. Phet's basic needs in his home environment.
- During these initial culture brokering activities, you actively evaluate strategies to resolve the identified breakdown, helping to maintain connections across the various health systems that may work with Mr. Phet.

accessed through http://www.tcns.org. Certification as a transcultural nurse can also be obtained through TCNS.

General Strategies for Developing Cultural Competence

An essential step toward developing cultural competence is to examine your own perceptions, prejudices, and stereotypes. It is helpful to suspend personal judgments in favor of learning more about the culture's history, migration, and immigration patterns. What specific cultural beliefs, values, practices, and healing traditions may relate to particular lifestyle habits (e.g., religion, gender, dietary patterns, use of alcohol and drugs, use of touch, use of time, etc.)? Be careful of your own ethnocentrism because culturally diverse groups may initially view you as foreign and uneducated regarding their proper forms of address, social customs, and appropriate methods for dealing with their concerns and health problems. If possible, attempt to identify issues related to access to health care for

Transcultural Nursing Society

Case Study: Culturally Sensitive Nursing

this cultural group as well. Such issues may include patterns of care, barriers to care (including accessibility, availability, and acceptability), and the use of social assistance services. Your Intervention Strategies outlines several helpful suggestions for working with culturally diverse clients and groups. Such strategies will help you to apply principles of cultural competence and sensitivity.

WHY I BECAME A PSYCHIATRIC— MENTAL HEALTH NURSE

Beth Moscato, RN, PhD

There is nothing more fascinating than human behavior. What people perceive, feel, say, and do never ceases to intrigue me. I am grateful for the unique opportunities I have had in psychiatric nursing in a federal hospital for the treatment of substance abusers, on a locked ward of an inpatient service, as an outpatient therapist in a state psychiatric facility, and as a psychotherapist and consultant in an interdisciplinary private practice group. Most recently, I challenged myself to expand the field of psychiatric epidemiology as a teacher of graduate students and as a researcher in the conduct of several international psychiatric studies. In addition, I am dedicated to volunteer international health projects in developing countries including Ecuador, British Guyana, and Ukraine.

For those of you starting on a path in psychiatric nursing: Respect and reinforce resiliency. Keep your focus on the issues that really matter to you—the issues that you feel passionate about. Develop a global perspective. Realize that resources are not limitless. Look into the eyes of the underserved and reinforce their dignity. Seek mentors who can support and enrich you and your practice. Remember that clients will teach you more about who you are and who you can become. Enjoy the journey. Gandhi said that a majority of one is all that is needed. Be that one.

Developing Cultural Competence With Specific Cultural Groups

Summaries of cultural health beliefs and practices for five major cultural groups (Hispanic, African-American, Native American and Alaska Native, Asian-American, and Pacific Islander populations) are in Partnering With Clients and Families on pages 172–173. Helpful suggestions to consider when working toward cultural competence are provided for each of these groups. It is advantageous to consult with family members, a professional interpreter, a cultural consultant, multicultural community resources, or a nurse anthropologist whenever possible to facilitate your development toward cultural competence with a particular cultural group. You may also wish to consult the bibliography at the end of this chapter for specific applications to clinical care and transcultural assessment and intervention.

Culturally Competent Health Care Promotion and Disease Prevention Programs

Nurses often may be able to plan, implement, and/or evaluate a program designed to meet the complex nursing needs of a specific cultural group. Examples of such community-based programs include the following:

- A community-level anger management program in an urban barrio to reach Mexican-Americans, using the media as part of a mental health campaign
- An HIV sexual-risk-reduction intervention among young African-American adults diagnosed with schizophrenia
- A "talking circle" program with Native Americans to reduce alcohol-related injuries and alcoholism

The first formal step of any program planning process is to involve those individuals affected by the problem. This principle of participation appears to be the most important component of any program development. Collaboration between planner and participants can be achieved only if there is respect for each other's values and for the agenda to be

YOUR INTERVENTION STRATEGIES   Applying Principles of Cultural Competence and Sensitivity

Remember to carry out these suggestions when working with a culturally diverse client or group.

- Learn about the culture of interest by making multiple visits to the community to become familiar with the community's way of life. Activities may include talking to community leaders and residents, eating at local restaurants, visiting cultural sites, and attending local events.
- Learn specifically about the culture's orientation to health, disease, health traditions, and traditional healing practices.
- Identify and learn about the traditional healers within the community. Note the healers' ease of access, medicines used, cultural acceptability, and cost of care.
- Be open and nonjudgmental regarding specific cultural practices that are not part of your cultural heritage.

- Add questions to your assessment tools that reflect these cultural beliefs, values, practices, and healing traditions.
- Practice cross-cultural communication skills.
- Learn how to work with a competent interpreter as necessary.
- Take time to explain Western concepts of health, disease, treatment, and prevention that are relevant and understandable to the culture of interest.
- Use educational materials that are culturally appropriate and relevant to this culture.
- Work with, and learn from, indigenous health care providers when addressing the needs of this culture.
- Learn how to work with peer educators from the community.
- Seek ways to improve access to services for multicultural groups with emphasis on availability, accessibility, and acceptability.

accomplished. As you become involved in any community-based program, remember to utilize the group's cultural uniqueness by incorporating how group members define health problems, identify proposed solutions, and select activities to be emphasized. Group members are invaluable participants in identifying how health-promoting behavioral changes, once achieved, can be sustained in that community.

CULTURAL RISK FACTORS FOR MENTAL DISORDER

A critical issue related to cultural diversity is that important factors reflecting varying cultures need to be assessed in clinical practice and research. Ethnicity, race, dietary patterns, the use of alcohol and drugs, health and healing practices, other lifestyle habits, religious or spiritual beliefs, the use of time, and migration patterns may differentially affect the experience, expression, reporting, and evaluation of mental disorders among culturally diverse groups. Past research has been criticized in retrospect for studying white males and, to a lesser extent, white females, and then generalizing the results to all other groups.

The notion of biopsychosocial risk factors is common in psychiatric literature. A **risk factor** is a factor whose presence is associated with an increased chance or probability of mental disorder. Some risk factors, such as age, cannot be modified. Other risk factors, such as personal lifestyle habits regarding the use of alcohol and tobacco, are susceptible to change. Note that the presence of one particular risk factor does not inevitably lead to the development of a mental disorder. Rather, a number of factors occurring in a defined time period may cause a disorder. *Multifactorial causation* is the term used to describe the requirement that a combination of causes or factors may be needed to produce the disorder.

A limited review of numerous risk factors associated with the occurrence of many psychiatric disorders as outlined by Bromet (2007) and others is given in the following sections.

Gender Differences

Differences in rates between males and females are found for substance abuse, anxiety disorders, and depression. Anxiety and depressive disorders are more commonly experienced by women and substance abuse disorders by men (Fleury, Grenier, Bamvita, Perreault, & Caron, 2011) who are also more likely to use a wider variety of substances (Torcholla, Okoli, Malchy, & Johnson, 2011). In a study investigating the effects of violence on adolescents, girls seemed to be especially vulnerable despite the fact that boys were more frequently exposed to violence (Zona & Milan, 2011). Exposure to violence predicted an increase in all types of symptoms for both genders; however, girls were more likely to experience dissociative symptoms.

Age

Age is associated with the occurrence of mental disorders. Young adults (ages 25–44) have the highest prevalence estimates for most disorders. Alcoholism is known to peak in the early forties. Heavy drinking associated with driving or fighting appears to peak in the early twenties.

Social Class and Poverty

Lower social class status and poverty are associated with increased rates of depression, alcohol and other substance abuse, and antisocial personality disorder. Although risk factors vary among mental disorders, studies indicate that adults in poverty are at higher risk for an episode of at least one mental disorder compared with adults not in poverty.

Ethnicity

Ethnicity appears to be indirectly associated with mental disorders because different ethnic groups share different social and physical environments. For major depression, Caucasian men tend to have higher rates than African-American men, while African-American women tend to have higher prevalence rates than Caucasian women. Caucasians of all ages have higher suicide rates than African-Americans, with Native American youth at increased risk for suicide. Be aware that racial–ethnic disparities do exist in mental health care and that mental health staff may have unconscious racially biased behaviors (Mallinger & Lamberti, 2010).

Marital Status

Marital status, especially being single, may be associated with psychiatric disorders such as schizophrenia. Married women are more depressed than nonmarried women. In contrast, married men are less depressed than unmarried men. The highest rates of depression occur among those recently divorced or separated.

Physical Health Status

The link between physical and mental health is noteworthy. Studies provide evidence that psychiatric clients may have an increased mortality rate. Medically hospitalized clients have increased rates of mental disorder as well. Major depression is associated with many chronic medical conditions and is predictive of shortened life expectancy.

Positive Family History

Depression, schizophrenia, and dementia of the Alzheimer's type (DAT) appear to be related to a history of such disorders in the family. Evidence points to a genetic vulnerability for developing alcoholism. Bipolar disorder and anxiety disorders are being studied extensively with regard to family history. Refer to Chapter 6∞ for recent developments in genetics that may contribute to further understanding of the contribution of family history to the development of mental disorders.

Season of Birth

Studies in some countries, including the United States, reveal that individuals with schizophrenia are more likely to be born during winter or spring. A study of suicide completers in Hungary (Dome, Kapitany, Ignits, & Rihmer, 2010), the country with one of the highest suicide rates in the world over the last century, found that completed suicide is more likely to occur among those born in the spring and summer. The association was highest among males.

Adverse Life Events

Higher levels of stress associated with natural disasters may be associated with increased rates of mental disorder. A study of tsunami-exposed women found increased rates of depression and decreased physical health 3 years after exposure to the natural disaster (Wickrama & Ketring, 2011). Single traumatic events, such as bereavement or unemployment, have been known to produce adverse mental health consequences. The diagnosis of post-traumatic stress disorder (PTSD) represents a response to an unusual, intense stressor. Adverse life events are known to contribute to some forms of depression as well as PTSD. A stressful family environment is an established risk factor for behavioral problems in children. What Every Nurse Should Know highlights some surprising cultural differences regarding the possible causes of mental disorder.

Physical Environment

High-level chemical exposures to mercury, carbon monoxide, carbon disulfide, and lead are related to serious central nervous system disturbances. Environmental exposure to lead is related to deleterious nervous system effects on children. When considering homelessness, rates of mental disorder among homeless adults and children are remarkably high.

Lifestyle Habits

Culturally diverse lifestyle habits—dietary patterns, use of alcohol and drugs, health and healing practices, religious and spiritual beliefs, use of time, and migration patterns—may influence the experience, expression, reporting, and evaluation of mental disorders.

CULTURE AND CULTURE-BOUND SYNDROMES IN THE DSM

Although discussions regarding the *Diagnostic and Statistical Manual of Mental Disorders* (DSM-IV-TR)—the means by which we categorize and classify mental disorders today—are incorporated throughout this textbook, DSM features relating to cultural diversity deserve emphasis in this chapter. A section for each disorder entitled "Specific Culture, Age, and Gender Features" systematically offers guidance concerning variations that may be attributable to one's cultural setting and provides information on prevalence rates related to culture.

Guidelines for a detailed cultural assessment are offered in the DSM to provide a systematic review of the client's cultural and ethnic background and to identify ways in which the cultural context influences care. The DSM's glossary of **culture-bound syndromes** describes locality-specific patterns of experience—localized folk diagnostic categories that explain repetitive and troubling behaviors to specific societies. Descriptions of some of the more common culture-bound syndromes that you may encounter are described in Box 9-1. We encourage you to familiarize yourself with these specific culture-bound syndromes as you strive for cultural competence in your clinical work.

WHAT EVERY NURSE SHOULD KNOW

Cross-Cultural Attitudes Toward Mental Disorder

Clients and their families from certain cultures may seek medical or psychiatric care only as a last resort and when absolutely necessary after other cultural treatments have been tried. Various cultures have very divergent views of the causes of mental disorder that may be surprisingly different from the biopsychosocial framework of this textbook. Becoming familiar with the common beliefs of a culture contributes to your cultural competence in everyday practice.

Many cultures often attribute mental disorder to spiritual or supernatural origins. Examples include: disruption in the spiritual world (Filipinos, Koreans), supernatural influences (Central Americans), a curse or spell (Dominicans), or evil spirits (Ethiopians, Samoans). Haitians often believe in supernatural causes (e.g., a hex or retaliation for not honoring protective spirits). Mexicans and Dominicans may view a mental disorder as a punishment for past misdeeds. Many East Indians and Pakistanis believe that psychosis may originate from an evil spirit or because of an enemy casting a spell. Perceived causes by Arabs may include sudden fearfulness, the devil's curse, God's wrath, or loss of country and family. It is common for Vietnamese to believe in possession by evil spirits, but bad karma from past mistakes (for Buddhists) and bad luck in family inheritance may also contribute to mental disorder. Causes of mental disorder among Native American groups may include loss of harmony with the environment, violation of taboos, and ghosts. It is important to assess both the client's and the particular tribe's degree of acculturation to determine how mental disorder is perceived. Families may seek spiritual advice first when the cause of disorder is perceived to be spiritual or supernatural in origin.

Family stigma and shame may accompany mental disorder. The client's family may fear stigmatization or actually be highly stigmatized when mental disorder is evident in a family member (Cubans, Puerto Ricans, West Indian/Caribbean islanders, Central Americans, Haitians, East Indians, Irish, Nigerians). Mental disorder in a family may be viewed as shameful (Greeks). In addition, seeking treatment may be perceived as bringing shame to the family (Arabs). In many cultures, the family may be concerned about the negative effect that mental disorder may have on matrimonial prospects. Some Colombians maintain that emotional problems in women result from love deceptions.

Several cultures associate the effects of war with the origins of mental disorder. Bosnians and Serbs seem familiar with PTSD as a result of the devastating impact of events related to war in their country. Cambodians believe that emotional problems resulted from the Khmer Rouge brutalities, and that evil spirits or ancestors may cause mental disorder. Jewish Holocaust survivors may have experienced psychiatric effects because of war atrocities. The Hmong appear to accept those who have depression and PTSD because these conditions are common among those who experienced war.

Be aware that these insights are generalities and may not necessarily reflect the uniqueness of people within their own countries.

Box 9-1   Culture-Bound Syndromes

- **Ghost sickness:** Various symptoms such as nightmares, weakness, feelings of impending doom, fainting, hallucinations, loss of consciousness, and a sense of suffocation, among others, along with a preoccupation with death are associated with the deceased and sometimes with witchcraft.
- **Mal de ojo:** This Spanish phrase means "evil eye." Common in other Mediterranean cultures, the evil eye can be a curse instituted by an enemy. Children are especially at risk; their symptoms include fitful sleep, crying without apparent cause, diarrhea, vomiting, and fever.
- **Nervios:** A term that means a distress of the nerves, common among Latinos in North America and Latin America. It includes a wide range of symptoms of emotional and somatic disturbance and refers to a general state of vulnerability to stressful life experiences. Other ethnic groups (such as *nevra* among the Greeks) have similar ideas about "nerves."
- **Shenkui:** In China and Taiwan, this folk label describes marked anxiety or panic symptoms accompanied by somatic complaints, frequent dreams, and sexual dysfunction (such as erectile dysfunction and premature ejaculation). It is attributed to excess semen loss through frequent intercourse, masturbation, and nocturnal emission. Excessive semen loss is feared because it represents the loss of vital essence and can be seen as life threatening.
- **Susto:** This folk illness is prevalent among some Latinos in the United States and among people in Mexico and Central and South America. Also known as "soul loss," it is thought to be caused by a frightening event that causes the soul to leave the body, resulting in unhappiness and sickness including appetite disturbances, feelings of sadness, lack of motivation, troubled sleep, feelings of diminished self-worth, headache, stomachache, and diarrhea.

ADVOCATING ISSUES OF CULTURAL DIVERSITY IN NURSING

Nurses need to make a conscious decision to acknowledge and value the diversity in others. Developing cultural competence and sensitivity needed for comprehensive care is based on new knowledge, personal self-assessment, supervised practice, mentoring experiences, experience in culturally diverse clinical practice settings, participation in discussions, and diversity training.

Nursing Practice

Nursing competencies must include the ability to actively and effectively work with culturally diverse clients. Look for opportunities for meaningful dialogue and relationship building across cultures. You may seek out practicing nurses of a particular cultural background to serve as resource consultants. You may mentor nurse colleagues from other cultures who work in your setting. You may seek information from transcultural health care nurses with experiences in developing countries, such as the nurses who sponsor http://www .culturediversity.org, which can be accessed through the Online Student Resources for this book. You may read transcultural journals (e.g., *Journal of Transcultural Nursing, Journal of Cultural Diversity*, etc.) to familiarize yourself with critical culture-based issues and opportunities. You may become a member of an organization such as TCNS or a certified transcultural nurse.

Make every attempt to openly discuss cultural conflicts in order to actively address suspicions and distortions. Avoiding conflict may result in chronic strained communication, insensitivity, and exclusion that thwart culturally competent care. Recognize the importance of fostering transcultural communication with other health care providers, and take into account the presence of a multicultural workforce.

Because most people with mental disorders never seek professional treatment, there is a need for more outreach to ensure availability, accessibility, reasonable cost, and quality of mental health services for all subgroups of the population. Psychiatric nurses may advocate for more outreach aimed at high-risk groups, such as the impoverished, the homeless, and those with comorbid conditions. We also encourage you to develop and expand your psychiatric–mental health nursing practice by continuing to familiarize yourself with global mental health issues.

Nursing Research

Nurses can use research training and development to seek collaboration, coalition, and compassion across cultures. Nursing research may define what knowledge is meaningful for a particular multicultural group. Through research, nurses can become informed regarding which interventions might be useful in specific community-based programs. Research may contribute to the development of more inclusive theories to account for behaviors observed in multicultural groups. Research may better identify important health-related distinctions among numerous cultural groups that are currently classified into one category (e.g., various values and traditions of specific Native American Indian Nations such as the Cherokee, Navajo, and Sioux).

The results from some epidemiologic studies suggest that the causes and consequences of high comorbidity should be the focus of continued research. More research on potential barriers to professional care seeking is needed, including care-seeking patterns that consider ethnic and cultural differences. There continues to be a lack of systematic, evaluative studies aimed at determining which treatments are most effective for which disorders in which groups at any given time. Research into productivity and efficiency is important: Many clients, especially those with severe or persistent mental disorders, have found a fragmented, underfinanced, uncoordinated, and frequently inaccessible system of care.

Nursing Education

Although the nursing profession remains a field dominated by white females, it is apparent that schools of nursing need to integrate content that emphasizes cultural diversity. Educators need to work within multicultural and multidisciplinary frameworks to tackle issues in the "real world." Yet, recruitment and retention of students from diverse cultures continue

EVIDENCE-BASED PRACTICE

Cultural Diversity in Nursing

Juireith is a 24-year-old African-American female beginning the baccalaureate nursing program at your local university. She was born in Jamaica and then moved to the Bronx, New York, to live with extended family. She now lives alone in your town, determined to earn a university degree in nursing. She sits with the few other African-American nursing students in class. As a student interested in the development of cultural sensitivity in professional nursing education and practice, you understand that racial and ethnic minority students have high attrition rates in nursing school. Loneliness and isolation, peers' lack of understanding of cultural differences, and coping with insensitivity and discrimination are some of the experiences that racial and ethnic minority students may have in nursing school. You practice specific strategies, based on the following research studies, as a way of demonstrating the personal value you place upon diversity. These strategies are as follows:

- Evaluate your assumptions, understand your attitudes, and learn about the differences in others to eliminate stereotyping.
- Listen to the concerns and issues of students from other cultures and become a mentor for them.

- Offer opportunities for participation in scholarly efforts to students from other cultures, thereby encouraging collaboration.
- Confront feelings of racism, because most individuals in mainstream U.S. culture may not be aware of passive racism. Using your culture brokering skills, emphasize that words or actions can be discussed and explained if misinterpreted.
- Acknowledge and appreciate cultural differences. Welcome and value change and a new approach.
- Contribute toward building a student learning environment that accommodates cultural differences.
- Encourage students from other cultures to directly interact with faculty members.

Baker, B. H. (2010). Faculty ratings of retention strategies for minority nursing students. *Nursing Education Perspectives, 31*(4), 216–220.

Kardong-Edgren, S., Cason, C. L., Brennan, A. M., Reifsnider, E., Hummel, F., Mancini, M., & Griffin, C. (2010). Cultural competency of graduating BSN students. *Nursing Education Perspectives, 31*(5), 278–285.

CRITICAL THINKING QUESTIONS

1. How would valuing cultural diversity enhance psychiatric–mental health nursing practice?
2. If someone from another culture comes to your school or your hometown, is it up to that person to adjust?
3. What specific actions could you take in a mental health setting that would show that you acknowledge and appreciate cultural differences?

to be problems in schools of nursing. Nursing faculty can recruit and mentor students from diverse cultures to serve as clinicians, managers, faculty, and leaders who can then serve as role models for other students. One way to attract and educate a diverse student group is to practice diversity in faculty recruitment. When considering nursing curricula, it is important to note that knowledge of a foreign language will be essential as we strive to meet global needs in the 21st century. Nursing students themselves also have a responsibility to their classmates from diverse cultures. The Evidence-Based Practice feature suggests practical strategies you can use in your relationships with classmates from other cultures.

Pearson Nursing Student Resources

Find additional review materials at
nursing.pearsonhighered.com

Prepare for success with NCLEX®-style practice questions,
interactive assignments and activities, web links, animations
and videos, and more!

REFERENCES

Baker, B. H. (2010). Faculty ratings of retention strategies for minority nursing students. *Nursing Education Perspectives, 31*(4), 216–220.

Bromet, E. J. (2007). Psychiatric disorders. In R. B. Wallace (Ed.), *Maxcy–Rosenau–Last Public health and preventive medicine* (15th ed.). Stamford, CT: Appleton & Lange.

Dome, P., Kapitany, B., Ignits, G., & Rihmer, Z. (2010). Season of birth is significantly associated with the risk of completed suicide. *Biological Psychiatry, 68*(2), 148–155.

Ember, C. R., & Ember, M. R. (2010). *Cultural anthropology* (13th ed.). Upper Saddle River, NJ: Prentice Hall.

Ferraro, G., & Andreatta, S. (2011). *Cultural anthropology: An applied perspective* (9th ed.). Albany, NY: Cengage Learning.

Fleury, M. J., Grenier, G., Bamvita, J. M., Perreault, M. & Caron, J. (2011). Typology of adults diagnosed with mental disorders based on socio-demographic and clinical and service use characteristics. *BMS Psychiatry, 11*(1), 67.

Gezon, L., & Kottak, C. (2011). *Culture.* New York, NY: McGraw-Hill.

Giger, J. N., & Davidhizar, R. E. (2008). *Transcultural nursing: Assessment and intervention* (5th ed.). St. Louis, MO: Mosby.

Huff, R. M., & Kline, M. V. (Eds.). (2008). *Health promotion in multicultural populations: A handbook for practitioners* (2nd ed.). Thousand Oaks, CA: Sage Publications.

Jezewski, M. A. (1993). Culture brokering as a model for advocacy. *Nursing and Health Care, 14*(2), 78–85.

Jezewski, M. A. (1995). Evolution of a grounded theory: Conflict resolution through culture brokering. *Advances in Nursing Science, 17*(3), 14–30.

Kardong-Edgren, S., Cason, C. L., Brennan, A. M., Reifsnider, E., Hummel, F., Mancini, M., & Griffin, C. (2010). Cultural competency of graduating BSN students. *Nursing Education Perspectives, 31*(5), 278–285.

Mallinger, J. B., & Lamberti, J. S. (2010). Psychiatrists' attitudes toward and awareness about racial disparities in mental health care. *Psychiatric Services, 61*(2), 173–179.

Miller, B. (2010). *Cultural anthropology* (6th ed.). Upper Saddle River, NJ: Prentice Hall.

Purnell, L., Davidhizar, R. E., Giger, J.N., Strickland, O. L., Fishman, D., & Allison, D. M. (2011). A guide to developing a culturally competent organization. *Journal of Transcultural Nursing, 22*(1), 7–14.

Spector, R. E. (2009). *Cultural diversity in health & illness* (7th ed.). Upper Saddle River, NJ: Prentice Hall.

Torchalla, I., Okoli, C. T., Malchy, L., & Johnson, J. L. (2011). Nicotine dependence and gender differences in smokers accessing community mental health services. *Journal of Psychiatric and Mental Health Nursing, 18*(4), 349–358.

Wickrama, T., & Ketring, S.A. (2011). Change in the health of tsunami-exposed mothers three years after the natural disaster. *International Journal of Social Psychiatry.* Advance online publication. doi: 10.1177/0020764010394279

Zona, K., & Milan, S. (2011). Gender differences in the longitudinal impact of exposure to violence on mental health in urban youth. *Journal of Youth and Adolescence.* Advance online publication. doi: 10.1007/s10964-011-9649-3

3 UNIT

PSYCHIATRIC–MENTAL HEALTH NURSING PROCESSES

After she lights two candles, GAVRIELLA (whose name means "God is my strength") recites the Shabbat blessing, bringing the spirit of Shabbat into her home in Jerusalem. Adding a silent prayer for her sister, Nava, Gavriella prays for Navas' recovery from schizophrenia. Like many Israelis, Gavriellas' mother and father, and Gavriella herself, feel a combination of guilt, shame, and self-blame for Navas' *machalal nefesh*, or disease of the soul. The term suggests that the essence of a person—one's hopes, dreams, loves, and decisions—are diseased.

Although there is greater awareness of mental health issues and the stigma attached to it in Israeli culture, in Gavriellas' ultra-Orthodox community the perception is that people with a mental disorder are unpredictable and violent and should be feared. The family unit is considered to be an extension of the person with mental disorder. They tried, but failed to hide Navas' symptoms from their neighbors and have been avoided and isolated.

In Israel, the focus of care has shifted from psychiatric hospitals to care in community-based facilities, and more Israelis with mental illness are living in the community. Despite this shift in care, stigma remains in housing, employment, and among mental health care providers whose behaviors and attitudes reflect dehumanization and paternalism, demonstrate a lack of respect for persons with mental illness, and result in coercive treatment.

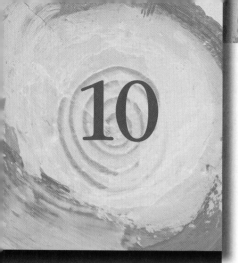

10

Therapeutic Communication

CAROL REN KNEISL

KEY TERMS

feedback *192*
illusion *185*
interpersonal
    communication *189*
intrapersonal
    communication *189*
mixed message *187*
neologism *187*
nonverbal
    communication *187*
overload *192*
perception *185*
subculture *186*
tangential reply *192*
underload *192*

LEARNING OUTCOMES

After completing this chapter, you will be able to:

1. Describe the factors that influence the process of human communication.
2. Explain why nonverbal communication is important in interpersonal relationships.
3. Identify the principles of therapeutic communication and explain why they are essential ingredients of interpersonal relationships.
4. Formulate a strategy for improving your personal ability to communicate therapeutically.
5. Employ the skills discussed here to foster relationships and communication in the psychiatric–mental health setting.
6. Explain how the skills discussed here foster relating and communicating in any health care setting.

CRITICAL THINKING CHALLENGE

You are about to embark on your first inpatient psychiatric nursing experience. You feel anxious because although you've read the therapeutic communication techniques described in this chapter, you feel uncomfortable about using them. They seem artificial, stilted, and "not you."

1. What can you do to decrease your discomfort and anxiety and help make your psychiatric–mental health nursing experience a positive learning experience for you as well as for your clients?
2. How would you modify the therapeutic communication techniques discussed in this chapter to match your own personal style?
3. What problems could you run into by overusing a communication technique?
4. How can therapeutic communication techniques be useful when communicating with classmates? Friends? Family members?

The mechanism for establishing, maintaining, and improving human contacts is interpersonal communication. Communication is a very special process and the most significant of human behaviors. Moreover, it is the main method for implementing the nursing process. When they tell "their story," clients explain themselves, the events of their lives, and the circumstances they face. As psychiatric–mental health nurses, we help clients tell their stories, explore the circumstances of their lives, and move in a more satisfying and mentally healthier direction.

For many students, like the student in the clinical example that follows, the instruction to use one's self therapeutically is mysterious jargon quite unlike the clear-cut step-by-step procedures for some physical treatments.

Clinical Example

I found myself watching my instructors and the nurses on the unit closely when they talked with clients. Somehow I thought that by imitating things that they did or said, I'd figure out what "being therapeutic" was supposed to mean. I knew it had something to do with things the nurse said or didn't say when she talked with clients. But it all got very fuzzy to me beyond that very elementary grasp of it. I used to latch on to ideas like "Agreeing is untherapeutic. So is giving advice or opinions." The only entries I felt safe putting down in my process recording were stiff-sounding reflections like "You sound angry."

Because the process of human communication is complex and has many dimensions, it cannot be reduced to a few simple steps that you can simply memorize and perform. However, there are some principles and techniques that we will teach you to use so that you can be comfortable and therapeutic at the same time. Effective communication is the cornerstone for all psychiatric–mental health nursing practice. Two other chapters correlate closely with this chapter on communication. Chapter 3 ∞ discusses the nurse's personal characteristics that are a basis for therapeutic use of self. Chapter 4 ∞ discusses the actual structure and process of the one–to–one relationship.

THE PROCESS OF HUMAN COMMUNICATION

As you will see in this chapter, communication is an ongoing, dynamic, and ever-changing series of events. Some people mistakenly believe that communication is simply the transfer of information or meaning from one human being to another. The truth is that meaning *cannot* be transferred; it must be mutually negotiated, because meaning is influenced by a number of significant factors.

Role of Perception

A person's perception of the world is an essential element in communicating. The term **perception** refers to the experience of sensing, interpreting, and comprehending the world in which one lives. Perception is a highly personal and internal act.

People process through their senses all the information they have about the world around them. However, seeing is not

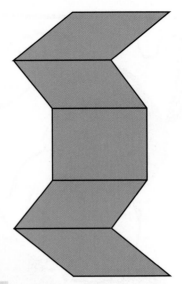

FIGURE 10-1 ■ A perceptual illusion.

always believing. Communication specialists have discovered that because of human physiologic limitations, the eye and brain are constantly being tricked into seeing things that are not really what they seem; these are called **illusions.** Before continuing to read, stare at FIGURE 10-1 ■ for 20 seconds. The illustration will appear to swing back and forth. You can verify that the movement is an illusion by checking your visual perception against your tactile sensations.

What people "see" or sense is strongly influenced by many factors. For example, past experiences have prepared us to see things, people, and events in particular ways. Also, we tend to observe more carefully when a purpose guides the observation. The nurse in an intensive care unit observes a cardiac surgery client differently than a family member does.

Finally, when understandings differ, you and I can look at the same object and see different things. Mental set helps determine how and what a person perceives. Before you read any further, look at the picture of the young woman in FIGURE 10-2 ■ on page 186. Do you see the silhouette of a young woman? Do you also see the face of an elderly woman? (Remember: Stop here and look at Figure 10-2 on page 186.) Using the phrase "the picture of the young woman in Figure 10-2" encouraged you to perceive the illustration in a particular way. Now you should also be able to see the elderly woman in the illustration.

As the illustrations demonstrate, the old axiom might be better stated: "Believing is seeing." Because we tend to perceive in terms of past experiences, expectations, and goals, perceptions may be a prime obstacle to communication. No two individuals perceive the world in exactly the same way, and the meanings of events differ because people's perceptions of them differ. Perceptions of other human beings are of particular importance because human communication is inevitably affected by how we perceive one another. To see others at all as they are, people need to know themselves and to know how the self affects their perceptions of others.

FIGURE 10-2 ■ The influence of mental set on perception.

Role of Values

Values are concepts of the desirable. People value what is of worth to them. Values influence the process of communication because people's values, like their perceptions, differ.

Value systems differ for a number of reasons. Age is one. Children's values shift when they become teenagers. The college or work experience generally influences values in yet other directions. Marrying or being a parent or grandparent may cause other value changes or shifts.

Psychiatric–mental health nurses must ultimately come to terms with the problem of values, because conflicting value systems among mental health professionals expose clients to uncertainty and confusion. Consider the following example.

Clinical Example

The parents of a 15-year-old girl were upset to find a small plastic bag of marijuana in her dresser drawer. She had been playing hooky from school and wore low-slung jeans that her parents considered too sexy. After a series of lengthy, angry discussions with her parents, she was confined to her room. During this period she refused to eat or drink. When the teenager was seen by a mental health treatment team, the members' opinions were divided. Some said that her behavior signaled an emotional disturbance. They labeled her antisocial, depressed, and anxious. Others believed the parents were old-fashioned and too rigid in attempting to force her to accept their values.

Clearly, these staff members were influenced by their own values.

The daily roles people take also influence their values. In any one day a man may be a student, husband, father, nurse, citizen, speaker, artist, son, and teacher.

Role of Culture

Each culture provides its members with notions about how the world is structured and what it means. These preconceptions, learned at an early age, are so subtle that they often go unrecognized. They nonetheless set limits on communication and interaction with others. Relying on culturally determined generalizations or stereotypes can have profound effects on one's relationships with others.

Communication is culture bound in a wide variety of ways. The culture and the **subculture** (the culture within the culture) teach people how to communicate through language, hand gestures, clothing, and even in the ways they use the space around them. When you overhear two clients talking about "angel dust" you need to know that the term refers not to something religious, but to PCP—an animal tranquilizer. In some cultures, belching after dinner is a compliment to the host. In other cultures, belching may be considered uncouth or an insult. Other interesting examples of cultural differences in communication are discussed in Developing Cultural Competence.

DEVELOPING CULTURAL COMPETENCE

Cultural and Gender Perspectives in Communication

We know, from research, that people interpret communication from their unique cultural perspectives. For example, facial expressions that convey sadness, happiness, anger, disgust, and surprise seem to be shared in most cultures. However, rules for displaying emotions may vary. In Japanese culture, the show of negative emotions is discouraged—it is more important to "save face" for one's self and others than it is to express a negative emotion. There seems to be more eye contact between Arabs, South Americans, and Greeks than between people from other cultures, and African Americans tend to look less often at others than Caucasians. The "okay" gesture made by forming a circle with the thumb and finger that we use in North America has sexual connotations in some South American and Caribbean countries. In France, the "okay" sign means "worthless." People from Greece, Italy, and South America come from high-contact cultures. They prefer closer distances, exhibit more touching behavior and expect more touching behavior, than people from Northern Europe and North America. Men tend to require more space around them than women and are more likely to use gestures, while women smile more often than men. Women also use their voices to communicate a wider range of emotions than do men.

CRITICAL THINKING QUESTIONS

1. What are the rules in your culture for the expression of emotion?
2. How might your preferences for interpersonal distance and touching behavior influence your nursing care?

These examples make it obvious that communicating with meaning requires that the participants take culture into account. How people communicate with others who do not share similar histories, heritages, or cultures is of critical importance in humanistic psychiatric–mental health nursing practice. Chapter 9 ∞ discusses the personal strategies you can use to develop cultural competence in your clinical work.

The Spoken Word

Problems arise when we discover that words mean different things to different people. That is, *words* do not "mean" something; *people* do. If communication between yourself and the client is to be mutually negotiated in order to be understood by both of you, then you must understand the four concepts discussed next.

Denotation and Connotation

A *denotative meaning* is the literal or restrictive meaning of the word. It is one that is in general use by most people who share a common language. A *connotative meaning* usually arises from a person's personal experience. That is, it has a personal and subjective meaning. While all Americans are likely to share the same general denotative meaning of the word *pig*, the word may have a completely different positive or negative connotation for a farmer, a consumer of meat, a person of the Muslim faith, someone who is Jewish, a prisoner, and a police officer. Connotative meanings can evoke powerful emotions.

Private and Shared Meanings

For communication to take place, meaning must be shared. People can use private meanings to communicate with others only when the parties agree about what the word means. The private meaning then becomes a shared meaning. It is common for families, two friends, or members of larger social groups (military personnel, drug users, adolescents) to use language in highly personal and private ways. Problems arise when the assumption is made that people who are outside the group share these meanings. For example, if you are not up-to-date on contemporary slang, you will not know that "fo' shizzle" means certainly, "wikidemia" is a term paper researched entirely on http://www.wikipedia.org, and "brodown" means boy's night out.

People with schizophrenia (refer to Chapter 16 ∞) may use language in an idiosyncratic way or may use a private, unshared language referred to as **neologisms**. Such people are unaware that others don't share this use of language. People who use neologisms, such as the young man in the following clinical example, expect to be understood and may become upset when they are not.

In trying to make private meanings shared, make an effort to reach mutual understanding of the client's message. It is insufficient, and quite possibly inaccurate, to attach meaning based solely on your (or the client's) interpretation of an event, a word or phrase, or a gesture.

Clinical Example

A young man who was hospitalized on a psychiatric unit complained to other clients and staff members that he had been odenated, and he became increasingly frustrated and anxious when it became apparent that he wasn't being understood. Rather than simply writing him off as confused, his primary nurse recognized that odenated most likely had a private meaning. With some help he was able to explain that he was upset about having been moved to a private room. The room was, he said, so dark and dingy that it looked like a cave. Animals live in caves that are called dens. In his view he had been o-den-ated—put into a cave.

Nonverbal Messages

Most researchers agree that **nonverbal communication** channels carry more social meaning than spoken words. That is, chances are that people are making inferences about you based on your nonverbal communication (Beebe, 2011).

There is a wide variety of nonverbal channels: body movements, including facial expressions and hand gestures; pitch, rate, and volume of the voice; the use of personal and social space; touch; and the use of cultural artifacts (such as clothing, jewelry, and cosmetics). Nonverbal cues help us judge the reliability of verbal messages more readily, especially in the presence of a **mixed message** (inconsistency between the verbal and nonverbal components) because nonverbal messages are the way we communicate our feelings and attitudes.

Body Movement

The study of body movement as a form of nonverbal communication is called *kinesics*. Facial expressions, gestures, and eye movements are the most common categories.

Facial expressions are the single most important source of nonverbal communication. They generally communicate emotions. The silent-film comedians—blank-faced Buster Keaton and comic Charlie Chaplin—and the great mime Marcel Marceau communicate not only isolated acts but complete sequences of behavior with kinesics alone.

Body movements and gestures provide clues about people and about how they feel toward others. For example, hand gestures can communicate anxiety, indifference, and impatience, among other things. Foot shuffling and fidgeting may express the desire to escape.

Body position gives cues about how open one person is to another person, or how interesting and attractive one person is to another. People tend to position their bodies according to their feelings about the person with whom they are communicating. Choosing to stand or sit close to another usually indicates attraction, whereas creating greater physical distance may signify an attempt at interpersonal distance.

Eye contact is another very important cue in communicating. For example, proper sidewalk behavior among Americans is for passers-by to look at each other until they are about 8 feet apart. At this distance, both parties look downward or away so they will not appear to be staring. Several common but unstated rules about eye contact are as follows:

- Interaction is invited by staring at another person on the other side of the room. If the other person returns the gaze, the invitation to interact has been accepted. Averting the eyes signals a rejection of the looker's request.
- A person's frank gaze is widely interpreted as positive regard.
- Greater mutual eye contact occurs among friends.
- People who seek eye contact while speaking are usually perceived as believable and earnest.
- If the usual short, intermittent gazes during a conversation are replaced by gazes of longer duration, the person looked at is likely to believe that the person gazing considers the relationship between the two people to be more important than the content of the conversation.

Keep in mind that nonverbal messages are often moderated by culture.

Voice Quality and Nonlanguage Sounds

Voice quality, such as pitch and range, and nonlanguage vocalizations, such as sobbing, laughing, or grunting—noises without linguistic structure—are other components we use to make inferences about other people.

Vocal cues can differentiate emotions. Who hasn't heard the injunction, "Don't speak to me in that tone of voice!" Sometimes people use vocal cues to make inferences about personality traits. For example, people who increase the loudness, pitch, timbre (overtones), and rate of their speech are often thought to be active and dynamic. Those who use greater intonation and volume and are fluent are thought to be persuasive. Status cues in speech are based on a combination of word choice, pronunciation, grammar, speech fluency, and articulation, among other factors.

Personal and Social Space

A pioneer in the study of proxemics—space relationships maintained by people in social interaction—was Edward T. Hall (1990). Proxemics includes the dimensions of *territoriality* (fixed and permanent territory that is somehow marked off and defended from intrusion, such as in the clinical example that follows) and *personal space* (a portable territory surrounding the self that others are expected not to invade).

Clinical Example

Norma was an avid bingo player. She played at the same bingo hall in Florida almost every day. Norma always carved out her territory. She put her purse on the chair to her left, her bingo cards in the middle of the table, her snacks and beverages on the left side of the table, and her bingo daubers on the right side of the table. In essence, Norma secured for herself the space normally shared by three people.

Figure 10-3 ■ illustrates the various relationships between intimacy and personal space.

Knowing something about proxemics is useful, for example, in planning the physical space in which communication is to occur. You can arrange furniture to increase or decrease interpersonal distance. A cozy, open seating arrangement encourages interaction; chairs in a row that face the front of a room discourage interaction. It is important to be especially sensitive to the constraints imposed on communication by physical objects. An understanding of proxemics coupled with paying attention to how others use interpersonal space will enhance your ability to decipher verbal communication.

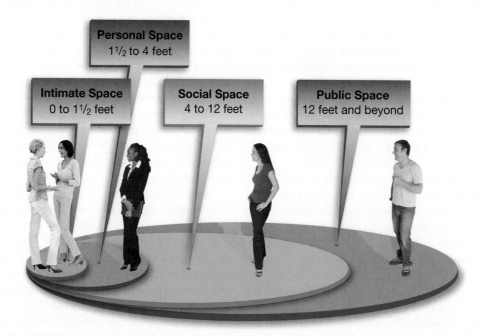

FIGURE 10-3 ■ Edward T. Hall's four zones of space.
Source: Beebe, S. A. (2011). *Interpersonal communication: Relating to others.* Upper Saddle River, NJ: Pearson Education, Figure 7-1, p. 200.

Touch

Touching behaviors, because they tend to personalize communication, are extremely important in emotional situations. In North American society, the use of touch is governed by strong social norms. Unwritten guidelines control who, when, why, and where people touch. For example, North American men are more uncomfortable with being touched by other men than women are with being touched by other women. Some people are high-touch-avoidance individuals—they simply do not like to be touched.

Most of the taboos against touching seem to stem from the sexual implications of touching behavior. However, although touching is a physical act, it may or may not be sexual in nature. A realization of the importance of touch and an understanding that touching is not necessarily a sexual behavior may make this channel of communication available to more people. It is equally important to be sensitive to the other person's disposition toward touching, so as not to alienate another by infringing on the person's right not to be touched. The use of touch in therapeutic work is discussed in Chapters 3 and 4 ∞.

Cultural Artifacts

Artifacts are items in contact with interacting people that may function as nonverbal stimuli: clothes, cosmetics, perfume, deodorants, jewelry, eyeglasses, body piercings, wigs and hairpieces, beards and mustaches, and so on.

Think about what information is communicated through artifacts such as a full-length mink coat, hair that is dyed purple, a gold band on the third finger of the left hand, a military uniform, or a Phi Beta Kappa key.

Verbal and Nonverbal Links

The verbal and nonverbal elements of human communication are inextricably linked. Six different ways in which verbal and nonverbal systems interrelate are discussed here.

1. A nonverbal cue may *repeat* a verbal cue but in a different way. The deep-sea fisherman who verbally describes the size of the sailfish he caught may also extend both hands to indicate its length. The gesture repeats the idea.
2. Nonverbal behavior may also *contradict* verbal behavior. Consider the woman who meets a college roommate she hasn't seen for some time. She says, "You haven't changed a bit," but her tone of voice and facial expression convey sarcasm. When verbal and nonverbal cues contradict one another, it is usually safer to put more faith in the nonverbal cues.
3. Nonverbal messages may *add to or modify* verbal messages. When a man says he is a "little" irritated about being kept waiting, his tone of voice and body actions may indicate a more profound anger.
4. Certain nonverbal cues *accent or emphasize* verbal cues. A woman shrugs her shoulders when she says she doesn't really care which movie she and her

companion see. A master of ceremonies holds up his hand when he asks for quiet. These gestures and body movements emphasize the words.
5. Cues that *regulate,* such as those that tell people when to start talking or when to stop talking, are usually nonverbal. A woman who keeps opening and closing her mouth briefly while others are talking is indicating that she wants a turn too.
6. Sometimes nonverbal cues are used to *substitute* for words. A wave from a friend at a distance replaces "hello." Applause at the end of a play tells the actors that they have pleased the audience.

BIOPSYCHOSOCIAL THEORIES AND MODELS OF HUMAN COMMUNICATION

Communication takes place on at least three different levels: intrapersonal, interpersonal, and public (such as communication through the mass media or giving a public speech). Psychiatric–mental health nurses are more concerned with intrapersonal and interpersonal communication. **Intrapersonal communication** occurs when people communicate within themselves. When you walk into a client's room and think, "The first pint of blood is almost finished. I'd better get the next one ready for infusion," you are communicating intrapersonally. **Interpersonal communication**, which this chapter discusses in depth, takes place in dyads (between two people) and small groups. This level of person-to-person communication is at the heart of psychiatric–mental health nursing.

One of the easiest ways to illustrate the nature of human communication and the elements of the process of human communication is through a model, or visual representation. People use models frequently for many purposes. They might use a map or their GPS, which are visual representations of a geographic location, to find their way to the community mental health center they plan to visit. Health professionals use electroencephalograms (EEGs) to see a visual representation of the electrical activity in the brain. However, models provide incomplete views—a map does not show all the trees, buildings, or park statues in the territory; an EEG tracing does not show the color, size, or blood supply of the brain. It is important to keep this in mind when looking at models. They sometimes make a process look simpler than it is.

Symbolic Interactionist Model

A symbolic interactionist model is based on a transactional perspective. It views human communication on the social–interpersonal level and accounts for the whole persons involved in the process. Communication is viewed as a process of simultaneous mutual influence, rather than as a turn-taking event. The participants are products of their social system and integral parts of it. In the communication, some events take place *within* the participants (they are intrapersonal), and some take place *between* the participants (they are interpersonal).

Participants are who they are in relationship to the other person with whom they are communicating. For example, in this dyadic (two-person) communication event between Jeff and Sarah, there are at least *six* perceptions involved:

1. Jeff's perception of himself
2. Jeff's perception of Sarah
3. Jeff's impression of the way Sarah sees him
4. Sarah's perception of herself
5. Sarah's perception of Jeff
6. Sarah's impression of the way Jeff sees her

Therefore, in addition to the *content* message, a *relationship* message also exists. Suppose Jeff passes Sarah in the corridor and Jeff says, "Hi, how are you?" Sarah answers, "Just fine, thanks," but moves down the corridor and away from Jeff as quickly as possible. Their subsequent communication will be affected by whether Jeff perceives Sarah as walking away because she wanted to get home before a rainstorm, or because he believes that Sarah is angry with him and her behavior is a comment on their relationship. The transactional model of the communication process illustrated in FIGURE 10-4 ■ helps explain what takes place between Jeff and Sarah.

A transactional approach is based on systems theory, which was discussed in Chapter 5 ∞. Recall that a system is a set of interconnected elements in which a change in any one element affects all the other elements. Therefore, in a transactional model of human communication, a change in any aspect of the communication system can influence all of the other elements in the system. Note in Figure 10-4 that both individuals are the source of communication as well as the receiver of communication and that messages involve feedback (the response to the message) as well as context (the psychological as well as the physical environment for communication). Note also that both individuals send and receive messages at the same time. Their communication is not linear and it is complex because all of the components occur simultaneously. Every element of communication is connected to every other element of communication.

Let us say that Jeff is attracted to Sarah and would like to get to know her better. Jeff first scans the information about himself and others (Jeff enjoys movies and remembers hearing Sarah tell a friend that she'd really like to see one particular movie) and then mentally rehearses possible actions to take (*role-playing*) and possible reactions of the other (*role-taking*). This gives Jeff the chance to think of four or five different ways to approach Sarah. In this rehearsal phase, Jeff decides what to say, how to say it, and even whether to send the message to Sarah at all. His decision is to ask Sarah to the movie.

Jeff's message ("Would you like to go to the movie with me?") serves as a stimulus for Sarah. Sarah thinks about Jeff's invitation, decides whether she wants to go to the movie with him, and considers what response to make to Jeff. Sarah's response provides feedback and serves as a stimulus for Jeff, and the interaction continues. Feedback (Sarah's response) allows the person an opportunity to determine whether he or she has made an error in the approach to the other and to make appropriate corrections. Jeff carefully considers Sarah's response. He listens to what she says and watches her behavior toward him. If her response is less than enthusiastic, he will try to determine what went wrong and how to correct it.

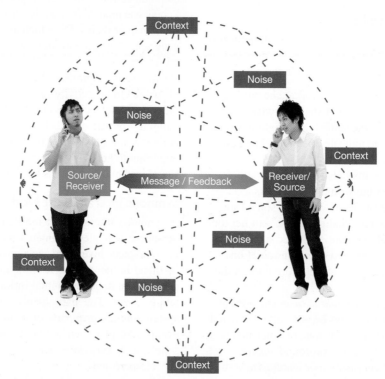

FIGURE 10-4 ■ A model for communication as a mutual transaction.
Source: Beebe, S. A. (2011). *Interpersonal communication: Relating to others.* Upper Saddle River, NJ: Pearson Education, Figure 1-3, p. 11.

In summary, the transactional view of communication includes the following concepts:

- People run through a series of internal trials in the process of organizing a message.
- People select and transmit the message that will, in their view, have the highest probability of success.
- Success depends on the accuracy and completeness of the cognitive map and the accuracy and efficiency of the intrapersonal and interpersonal feedback loops.
- Communication is a dynamic (ever-changing) process that is unrepeatable and irreversible.
- Communication is complex.
- The meaning of messages is not transferred; it is mutually negotiated.

Communication is, at the very least, a very complicated process.

Neurobiologic Factors

Looking at communication in its broadest sense requires us to go beyond the spoken word, the written word, and motor activity to the molecular level. In this broad view, communication can also be thought of as the movement of neurotransmitters within a synapse between neurons. Neurobiology researchers believe that energy and movement at the molecular level may be the root of all brain functioning, including communication.

The neuron, the functional unit of the brain, differs from other cells in the body in that it is specialized for the function of information processing. The flow of information from one nerve cell to another involves the passage of electrically charged chemical particles—sodium, potassium, calcium, and chloride—across the cell membrane of the neuron. Neurotransmitters released by the presynaptic membrane of the axon cross the synaptic cleft and bind to their receptors on the postsynaptic membrane of the dendrite of the target cell. This process is more fully described in Chapter 6 ∞.

Therefore, brain activity can also be thought of in terms of messages and receptors. It makes sense to acknowledge that when communication is disrupted at one level—for example, when a crucial chemical in the brain undergoes an alteration—the end result can be felt at other, more obvious communication levels of the individual (such as verbal and nonverbal communication and intrapersonal and interpersonal communication). To put this into perspective, your understanding of the words on this page is related not only to your understanding of written English but also to the chloride ion channel activity on the membranes of millions of your brain cells.

The neurobiology of human communication is very complex and not yet fully understood. For example, we know that there is a speech circuit in the brain between the auditory cortex on the left, which passes to Wernicke's area in the temporal cortex, and from there to Broca's area in the left frontal lobe via the arcuate fasciculus (a pathway composed mainly of axons that synapse with other neurons). This speech circuit is detailed in FIGURE 10-5 ■.

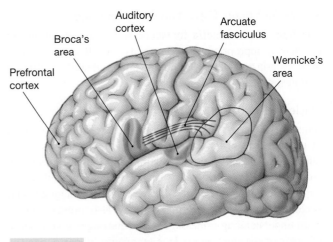

FIGURE 10-5 ■ The speech circuit.
Source: Smock, T. K. (1999). *Physiological psychology: A neuroscience approach.* Upper Saddle River, NJ: Prentice Hall.

However, knowing about the speech circuit does not go far enough in explaining the complexities of the neurobiologic basis of human communication. Some elements of the communication process are distributed more widely in the brain than was previously believed. To add to the complexity, these areas are not the same in all of us. Therefore, there is no specific map of the brain that can locate specific communication functions with absolute certainty. Nor does it mean that damage in a specific region will necessarily cause a deficiency in a function thought to be contained in that region.

Therapeutic Communication Theory

In the view of psychiatrist Jurgen Ruesch (1961), communication includes all the processes by which one human being influences another. Ruesch's theory takes into account the perceptions and interpretations that influence one person's view of the other. Further, Ruesch assumes that, to survive, the individual must communicate successfully.

According to Ruesch, communication is one of the most difficult human skills to master. It takes a long time to learn because it occurs in a series of steps, each building on the previous one. To communicate effectively requires decades of continuous practice. It is believed that interference hampers development and leaves an indelible mark.

Basic Concepts

The basic concepts of Ruesch's theory are as follows:

- Communication occurs in four different settings: intrapersonal, interpersonal, group, and societal.
- The ability to receive, evaluate, and transmit messages is influenced by perception, evaluation (which involves memory, past experiences, and value systems), and the transmission quality of messages (amount, speed, efficacy, and distinctiveness).
- Messages achieve meaning when they are mutually validated or verified between the two parties.
- Correction through feedback is basic to adaptive, healthy behavior and successful communication.

Successful Versus Disturbed Communication

The four formal criteria for successful communication are efficiency, appropriateness, flexibility, and feedback. When these criteria are not met, communication is disturbed (Ruesch & Bateson, 1968).

Efficiency

Simplicity, clarity, and correct timing are all components of efficient messages. Psychiatric–mental health nurses and other mental health professionals may find themselves using complex and scientific words or professional mental health jargon to convey messages. Obscure or clumsy language and irrelevant or useless information may also prevent others from understanding a message. Clear messages give a sense of order or structure and reduce ambiguity by narrowing the number of possible interpretations of meaning. Emphasizing the important ideas helps.

Proper timing is also important. It is best to give messages when the other person is able to "hear" them, when there are no intervening noises or inputs, and when the other person can interpret them without undue haste. Problems occur if the interval between the messages is either too short or too long.

Appropriateness

Messages are appropriate when they are relevant to the situation at hand and when there is mutual fit of overall patterns and constituent parts. Communication is inappropriate when it does not fit the circumstance, is irrelevant, or is misconstrued.

Communication can also be inappropriate in amount. Because every individual has both high and low tolerance levels for stimulation, a person's ability to cope with ideas, make decisions, and act is affected by the amount and rate of sensory input received. Exceeding a tolerance level is called **overload**. A person who is overloaded by too many messages or by messages too closely spaced cannot handle incoming messages. **Underload** occurs when delay or lack of information interferes with a person's ability to comprehend the message of another.

The **tangential reply** is another example of inappropriateness. A tangential reply to a statement disregards the content of the message and is directed toward an incidental aspect of the initial statement, the type of language used, the emotions of the sender, or another facet of the same topic. It indicates that the other person is not attending to your message.

Flexibility

People cannot always be sure how a message will be received, because each person with whom they communicate is unique and changing. Because they cannot expect constancy from others, people need to be flexible. In communication, lack of flexibility manifests itself as either exaggerated control or exaggerated permissiveness. Both extremes increase the likelihood of frustrating, ungratifying, or disturbed communication.

Maintaining flexibility can be difficult if doing so requires a person to abandon or temporarily lay aside a carefully planned goal. To be flexible, a person must have the ability to set new priorities and to move to meet immediate goals.

People who practice humanistic psychiatric–mental health nursing work to achieve flexibility in their relationships with clients and colleagues.

Feedback

Feedback is the response to the message (Beebe, 2011). It is the process by which performance is checked and malfunctions corrected. It performs a regulatory function in the communication process. One example of how feedback can help to correct a system malfunction is illustrated in Evidence-Based Practice. Feedback allows people to decide which messages have been understood as intended. It requires the cooperation of two people—one to give it and one to receive it. Giving helpful feedback is discussed further later in this chapter.

Under certain circumstances of disturbed communication, feedback either fails or functions poorly. When messages do not get through or are distorted, appropriate replies cannot be obtained, and corrective feedback does not occur. Content that elicits anxiety, fear, shame, or any of several other strong emotions is likely to hamper feedback.

Behavioral Effects and Human Communication Theory

Watzlawick, Beavin, and Jackson (1967) base their theory of human communication on the assumption that communication is synonymous with interaction. These authors maintain that, in the presence of another, all behavior is communicative. This theory is concerned with the pragmatics, or the behavioral effects, of human interaction. What makes this theory particularly useful to you is its conception of human communication as a reciprocal process.

Communication Levels

According to this theory, one cannot *not* communicate. Both activity and inactivity, verbalizations and silences, convey messages. This communication occurs on two levels. The *content level* of a communication is the report aspect, in which information is conveyed. The *relationship level* is communication about a communication.

All interchanges can be viewed as either *symmetric* (based on equality) or *complementary* (based on difference). In symmetric relationships, the partners usually mirror each other's behavior, thus minimizing difference. Complementary relationships, in contrast, maximize difference.

Communication Disturbances

Communication can be disturbed when a person attempts *not* to communicate. As an example, in this framework, the basic dilemma occurs when a person attempts not to communicate. However, because it is impossible not to communicate, the attempt to not communicate is a communication in itself.

Another disturbance occurs when a person communicates in a way that invalidates the messages sent to or received from the other person. Such communications, called *disqualifications,* include a wide range of behavior such as self-contradictions, inconsistencies, subject switches, incomplete sentences, and misunderstandings.

EVIDENCE-BASED PRACTICE

Feedback Helps Create a More Human Setting

Julie Rodriguez, a staff nurse in the psychiatric emergency department of a large metropolitan hospital, has been concerned because of the unfavorable evaluations left in the comment box by visitors to the emergency department. Although the waiting room has been newly remodeled and has comfortable seating, visitors to the department feel they are ignored for long periods of time while waiting to be seen. Their view of the staff is that staff members are very busy and seem to be working very hard. This doesn't seem to make up for the visitors' feelings that nurses and other staff are emotionally distant or "just there to do a job." The majority of visitors believe they have waited longer to be seen than what the documented records show; for them, time seems to pass very slowly.

Julie believes the emergency department staff should be rated as highly as the physical environment. To achieve this goal, Julie has come up with the following plan, which she presented to her colleagues in their weekly meeting:

1. Provide a staff member presence at intermittent intervals—a nurse attuned to client needs and concerns related to their condition or to their care, and a volunteer to assist visitors with other questions or concerns such as those related to insurance, transportation, hospital admission, and so on.
2. Provide relaxing music, educational videos, books and puzzles, magazines and newspapers, and games for visitors'

use. The volunteer would be responsible for maintaining these activities.

Julie's rationale for her proposal is that providing more than a physical presence in the waiting room avoids the perception that staff members are emotionally distant or just there to do a job and, in conjunction with the additional activities, transforms a technical, potentially impersonal setting into a more human place. Her rationale is based on knowledge she gained from several research articles, including:

Chang, G., Weiss, A. P., Orav, E. F., Jones, J. A., Finn, C. T., Gitlin, D. F., . . . Rauch, S. L. (2011). Hospital variability in emergency department length of stay for adult patients receiving psychiatric consultation: A prospective study. *Annals of Emergency Medicine.* Advance online publication. Retrieved January 10, 2011 from http://www.annemergmed.com/article/S0196-0644%2810%2901835-4/abstract

Shafiei, T., Gaynor, N., & Farrell, G. (2011). The characteristics, management and outcomes of people identified with mental health issues in an emergency department, Melbourne, Australia. *Journal of Psychiatric and Mental Health Nursing, 18*(1), 9–16.

CRITICAL THINKING QUESTIONS

1. What personal steps could busy nurses take to reduce emotional distance between themselves and clients or themselves and family members?
2. Clients and family members waiting to be seen in an emergency department often feel anxious. If anxiety is interpersonally communicated (see Chapter 8 ∞), what staff behaviors in this example could add to their anxiety?
3. Which verbal and nonverbal therapeutic communication skills are likely to help reduce their anxiety?

A person may communicate in a way that confirms, rejects, or *disconfirms* the other person's view of self. Confirmation of one person's self-view by another is thought to be the greatest single factor in ensuring healthy mental development and stability. Rejection of the other's definition of self essentially conveys this message: "You're wrong." Disconfirmation causes others to value themselves less by conveying this message: "You don't exist." Disconfirmation questions the other's authenticity. Disconfirmation leads to alienation and has been found to occur with some regularity in the experiences of people with schizophrenia.

Although all relationships are necessarily either symmetric or complementary, *runaways* (exaggerations to the point of disturbance) may occur in either of the patterns. For example, the danger of competitiveness is ever-present in symmetric relationships. Symmetric interactions that lose their stability may enter a spiral in which each individual attempts to be just a little bit "more equal" than the other. Runaways are seen in quarrels between people or wars between nations, behaviors that are relatively open. Rejection of the other's self generally occurs when a symmetric relationship breaks down.

Breakdowns in complementary relationships, however, are generally characterized by disconfirmation of the other. For this reason, they are usually viewed as more serious (Watzlawick, 1993).

Neurolinguistic Programming Theory

Neurolinguistic programming (NLP) is a communication model developed in the early 1970s by Richard Bandler and John Grinder. The model is derived from theory in linguistics, neurophysiology, psychology, cybernetics, and psychiatry (Bandler, 1993).

Bandler and Grinder first observed psychotherapists who were known as expert communicators to discover what made them effective as therapists (Dilts, Bandler, & Bandler, 1990). They concluded that people take in, or *access*, information in three sensory modalities:

1. Auditory
2. Visual
3. Kinesthetic

Further, each person prefers one mode over the others. Sounds may facilitate communication with one person, while sight or touch may be more effective with another person. In addition, people process information, or make sense out of it, according to the representational system (the NLP phrase for sensory modality) through which they receive it.

They also found that the expert communicators they observed were able to adapt themselves to match the client's representational system and to imitate the client in a natural and respectful way. Bandler and Grinder theorized that by tuning in to and then using the other person's preferred sensory mode, one could greatly enhance the ability to establish rapport. The most effective communicators, according to NLP theory, are those who can use all three modalities and easily move from one representational system to another.

Determining the Sensory Modality

To determine whether a client's representational system or sensory modality is auditory, visual, or kinesthetic, one identifies the client's:

- Preferred predicates (verbs, adjectives, adverbs that tell something about the subject)
- Eye-accessing cues
- Gross hand movements
- Breathing pattern
- Speech pattern and voice tones

Preferred Predicates A necessary first step before attempting to link words with nonverbal behavior is observing the client to see which set of predicates is preferred. Sample preferred predicates of the auditory, visual, and kinesthetic types are listed in Your Assessment Approach.

Eye-Accessing Cues Eye-accessing cues correlate with an individual's thinking process. People who are visualizing generally turn their eyes upward or look straight ahead, focusing on nothing. Someone processing auditory information usually moves the eyes from side to side. A person engaging in intrapersonal communication usually focuses the eyes

down in the direction of the nondominant hand. A person in the kinesthetic mode looks down toward the dominant hand when experiencing sensations or emotions.

Gross Hand Movements Gross hand movements also give clues to the client's sensory mode. People have a tendency to point toward or touch the sense organ that matches their current sensory mode. The person in a visual mode often points toward the eye, and the person in an auditory mode often points toward or touches the ear.

Breathing Pattern Assessing the breathing pattern helps the observer understand the client's representational model. Shallow, thoracic breathing is often associated with visual accessing. Even breathing or prolonged expiration is associated with auditory accessing, and deep abdominal breathing is associated with kinesthetic accessing.

Speech Pattern and Voice Tones Visual accessing often correlates with quick bursts of words that are high pitched, strained, or nasal. Auditory accessing is often associated with a clear, midrange voice tone or with a rhythmic tempo and clearly enunciated words. Kinesthetic accessing is associated with a slow voice and a low volume or deep tone, or with a breathy tone and long pauses.

Therapeutic Use of NLP

Using NLP theory in psychiatric–mental health nursing practice can enhance our interactions with clients (Thomson & Menzies, 2010). It gives us yet another way to empathize with clients by "trying on" their style. People tend to be less anxious with the familiar. Those of us who mirror the client's sensory mode are likely to be experienced as more comfortable and safer to be with, conditions that facilitate rapport.

We can use mirroring to help the client follow our lead. For example, with an anxious client, we might begin by mirroring the behaviors that indicate the client's anxiety and then shift into a more relaxed posture and less anxious behaviors. It is easier to lead the client from a more anxious state to a less anxious state by employing the NLP principles discussed here. NLP has even been used to help claustrophobic clients about to undergo magnetic resonance imaging (Bigley et al., 2010).

An important benefit of the NLP approach is that it allows us to assess the client's style and preferred sensory mode and to communicate more effectively by using both verbal and nonverbal communication in the client's preferred mode. The following examples express the same nursing intervention with different predicates, depending on the client's preferred mode:

> Visual—"Yes, I can *see* that you are much better. You *look* good, your eyes are *clear,* your *appearance* has certainly changed."
>
> Auditory—"Yes, I can *hear* from the *sound* of your voice that you are better. *Talking* with you today is quite different from yesterday."
>
> Kinesthetic—"Yes, you do seem to be *feeling* much better today, you're *holding* your head up, and your *grasp* is certainly *firmer* than yesterday."

YOUR ASSESSMENT APPROACH
Preferred Predicates

Auditory	Visual	Kinesthetic
Argue	Appear	Attach
Chant	Bright	Breathless
Debate	Colorful	Calm
Eavesdrop	Glimpse	Excite
Hassle	Image	Fondle
Hear	Observe	Hurt
Listen	Pretty	Rough
Overhear	Scan	Sharp
Praise	Sight	Soft
Quiet	Spy	Sore
Scream	Stare	Support
Silent	Ugly	Tension
Tell	View	Throw
Whine	Watch	Touch
Whisper	Wink	Warm

By expanding our abilities to communicate with clients in all three modes, we can become more effective communicators.

FACILITATING COMMUNICATION AND BUILDING A RELATIONSHIP

Therapeutic communication aims at initiating, building, and maintaining fulfilling and trusting relationships with other people. Communicating ideas and feelings with clarity, efficiency, and appropriateness helps a person to be interpersonally effective. In reading the rest of this chapter, try to relate the therapeutic communication principles and practices discussed earlier to these ideas about facilitating communication.

Don't forget about using appropriate nonverbal skills. Your verbal and nonverbal messages should be consistent with one another. Nonverbal messages should enhance, not detract from, verbal messages. Your Self-Awareness presents some guidelines for you in achieving this goal.

Superficiality Versus Intimacy

Most relationships between people begin at the level of social superficiality. In a nurse–client relationship, we try to develop facilitative intimacy, which differs from social intimacy. For example, the interdependence that characterizes the social relationship is greatly reduced. In social relationships, participants may "tell their stories" to one another. In relationships that have therapeutic goals, only the client is engaged in storytelling with the nurse. (If necessary, review the section on self-disclosure in Chapter 3 ∞.) The process is specifically focused. Clients not only explain themselves, the events of their lives, and the circumstances they face, they do so with a purpose in mind—understanding the circumstances through exploring them and moving to improve their lives.

Movement toward therapeutic intimacy may be difficult at first. For one thing, such intimacy violates certain social taboos. For example, at a party it may be socially incorrect to comment on a person's anxiety, stuttering, or facial tic. When communication has a therapeutic goal, all messages, including these nonverbal ones, are heeded and may be discussed. Therapeutic intimacy also requires that the participants move beyond social "chitchat" into meaningful areas of concern for the client. Therapeutic intimacy requires high involvement and commitment.

Facilitating Intimacy

Several interpersonal principles and practices are essential to facilitating intimacy.

Responding With Empathy

Most theorists believe that empathy is the most important dimension in the helping process. Without a high level of empathic understanding, nurses have no real basis for helping. Empathy facilitates interpersonal exploration. A more complete discussion of empathy follows in the section on Therapeutic Communication Skills.

Responding With Respect

Responding with respect demonstrates that you value the integrity of the client and have faith in the client's ability to solve problems, given appropriate help. By encouraging clients to put forward possible plans of action, you convey respect for their ability to take charge of their own destiny. Giving advice, by contrast, conveys a directly opposite message.

Responding With Genuineness

Genuineness refers to the ability to be real or honest with another. To be effective, genuineness must be timed properly and based on a solid relationship. Honesty is not always the best policy, especially if it is brutal or if the client is not capable of dealing with it.

Clients who can experience your authenticity can risk greater genuineness and authenticity themselves. The nurse who is genuine is more likely to deal with and eventually help the client resolve all problems, rather than just those that are safe or socially acceptable.

Responding With Immediacy

Responding with immediacy means responding to what is happening between the client and yourself in the here-and-now. Because this dimension may involve the feelings of the client toward you, it can be one of the most difficult to achieve. For example, the client may confront you with overt or implied criticism of your role or competence. If you respond in a defensive or evasive way, the relationship may be threatened. If you are open, reasonable, and concerned, the relationship may be strengthened.

YOUR SELF-AWARENESS
Guidelines for Improving
Nonverbal Communication

1. **Relax.** The simple act of relaxing makes it easier for others to be relaxed and more open. Remember, anxiety is interpersonally communicated (see Chapter 8 ∞). Take some deep breaths, do a quick body scan, and allow the tension to flow out of your body (see Chapter 33 ∞ for directions for these relaxation techniques).
2. **Use facial, hand, and body gestures judiciously.** Nonverbal gestures that are used indiscriminately lose their effectiveness. Overdoing a gesture—constantly smiling, constantly nodding your head—may become annoying to others and make it more difficult for them to talk with you.
3. **Ask for feedback on your nonverbal communication.** Your classmates and instructors are sources of feedback. Ask them to comment on the facial expressions and body gestures that you use when you converse with them. Consider being videotaped so that you can see for yourself any mannerisms or gestures that intrude on your ability to be an effective communicator.
4. **Practice.** Once you've identified any intrusive facial expressions or body gestures, practice blending your verbal message with appropriate nonverbal cues such as hand gestures, body posture, facial expression, and tone of voice. Then, role-play with your classmates and ask them to comment on your effectiveness.

Care Plan: Developing the Nurse-Client Relationship

WebLink Application: Communicating with Special Populations

Responding With Warmth

Warmth is so closely linked with empathy and respect that it is seldom communicated as an independent dimension. It is important, however, to note some additional points about the expression of warmth. Effusive, chatty, "buddy-buddy" behavior should not be confused with warmth. Warmth is most often conveyed in communications of respect and empathy.

Be aware of and accept the client's right to maintain distance (refer back to Figure 10-3 on page 188). Warmth and intimacy cannot be forced. Initially, high levels of warmth can be counterproductive for clients who have received little warmth from others in their lives, are suspicious, or have been taken advantage of by others. Warmth alone is insufficient for building a relationship and solving problems.

THERAPEUTIC COMMUNICATION SKILLS

Think of the communication techniques presented here as having the potential to foster effective communication. You must make them your own and adapt them individually for each human encounter. Blend them with the understanding you have gained from the interpersonal communication principles and practices discussed earlier in this chapter and the dimensions of self-knowledge that you examined in Chapter 3 ∞.

Be aware that using a set of communication skills as a sort of relationship "magic" will probably doom you to failure. Relationships, and the people in them, are unique and much too complex to rely on a communication formula that can be applied to all people and all situations. Remember that a holistic approach is inconsistent with the rigid, inflexible application of communication techniques.

Speaking to the Hard of Hearing

Be considerate and respectful when a client is hard of hearing. Here are some suggestions based on the work of Dreher (2001) for communicating with a client who is hard of hearing:

1. Move close enough to the client so that you are speaking from a distance of 3 to 6 feet.
2. Determine if the client hears better through one ear than the other. If so, speak into the good ear.
3. Choose an environment that is free of competing noise and turn off television sets, radios, and so on.
4. Place yourself so that the client can see you clearly, preferably with light on your face.
5. Make sure the client can see your lips and be careful not to obscure them with gestures or articles of clothing.
6. Speak at a natural rate. People comprehend faster than they speak, so it is not necessary for you to slow down unless the client does not understand.

If you fail to recognize and compensate for a client's hearing problem, you risk miscommunication.

Empathizing

Psychiatric–mental health nursing students are taught the skills of active listening. But listening without *empathy* is not enough. Empathic understanding not only increases your grasp of the client's difficulties but also helps you offer feedback on how the client affects others. Empathy can best be understood as a process through which people feel with one another. They are able to sense the feelings of another because they have evoked in themselves the attitude of the person to whom they are relating (in other words, they have engaged in role-taking, discussed earlier in this chapter). Central to learning the skill of empathizing is embracing the idea that what the client has to say or what the client feels is important (to the client) and deserves acknowledgment. A recent study of what it means to individuals with mental illness to be understood revealed three predominant themes: "I was important," "It really made us connect," and "They got on my level" (Shatell, McAllister, Hogan, & Thomas, 2006). Being empathic helps to connect with clients and validates their importance.

Empathic involvement with troubled clients can have a number of stressful consequences. Problems can arise at any phase in the empathy process. The obstacles to achieving an empathic concern for clients can be understood as a failure to cope with one of the four phases of achieving empathy. These four phases are discussed in Box 10-1. Be careful not to over-identify and lapse into sympathy for the client. By doing so, you may fail to incorporate the client's feelings and instead project personal ones. Bypassing the reverberation phase and substituting gut-level intuitions for rational problem solving can be another problem. Be sure to guard against overdistancing or burnout.

The term *empathy* is often mistakenly used synonymously with *sympathy*. Empathy contains no elements of condolence, agreement, or pity. When we sympathize rather than empathize, we assume that there is a parallel between our feelings and those of the client. The perceived similarity makes professional judgment and objectivity difficult. Sympathy can also be an appropriate response given the right circumstances. What Every Nurse Should Know discusses how to respond appropriately with sympathy.

Box 10-1 Four Phases of Therapeutic Empathizing

The process of empathic understanding has four phases:

1. **Identification.** Through the relaxation of conscious controls, we allow ourselves to become absorbed in contemplating the client and the client's experiences.
2. **Incorporation.** We take in the experiences of the client rather than attribute our own experiences and feelings to the client.
3. **Reverberation.** We interplay the internalized feelings of the client and our own experiences or fantasies. While fully absorbed in the client's identity, we still experience ourselves as separate personalities.
4. **Detachment.** We withdraw from subjective involvement and totally resume our own identity. We use the insight gained from the reverberation phase as well as reason and objectivity to offer responses that are useful to the client.

WHAT EVERY NURSE SHOULD KNOW

Expressing Sympathy to the Bereaved

Although empathizing is preferable to sympathizing when you are serving in a professional role, there are occasions in which sympathy is not only appropriate but helpful. One such example is when a client you are taking care of dies, or a friend, colleague, or acquaintance has just lost a loved one and you wish to reach out and offer support to the bereaved individual or family. Many people worry about finding the right words or worry that they will say the wrong thing. It is hard to go wrong if you are sincere in offering support. Remember that nonverbal messages enhance verbal messages and your sincerity when acknowledging the bereaved person's feelings will temper any words that are not quite perfect. Here are some suggestions for expressing sympathy in a therapeutic way:

- Celebrate the deceased person's life rather than dwell on the death. Not everyone gains comfort from hearing that a death "was a blessing" or that the deceased is "in a better place."
- Invite the bereaved person to talk, and listen carefully. Talking often helps the bereaved person feel better. Inviting the bereaved person to share stories about the deceased's life can be a healing experience.
- Share a good memory that you have about the deceased. Sharing memories, mementos, and photographs of the person who died may help spark happy memories.
- Be proactive in providing help. People in mourning may find making decisions taxing. Rather than asking if they would like help—making a dish, mowing the lawn, walking the dog, doing the food shopping—just go ahead and declare that you will do it.
- Keep checking in. There is often a rush of support from people wanting to help, but typically, support wanes quickly. Keep in mind that holidays and anniversaries of the person's death can be especially difficult and make an effort to let the person know that you care.

Doing something to provide comfort is much preferable to doing nothing because you are unsure of what to say.

Active Listening

Most of us assume that we are good listeners. The truth is that active listening requires *mindful* listening, which is more difficult than you might think. Mindfulness is the ability to consciously think about what you are doing and experiencing. It is more than being quiet while the other person talks—it requires paying undivided attention to what the client says, does, and feels, and putting aside your own judgments and ideas long enough to really hear. Mindful listening requires intention—that is, when you intend to really hear what another is saying, and what that other person thinks, feels, and needs, the better you can understand that person and his or her needs. If you don't listen mindfully, you won't be able to comprehend the message. If you don't comprehend the message, you

will not be able to effectively use the therapeutic communication techniques that follow.

There are several blocks to listening that may prevent you from hearing what the client is saying and convey the message that what he or she is saying is not very important:

1. Rehearsing: Being too busy planning what you are going to say next
2. Being concerned with yourself—your intelligence, your level of competence, your feelings, or your accomplishments
3. Assuming: Thinking that you know what the client "really means" because of your assumptions and hunches
4. Judging: Framing what you hear or what you see in terms of your judgment of the client as being wrong, immature, anxious, paranoid, or depressed
5. Identifying: Focusing on your own similar experiences, feelings, or beliefs when what the client says triggers your own memories or concerns
6. Getting off track: Changing the subject or making light of it when you become uncomfortable, bored, or tired
7. Filtering: Tuning out certain topics or hearing only certain things, perhaps because of anxiety, regardless of what else is said

Mindful listening is best accomplished when environmental distractions are minimized. Consider finding a quiet place, turning off the television, or closing the door if it is appropriate and safe. Avoid taking notes; they take your attention away from the client, and you will miss some of what is being said on the verbal level and done on the nonverbal level.

Face the client, use eye contact, show interest, and listen objectively while minimizing your own personal responses. Remaining silent while clients express themselves is a sign of respect and interest. Avoid interrupting the client because you feel the need to say or do something. Specific circumstances in which it is appropriate, for therapeutic reasons, to interrupt the client or steer the conversation in another direction are discussed in the chapters in Unit 3 ∞.

When listening, pay attention not only to what the client says (the verbal communication) but also to what the client does and how the client looks (the nonverbal communication). Nonverbal cues often shed light on what the client says. Although listening enables you to observe the client's nonverbal messages, it does not follow that you will necessarily interpret the nonverbal cues accurately. You should validate nonverbal cues with your clients.

Using Silence

Do not feel obligated to respond after every statement a client makes. *Using silence* goes beyond mindful listening and can be a very effective therapeutic technique when it encourages the client to communicate, when it allows the client time to ponder what has been said or a connection the client has made, when it allows the client time to collect his or her thoughts, or when it allows the client time to consider alternatives. Looking interested while maintaining an open posture or a questioning look will encourage the client to use the time effectively.

Break and analyze any uncomfortable silences. You would not want a client to become increasingly anxious or resistive. (See Chapters 8 and 18 ∞ for suggestions on handling anxiety and Chapter 4 ∞ for suggestions on handling resistance.)

Remember, silence is an effective communication technique only when it is used as an appropriate and purposeful therapeutic intervention. For example, clients who are depressed and feel pressured to interact will benefit from your silent, undemanding presence. Nurses who are silent because they are uncomfortable or because they lack the knowledge or the skill to communicate effectively must seek an experienced clinical supervisor to help them analyze their own personal and professional growth needs.

Reflecting

Reflecting is repeating the client's verbal or nonverbal message for the client's benefit. It encourages the client to become more actively involved. Reflecting also actively acknowledges what you have heard or seen.

Reflecting Content

Reflecting the *content* of the message basically repeats the client's statement. This gives clients the opportunity to hear and mull over what they have told you. Following are some examples:

- "The nurse believes things will be better soon."
- "The nurse thinks it would be better to take a part-time job."

Content reflection is perhaps one of the most misused and overused methods in mental health counseling. Use it judiciously. It loses its effectiveness when used for lack of other choices.

Reflecting Feelings

Reflecting *feelings* is verbalizing the implied feelings in the client's comment. Remember to respect the client's right to his or her opinion and feelings even when you may disagree with them. Following are some examples:

- "Sounds like you're really angry at your brother."
- "You're feeling anxious about being discharged from the hospital."

In reflecting feelings, you attempt to identify latent and connotative meanings that may either clarify or distort the content. Reflection is useful because it encourages the client to make additional clarifying comments.

Imparting Information

Imparting information helps the client by supplying additional data. This encourages further clarification based on new or additional input. Following are some examples:

- "Group therapy will be held on Tuesday evening from 6:30 until 8:00."
- "I am a nursing student."

It is not constructive to withhold useful information from the client or to reply "What do you think?" to a straightforward, information-seeking question. However, be careful not to cross the line between giving information and giving advice, or giving information as a way of avoiding an area of interpersonal difficulty. Also, by giving personal, social information you will likely move out of the realm of therapeutic intervention (see the discussion of self-disclosure in Chapter 3 ∞). Information that is important to disclose to the client to protect the client's rights includes your title and position. Resist the temptation to deny you are new to the field—it may only cause mistrust.

Remember that clients' participation in decision making begins when they take in and understand information about their own condition. The goal of imparting information should be to provide effective education that empowers clients and their families. Studies have shown that an educated, empowered client is more likely to achieve positive mental health outcomes and less likely to need admission or readmission to an acute care facility. You can help clients by using each teachable moment.

Avoiding Self-Disclosure

When you choose to avoid self-disclosure in a given instance (such as those discussed in the section on self-disclosure in Chapter 3 ∞), several communication techniques may be helpful. For instance, a client might ask you to disclose marital status, home address, religious affiliation, or a pressing personal problem. The following list offers practical and therapeutic ways to deflect a request for self-disclosure:

- *Use honesty.* "I don't share my home address with clients."
- *Use benign curiosity.* "I wonder why you're asking me this today?"
- *Use refocusing.* "You were talking about how your father treats you. I wonder why you changed the topic? You were saying that. . . ."
- *Use interpretation.* "I notice that every time you talk about your father, you change the subject and ask me a question." (pause)
- *Seek clarification.* "You keep asking me my home address. I wonder what concerns you might have about me today."
- *Respond with feedback and limit setting.* "I'm really uncomfortable when you ask me who pays my tuition. Talking about my finances isn't part of our agreement to work together." Adding "The last time we met, you were deciding if you were going to call your boss on the phone . . ." helps restructure the situation.

Use these communication techniques in the context of the therapeutic relationship, and assess and evaluate client responses in an ongoing manner with an instructor or clinical supervisor.

Clarifying

Sometimes, even though you've listened carefully, you're still not totally clear. In this situation, it is important to ask for clarification. *Clarifying* is an attempt to understand the basic nature of a client's statement. Following are some examples:

- "I'm confused about exactly what is upsetting to you. Could you go over that again, please?"
- "You say you're feeling anxious now. What's that like for you?"

Asking the client to give an example to clarify a meaning helps you understand the client's intended message better. A person who describes a concrete incident is more likely to see the connections between it and similar occurrences. Illustrations or examples are also very useful qualifiers.

Paraphrasing

The only way to know whether or not you have understood another person's message is to check your understanding of the facts and ideas by paraphrasing your understanding. In *paraphrasing,* you assimilate and restate in your own words what the client has said. Following are some examples:

- "In other words, you're fed up with being treated like a child."
- "I hear you saying that when people compliment you, you feel embarrassed. If they knew the real you, they'd stay away."

Paraphrasing gives you the opportunity to test your understanding of what a client is attempting to communicate and can dramatically reduce misunderstandings. It is reflective in nature, in that it lets the client know what you heard and how you understand what has been said. It also gives the client the opportunity to clarify content or feelings. People are more likely to trust and value those who paraphrase the content and their feelings (Beebe, 2011).

Checking Perceptions

Checking perceptions means sharing how one person perceives and hears another. After letting the client know what your perceptions of the client's behaviors, thoughts, and feelings are, ask the client to verify the perception. Asking someone to confirm your perception actively demonstrates that you are committed to understanding his or her behavior. It gives the other person the opportunity to correct inaccurate perceptions and allows you to avoid actions based on false assumptions about the client. Following are some examples:

- "Let me know if this is how you see it too."
- "When I see you fidgeting in your chair and tapping your foot, I get the feeling that you're uncomfortable when we're silent. Does that seem to fit?" or, "I know you said it doesn't matter, but when you frown, won't look at me, and fold your arms across your chest, it seems as if you're upset. Are you feeling angry?"

Perception checks are equally important in relationship to nonverbal behavior. When you observe a client's eye contact, posture, facial expression, gestures, or tone of voice you interpret what you think the client is expressing. Be sure to check the validity of your interpretation with the client by asking if it is accurate as in the examples in the bulleted list just provided.

Questioning

Questioning is a very direct way of speaking with clients. But when used to excess, questioning controls the nature and range of the client's responses. Questions can be useful when you are seeking specific information as in a structured mental health assessment (see Chapter 11∞) or when you are assessing a client for suicidal thoughts (see Chapter 23 ∞). When your intent is to engage the client in meaningful dialogue, however, you should limit questions.

When you do use questions, it is best to make them open-ended rather than closed. An *open-ended question* focuses the topic but allows freedom of response. Following are some examples:

- "How were you feeling when your mother said that to you?"
- "What's your opinion about . . . ?"

Asking a *closed-ended question* limits the client's choice of responses, generally to "yes" or "no" ("Were you feeling angry when your mother said that?"). Closed-ended questions limit therapeutic exploration. However, clients whose thinking is disorganized may need to be guided by closed-ended questions.

"Why" questions usually have the same effect. They are often impossible to answer and rarely lead to a clearer understanding of the situation. However, questions that include "who," "what," "when," and "how" may be helpful when used judiciously.

Be careful when questioning not to steer the client to answer in a certain way. For example, "You don't drink alcohol to excess, do you?" suggests that the client should answer "no."

Structuring

Structuring is an attempt to create order or evolve guidelines. It helps the client become aware of problems and the order in which the client might deal with them. Following are some examples:

- "You've mentioned that you want to improve your relationships with your wife, your sister, and your boss. Let's put them in order of priority."
- "No, I won't be giving you advice, but we can discuss some possible solutions together."

Structuring is particularly useful when clients introduce a number of concerns in a brief period and have little idea of where to begin. Use structuring not only to explore content but also to delimit the parameters of the nurse–client relationship and to identify how you will participate with the client in the problem-solving process.

Pinpointing

Pinpointing calls attention to certain kinds of statements and relationships. For example, you may point to inconsistencies among statements; to similarities and differences in the points of view, feelings, or actions of two or more people; or to differences between what one says and what one does.

- "So, you and your wife don't agree about how many children you want."
- "You say you're sad, but you're smiling."

Linking

In *linking,* you respond to the client in a way that ties together two events, experiences, feelings, or people. You can use linking to connect past experiences with current behaviors. Another example is linking the tension between two people with current life stress, as shown in the following examples:

- "You felt depressed after the birth of both your children."
- "So, the arguments didn't really begin until after you got your promotion."

Giving Feedback

Giving *feedback* is telling the other person your reaction to what he or she has said. It helps clients become aware of how their behavior affects others and how others perceive their actions. Responding with feedback is therapeutic self-disclosure on your part. It allows you to offer clients constructive information

that makes them aware of their effect on others. However, total self-disclosure by the nurse (discussed in greater detail in Chapter 3 ∞) is inappropriate in the nurse–client relationship. It places a burden of interdependence on the client and limits the time and energy available to work on the client's concerns. Reciprocal self-disclosure is more appropriate in friend and colleague relationships.

Effective feedback should be immediate (given as soon as possible), honest (giving your true reaction), and supportive (given in ways that are tolerable to hear and not hurtful or brutal). Following are some examples:

- "When you wring your hands, I feel your anxiety."
- "Sometimes when you turn your head away from me, I think you're angry."

It is important to give feedback in a way that does not threaten the client and result in increased defensiveness. The more defensive the client, the less likely the client will hear and understand the feedback. Feedback that is harsh, hurtful, or cruel, or appears to reject the client, creates barriers between yourself and the client. You want to do your best to prevent the client from experiencing your feedback as a personal rejection. Your Intervention Strategies lists strategies and rationales for giving helpful, nonthreatening feedback.

YOUR INTERVENTION STRATEGIES   Giving Helpful, Nonthreatening Feedback

Strategy	Rationale
Focus feedback on behavior rather than on client.	Refer to what client actually does rather than how you imagine client to be.
Focus feedback on observations rather than inferences.	Refer to what you actually see or hear client do; inferences refer to conclusions or assumptions you make about client.
Focus feedback on description rather than judgment.	Report what occurred rather than evaluating it in terms of good or bad, right or wrong.
Focus feedback on "more or less" rather than "either/or" descriptions of behavior.	"More or less" descriptions stress quantity rather than quality (which may be value-laden).
Focus feedback on here-and-now behavior rather than there-and-then behavior.	The most meaningful feedback is given as soon as it is appropriate to do so.
Focus feedback on sharing information and ideas rather than advice.	Sharing ideas and information helps client make decisions about own well-being; giving advice takes away client's freedom to be self-determining.
Focus feedback on exploration of alternatives rather than answers or solutions.	Focusing on a variety of alternatives for accomplishing a particular goal prevents premature acceptance of answers or solutions that may not be appropriate.
Focus feedback on its value to the client rather than on catharsis it provides you.	Feedback should serve client's needs, not your own.
Limit feedback to the amount of information client is able to use rather than the amount you have available to give.	Overloading will decrease effectiveness of feedback.
Limit feedback to the appropriate time and place.	Excellent feedback presented at an inappropriate time may be ineffective or harmful.
Focus feedback on what is said rather than why it is said.	Focusing on why things are said or done moves away from observations and toward motive or intent (which can only be assumed, unless verified).

Be aware that clients express not only information about themselves when they interact with you; but also information about how they perceive you. Cues about how your words and your behavior affect clients are there if you look for them. Be open and receptive to these unsolicited cues—the client's feedback to you—that can help you to become a more effective psychiatric–mental health nurse. The Your Self-Awareness feature in this section will help you to engage in self-reflection.

Confronting

Constructive confrontations often lead to productive change. *Confronting* is a deliberate invitation to examine some aspect of personal behavior that indicates a discrepancy between what the person says and what the person does. Confrontation requires careful attention to nonverbal communication and the discrepancies between nonverbal and verbal messages.

Confrontations may be informational or interpretive, and they may be directed toward both the resources and the limitations of the client. An *informational confrontation* describes the visible behavior of another person. Following is an example:

- "You say you're 'the dummy in the family,' yet none of your brothers or sisters made the honor roll like you did."

An *interpretive confrontation* expresses thoughts and feelings about the other's behavior and draws inferences about the meaning of the behavior. Following is an example:

- "Ever since Sally and Joe criticized the way you conducted the meeting, you haven't spoken to them. It looks like you're feeling angry."

YOUR SELF-AWARENESS
Reflecting on Feedback from Your Clients

Input—both positive and negative—from clients, classmates, instructors, staff, and family members and friends can help you to become aware of your "blind spots," the characteristics about yourself that you ignore, deny, or defend. Protecting oneself through self-deception interferes with both relating and communicating. To become more self-aware, do the following:

- Think about a recent interaction with a client and how that client responded to you.
- Identify the positive/negative elements in the interaction.
- Try to determine what the client was telling you about yourself in this interaction, that is: What characteristic(s) do you have that enables clients to openly express their thoughts and feelings? What characteristic(s) do you have that prevents clients from openly expressing their thoughts and feelings?
- Discuss the interaction and your interpretation of it with an instructor.
- Ask for feedback on your behavior from others—family members, classmates, staff, friends.

Six skills to be incorporated in constructive confrontations are as follows:

1. Use of personal statements with the words *I, my,* and *me*
2. Use of relationship statements expressing what you think or feel about the client in the here and now
3. Use of behavior descriptions (statements describing the visible behavior of the client)
4. Use of description of personal feelings, specifying the feeling by name
5. Use of responses aimed at understanding, such as paraphrasing and perception checking
6. Use of constructive feedback skills (see Your Intervention Strategies)

Summarizing

Summarizing highlights the main ideas expressed in an interaction. It shows the client that you understand. Both you and the client benefit from this review of the main themes of the conversation. Summarizing is also useful in focusing the client's thinking and aiding conscious learning. Following are some examples:

- "The last time we were together you were concerned about . . . ?"
- "You had three main concerns today."

You can use this technique appropriately at different times during an interaction. For example, it is useful to summarize the previous interaction in the first few minutes you and the client spend together. Early summarizing helps the client recall the areas discussed and gives the client the opportunity to see how you have synthesized the content of a previous session. Summarizing is useful because it keeps the participants directed toward a goal.

Injudicious use of summarizing is a common pitfall. You may rush to summarize despite other, more pressing and immediate client concerns. In this instance, summarizing is likely to meet your needs for structure but does nothing to address the client's here-and-now concerns.

Processing

Processing is a complex and sophisticated technique. Process comments direct attention to the interpersonal dynamics of the nurse–client experience—in the content, feelings, and behavior being expressed.

- "It seems that important things that need to be taken care of come up in the last 5 minutes we have together."
- "Today is the first day our time together has started out with silence. Last week it seemed there wouldn't be enough time."

As you can see, processing is an advanced skill. Processing is most useful when therapeutic intimacy has been achieved.

WHY I PLAN TO BECOME A PSYCHIATRIC–MENTAL HEALTH NURSE

Belinda's Story: I've known for 5 years that I want to be a psychiatric–mental health nurse. When I served in the Marine Corps, I was trained as a field medic and did two tours of duty in Afghanistan and then at the Pensacola Naval Hospital's outpatient psychiatric clinic. In both places, I saw several Marines who had big problems—they couldn't relax, they couldn't sleep, they had nightmares all the time. A lot of the veterans we saw started drinking too much and too often. They moved from marijuana to harder drugs, and some lost their jobs and their families. That's when I made up my mind to go into nursing school and learn as much as possible about stress and how it affects people. I have one more semester to go, and when that's done I'm going back into the service. I'll be joining the Army Nurse Corps and go to Officer Candidate School.

COMMON MISTAKES

When we are experiencing discomfort or strong negative feelings, it becomes difficult to empathize and to communicate with clients in a therapeutic way. Some common mistakes to guard against are as follows:

- *Giving advice.* Giving advice ("You should . . . ," "Why don't you . . . ," "It would be better if you . . .") carries the implicit message that the client is incapable of solving his or her own problem.
- *Minimizing or discounting feelings.* Telling a client that he or she is over-reacting, that there is nothing to be afraid of, or not to worry are attempts at reassurance that minimize and discount the client's feelings.
- *Deflecting.* Hearing clients express their pain can be anxiety provoking. Changing the subject or making a joke are attempts to move to something less painful. This is not a positive shift of focus—rather, it gives the client the message that you cannot or do not want to cope with the pain the client is feeling.
- *Interrogating.* Asking a barrage of questions implies that you are more interested in gathering information than you are in listening to the client.
- *Sparring.* No matter what the client says, you know better. Debating or disagreeing with the client prevents you from listening to the client.

CIRCUMVENTING POTENTIAL CULTURAL BARRIERS TO COMMUNICATION

When English is not the client's primary language and you are a monolingual provider, it will help if you select the words you use carefully, avoiding buzz words, slang, and technical jargon. Show respect by speaking clearly and directly to the client, pacing yourself to be neither too fast nor too slow. Words that are slurred, have many syllables in them, or are too technical make communication more difficult. Speaking too fast may overload the client and make it difficult for the client to follow. Speaking too slowly may lose the client's attention.

Select the gestures you use with care, using your nonverbal behavior to underscore your words and your actions. The proper use of gestures can clarify a message, and drawings can sometimes be helpful. Be careful however; as discussed earlier in this chapter, not all gestures mean the same thing in all cultures and some body language may be offensive or misunderstood.

Listen to your client's words and watch your client's gestures carefully. Do your best to understand and validate the meaning they have for you. Listening carefully to the client helps you avoid focusing on what you will say or do next and demonstrates your genuine concern for the client's distress.

If the client attempts to speak English, his or her thoughts may appear distorted when language is the real problem. There have been a number of documented instances in which people have been diagnosed as mentally disordered and confined to a mental hospital because mental health professionals erroneously diagnosed a language problem or value difference as disordered thinking or psychosis. Use open-ended questions and rephrase them in several ways to obtain accurate information.

An interpreter may be necessary if language is a barrier. If the client does not have his or her own interpreter, you may be able to enlist the aid of a bilingual staff member. For the sake of confidentiality and the client's privacy and reputation, avoid using family members as interpreters. Clients may not want family members privy to personal information (Martin & Nakayama, 2006), for example, sexual preference, drug or alcohol use, or content of hallucinations (what the voices say). Health and social services departments, international institutes, college language departments, neighborhood houses, or cultural centers will often know of people who are willing to volunteer as interpreters. Most health care facilities have contracts with interpreter services using a variety of technologies (three-way phones, computers, and videophone, etc.). Remember to always speak directly to the client and not to the interpreter.

Being aware of cultural phenomena that affect etiquette will be appreciated by the client. Spector (2009) suggests the following strategies:

1. Use the proper form of address for a given culture.
2. Know the ways by which people from that culture welcome one another, that is, when a handshake or embrace is expected as well as when physical contact is prohibited.
3. Be aware of when smiling indicates friendliness or is taboo, and when eye contact is a sign of respect or aggression.
4. Remember that gestures do not have universal meaning.

Emphasizing similarities can help to form a therapeutic relationship. Differences may serve as topics for discussion. An open, ongoing dialogue is beneficial for both parties because it promotes understanding.

Pearson Nursing Student Resources
Find additional review materials at
nursing.pearsonhighered.com
Prepare for success with NCLEX®-style practice questions,
interactive assignments and activities, web links, animations
and videos, and more!

REFERENCES

Bandler, R. (1993). *Time for a change*. Denver, CO: Meta Publications.

Beebe, S. A. (2011). *Interpersonal communication: Relating to others*. Upper Saddle River, NJ: Pearson Education.

Bigley, J., Griffiths, P. D., Prydderch, A., Romanowski, C. A., Miles, L., Lediard, H., & Hoggard, N. (2010). Neurolinguistic programming used to reduce the need for anesthesia in claustrophobic patients undergoing MRI. *British Journal of Radiology, 83*(986), 113–117.

Chang, G., Weiss, A. P., Orav, E. F., Jones, J. A., Finn, C. T., Gitlin, D. F., . . . Rauch, S. L. (2011). Hospital variability in emergency department length of stay for adult patients receiving psychiatric consultation: A prospective study. *Annals of Emergency Medicine*. Advance online publication. Retrieved January 10, 2011 from http://www.annemergmed.com/article/S0196-0644%2810%2901835-4/abstract

Dilts, R., Bandler, R., & Bandler, L. C. (1990). *Neurolinguistic programming*. Denver, CO: Meta Publications.

Dreher, B. B. (2001). *Communication skills for working with elders* (2nd ed.). New York, NY: Springer.

Hall, E. T. (1990). *The hidden dimension*. New York, NY: Knopf Doubleday.

Martin, J. N., & Nakayama, T. K. (2006). *Intercultural communication in context* (4th ed.). Philadelphia, PA: McGraw-Hill.

Ruesch, J. (1961). *Therapeutic communication*. New York, NY: Norton.

Ruesch, J., & Bateson, G. (1968). *Communication: The social matrix of psychiatry*. New York, NY: Norton.

Shafiei, T., Gaynor, N., & Farrell, G. (2011). The characteristics, management and outcomes of people identified with mental health issues in an emergency department, Melbourne, Australia. *Journal of Psychiatric and Mental Health Nursing, 18*(1), 9–16.

Shatell, M. M., McAllister, S., Hogan, B., & Thomas, S. P. (2006). "She took the time to make sure she understood": Mental health patients' experiences of being understood. *Archives of Psychiatric Nursing, 20*(5), 234–241.

Spector, R. E. (2009). *Cultural care: Guide to heritage assessment and health traditions* (6th ed.). Upper Saddle River, NJ: Prentice Hall.

Thomson, G., & Menzies, S. (2010). Effective interaction. Interview by Mary-Claire Mason. *Nursing Standard, 24*(31), 25.

Watzlawick, P. (1993). *The language of change: Elements of therapeutic communication*. New York, NY: Norton.

Watzlawick, P., Beavin, J., & Jackson, D. (1967). *The pragmatics of human communication*. New York, NY: Norton.

11

Psychiatric–Mental Health Assessment

EILEEN TRIGOBOFF
CAROL REN KNEISL

LEARNING OUTCOMES

After completing this chapter, you will be able to:

1. Perform an ongoing psychiatric–mental health assessment of clients in your care.
2. Determine how and when to apply assessment principles in professional practice.
3. Elicit a psychiatric history from a client and the client's family.
4. Conduct a mental status examination on a client.
5. Describe the essential components of physiological assessment, neurologic assessment, psychological testing, and psychosocial assessment.
6. Explain the importance of each of the five axes of the DSM multiaxial system to the overall assessment of clients and their families.
7. Incorporate the result of the GAF Scale in a nursing care plan for a client with a mental disorder.

CRITICAL THINKING CHALLENGE

You are responsible for an intake assessment with Jared, a 35-year-old male client. He is being admitted to inpatient care from an emergency department after driving his car off a highway into a building. His psychiatric diagnosis is major depression with psychotic features, and he has had prior hospitalizations for "suicidal gestures," as noted in his medical record. Most guidelines for conducting a mental status intake examination emphasize the importance of a suicide assessment, which includes questions such as "Have you ever thought of ending it all?", "Have you ever considered suicide?", or "Do you plan to hurt yourself?" In your interview, you ask if he is considering hurting himself again, and he says, "No."

Jared seems anxious and does express feeling, "down all the time." He mentions that, "You have better things to do than waste your time on just me."

1. You know he is not currently lethal, so what would your assessment focus on as the next priority?
2. When in your assessment would you discuss the types of antidepressants and other medications Jared is taking?
3. Would you consider Jared's statements evidence of a thought process disorder?

The systematic scientific approach known among nurses as the *nursing process* has evolved as the cornerstone of clinical practice. The nursing process begins with assessment, an ongoing action, that collects and analyzes objective and subjective data about the clients with whom we work.

THE NURSING ROLE IN ASSESSMENT

A comprehensive assessment will enable you to make sound clinical judgments and plan appropriate interventions. The primary sources of client data in most instances are the clients themselves. Nurses' documentation, psychological evaluations and tests, physicians' orders, social workers' information, and other secondary data sources can enlarge, clarify, and substantiate data obtained directly from the client.

Your assessment skills are essential and will be utilized throughout an individual client's care. Because nurses assess on an ongoing basis, success of a treatment regimen in every setting depends on a nurse's continual assessment.

PSYCHIATRIC EXAMINATION

Systems of data collection and assessment vary among mental health agencies. The psychiatric examination consists of two parts: the psychiatric history and the mental status exam. It is most often done during initial or early interactions with a client. The traditional psychiatric examination is discussed in this chapter because it is still used in settings where psychiatric nurses work and is considered the counterpart of the physical examination and history.

Psychiatric History

The **psychiatric history** gathers information about the client's current condition and previous diagnoses, interventions, and treatment, along with a family history.

Data Sources

Not all data gathered during psychiatric history taking are obtained from the client. There are several other sources. Family, friends, police, mental health personnel, neighbors, and others may contribute data to the psychiatric history. When the sources are varied, the psychiatric history focuses on the perceptions of others: how they see the client and the circumstances of the client's life. Always clearly indicate the sources of the information in the psychiatric history and their relationship to the client. Review and understand information given by these collateral sources in terms of that relationship.

The psychiatric history generally includes the following categories of data:

- *Complaint:* the main reason the client is having a psychiatric examination. The client may have personally initiated the psychiatric examination, or others (such as courts, hospital staff, family, referral from school or employer) may have initiated it. Record the "chief complaint" verbatim and use with quotation marks ("I just don't want to live any longer" or "I know these are crazy thoughts but I can't stop them. They're too strong.").

- *Present symptoms:* the nature of the onset and the development of symptoms. These data are usually traced from the present back to the last period of adaptive functioning.

- *Previous hospitalizations and mental health treatment:* information from the client, closed facility records, ancillary information.

- *Family history:* generally, whether any family members have ever sought or received mental health treatment.

- *Personal history:* the client's birth and development; past and recent illnesses; schooling and educational problems; occupation; sexual development, interests, and practices; marital history; the use of alcohol, drugs, caffeine, and tobacco; trauma history; and religious, spiritual, or cultural practices.

- *Personality:* the client's relationships with others, moods, feelings, interests, and leisure activities.

Input from family and friends can give you a better perspective of the client as well as insight into the psychosocial aspects of the circumstances in which the client lives. This input includes perceptions of the client by others (how they see the client), how symptoms are expressed in that environment, and patterns of interaction. Keep in mind that family and friends have their own perspectives through which they filter events. All information from family and friends is treated as important data to be contributed to the whole assessment and not necessarily a total picture of the client.

The main purpose of history taking is to gather information, although it is often also effective in establishing rapport with a client. The information the client offers will not likely emerge in the exact order of the forms you will complete. You can shape and guide the interview while allowing the client to provide information at a comfortable pace. You can also promote rapport by avoiding an interrogative approach and allowing the client's story to unfold naturally. For the most part, the assessment process involves inserting all collected data for documentation without maintaining a rigid structure.

Assessing for psychological symptoms is not substantially different for nurses in varying specialty areas. It may be more demanding to be an emergency department nurse and have to assess for emergent physical situations in addition to psychological symptoms; however, the basics remain the same. See What Every Nurse Should Know for an example of how you would assess in those circumstances.

Mental Status Examination

The **Mental Status Examination (MSE)** is usually a standardized procedure in agencies that use it. The primary purpose of the MSE is to help the examiner gather more objective data to be used in determining etiology, diagnosis, prognosis, and treatment, and to deal immediately with any risk of violence or harm. The sections of the MSE that deal with sensorium and intellect are particularly important in establishing the existence of delirium, dementia, amnestic, and other cognitive disorders. The purpose of the MSE differs

WHAT EVERY NURSE SHOULD KNOW

Assessing a Mentally Ill Client in the Emergency Department

People move quickly in the emergency department (ED). Lives hang in the balance; speed can make all the difference. Bringing a mentally ill client into this fast-paced environment requires adjustments in order to assess properly and provide good nursing care.

Verbal interactions are the main approaches appropriate for interacting with a mentally ill client in the ED, as opposed to the algorithms for physical care. Your assessment of a client with chronic psychiatric difficulties focuses on why the client is in the ED at this time. Something happened to make today different from yesterday, when the client was not in the ED. Ask questions about the current situation and what has changed for the client.

Other considerations for ED assessments of a mentally ill client include allowing for greater personal space than you would with someone receiving physical care. Physical contact may be interpreted entirely differently than usual, especially normally supportive gestures such as hand holding or shoulder touching.

Keep in mind that speed is not an asset under these circumstances. People who have psychiatric illnesses likely have cognitive difficulties, cannot absorb information quickly, have trouble concentrating and remembering, and need a quieter environment to reduce distractions. Using your assessment skills can promote client safety and enhance the movement of the client through the system in a timely manner (referred to as *ED throughput*).

from that of the psychiatric history in that it identifies the person's present mental status. The categories of information (not necessarily in the sequence presented here) follow in the next section.

General Behavior, Appearance, and Attitude

Provide a complete and accurate description of the client's physical characteristics, apparent age, manner of dress, use of cosmetics, personal hygiene, postures, gait, gestures, facial expression, mannerisms, general activity level, and responses to the MSE examiner.

For descriptive purposes, we will use excerpts from the MSE of Andrew, a client requesting services at a mental health clinic as a Clinical Example throughout this section.

Clinical Example

Andrew, a 35-year-old white male, appears stated age, dressed in torn, disheveled jeans. He presents with a tense facial expression, rigid posture, and a stiff gait. He has an elevated activity level in that he moves quickly and uses abrupt gestures.

Other descriptors that may be used include frank, friendly, irritable, dramatic, evasive, indifferent, and so forth. Details should be sufficient to identify and characterize the client.

Characteristics of Speech

The form, rather than the content, of the client's speech is described here. Speech is described in terms of how loud it is, and its flow, speed, quantity, level of coherence, and logic. You may include a sample of the client's conversation in quotation marks. The goal is to describe the quantity and quality of speech to discern difficulties in thought processes. In particular, note the following patterns, if present.

Mutism The client has no verbal response despite indications that the client is aware of your questions.

Circumstantiality The client's speech is cumbersome, convoluted, and has unnecessary detail in response to questions.

Perseveration This is a pattern of repeating the same words or movements despite apparent efforts to make a new response.

Flight of Ideas These are rapid, overly productive responses to questions that seem related only by chance associations between one sentence fragment and another; with flight of ideas, you might hear rhyming, clang associations, punning, and evidence of distractibility.

Blocking *Blocking* is a pattern of sudden silence in the stream of conversation for no obvious reason but is often thought to be associated with intrusion of delusional thoughts or hallucinations.

Andrew's speech is described in the following Clinical Example.

Clinical Example

He was cooperative. His speech was loud and he used an excessive number of words in his responses. There was some disjointed speech, with a pattern of topic shifts from himself to his ex-wife.

Emotional State

The person's pervasive or dominant mood or affective reaction is recorded here. Both subjective and objective data are included. Subjective data are obtained through the use of non-leading questions, for instance, "How are you feeling?" If the client replies with general terms, such as *nervous*, ask the client to describe how the nervousness shows itself and its effect, because such words may have different meanings to different individuals.

Observe objective signs, such as facial expression, motor behavior, the presence of tears, flushing, sweating, tachycardia, tremors, respiratory irregularities, states of excitement, fear, and depression. The attitude of the client toward the MSE examiner sometimes offers valuable clues. Note any hostility, suspiciousness, flirtatiousness, a desire for bodily contact, or outspoken criticism.

The psychiatric client is apt to have a persistent emotional trend reflective of a particular emotional disorder, such as depression. If this is true, probe further to discover the intensity and persistence of this reaction, in keeping with *Diagnostic and Statistical Manual of Mental Disorders,* 4th edition, Text Revision (DSM-IV-TR) criteria.

If possible, record verbatim the replies to questions concerning the client's mood. The relationship between mood and the content of thought is particularly significant. There may be a wide divergence between what clients say or do and their emotional state as expressed by attitudes or facial expressions.

Note whether intense emotional responses accompany discussion of specific topics. *Flat affect* is an insufficiently intense emotional display in association with ideas or situations that ordinarily would call for a stronger response. Dissociation or disharmony is often indicated by an inappropriate emotional response, such as smiling or silly behavior, when the attitude should be one of concern, anxiety, or sadness. It is difficult to evaluate emotional reactions in clients who use simulation or play-acting. Clients who are trying to cover up a deep depression may feign cheerfulness and good spirits.

The client's emotional reactions may be constant or may fluctuate during the examination. Try to specify the ease or readiness with which such changes occur in response to pleasant or unpleasant stimuli. You can use the following terms to describe intensity of response:

- Composed, complacent, frank, friendly, playful, teasing, silly, cheerful, boastful, elated, grandiose, ecstatic
- Tense, worried, anxious, pessimistic, sad, perplexed, bewildered, gloomy, depressed, frightened
- Aloof, superior, disdainful, distant, defensive, suspicious
- Irritable, resentful, hostile, sarcastic, angry, rageful, furious
- Indifferent, resigned, apathetic, dull, affectless

Pay attention to the influence of content on affect, and note especially disharmony between affect and content. Also important is constancy or change in the emotional state. The following Clinical Example continues with Andrew's MSE:

Clinical Example

His affect was slightly tense. His mood frustrated. "I really get upset when she doesn't inform me of stuff." There was a pessimistic tone to his descriptions, although this may be a recent change to his perspective.

Content of Thought

Special preoccupations and experiences such as *delusions,* illusions, or hallucinations, depersonalizations, obsessions or *compulsions,* phobias, fantasies, and daydreams are documented here. You can elicit these data by asking such questions as "Do you have any difficulties?" or "Have you been troubled or ill in any way?"

Delusions are false beliefs held even in the face of contradicting or no evidence. If the client has delusions of someone or something in the environment paying extra attention to him or her, some of the following questions might reveal them: "Do people like you?" "Have you ever been watched or spied on or singled out for special attention?" "Do others have it in for you?" If you suspect the client has delusions of being controlled by someone or something, ask the client such questions as "Do you ever feel your thoughts or actions are under any outside influences or control?" or "Are you able to influence others, to read their minds, or to put thoughts in their minds?" Chapter 16 ∞ discusses these psychotic symptoms in more detail. See both Rx Communications in this chapter for examples and rationales for these interactions.

Hallucinations are false sensory impressions with no external basis in fact. Hallucinations occur with the five senses of hearing, seeing, smelling, tasting, or touching. Try to elicit details of the experience—for example, the source of sounds or voices (from outside or inside the head), the clarity and distinctness of the perception, and the intensity. Be subtle when approaching the client for evidence of hallucinatory phenomena, unless the client is obviously hallucinating. In the case of obvious hallucinations, it is appropriate to ask direct questions.

Obsessions are insistent thoughts recognized as arising from the self. The client usually regards them as absurd and relatively meaningless, yet they persist despite endeavors to get rid of them. *Compulsions* are repetitive acts performed through some inner need or drive but supposedly against the client's wishes; yet not performing them results in tension and anxiety. *Fantasies* and *daydreams* are preoccupations that are often difficult to elicit from the client. The difficulty may be that the client is not sure what you want in terms of detail or is ashamed to discuss fantasies and daydreams because of their content. Fantasy is discussed in Chapter 8 ∞ .

Clinical Example

Although Andrew denied delusions or hallucinations, he seemed to be distracted during the interview. When asked a question he would pause and tip his head, mumble indistinctly, then answer the question. Andrew endorsed the distraction but stated there were sounds and noises in the room that, "You probably can't hear because I have super strong hearing." He denied current and past lethality.

R℞ COMMUNICATION

Assessing Your Client

CLIENT: "I don't trust you. You are just another one of those cogs in the big wheel meant to crush my spirit."

NURSE RESPONSE #1: "You're very uncomfortable, so let's get this done efficiently."	**NURSE RESPONSE #2:** "That tells me how hard this is for you, but let's put it into your words."
RATIONALE: Empathic reflection, redirection, guidance, and limit setting	*RATIONALE:* Accurate empathy, therapeutic reframing

R_X COMMUNICATION

Assessing Your Client

CLIENT: "They're all out to get me. I can't get a day without being interfered with and manipulated. I hear them talking about me even now."

NURSE RESPONSE #1: "You think that others have it in for you?"	**NURSE RESPONSE #2:** "Tell me the ways you've been coping so we can figure out what would be best for you."
RATIONALE: Focus on process, ventilation/catharsis of feelings.	*RATIONALE:* Focus on emotional process, seeking details of client's behaviors and planned actions.

Orientation

Document the client's orientation in terms of time, place, person, and self or purpose; it helps determine the presence of confusion or clouding of consciousness. You may ask, "Have you kept track of the time?" If so, "What is today's date?" Ask clients who say they do not know to estimate or guess the answer. Many clinicians begin the MSE with these questions because disorientation would raise the question of the validity and reliability of data obtained subsequently.

Clinical Example

Oriented to person, but not to time (stated the year as 2 years before), or place (did not know where he was). Reported having trouble because "I get so mad I get confused" and those incidents were related to mood. Denied alcohol abuse or substance use.

Memory

Attention span and ability to retain or recall past experiences in both the recent and remote past are tests of memory. If memory loss exists, determine whether it is constant or variable, and whether the loss is limited to a certain time period. Be alert to *confabulations*—memories invented to take the place of those the client cannot recall. It is useful to introduce questions relating to memory with some general question such as "How has your memory been?" Then you can move on to more specific questions such as "Have you had difficulty remembering where you put things or appointments?"

- *Recall of remote past experiences:* Ask for a review of the important events in the client's life. Then compare the response with information obtained from other sources during the history taking.
- *Recall of recent past experiences:* Ask for the events leading to the present seeking of treatment.
- *Retention and recall of immediate impressions:* Ask the client to repeat a name, an address, or a set of objects (for example, rose, teacup, and battleship) immediately and again after 3 to 5 minutes. Another test is to have the client repeat three-digit numbers at a rate of one per second, or repeat a complicated sentence.
- *General grasp and recall:* You might ask the client to read a story and then repeat the gist of the story to you with as many details as possible.

Clinical Example

Andrew's memory functions appeared grossly intact. Three objects named at the beginning of session were recalled without difficulty.

General Intellectual Level

This is a nonstandardized evaluation of intelligence. You are exploring the person's ability to use factual knowledge in a comprehensive way.

- *General grasp of information.* The client may be asked to name the five largest cities of the United States, the last four presidents, or the governor of the state.
- *Ability to calculate.* Tests of simple multiplication and addition are useful for this purpose. Another test consists of subtracting from one hundred by sevens until the person can go no further (serial sevens test).
- *Reasoning and judgment.* A common test of reasoning is to ask what the client might do with a gift of $10,000. Examiners must be particularly careful to correct for their own biases and values in assessing each client's answer.

Abstract Thinking

In this section of the MSE, you are asking the person to make distinctions between abstractions, for example asking what the difference is between poverty and misery or idleness and laziness. It is common to ask the client to interpret simple fables or proverbs such as "Don't cry over spilled milk."

Insight Evaluation

This section of the MSE determines whether clients recognize the significance of the present situation, whether they feel the need for treatment, and how they explain the symptoms. Often, it is helpful to ask clients for suggestions for their own treatment.

Summary

Summarize the important psychopathologic findings and a tentative diagnosis. Add to the summary any pertinent facts from the medical history and/or physical examination.

Mini-Mental State Exam

If there is not enough time to complete a full MSE, it is possible to fairly accurately assess and evaluate a client's functioning in a streamlined manner. The **Mini-Mental State Exam**

Box 11-1 MMSE Sample Items

- Orientation to Time—"What is today's date?"
- Registration—"Listen carefully, I am going to say three words. You say them back after I stop. Ready? Here they are: APPLE [pause], PURPLE [pause], SPOON [pause]. Now repeat those words back to me." [Repeat up to 5 times, but score only the first trial.]
- Naming—"What is this?" [Point to a wristwatch.]
- Reading—"Please read this and do what it says." [Show examinee a piece of paper with the following instruction written on it, "Close your eyes."]

Source: Mini-Mental State Examination, by Marshal Folstein and Susan Folstein, Copyright 1975, 1998, 2001 by Mini Mental LLC, Inc. Published 2001 by Psychological Assessment Resources, Inc.

(MMSE) (Folstein, Folstein, & McHugh, 1975) provides a framework for such an assessment. The main focus of the exam is cognitive functioning, although you can ascertain the client's mood in the process.

For the test to be efficient and valid, you must ask the questions in the order they are listed. Box 11-1 shows four sections of the MMSE and the general area of information the questions address. A total of 11 questions cover the scope of a client's thinking and reactions. Scores are assigned to each question, and the total score indicates the likelihood and level of cognitive decline. The maximum score is 30 points, and the score is represented as a fraction with the actual points scored as the numerator and 30 points as the denominator (e.g., 28/30, 20/30, etc.).

It is important to note that there are limitations to using the MMSE with people who have certain disabilities with sight or motor movement related to writing. If a client is not able to perform one of the activities, it may be necessary to conduct a full MSE or to document the results of the relevant aspects of the MMSE without a score.

Nurses' Observation Scale for Inpatient Evaluations

An assessment tool designed specifically for use by inpatient nurses is the **Nurses' Observation Scale for Inpatient Evaluations (NOSIE).** Developed and determined to be a valid and reliable tool in 1966 (Honigfeld, Gillis, & Klett, 1966), it has been useful in quickly assessing client functioning on positive features and negative features. Because you can complete this by observing and assessing, it is extremely useful with individuals who refuse to divulge information or are so agitated that closer interactions would not be safe or productive. The NOSIE comes in a long and short version and takes place within a specific time period, typically within 3 days of admission.

PHYSIOLOGICAL ASSESSMENT

As the summary of the MSE suggests, carefully consider the possibility that a client's symptoms may have a physiological or, in particular, a neurologic basis. In some reported instances, clients with brain tumors or bromide intoxication have been hospitalized on psychiatric units and treated exclusively for their apparent psychiatric symptoms. Such a critical oversight obviously delays and seriously hampers appropriate treatment

of the correct biologic or neurologic problem. We cannot overemphasize the value of careful assessment regarding general health issues and screening for biologic disorders. In many community settings, psychiatric–mental health nurses are the only mental health care providers prepared to undertake a biologic and neurologic assessment and interpret the results.

The objectives of a biologic and neurologic assessment are as follows:

1. Detection of underlying, and perhaps unsuspected, organic disease that may be responsible for psychiatric symptoms
2. Understanding disease as a factor in the overall psychiatric disability
3. Appreciation of somatic symptoms that reflect primarily psychological rather than physiological problems

Biologic History Taking

Taking the client's history is an important procedure among several that can contribute to a fuller understanding of the biologic aspects of psychiatric symptoms. Inquire into three primary areas of a client's biologic history:

1. Facts about known physical diseases and dysfunction
2. Information about specific physical complaints
3. General health history

Information about previous illnesses may provide essential clues. Clients with comorbidities of substance abuse and mental disorder are particularly challenging. For example, suppose a client's presenting symptoms include paranoid delusions and the client has a history of similar episodes. During each previous episode, the client responded to diverse forms of treatment and demonstrated no residual symptoms. This history suggests a strong possibility of amphetamine- or other drug-related psychosis, and a drug screen laboratory test may be indicated. An occupational history may provide information about exposure to inorganic mercury, leading to symptoms of psychosis, or exposure to lead, resulting in mental disorder.

The second area of emphasis in biologic history taking is eliciting information from the client about specific physical complaints. Again, it is crucial to consider symptoms in terms of both psychiatric conditions and physical diseases. Symptoms that are atypical of psychiatric disorders are particularly revealing clues. For example, suppose a client with hallucinations and delusions also complains of a severe headache at the onset of the symptoms. All symptoms together suggest possible brain disease and call for careful and repeated neurologic assessment and use of brain imaging techniques.

History taking should also include information about medications the client is currently taking. Digitalis intoxication may result in visual distortions that may be interpreted as hallucinations. Reserpine may produce symptoms generally considered psychiatric in nature. Complications such as ataxia and slurred speech could arise from combining the antidepressant medication category selective serotonin reuptake inhibitor

YOUR ASSESSMENT APPROACH   Basic Sleep Pattern Assessment

Sample questions for assessing a client's basic sleep patterns are as follows.

Sleep–Wake Schedule

What time do you usually go to bed?

How long does it usually take you to fall asleep after you have turned off the light?

What time do you usually wake up?

What is different about your sleep–wake schedule on the weekend/days off?

How often do you take naps? (Be alert here for cultural influence, such as taking siestas, or occupational influence.) Under what circumstances?

Getting to Sleep

What helps you get to sleep?

What makes it difficult for you to get to sleep?

Staying Asleep

On average, how many times do you wake up during the night?

What seems to waken you?

How long does it usually take to get back to sleep?

What do you do if you are having trouble getting back to sleep?

Waking Up

How difficult is it for you to wake up?

How soon after waking up do you usually get up?

How do you feel when you first get up?

Daytime Functioning

At what time of day do you usually feel most energetic?

At what time of day do you feel most sleepy?

Would you call yourself a "morning person" or an "evening person"?

Satisfaction With Sleep; Potential Problems

How satisfied are you with the sleep you usually get?

Do you think you get enough sleep on average? How do you know?

How has your sleep been during the past 2 weeks in comparison to what is normal for you?

Are you concerned about any of the following things?

- Getting to sleep
- Waking up too many times during the night
- Waking up too early
- Having to fight sleepiness during the day
- Snoring, restlessness, talking or walking in your sleep
- Bad dreams
- Drinking too much coffee (or other caffeine/nicotine sources)

When do you enjoy sleep the most?

(SSRI) with a naturally occurring monoamine oxidase inhibitor (MAOI), which is the herb St. John's wort (Fontaine, 2011).

The third area is the general health history. As mentioned earlier, psychiatric nurses need to assess for a variety of general health problems and must therefore have medical–surgical nursing skills. During your assessment of any client, assess for medical problems as well as the psychiatric symptomatology. A good gauge of a client's health and psychiatric status is the client's sleep patterns. Consider asking the questions on the Your Assessment Approach feature to determine if a problem exists. Keep in mind that some medical problems are masked by psychiatric symptoms and that psychiatric symptomatology can be the result of a medical disorder. Chapter 8∞ has a discussion of psychological factors affecting medical conditions.

Observation

Observation also yields important data bearing on the possible presence of organic disorders. Some examples follow:

- An unsteady gait may suggest diffuse brain disease or alcohol or drug intoxication.
- Asymmetry—dragging a leg or not swinging one arm—might be a sign of a focal brain lesion.
- Although inattention to proper hygiene and dress, particularly mismatched socks or shoes, is common in people with emotional disorders, it is also a hallmark of dementia.

- Frequent, quick, purposeless movements are characteristic of anxiety, but they are equally characteristic of chorea and hyperthyroidism.
- Tremors accompanied by anxiety may point to Parkinson's disease.
- Recent weight loss, although often encountered in depression and schizophrenia, may be due to gastrointestinal disease, carcinoma, Addison's disease, and a number of other physical disorders.

Observe skin color, pupillary changes, alertness and responsiveness, and quality of speech and word production, keeping in mind the possibility of delirium, dementia, substance intoxication, or other medical conditions.

NEUROLOGIC ASSESSMENT

A careful neurologic assessment is mandatory for each client suspected of having brain dysfunction. Its goal is to discover signs pointing to circumscribed, focal cerebral dysfunction or diffuse, bilateral cerebral disease.

Brain Imaging Techniques

As described in Chapter 6∞, a range of brain imaging techniques are now available for viewing the living brain to detect seizure activity; evaluate sleep disorders; detect disorders such as multiple sclerosis; detect tumors, trauma, and strokes; examine the blood flowing to the brain; and identify cerebral

(a)   (b)

FIGURE 11-1 ▪ This frontal lobe glioblastoma multiforme, a primary tumor, is metabolically very hot. (a) Note the large red area of the tumor. (b) The same tumor at a different level in the brain.

Photo courtesy of Dr. Giovanni DiChiro and Dr. Ramesh Raman of the Neuroimaging Branch, National Institute of Neurological Disorders and Stroke, National Institutes of Health.

atrophy, cerebral hemorrhage, cerebral infarct, hematomas, and abscesses. All of these conditions may present as psychiatric or behavioral symptoms. The most frequently used brain imaging techniques are described in Box 6-1, "Tools of Psychobiology," in Chapter 6 ∞ (page 91). The positron-emission tomography (PET) scan brain image (see FIGURE 11- 1 ▪) shows two scans of the same brain tumor (glioma) at different areas (levels) of the brain.

Mental health practitioners understand the need for thorough biologic and neurologic assessment of clients seen in psychiatric settings. The psychiatric literature abounds with accounts of clients whose symptoms were initially considered exclusively psychiatric but ultimately proved medical, especially neurologic. Assessment errors occurred not because the symptoms did not suggest medical disease but because such symptoms were given too little weight or were misinterpreted. Changes in the American Psychiatric Association's (APA's) DSM-IV-TR (2000) require that both medical condition and substance abuse be ruled out as conditions resulting in psychiatric symptoms.

PSYCHOLOGICAL TESTING

Clinical psychologists administer and interpret a wide variety of psychological tests. There are two categories—those concerned with personality and those concerned with cognitive function.

Personality Tests

There are objective and projective personality tests.

Objective Personality Tests

Objective personality tests provide data on various aspects of the client's personality, which are scored or analyzed using empirically derived criteria.

- **Minnesota Multiphasic Personality Inventory–2 (MMPI–2)** is a true–false test. There are 10 major clinical scales measured in this test that include paranoia, schizophrenia, depression, mania, and anxiety.
- **State–Trait Anxiety Inventory** is a self-report instrument. It measures state anxiety (a transitory emotional state characterized by consciously perceived feelings of tension and apprehension and heightened autonomic nervous system activity) and trait anxiety (relatively stable individual differences in vulnerability to anxiety) (Spielberger, 1976).
- **Millon Clinical Multiaxial Inventory–II (MCMI–II)** consists of true–false questions. This test can provide valuable assistance in clarifying underlying consistent personality features.
- **Beck Depression Inventory** consists of questions that ask the client to rate the presence and intensity of various symptoms of depression.

Projective Personality Tests

Projective personality tests involve presenting the client with a somewhat ambiguous stimulus, often a visual one, to which the client responds with his or her own perception. It is thought that in this process the client projects something of himself or herself into the response.

- The **Rorschach Test** consists of 10 standardized inkblots on separate cards. Clients are asked to state what the inkblots look like to them, and why.
- The **Thematic Apperception Test (TAT)** cards are pictures of people in various situations. Clients are asked to describe what seems to be happening in the

picture, what the people are feeling and thinking, and how the situation will be resolved. Because the pictures are ambiguous, the responses are thought to reveal aspects of the clients' own emotional lives.

- The **Sentence Completion Test** asks clients to complete an extensive series of incomplete sentences with the first thoughts that come to mind.

Cognitive Function Tests

Cognitive function tests generally measure how well, or how poorly, a person is able to think and process information. The information processed contributes to intellectual functioning and is counted as a gauge of intelligence.

Common Cognitive Function Tests

Common cognitive function tests are as follows:

- The **Wechsler Adult Intelligence Scale–IV (WAIS–IV)** consists of a number of subtests for the derivation of intelligence quotient (IQ) scores.
- **Raven's Progressive Matrices Test** asks the client to solve two-dimensional visual–spatial problems of increasing difficulty, problems that are relatively culturally unbiased.
- The **Benton Visual Retention Test** is an example of a neuropsychological assessment instrument and is sometimes used as a quick screening device to see if the test taker may be manifesting signs of cognitive dysfunction. The test taker is asked to reproduce various geometric designs after examining the designs for a few seconds.

PSYCHIATRIC DIAGNOSTIC PRACTICE ACCORDING TO THE DSM

As Chapter 1∞ demonstrated, determining that someone is mentally ill is often a matter of judgment. Individual perceptions and social context influence how we distinguish normality from abnormality. A now classic study that voiced doubts about the validity of psychiatric diagnosis is at least partly responsible for revamping the system of psychiatric diagnosis.

In this study, David Rosenhan (1973) enlisted the assistance of 8 pseudopatients who sought admission to a variety of mental hospitals in 5 states. The pseudopatients arrived at the hospitals complaining of one false symptom—hearing voices. Other than this false symptom, they acted as they normally would and gave accurate information when interviewed for a psychiatric history and mental status examination. All were admitted to the mental hospitals to which they applied. There were a total of 12 admissions (some pseudopatients did it twice). In all but one case, the admitting diagnosis was schizophrenia.

Once in the hospital, the pseudopatients stopped simulating the symptom (hearing voices) and behaved in their usual manner. The average length of stay was 19 days; the range was 7 to 52 days. While in the hospital, the pseudopatients openly took notes on their experiences. Their note taking was not hidden from the staff or the other clients. An examination of their charts after the study was concluded revealed that the staff viewed the note taking solely as a symptom of the pseudopatients' mental disorder. They were discharged with a diagnosis of schizophrenia in remission (indicating that the disorder is currently under control). In other words, the normality of the pseudopatients was unrecognized even when they were released after ample opportunity for observation by the staff.

Interestingly, the other clients recognized the normality of the pseudopatients more frequently than did the professional staff. Many clients told them something like, "You're not crazy. You're a journalist or a professor checking up on the hospital." On the other hand, the pseudopatients were impressed by the largely normal quality of the real clients' behavior. They also revealed that the staff spent surprisingly little time interacting with the clients and concluded that people with mental illness act in a deviant manner only a small fraction of the time. This lack of interaction presumably contributed to the staff's failure to detect that the pseudopatients were normal.

Rosenhan's study provoked a great deal of controversy. In defense of the hospitals and their staffs, critics of the study argued that it would have been inhumane to turn an individual away who was hearing voices and that hearing voices made schizophrenia the most probable diagnosis. This is undeniably true. However, it overlooks the fact that the hospital staffs did not have to make an immediate diagnosis based on one symptom alone. They could have deferred a diagnosis pending further observation and assessment.

The subsequent revisions of the DSM led to substantial increases in diagnostic consistency. Let us look at how this system has evolved into its current form. The American Psychiatric Association (APA) published the first edition of the DSM in 1952. The DSM-IV-TR (the "TR" stands for Text Revision), published in 2000, represents the current state of knowledge about diagnosing mental disorders. DSM-5 (the Roman numeral is being replaced with the Arabic number) is nearing publication at this writing. The continual evolution of this specialty area is represented in the changes made from the original DSM. It is composed of a list of all the official numeric codes and terms for all recognized mental disorders, along with a comprehensive description of each and specified diagnostic criteria that must be present in order to make each diagnosis. Each edition contains updated information regarding numerous clinical issues such as prevalence and comorbidity, among others. (For a complete list of codes and diagnoses according to the DSM-IV-TR, see this text's Appendix A ∞ .)

The DSM uses a language describing mental health and disorders that is used by many specialty disciplines in psychiatry–mental health. Nurses use the DSM in two primary ways: We use the diagnostic categories to communicate with other professionals using a common framework, and we use the research presented for causes and prevalence in discussions with clients and their families. Read the Your Self-Awareness feature to determine your abilities to communicate. Details on the specific theories of mental health and disorders are in Chapter 5 ∞ .

YOUR SELF-AWARENESS
Evaluating Your Own Assessment Skills

Evaluate your assessment skills by responding to the following:

1. Can you ask an open-ended question and not anticipate the answer?
2. Are you able to remain silent during an interview without being uncomfortable?
3. Do you accept information given to you without criticism or judgment?
4. Can you show empathy, not sympathy, for others' problems?
5. Gauge your tolerance for unusual or abnormal behavior.
6. Evaluate how aware you are of other cultures and their expressions of distress.
7. What is your skill level for understanding the content of what is said to you as well as the process (how things are said, not said, done, and not done)?
8. Do you have success getting your message across to others?
9. Have you been able to make necessary changes when you received feedback on your interactions?
10. Rate your skills for assessing someone accurately on a scale of 0 to 10, with 0 being the lowest level and 10 being the highest. (For example, use a brief interaction with a new colleague and then discuss your assessment with the colleague.) Discover your weak assessment areas and work on improving them (and raising your score). Repeat regularly.

Basic Principles of the Multiaxial System

In the DSM multiaxial system, every person is evaluated on five axes, each dealing with a different class of information about the client. DSM's multiaxial assessment is congruent with holistic views of people, recognizes the role of environmental stress in influencing behavior, and requires that the clinician collect data about client adaptive strengths as well as about symptoms or problems. One of the most important features of the DSM is increased interclinician reliability resulting from the use of specified observable criteria that have been field tested for inter-rater reliability. Its multiaxial approach is of significance to psychiatric–mental health nursing because it expresses the multidimensionality of human responses to environment, one of the hallmarks of the nursing process.

The following example illustrates the principle behind a multiaxial system.

Clinical Example

A 54-year-old woman came to an outpatient mental health clinic for evaluation and treatment of severe fear and avoidance of flying that amounted to a phobia. However, she also had a long-term personality disturbance and had noticeable eczema.

Suppose three different clinicians were asked to evaluate this woman. A biologically oriented clinician would certainly diagnose the eczema but might fail to notice the personality disturbance and make little of the phobia. A psychodynamically oriented clinician would be sure to diagnose the personality disorder but might overlook the eczema and the phobia, considering them to be merely manifestations of the underlying personality disturbance. Finally, a clinician who was behaviorally oriented would notice the phobia but might not diagnose the personality disturbance and the eczema. It is clear, then, that because of their differing theoretic orientations, these clinicians have a rather high likelihood of diagnostic disagreement.

Now suppose the same three clinicians were required to evaluate her in each of three different areas of functioning: behavioral or psychological, personality, and physical functioning. In this case, all three clinicians would be much more likely to diagnose all three conditions and thus, their evaluations are much more likely to be congruent.

The DSM multiaxial system includes the five axes described below. Axes I and II include all the mental disorders in the DSM and therefore might be said to represent the intrapersonal or *psychological* area of functioning. Axis III is for recording general medical conditions related to understanding the cause of psychiatric symptoms and treating the individual and thus represents the area of physical functioning. Axes IV and V, for identifying psychosocial and environmental problems and the Global Assessment of Functioning (GAF) scale, include an assessment of social functioning. In this sense, the multiaxial system provides a comprehensive biopsychosocial approach to assessment.

Description of the Axes

The following are the components of the multiaxial system.

Axis I: Clinical Disorders Axis I includes all of the Adult and Child Clinical Disorders. Axis I also contains other conditions that may be a focus of clinical attention, but it is not universally agreed that these conditions actually constitute clinical syndromes. Nevertheless, the symptoms elucidated in these conditions are observed often enough to warrant their inclusion in the diagnostic array available to clinicians. These include psychological factors that would affect a physical condition, medication-induced movement disorders, and relational problems. More specific examples include such conditions as marital problems, occupational problems, and parent–child problems, in which the problem being evaluated, or for which clinical care is sought, is not due to a mental disorder.

A mental disorder is differentiated from other problems as a clinically significant behavioral or psychological syndrome or pattern that occurs in an individual. A mental disorder is associated with either a painful symptom (distress) or impairment in functioning (disability), or with an increased risk of suffering, death, pain, disability, or loss of freedom. Further, the distress or disability does not primarily reflect a sanctioned response to an event, deviant behavior, or conflict between an individual and society.

Clinical Example

A man with bipolar disorder that has been in remission for many years develops marital difficulties for reasons unrelated to his psychiatric history or condition. He and his wife have been arguing about her intent to resume a career.

Both "marital problem" and "bipolar disorder in remission" could be recorded on Axis I. If, however, the bipolar disorder is not in complete remission, and marital conflict develops as a result of the client's changeable moods and other symptoms associated with the mental disorder, the marital problem would not be recorded in addition to the bipolar disorder, because the marital problem in this case is due to the client's mental disorder.

Axis II: Personality Disorders Axis II contains the personality disorders, usually diagnosed in adults, and developmental disorders including **intellectual disability** (formerly labeled *mental retardation,* and describes impaired cognitive functioning and adapting), diagnosed in children and adolescents. Axis II is also used to report maladaptive personality traits. All the remaining mental disorders of adults and children and associated conditions are recorded on Axis I.

The classes of disorders on Axis II were given their own axis because their usually mild and chronic symptoms are often overshadowed by a more problematic Axis I condition. DSM clarifies the distinction between Axis I and Axis II by noting that Axis II conditions have an early onset and a stable, not episodic, course. Axis II also has options for describing the lack of a diagnosis or condition on the axis.

Axis III: General Medical Conditions Clinicians use Axis III to record physical disorders and medical conditions that must be taken into account in planning treatment, or that are relevant to understanding the etiology or worsening of the mental disorder. A clinician might also want to record other significant physical findings, such as "soft" neurologic signs or even a single symptom (such as vomiting).

If there is a lack of information on Axis III, you should state that fact as: "No information," or "Diagnosis deferred—not evaluated," or "Referred to Dr. Smith for her evaluation." In any event, you should note *something* on this axis; omitting it for lack of information undermines the purpose of a holistic, multiaxial system. Of course, recent advances in psychobiologic knowledge make Axis III findings particularly important for psychiatric–mental health nursing.

Axis IV: Psychosocial and Environmental Problems Axis IV is used to identify psychosocial problems that may affect the diagnosis and treatment of mental disorders. General categories of psychosocial problems are listed in Appendix A∞ on page 772. In addition to identifying the type of problem(s), evaluators should also note in their own words the specific problems they consider pertinent.

Axis V: Global Assessment of Functioning Axis V, the **Global Assessment of Functioning (GAF)**, reports on the client's overall level of functioning. This information is useful in planning treatment and measuring its impact, and in predicting outcomes. You can perform the reporting of overall functioning on Axis V using the GAF Scale as shown in Appendix A∞ on page 772. The GAF Scale gives the clinician an opportunity to examine the overall impact of the client's circumstances on psychological, social, and occupational performance. The ratings on this scale fall within decile ranges and track both symptom severity and functional level. When symptoms and functioning are at different levels, the worse of the two is shown through the score. For example, if a client has moderate symptoms and severe problems functioning, the rating would demarcate the severe problems in functioning. If a client's functioning is basically unimpaired but the symptoms experienced are significant, the symptom level would be represented in the GAF rating. Generally, ratings on the GAF Scale reflect the client's current level of functioning, meaning the lowest level of functioning within the previous 7 days.

One of the most accurate indicators of clinical outcome is the individual's sustained level of premorbid functioning. For this reason, the GAF Scale can be used to rate the highest level of psychological, social, and occupational functioning that an individual was able to sustain for at least a few months during the previous year as well as at the time of evaluation.

PSYCHOSOCIAL ASSESSMENT

Psychosocial assessment is a dynamic process. It begins during the initial contact with the client and continues throughout your nurse–client experience. Individual psychosocial assessments are an option, as are family or group psychosocial assessments. Family and group assessments are discussed in Chapters 28 and 29∞. In every case, they begin with the identifying characteristics, such as name, gender, age, marital status, and ethnic and cultural origins. Problem identification and definition are also necessary phases in the assessment process.

Individual Assessment

During the individual assessment, consider the following factors:

1. Physical and intellectual
   a. Presence of physical illness and/or disability
   b. Appearance and energy level
   c. Current and potential levels of intellectual functioning

d. How the client sees his or her personal world and translates events around self; client's perceptual abilities

e. Cause-and-effect reasoning; ability to focus

2. Socioeconomic factors

a. Economic factors—level of income and adequacy of subsistence, and their effect on lifestyle, sense of adequacy, and self-worth

b. Employment and attitudes about it

c. Racial, cultural, and ethnic identification; sense of identity and belonging

d. Religious identification can be linked to significant value systems, norms, and spiritual practices. Spirituality and its meaning for the client are a part of the Psychosocial Assessment. Attachment to a system of meaning, whatever that system may be, can be an asset. (See the Caring for the Spirit feature for sample questions that you can use during a spiritual health assessment.)

3. Personal values and goals

a. Presence or absence of congruence between values and their expression in action; meaning of values to individual

b. Congruence between the individual's values and goals and the immediate systems with which the client interacts

c. Congruence between the individual's values and the assessor's values; how agreement or divergence regarding values impacts intervention

4. Adaptive functioning and response to present involvement

a. Manner in which the individual presents self to others—grooming, appearance, posture

b. Emotional tone and change or constancy of levels

c. Style of communication—verbal and nonverbal; ability to express appropriate emotion, follow train of thought; factors of dissonance, confusion, uncertainty

d. Symptoms or symptomatic behavior

e. Quality of relationships the individual seeks to establish—direction, purposes, and uses of such relationships by the individual

f. Perception of self

g. Social roles that are assumed or ascribed; competence in fulfilling these roles

h. Relational behavior:
- Capacity for intimacy
- Degree of dependence or independence on a continuum from one extreme to the other
- Power and control conflicts
- Exploitative nature
- Openness

5. Developmental factors

a. How role performance equates with life stage

b. How developmental experiences have been interpreted and used

c. How past conflicts, tasks, and problems have been handled

d. Whether the present problem is unique in the person's life experience

The Place of Assessment in Practice

Assessment is essential in clinical practice and serves several purposes:

- Identifying problems
- Identifying client motivations, strengths, and resources
- Identifying forces (both internal and external to the client) that may hinder the team's therapeutic plan

---

CARING FOR THE SPIRIT

Spiritual Health Assessment

For these first five statements, indicate whether you *never*, *sometimes*, *often*, or *nearly always* agree.

1. I trust myself.
2. I feel my life has meaning and purpose.
3. Other people give meaning to my life.
4. I trust other people.
5. I have close friends.
6. I have experienced the following in my life:
   Loss _____ Separation _____ Divorce _____
   Geographic moves _____ Rejection _____ Death _____
7. Do *religion* and *spirituality* mean the same thing to you? If not, what are the differences to you?
8. With 1 being the lowest and 10 the highest, place an X on the following scale to indicate your relationship with your higher power, and circle the place on the scale that you feel would be ideal for your relationship with your higher power. Explain why you chose each of these points.

(no relationship)		(turn only problems over)		(turn total self over)	
1 2 3		4 5 6 7		8 9 10	

9. My religious upbringing and background can be described as (check as many as apply):
   Nurturing _____ Helpful _____ Strict _____
   Conservative _____ Liberal _____ Punishing _____
   Negative _____ Had very little _____ Had none _____

- Setting reasonable goals with the client, given who the client is at this time
- Determining appropriate intervention strategies
- Providing continuous evaluation of the process and indicating when the therapeutic plan should be changed

Assessment is an ongoing, dynamic process that utilizes all your senses and all your skills. Your observations, combined with all the information you receive from the client, interdisciplinary team members, and collateral sources provide an opportunity to engage in a partnership based on mutual definition of problems and goals. If a client says, "I'd be better off dead," you must assess the lethality risk and intervene to prioritize the client's safety. If you see physical signs of abuse such as bruises in various stages of healing without adequate explanation, your assessment warrants a private interview with the client during which you can ask, "Does anyone ever hurt you?" If treatment does not seem to be addressing the main symptoms or side effects from medications seem to cause flagging focus on continued adherence, assess the client's reactions and discuss options (Adams, Holland, & Urban, 2011).

Assessment is the solid base upon which you build your practice and perform your interventions. See the Evidence-Based Practice feature for an example of how assessment of the client and the environment are vital to good nursing care. Information and services that help nurses, physicians, consumers, other providers, and health plans navigate the complexity of the health care system can be found at Web MD, http://www.webmd.com, and can be accessed on the Online Student Resources for this book.

Nursing Care Plans

Nursing care plans are a means of providing nursing personnel with information about the needs and therapeutic plans for each client. They are of major importance when an agency uses source-oriented documentation, because they provide an ongoing, up-to-date record of goal-directed, individualized nursing care. When problem-oriented documentation is used, nursing care plans may be an outgrowth of that documentation.

Critical Pathways

Critical pathways are another way to represent a nursing plan of care. Their use varies geographically and with facility procedures. They are usually formatted in columns and emphasize client outcomes tied to target dates. Critical pathways in general specify the following categories of information:

1. Daily client outcomes (short-term goals)
2. Assessments, tests, and treatments
3. Knowledge deficit (daily prescriptions for nursing interventions focused on client teaching)
4. Diet (daily prescriptions)
5. Activity (daily prescriptions for nursing interventions)
6. Psychosocial considerations (daily prescriptions for nursing interventions)

The precise format for critical pathways may vary from setting to setting or may be based on the client's condition. As is the case with nursing care plans, critical pathways are not set in stone; you must modify them based on changes in client assessment data. Furthermore, you should always individualize standardized critical pathways for individual clients.

EVIDENCE-BASED PRACTICE

Assessment of an Older Adult and Her Caregiving Family Members

Jane is an 84-year-old woman whose 87-year-old husband and other family members provide caregiving services in her home for end-stage heart disease. Even though she enjoys having her family care for her, there are many times when Jane feels stressed by the reactions of her family to the inevitability of her health status. Fatigue and shortness of breath have been the main symptoms Jane experiences, although she has been sad and feeling unsupported lately. Jane has not told anyone about these feelings.

Your assessment of Jane's situation is based on current research results. Your research review highlights quality-of-life issues for end-of-life care and the contribution of psychological distress for the caregivers when higher levels of care are needed. You learned that Jane, and possibly her husband, will likely have psychosocial symptoms. A discussion with Jane and her husband may help both of

them voice their feelings and consider the interplay of physical and emotional symptoms. Assessing physical and psychosocial symptoms allows a complete picture of the status of a client and directs interventions.

The professional involved in Jane's care discussed the information you gathered during your assessment. The plan is to incorporate feeling identification, support system structures, and ongoing assessment of symptoms of depression into the overall care that Jane receives. Intervening with Jane's caregivers is similarly important.

You should base action on more than one study, but you would find the following research helpful in this situation.

Pinquart, M., & Sörensen, S. (2011). Spouses, adult children, and children-in-law as caregivers of older adults: A meta-analytic comparison. *Psychology and Aging, 26*(1), 1–14.

CRITICAL THINKING QUESTIONS

1. How could you use the Global Assessment of Functioning Scale to develop a plan of care for Jane?
2. Why would you approach Jane and her family members to discuss these issues?
3. What specific communication techniques (based on the information in Chapter 10 ∞) would be helpful in obtaining an accurate assessment and encouraging Jane and her family to talk with you about their concerns?

WHY I PLAN TO BECOME A PSYCHIATRIC–MENTAL HEALTH NURSE

Anna's Story: During the first 3 years of nursing college I became convinced I would become a critical care nurse. Every rotation where I was involved in the care of someone who had an emergency or a major system failure, I became convinced that critical care would be my specialty. My plan was to be a critical care nurse when I graduated.

Then I took care of a woman whose abdominal incision would not close. She remained fairly stable through painful procedures and restricted movement. One day she told me she was hearing puppies barking and she couldn't get any rest because of the noise. She begged me to please remove the puppies from the unit. There were no sounds that could be misinterpreted as a dog's bark in the environment. My suspicion of ICU psychosis was verified when the liaison nurse came to assess this client.

This experience changed my plans as I became fascinated with how something unseen and basically hidden from me (the client's thought processes) could have such a major effect on her functioning. This was not a wound to dress, a task to complete, or a bone to set—this was a brain thinking and feeling and experiencing the world. The liaison nurse, a clinical nurse specialist in psychiatric–mental health nursing, asked questions I would not have thought to ask and got answers I did not expect. It was intellectually stimulating for me. My current plan to become a psychiatric–mental health nurse stems from accepting the challenge of combining the nursing skills around human physiology and psychological complexities.

Algorithms

Algorithms are behavioral steps, or step-by-step procedures, for the management of common problems. Algorithms have proved to be useful protocols, particularly in settings that employ large numbers of paraprofessionals. At intake points in community mental health settings, such as walk-in neighborhood clinics, mental health workers often make the initial psychosocial assessment and may plan and implement treatment strategies.

Clinical algorithms for common mental health problems provide structured, standardized guidelines for decision making. Professional nurses in nonpsychiatric settings find clinical algorithms particularly useful when assessing psychiatric symptoms. Algorithms for depression and suicidal lethality have been found to be reliable and valid in these circumstances.

QUALITY ASSURANCE

Quality assurance is known by many names, including performance improvement (PI), quality management (QM), continuous improvement (CI), and continuous quality improvement (CQI). (For our purposes we will use the term quality assurance [QA] in this text.) No matter what name is used, the basis of QA is to ensure that quality is maintained through an ongoing effort to find new and better ways of conducting care and achieving better results.

When QA is properly conducted, it involves the entire organization, whether a large bureaucratic hospital setting or a small private practice. All members of the workforce are involved in evaluating procedures, looking for ways to improve them, and then improving them. In fact, QA is best conducted by the people doing the work rather than by supervisors and administrators.

You will hear QA referred to as a process. This is because QA is evolving as it improves clinical practice. It is not a fixed or rigid plan. QA involves four basic steps—Plan, Do, Check, and Act—that are continuously progressing (see FIGURE 11-2 ■). (Hence the word "continuous" in the terms *Continuous Improvement* and *Continuous Quality Improvement*.)

Quality assurance is about asking questions, using perception surveys and questionnaires, and listening carefully to both compliments and complaints from the people involved in the process. The recipient of your clinical services can be viewed as your customer, someone who can make choices to a certain extent about from whom they receive services. And customers are the best judges of quality. They know best whether their needs and expectations are being met.

When you assess a client, are your procedures the best they can be? Have you utilized all possible and available resources to form the most comprehensive impression of this individual and how to approach treatment? One useful strategy for applying QA to assessment procedures is to compare the outcome of a clinical case with the assessment. Were the recommendations for treatment from the assessment helpful in treating the individual? The involvement of several clinicians in this effort can shape more and more advantageous procedures. If you follow a QA format when examining your practices, then you are more likely to be able to create a truly quality assessment.

The *psychiatric audit* is one way to evaluate the quality of mental health services that consumers receive. An audit consists of a review of the client's treatment record to compare criteria for quality care with actual practice. Problem-oriented documentation provides the descriptive documentation necessary for such QA programs. Although documentation may not always accurately indicate the quality of the care given, it is an important part of the process that keeps mental health care workers accountable to consumers of their services.

When QA is utilized in this way, it benefits everyone. Recipients and their families have an opportunity to receive a higher quality of care, which means better health and greater

FIGURE 11-2 ■ The quality assurance cycle of activities. The four steps of quality assurance are labeled Plan, Do, Check, and Act and are performed in a cyclic fashion.

satisfaction with treatment. You and your coworkers find better ways of providing nursing care, which can lead to greater job satisfaction. The treatment setting benefits from QA as an ongoing focus on improving quality, which helps the facility fulfill its mission and do its job.

Accurate problem identification and intervention strategies often depend on the quality of the assessment. Mental health client information is gathered, assessed, and communicated through the various interdisciplinary assessments. The primary purpose of your assessment is to gather data to formulate a psychiatric diagnosis, prognosis, and treatment plan. If the assessment of a client is based on incomplete, misinterpreted, or inaccurate information, the psychiatric diagnosis, prognosis, and treatment plan may be faulty.

Pearson Nursing Student Resources
Find additional review materials at
nursing.pearsonhighered.com
Prepare for success with NCLEX®-style practice questions, interactive assignments and activities, web links, animations and videos, and more!

REFERENCES

Adams, M.P., Holland, L.N., & Urban, C.Q. (2011). Pharmacology for nurses (3rd ed.). Upper Saddle River, NJ: Pearson Education.

American Psychiatric Association. (2000). *Diagnostic and statistical manual of mental disorders* (4th ed., Text Revision). Washington DC: Author.

Folstein, M., Folstein, S., & McHugh, P. (1975). Mini-mental state: A practical method for grading the cognitive state of patients for the clinician. *Journal of Psychiatric Residents, 12,* 189.

Fontaine, K.L. (2011). Complementary and alternative therapies for nursing practice (3rd ed.). Upper Saddle River, NJ: Pearson Education.

Honigfeld, G., Gillis, R.D., & Klett, C.J. (1966). NOSIE-30: A treatment-sensitive ward behavior scale. *Psychological Reports, 19,* 180–182.

Pinquart, M., & Sörensen, S. (2011). Spouses, adult children, and children-in-law as caregivers of older adults: A meta-analytic comparison. *Psychology and Aging, 26*(1), 1–14.

Rosenhan, D.I. (1973). On being sane in insane places. *Science, 179,* 250–258.

Spielberger, C.D. (1976). The nature and measurement of anxiety. In C.D. Spielberger & R. Diaz-Guerrero (Eds.), *Cross cultural anxiety* (pp. 3–12). Washington, DC: Hemisphere/Wiley.

Ethics, Clients' Rights, and Legal and Forensic Issues

CAROL REN KNEISL

LEARNING OUTCOMES

After completing this chapter, you will be able to:

1. Relate the six principles of bioethics to the practice of psychiatric–mental health nursing.
2. Apply ethical guidelines in reconciling crucial ethical dilemmas.
3. Describe how psychiatric–mental health nurses can avoid indirectly contributing to the stereotypes associated with psychiatric diagnostic categories.
4. Explain why psychiatric–mental health nurses need to be knowledgeable about the mental health statutes and regulations in the state in which they practice.
5. Compare admission and release procedures for voluntary admission and involuntary commitment.
6. Deliver psychiatric–mental health nursing care in a manner that preserves and protects client rights, dignity, and autonomy.
7. Partner with clients and their families in developing psychiatric advance directives.
8. Assist clients and families to develop skills for self–advocacy.

CRITICAL THINKING CHALLENGE

Sue Aberdeen is a client of a mental health outreach clinic. She was diagnosed with bipolar disorder more than 20 years ago. At one time or another during this period, various mental health care providers have prescribed several different medications for Sue. Most have been only slightly helpful or ineffective. Most recently, Sue has been taking lithium, which seems to be the most helpful. Her long-time friend brought Sue to the clinic because Sue has not been taking her medication. She has been unable to sleep and is distracted and agitated. Sue has been to a different bar every night this week, and has gone home with and had sex with a different man each night. The nurse assigned to her case has been attempting to persuade Sue to take her lithium. Sue has continued to refuse, and the nurse has continued to explain and cajole. Finally, Sue shouted: "You just don't get it, do you? Buzz off, you bitch!" and stomped out of the clinic.

1. How can you reconcile the desire and duty to help with a client's refusal for treatment?
2. When do you think it is acceptable for a client to refuse to be treated?
3. What are the options for handling a client's refusal to cooperate with treatment?

Ethical, judicial, legislative, political, and economic decisions profoundly influence mental health practice and bring about changes in the understanding and practice of mental health intervention. These changes challenge the psychiatric–mental health nurse to examine central issues, such as the following:

- How does one balance the common and the individual "good" in health care?
- What are nurses', mental health consumers', and society's rights, liability, and accountability?

An examination of these issues generally improves care, but it often confuses the boundaries of ethical behavior, mental health practice, and the law. This confusion entraps mental health care professionals, mental health consumers, families, lawyers, and the public in a muddle of conflicting policies and procedures. In addition, a client's right to privacy, to receive and refuse treatment, and to define happiness and growth pivot on society's values.

This chapter will bring some clarity to the ever-changing relationship between ethics, the law, and mental health services so that you can practice ethically and with confidence, and also exercise your power as citizens, professionals, and advocates to influence the direction of mental health care.

ETHICS

Having a good foundation in ethics in important in psychiatric–mental health nursing. You may find yourself having to identify alternative courses of action and decide what to do when there is a conflict of rights and obligations between clients and families, between yourself and other mental health care workers, between yourself and the mental health agency or institution, or between the client's good and the community or social good.

Ethics is a branch of philosophy that deals with the values that are related to human conduct, the rightness or wrongness of actions, the goodness and badness of one's motives, and the goodness and badness of the results of one's actions. *Bioethics* is a field that applies ethical reasoning to issues and dilemmas in the area of health care. Ethical conflicts involve complex ethical issues and dilemmas that are tempered by the need to provide culturally congruent care.

Ethical Analysis

One of the major difficulties in ethical analysis is that there are no definite, clear-cut solutions to ethical dilemmas. For centuries, moral philosophers—beginning with Socrates, Plato, and Aristotle—have struggled with two main ethical questions: What is the meaning of right or good? and What should I do?

Taking a stand on an ethical issue involves much more than merely accepting the moral position or personal values of another. It requires an understanding of the principles of bioethics. To identify, clarify, define, and defend a stand on an ethical issue, we must engage in a process of ethical reasoning. Carefully consider the content in Mental Health in the Movies. Which of the following ethical principles may have been violated in the circumstances described there?

Principles of Bioethics

The six principles of bioethics discussed here are autonomy, beneficence, fidelity, justice, nonmaleficence, and veracity. Nurses in psychiatric–mental health settings continually balance the principles of beneficence and nonmaleficence with autonomy (Chiovitti, 2011).

Autonomy

Autonomy is the freedom to choose a course of action, to act on that choice, and to live with the consequences of that choice. Helping clients, their families, and their significant others make choices fosters autonomy. You help clients by providing them with the information they need in order to choose, helping them to understand and sort through the information, and supporting their choice, even when that choice is one that

---

MENTAL HEALTH IN THE MOVIES
Sybil

Sybil, the pseudonym for an actual person in treatment for dissociative identify disorder (DID; known then as multiple personality disorder), was one of the most famous psychiatric clients known to the general public. Her life and treatment became worldwide knowledge with the publication of a book by Rita Schreiber that became a made-for-television movie in 1976 (starring Sally Fields as Sybil and Joanne Woodward as her psychoanalyst) and once again in 2007. The movie portrayed Sybil's harrowing childhood and her dissociation into 16 different personalities in her attempts to cope. Sybil's personalities varied from self-assured and sophisticated, fearful, angry, intensely religious, to perpetual teenager, and even a less well-developed baby.

Sybil's psychiatrist used amobarbital and hypnosis in her attempts to reintegrate Sybil's various selves and merge them together.

In 1998, newly found 25-year-old audiotapes suggested that Sybil's personalities may have actually been implanted by her doctor. Before the first movie was made, there were fewer than 80 known cases of DID. Once Sybil's case became widely known, mental health professionals began to diagnose DID at an alarming rate—more than 20,000 by 1990, with some clinicians estimating that 2 million more cases were in existence. Some mental health professionals (but not all) believe that DID is actually a misdiagnosis of borderline personality, or some form of anxiety disorder. Because Sybil's psychiatric files are sealed and both Sybil and her psychoanalyst are deceased, we may never know the truth to this story. DID remains a controversial diagnosis.

Photo courtesy © Everett Collection.

you may not have made. Professional autonomy for you, as a psychiatric–mental health nurse, means having to account for and accept the consequences of professional decisions and actions. Nursing professionals must balance the goal of greater autonomy with efforts to achieve what providers and consumers determine are the common and the individual good in health care.

Beneficence

Beneficence is the principle of attempting to do things that benefit others or promote the good of others. You operate under the principle of beneficence whenever you help clients who cannot decide for themselves or are incapacitated or incompetent. Protecting clients from harming themselves because of thoughts, feelings, or behaviors that lead to self-harm is done in a spirit of beneficence. Beneficence is also the principle that motivated the paternalism in health care that was common until recently (Parks & Wike, 2010)—that is, wanting to do good for clients meant to some health care providers that lying to them ("You do not have cancer"), or withholding information ("You have a tumor," but failing to say that the tumor is malignant), or dictating treatment ("You must have a radical mastectomy," but failing to offer options such as lumpectomy, chemotherapy, or radiation) was in the client's best interest.

Fidelity

Fidelity means that you maintain loyalty and commitment to your clients and are faithful to your promises, duties, and obligations. Fidelity is crucial to establishing trusting relationships with clients, their families, and other mental health workers. Fidelity also means that you do not make promises you will not or cannot keep.

Justice

Justice is the principle of treating others fairly and equally. It is the fair and equitable distribution of burdens and benefits. The principle of justice has always been a cornerstone of bioethics and has become even more important when considered in issues related to health care reform and managed care. The principle of justice raises questions such as the following:

- Should indigent persons who are schizophrenic be treated with older traditional medications with uncomfortable side effects, but those who can afford it be treated with newer and costly psychotropic drugs that have fewer side effects?
- Is insurance coverage for psychiatric–mental health services a basic service or a luxury?
- Should mental health care be given to those who need it or only to those who can pay for it?

Nonmaleficence

Nonmaleficence is the intention to do no wrong. Your motives for actions should be in the direction of helpfulness based on sound knowledge of psychiatric–mental health theory. Nonmaleficence requires you to be self-aware and is the principle behind the Your Self-Awareness features throughout this text.

Veracity

Veracity is the intention to tell the truth. Veracity is critical to establishing trust with clients, their families, and other mental health care workers. If you cannot be trusted to do what you say you will do or to tell the truth, you cannot be depended on; what you do and what you say will be open to suspicion. Veracity means that you do not lie to clients to "humor" them.

Neuroethics: An Emerging Field

The field of neuroethics is emerging from a 21st-century partnership between bioethics and neuroscience. Rapid advances in neuroscience, brought about by brain research, have raised critical ethical, social, and legal issues about neuroimaging, psychopharmacology, deep-brain stimulation, and psychosurgery (deep-brain stimulation and psychosurgery are discussed later in this chapter). The critical questions revolve around the prediction of disease (including mental disorders in certain instances); questions of privacy and confidentiality; concerns about the effects on an individual's autonomy; and the influences of neuroimaging, psychopharmacology (Mohamed & Sahakian, 2011), deep-brain stimulation (Clausen, 2010), and psychosurgery on an individual's concept of self and personal identity.

Despite the myriad of new neuroscience information and the creation of a new journal in 2008 (*Neuroethics*), the brain remains the most complex and least understood of all the organs in the human body. Mapping the neural correlates of the mind through brain scans and altering these correlates through surgery, stimulation, or psychopharmacologic interventions can affect people in both positive and negative ways. Neuroscientists and mental health professionals must carefully weigh and actively debate the potential benefits of this knowledge and technology against their potential harm.

Ethical Guidelines for Psychiatric–Mental Health Nurses

Most professions develop guidelines for the behavior of their members. Ethical guidelines for psychiatric–mental health nurses stem from two sources. The first source is the standards for psychiatric–mental health nursing practice published by the American Nurses Association (ANA) (2007). (These standards are reproduced and discussed in detail in Chapter 2∞.) The standard of professional performance that deals specifically with ethics for psychiatric–mental health nurses is Standard 12. You are most likely familiar with the second source from your nursing fundamentals course—the general code of ethics for nurses, also developed by the ANA (Fowler, 2010). If you need to refresh yourself on the ANA Code of Ethics, refer to a nursing fundamentals text. Use these sources to make clinical judgments and to engage in ethical reasoning. You may also find ANA's online journal of issues in nursing (OJIN) helpful in your practice. The journal can be accessed through the Online Student Resources for this book.

Clinical Judgment and Ethical Reasoning

Psychiatric–mental health nurses are frequently faced with the following two goals:

1. Responding to the therapeutic needs of individuals
2. Serving society by preserving social order

Often, these two goals are in conflict, and nurses face the dilemma of placing one above the other, especially in circumstances in which a mentally ill individual behaves in a threatening or violent manner (Mariano et al., 2011).

Nurses are necessarily guided in therapeutic work by a belief system—some vision of what kinds of changes would improve a client's life. Nurses are further guided by some moral principles that limit the extent to which they will help a client obtain happiness at the expense of others, and the extent to which they will participate in the oppression of an individual in the interests of societal control. Anyone who is responsible for moral choices is obliged to recognize the reason, virtue, ideal, rule, or principle on which he or she makes a decision. Laws represent yet another source of limits. They are discussed later in this chapter in the section on clients' rights.

Ethical Dilemmas in Psychiatric–Mental Health Nursing

Ultimately, nurses must reconcile a number of crucial ethical dilemmas with their personal and professional values. Among these issues are the following:

- The potential stigma of psychiatric diagnostic labels
- Psychiatry's right to control individual freedom
- The justification for involuntary treatment
- The use of restrictive treatment interventions
- The client's right to suicide
- The client's right to privacy

Practicing psychiatric–mental health nursing requires ethical responsibility, a measure of professional excellence. However, problems arise when there is conflict about the ground rules for behavior, whether the conflict is between client and social group, nurse and profession, or nurse and agency. As Davis and her associates put it, nurses are agents for both the institution or agency and the client (Davis, Fowler, & Aroskar, 2010). These problems are phrased in the ethical language of right and wrong. Circumstances likely to give rise to such problems include the following:

- The professional and the client are from different cultures and may have different values.
- The voluntary nature of the client's participation is compromised.
- The client's competence to enter into an agreement about intervention is questionable, or the client does not realize that certain interventions are being implemented.
- External factors (lack of time, lack of staff, high demands) prevent the professional from doing what is best for the client.

It has been suggested that having moral insight, virtue, and ethics in nursing can be taught through appropriate experience, habitual practice, and good role models (Begley, 2006). Look for an experienced nurse mentor who can supervise your ethical practice and serve as a good role model.

Every nursing relationship begins with an unusual burden of ethical responsibility. The following sections explore some of these moral issues.

Stigma of Psychiatric Diagnoses

The list of stereotypes associated with psychiatric diagnostic categories is well known to most nurses. Equally familiar are the consequences to people with these diagnoses. As Chapter 1∞ points out, people labeled as drug addicts, alcoholics, convicts, paranoids, and so on acquire a discredited social identity because of the character flaws often associated with the labels. To much of society, the labels used in psychiatry suggest decadence, immorality, and wanton disregard for society's values. It is important to consider how and when psychiatric–mental health nurses, while advocating humane treatment for clients, indirectly contribute to discrediting a client's social identity by participating in the arbitrary use of oppressive labels. Keep this in mind while you review the content in Your Self-Awareness.

Need for Diagnostic Labels Diagnosis has considerable value in psychiatric practice, as Chapter 11∞ points out. Putting clients into diagnostic categories makes it easy for health care professionals to communicate with each other

---

YOUR SELF-AWARENESS
Does Standardized Terminology Conflict With Individualized Client Care?

This textbook challenges psychiatric–mental health nurses to engage in reflective and creative responses to complex mind–body–spirit problems. We are challenged to face issues of global mental health with intelligence, stamina, creativity, and moral courage. The word *courage* is rooted in a French word meaning "heart." In many of the chapters in this book, you are presented with a vocabulary of standardized language including NANDA, NIC, NOC, and DSM. As you know, language and symbols are critical in creating the assumptions, emotional climate, and behavioral norms that define people and their environments and what is possible within them. Reflect on your own ideas about the following questions:

- Do you believe that any standardized vocabulary dismisses the unique stories of clients and their families?
- What do you think are the advantages and disadvantages of using an accepted language or vocabulary when working as a mental health team member?
- When evaluating the categories and language in NANDA, NIC, NOC, and DSM, do you think they adequately portray the diversity of people's lived experience and contribute to a nurse's ability to plan effective care?
- Do you think that standardized language systems are compatible with bringing "heart" to psychiatric–mental health nursing?

about the client. The diagnosis often dictates a particular course of treatment and enables the mental health team to prognosticate about a client's recovery. Diagnostic categories enable nurses to plan comprehensively for client care and to conduct research.

Nurse's Moral Stance on Diagnoses Take time to consider carefully how you would answer the following questions:

- Does labeling with psychiatric diagnoses merely provide psychiatric professionals with some additional sense of control in their dealings with clients?
- Is it true that a diagnosis gives staff members an increased sense of being able to predict client behavior and a way of calmly viewing what might otherwise be upsetting behavior? For example, "That's just her hysterical personality coming out," or "Those complaints are just paranoid delusions."

The consequences of psychiatric labels for clients and their families, however, raise moral questions about their legitimacy (refer back to the Rosenhan study in Chapter 11∞ on page 212) when they are used arbitrarily or without current knowledge of diagnostic criteria.

Nurses have a moral responsibility to question practices that exact a price from clients far in excess of the benefits. Every moment of moral injustice takes its toll on us, as well as our clients. Every moment of moral responsibility strengthens our own, as well as our clients', sense of personal integrity.

Control of Individual Freedom

Involuntary hospitalization and treatment of psychiatric clients are usually considered humanitarian efforts. Yet, any practice that directly and coercively deprives a person of freedom has political implications. In some states, clients have no guarantee that they will ever be released from the hospital. This ethical issue is further complicated by the fact that psychiatric professionals can no longer argue that involuntary hospitalization is necessary to restore mental health. Instead, the confinement must be justified as necessary to protect the client or others from harm.

Violence Against Others Psychiatric–mental health nurses are faced with the dilemma of trying to be both healer-helpers and agents of social control. Dealing with violently destructive clients requires balancing the value of life against the value of liberty. A thorough discussion of violence in the psychiatric setting is in Chapter 35∞.

Suicide Traditionally, nurses have felt that they should do everything possible to preserve life. We have relied on this imperative to justify intervention in suicide attempts as well as heroic technical measures to avert impending deaths. Psychiatry, in general, rejects the notion of rational suicide and assumes that suicidal ideation is an irrational belief resulting from mental disorder. Further, we assume that a person without a mental disorder would not choose suicide. Thus, we seek to prevent suicide on the basis that this is what the client would choose if the client were mentally capable of choosing. In this, as well as in many areas of psychiatric–mental health

nursing practice, there are contested matters and areas of differing opinion.

The treatment given to dying clients is often in conflict with the treatment they desire. For example, a physician may disregard a client's protests against treatment. The physician may assert that the client's medical condition is causing the client to behave irrationally. There is not necessarily an ethical difference between clients dying of physical deterioration and clients dying of emotional or mental deterioration. Many of the same ethical questions emerge about the suicidal client, as in the following examples:

- How is *quality of life* defined?
- Is the definition limited to physical factors?
- Who should have the right to make the definition?
- How is rationality to be measured?
- Are people always in conscious control of their choices?

A thorough discussion of suicide is in Chapter 23∞.

An individual's right to choose when and how to die is a complex biomedical issue. The thoughtful professional nurse needs to clarify the issues, give them careful consideration, and search for a personal position. There are many ways in which people can deliberately shorten or end their own lives. They can destroy themselves quickly with a gun, or slowly through the chronic use of drugs such as tobacco or alcohol. When is coercive intervention by psychiatric practitioners justified?

Psychosurgery The most dramatic of restrictive measures is *psychosurgery,* the surgical removal or destruction of brain tissue with the intent of altering behavior even though there may be no direct evidence of structural disease or damage in the brain. Psychosurgery has become the subject of marked controversy on ethical grounds (Lipsman, Mendelsohn, Taira, & Bernstein, 2010). Advocates claim that it is done to restore rather than destroy individual freedom. They argue that before psychosurgery, the client is crippled by mental illness and individual autonomy is compromised by the client's bizarre behavior or internal psychological state. After the surgery, clients supposedly are more autonomous than before, by their own and others' criteria. Advocates of the selective use of psychosurgery, even against the client's will, outline the following three conditions that must be met to justify it:

1. The illness being treated is seriously disabling and untreatable by nonsurgical means such as medication or psychotherapy.
2. The treatment is undertaken with some sort of systematic investigative protocol; it is accompanied by evaluation research.
3. The treatment occurs in settings with as many safeguards as possible to arrive at informed consent, if possible, perhaps using a client advocate during the procedure.

The most common psychosurgery in the mid-1900s was prefrontal lobotomy (severing of the prefrontal tracts in the cortex) to treat schizophrenia. Although prefrontal lobotomy has been discredited after having been found to be ineffective in treating schizophrenia and because of its untoward aftereffects—memory loss, personality changes, the absence of emotional responses—less destructive psychosurgery is once again a growing field.

Today, the case for psychosurgery is most likely to be made in instances of severe and resistant depression (Schoene-Bake et al., 2010), or when obsessive–compulsive disorder is not helped by behavior therapy or psychotropic medications and is severely disabling (Mendelsohn, Lipsman, & Bernstein, 2010). These are conditions called *treatment-refractory* mental illness. In this instance, *cingulotomy,* a surgical procedure in which small, precisely pinpointed regions of the brain are selectively destroyed, may be employed. Another procedure, *stereotactic amygdalotomy,* the purposeful production of lesions in the amygdala, has been performed for the treatment of severe aggressive behavior disturbances and for self-mutilation disorder refractory to treatment. *Deep-brain stimulation,* the implantation of a brain pacemaker to send electrical impulses to specific parts of the brain, has been used to treat major depression and obsessive–compulsive disorder. While it has a long history as a treatment for Parkinson's disease, chronic pain, tremor, and dystonia, there is insufficient evidence at this time for its use as a therapeutic modality for mental illness (Lipsman et al., 2011). There is potential for serious complications and side effects. Although these procedures are not as destructive as prefrontal lobotomy, there is potential for serious complications, side effects, and irreversible brain damage.

Psychotropic Medications The discovery that certain medications can radically alter the expression of human emotions has had an enormous impact on psychiatry. The mental hospital is no longer seen as a "warehouse" for storing society's deviants; it is now a "clearinghouse" where clients are sorted, renovated, and dispatched back into their communities with symptomatic behavior under control through one or another of the current psychiatric medications.

Mental health professionals have associated the advent of psychotropic medications with a new optimism and less fear about working with people labeled mentally ill. Furthermore, it might be argued that medications have helped keep people out of the hospital and have decreased the need for other more dramatic measures, such as restraint and seclusion. Medications that make people feel better, however, can lessen their motivation to confront an oppressive situation. This can have serious implications for the political and moral climate of society. It is conceivable that pills could be developed to keep a person quietly enslaved. Suppose drugs were coercively given to anyone whose unhappiness was rooted in social oppression?

The cautious and judicious use of drugs with the client's consent can be helpful. Used irresponsibly, they can close off moral and political confrontations. Decisions about the use of drugs are made in the context of the social situation and environment. In hospital settings, medications are regularly used to reduce symptoms and make client behavior more manageable. Most staff members justify their use of chemical controls by defining violent or bizarre behavior as an indirect request for limits, as in the clinical example that follows.

Clinical Example

After pacing angrily up and down the hall in front of the nurses' station for 20 minutes or so, Carlotta kicks over some mops in a bucket. A male staff member shouts to the nurse to get her PRN medication ready and strides into the hall telling the client to stop it. Carlotta cries and shouts, and they begin struggling. Several other staff members rush over to assist. They drag and carry Carlotta into her room, where she is given 10 mg of haloperidol (Haldol). She continues fighting and screaming. Staff members continue to wrestle with her in her room. Finally they decide to transfer her to the unit downstairs, where she can be put into a seclusion room. In a report, a staff member describes the incident as: "Carlotta blew up and needed controls."

By assigning this meaning to the use of drugs, practitioners can feel that their actions to suppress symptoms are based on the client's needs rather than on the staff's management motives. It is possible that all these controls would not have been necessary had a staff member responded to the nonverbal cues of mounting tension (see Chapter 35∞) before the client kicked over the mops.

Restraints Even the physical characteristics of psychiatric inpatient settings convey the notion that clients are not expected to be capable of self-control and that staff members have the responsibility for providing it. From the client's perspective, physical restraints have a negative psychological impact, are traumatizing, are perceived by clients as unethical behavior on the part of staff members, and result in clients feeling as if their spirit is broken (Strout, 2010). Many clients view these interventions as forms of abuse, while the staff sees them as "helping people who can't take care of themselves."

All the judgments made about restraining clients involve moral decisions such as:

- What other techniques have been tried?
- Is the client obviously out of control?
- How does the nurse decide when restraints are necessary?
- Is the client cognitively compromised?
- What will be the effects on the client of such a dramatic intervention?
- What are the effects on others in the milieu?

Legal factors that influence judgments about restraints are discussed later in this chapter. Clinical factors that influence judgments about restraints are discussed in Chapter 35∞.

Client Privacy and Confidentiality

When people seek psychiatric help, they often reveal highly personal, possibly embarrassing, and potentially damaging information about themselves. Almost all modes of therapeutic intervention rely on the client's willingness to talk openly and honestly about personal concerns, feelings, or problems. The solo therapist in private practice with voluntary clients is usually able to avoid compromising the client's right to confidentiality. In fact, many private therapists view themselves as vigilant protectors of their clients' privacy. You, however, may encounter a serious ethical conflict in being both the confidante of the client and the employee of the organization. Nurses have dual allegiances—to the client and to the agency. Be aware that clients who do not trust that you will respect their privacy are likely not to be forthcoming.

Clients usually assume that health care professionals have no other purpose than to help them. They lose sight of the fact that nurses are often asked to collect data about them that might be highly influential in determining their medications, their disposition, and even their civil rights. While it is often the psychiatrist who makes final pronouncements about a client's mental health status, diagnosis, prognosis, and the like, such pronouncements rest on information collected and communicated to the physician by nurses. This information-gathering process merits serious scrutiny.

Information gathering and sharing are part of your role. Thoughtful handling of client confidentiality is facilitated by the following three safeguards:

1. Convey to clients the limit of confidentiality in your exchanges—that is, what you do with the information a client shares.
2. Attempt to portray accurately to others the reliability, validity, and representativeness of the data you communicate about a client.
3. Recognize that strict confidentiality may have to be violated when an innocent third party is endangered (see the Tarasoff decision discussed later in this chapter).

Confidentiality is discussed further in this chapter in the section on client rights.

LEGISLATION, COMMITMENT, AND HOSPITALIZATION ISSUES

In the last 30 years, the courts have had significant impact on the direction of mental health legislation and state statutes. As a review of history tells us, the courts have traditionally been concerned with the possibility of wrongful commitment. Little attention was paid to the restrictions placed on the legal and civil rights of an individual once hospitalized. In recent years, however, the courts have become more concerned with the substantive rights of psychiatric clients whether hospitalized or not, including the right to treatment, the right not to perform institutional labor, and retention of civil rights such

as the rights to communication, visitation, religious activities, and medical self-determination. This is reflected in many state statutes, along with an emphasis on procedural safeguards. One of the most prominent voices for improving the lives of people with mental illnesses through changes in policy and law has been Judge David L. Bazelon. His Bazelon Center for Mental Health Law is committed to providing the ability to exercise their own life choices to people with mental disabilities.

A review of mental health laws and judicial decisions underscores the fact that there is *great variability from state to state;* thus, an exploration of the mental health laws of each and every state is beyond the scope of this chapter. Because of this variability, it is critical to safe practice that you are knowledgeable about the mental health statutes and regulations in the state in which you practice. Most mental health agencies and psychiatric facilities maintain copies of these statutes, as do local law libraries. You may also refer to the agency in your state that oversees mental health care.

Admission and Commitment Categories

The two major categories of hospitalization are voluntary admission and involuntary commitment. Admission and release procedures differ accordingly. They are described in the following section and compared in TABLE 12-1 ■.

Voluntary Admission

Voluntary admission comes about by written application for admission by prospective clients, or someone acting in their behalf, such as a parent or guardian, a partner, or a mental health agent appointed through a psychiatric advance directive (discussed in a later section of this chapter). As the word *voluntary* implies, the client has a right to demand and obtain release. Depending on the state, the client agrees to give notice, usually in writing, of the intention to leave during a grace period from 24 hours to 15 days. It is justified on the grounds that the hospital staff needs time to examine the client to determine whether a change to involuntary status is indicated. The extra time also gives family and staff the opportunity to persuade the client to remain voluntarily. This "conditional provision" is seen by some as a covert form of involuntary hospitalization. In most states, there are now statutory assurances that voluntary clients must be adequately informed of their rights and status.

TABLE 12-1 ■ Voluntary Admission and Involuntary Commitment Compared

	Voluntary Admission		Involuntary Commitment			
	Informal	Voluntary	Emergency	Temporary	Extended	Outpatient
Release	Anytime	Usually conditional	Average after 3–5 days	48 hours to 6 months	After 60–180 days or an indeterminate time	Can be indeterminate
Use	Limited	Increasing	Increasing	Increasing	Decreasing	Increasing
Criteria for admission	Client request	Client request	Usually client dangerousness	Client dangerousness or need of care and treatment	Client dangerousness or need of care and treatment	Client condition deteriorating or client in need of treatment

Informal voluntary admission, an alternative to the structure and personal concessions required in voluntary admission, is an option in several states. This procedure is similar to that required in a medical admission. The prospective inpatient verbally requests admission and is free to leave the institution at any time. Informal voluntary admission procedures are more likely to be an option in general hospital psychiatric units and private facilities than in state institutions, and they account for a small percentage of all admissions in states that have this provision.

Involuntary Commitment

Involuntary commitment can come about if the designated body, such as a court, an administrative tribunal, or the required number of physicians find that the prospective client's mental state meets the statutory criteria for involuntary commitment. The state's ability to hospitalize or commit an individual involuntarily is sanctioned by one of the following two state powers:

1. Police power enables the state to hospitalize people who are considered dangerous to others because of their illness.
2. *Parens patriae* power enables the state to take on the role of protector and assume responsibility for people considered dangerous to themselves or unable to care for themselves in a potentially dangerous situation because of a mental disability.

Most states provide for more than one involuntary hospitalization procedure. The criteria vary from state to state according to the type of involuntary hospitalization. However, all state involuntary commitment statutes can be expected to include one or more of the following criteria:

- Dangerous to self or others
- Unable to provide for basic needs
- Mentally ill

In an increasing number of states, involuntary commitment is justified only if the individual presents a danger to self or others because of a mental disorder. Nevertheless, involuntary commitment can produce ethical conflict—the duty of beneficence toward others versus personal autonomy (Cherry, 2010). The remaining states augment the argument for involuntary commitment by stating that the client's need for care and treatment may also justify commitment. There is a growing movement for involuntary treatment for drug and alcohol dependence because the availability of third-party funding for the voluntary treatment of individuals with substance use disorders has decreased (Nace et al., 2007).

Involuntary commitment can be divided into the following four categories:

- Emergency
- Temporary or observational
- Extended or indeterminate
- Outpatient commitment

Emergency   Emergency involuntary hospitalization is available in almost all states. It is a temporary measure with limited, short-range goals, and it deals largely with the prevention of behavior likely to create a "clear and present" danger to the client or others. Under common law, any official or private person has the right to detain a dangerous mentally disordered person.

Some formal application is required to initiate emergency detention. In some states, any citizen may make the application. In others, it is limited to police officers, health officers, and physicians. Because this type of involuntary admission is an emergency measure and is warranted only until the appropriate legal steps can be taken, the statutes limit the amount of time an individual can be detained. The usual practice is to allow detention for 3 to 5 days, although some states set a limit of 24 hours.

Temporary or Observational   Temporary or observational involuntary hospitalization is the involuntary commitment of an allegedly mentally disordered individual for a specified period of time to allow for adequate observation so that a diagnosis can be made and treatment instituted. The actual time period can vary from 48 hours to as long as 6 months.

In some states, any citizen can make an application for the temporary hospitalization of a person in need of aid. Others require a family member or guardian, a health or welfare officer, or a physician to apply. Temporary hospitalization may be brought about by the medical certification of one or two physicians, or it may require further approval by a judge, justice, or district attorney in some jurisdictions.

At the end of the observation period, several options are available. The treating physician may (a) discharge the client, (b) encourage the client to stay voluntarily, or (c) file an application for extended hospitalization. In some states, observational hospitalization is mandatory before a court ruling may be made in favor of extended hospitalization.

Extended or Indeterminate   Extended or indeterminate involuntary hospitalization can come about through either judicial or nonjudicial procedures. Judicial hospitalization procedures require that a judge or jury determine whether the person is mentally ill to a degree that requires extended hospitalization. If so, the court orders the client hospitalized for an extended period (60 to 180 days) or an indeterminate time.

Proceedings are usually initiated by an application for hospitalization of an allegedly mentally ill person. About half the states permit any responsible person or citizen to make or swear to the application. Others allow only one or more of the following groups: relatives, public officers, physicians, and hospital superintendents. Supporting medical evidence may or may not be required at the time of application.

Most states having judicial hospitalization procedures make some provision for a prehearing medical examination in addition to the medical certification required to support the application. In all jurisdictions having judicial hospitalization procedures, it is mandatory to notify the person who is proposed to be hospitalized of the hearing. Most states also require notice to the client's attorney, family, or guardian.

A hearing is mandatory in most states, although a few states leave it to the client to request it. While the client's presence is required at the hearing in a few states, most states merely permit attendance if it is not thought to be harmful to the client's condition or if the client in fact demands it. Few states require the hearing to be held in a courtroom. Most say the choice of site is entirely discretionary. Jury trials are no longer mandatory in any state, although a few states still have provisions for the use of a jury to decide the question of hospitalization.

Nonjudicial hospitalization procedures for extended or indeterminate involuntary hospitalization include both administrative and medical certification, but such procedures are now much less prominent on the statute books. Extended hospitalization brought about by an administrative board follows the same procedure used in judicial hospitalization.

Involuntary hospitalization by medical certification, an alternative to the more traditional judicial commitment, is usually advocated for clients who are incapable of consenting to voluntary treatment, although they do not protest hospitalization. The need for hospitalization is usually determined by an examination by one or more physicians and documented by a medical certificate. All states having medical certification provide either for judicial proceedings (if the client contests the hospitalization at any time after certification), or for expanded habeas corpus proceedings, described later in this chapter in the section on client rights.

Involuntary Outpatient Commitment

In response to several highly publicized and dramatic instances of violent acts by mentally disordered persons, most states have modified their statutes and regulations to allow for court-ordered outpatient treatment. In most states allowing for involuntary outpatient commitment (IOC), the criteria are similar to that necessary for inpatient commitment: proof of mental illness and dangerousness. A few states have passed statutes permitting preventive commitment. In these instances, IOC is intended to avert a further deterioration of the person's mental health that would require inpatient hospitalization. IOC has also been used to ensure that mentally ill offenders follow through with outpatient treatment once they are released from prison. Conditional release, a concept related to IOC, is discussed later in this chapter.

Thought to be a way to ensure adherence to a medication regimen, the ethicality of IOC has been questioned because of its coercive nature. Its effectiveness has been questioned by critics who say that it may actually accomplish the opposite, that is, drive people away from treatment. The Bazelon Center is opposed to outpatient commitment on the basis that building a responsive mental health system with services such as mobile crisis teams, assertive community treatment teams, and supported housing is the best strategy. They believe that when people are dangerous, they should be hospitalized, and when safety is not an issue, then treatment should be voluntary. Outpatient commitment reflects a failure in community treatment that could have been avoided by early and effective interventions (Bazelon Center for Mental Health Law, 2011).

A search of the literature indicated that IOC may not be better than standard care in relationship to social functioning or quality of life, although IOC clients are less likely to be victims of crime (Kisely, Campbell, & Preston, 2011). IOC may also be vulnerable to legal challenges on the basis of constitutional standards.

Ethical Dilemmas of Involuntary Hospitalization

Involuntary hospitalization is an exercise of power, and like all forms of power, it can be abused. Because of this potential for abuse, commitment criteria are important. In this country, a person's loss of liberty can be justified only under certain circumstances.

As the review of mental health statutes shows, a degree of "dangerousness" is the favored justification for loss of liberty by involuntary hospitalization. The "dangerousness" criterion is not without its inherent problems (King & Robinson, 2011). Some of these problems are as follows:

- Definitions of "dangerousness" vary from state to state.
- It is impossible to predict dangerous behavior reliably.
- In the absence of other criteria, "dangerousness" will be overused to justify admission.
- The stigma of *dangerous* will be added to that of *mentally ill.*
- The stereotype of *mentally disabled* will be reinforced and thus will work against the development of community programs.
- The media will be encouraged to continue selective reporting of instances in which mental illness and criminal behavior appear to be linked.
- Clinical practice shows that "dangerous" individuals are often not treatable, while the most treatable individuals are not dangerous.

Discharge or Separation Categories

A client can separate from a mental institution in one of three ways: discharge, transfer, and escape.

Discharge

Like admission, discharge from a mental hospital can have various layers of complexity. Discharges occur in one of two ways—conditionally or absolutely.

Conditional As implied by the word *conditional,* complete discharge in this situation depends on whether the person fulfills certain conditions over a specified period of time, usually 6 months to 1 year. Adherence to outpatient care, demonstrated ability and willingness to take medications, and the ability to meet the needs of daily living are a few of the many possible prerequisites.

A person who is unable to meet the specified conditions can be reinstitutionalized without going through any legal admission procedure. An individual committed for an extended or indeterminate time is more likely to be a candidate for conditional, rather than absolute, discharge.

Absolute The legal relationship between the institution and the client is terminated by an absolute discharge. If the client should require readmission to the hospital at any time, even a few hours after discharge, a new hospitalization proceeding would be required.

An absolute discharge can be achieved in the following three ways:

1. An administrative discharge is issued by hospital officials.
2. A judicial discharge is ordered by the courts.
3. A writ of habeas corpus is ordered by the courts on the client's application.

As a rule, the authority for discharging involuntary clients rests in the hands of the hospital director, and these clients are given administrative discharges. However, a few statutes extend this power to the central agency responsible for supervising mental institutions in the state, such as the Department of Mental Health. The client has no formal method of initiating an administrative discharge.

The majority of states have provisions for judicial discharge, which is initiated by an application to the court by the client, the client's family, or any citizen who is in disagreement with hospital authorities over the client's need to be hospitalized. A few states require the application to be accompanied by a medical certificate supporting the idea that the client is ready for discharge. In many states, judicial discharge does not depend on complete recovery. A degree of improvement may be sufficient. Some states guard against frequent applications for discharge by the same clients by imposing a 3-month to 1-year waiting period between requests.

Transfer

Transfers account for a small number of separations from a mental health care facility. Most are transfers within state and county mental health systems. A smaller number are transfers from state to federal facilities or from one state to another.

Escape

A client may take the initiative and decide to terminate the relationship with the institution by informally leaving the hospital grounds. This is commonly called *escape, elopement,* or being *AWOL* (absent without leave). Voluntary clients cannot generally be returned to the hospital against their will. However, involuntarily committed clients may be brought back to the hospital against their will with the assistance of the police, if necessary.

PSYCHIATRY AND CRIMINAL LAW

Our legal system in the United States is based on the assumption that the majority of criminal offenders chooses to commit crimes for rational reasons. The assumption is that offenders commit these crimes of their own free will and deserve to be punished for their acts. However, some offenders are mentally disturbed, irrational, or unable to control their behavior.

Clinical Example

Carolyn has a 12-year history of bipolar disorder and had not been taking her medication since being discharged from a psychiatric hospital. Two weeks prior to the alleged offense, Carolyn began having difficulty sleeping, her behavior became erratic, and she spent most nights walking up and down the streets in her neighborhood. Two nights ago, neighbors called the police after they saw her removing items from garages and painting driveways with colorful rainbows. Carolyn was arrested and charged with burglary and malicious mischief.

Only a minority of criminal offenders is mentally disturbed—fewer than 4% of mentally ill offenders pursue a defense of legal insanity, and even fewer, 1%, are eventually acquitted by reason of insanity (Bazelon Center for Mental Health Law, 2007).

Determining Legal Sanity

Legal sanity differs from *clinical sanity,* which is the absence of a major mental disorder. **Legal sanity** is defined as an individual's ability to know right from wrong with reference to the act charged, the capacity to know the nature and quality of the act charged, and the capacity to form the intent to commit the crime. Legal sanity is determined for the specific time of the act, as determined by the court order. It may be the brief period of a physical assault or the length of a crime spree over several days.

In most states, the presence of a major mental disorder is a prerequisite for a finding of legal insanity. State insanity laws may have wording variations, but will cite the "presence of mental disorder or defect." Either can be used toward a finding of legal insanity. The term *mental disorder* usually refers to a major mental illness, such as that described in the clinical example that follows; while *mental defect* usually refers to developmental disability or some physiological condition affecting cognition, such as a head injury, brain tumor, or dementia.

The burden of proving legal insanity has shifted to the defense as a result of the Hinckley case (John Hinckley is the person who shot President Ronald Reagan in 1981). In the Hinckley trial, the prosecution failed to prove that Hinckley was sane beyond a reasonable doubt (the practice at that time in the federal courts). Most states now place the burden of proof on the defense. In federal courts, the defense now must prove a defendant's insanity rather than the prosecution having to prove that the defendant is sane. (See Mental Health in the News on John Hinckley in Chapter 13∞ on page 257.)

Proof of criminal guilt must be determined "beyond a reasonable doubt" (i.e., it is about 90% to 95% likely that the defendant committed the act). The need for civil commitment in mental health law is based on "clear, cogent, and convincing" evidence (somewhere between 51% and 90%, usually around 75%). Legal insanity is determined by "a preponderance of the evidence" (at least 51%) (American Bar Association, 1995). The situations in which a legal insanity defense is usually raised are listed in Box 12-1.

Box 12-1 Reasons for Raising an Insanity Defense

A legal insanity defense is raised most often because of the following:

- Presence of or history of mental disorder
- Depression with suicidality
- Developmental disability
- Sexual deviance
- Amnesia and dissociative states, including a claim of multiple personality
- Medical issues such as brain tumor or other conditions that affect behavior
- Factitious disorder by proxy (formerly known as Munchausen syndrome by proxy; see Chapter 19∞)
- Medications that affect behavior
- Personality disorder
- Substance addiction

In criminal cases in which the question of legal sanity is raised, the possibility of malingering a mental disorder will also be raised. Malingering a mental illness (intentionally producing false or exaggerated psychological symptoms) is not uncommon. The *Diagnostic and Statistical Manual of Mental Disorders,* published by the American Psychiatric Association (APA), states that facing a forensic evaluation is a strong indicator for suspecting the malingering of a mental illness (2000). Malingering is discussed in Chapter 19∞.

The legal standards most commonly used to determine legal sanity are discussed in the following section.

M'Naghten Rule

In most jurisdictions, the determination of legal sanity is based on the *M'Naghten Rule,* which was the result of a famous case in England.

Clinical Example

Daniel M'Naghten was a Scottish carpenter who believed that Jesuits and Tories were tormenting him. He told his family that spies for the government were following him and laughing at him. He was evicted from his boardinghouse because of his bizarre behavior. In 1843 he stalked Prime Minister Sir Robert Peel, eventually shot Peel's secretary, and was charged with the death. Nine physicians who were experienced in the care of persons with mental disorders testified at the trial (three for the defense, three for the prosecution, and three who listened to the evidence and observed M'Naghten's behavior in the courtroom). All nine agreed M'Naghten suffered from monomania (probably paranoid schizophrenia today) and was not legally sane, according to the legal tests at the time. The jury huddled in the courtroom for 2 minutes and then found him to be legally insane. He was sent to the local mental institution, Bethlehem Hospital. The public was outraged, believing hospitalization to be too lenient. The queen ordered a task force in the House of Lords to review the case and come up with a new legal standard.

Although the M'Naghten Rule was not applied in this famous case, it was a result of its conclusion. The M'Naghten Rule established the "right from wrong" principle for determining insanity. That is, if a mental disease or defect prevents a criminal from knowing the wrongfulness of his or her actions, the criminal can be found to be **not guilty by reason of insanity (NGRI)**. Subsequent developments first broadened, then later narrowed, the grounds for determining legal sanity.

Irresistible Impulse

A volitional component was added to the cognitive component of the M'Naghten Rule in 1929. This became known as the *Irresistible Impulse Test,* which holds that a defendant is exculpated (freed from blame) even if the defendant knew the criminal act was wrong but could not restrain his conduct because of mental disease or defect. A modern interpretation of the standard is known as *The Policeman at the Elbow Test.* That is, would the defendant have committed the act had he known he was being observed by a police officer?

American Law Institute Model Penal Code

The Model Penal Code was approved in 1962 to serve as a guide for states wishing to reform their criminal law. It suggests that a person is not responsible for criminal conduct if, at the time of such conduct, the person, because of mental disease or mental defect, lacked substantial capacity either to appreciate the criminality (wrongfulness) of his conduct or to conform his conduct to the requirements of the law. The code specifies that the terms *mental disease* and *mental defect* do not include abnormal thinking that is manifested by only repeated criminal or otherwise antisocial conduct. The intent of the wording was to preclude the use of personality or character disorders in an insanity defense, especially antisocial personality disorder.

Guilty but Mentally Ill

The insanity defense periodically comes under fire from a public who believes that it is too lenient a response to violence. Some states have opted to use another option—**guilty but mentally ill (GBMI)**—in an attempt to reform the insanity defense (American Bar Association, 1995). Defendants can be found GBMI if they are guilty of the crime and were mentally ill but not legally insane at the time the crime was committed. The defendant's psychotic state is acknowledged and the defendant is sentenced in the same manner as any criminal. A judge may impose any sentence under the law for the crime in question (Schmalleger, 2009). The defendant may also receive court-ordered treatment for the mental disorder as well. Once stable, the defendant is transferred to a prison for the remainder of the sentence.

Diminished Capacity

Diminished capacity is an element of the insanity law that refers to an individual's capacity to form the intent to commit a specific act. There are four levels of intent—purposely, knowingly, recklessly, or negligently—and a court may order an evaluation specific to one level, depending on the degree of crime charged. A finding of diminished capacity is based on legal criteria in each state. For example, in some states, the cause of the inability to form intent must be a mental disorder, not amounting to insanity, and not emotions like jealousy, fear, anger, or hatred. The mental disorder must be causally connected to the lack of specific intent, not just reduced perception, awareness, understanding, or over-reaction.

Competence to Stand Trial

No person may be tried if he is incompetent. The conviction of an incompetent defendant is a violation of the Fourteenth Amendment—the right to due process. Therefore, a court will remand (send) the incompetent defendant to a "suitable facility" (usually a locked unit in a mental hospital) for treatment to regain competency. Because courts have held that defendants cannot be hospitalized or incarcerated indefinitely, court orders stipulate a specific period of time in which the defendant is given treatment.

While legal insanity is a test of culpability, competence to stand trial is an issue of ability to stand trial. It is defined as having the capacity to understand the proceedings and to assist one's attorney. The presence of a developmental disability, symptoms of a mental disorder, or a history of mental disorder does not necessarily preclude one's competence to stand trial. For example, the presence of delusions may or may not have an impact. It depends on whether the delusion is related to the courtroom, the crime, or the proceedings. The specific content of the delusion, and the degree to which the symptoms affect the abilities and skills needed to be competent, are the important factors. National standards for determining competence to proceed, such as the McGarry Checklist, are available for assessing competence.

PSYCHIATRIC FORENSIC NURSING

Psychiatric forensic nursing can be defined as the psychiatric nursing assessment, evaluation, and treatment of individuals pending a criminal hearing or trial. The defendant is the client, and the client's thinking and behavior prior to, and during, the commission of the crime are the primary focus of the nurse–client relationship. Several other roles for psychiatric forensic nurses are identified and discussed later in this section. Forensic nurses may also care for victims of violence.

Psychiatric forensic nursing as an expanded role is evolving into an advanced practice role. However, some role functions can be undertaken by nurses at the generalist level, usually those who work in correctional mental health settings in a jail, a prison's psychiatric unit, or in a forensic psychiatric hospital's long-term unit where persons who are not guilty by reason of insanity are treated. TABLE 12-2 ■ differentiates forensic psychiatric nursing from correctional mental health nursing.

Dimensions of Practice

The dimensions of practice in psychiatric forensic nursing are affected both by the nature of the client and the client's current involvement with the criminal justice system. While the core of practice is psychiatric–mental health nursing, the relationship between nurse and client is markedly different from that in a psychiatric–mental health nursing role because of the alternative social context of the situation that precipitates their interaction. In addition, the setting—a crime scene, a courtroom, a forensic treatment setting, or a correctional facility—influences the forensic nurse's practice.

TABLE 12-2 ■ Differentiating Psychiatric Forensic Nursing and Correctional Mental Health Nursing		
Variables	**Correctional Mental Health Nursing**	**Psychiatric Forensic Nursing**
Who is the client?	Jail/prison inmate	Attorney
	Client committed to forensic hospital following "not guilty by reason of insanity" plea	The court
Mindset of nurse	Supportive	Objective
	Accepting	Neutral
	Empathic	Detached
Focus of the nurse–client relationship	Inmate or client's current and future needs with eye to reintegration into community	Defendant's behavior and thinking at time of crime
Location	Psychiatric unit within a jail/prison	Community
	Long-term unit within a forensic hospital	Jail or prison
		Hospital ward
Primary purpose of relationship	Psychiatric nursing care of client's (inmate's) present mental health needs	Pretrial completion of court-ordered sanity/competency evaluation
Examples of nursing role functions	Medication teaching	Evidence collection
	Therapeutic groups	Report to court
	One–to–one counseling	Court testimony
Timing	Length of court-ordered commitment, after adjudication	Pretrial

Role Credibility

The psychiatric forensic nurse must be highly skilled in interpersonal relations and communication. Developing collegial relationships with other disciplines is central to the role because of the intersections of practice that overlap with the domain of other disciplines (forensic science, criminal science). The prerequisite to this expanded role is educational preparation—a graduate degree in forensic nursing or a graduate degree in psychiatric–mental health nursing with additional training in forensic nursing. Several colleges and universities offer degree programs as well as certificate courses in forensic subspecialties.

The International Association of Forensic Nurses (IAFN) has developed certification examinations for sexual assault nurse examiners. You can check on the status of the development of other certification programs through the IAFN website, http://www.iafn.org, which can be accessed on the Online Student Resources for this book. Credibility is substantiated by membership or certification in such organizations as the IAFN, the American Academy of Forensic Sciences (http://www.aafs.org), and the American College of Forensic Examiners (http://www.acfei.org), which has a board of forensic nurse examiners. Information on these memberships and certifications can be found on the Online Student Resources for this text. Psychiatric forensic nurses are guided by the standards of forensic nursing practice developed by the American Nurses Association and the International Association of Forensic Nurses (2009).

Roles and Functions

Psychiatric forensic nursing combines elements of nursing science, forensic science, and criminal justice. Psychiatric forensic nursing appeals to a particular type of nurse (male or female) who thrives on the opportunity to work in a stimulating intellectual environment, and who seeks out the opportunity to apply clinical skills to complex legal problems. Psychiatric forensic nurses work as forensic examiners, competency therapists, expert witnesses, and consultants to law enforcement, attorneys, or the criminal justice system. The wide range of possible psychiatric forensic nursing role functions are listed in Box 12-2.

Forensic Examiner

The forensic examiner conducts court-ordered evaluations of legal sanity or competency to proceed, answers any specific medicolegal questions as directed by the court, and renders an expert opinion in a written report or courtroom testimony. Court-ordered sanity or competency evaluations can be requested by the defense, the prosecution, or the court. They are usually initiated because of the defendant's history or behavior at the scene, in jail, or in the courtroom. A thorough and complete forensic examination includes face-to-face interviews, review of police reports, and thorough psychosocial history. The ethical forensic examiner's expert opinion is based on the scientific processing of the following:

- Collected pertinent clinical data
- Observed client behavior

> **Box 12-2 Psychiatric Forensic Nursing Roles**
>
> - Forensic evaluation for legal sanity or competence to proceed at trial
> - Assessment of capacity to formulate intent
> - Assessment of potential for violence or to reoffend
> - Parole/probation considerations
> - Assessment of racial/cultural factors during crime
> - Consultation on countermeasures to violence
> - Assisting in jury selection
> - Investigation of criminal history
> - Sexual predator screening and assessment
> - Courtroom consultation to attorneys
> - Competency therapy
> - Formal written reports to court
> - Expert witness services
> - Police training
> - Review of police reports
> - On-scene consultation to law enforcement

International Association of Forensic Nurses

- Forensic evidence in police reports and laboratory reports
- Results of psychological testing
- Thorough psychosocial history

As a forensic examiner, you are expected to be able to verbalize an exceptional understanding of major mental illnesses and personality disorders. It is also expected that you will keep abreast of theories being developed on social deviancy and interpersonal violence, and keep current on social trends (for example, changes in drug use, growth of gang activity, or cult participation) both nationally and in your own jurisdiction. The successful forensic examiner is able to:

- *Separate personal opinion from professional opinion.* Personal opinion is based on your background, upbringing, education, and values. Professional opinion is based on scientific principle, advanced education in a specific field of endeavor, and the unbiased standards set by research in that area.
- *Isolate personal feelings in dealing with cases of criminal violence.* Sexual deviance, ethnic norms, or cultural behaviors that may not reflect your own personal value system may be integral to the questioning.

Competency Therapist

Competency is the ability to cognitively understand the situation one is in and the implications of treatment. Traditionally, treatment for incompetency meant little more than the prescribing of antipsychotic or other medications. With registered nurses moving into this role, a more holistic approach is being taken—one that encompasses the client's physical, emotional, and spiritual needs. Psychiatric forensic nursing role functions for the competency therapist include the following:

- Administration of assessment tools
- Assessment of competence and mental disorder
- Forensic interview

- Documentation of the client's progress toward competence
- Completion of formal reports to the court
- Expert witness testimony

Competency therapists work with defendants on one–to–one and group levels. It is important that the competency therapist retains objectivity and does not confuse competency therapy with psychotherapy. Competency therapy is education/training-based. The focus of the relationship is on the defendant's thinking and behavior at the time of the crime, not, for instance, on the defendant's history of abuse or failed interpersonal relationships. The client of the competency therapist is the court, not the defendant, and the goal is a competent defendant and completed report.

Expert Witness

By license, any registered nurse can be subpoenaed to court as a *fact witness*. In this role, you testify as to what you personally saw, heard, performed, or documented related to a particular client's care. You are questioned as to these firsthand experiences, and then excused from the courtroom.

An **expert witness** is recognized by the court as having a high level of skill or expertise in a designated area in order to render an opinion on a legal matter in court. As an expert witness, you will be subpoenaed to court to testify on your involvement with the defendant. You will testify as to the role functions you performed and to your documentation. At this point, the court will allow you to give additional testimony in the form of your professional opinion, based on your conclusions, as to the defendant's legal sanity, competence to proceed, future dangerousness, or likelihood of committing future felonious acts.

To establish credibility as an expert and to have one's opinion given equal weight in court opposite a psychiatrist, the forensic nurse specialist must have the following:

1. *Expertise.* Expertise is established by your credentials.
2. *Trustworthiness.* Trustworthiness is the degree of honesty exuded in your demeanor and opinion, as perceived by the judge or jury.
3. *Presentation style.* Presentation style is how you come across to others. You may be credible, trustworthy, and an authority in a specialty area, but without the ability to communicate in a concise and convincing fashion, the value of your testimony is limited.

Consultant to Attorneys

Psychiatric forensic nurses may be called on as a resource for education and information about mental illness by either side of the courtroom. Or you may be asked to attend the hearing as a courtroom observer who listens to other witness testimony for the purpose of guiding further cross-examination. You may also be asked to assist in preparation for trial by giving information about mental illness, personality disorders, or paraphilias, give suggestions for cross-examining a

defendant, or evaluate potential jurors. You may be asked to testify regarding mental health treatment options, medications, and community resources.

Consultant to Law Enforcement

Interagency cooperation between mental health agencies and law enforcement has increased over the last decades, partly due to community need caused by deinstitutionalization. The mental health personnel summoned in those situations function as advocates for the defendant, whose well-being is the focus of the interaction that may result in civil detention and admission to a hospital. Community mental health nurses have traditionally acted in this role.

Psychiatric forensic nurses are expanding their scope of practice by working as consultants to law enforcement in hostage negotiation and criminal profiling. In addition to giving suggestions on how to interview a subject, psychiatric forensic nurses may be involved in actual hostage negotiation or criminal profiling. Over half of all hostage incidents involve hostage takers who are classified in law enforcement as mentally disturbed. Criminal profiling is an educated attempt to provide law enforcement with specific information on the type of individual who would have committed a certain crime after studying behavioral and psychological indicators left at a violent crime scene. These roles differ from that described earlier in purpose and philosophy.

Correctional Mental Health Nursing

Correctional mental health nurses care for inmates housed in a jail or prison's psychiatric unit, or in a forensic psychiatric hospital's long-term ward where persons adjudicated (by judicial procedure) as NGRI are treated. However, the nature of their relationship with the client remains focused on the client's present needs rather than on his or her thinking or behavior in the past (at the time of the crime). Correctional mental health nurses perform psychiatric nursing skills rather than forensic nursing skills. Jails and prisons today house many seriously mentally ill citizens who in prior decades were treated in mental hospitals and community mental health programs (Bloom, 2010). Refer back to Table 12-2 on page 230, which illustrates the differences in forensic psychiatric nursing and correctional mental health nursing.

Correctional mental health nurses make substantial and valued contributions to the care, treatment, rehabilitation, and management of individuals in secure facilities who are deemed legally insane. It is a difficult and challenging client population to work with (Shelton, Weiskopf, & Nicholson, 2010), and personal safety is an issue during every shift. The dedication of correctional mental health nurses has significantly increased the quality of care for their clients. There are high expectations for this specialized area of practice that continues to contribute to the growing fund of nursing knowledge. Correctional mental health nurses are guided by the standards of nursing practice in correctional facilities developed by the American Nurses Association (2007).

CLIENT RIGHTS

The current concern for client rights did not develop overnight. It actually has been evolving since the 1960s, when there was an increased interest in under-represented minority groups, the poor, women, and the mentally disabled.

In 1980, the United States Congress passed the Mental Health Systems Act, which included a model mental health client's bill of rights. This piece of legislation can be thought of as a set of recommendations; it is not a requirement that individual states follow them. In 1990, the American Hospital Association published a Patient's Bill of Rights that many health care settings throughout the United States have adopted. Consumer groups and professional organizations have, at various times, published their own versions of a bill of rights. A mental health consumer's bill of rights has been developed and supported by 15 professional organizations, including nursing, for those seeking mental health and substance abuse treatment. This particular bill of rights can be accessed through the Online Student Resources for this book.

However, there is no one standard mental health client bill of rights at the national level, and the variability among states is great. Some states guarantee several important rights, while some states guarantee only a few. In other words, there is no consistency among states. It is important to understand the basic rights to which psychiatric clients are entitled in the state in which you practice (Cady, 2010). Agency legal and risk management teams can help you to understand the laws in your particular state.

The rights that mental health consumers should have in practice and that you should consider when planning your interventions are outlined in Your Intervention Strategies. A discussion of several of these important rights follows. One means of helping clients protect some of their rights is through the execution of a psychiatric advance directive discussed later in this chapter.

Right to Informed Consent

A client has the right to understand the treatment process prior to consenting to treatment. This is called **informed consent** and is required by all states. The main purpose of the doctrine of informed consent is to encourage individual autonomy and sound decision making. Client self-determination is the basic principle of informed consent.

Key elements of informed consent are competency, information, and voluntariness (Lim & Marin, 2011). If a client's competency is in question, a mental status examination may be necessary. You may need to review the medication record to determine if the client received medication that might interfere with cognitive ability. Take into account any deficits in the client's reception and processing of information. The client must be competent to understand the problem, along with the negative and positive effects from the proposed treatment, and the likely outcome with and without treatment.

Many illnesses impair the ability to acquire new information. In some cases, this is a response to the biologic components of the illness or the effects of medication. In other cases, there may be an educational deficit. For some long-term clients, the presence of a mental illness may have affected the educational experience. This does not mean that intelligence is affected, but that reading and writing skills may not be consistent with chronologic age. Developing plans for offering information that would be needed in the decision-making process helps to ensure a client's right to informed consent. It may be necessary to present information in small pieces using simple language and pictures. Several short presentations may be required, with some mechanism to assess learning to determine whether the client understands the proposed treatment.

Offer all clients choices and give them the advantages and disadvantages of each. While members of the mental health team can offer suggestions, it must be made clear to the client that there is no self-serving bias on the part of the treatment team for one choice or another. Provide the client with the opportunity to ask questions or gain a second opinion. Do not rush or coerce the client into giving consent.

You must document informed consent in writing through the use of a specific form signed by the client, or by an entry into the client's medical record. While written documentation of informed consent will likely fulfill the legal obligation, it is helpful to think of informed consent as more of a recurring process. While hospitalized, you should offer clients many chances to participate in their own care.

Mental Health Consumer's Bill of Rights

YOUR INTERVENTION STRATEGIES   The Rights of Mental Health Consumers

Keep the following rights in mind when planning and implementing nursing interventions:

- Right to informed consent
- Right to treatment
- Right to refuse treatment
- Right to treatment in the least restrictive setting
- Right to communicate with others
- Right not to be subjected to unnecessary mechanical restraints
- Right to privacy
- Right to periodic review of status

- Right to independent psychiatric examination
- Right to participate in legal matters including making a valid contract, executing a will, marrying or divorcing, voting, driving a motor vehicle, practicing a profession, suing or being sued, managing or disposing of property
- Right to habeas corpus
- Right to legal representation
- Right to keep clothing and personal effects
- Right to religious freedom
- Right to education
- Right to civil service status

In assessing whether informed consent has been obtained, you must determine whether the client:

- Is of the age of consent
- Is deemed mentally competent
- Can state that he or she is acting voluntarily
- Can repeat the elements of the condition
- Can repeat the treatment options
- Can repeat the benefits and consequences of each treatment
- Can repeat the consequences of inaction
- Is not impaired by alcohol or other drugs
- Can complete specific written forms such as consent forms, treatment plans, and discharge plans

At times, it may become clear that the client lacks the ability to offer consent. In this case, it is important to interact with legal counsel to determine what should be done. Some states allow legal relatives to participate for a client who cannot consent. Other states demand that the client have an advocate appointed to serve as decision maker. A summary of informed consent requirements is in Your Assessment Approach.

Right to Treatment

The first argument for a right to treatment for involuntarily committed individuals came from Morton Birnbaum, a lawyer and physician, in an article published in 1960. However, the groundbreaking cases did not come from the familiar circles of civil commitment but from people who had been sidetracked from the prison system into hospitals.

Clinical Example

Instead of being convicted for carrying a dangerous weapon and receiving a maximum sentence of 1 year, a man in Washington, D.C. who pleaded not guilty by reason of insanity was sent to the maximum security unit of a federal psychiatric hospital for treatment on an involuntary commitment basis. Four years later, he questioned his detention on the basis of not having received any psychiatric treatment.

A man indicted for murder was sent to a Massachusetts state hospital after having been found incompetent to stand trial. He requested transfer to another facility on the grounds that he was not receiving adequate treatment. Through the testimony of experts, his attorneys were able to show that he was simply receiving custodial care.

An involuntary client in a Florida mental hospital for over 14 years brought suit against the hospital director, claiming that he had been deprived of his constitutional right to liberty. At trial, the jury found that (a) he had received not merely inadequate treatment but no treatment at all; (b) he was not dangerous; (c) acceptable community alternatives were available; and (d) because the hospital director knew all this, he had "maliciously" deprived him of liberty.

In these instances, the courts found a constitutional rationale for treatment. Depriving a citizen of liberty on the altruistic theory that the loss of liberty is for the purpose of therapy, and then failing to provide adequate therapy, violates the rights of citizens guaranteed by the Constitution.

Right-to-treatment issues also have to do with inappropriate releases, or passes to leave a hospital when prudent care would indicate that freedom was inappropriate.

Clinical Example

Eight days after admission to a New Orleans hospital for severe depression, a client was given a weekend pass, during which she attempted suicide. She sued the hospital and psychotherapists for allowing her to leave the hospital when she was not in a fit mental condition.

In Washington, D.C., a client who had been committed to a hospital after being acquitted of murder by reason of insanity left the hospital grounds and stabbed his wife. The hospital was found liable based on its failure to take reasonable measures to ensure that the client did not leave the hospital grounds.

The concept of right to treatment is an outgrowth of the philosophic point of view that the deprivation of liberty, whether voluntary or involuntary, must have an over-riding purpose. A review of court cases indicates that the right to treatment came about because there was no over-riding purpose: Because of overcrowded conditions, inadequate staffing, and financial and programmatic deficiencies, there were not enough resources to deliver the bare minimum of treatment. "Right to treatment" ensures that clients are not in a treatment setting for custodial purposes only. The necessary elements in a treatment-oriented program are listed in Your Intervention Strategies.

Be sure that your facility's program includes the following:

- Physical examination and psychosocial assessment on admission and then as indicated
- Treatment plans with clear objectives and interventions
- Evidence of client participation in treatment planning and consent for all treatment methods
- Up-to-date medical records
- Treatment in as normal an environment as possible
- Staff in adequate numbers and with sufficient training to provide quality care

- Availability of treatment that meets client needs as identified in the treatment plan
- Necessary support services such as dental, speech, physical, and rehabilitation therapy
- Ongoing treatment plan evaluations
- Programs to help clients develop skills needed for independent versus institutional living
- Adequate planning for discharge to a less restrictive setting, according to client needs

Right to Refuse Treatment

At some time in their lives, all people experience the kind of excessive stress that makes them feel miserable or even desperate. But some people communicate these feelings in ways that are inappropriate, troublesome, unreasonable, or frightening to others. A young woman who in times of stress mutilates her body by burning it repeatedly with cigarettes; a teenager who breaks everything in sight during violent, destructive outbursts; and a belligerent man who initiates physical fights with anyone and everyone without provocation—all usually become candidates for *symptomatic treatments*, behavioral control measures often used against a person's will. However, all clients have the right to refuse treatment. The clinical example that follows demonstrates how the right to refuse treatment has been upheld by the courts.

Clinical Example

One of the first cases against restrictive treatment was brought in Minnesota in 1976. In this case, electroconvulsive therapy (ECT) was felt to be an "intrusive" treatment and was not allowed to be given against a competent client's wishes.

An involuntarily committed client at a New Jersey state hospital claimed that forcibly administering medications violated his constitutional rights. He objected to the side effects produced by chlorpromazine (Thorazine) and lithium carbonate. The judge ruled in the client's favor, noting that a person subjected to the harsh side effects of psychotropic drugs should have control over their administration.

Clients at a Massachusetts state hospital initiated a class action suit contending that their constitutional rights were being violated by the hospital's practice of using forced seclusion and medication in nonemergency situations. The court granted competent clients and guardians of incompetent clients an absolute right to refuse medication in nonemergency situations.

An issue that captured public attention was the notorious case of a homeless New York woman forcibly removed from the streets because of her self-neglect and provocative behavior. She was judged competent, however, to refuse medication despite her status as an involuntary client.

In another case, the court found that a nurse who forcibly administered medication to a competent adult client had committed an intentional tort (a wrongful act). The client was involuntarily committed to a mental hospital. She was a practicing Christian Scientist and refused medication. The court held that medication could be given over the client's religious objections only if she were harmful to herself or others. The court allowed her damages for assault and battery.

A more recent trend in some states is toward assisted outpatient treatment (AOT), spurred by New York's Kendra's Law.

Clinical Example

Kendra was a young woman pushed to her death from a subway platform by a man with schizophrenia who had a documented history of assaults and failed to follow prescribed medication regimens. Kendra's parents and other advocates pushed for a statewide law in New York to ensure that persons who are deemed a danger to themselves and others are given assistance in adhering to prescribed medication regimens.

Since Kendra was pushed to her death, almost all states now have some form of statewide AOT that is court ordered for medication nonadherence. Securing the common good is undoubtedly the basis for this form of legislation.

In almost all states, ECT is closely regulated by statute. Most state statutes specify that ECT can be administered only if informed consent is obtained from the client. In the case of an incompetent client, consent must be obtained from the guardian or next of kin. The client's right to refuse ECT is specifically mentioned in many state statutes.

Psychosurgery, referred to in various state statutes as "brain surgery," "lobotomy," or "experimental" or "hazardous" procedures, is also closely regulated by state statute. Most state statutes specify that psychosurgery can be performed only if informed consent is obtained from the client. In several states, psychosurgery can be performed only upon a court order if the client is incompetent. The client's right to refuse psychosurgery is also specifically mentioned in many state statutes.

If written consent is withheld by a client already declared "legally incompetent" by the court or certified "functionally incompetent" by a treating psychiatrist, the decision to medicate forcibly would be referred to a client advocate. It would be up to the client advocate's discretion to request a hearing before an independent psychiatrist. In the case of a competent though involuntarily hospitalized person, a hearing before an independent psychiatrist would be required at which the client would have the right to legal counsel. It is vital to remember that over-riding a client's right to refuse treatment is legally complicated and related to safeguards that are in place to manage such situations. These legal safeguards serve to protect the rights of all people.

Ethical Dilemmas

There are a number of areas of judicial disagreement in the right to refuse treatment that can create dilemmas for the mental health care professional. For example, there is no common definition of the term *psychiatric emergency*. The traditional definition of *emergency* refers to an overt and immediate threat to a person's life. The contemporary definition is less clear and focuses on the immediate, impending, and significant deterioration of the client's condition. Another area of controversy is: At what point can the state over-ride an involuntarily committed client's right to refuse psychotropic medication in a nonemergency? Is it only when a person has been judged incompetent, or does danger to self or others provide a legitimate reason under the state's police power to administer treatment?

In the case of an incompetent individual, there is disagreement over who should decide for the person and what standard should be used. Is it to be a guardian, the hospital staff, or the judiciary? Is the standard what the best interests of the client seem to be, as judged by an informed outsider, or is it what the client would want if competent to make the choice?

The following are some criteria a court is likely to use in ruling on a case involving the right to refuse treatment:

- *Client competency.* If the client is competent, informed consent is possible.
- *Intrusiveness of treatment.* As the intrusiveness increases, so does the court's scrutiny.

- *Permanence of treatment effect.* If side effects are adverse and permanent, the court is less likely to over-ride refusal.
- *Experimental nature of treatment.* The treatment must have scientific merit, and the client must give informed consent.
- *Risk–benefit ratio.* The benefits of treatment must outweigh the risk.
- *Motivation for treatment.* The treatment cannot be used to punish or "quiet" the client for the staff's benefit.
- *Motivation for refusal.* Religious objections are usually upheld.

Despite the difficulties and issues raised by the client's right to refuse treatment, following are some very real positive outcomes:

- Clients must be involved in treatment choices, process, and outcome.
- Clients must be informed of choices and offered alternatives.
- Staff members must acquire a second opinion on potentially harmful procedures.

Consider the other dilemmas outlined in Your Self-Awareness.

Right to Treatment in the Least Restrictive Setting

The idea of least restrictive setting or least restrictive alternative has become an important component of both the

YOUR SELF-AWARENESS
Right to Refuse Treatment

To increase self-awareness of your own opinions about a client's right to refuse treatment, think about the following questions:

- How do I feel when a client's legal right to leave a treatment setting is deemed more important than the client's need for treatment?
- Should clients whose behavior disrupts and frightens other clients be allowed to refuse treatment even when interventions such as medication would definitely reduce their symptoms?
- In the case of a client judged to be mentally incompetent, what standard should be used to make decisions about treatment? Should it be what the hospital staff wants? What a guardian wants? What is in the best interests of the client? What the client would want if competent to make the choice?
- Does society have an obligation to care for a seriously mentally ill person even if this requires limiting that person's freedom to refuse treatment?
- Do we need to protect rights vigorously or is the duty to treat a greater obligation?
- Should a person on the street who is gesturing and talking to herself and carrying a few belongings in a plastic bag be allowed to continue living on the street or be mandated into outpatient commitment?

deinstitutionalization and client rights movements. The term **least restrictive setting** generally refers to the placement of clients in the therapeutic setting that will provide care while allowing maximum freedom. By extension, it also means providing for the least amount of limitation or interference in an individual's thought and decision making, physical activity, and sense of self as necessary to provide for safety.

Clinical Example

A 61-year-old District of Columbia woman had difficulty caring for herself because of confusion secondary to arteriosclerotic brain disease. While not considered a danger to others, she did wander when confused and was subsequently admitted to the federal psychiatric hospital. The court ruled that she did not need 24-hour psychiatric supervision and that a less restrictive form of treatment should be found. Today, such clients can be supervised in assisted living facilities for the cognitively impaired.

The American Nurses Association's standards of psychiatric–mental health nursing practice (2007) direct the nurse to choose the least restrictive limit and use it only for as long as it is necessary for the safety of the client and others.

Treatment Setting

A treatment setting is evaluated on such criteria as the limitations it places on physical freedom (locked or unlocked), choice of activities, and the presence of "adult status" as shown by locked bedrooms and the unsupervised use of private bathroom facilities. In this scheme, inpatient psychiatric settings would be considered the most restrictive, halfway houses less so, and family or independent living the least restrictive.

Institutional Policy

Institutional policy is the degree of restriction imposed by the rules and regulations necessary to run the treatment setting. Criteria to evaluate a setting would include such items as the amount of supervision in daily living tasks, the amount of client involvement in treatment planning, and the priority of activities that increase the client's autonomy.

Enforcement

The enforcement dimension includes the methods sanctioned to enforce the treatment setting's rules. Is coercion or threat of punishment used? Is the standard for socially acceptable behavior higher in the treatment setting than it would be in the client's own environment? How readily and to what extent is the client's autonomy compromised to meet organizational needs?

Treatment

The treatment dimension has to do with the intrusiveness of the treatment used. Psychosurgery and ECT would be considered more intrusive than medication. Long-acting medication such as fluphenazine decanoate would be considered more intrusive than oral medication. The clarity of treatment goals is also a consideration. Nebulous or nonexistent goals increase restrictiveness.

Client Characteristics

The client's illness characteristics are seen by some as restricting behavior to a much greater degree than any locked door. Some believe it is simplistic to think that moving a client from an inpatient setting to the community will automatically result in less restriction. Without effective community-based treatment, including safe housing, many seriously and persistently mentally ill clients frequently end up on the streets (see Chapter 32∞).

Right to Communicate With Others

The basis for laws granting communication rights is that such communication can expose cases of wrongful hospitalization. Generally, communication is unrestricted or guaranteed to named public officials or the central hospital agency for the state. Most states extend this guarantee to include correspondence with attorneys. Most states also require that any correspondence limitation be part of the client's clinical record. Approximately half the states require the client to have reasonable access to writing materials and postage.

Most states have some statutory provisions concerning visitation. However, hospital authorities are generally given broad discretionary powers to curtail this right. Before implementing any restriction in communication or visitation, you should ask: Is it fair and reasonable? Could I defend it to a noninvolved professional?

Right Not to Be Subjected to Unnecessary Mechanical Restraints

Though improvements in treatment have decreased the use of mechanical or physical restraints, such restraints still play a role in some treatment programs. The use of restraints is a complex and multifaceted problem because principles of ethics can be in conflict with each other (Mohr, 2010). Most states have attempted to regulate their use by statute through specifying that restraints can be used only in emergency situations, and only as a measure of last resort, when the client presents a risk of harm to self or others. In those states not having statutory provisions regarding restraints, the procedures to be followed are usually found in the administrative regulations.

Many states and mental health facilities have statutes or protocols that relate to manual restraint. Manual restraint includes holding or restraining an individual against his or her will, regardless of the intent or purpose. For example, holding a person's arm or hand while the person receives an injection or has blood drawn can be considered manual restraint against the person's will unless the person requests physical contact or accepts it when it is offered.

Half the states have laws relating to seclusion. Prevention of harm to self or others is the most common criterion, followed by treatment or therapeutic reasons. You must document the use of either restraints or seclusion in the client's medical record. Nursing organizations such as the American Psychiatric Nurses Association (APNA) and mental health consumer advocacy groups such as the National Alliance on Mental Illness (NAMI) have developed position statements on the use of seclusion and restraint. The position statements are available at the APNA website at http://www.apna.org/i4a/pages/index.cfm?pageid=3504, and at http://www.nami.org, the website for NAMI. Both websites can be accessed through the Online Student Resources for this book. See also Chapter 35∞.

It has become clear that changes in a unit's philosophy can reduce the incidence of the use of seclusion and restraint. A unit with a culture of structure, calmness, negotiation, and collaboration (Delaney & Johnson, 2006) in which staff assess early changes with clients and intervene early with less restrictive measures—verbal and nonverbal communication, reducing stimulation, active listening, diversionary techniques, limit setting, and the judicious use of PRN medication (Johnson & Delaney, 2007)—more clearly safeguard the rights of clients.

Right to Privacy

Almost all states have a specific statute regarding the mental health consumer's right to keep personal information secret, and the specific steps to be taken for release of that information. The confidential nature of the client information is also cited in the American Nurses Association Code of Ethics—maintaining client confidentiality within ethical, legal, and regulatory parameters—as it is in most professional codes.

The goal of confidentiality is to ensure the client's privacy. A significant amount of stigma is attached to being the recipient of psychiatric treatment. Though professionals may argue that this is unfair, it is a fact. Because of this, it is important that clients are the ones to give out information about themselves. You should not discuss the client's name outside of the treatment area unless it is a secure environment and the discussion is among treatment providers for that client. Instructors, students, supervisors, or team members who receive information about a client in the course of supervision or in providing treatment for the client are also obligated to treat this material as confidential.

In order for the disclosure of information to occur, a client must sign a release form. To be a valid release, tell the client as specifically as possible what information is to be released. The client should know the following prior to signing:

- What information is going to be released?
- Who needs it?
- Why do they need it?
- When will they need it?
- How will it be used?

Certain situations require signed consents. FIGURE 12-1 ■ illustrates situations in which signed consents are necessary. Be especially careful to be aware of when written consent is necessary (Rippee, 2010).

Emergency situations may arise. For example, a client may be in a car accident or take an overdose and require treatment in a hospital emergency room. In these situations, the release of information can occur without the client's approval. It is important to document such a breach of confidentiality.

Guidelines for the Use of Restraint and Seclusion

Is a signed written consent required
for the release of personal
information about a client?

NO

Involved treatment
team members; staff
supervisors; involved
mental health care
students and faculty;
mental health care
consultants

YES

Insurance companies;
HMOs; uninvolved
staff members, mental
health care students
and faculty; support
staff; family; lawyers;
law enforcement
agencies

FIGURE 12-1 ■ When a written consent from a mental health consumer is required for release of personal information.

Confidentiality of information is not easy to maintain. Medical records are generally kept not in locked files, but at an easy access point in the nurses' station. Medical files usually travel all over the hospital with the client and are often available for the perusal of others not directly involved in the client's treatment. The increased use of computers for communication and data storage, along with the information requested by the government, third-party payers, and employers, often poses a threat to a client's privacy. More mundane, but equally serious, incidents of breaches of confidentiality occur when staff members talk about clients in the halls, elevator, and cafeteria.

Privileged Communication

Privileged communication is a narrower concept than confidentiality. It is established by state statute to protect possibly incriminating disclosures made by the client to specified professionals.

Clinical Example

A minister brought suit because his former psychiatrist disclosed confidential information about him to his clerical superiors. The court held that unless a client poses a serious threat to himself or to others, the psychiatrist owes a duty of confidentiality. The client was able to recover damages for lost earnings, harm to his reputation, and emotional distress.

YOUR INTERVENTION STRATEGIES
When the Right to Privacy Can Be Breached

The release of information without the client's consent can be made under the following conditions:

■ When acting in the client's best interests in an emergency situation
■ When acting to protect third parties
■ During commitment proceedings
■ When making a court-ordered evaluation or report
■ When a client is incompetent and consent is given by a guardian, or when the guardian is not available
■ When reporting child abuse, gunshot wounds, or contagious diseases, as required by state law
■ During criminal proceedings
■ In child custody disputes
■ During child abuse proceedings
■ When a client introduced a defense of mental illness into litigation proceedings

Privileged communication has traditionally existed between husband and wife, attorney and client, clergy and church member, and physician and client. In some states, communication between psychologist and client is also accorded privileged status. Only a few states recognize privileged communication between nurse and client. Be sure that you are informed about the law in your state. The privilege is the client's and can be claimed only if a therapeutic relationship exists. The professional can reveal the information at the client's request.

Each state that grants a privilege also specifies exceptions to that privilege. Instances in which the right to privacy can be breached are discussed in Your Intervention Strategies.

Disclosure to Safeguard Others

An exception to confidentiality and privilege that has developed from a California Supreme Court decision illustrates the competition between two responsibilities of the mental health care professional: (1) confidentiality to the client, and (2) protection of the public from the "violent" client. This landmark case is often referred to as "the Tarasoff decision" among mental health professionals. In the **Tarasoff decision**, the court's ruling underlined the mental health care professional's responsibility to

MENTAL HEALTH IN THE NEWS

The Tarasoff Decision

The parents of a young woman, Tatiana Tarasoff, successfully sued the University of California, claiming that a psychotherapist from the student counseling center had a responsibility to warn their daughter that his client had threatened to kill her. At the time, the psychologist did notify campus security officers that he believed his client was dangerous and should be involuntarily committed for observation and treatment. However, the man appeared rational to the police and promised them he

would stay away from the young woman. He then terminated treatment, and 2 months later killed her. The California Supreme Court said that, despite the unsuccessful attempt to confine the client, the therapist knew that he was at large and dangerous and had a duty to warn the young woman of the danger. The court recognized the client's right to confidentiality but said this must be weighed against the public's need for safety against violent assault, especially when an individual in danger can be identified.

Photo courtesy of AP PHOTO.

Care Plan: Duty to Warn

balance confidentiality with the "duty to warn" and the "duty to protect." The circumstances that gave rise to the Tarasoff decision are discussed in Mental Health in the News.

In a number of cases, therapists were held liable for not taking some action to protect potential unidentified victims. Your Intervention Strategies shows a model to help mental health caregivers decide on a course of action in implementing the duty to warn or protect.

The duty to warn has stirred up controversy in the mental health community. There is a concern that clients with aggression problems will drop out of therapy, not use it effectively, or be less likely to seek treatment for fear of being betrayed. Remember also that no mental health care professional can reliably predict the future violence of a mentally disordered person.

Right to Periodic Review

Most states have some provision for periodic review of involuntary clients. Periodic review provides some protection for the individual against spending more time than necessary in the hospital. Review is required every 30 days in some states, every year in others. A few states require review "as frequently as necessary," or "from time to time." The actual scope of the review is usually not governed by statute. The trend in recent years has been away from hospitalization for indeterminate periods of time. In New York and California, short-term commitment is the rule, and court review is necessary to extend commitment for another short period.

Right to Independent Psychiatric Examination

Mental health consumers have the right to an independent psychiatric assessment by a physician of their own choosing. The client must be released if the physician determines the client is not mentally ill.

Right to Participate in Legal Matters

Mental health consumers have rights to participate as citizens in legal matters.

Contracts

Clients committed to a mental hospital generally maintain their right to make a valid contract, unless they have also been judged incompetent. In most states, commitment proceedings are separate from those for competence. Therefore, an individual who is legally incompetent is not necessarily subject to commitment, and an individual committed to an institution is not automatically legally incompetent. Even though the issue of contracts may seem clear-cut, in reality a client's right to contract may be restricted by the administrative regulations of hospitals and state mental health agencies. A contested contract would most likely be a matter for the court to decide.

Wills

To make a valid will, a person must:

- Be aware of making a will.
- Be familiar with the property being disposed of.
- Know the names, identities, and relationships of the people named in the will.

A person with a psychiatric diagnosis, whether in or out of the hospital, can make a valid will as long as these requirements are met. Psychosis with accompanying delusions does not by itself negate a valid will. The delusions have to produce a significant distortion of the person's perception of the property, family, or personal relationships to invalidate the will.

Marriage and Divorce

According to statute and common law, a valid marriage contract hinges on the individual's possession of sufficient mental

---

YOUR INTERVENTION STRATEGIES
A Model for Implementing the Duty to Warn or Protect

Action	Implementation
Assess dangerousness	Compare data to factors believed to correlate with dangerous behavior such as increasing use of drugs and/or alcohol, current and past threats of violence and/or assaultive behavior, and presence of command hallucinations.
	Be sure to review past and current treatment records. Interview client, family, and significant others.
	Ask: Is the threat serious? Are the threats repeated? Are the means to carry out the threat available? Can the victim be identified? Is the victim accessible?
Select a course of action to protect the victim	Consider voluntary hospitalization, or, if necessary, initiate involuntary commitment.
	If the client is already hospitalized, is a more secure unit needed to prevent escape?
	If the client is an outpatient, is medication needed? Are more frequent visits needed? Is a more intensive outpatient care needed, such as a day program?
	Because threats often involve family members, is intensive, systems-oriented therapy indicated to include the intended victim?
	If containment or control is not possible, contact the identified victim. Consider also alerting the police.
Implement decision	Continue to monitor: If the initial course of action fails, take other measures. Be sure to document this decision-making process in the client's record.

capacity to give consent. Sufficient mental capacity implies that the person:

- Understands the nature of the marriage relationship
- Knows the duties and obligations involved

The statutes of a small number of states prohibit marriage by mentally disordered people because they are believed to be incapable of making a contract. More states, however, prohibit marriage by the mentally disordered on the grounds that they are "insane" or "of unsound mind," without specifically defining these terms. Despite these prohibiting statutes, few states even try to enforce the prohibition outside mental institutions.

Most states also have provisions for annulment or divorce on the grounds of prenuptial mental disability. Divorce on the grounds of postnuptial mental disability has been incorporated in the statutes of most states.

Voting

People with psychiatric disabilities are often denied the opportunity to vote on the grounds that they are not competent (Bazelon Center for Mental Health Law, 2011) despite the fact that most states do not actually prohibit them from voting. The hospitalized client's right to vote is probably more restricted by caretaker and community apathy or by poll workers, election officials, and service providers who prevent them from voting, than it is by statute. Under federal law, a person cannot be barred from voting except in very limited circumstances.

Right to Drive

Statutes on driving privileges are difficult to interpret. Most states do not issue a driver's license to mentally disturbed people. In some states, this restriction also applies to people with seizure disorders or substance abuse problems. Several states suspend a driver's license as soon as the individual enters a mental institution. Other jurisdictions limit the restriction to those admitted involuntarily, while still others base suspension on legal competency.

Right to Practice a Profession

The ability of a hospitalized client to practice a profession is usually impaired simply by the physical confinement. However, most states have some statutes prohibiting the practice of a profession by a mentally disturbed person. The vagueness of the statutes often makes it difficult to know when they are applicable. As a rule, it is up to the professional licensing board to suspend or revoke the license of a member who is believed to be too mentally incapacitated to practice a profession safely, even though not hospitalized.

Right to Habeas Corpus

Mental health consumers in all states have the protection of the constitutional right of **habeas corpus**. Habeas corpus requires the speedy release of any person who has been illegally detained. Any client can petition for release on the grounds of being sane. If the client is found sane in a hearing, the client must be discharged.

Rights of Children or Minors

The rights of children have been the subject of much judicial and legislative action. In most states, an individual is considered a minor or juvenile if younger than 18 years of age. As a minor, the person is considered legally incompetent. Legal consent for medical treatment must come from parents or a guardian. There are, however, a number of exceptions to this general rule of presumed legal incompetency in some state statutes. These include the rights to:

- Seek treatment for drug abuse.
- Consent to contraception or abortion.
- Seek psychiatric treatment.

Other factors, such as military service, marriage, emancipation, pregnancy, and parenthood, may also affect the age at which a minor may be considered competent.

The most controversial issue of a minor's role in the mental health system involves involuntary commitment. Like adults, minors can be committed to a mental hospital against their will. But, unlike adult admissions, the admission of a minor who objects is considered "voluntary" if the parents have authorized it. Because of the realization that parents may not always be acting in the best interests of the child, a number of lawsuits challenging this practice were filed. It was argued that the "voluntary" admission of minors without procedural safeguards was unconstitutional, and that a court hearing should always be held to determine if commitment is warranted. The United States Supreme Court upheld the rights of parents to admit their children to psychiatric facilities as long as a "neutral factfinder" (physician) believes medical standards for admission have been met.

The trend for inclusion of procedural safeguards continues as an increasing number of states have modified their "voluntary" parental commitment statute by one or more of the following factors:

- Lowering the age of required consent: the majority of states specify age 16 to 18
- Requiring the consent of the child
- Providing for a court hearing if the child protests
- Providing for self-initiated institutionalization for minors

PSYCHIATRIC ADVANCE DIRECTIVES

Psychiatric advance directives (PADs) are modeled after advance directives for end-of-life care. They are legal instruments that allow competent persons to document their preferences regarding mental health treatment. Any person can prepare a PAD as a contingency plan to put in place should the person be incapacitated, found to be incompetent, or unable to make reliable decisions about psychiatric care. Some people *expect to become incapacitated* in the future—for example, a person with symptoms of early Alzheimer's or Pick's disease (see Chapter 14∞). Others may simply *anticipate the possibility of becoming incapacitated* in the future—for example, a person with a family history of Alzheimer's or Pick's disease. Still others have experienced an episode of mental disorder—perhaps depression requiring a period of hospitalization during which they received ECT—and wish to register their preferences for any future psychiatric intervention.

A written PAD allows a person to do the following:

1. Register refusal of certain psychiatric interventions such as ECT, psychotropic medications, psychosurgery, and the like.
2. Register consent and desire for certain psychiatric interventions.
3. Specify the conditions under which these interventions are acceptable.
4. Appoint a trusted surrogate decision maker, a person(s) authorized to give consent on the person's behalf.
5. Register whether the person is willing or unwilling to participate in psychiatric research studies.
6. Improve communication between the person and the mental health care provider.
7. Possibly shorten a hospital stay (Bazelon Center for Mental Health Law, 2011).

Increasing numbers of mental health professionals favor PADs because in addition to guiding family members, significant others, and professionals, they respect the client's autonomy. In addition, they help engage the client in treatment, increase the client's satisfaction with treatment, and enhance the therapeutic alliance with mental health care providers (Van Dorn, Scheyett, Swanson, & Swartz, 2010). Advance directives become even more important when the surrogate decision maker is other than the client's next of kin (see Evidence-Based Practice). In this instance, a PAD can also reduce the use of court proceedings.

While PADs are becoming more popular (they first came into existence in the 1990s), they are still not in common use.

A survey of 1,011 psychiatric outpatients in five U.S. cities indicated that only 4% to 13% of participants had completed a PAD, but between 66% and 77% reported wanting to complete one if given assistance (Swanson, Swartz, Ferron, Elbogen, & Van Dorn, 2006). Some 22 states have created specific forms for PADs. They can be accessed through a resource center created in 2006, the National Resource Center on Psychiatric Advance Directives (NRC-PAD), which can be accessed through the Online Student Resources for this text or at http://www.nrc-pad.org. Persons in states that do not have a specific PAD form can use the Bazelon Center for Mental Health Law template at http://www.bazelon.org. All states have a provision for a durable power of attorney for health care to which a PAD can be attached.

Mental health consumers who are now using these documents find that a PAD is a tool for empowerment and self-determination. At the same time that mental health consumers anticipate the likelihood that mental health care providers, hospitals, and judges honor their choices, they are concerned about the limited knowledge of PADS among mental health service providers (Kim et al., 2007). An advance directive such as a PAD provides written direction for ethically sensitive judgment on the part of professionals and surrogates even in states in which they are not legally recognized. FIGURE 12-2 ■ illustrates the elements that comprise a PAD and a step-by-step process that you can use to help a client develop and implement a PAD.

LIABILITY AND THE PSYCHIATRIC–MENTAL HEALTH NURSE

Criminal and civil are the two main classes of law. *Criminal law* pertains to behavior considered to be a threat to the order of society as a whole, such as murder, assault, and robbery. *Civil law* is concerned with the legal rights and duties

EVIDENCE-BASED PRACTICE

Acting as a Client Advocate

Heather Adams is a neighbor in your apartment building. On weekends, the two of you sometimes get together for morning coffee. Last weekend, Heather shared with you a concern that has been troubling her for a few weeks. She is 31 years old, unmarried, and lives alone. Her father died 3 years ago in a construction accident. Since that time, Heather's mother has become increasingly incapacitated with Alzheimer's disease and is now a resident in a long-term care facility for the cognitively impaired. When she was in her early 20s, Heather was hospitalized and treated for depression. Heather's next of kin is her brother, Ed, from whom she has been estranged for 5 years. Her fear is that, should she become incapacitated again with depression, the brother whom she actively dislikes and with whom she does not get along will make treatment decisions as next-of-kin.

You have decided to invite Heather for coffee on Saturday. Because Heather seems to be a person who would benefit from a formal PAD, you intend to educate her about her choices. You plan to use

Figure 12-2 as the basis for a discussion with Heather and to help her formalize her wishes concerning any possible future psychiatric treatment such as medication and ECT, treatment setting, the selection of a trusted surrogate, and whether or not she is willing to participate in psychiatric research studies. The next step is to obtain a sample PAD from the Bazelon Center for Mental Health Law (see the References at the end of this chapter) for Heather to review. This way, as suggested in the following studies, you can serve as an active resource for Heather.

Caldwell, B. A., Sciafani, M., Swarbrick, M., & Piren, K. (2010). Psychiatric nursing practice and the recovery model of care. *Journal of Psychosocial Nursing and Mental Health Services, 48*(7), 42–48.

Van Dorn, R. A., Scheyett, A., Swanson, J. W., & Swartz, M. S. (2010). Psychiatric advance directives and social workers: An integrative review. *Social Work, 55*(2), 157–167.

CRITICAL THINKING QUESTIONS

1. On what basis do you act as an advocate for Heather?
2. Is it ethical for you to serve as the surrogate decision maker?
3. Why might some mental health professionals have negative attitudes about PADs?

FIGURE 12-2 ■ Helping a client develop and implement a psychiatric advance directive.

of private parties. Most legal actions against nurses are civil actions.

An important division of civil law is known as *tort law*. A tort is a wrongful act resulting in injury for which the injured party files a civil suit requesting legal redress, usually in the form of monetary damages. Torts may be intentional, as in assault, battery, defamation of character, invasion of privacy, false imprisonment, fraud, and misrepresentation; or unintentional, as in negligence. Under tort law, nurses can be held responsible for their own actions. Therefore, all nurses should carry their own malpractice insurance.

Negligence

The concepts of duty and responsibility permeate human relationships. In healthy relationships, expectations are negotiated between individuals that delineate the responsibilities of each person. People who experience times of stress and illness may have difficulty forming realistic expectations, accepting responsibility for actions, and understanding the roles and limits of those who would like to help.

There are times when two people may experience problems understanding and meeting the duties and responsibilities of the relationship. The resolution of such problems is often a therapeutic issue. At times, however, the legal system may become involved. This is particularly true if the client, or the client's family, perceives that the nurse failed to provide the quality of care expected.

All nurses are responsible for determining the quality of care as experienced by their clients. You should address any lapses in the quality of care. The term **negligence** is used whenever a nurse fails to act in a manner in which most reasonable and prudent people would act or when a nurse acts in a way that a reasonably prudent person would not act under similar circumstances. How does one determine what is reasonable and prudent? First, you are accountable to external legal authorities such as the nurse practice act of the state in which you practice, as well as civil and criminal codes. You are also accountable to maintain the standards of psychiatric–mental health nursing practice (2007) published by the American Nurses Association, and to the employing agency or hospital. You are also accountable for familiarizing yourself with current journal and textbook information related to the care of mental health clients.

Conditions for Establishing Negligence

A simple breach in the quality of care does not necessarily mean that a nurse was negligent. Certain conditions must be met to determine negligence and hold the nurse accountable. These conditions are discussed in the following section and summarized in Box 12-3.

Contract for Care A contract for care must have been established between the nurse and the client. A nurse may also begin this contract by accepting a client assignment, having a discussion with the client, offering information or education, providing treatment, serving as a group leader, accepting a client into an activity, or supervising the activities of a mental health worker. It is important to note that entering into a therapeutic relationship creates a legally binding contract between the nurse and the client.

Duty of Care There must be identifiable, explicit, and manifest duty of care in which the intentions of the nurse are to help the client. This intention to help is termed *good faith*. One example is the "good faith" use of the nursing process, including pertinent and timely assessment, planning, outcome

identification, intervention, and evaluation of the client. Another example is a nursing care policy that indicates a course of action. A policy of a given mental health agency might state that each nurse must perform an assessment that includes information related to the emotional, physical, and social health of each client. Failure to use the nursing process and to follow the procedure to provide such an assessment (and take actions based upon this assessment) might be grounds for a charge of negligence.

Ignorance of a policy or procedure is not an acceptable rationale for not following a policy or procedure. For example, all nurses are expected to assess clients for the potential to commit suicide. All reasonable, prudent nurses perform an assessment for suicide potential. The nurse must act to safeguard the life of the client within the limits of the law. Failure to perform such an assessment or take actions to protect the client might be deemed negligent, if harm is present.

Presence of Harm The client must suffer harm that can be directly linked to the failure of the nurse to act in a reasonable and prudent manner. A nurse who fails to assess for suicide potential, thus failing to protect the client, can be held negligent only if the client suffers harm in a suicide attempt or dies as a result of self-inflicted action.

Common Practice There may be no written policy or procedure, nor a law to guide a practitioner in acting, but there is strong indication for action based on what is generally considered *common practice*. Consider a client who lacks any contact with reality. The client cannot perform activities of daily living such as eating, bathing, toileting, or making decisions about safety. It is common practice, in this situation, to perform the activities of daily living for the client. Conversely, it is common practice to encourage clients to do as much for themselves as possible.

Boundary Violation Another example concerns the boundaries of personal relationships between clients and mental health care professionals. Some states fail to define the boundaries of personal relationships between clients and mental health care professionals. In these cases, each nurse must define the nature of the nurse–client relationship. Nurses do not form social relationships with mental health clients with whom there is or has been a professional relationship. This implies that nurses do not date nor engage in sexual activity with a client. Any suggestion or promise that the relationship might be personal can be considered negligence—the failure to explain the limits of the relationship to the client and to act within the boundaries of that relationship. (Boundaries are also discussed in Chapter 4∞.)

Acting Against the Nurse's Advice Clients sometimes contribute to the harm they suffer. A client may be informed of the dangers of certain actions and yet may decide to act against the advice of the nurse. Each client maintains the civil rights of freedom of speech, movement, and action unless there are grounds to curtail these rights, as in the case of harm to self and others. Consider the following clinical example.

Box 12-3 Determining Negligence

- Did a contract for care exist?
- Was the care reasonable and prudent?
- Did the care follow guidelines suggested by external sources such as nurse practice acts, the ANA Code of Ethics, the ANA Standards for Psychiatric–Mental Health Nursing, and the state Mental Health Act?
- Was the care consistent with internal sources such as policies and procedures of the agency or physician orders?
- Was there evidence of thorough assessment of the client, including old records and interviews with family members?
- Did the action taken reveal appropriate ongoing monitoring of the client's condition?
- Did harm result to the client?
- Was the harm due to violation of the duty to care?

Clinical Example

A client had been beaten by her boyfriend. The pattern of escalating abuse was pointed out to her, and she was given the phone numbers of agencies that were available on a 24-hour basis, encouraged to form a safe plan, and offered alternative living arrangements. She decided to return to her boyfriend and suffered paralysis from another beating. She claimed the staff did not act to protect her.

Refer back to Box 12-3 to consider whether the staff was negligent in this case.

Malpractice

Malpractice refers to the negligent acts of health care professionals when they fail to act in a responsible and prudent manner in carrying out their professional duties. The most common sources of liability in psychiatric–mental health services are identified in Box 12-4.

Need to Document

The following cases illustrate a breach of the ANA's standards of psychiatric–mental health nursing practice and emphasize the importance of written communication between nurse and physician.

Clinical Example

A man was admitted to a hospital after becoming increasingly depressed and suicidal secondary to the medication used to treat his hypertension. As a new client, he was not allowed to leave the unit. Four days later, the nursing staff assumed without a verifying written medical order (later a verbal order would be claimed) that he was allowed to leave the unit, unescorted, to attend Mass with permission of the nurse on duty. The following morning he was allowed to go to breakfast unescorted. This time, however, he committed suicide by jumping from a seventh-floor window. The court ruled that the nurse involved with his care breached the standard of care due under Alaska law. The nurse failed to exercise reasonable care to protect a suicidal client against foreseeable harm to himself.

Another case shows the importance of nursing observation and documentation, even though in this case it did not prevent a tragedy.

Box 12-4 Common Sources of Liability in Psychiatric–Mental Health Services

- Client suicide
- Improper treatment
- Misuse of psychotropic medications
- Breach of confidentiality
- False imprisonment
- Injuries or problems related to ECT
- Sexual contact with a client
- Failure to obtain informed consent
- Failure to report abuse
- Failure to warn potential victims

Clinical Example

Distraught with problems and a pending divorce, a 35-year-old man was voluntarily admitted to a psychiatric hospital. During this admission, he expressed thoughts of suicide and also thoughts of killing his wife and her mother. Three weeks after his discharge, he was readmitted voluntarily after a suicide attempt. Nurses' notes revealed his repeated homicidal threats. Three weeks after his second admission, he was given a pass. He subsequently secured a gun and shot and killed his wife and her friend. He was tried and convicted on two counts of murder. The children brought a wrongful death action against the hospital, seeking damages for the murder of their mother by their father. The court granted substantial damages to the children. No liability was attributed to the nurses involved, but the physician was judged negligent.

It is important to remember the nature and purpose of hospital records and to follow prudent, appropriate, and ethical procedures in record maintenance. Records that have been changed for whatever reason need to include the date, the reason for the change, and the signature of the person making the change. A dishonest change could result in the charge of fraud or misrepresentation, as occurred in the next example.

Clinical Example

A 23-year-old woman was admitted with a diagnosis of schizophrenia. She spent 3 days in a bare, quiet room for safety reasons. On the fourth day the bed was returned to the room, but no rationale was noted in the chart. A few days later, an order on the client's chart for an antipsychotic medication was not noted, and the client was without medication for 3 days. The client was later found in a semicomatose condition with her head lodged between the side rails and mattress. Subsequently, the nursing director ordered the nursing staff to "rewrite" the nursing notes. The substituted record clearly conflicted with other records and staff testimony. A $3.6 million verdict against the hospital was upheld.

Many factors contribute to the initiation of a malpractice suit by a client. As long as you are involved in practice, lawsuits are a possibility.

CLIENT ADVOCACY

Despite the prevalence of mental disorder in the United States, mental health services remain poorly funded, mental illness remains misunderstood, and individuals with recurring mental illness live lives characterized by isolation, underemployment, stigma, and denial of rights (Caldwell, Sciafani, Swarbrick, & Piren, 2010). The gap between the rights clients have in theory and in practice may be the result of a knowledge deficit on the part of treatment providers. If so, the remedy is simple: Educate the treatment providers so that they in turn can educate their clients. Another possibility that may not be so amenable to an easy solution is that direct care providers are threatened by the expansion of client rights. Mental health staff members have been heard to say that new regulations not only hampered treatment but made their job both more difficult and more dangerous.

The federal government has encouraged states to develop ombudsmen (persons who speak for or champion the cause of others) or advocacy programs and nurses have advocated for the protective empowering of their clients (Chiovitti, 2011). State advocacy programs have the authority to investigate reported incidents of neglect and abuse to the mentally ill in public or private mental health treatment settings, research facilities, and nursing homes.

Two recent pieces of federal legislation have implications for the rights of clients. In 1990, the Americans with Disabilities Act (ADA) extended federal protection to individuals with physical and/or mental health disabilities for access to public services, employment, and benefits. In an effort to increase the involvement of individuals in directing their own medical care, the Patient Self-Determination Act (PSDA) of 1991 was ratified by Congress as part of the Omnibus Budget Reconciliation Act. The PSDA was designed to inform competent clients at the time of their admission to a hospital of their rights to accept or reject aspects of their medical care.

Although laws can protect certain aspects of human rights, there is a far greater area that laws cannot protect. Laws rarely have a direct effect on a person's beliefs, values, and attitudes, which to a great extent determine whether the letter or the spirit of the law will be carried out. Remember that while the letter of the law may require reading clients their rights on admission, the spirit of the law may not necessarily be satisfied. Clients may not understand the information, remember it, or be able to take it in because anxiety may be causing selective inattention (see Chapter 8∞). Wariness of staff may also cause client discomfort, such as occurred in a study of adult clients with PADs who experienced psychiatric crises. Some clients revealed their discomfort in acknowledging that they had a PAD because they feared a negative response from staff or even involuntary treatment (Kim et al., 2007). Psychiatric–mental health nurses practicing from a humanistic perspective are often in a position to advocate both the letter of the law and the spirit of clients' rights.

Physical and Psychological Abuse of Clients

Clients are particularly vulnerable to both physical and psychological abuse and often do not have the ability or power to defend themselves. There is little actual information on how much client abuse exists in treatment settings. One advocate group ranked client abuse as the most frequent rights-violation complaint. Another ranked it third. The following are the types of abuse reported to occur with some frequency:

- Supplying clients with drugs or alcohol in return for favors
- Making privileges contingent on favors from clients
- Slapping and kicking clients when staff members felt frustrated
- Using restraints when other less intrusive alternatives were available
- Verbal harassment, including threats, sarcasm, and other "put-downs"
- General threats of harm if clients do not behave "appropriately" or as they are told
- Inhumane physical facilities

Sexual conduct with clients is also a form of abuse as well as a boundary violation.

Advocacy Interventions

Psychiatric–mental health nursing advocacy interventions would be directed at some of the identifying causes that may lead to client abuse, including the following:

- Unsuitability of certain staff members who do not have the patience or understanding to work with clients having trouble with control
- A buildup of stresses that have reduced both the staff's patience and ability to problem solve (burnout)
- An actual lack of knowledge of other means of interacting with clients in a high-stress situation

The clinical example that follows demonstrates all three causes.

Clinical Example

John had akithesia, a side effect of his medication, that caused extreme restlessness. John was unable to sit still or to stay in one place for any length of time. Psychiatric attendants, who were charged with keeping an eye on John for his own safety, were often frustrated by what they saw as their need to keep him contained. Two nursing students observed one of the attendants roughly pulling on John and slinging him into a chair in the dayroom. The students reported their observations to their clinical instructor. The three of them approached the charge nurse to complain about the attendant's treatment of John. The result was a team meeting in which the professional staff developed a plan of care for John that included a medication change as well as behavioral training for the staff that incorporated a humane treatment plan based on an increased understanding of the reasons for John's restlessness.

Make no mistake about it; advocating for clients can have positive effects. Do not hesitate to bring to awareness any instances that you observe of physical or psychological abuse. Other areas of advocacy include the following:

- Educating clients and their families about their legal rights
- Monitoring treatment planning and delivery of service for the abuse of client rights
- Evaluating policies and procedures regarding client rights infringement
- Making sure clients have the necessary information to make an informed decision or give informed consent
- Questioning other health care professionals when their care is based more on stereotypic ideas than on an assessment of the client's needs
- Speaking out for safe practice conditions when threatened by budget cutbacks
- Supporting a private advocacy organization such as the Bazelon Center for Mental Health Law that defends the rights of children and adults with mental disabilities through policy advocacy

Duty to Intervene

In medical–surgical nursing, it is often very easy to determine when and how to help clients. If a client has low blood sugar, you offer food to increase the blood sugar level. In psychiatric–mental health nursing, it is often difficult to determine when and how to intervene in particular situations. What is my responsibility? What should be done? Who should do it? What are the appropriate legal choices? What is an appropriate ethical response? Am I going to get sued for doing this? Am I going to get sued if I don't?

Contract for Care

A contract for care implies that the client has a need for help and that the nurse has agreed to act in good faith for the interest of the client. Nurses form this contract when they accept the duty to care for a client during the process of working on a mental health unit. This contract focuses on the nurse's professional perception that there is an issue that requires management.

Notice that the client may not have asked for help. There are many times when the client is so ill that asking for help is not a reasonable expectation. When working with mental health clients, one general rule applies: Once a situation has come to your awareness, it is important that you take all reasonable and prudent actions to intervene to be helpful to the client.

The process of admission should prepare a client for the actions that will be taken given certain situations such as suicidal threats or acts of violence. Most mental health units have a list of client rights and administrative policies and procedures. For example, material that is confidential is explained and material that must be shared is discussed. At times, clients may attempt to use the mental health unit as a shield against facing legal charges. In these instances, make relevant policies explicit to the client.

Assessment

All interventions must follow a thorough assessment. Inform the client that staff members will perform ongoing assessments to facilitate care. When clients are unable to cooperate with assessments because of cognitive impairment, it is vital to obtain information from other sources including records from previous hospitalizations, family members, or community therapists (with client permission). The staff may need to review lab work to explore the level of reliability in the information presented by clients with respect to drug or alcohol use, for example.

Lying on the part of the client has several aspects with legal implications. A client may deliberately mislead the staff member by telling stories that the client knows are not true. This is best dealt with through respectful confrontation. A client may not actually lie but may frame a situation so that the client is viewed as a victim, without including details pertinent to a full understanding of the situation. In this case, it may be helpful to walk through the situation several times, with more than one interviewer, and ask for further details.

Some mental disorders affect the perception and memory of events so profoundly that only a third party such as a family member can offer an accurate view. You must make a good faith effort to perform a full assessment of a client before intervening. Record this information in the chart with statements not only related to information you were able to obtain but also actions you took to obtain information. Failure to assess the client and the situation may result in errors in judgment. It is essential to take the time to collect information essential for decision making. This process requires expert communication skills not only with the client but with others involved in the client's care.

Responsibility to Communicate and Collaborate

The duty to intervene requires that information be communicated clearly to others, particularly those who participate in the decision-making process. You are responsible for informing all individuals involved in the care of a client of the results of the assessment and of the considerations for the intervention phase.

Providing optimal care to clients requires cooperation and collaboration with others. No one professional can make decisions without consultation with others. You must be able to communicate effectively within the established protocols of the agency of employment. These policies and procedures are often called the *chain of command*. The chain of command is the expected pattern of communication surrounding the care of clients. Several aspects of the chain of command are important to remember.

1. Nurses are often responsible for the care provided by others. The nurse may work with several nursing assistants or mental health technicians or psychiatric attendants. The nurse must make clear to nonprofessionals the situations that demand immediate attention. The paraprofessionals working on a psychiatric–mental health nursing unit must be able to recognize situations that should be immediately reported.
2. The nurse often serves as a liaison to other departments. The nurse practice act in the state in which you work will determine the dependent, independent, and interdependent roles of the nurse. Often these roles need to be explained to other professionals.
3. The ANA's standards for psychiatric–mental health nursing practice (2007) provide standards of care. Many professionals do not know that the psychiatric nurse must judge her or his practice based on these guidelines. The hospital or mental health agency will provide guidelines for notification and decision making that must be followed. It is vital to know the policies of the institution.

These three elements form a framework for your actions. Once an event has occurred, notify team members who may not be present on the unit. Usually, you must notify the nurse manager or supervisor, physician, psychologist, social worker, security department, and at times the family, a person who has been threatened, or the police.

Formulating a Plan to Intervene

It is vital to formulate a plan before making a decision to intervene. Nurses often complain of not having "think time," time to consider all options before acting. Many nurses indicate that they respond based on past experience or intuition. While this may work for many expert nurses, beginning nurses need to carefully think through options and learn to assess the clinical and legal implications of actions in a methodical fashion.

Illegal, Immoral, or Unethical Activities of Professionals

At times, you may notice that peers are engaging in illegal activities. It is vital that every nurse understands the legal mandate that requires a response from any professional who has knowledge of illegal, immoral, or unethical activities. Normally, this response is to report the activity to others in the agency, using the chain of command. At other times, you may need to seek the guidance of the State Board of Nursing or the American Nurses Association.

Nurse impairment is perhaps the most common situation encountered by professional staff. A nurse may be impaired through addiction to alcohol or narcotics, or through an event of personal experience with emotional illness. This impairment may be linked with other illegal acts such as theft of drugs or a client's personal property. Each nurse is first responsible to the client and must report such impairment to an immediate supervisor in a reasonable, prudent, and timely manner. Although some nurses erroneously view this intervention as an invasion of privacy or "tattling," prompt, efficient action may safeguard the client from harm while offering the impaired nurse a chance at recovery. Most hospitals have programs to assist impaired nurses to recover. Many state nursing boards or state professional associations have programs to assist the nurse addict or emotionally impaired nurse.

Pearson Nursing Student Resources

Find additional review materials at nursing.pearsonhighered.com

Prepare for success with NCLEX®-style practice questions, interactive assignments and activities, web links, animations and videos, and more!

REFERENCES

American Bar Association. (1995). *Mental disability law* (5th ed.). Washington, DC: Author.

American Nurses Association. (2007). *Corrections nursing: Scope and standards of practice.* Silver Spring, MD: Nursesbooks.org

American Nurses Association, American Psychiatric–Mental Health Nurses Association, and International Society of Psychiatric–Mental Health Nurses. (2007). *Psychiatric–mental health nursing: Scope and standards of practice.* Silver Spring, MD: Nursesbooks.org.

American Nurses Association & International Association of Forensic Nurses. (2009). *Scope and standards of forensic nursing practice.* Washington, DC: Author.

American Psychiatric Association. (2000). *Diagnostic and statistical manual of mental disorders* (4th ed., Text Revision). Washington, DC: Author.

Bazelon Center for Mental Health Law. (2007). *Power in planning: Self-determination though psychiatric advance directives.* Washington, DC: Bazelon Center.

Bazelon Center for Mental Health Law. (2011). *Outpatient and civil commitment.* Retrieved from http://www.bazelon.org

Begley, A. M. (2006). Facilitating the development of moral insight in practice: Teaching ethics and teaching virtue. *Nursing Philosophy, 7*(4), 257–265.

Bloom, J. D. (2010). The "incarceration revolution": The abandonment of the seriously mentally ill to our jails and prisons. *Journal of Law and Medical Ethics, 38*(4), 727–734.

Cady, R. F. (2010). A review of basic patient's rights in psychiatric care. *JONA's Healthcare Law and Ethics and Regulation, 12*(4), 117–125.

Caldwell, B. A., Sciafani, M., Swarbrick, M., & Piren, K. (2010). Psychiatric nursing practice and the recovery model of care. *Journal of Psychiatric Nursing and Mental Health Services, 48*(7), 42–48.

Cherry, M. J. (2010). Nonconsensual treatment is (nearly always) morally impermissible. *Journal of Law and Medical Ethics, 38*(4), 789–798.

Chiovitti, R. F. (2011). Theory of protective empowering for balancing patient safety and choices. *Nursing Ethics, 18*(1), 88–101.

Clausen, J. (2010). Ethical brain stimulation—Neuroethics of deep brain stimulation in research and clinical practice. *European Journal of Neuroscience, 32*(7), 1152–1162.

Davis, A. J., Fowler, M. D., & Aroskar, M. A. (2010). *Ethical dilemmas & nursing practice* (5th ed.). Upper Saddle River, NJ: Pearson Education.

Delaney, K. R., & Johnson, M. E. (2006). Keeping the unit safe: Mapping psychiatric nursing skills. *Journal of the American Psychiatric Nurses Association, 12*(4), 1–10.

Fowler, M. D. M. (2010). *Guide to the code of ethics for nurses: Interpretation and application.* Silver Spring, MD: American Nurses Association.

Johnson, M. E., & Delaney, K. R. (2007). Keeping the unit safe: The anatomy of escalation. *Journal of the American Psychiatric Nurses Association, 13*(1), 42–52.

Kim, M. M., Van Dorn, R. A., Scheyett, A. M., Elbogen, E. E., Swanson, J. W., Swartz, M. S., & McDaniel, L. A. (2007). Understanding the personal and clinical utility of psychiatric advance directives: A qualitative perspective. *Psychiatry, 70*(1), 19–29.

King, R., & Robinson, J. (2011). Obligatory dangerousness criteria in the involuntary commitment and treatment provisions of Australian mental health legislation. *International Journal of Law in Psychiatry, 34*(1), 64–70.

Kisely, S. R., Campbell, L. A., & Preston, N. J. (2011). Compulsory commitment and involuntary outpatient treatment for people with severe mental disorders. *Cochrane Database of Systematic Reviews 2011* (2). Art. No.: CD004408. doi: 10.1002/14651858.CD004408.pub3

Lim, T., & Marin, D. B. (2011). The assessment of decisional capacity. *Neurology Clinics, 29*(1), 115–126.

Lipsman, N., Mendelsohn, D., Taira, T., & Bernstein, M. (2011). The contemporary practice of psychiatric surgery: Results from a survey of North American functional neurosurgeons. *Stereotactic and Functional Neurosurgery, 82*(2), 103–110.

Mariano, M. T., Grace, J. J., Trigoboff, E., Di Stefano, D. J., Olympia, J. O., & Watson, T. H. (2011). Individuals with threatening or violent criminal behavior: Civil commitment or release after incarceration. *Innovations in Neuroscience, 8*(6), 29–34.

Mendelsohn, D., Lipsman, N., & Bernstein, M. (2010). Neurosurgeons' perspectives on psychosurgery and neuroenhancement: A qualitative study at one center. *Journal of Neurosurgery, 113*(6), 1212–1218.

Mohamed, A. D., & Sahakian, B. J. (2011). The ethics of elective psychopharmacology. *International Journal of Neuropsychopharmacology.* Advance online publication. doi: 10.1017/S146114571100037X

Mohr, W. K. (2010). Restraints and the code of ethics: An uneasy fit. *Archives of Psychiatric Nursing, 24*(1), 3–14.

Nace, E. P., Birkmayer, F., Sullivan, M. A., Galanter, M., Fromson, J. A., Frances, R. J., . . . Westermeyer, J. (2007). Socially sanctioned coercion mechanisms for addiction treatment. *American Journal of Addictions, 16*(1), 15–23.

Parks, J. A., & Wike, V. S. (2010). *Bioethics in a changing world.* Upper Saddle River, NJ: Prentice Hall.

Rippee, S. M. (2010). Talking to lawyers about patients: When is it really okay? *Journal of the Mississippi State Medical Association, 51*(9), 273–274.

Schmalleger, F. (2009). *Criminal justice today.* Upper Saddle River, NJ: Pearson Education.

Schoene-Bake, J. C., Parpaley, Y., Weber, B., Panksepp, J., Hurwitz, T. A., & Coenen, V. A. (2010). Tractographic analysis of historical lesion surgery for depression. *Neuropsychopharmacology, 35*(13), 2553–2563.

Shelton, D., Weiskopf, C., & Nicholson, M. (2010). Correctional nursing competency development in the Connecticut Correctional Managed Health Care program. *Journal of Correctional Health Care, 16*(4), 299–309.

Strout, T. D. (2010). Perspectives on the experience of being physically restrained: An integrative review of the qualitative literature. *International Journal of Mental Health Nursing, 19*(6), 416–427.

Swanson, J., Swartz, M., Ferron, J., Elbogen, E., & Van Dorn, R. (2006). Advance directives among public mental health consumers in five U.S. cities: Prevalence, demand, and correlates. *Journal of the American Academy of Psychiatry and the Law, 34*(1), 43–57.

Van Dorn, R. A., Scheyett, A., Swanson, J. W., & Swartz, M. S. (2010). Psychiatric advance directives and social workers: An integrative review. *Social Work, 55*(2), 157–167.

13

Creating Hospital and Community-Based Therapeutic Environments

CAROL REN KNEISL

LEARNING OUTCOMES

After completing this chapter, you will be able to:

1. Identify the types of hospital-based and community-based settings in which psychiatric–mental health nurses practice.
2. Minimize external factors that negatively affect the degree of cohesion and involvement of clients in inpatient settings.
3. Maximize the common good of all clients in a hospital setting while maintaining the privacy and autonomy of individual clients.
4. Discuss the specific challenges that psychiatric home care nurses face.
5. Coordinate a client's care with a wide diversity of providers in a complex mental health system by incorporating the principles of the case management role.
6. Explain how managed mental health care organizations influence the delivery of psychiatric–mental health care.

CRITICAL THINKING CHALLENGE

At a nursing care conference, you and your nurse colleague, Sylvia, disagree about the future direction of mental health care for Tommy, a client at the outpatient clinic of the community mental health center where you both work. Tommy, now 53 years old, has been in and out of psychiatric hospitals since he was 18. He now lives in an adult foster care home and visits the clinic monthly for follow-up purposes. Sylvia believes that the number-one nursing goal should be to provide support to Tommy so that he can maintain his current level of functioning. You believe that the number-one nursing goal should be for Tommy to achieve a more independent, higher level of functioning.

1. Can these two different stances be reconciled? How?
2. Do you see this issue as a matter of psychiatric nursing practice or as a question of moral beliefs? Why?
3. Is it possible to provide support for Tommy while helping him to become more independent at the same time?

Economic, political, technologic, legal, and demographic forces are propelling reform and change in the provision of mental health care. Great strides continue to be made in the treatment of mental illness along with a commitment to comprehensive service delivery and innovations in multidisciplinary approaches to care. At the same time, concerns about gaps in coverage for mental health treatment are being voiced. Continued high out-of-pocket expenses for mental health treatment may impede access to mental health treatment, especially when decisions are made on the basis of cost rather than on need (Hall, Carroll, & Moore, 2010). Families with one or more members with mental illness have a 37% out-of-pocket burden for mental health treatment in a single month (Zuvekas & Seiden, 2010).

Our clients and their care are increasingly located in the larger community of which they are a part. In fact, pockets of mentally ill in the community refuse to, or are unable to, seek care within the confines of the four walls of a psychiatric hospital, a comprehensive community mental health center, or even a walk-in clinic in a storefront. Intensive outreach programs currently lead community mental health efforts. The shift away from institution-based care began with what is known as the community mental health movement.

This chapter discusses the wide variety of hospital- and community-based mental health treatment services and programs available today and the high-risk populations most likely to use them. Managed care, case management, and establishing therapeutic environments are discussed as processes by which the goals of services and programs are met. In addition to this chapter, each disorder chapter in Unit 4 of this text discusses home care, community-based care, and case management and Chapter 32∞ discusses psychiatric rehabilitation and recovery processes.

DEINSTITUTIONALIZATION AND THE COMMUNITY MENTAL HEALTH MOVEMENT

From the early 19th century until the 1960s, state and county mental hospitals constituted the major treatment resource for the mentally ill (see FIGURE 13-1 ■) and were likely to become their permanent residence. As it most often turned out, these hospitals (such as the one in the clinical example) served as the mentally ill client's long-term, and sometimes permanent, residence.

Clinical Example

In the 1950s, Kings Park Psychiatric Hospital in Long Island, New York, was the largest mental hospital in the country. More than 9,000 mentally ill people lived there. It had its own power plant, farm, laundry, and railroad spur, and housed staff on site. As part of their therapy, clients were expected to feed livestock, grow food, and work in the laundry and on the farm. Large total institutions such as Kings Park were no longer needed once chlorpromazine (Thorazine), the first widely used medication for the treatment of psychosis, made it possible for clients to live outside of mental institutions.

Today, most clients do not live in a mental hospital; instead, they are being treated in the communities in which they live. **Deinstitutionalization**, bringing mental health clients out of

FIGURE 13-1 ■ One of the first 10 mental hospitals in the country, the Insane Asylum of the State of Louisiana (now East Louisiana State Hospital) was built in the 1840s. Once housing over 5,000 people before deinstitutionalization, this national historic landmark, an example of Greek Revival architecture, has a current hospital population of 260.
Photo courtesy of Kay R. Hanks RN who has 18 years of service with the East Louisiana State Hospital.

WebLink Application: Deinstitutionalization

the hospital and into the community, began in the post–World War II period, when large public mental hospitals were overcrowded, had fallen into disrepair, and were widely criticized among humanitarians for "warehousing" their residents.

With the development of psychotropic drugs in 1954 and the enactment of state statutes that restricted involuntary detainment in psychiatric facilities, the resident population of state and county mental hospitals declined. By the late 1970s, only one third as many people were hospitalized in psychiatric hospitals. This phase-down of large bureaucratic institutions occurred within the context of a much broader community mental health movement that reached its apex in the 1960s. When federal funds first became available in the 1960s for the construction of community mental health centers and the provision of acute care and ambulatory services in the community, it was assumed that equal access to all levels of mental disorder prevention and treatment would exist.

In theory, it seemed like a good idea to close public mental hospitals. However, unforeseen problems and several disturbing trends cast this assumption into doubt (Torrey, 2010). Many residents of mental hospitals had no family or home to which they could return. Hospital care remained the main treatment modality for the severely mentally ill with repeated readmissions replacing long-term institutional residence. Community mental health centers were often insufficiently funded and unable to provide necessary services when national priorities shifted during the 1980s. New populations of the mentally ill in the community—the homeless, crack cocaine addicts, mentally ill criminal offenders, and the persistently and seriously mentally ill—were unable or unwilling to use the provided services. There is an insufficient number of aftercare facilities—live-in facilities that serve as a home base for those discharged from an inpatient facility—known as board-and-care homes, transitional facilities, or half-way houses even though a review of the psychiatric and psychological literature found that residential care is a viable alternative to hospitalization (Lichtenberg, 2011). Those that do exist are often substandard and poorly regulated.

Many clients are discharged but are not ready for community living. Many who are discharged are not followed up sufficiently or often enough to ensure successful adaptation to community living (Butcher, Mineka, & Hooley, 2010). We find that they fall "between the cracks." It became apparent that aggressive outreach services were needed in order to make both hospital-based and community-based treatments and programs accessible to those individuals who needed them. Nurses have been especially interested in integrating primary care and mental health care services through community partnerships (Davis et al., 2011). The greatest problems have been in creating adequate and accessible community resources.

THE THERAPEUTIC ENVIRONMENT IN HOSPITAL-BASED CARE

The **therapeutic environment** is the purposeful use of people, resources, and events in the client's immediate environment to:

- Ensure safety.
- Promote optimal functioning in the activities of daily living.
- Develop or improve interpersonal skills.
- Enhance the capacity to live independently outside the institutional setting.

Various terms such as *therapeutic milieu, therapeutic community,* and *milieu therapy* have been used to identify treatment environment philosophies. The terms are often used interchangeably and refer to the impact of the authority structure and the roles and relationships that affect decision making and client interactions. Mental Health in the Movies provides an example of a treatment environment that highlights the negative impact of the authority structure in an institution.

In milieu therapy models, organizational hierarchy is flattened, therapeutic potential is seen in multiple relationships, and the client assumes personal responsibility for behavior. Originally, therapeutic milieu programs were at least several months long and had homogenous client populations. The inpatient psychiatric milieu remains an important, but often neglected, component of psychiatric treatment (Thibeault, Trudeau, d'Entrement, & Brown, 2010). Although we discuss milieu therapy principles in this section on hospital-based care, we wish to emphasize the importance of incorporating milieu therapy principles in all treatment settings.

Admission Criteria

Clients admitted to inpatient settings must meet admission criteria. The admitting diagnosis is often one that is life threatening. Overall effectiveness of functioning using the DSM Axis V global assessment of functioning scale (GAF; see Appendix A∞, page 772) determines the acuity of the illness. In most instances, impairment in functioning must be in the 10 to 50 range to qualify for admission. Clients experiencing this degree of discomfort require intense, skilled nursing care to provide for safety needs. For example, a GAF score of 30 indicates that behavior is strongly influenced by delusions or hallucinations, serious impairment in communication or judgment, or an inability to function in almost all areas. Some managed care organizations (MCOs) have designed their own criteria that require ratings of functioning, physical impairments, family support, and other elements as part of a preadmission assessment.

You can easily see how your role as a nurse in the inpatient psychiatric setting is similar to that of the critical care nurse in the general hospital. Clients who are admitted to the psychiatric unit with active suicidal ideation, who are psychotic, or who are experiencing withdrawal symptoms require intensive nursing care and case management.

MENTAL HEALTH IN THE MOVIES
One Flew Over the Cuckoo's Nest

Randle Patrick McMurphy (Jack Nicholson) is a criminal sentenced to a short prison term who voluntarily commits himself to a mental hospital believing that he can avoid hard labor and serve out his term in relative comfort. McMurphy's rebellious antiauthority ways pit him against the cold, cruel, and dictatorial Nurse Ratched (Louise Fletcher) at the same time that he inspires and rallies the other clients on the ward. Under his leadership, the others throw off their dejected, cowed demeanors and become more difficult for Nurse Ratched to manage, despite the electroshock therapy (ECT) they are given as punishment for their rebellious behavior.

When McMurphy realizes that being released is not a certainty and that the institution has the power to keep him committed indefinitely, he plans his escape. After a night of debauchery when McMurphy manages to smuggle two young women and whiskey into the ward, Nurse Ratched comes down hard on Billy, a severely anxious young man, who breaks down. When left alone momentarily, Billy commits suicide. Enraged, McMurphy attempts to strangle Nurse Ratched. The ultimate tragic punishment for McMurphy—under the guise of treatment—is lobotomy.

The film had several consequences. It put psychiatric care and psychiatric nurses into a most unfavorable light, stigmatizing mental institutions and those work who work in them. It also contributed to the mounting criticism of ECT. As a result, the treatment was all but eliminated in most mental hospitals. The negative views of ECT remain in the public consciousness despite the fact that today, ECT is a much more benevolent and humane procedure. The film also raised the question of whether voluntarily renouncing one's freedom is a price anyone should pay.

Photo courtesy of Everett Collection.

A Unique Role for Nurses

In inpatient treatment settings, the nursing staff has 24-hour daily contact with clients. This provides a unique opportunity for creating and managing the therapeutic environment as a special domain (see FIGURE 13-2 ■). No other discipline literally shares with clients the living space of the treatment unit. Nurses individually influence the environment through their presence. Remember that the holistic care of clients in the therapeutic milieu also requires attention to clients' physical needs that may be neglected in inpatient settings (Howard & Gamble, 2011). Although most mental health nurses recognize that they have a responsibility to the physical health needs of people in acute inpatient care settings, their actual clinical practice may not always reflect this perception.

Nurses provide human contact, support, therapeutic interactions, and direction for clients and they share philosophy and values with a multidisciplinary staff with whom they establish collaborative work relationships. Nurses can indirectly influence client behavior by the assessment and manipulation of both the physical and social environments. These responsibilities make it increasingly important that you review and explore your attitudes about organizational rules and client autonomy and self-determination. Your Self-Awareness lists some questions that merit your thoughtful consideration.

While many milieu principles remain relevant in current treatment environments, trends such as short lengths of stay, high client acuity, and resurgence of the biomedical model require re-examination of the relevance of the assumptions of the therapeutic community in acute inpatient care. The emergence of subacute treatment settings and community-based rehabilitation programs also offers new arenas to implement therapeutic environment principles. A continuing challenge of psychiatric–mental health nursing is to synthesize a new model that includes the best aspects of both the psychobiologic and therapeutic milieu models.

FIGURE 13-2 ■ Psychiatric nurses in 1901 in a typical ward at the Buffalo State Hospital (now the Buffalo Psychiatric Center). At this time, it was believed that architecture could influence the course of mental illness. For example, depressed persons were housed in wards with high ceilings such as this one to elevate their spirits.
Photo courtesy of Buffalo Psychiatric Center, Buffalo, New York.

YOUR SELF-AWARENESS
Your Attitudes About Organizational Rules and Client Autonomy

To increase self-awareness of your own attitudes about organizational rules in a treatment setting, ask yourself the following questions:

- Which client behaviors make me uncomfortable?
- Which client behaviors make me angry?
- Which unit rules are most important?
- Which unit rules could be easily eliminated?
- How do I feel when a client breaks a unit rule?
- What do I do in response to a client who breaks a unit rule?

External Factors Affecting the Treatment Environment

A variety of external factors, discussed in Box 13-1, affect the therapeutic environment. These issues have an impact on the treatment environment in several ways. It is more difficult to develop group cohesiveness and involvement with other clients' progress when group membership changes frequently. Symptom acuity may also limit a client's ability to be actively involved with the treatment issues of others. Staff roles may be more traditional and typical of medical care settings, and this may create more hierarchical relationships. In actual practice, these factors will be influenced by the program's attitude toward privacy, autonomy, safety, and group well-being.

Box 13-1 External Factors That Affect the Therapeutic Environment

Following are some external factors, both positive and negative, that affect the therapeutic environment:

- Client groups are not homogenous.
- Clients frequently have dual diagnoses, such as psychiatric and substance abuse problems or psychiatric and medical problems.
- The length of inpatient stays has decreased to an average of about 7 days.
- Treatment is closely monitored to determine the need for medication, seclusion, restraint, or other intensive supervision.
- Case managers quickly assess discharge planning needs and obstacles and coordinate access to other levels of services.
- There has been a resurgence of the biologic model of care as psychopharmacology and other somatic treatments offer specialized treatment approaches to symptom reduction.
- Clients with multiple medical problems and dementias may also require more traditional medical interventions.
- Staff members now have diverse and specialized training and are expected to work as multidisciplinary teams to address individualized treatment goals.
- Regulatory agencies, client rights groups, and professional practice standards establish criteria for the therapeutic environment.
- Managed mental health care organizations increasingly limit access to inpatient care to those who are a danger to themselves or others.

Privacy

Individuals routinely vary their patterns of contact with and withdrawal from others, as well as the information they share about themselves. The very nature of psychiatric hospitalization conflicts with the need for privacy. Intimate personal details are examined and discussed, and there may be no opportunity to escape staff surveillance or social contact. Nurses must respect a client's privacy by keeping surveillance and monitoring to the minimum necessary for client safety, honoring the confidentiality of personal information, and maintaining routine social practices such as knocking on the door and waiting for an answer before entering a bedroom or bathroom.

Autonomy

The rules and schedules that characterize psychiatric–mental health treatment settings usually promote the efficient and safe management of groups of people and may interfere with the personal decision making and autonomy of the individual client. Regulatory oversight by, for example, the Centers for Medicare and Medicaid Services, force the staff of acute care hospitals to face the moral complexity of balancing a client's right to autonomy with the regulatory demands of the federal government (Hannon-Engel, 2011). Although the ability of clients with mental disorders to carry out age-appropriate roles may be significantly impaired, a therapeutic environment provides opportunities for normal functioning according to each client's abilities.

Safety

Mentally disordered clients may pose significant safety hazards to themselves or others because of suicidal or assaultive behaviors, poor judgment, or confusion. Efforts to maintain client safety may deprive clients of privacy and autonomy. For example, clients requiring close surveillance have little or no privacy; nurses may intervene to over-ride decisions made by clients whose judgment is impaired.

Group Well-Being

A client's behavior may be disruptive or detrimental to the overall well-being of other clients. Nurses may need to monitor or manage certain clients to maximize the common good. As with the concept of safety, the individual's privacy and autonomy may be violated when group well-being is considered primary. (Some philosophers, however, consider that the group's well-being enhances the individual's autonomy.) Individual autonomy, individual well-being, and group well-being are often conflicting issues. Nurses must be sensitive to situations in which clashes occur.

Therapeutic Environment Principles

Some of the current ideas about the therapeutic environment, particularly the philosophic values, do not easily lend themselves to quick evaluation or manipulation. Staff must consider the clients' levels of functioning as well as the discrete features of the structural environment. What is suitable for one group of clients may be too strict or too lenient for another. Some general guidelines for incorporating therapeutic environment principles in your work with clients are in Your Intervention Strategies. You can apply these principles in any setting or specialty area in which you work. Selected guidelines are discussed later in this chapter.

Restrictiveness

The restrictiveness of the treatment environment is characterized according to physical, psychological, and social dimensions. The physical environment includes the location in the community, security, and options for behavior control (e.g., seclusion, quiet rooms, etc.). The psychological environment is composed of staff and client backgrounds, behavior, attitudes, and values. The social environment consists of the rules and regulations that govern the operation of the setting as well as the treatment standards for managing client behavior.

The importance of evaluating a program's restrictiveness stems from mental health legislation mandating care according to the least restrictive alternative. This concept is heavily influenced by ethical and legal theories that hold individual autonomy paramount. Thus, program rules or staff attitudes that interfere with a client's autonomy are considered more restrictive than a program that supports autonomy and self-determination. (See Chapter 12∞.)

A facility's physical structure is a major focus of attention in pursuing the least restrictive alternatives for treatment. Physical restrictiveness is ranked according to the degree of interference with client independence. The physical structure of many institutions—such as locked doors, communal living arrangements, and limited access to community resources—interferes with client freedom of movement and individuality. Thus, facilities located in huge hospital complexes—which do not interface with the community's shopping, religious, or entertainment activities or provide for client privacy—have a more restrictive environment than community-based settings. Facilities located away from the urban centers from which most clients and their families come, or those that are difficult to reach by public transportation, are also more restrictive environments.

Orienting the Client and Family

Inform clients and their families or significant others about all aspects of the therapeutic environment. Encourage them to verbalize their concerns and questions about what to expect during the treatment experience. Be sure to accomplish the following:

1. Orient and educate client, family, and significant others about hospitalization and treatment by reviewing the clinical problems, treatments, and behavioral outcomes that are the focus of hospitalization or treatment in the facility.
2. Engage clients, family, and significant others in the treatment process by encouraging them to identify personal goals and participate in evaluating the course of treatment.

Partnering with Clients and Families lists questions they may ask. Be sure to include information on all unasked questions in your health teaching orientation activities.

YOUR INTERVENTION STRATEGIES   Guidelines for Working With Clients
in the Therapeutic Environment

Strategy	Rationale
Safety and the Structural Environment	
■ Assess appropriate structural security, including locked doors, nonbreakable glass, seclusion room, silent alarms, and devices such as concave nonbreakable mirrors to view blind spots.	■ Security must be appropriate to client acuity and type of treatment program.
■ Provide unit rules and staff policy related to acceptable conduct.	■ Rules should be clearly stated.
■ Implement procedures and training for use of time-outs, seclusion, restraint, special precautions, and search and management of client personal belongings.	■ Staff training promotes consistency and safe implementation of security and client management techniques.
Structure	
■ Orient client to behavior expectations through multiple sources, including handbook, bulletin boards, community meeting, and identification of a primary nurse.	■ Clients are unfamiliar with expectations; new information may need to be repeated.
■ Delineate program schedule and expectations for client participation.	■ Clear expectations and written schedule promote client independence.
Support	
■ Guide and monitor client activities by being visible and available.	■ Demonstrates role-modeling skills and provides an opportunity for informal assessment and interaction.
■ Implement least restrictive interventions such as confirming messages, calming, personal control, setting limits, and medication to minimize the need for more restrictive behavior management.	■ Least restrictive interventions promote client autonomy and demonstrate respect.
■ Enhance normality of the environment through use of clocks, calendars, and furniture.	■ Reduces the institutional qualities of environment.
■ Promote opportunities for self-care decision making, and activities that prepare for return to community.	■ Reduces dependence on hospital; promotes positive transition to community.
■ Integrate client's existing social supports, including family and spiritual support system to reinforce goals and interventions.	■ Promotes family involvement and empowerment; extends opportunities for positive outcome by involving social supports.
■ Monitor and discuss staff concerns to promote communication, identify parallel issues, and ensure a positive social climate.	■ Staff interactions affect the general atmosphere and capacity for therapeutic interventions.
■ Support cultural diversity and staff self-awareness related to issues of client rights and social control.	■ Demonstrates respect and supports client autonomy and independence.
Socialization	
■ Orient client and family to the steps and process of psychiatric treatment.	■ Clients and family may be unfamiliar with psychiatric treatment; may have misinformation.
■ Identify fears and stereotypes client/family may have about "brain surgery, shock treatment, or padded cells," as well as concerns about how psychotherapy works.	■ Reduces fear and encourages engaging in treatment.
■ Educate client/family about legal rights of psychiatric clients and confidentiality of information.	■ Engages client and family in treatment process.
■ Encourage client participation in determining and evaluating treatment goals.	■ Promotes involvement and empowerment.
Self-Understanding	
■ Encourage formal and informal group participation.	■ Provides opportunities to gain social skills.
■ Emphasize commonalities of experience.	■ Reduces sense of isolation and hopelessness.
■ Identify skills gained through hospital experience.	■ Offers hope and focuses on the future.
■ Instill hope and social connectedness.	■ Reduces isolation.
■ Encourage client feedback about satisfaction with treatment and hospital experience.	■ Promotes empowerment.

PARTNERING WITH CLIENTS AND FAMILIES

Orientation to the Unit/Setting

When you orient clients and their families to the therapeutic environment, be prepared to answer their questions. Individualize your answers to reflect each unit's treatment philosophy and the specific legal rights of the client according to the state in which you practice. Following are some typical questions asked by clients and family members.

1. What psychiatric treatment can I expect to receive?
2. Will I receive medications? Do I have to take the medications?
3. Do I have to share a room with someone else?
4. Will I have to tell other clients about my problems?
5. Will you write down information that I tell you about myself or my family?
6. Is this unit a safe place for me?
7. Can I leave the unit on passes?
8. What happens if I no longer want to be a client in this hospital?
9. What happens if I have a disagreement with someone?
10. Who are the staff members here? Who can I talk to if I have questions?
11. Can I smoke?
12. When is bedtime?
13. What time are the meals? Can I keep my own snacks?
14. Is there a way for me to wash my own clothes?
15. Is there a telephone I can use?
16. When are the visiting hours?
17. Can I write letters and get mail?
18. Can I keep my money with me? Is my personal property safe?
19. Are religious services available?

Care Plan: Therapeutic Environment

Safety and the Structural Environment

Although building features are beyond your ability to influence, other aspects of the physical structure are open to your interventions. As the nurse, you should do the following:

1. Evaluate whether security is sufficient.
2. Assess the advantages and necessity of the security.
3. Assess whether the security has any detrimental impact.
4. Consider whether the security advantages could be accomplished through some other intervention that does not have a detrimental impact.
5. Re-evaluate structural controls implemented for specific reasons to determine whether they are no longer relevant and should be discontinued.

The following clinical example illustrates a structural control based on an unclear rationale.

Clinical Example

A 15-bed unit in an inpatient setting had laundry facilities for clients to care for their own clothes. A psychotic and confused client put a potted plant through a wash cycle, causing major damage to the washing machine. Staff members locked the laundry facilities to prevent future damage to the machines. The doors remained locked even after the client was discharged, preventing any independent client access to the facilities. Preventing possible future damage to machines became a predominant staff concern. While locking laundry room doors was intended as a short-term structural solution to avoid further environmental damage, the solution itself created a new problem of interference with self-care performance by more independent clients.

Seclusion and restraint are interventions that use structure to control client behavior in order to implement safety measures. Because seclusion and restraint are highly restrictive interventions that interfere with client autonomy and freedom of movement, it is important to implement alternative steps whenever possible. Chapter 12 ∞ discusses the ethical and legal facets of seclusion and restraint, and Chapter 35 ∞ discusses how and why seclusion and restraint may be used in clinical settings.

The structural environment should not dehumanize its inhabitants; moreover, it should actively contribute to their improved functioning and comfort. Reality-oriented resources such as the following contribute to a sense of normality:

1. Clocks and calendars to promote time orientation
2. Newspapers to encourage an awareness of social events
3. Ramps and rails to facilitate mobility and movement
4. Furniture arranged to promote interpersonal interaction

Healthy people may take these for granted, but they are critical resources to the impaired client.

Program Structure

Program structure, another aspect of the therapeutic environment, is composed of the schedule and expectations for client treatment and participation. Nurses have a number of opportunities to communicate expectations and to address issues that arise. How expectations are communicated and issues assessed and addressed are strongly influenced by the individual nurse's attitudes toward organization rules in a treatment setting (refer back to Your Self-Awareness on page 251).

Program Rules Give all clients the regulations of the setting either before or as soon after admission as possible. Although written expectations do not automatically ensure that clients pay attention to the program rules, they provide a clear baseline, serve as reminders, and provide structure for clients. These rules reinforce the staff's commitment to basic safety and specify obligations for all members of the setting. Written expectations may be presented to clients at the time of admission, discussed in community meetings, and used as a reference if a client violates a rule. In some instances, individualized behavioral contracts with specific clients may be necessary. Individualized behavioral contracts are discussed in Chapter 30∞.

While all programs have a set of rules and regulations, not all use community meetings or client government as an integral part of the program. Client government is more likely in therapeutic communities for children and adolescents or those with eating disorders or substance abuse.

Community Meetings Client groups provide an opportunity for clients to solve problems of conflicting interests, experience cooperation with others, share responsibility, and experience leadership in the group. The most common milieu-oriented group in long-term facilities is the community meeting. Its functions include the following:

- Welcoming new members
- Identifying and discussing unit rules (expectations)
- Discussing aspects of the unit environment such as cleanliness, privacy, radio and television use, or other interpersonal problems that may interfere with the quality of life for the group
- Planning activities

Clients usually chair the community meeting and report on assignments, such as checking for cleanliness of areas of responsibility (e.g., the kitchen or bedrooms). The community meeting is also used to solve problems related to living with a large group of people or living in the hospital unit.

Clinical Example

Clients on a 25-bed unlocked unit had access to two pay telephones. Both telephones, however, were near the nurses' station, and the nurses could easily overhear conversations. Clients complained in community meeting of the lack of privacy, and a nurse intervened to help them write a letter to the hospital administration. The administration purchased a new cordless telephone that allowed clients to make and receive calls in any area of the unit.

Client Government Some client community groups also grant clients privileges for demonstrating certain behaviors in the community living groups. Clients are expected to take responsibility for themselves and each other and to learn the consequences of their actions. Involving clients in the management of the unit and in therapeutic activities with one another allow opportunities for participation, corrective learning experiences, and the development of new behavior patterns. Feedback is an essential technique for increasing insight and promoting learning. This type of community group, known as **client government**, may be most suitable to intermediate and long-term care settings, where the client group is stable and a group culture evolves over time.

Clinical Example

The community meeting group of a 20-bed adolescent program bases recommendations for weekend passes on members' requests and the individual's functioning in the client community. Lisa, 14 years old, has a history of running away from home, lying, drug and alcohol abuse, prostitution, and suicide threats. She requested a Saturday day pass, although she did not have specific plans for how she would spend the time. Other clients commented that Lisa had not completed her ward job of checking the cleanliness of the kitchen, and the staff noted that she continued to withdraw from social contacts. The group agreed that Lisa should not receive a pass until she could demonstrate some improved ability to structure her time and interact with others.

Supportive Social Climate

According to clients themselves, the opportunity and ability to form relationships with other clients and staff appears to be the most significant factor in determining the success of the inpatient experience (Nolan, Bradley, & Brimblecome, 2011). Clients want person-centered help to better manage their lives.

The multiple influences on individual and group behavior may come from external sources such as professional practice standards, regulatory agencies, and laws. Staff members and clients' attitudes, beliefs, and behaviors, as well as styles of interaction between people, have a major impact on the therapeutic environment.

Nursing routines that limit client self-care can be detrimental to the unit atmosphere, signaling overinvolvement and loss of client autonomy.

Clinical Example

Acutely psychotic and severely and persistently mentally ill men and women are admitted to a 20-bed locked unit in a large county hospital. Nurses on this unit seem rushed and complain of having no time to discuss nursing care issues or write nursing care plans. A nurse consultant observed work patterns for several days and noted that the staff members were involved (frequently unnecessarily) in intimate details of the clients' daily activities. This involvement extended to lighting matches for cigarettes and squeezing toothpaste onto toothbrushes. Simple routines that interfered with client autonomy also controlled the staff by preventing professional performance and relationships.

The nurse consultant in the clinical example assessed that the staff's involvement in the daily details of client activities actually created self-care deficits for clients. The consultant recommended that the staff promote clients' self-care skills in accordance with their actual ability. This resulted in greater client independence and improved staff performance and morale.

Spirituality

Nurses can use the spiritual beliefs of clients to enhance the therapeutic environment. Specific assessment of a client's spiritual beliefs and practices provides the nurse an opportunity to understand their clinical impact and to use spiritual resources available to the client to enhance wellness and coping. Of 48 persons in a psychosocial rehabilitation program, 20 participated in an optional spirituality group, while the other 28 did not. Within 6 months, 100% of the spirituality group participants attained their treatment goals, and 57% in the control group did not (Wong-McDonald, 2007). In another study, 71% of the study population participating in a psychiatric rehabilitation program reported that their spiritual life played a significant role in their recovery (Bussema & Bussema, 2007). Caring for the Spirit lists some specific strategies you can use to incorporate spirituality into the therapeutic environment.

Discussing beliefs enables you to reassure clients who fear that their beliefs will be challenged or minimized in a psychiatric environment. For example, the staff in an inpatient setting could develop a psychoeducation program geared to their specific client population. One setting with a large number of orthodox Jewish clients used the *beit midrash* concept, a study hall for religious studies (Shor & Aivhod, 2011), as the basis for their psychoeducation program. Common principles of psychiatric rehabilitation were integrated and emphasized through the discussion of socially-oriented religious texts.

Finally, acknowledging the significant influence of spirituality in American life encourages us to recognize and explore our own beliefs in order to minimize the impact of bias in our interactions with our clients. Remember also that clients come from various cultural backgrounds and their beliefs about spirituality or religion may vary from culture to culture and will be influenced by their degree of cultural assimilation. Strive to provide spiritual resources that are both culturally congruent and culturally competent.

Encouraging a Partnership With Clients and Families

It is important to recognize that, in addition to educating the client and family about the client's illness and treatment, you also have a responsibility to teach them how to implement the principles of the therapeutic environment outside the treatment setting when the client is away from the hospital on pass, or in preparation for discharge. The goal is to partner with the client and family to reach a mutually agreeable plan for a safe, secure, and supportive living arrangement that meets their needs. Recognize that movement from inpatient care to the greater freedom that comes with community care can be quite unsettling for clients (Nolan et al., 2011).

Establishing a Daily Schedule A routine helps clients keep on track and organize their thinking as well as their activities. Suggest that clients do the following:

- Have a routine for waking up, eating, accomplishing daily activities, and resting.
- Identify specific tasks that need to be accomplished that day, or skills that need to be performed.
- Complete tasks in small, manageable increments.
- Take medications as prescribed.

Using Positive Communication Skills Misunderstandings and resentments between clients and their family members often result from inadequate, incomplete, or negative communication. Suggest to family members that misunderstandings and resentments can often be eliminated or reduced by following these guidelines as well as those presented in Chapter 10 ∞:

- Give instructions or directions at the level of the client's ability. This may include verbal prompting along with physical assistance, verbal prompting alone, and, especially, praise for independent performance.
- Avoid criticism, argument, and negative reinforcement (see Chapter 5 ∞ for a discussion of negative reinforcement).
- Be empathic by putting yourself in the client's shoes.

Identifying and Participating in Support Groups Support groups help both clients and families to cope. Families need to recognize signs of family stress and have a plan for respite, perhaps by trading off responsibilities with other

---

CARING FOR THE SPIRIT

Incorporating Spirituality into the Therapeutic Environment

Incorporate spirituality into the therapeutic environment by doing the following:

- Provide opportunities for ceremonies, such as weekly services or holiday celebrations.
- Facilitate group discussions based on sharing religious or spiritual beliefs.
- Demonstrate tolerance and acceptance of differing beliefs and rituals.
- Encourage the social support that can be provided by acceptance in a community that shares similar beliefs.

- Be aware of how one's own beliefs may influence client interactions.
- Define a negative life event in terms of an opportunity for spiritual growth.
- Use spiritual music or ceremonies to promote relaxation and reduce anxiety.
- Collaborate with clergy or a representative of the client's faith who is accepted by the client to (a) correct misinterpretations of spiritual information that the client may be using in a maladaptive way; (b) translate to clinicians spiritual aspects of a client's decision making; or (c) identify options and alternatives consistent with the faith that support adaptive resolution.

family members or significant others, or arranging for client day care or respite care. Families need to take the following steps:

1. Gather information about resources for the client and the family, including social, health care, and long-term financial resources.
2. Choose mental health care workers on the basis of their abilities and the degree of comfort in relating to them.
3. Evaluate the client's options for living arrangements and rehabilitation.

Recognizing Illness Relapse or Exacerbation Clients' symptoms can return (relapse) or worsen (exacerbate). Clients and their families should have the following:

- A plan for managing symptoms. This might include reducing schedule demands and/or contacting the

mental health team or case manager for assistance (see Chapter 32∞).

- A plan for emergency behavior management for possible instances of suicide or violence (see Chapters 23 and 35∞).

THE THERAPEUTIC ENVIRONMENT IN COMMUNITY-BASED CARE

There are a wide variety of community-based treatment settings. Their availability has been found to correlate with lower rates of psychiatric hospitalization (Wanchek, McGarvey, Leon-Verdin, & Bonnie, 2011). Box 13-2 provides several examples of community settings in which psychiatric–mental health nurses practice, some of which are discussed next. Several others are discussed in other sections of this chapter. Conflict between a client's desire for community-based care and the public need for protection from potentially violent clients is the theme of Mental Health in the News.

Box 13-2 Community Treatment Settings

Examples of community-based treatment settings are:

- Adult day care settings
- AIDS support programs
- Assisted living facilities
- Child day care centers
- Client's own home
- Community mental health centers
- Correctional facilities (jails, prisons, detention centers)
- Courts (mental health evaluation, mentally ill offenders, victims of violence)
- Crisis services
- Day treatment centers
- Emergency departments of hospitals
- Ethnic cultural centers
- Foster care homes for adults and youths
- Group homes
- Halfway houses
- Hospices

- Houses of worship (churches, synagogues, mosques, temples)
- Immigrant centers
- Industry and business centers
- Mobile outreach teams
- Nursing homes
- Rural mental health clinics
- Partial hospitalization programs
- Primary care centers
- Private practice offices (psychiatric–mental health nurses, psychiatrists, psychologists, social workers)
- Residential facilities for cognitively impaired
- Schools
- Senior centers
- Sheltered workshops
- Shelters and residential services (battered women, homeless, youths, people in crisis)
- Substance abuse programs
- Youth centers
- YMCAs/YWCAs

MENTAL HEALTH IN THE NEWS

John Hinckley

In 1981, John Hinckley, Jr. shot President Ronald Reagan in the chest and wounded three others in what he said was an attempt to impress actress Jodie Foster. Found Not Guilty By Reason of Insanity, Hinckley was remanded by the court to St. Elizabeths Hospital in Washington, DC, the most famous mental hospital in America, where he has lived for 30 years. Hinckley's community involvement is minimal. He is allowed to leave the hospital for short visits in his mother's custody. He has been granted a driver's license but must carry a GPS tracking device when out of the hospital. His goal is to have increased release time from the hospital and to do volunteer work in his mother's home town of Williamsburg,

Virginia. To that end, Hinckley is applying to the courts for extra time away from St. Elizabeths.

The Justice Department objects to more freedom in the community for Hinckley despite an evaluation by hospital staff that indicates that his psychosis is in remission. The Justice Department argues that he has inappropriate, infatuated, and counterproductive relationships with women (both clients and staff at the hospital), has thoughts of violence, continues to be obsessed with Jodie Foster, has attempted suicide at least three times, is secretive and deceptive and holds back information from the hospital staff that would demonstrate he is a danger to himself and others and remains mentally ill.

Photo courtesy © Bettmann/CORBIS.

Community Mental Health Centers

Community mental health centers (CMHCs) vary considerably in their appearance (see FIGURE 13-3) and in the services they offer. Services offered in CMHCs include the following:

- Emergency services
- Medication management clinics
- Psychoeducation groups
- Vocational rehabilitation
- Consultation services to hospitals, nursing homes, and primary care centers
- Other specialty services as determined by the population they serve (programs for the severely and persistently mentally ill, mental health clinics for the homeless, dual diagnosis services for chemically dependent mentally ill clients, elder services, etc.)

In large metropolitan areas, CMHCs often include additional services such as the following:

- Inpatient hospital-based care
- Partial hospitalization programs that include: day care services for those who need supervision and assistance during daytime hours, and night treatment services for those who are able to maintain employment during the day but need supervision and assistance during night-time hours

Mobile Outreach Units

Mobile treatment teams go out into the community by car or on foot to deliver services in whatever setting makes the client comfortable—a public place, a jail, a home, a shopping mall, a fast-food restaurant, under a bridge, or in an alley. Following are common treatment goals of mobile outreach units:

- Bringing community-based treatment programs to homeless clients and to those who would not otherwise seek mental health services or have little or no access to mental health care
- Providing medication management prescribed by another mental health professional to clients who have problems in adhering to treatment by psychotropic medications
- Preventing relapse and hospitalization
- Identifying and assessing persons in the community in need of mental health care and facilitating their entry into a mental health service program
- Providing emergency intervention or crisis prevention services to mental health consumers, police, employers, landlords, business owners, and so on
- Satisfying the requirements of court-ordered treatment

Mobile treatment teams have also been able to reduce the need for hospitalization in many instances. Following are major mental health consumer characteristics that relate to the likelihood of hospitalization:

1. Being young and homeless and experiencing acute problems
2. Having been referred by psychiatric hospitals, the legal system, or other treatment facilities

(a)

(b)

(c)

FIGURE 13-3 ■ A community mental health center is more a concept than a place. Community mental health centers cannot be recognized by appearance alone.
(a) A university-based medical center with a community mental health center and a neuropsychiatric inpatient unit.
(b) An inner-city mental health outreach clinic.
(c) A rural mental health outreach clinic and day treatment program.
Photo courtesy of Holly Skodol Wilson, PhD.

3. Showing signs of substance abuse
4. Being unemployed (Schmutte, Dunn, & Sledge, 2010), or having no income
5. Having had a previous admission for psychiatric hospitalization
6. Nonadherence to an antipsychotic treatment regimen (Lang et al., 2010)

Mobile mental health teams have also been effective in contacting suicidal persons released from emergency departments in a randomized controlled trial (Currier, Fisher, & Caine, 2010). Contact is important because these clients are likely to be significantly symptomatic and at risk for repeated emergency department visits.

Assertive Community Treatment (ACT)

Assertive programs have shown much promise in terms of service delivery to high-risk groups and are believed to prevent psychotic relapse and rehospitalization and reduce arrests, emergency room visits, and homelessness of clients with severe and persistent mental illness. Clients in an ACT program are also more likely to maintain contact with treatment providers than those receiving standard community care (Marshall & Lockwood, 2011). They are less likely to be admitted to the hospital, and if they are, they spend fewer days in the hospital. These are expensive, sophisticated programs that are believed to be cost effective because they offset still more expensive hospital episodes. Assertive programs are known by names other than ACT—Continuous Treatment Teams (CTTs), Intensive Case Management (ICM), and Programs for Assertive Community Treatment (PACT) are some of them.

These teams may include interdisciplinary groups of 7 to 12 staff members—nurses, psychiatrists, social workers, peer specialists who are mental health consumers, and mental health paraprofessionals—who deliver service in the client's own environment. Treatment teams not only provide a mobile outreach capacity, they also provide consumers with access to multidisciplinary providers and comprehensive services.

The team structure is believed to reduce stress and burnout of individual case managers by sharing the load of difficult clients. The client benefits from both reduced dependence on an individual clinician and the support of a large multidisciplinary group for backup during crisis. In addition, clients benefit because staff members in these teams must be clinically sophisticated and capable of managing acute care in the community. Evidence-Based Practice provides an example of how a multidisciplinary team can assist clients in a crisis.

Concerns about coercion have arisen with ACT treatment programs. A review of the literature points to controversy about whether ACT actually decreases health services use and increases clinical outcomes and social functioning and the need to assess this type of legislation because of its

EVIDENCE-BASED PRACTICE

Assertive Community Treatment

Angie is a 42-year-old woman who has been hospitalized several times for acute schizophrenic episodes. Each episode has been preceded by a period in which Angie stopped taking her medication. Angie usually becomes argumentative, hallucinates, fails to pay attention to her personal care, does not show up for her job, and withdraws from others, staying in her apartment in the dark. This time, Angie, who has a key to her boyfriend's apartment, entered his apartment when he wasn't there and locked herself in. She played a CD over and over at such a high volume that the neighbors next door and in the apartment below complained to the building superintendent.

When the building superintendent knocked on the door, Angie refused to let him in. His pleas with her to keep the noise down were met with increasing rage. Angie began throwing things in the apartment, broke a window, and damaged the walls. Fortunately, Angie's boyfriend arrived on the scene and called the mental health clinic where Angie was registered as a client. Soon after, the police arrived in response to calls from neighbors. Angie refused to open the door for them.

When the mobile mental health team from the mental health clinic arrived on the scene, they were able to persuade Angie to let them into the apartment. They negotiated an agreement among Angie, her boyfriend, the building superintendent, and the police that charges would not be filed against Angie, providing that she agreed to assertive community treatment that would involve involuntary outpatient commitment including medication management. Angie's boyfriend agreed to repair the window and any damaged walls. The goals were to avoid hospitalization for Angie, to avoid criminal charges, to help her adhere to a medication regimen, and to keep close contact with her and pre-empt future violent behavior. The mobile mental health team considered the following research studies in developing a plan of action for Angie:

Kisely, S. R., Campbell, L. A., & Preston, N. J. (2011). Compulsory commitment and involuntary outpatient treatment for people with severe mental disorders. *Cochrane Database of Systematic Reviews 2011*(2). Art. No.: CD004408. doi: 10.1002/14651858.CD004408.pub3

Marshall, M. & Lockwood, A. (2011). WITHDRAWN: Assertive community treatment for people with severe mental disorders. *Cochrane Database of Systematic Reviews 2011*(4). Art. No.: CD001089.

CRITICAL THINKING QUESTIONS

1. Which actions of the mobile mental health team could be considered coercive?
2. Because Angie caused the damage, shouldn't she be the person financially responsible for repairing the damages to her boyfriend's apartment?
3. Does Angie's behavior warrant her arrest by the police to protect public safety? Why or why not?
4. Angie has stopped taking her medication. Does that warrant hospitalization? Why or why not?

power (Kisely, Campbell, & Preston, 2011). A major concern has been that ACT teams often become actively and directly involved in many areas of the client's life and may control access to resources such as housing and money in return for adherence to medication and treatment programs through outpatient commitment. This paternalism interferes with the client's personal autonomy. Members of ACT teams must be sure to look for opportunities such as encouraging independent living (Marshall & Lockwood, 2011) to enhance clients' quality of life through personal goal setting and decision making to the extent possible for each individual client.

Guidelines and standards developed by the **National Alliance on Mental Illness (NAMI)** and recommended for assertive community treatment teams are available at http://www.nami.org/about/pactstd.html and can be accessed through the Online Student Resources for this book.

Psychiatric Home Care

Psychiatric home care nursing has a long history in community mental health. Some of the most successful programs for the severely mentally ill in the early years of community mental health employed visiting nurses to deliver home-based services. Today, there is growing demand for psychiatric home care nursing as a cost-effective alternative to hospitalization. Medicare, Medicaid, managed care organizations, and private health insurance all fund psychiatric home care at different levels and with different requirements for reimbursement.

Clients with a primary psychiatric diagnosis should be cared for in the home by an experienced psychiatric–mental health nurse. Advanced-level nurses may also provide direct psychiatric care or function as intensive case managers and consultants to staff as well as mental health consumers.

Other requirements for Medicare reimbursement are homebound status and the presence of a diagnosed psychiatric disorder. Homebound status for psychiatric home care would include clients who are immobilized by depression or anxiety attacks, clients who are disoriented or confused, clients with hallucinations or delusions that compromise their safety, or clients whose physical health prevents them from going to other locations where mental health services are offered.

Psychiatric home care is more likely to be used for clients recently discharged from a psychiatric hospital, the homebound elderly, persons with dementia, young adults with severe and persistent mental illness, or clients who have an associated medical condition. As clients are discharged from hospitals more quickly, the nurse who is providing home care may be providing services that traditionally would have been delivered in a hospital setting. For example, the medication clozapine (Clozaril), used to alleviate symptoms of schizophrenia, requires frequent blood tests to monitor for side effects. The home care nurse draws the blood and monitors the medication protocol in the home setting. Alcohol-related complications such as diabetes may require extensive family teaching to enable family members to successfully manage a chronic alcoholic family member who is also diabetic.

You might encounter your clients in personal care homes or transitional care facilities. In some personal care homes,

you may be the only professional who visits an elderly client. In these instances, part of your teaching plan is to work with ancillary staff members who are responsible for running the personal care home or transitional care facility. We cannot overemphasize the importance of medication adherence for a severely, persistently mentally ill person. Your method of ensuring that clients in personal care homes receive their medication as ordered is often to teach the managers of these facilities about the medication and its effects on behavior.

If you encounter your clients in retirement complexes, your teaching emphasis may be with an aging spouse. This person may not be able to carry out instructions and may require repetitive teaching plans and other aids to ensure that your client follows treatment protocols. In these instances, your skills in family systems will be useful aids in planning appropriate interventions (see Chapter 29∞).

In some home care agencies, there has been a lack of psychiatric services, reluctance to address behavioral problems, a failure to identify undiagnosed disorders, and a bias against accepting individuals with primary psychiatric disorders. Clearly, such agencies fail to meet the needs of clients with psychiatric diagnoses or behavioral problems. Providing direct psychiatric home care services requires that you are sensitive to several factors. They are outlined in What Every Nurse Should Know.

MANAGED MENTAL HEALTH CARE

Managed mental health care, a method for capping the rate of increase in the cost of mental health care while ensuring access to quality mental health care services, has become an increasingly important force. As a service delivery system, managed mental health care creates a rich climate for nurses to become actively involved in primary prevention and education.

Managed Care Settings

Managed care settings include both inpatient and outpatient care. Clients are admitted to hospitals in later stages of disease or illness, or perhaps not admitted at all. Criteria for hospitalization are based on medical necessity. For instance, the once-standard 28-day program for substance abuse treatment has given way to innovative and shorter models for detoxification services and outpatient treatment that meet the lifestyle needs of clients and their employers. Employer demands, coupled with cost containment, have created an entire range of ambulatory care services that at one time would have been considered ineffective. Substance-dependent clients may have options of day, evening, or weekend partial hospitalization programs. Some programs adhere to a Monday-through-Friday schedule of 4 to 6 hours per day or evening. Weekend programs are usually 8 hours on Saturday and 8 hours on Sunday.

Inpatient Settings

The admission criteria for inpatient care have been discussed earlier in this chapter. These goals are achieved through shorter, more intense hospital stays and the use of critical pathways and case management.

Shorter, More Intense Stays A focus on shorter, more intense stays came about through the emphasis in MCOs on

WHAT EVERY NURSE SHOULD KNOW

Challenges of Psychiatric Home Care

- Remember that you are a guest in the client's home and that the client has the right to refuse your admittance to that home.
- As a guest in the client's home, be aware of the client's cultural background and strive to be culturally sensitive. Incorporating the client's cultural beliefs into the care you give will not only enhance your relationship with the client and family, but will also positively influence the client's participation in the treatment process.
- Be sensitive to the factors that can influence a client's behavior, such as the physical environment, finances, or the presence of family and friends. For example, the presence of family and friends may raise concerns of confidentiality.
- Work collaboratively with the psychiatrist, other mental health professionals, or the client's primary medical care provider to provide in-depth psychiatric home care.
- Be sensitive to changes in the client's behavior that may indicate relapse or a worsening of symptoms.
- Remember to assess for medical problems that may compound or be compounded by the mental disorder.
- Provide psychoeducation, especially concerning psychotropic medications even for clients who have been on the same medication for years (medication nonadherence accounts for the majority of psychiatric hospital readmissions). Do not assume that clients received adequate instruction, or that they remember the instruction.
- Empower your clients and encourage increasing independence by involving them in the treatment plan.
- Be aware of any factors in the environment that threaten either the client's or your safety. Take a colleague with you on high-risk visits and leave the door open. Leave the client's home if your safety seems to be in question (see also Chapter 35∞) and inform family, caregivers, or other involved mental health professionals or community resources.

the need to maximize value for the mental health consumer and to keep costs down through the judicious use of available resources. These goals are achieved through the use of critical pathways and case management. Case management is discussed in detail later in this chapter in the section on creating a therapeutic environment. Case management for clients with specific mental disorders is discussed in the nursing process sections of each chapter in Unit 4∞.

Critical Pathways Critical pathways, or road maps of expected outcomes described earlier in Chapter 11∞, are valuable tools for helping nurses deliver care within managed-care frameworks. When a client "falls off the map" or fails to meet the desired outcomes, this information can be fed to a quality-improvement program to avoid such deviations in the future. However, because critical pathways are the tools by which MCOs achieve their goals, they have become increasingly important.

Primary Care Centers

Alternatives to hospitalization and accelerated discharge to ambulatory care settings create a demand for sophisticated, comprehensive, and well-coordinated services in the primary care setting. Managed care sites can offer rich concentrations of primary care resources to meet client needs. Such a setting is conducive to delegating responsibility to the most cost-effective, medically appropriate provider. The ambulatory care facilities of MCOs are ideal settings for psychiatric–mental health nurses to function in the role of primary mental health care provider.

Generally, psychiatric–mental health nurses in MCOs perform mental health assessments, monitor clients who are severely and persistently mentally ill, provide direct care for clients who are acutely ill, and facilitate health-promotion groups. Examples of some of the health-promotion activities nurses can initiate in primary care settings are stress management, parenting education, violence prevention, bereavement counseling, suicide prevention, and teen pregnancy prevention.

Triage Services

Psychiatric–mental health nurses provide effective *triage* services in the ambulatory care and primary care settings. Triage involves determining the severity of the illness and the need for immediate care in order to direct care and ensure the efficient use of medical and nursing staff and facilities. In the triage role, you often act as the *gatekeeper* of the system. You essentially decide who will use the system and at what level of care. The gatekeeping function is discussed in the case management section of this chapter.

Many factors need to be considered in the role of triage nurse. The common denominator in all instances is allocation of resources for ensuring quality and cost effectiveness. You may be performing face–to–face assessments or telephone triage. One of the most important required skills is good listening ability, coupled with an ability to collect information for making a decision about appropriate intervention. Information may be fragmented, and interviews with several people may be required to provide a comprehensive view of the client's presenting problem.

Triage clinicians in mental health care settings provide short-term, episodic intervention to members enrolled in the plan and simplify access to appropriate points of service in the system. Collaboration and consultation are important processes nurses use when performing this first-point-of-contact service. When triaging, you use a variety of nursing skills to evaluate the client's presenting problem. Using listening skills, you combine verbal and nonverbal data with information available in the client's medical record, as in the clinical example that follows.

Clinical Example

Margaret, a 35-year-old woman, is referred after several visits for minor medical problems. You note from the record a pattern of medication refills for antianxiety medication from the primary care provider. You also notice she has been referred for mental health care on two other occasions but has failed to keep these appointments. This information is valuable as you begin your assessment.

After completing the assessment, your next step is to decide a course of action. Using the nursing process, you begin to plan appropriate interventions. Choices include no intervention, immediate intervention, intervention within 24 hours, or routine appointment. Your further options include referral to a private mental health provider's office, a public clinic, or a hospital emergency room.

Employer-Based Clinics

As managed health care continues to develop new models, employers are becoming increasingly sophisticated in developing systems to meet the needs of their employees. Employers may establish on-site clinics with an MCO. The office is staffed with MCO employees. Here, the psychiatric–mental health nurse might be asked to serve as a consultant, counseling at the site a day or two per week, or seeing clients referred through the primary care providers in the employer-based clinic.

Unique Aspects of MCOs

There are several other aspects of practicing in managed care settings in mental health that are unique to this delivery system. These include legal issues, treatment and medication adherence, and continuity of care.

Legal Issues

In traditional fee-for-service practice, when a judge mandates treatment, there is usually acceptance of the client into the system for service. Service is delivered on demand, and then a charge is issued to the client. In MCOs, court-ordered treatment is negotiated on a case-by-case basis. What this means is that not every person with a request for court-ordered treatment will automatically receive this service.

Clinical Example

A transportation worker who has received his third DUI (driving under the influence) citation requests service. The member has already received two previous episodes of treatment and is not covered for services in the current calendar year.

A decision must then be made about how to respond to this request. These sometimes thorny and difficult legal cases are often referred for individual case review to the medical director.

A decision may be made to allow for a "flexing" of benefits or authorization of out-of-plan services. In flexing, an outpatient mental health care benefit may be converted to an inpatient benefit to allow for the needed hospitalization. The psychiatric–mental health nurse sometimes plays the role of client advocate, helping negotiate uncharted territory in these unusual circumstances.

Treatment Adherence

Issues of compliance or adherence (the term we use in this text) are more readily observed in MCOs, particularly in closed panel systems where appointment clerks, clinicians, and pharmacists may work side by side. Perhaps because services are prepaid, MCO consumers find it easier not to keep scheduled appointments. This is sometimes called DNKA (did not keep appointment). In mental health care, this behavior has clinical and administrative significance. It is important to note that different MCOs deal with this problem in different ways. One alternative is to set strict limits and not allow future appointments to be scheduled until the client makes copayment for all missed appointments. Another is to require clients to wait their turn in line for the next available appointment. Finally, the DNKA must be handled as a therapeutic issue in the therapy.

When missed appointments occur following hospitalization for a major psychiatric episode of illness, the clinician must aggressively maintain contact with the client. The importance of adhering to an after-care plan to avoid relapse is crucial. Phone calls, letters, or catching clients while they are visiting another department in the facility are all useful interventions. Some MCOs have developed transportation systems such as a free bus to ensure that clients keep appointments and follow after-care plans.

Medication Adherence

Encouraging medication adherence follows many principles used in other settings. Nurses in MCOs often work in collaborative relationships with other providers to ensure adherence, especially when uncomfortable side effects are responsible for a client's failure to adhere. When medication copayments are low, appointments are available, and transportation is accessible, the likelihood of adherence is increased. In the MCO setting, the primary care provider is an ally of the mental health care team. Primary care providers who see clients for routine medical problems are in a position to reinforce the importance of staying on psychotropic drugs. Often, a discussion of side effects eliminates confusion and increases understanding of the medicine's effect. When side effects are a problem, MCO nurses often contact the prescriber to arrange for a change in medication. Managed-care pharmacists can also help the mental health team ensure that clients adhere to their medication regimens.

MCO Member Expectations

Members' understanding of the managed care philosophy is crucial for effective and responsible health behaviors, including expectations of available services. The member's entitlement expectation is the member's understanding of the care he or she expects to receive. Entitlement expectations often differ from the specific provisions of the health plan contract. Health plan members often do not consider what type of mental health benefits they have purchased until they are in crisis. Your role as consumer educator is crucial to helping your clients understand how to use their managed-care plans in a manner that is satisfactory for all concerned. Examples of excluded mental health services of several large MCO contracts appear in Box 13-3.

Continuity of Care

Some MCOs are seamless delivery systems. In other words, consumers can move from one level of care to the next while remaining in the same delivery system. In this sense, members of an MCO can be considered to be in continuous therapy. This has clinical implications that require new conceptual frameworks for treatment. Primary care services tend to focus on the present impasse, while secondary care services are geared to examine the underlying obstacle. It is essential to the healing process that both are coordinated.

Box 13-3 Mental Health Services Often Excluded from Typical Managed Care Plans

Following are some examples of mental health services that are not included in typical MCO plans:

- Psychiatric or substance abuse therapy on court order, unless plan-approved as medically necessary
- Psychological testing, except for diagnosis or treatment of a psychiatric disorder
- Marriage counseling or treatment for stress, except when connected to treatment for a DSM psychiatric disorder
- Smoking cessation, obesity treatment, weight reduction, aversion therapy, custodial care, V code conditions (non–DSM conditions that may be a focus of clinical attention such as noncompliance with treatment, malingering, age-related cognitive decline, etc., as discussed in Appendix A∞), autism, learning disabilities, mental retardation, congenital disorders
- Experimental treatment (psychosurgery, megavitamin therapy, codependence therapy, or treatment for sexual addiction)

Ethics in Managed Mental Health Care

In effect, managed mental health care creates a situation in which the mental health professional no longer controls decisions about the type of treatment or the setting (inpatient versus outpatient). The autonomy and independent judgment of the nurse can be limited in managed care environments. Instead, decisions—such as two therapy sessions each week or outpatient drug rehabilitation—are monitored by an agent employed by insurers. Therapists in managed mental health care settings speak of a culture clash between themselves and managed care companies (Cohen, Marecek, & Gillham, 2006). They feel that some practices undermine therapeutic work and the therapist–client relationship and violate their standard of care and professional ethics. Clearly, managed psychiatric care raises serious ethical issues related to client autonomy of choice (see Chapter 12∞) regarding therapist and site, the integrity of the nurse–client relationship, and the risk that nonadherent psychiatric clients may be denied access to additional treatment.

Following are four principles to guide you through the ethical dilemmas posed by managed mental health care systems:

1. Recognize that as a clinician, you are dedicated to caring for clients in a relationship of fidelity and, at the same time, must act as a steward of society's scarce mental health care resources.
2. Recognize that it is ethically correct to recommend the least costly treatment unless you have evidence that a more costly intervention will yield a superior outcome.
3. Recognize that you need to advocate for the ethical principle of justice in managed mental health care situations so that cost savings with one client are used to meet the mental health care needs of another, not pay off an insurance company's debts.
4. Recognize that it is your responsibility to discuss the situation openly with your clients so that they understand the reimbursable parameters of their care and can act in their own interests.

A mental health consumer's bill of rights developed by the American Psychiatric Association that also examines insurance coverage and managed care plans in light of the principles identified in the bill can be accessed through the Online Student Resources for this book.

There is an ongoing moral debate about the ethics of applying managed care to psychiatric clients. Be prepared to sharpen your ethical reasoning skills and tools.

CASE MANAGEMENT

Rapid changes in the health care system have contributed to client feelings of being overwhelmed and confused about how to use services effectively. In many systems, clients no longer rely on a single provider or institution to shepherd them through an episode of illness. **Case management** is one strategy that has evolved in response to the shift in focus from inpatient to community care. Case management is most often employed when clients have been discharged from an inpatient to a community setting. However, the case manager role is also useful for long-term clients on inpatient units where it has been found to improve clients' day-to-day functioning on the unit (Elbaz-Haddad & Savaya, 2011). In this instance, a case manager is selected out of the inpatient staff. The central element that differentiates case management from other types of care is the coordination of one episode of care across the multiple settings of the care continuum. Each chapter in Unit 4∞ discusses specific case management strategies for each mental disorder.

The fundamental focus of case management is to integrate, coordinate, and advocate for individuals, families, and groups requiring extensive services. Like the nursing process, case management focuses on the following elements:

- Assessment and problem identification
- Planning
- Procurement, delivery, and coordination of service
- Monitoring to ensure that the multiple service needs of the client are met

The process of case management enhances quality by preventing unnecessary hospitalization, focusing treatment goals in least-restrictive settings, and preventing the duplication and fragmentation of services.

Recently, however, case management has come under fire. A very recent systematic review of the literature has indicated that case management may be of questionable value (Marshall, Gray, Lockwood, & Green, 2011). The literature review found that while case management may improve adherence to a program of treatment, it increases health care costs and does not produce clinically significant improvement in mental state, social functioning, or quality of life.

Case Manager Role

Nurses who perform the case manager role must be vested with the authority and accountability necessary to negotiate with complex systems and a wide diversity of providers and populations. Nurses are particularly prepared to function in this role by the very nature of the profession. This is especially evident in the managed care setting where clients from diverse backgrounds sometimes struggle to negotiate a new system of health care delivery. We know that race and poverty are factors that impede a client's access to mental health services and that race and ethnicity affect how clients use mental health services. Our racial diversity as a nation is increasing, and case management can help individuals and families who bring unique needs and cultural experiences to the managed care setting.

As case managers, nurses can provide physical assessment or illness-detection skills. An additional role because of the increased emphasis on psychobiology and pharmacology is helping clients cope with alterations in their mental health.

Gatekeeping and Facilitating

The service you provide as a case manager is one of gatekeeping and facilitating. As gatekeeper, you serve as the client's initial contact for care and referrals, as in the clinical example that follows.

Clinical Example

James, the case manager for Jerrod, a client with bipolar disorder, was contacted when Jerrod arrived at an emergency department in a manic state. Because James had knowledge of Jerrod's prior history and treatment, he was able to determine if inpatient care was required. James also had access to recent laboratory studies regarding Jerrod's lithium carbonate levels and also had an established relationship with family members.

In other words, case management helps clients and their caregivers make informed decisions, such as whether the client needs hospitalization, based on client needs, abilities, resources, and personal preferences.

In a case of recurring substance abuse, the nurse case manager can help a family make informed decisions, taking into consideration the client's health status and diagnosis, treatment plan, payment resources, and health care options. This facilitation aspect of case management ensures that clients receive care that is appropriate, individualized, cost effective, and has optimal outcomes.

Client Advocacy

Agencies that provide client services must have clear statements regarding client rights and responsibilities. The case manager often refers to these in negotiating with both client and system regarding appropriate referrals and authorizations for treatment.

The most fundamental aspect of the case manager role is that of being a client advocate. While there are many and varied models of case management, the nurse who defines this role as client advocate will have the greatest chance of success. When you carry out your case manager role, you bring to the multidisciplinary team skills and knowledge that extend beyond biologic or pathologic aspects of care. You view the client through a holistic perspective. You piece together the fragmented pieces of the client's care. This cannot be done in the isolation of an office or simply by telephone. It requires active,

on-site presence, interviews, meetings, attendance at treatment planning conferences, and appropriate documentation.

In the role of case manager, the nurse may be caught in the middle of conflicting value systems. For example, clients with alcoholism or bulimia have been treated traditionally with intensive, extended inpatient treatment programs. Some insurance plans may authorize this treatment only in an outpatient setting. The nurse must respond to clients' need for autonomy in making decisions regarding treatment as well as negotiate within the limitations of the plan. Case managers must use creativity and flexibility in negotiating among the conflicting needs of several parties. Clients and families who are accustomed to specific treatment models for illnesses with relapse potential often feel confused and misunderstood when new treatment approaches are suggested that appear economically motivated, that is, an attempt by the MCO or insurance company to save money by choosing a less expensive, but also less effective or more uncomfortable treatment approach.

Assessment Phase Challenges

Nurses who function as case managers must interact with all members of the health care team. Trust, mutual support, and clear communication among team members are necessary before you can implement case management services. When meeting with administrative personnel, employ tactful systems-entry strategies while laying the groundwork for a case management program. Careful introduction of the case management role, which differentiates it from medical care management, is necessary in clarifying role responsibilities. Other members of the team may feel threatened by the addition of a case manager and view it as an indictment of their own role performance. When staff members are oriented to the case manager's role, there is a higher level of acceptance of the service as augmenting client care rather than interfering with it.

Planning Phase Challenges

In this phase of care, you can bring valuable information concerning benefits, limits, family resources, expectations, and other pertinent data to the treatment planning table. Using the formal and informal support systems, the treatment team is able to set mutually agreed-upon goals with desired outcomes and can begin to plan action steps using intended time frames or critical pathways as a guide.

Implementation Phase Challenges

The next phase of the case management process is to ensure that the client gets needed care. In some systems, the case manager may be asked to deliver care. However, this approach is not in the best interest of the client because the case manager's role is to remain the objective, internal consultant, looking at the whole picture. When pulled into delivering the care, the case manager loses perspective and may find important issues clouded. For example, a case management nurse who is asked to function as the client's primary therapist because the primary nurse is overloaded will sacrifice time and resources needed to monitor the quality of care delivered and perhaps lose objectivity.

Keep in mind during the implementation phase that your role involves conflict resolution. To set limits tactfully, arbitrate differences, and maintain successful outcomes for all, you need patience, maturity, and experience. The case manager is also called on to provide additional data or client/family education where a denial or extension of service is in question. As client advocate, you may identify gaps in care that require action in the community, in a treatment facility, or within the nursing system. Nurse case managers are among the best consultants to nursing departments for improving quality because they view problems in the system from the client's perspective.

Evaluation Phase Challenges

The case manager's role in evaluation consists of continuous monitoring of intervention responses and progress toward desired outcomes. This may include medication monitoring for dosage and adherence, as well as monitoring client response to other therapies. You may interview the client directly to gather this information, and then compare it with what is recorded in the medical record. Inconsistent data are always a red flag for intervention by the case manager. Or perhaps the process is moving too slowly or the client is not an active participant in the care plan.

Once outcomes are achieved and the client is discharged, there must be a mechanism for ongoing quality improvement based on recommended standards of nursing practice. Communicate critical incidents and inconsistencies in the care in an ongoing, systematic program of continuous quality improvement. This information is ultimately used to measure provider and facility performance for contract renewal decisions.

Pearson Nursing Student Resources

Find additional review materials at
nursing.pearsonhighered.com

Prepare for success with NCLEX®-style practice questions, interactive assignments and activities, web links, animations and videos, and more!

REFERENCES

Bussema, E. F., & Bussema, K. E. (2007). Gilead revisited: Faith and recovery. *Psychiatric Rehabilitation Journal, 30*(4), 301–305.

Butcher, J. N., Mineka, S., & Hooley, J. M. (2010). *Abnormal psychology* (14th ed.). Boston: Allyn & Bacon.

Cohen, J., Marecek, J., & Gillham, J. (2006). Is three a crowd? Clients, clinicians, and managed care. *American Journal of Orthopsychiatry, 76*(2), 251–259.

Currier, G. W., Fisher, S. G., & Caine, E. D. (2010). Mobile crisis team intervention to enhance linkage of discharged suicidal emergency department patients to outpatient psychiatric services: A randomized controlled trial. *Academic Emergency Medicine, 17*(9), 38–43.

Davis, K. E., Brigell, E., Christiansen, K., Snyder, M., McDevitt, J., Forman, J., . . . Wilkniss, S. M. (2011) Integrated primary and mental health services: An evolving partnership model. *Psychiatric Rehabilitation, 34*(4), 317–320.

Elbaz-Haddad, M., & Savaya, R. (2011). Effect of a psychosocial intervention model for persons with chronic psychiatric disorders in long-term hospitalization. *Evaluation Review.* Advance online publication. doi: 10.1177/0193841X11406080

Hall, J. P., Carroll, S. L., & Moore, J. M. (2010). Health care behaviors and decision-making processes among enrollees in a state high-risk insurance pool: Focus group findings. *American Journal of Health Promotion, 24*(5), 304–310.

Hannon-Engel, S. (2011). Regulatory oversight: Do psychiatric patients have the right to refuse active treatment? *Volume, 25*(1), 21–23.

Howard, L., & Gamble, C. (2011). Supporting mental health nurses to address the physical health needs of people with severe mental illness in acute inpatient care settings. *Journal of Psychiatric and Mental Health Nursing, 18*(2), 105–112.

Kisely, S. R., Campbell, L. A., & Preston, N. J. (2011). Compulsory commitment and involuntary outpatient treatment for people with severe mental disorders. *Cochrane Database of Systematic Reviews 2011* (2). Art. No.: CD004408. doi: 10.1002/14651858.CD004408.pub3

Lang, K., Meyers, J. L., Korn, J. R., Lee, S., Sirica, M., Crivera, C., . . . Menzin, J. (2010). Medication adherence and hospitalization among patients with schizophrenia treated with antipsychotics. *Psychiatric Services, 61*(12), 1239–1247.

Lichtenberg, P. (2011). The residential care alternative for the acutely psychotic patient. *Psychiatric Quarterly.* Advance online publication. doi: 10.1007/s11126-011-9176-0

Marshall, M., Gray A., Lockwood, A., & Green, R. (2011). WITHDRAWN: Case management for people with severe mental disorders. *Cochrane Database of Systematic Reviews 2011*(4). Art. No. CD000050.

Marshall, M., & Lockwood, A. (2011). WITHDRAWN: Assertive community treatment for people with severe mental disorders. *Cochrane Database of Systematic Reviews 2011*(4). Art. No.: CD001089.

Nolan, P., Bradley, E., & Brimblecome, N. (2011). Disengaging from acute inpatient psychiatric care: A description of service users' experiences and views. *Journal of Psychiatric and Mental Health Nursing, 18*(4), 359–367.

Schmutte, T., Dunn, C. L., & Sledge, W. H. (2010). Predicting time to readmission in patients with recent histories of recurrent psychiatric hospitalization: A matched-control survival analysis. *Journal of Nervous and Mental Disorders, 198*(12), 860–863.

Shor, R., & Aivhod, G. (2011). The conceptual model and guiding principles of a supported-education program for orthodox Jewish persons with severe mental illness. *Community Mental Health Journal.* Advance online publication. doi: 10.1007/s10597-011-9387-8

Thibeault, C. A., Trudeau, K., d'Entremont, M., & Brown, J. (2010). Understanding the milieu experiences of patients on an acute inpatient psychiatric unit. *Archives of Psychiatric Nursing, 24*(4), 216–226.

Torrey, E. F. (2010). Documenting the failure of deinstitutionalization. *Psychiatry, 73*(2), 122–124.

Wanchek, T. N., McGarvey, E. L., Leon-Verdin, M., & Bonnie, R. J. (2011). The effect of community mental health services on hospitalization rates in Virginia. *Psychiatric Services, 62*(2), 194–199.

Wong-McDonald, A. (2007). Spirituality and psychosocial rehabilitation: Empowering persons with serious psychiatric disabilities at an inner-city community program. *Psychiatric Rehabilitation Journal, 30*(4), 295–300.

Zuvekas, S. H., & Seiden, T. M. (2010). Mental health and family out-of-pocket expenditure burdens. *Medical Care Research Review, 67*(2), 194–212.

4
UNIT

CLIENTS WITH MENTAL DISORDERS

JUSTIN's platoon lost several soldiers during his second deployment to Iran (U.S. military serve longer and more frequent tours of duty than their counterparts from Great Britain and other countries), and his best friend is on his way back to Fort Bragg after a suicide attempt. Twenty-five American soldiers killed themselves in April, 2011, equal to about half the deaths in Afghanistan that month. Nightmares prevent Justin from having a restful night's sleep and he daydreams about the deaths of the members of his platoon. His platoon sergeant has cautioned Justin, who hopes to make the military his career, to keep his nightmares, anxiety, and daydreams hidden from his comrades who could perceive him as weak, and from his commanding officer who could negatively affect his career promotion and advancement.

Men and women who have returned home from Iran and Afghanistan have suicide rates that surpass those of the general public. In addition, there are other disturbing trends—family violence, substance abuse, post-traumatic stress disorder, and depression. Worries about stigma and discrimination cause many soldiers to avoid asking for mental health treatment at the same time that they face an increase in the duration and frequency of military deployments. Because he has kept his symptoms hidden, Justin has been unable to take advantage of Department of Defense anonymous mental health and substance abuse self-assessments and referrals that are available online or on the phone, or supportive programs such as the Real Warriors Campaign for psychological health and traumatic brain injury.

14

Cognitive Disorders

EILEEN TRIGOBOFF

LEARNING OUTCOMES

After completing this chapter, you will be able to:

1. Examine the biopsychosocial theories that explain delirium, dementia, amnestic disorders, and other cognitive disorders.
2. Differentiate among the various types of cognitive disorders.
3. Analyze the differences between delirium, dementia, and depression.
4. Compare possible assessment findings in delirium and dementia.
5. Compare and contrast the nursing interventions and their rationales for clients with delirium and dementia.
6. Incorporate psychiatric–mental health nursing strategies that support optimal memory and cognitive functioning in the care of clients with cognitive disorders.
7. Predict the difficulties caregivers may face when working with clients who have cognitive disorders.
8. Determine your own personal feelings and attitudes that are likely to interfere with your ability to care for cognitively impaired clients.

CRITICAL THINKING CHALLENGE

You are the community mental health nurse for Mrs. Downston, an elderly widow with dementia of the Alzheimer's type (DAT). This client has lived with her daughter Dolores, her son-in-law Don, and their two teenage daughters in their suburban home for the past 3 years. You have been involved with this case throughout. It is notable how the stress of Mrs. Downston's deterioration is affecting the entire family. Dolores and Don have been rearranging and strictly limiting their social activities to make sure Mrs. Downston is supervised. Their care load is increasing, and they both have physical problems that will soon make rendering this care difficult, if not impossible. Because Mrs. Downston is frightened by newcomers and screams in terror, her teenage granddaughters have been unable to invite their friends to the house.

Psychiatric practitioners frequently advocate institutionalizing clients with DAT. Family caregivers, on the other hand, often have difficulty with this decision and may even take offense at this suggestion despite feeling mentally and physically exhausted.

1. What suggestions or alternatives would you propose to Mrs. Downston's family?
2. At what point, if ever, should a professional exert pressure on family caregivers to institutionalize their loved one?

As a result of the aging of the U.S. population, psychiatric–mental health nurses are increasingly in contact with clients who have delirium, dementia, amnestic disorder, and other cognitive disorders. Clients with these disorders provide a special challenge because they may perceive themselves and their environment differently than we do and often have problems in receiving communication and expressing themselves. These are similar to challenges psychiatric–mental health nurses face when communicating with a client who has a florid (occurring in fully developed form) psychosis. Discovering how to communicate, how to assess how they feel, and how to care for them are vital nursing skills.

In addition to family caregivers, nurses are the most logical advocates for these clients. Frequently, we are in charge of day treatment centers or long-term care facilities, or we facilitate support groups. Families look to us for suggestions to ease their burdens, for strategies to cope with difficult behavioral symptoms, for education to explain unpredictable behavior, and for resources that might alleviate their situation.

Your knowledge of psychobiology and your holistic approach to client care are unique assets essential to providing quality care for clients with cognitive disorders. Before the 20th century, all organic brain disorders of older adults were categorized as senile dementia. At the turn of the 20th century, neuropathologists doing autopsy work distinguished senile dementia from arteriosclerotic conditions and neurosyphilis. Arteriosclerotic brain disease was then considered the primary cause of confused states in older adults and the result of diseased cerebral vessels.

By the middle of the 20th century a new category, organic brain disease (OBD), was added. This category was broader, allowing for a defect both in the vessels and in the brain itself. The category organic brain syndrome (OBS) then followed, which recognized the need for a diagnosis that included symptoms without a known cause. A few years ago, the term *organic mental syndrome* (OMS) referred to a group of psychological or behavioral signs of unknown or unclear etiology, while *organic mental disorder* (OMD) referred to a particular syndrome whose etiology was known or presumed. The terms are no longer used; the term *cognitive disorder* is preferred.

DELIRIUM

Older adults, especially those with dementia, are prone to transient cognitive disorders usually called either *delirium* or *acute confusional state*. There is a wide range (11% to 89%) to the estimation of how many older general medical clients experience a life-threatening acute confusional state (Rudolph & Marcantonio, 2011; Voyer, Richard, Doucet, & Carmichael, 2011). If hospitalized, they remain in the hospital twice as long as clients without delirium, and one fourth of these older adults with delirium die within 1 month of admission. Residents over 75 years of age in long-term care facilities are at particular risk and significant numbers may be delirious at any time.

Delirium is an abrupt-onset type of confusional state marked by the following:

1. Fluctuations in level of confusion
2. Inability to pay attention during interactions
3. Disorganized thinking
4. Changes in consciousness
5. Agitation or quiet and hypoactive behavior (such as quickly falling back to sleep)

Additional elements include diminution of all mental activity. Rage, depression, fear, apathy, and incontinence are common.

Differentiating delirium from dementia can be a difficult process for nurses and physicians; however, failure to recognize delirium in clients can delay appropriate treatment, with serious health consequences. See DSM Essential Features for the taxonomy of delirium.

Signs of Delirium

Detecting delirium involves examining how the person thinks (cognition), as well as the ability to pay attention, degree of wakefulness, and psychomotor behavior.

Cognition

The three components of cognition—perception, thinking, and memory—are all disrupted in delirium:

1. *Perception.* The person shows a reduced ability to distinguish and integrate sensory information and to differentiate it from hallucinations, dreams, illusions, and imagery.
2. *Thinking.* The thinking process is fragmented and disorganized to the extent that the person is unable to reason, judge, abstract, or solve problems.
3. *Memory.* Memory is impaired in all three aspects; the person is unable to form memories or store and retrieve (register, retain, or recall) information.

DSM ESSENTIAL FEATURES

Cognitive Disorders

Delirium: Delirium is a disturbance of consciousness with reduced ability to focus, sustain, or shift attention. There is a change in cognition and the disturbance develops over hours to days and tends to fluctuate during the day. A medical condition also contributes to the difficulties.

Dementia of the Alzheimer's Type (DAT): DAT involves multiple cognitive deficits with memory impairment and aphasia, apraxia, agnosia, and/or a disturbance in organizing. This causes impairment and lower functioning in important areas. It starts gradually and is progressive and problems are not due to other sources.

Attention and Wakefulness

Attention is impaired in all three areas. The person has difficulty with the following:

- Alertness, or maintaining vigilance
- Selectiveness, or the ability to focus and filter out or selectively attend to stimuli at will
- Directiveness, or the ability to pull oneself back to a task or direct and focus one's mental processes

Wakefulness is usually reduced during the day, leading to drowsiness and naps. The person often experiences sleeplessness, restlessness, and agitation at night. There is a disturbed sleep–wake cycle, with hour-to-hour variation. Interestingly, delirium and dreaming are both characterized by the same electroencephalographic (EEG) changes. The person with delirium is then caught between dreaming and hallucinating, sleeping and wakefulness.

Psychomotor Behavior

The delirious client is either hyperactive or hypoactive, often alternating between the two extremes. Speech may be slurred and disjointed, with aimless vocalizations and repetitions. Tremors and irregular spasmodic (choreiform) movements may be present, as illustrated in the following clinical examples of delirium.

Clinical Example

A 55-year-old man, Mr. Bruener, was in the midst of a difficult divorce and went drinking with his friends. He drank numerous "straight shots" and shortly thereafter began screaming, crying, and acting aggressively toward others in the bar. At one point he tried to choke a man, and later picked up a chair and threw it. The police took him to jail and, when he began to convulse, to the hospital.

Mrs. Weinstein, a 65-year-old woman, was in the hospital with renal problems. Although previously alert, she rapidly became agitated and confused about where she was. She was unresponsive to the nurse's efforts to orient her and refused to cooperate during her morning care. Within hours after this extreme agitation, she lapsed into a stupor and then a coma.

DIFFERENTIATING DELIRIUM FROM DEMENTIA AND DEPRESSION

The following criteria distinguish delirium from dementia:

- *State of consciousness.* People with delirium have fluctuating consciousness, but people with dementia are as attentive as they can be and do not have clouded consciousness until terminal stages.
- *Stability.* In clients with delirium, the ability to pay attention and respond changes from hour to hour. Clients with dementia pay attention and respond at a particular level in a relatively stable manner.
- *Duration.* Delirium can be short lived; dementia is prolonged.
- *Rate of onset.* Delirium develops rapidly, whereas dementia is usually an insidious, gradual process.
- *Cause.* Delirium may be traced to a recent source, whereas dementia cannot be linked to another cause.

For a summary of the characteristics of delirium and dementia, and the differentiation between them and depression, see TABLE 14-1 ■. Depression is discussed in Chapter 17∞.

DEMENTIA

The prevalence of dementia may be different in various racial/ethnic groups; however, research arrives at an approximate level of 6% to 7% in the United States (Chin, Negash, & Hamilton, 2011). The Alzheimer Association reports that 5.4 million Americans are living with Alzheimer's disease—5.2 million aged 65 and over. By 2050, as many as 16 million Americans will have the disease. It is the fifth leading cause of death in those 65 years of age and older. Be alert in every clinical setting for the presence of symptoms that could indicate an early form of dementia. What Every Nurse Should Know gives an example that may pique your interest.

Dementia of all types is becoming fairly common. With the rate of DAT in the elderly 11% for men and 17% for women, chances are you will be involved in the care of someone with any type of dementia during your career as a nurse. See Mental Health in the News on page 275 for examples of the many people who had some type of dementia.

Long-term care facilities have large populations of people with diagnoses of dementia. A now common clinical syndrome, dementia is marked by the following:

- Global cognitive impairment extending to the areas of abstract thinking, judgment, insight, complex capabilities (language, tasks, recognition), and personality change
- Memory impairment
- Decline in intellectual function
- Altered judgment, in awake and alert states
- Altered affect
- Spatial disorientation

WHAT EVERY NURSE SHOULD KNOW

A Family Member's Cognitive Skills

Imagine you are a community health nurse. You will have contact with a number of people who are aged but still living independently in their own community living situations. When you make a home visit to an elderly couple to treat the husband's surgical incision site, you also notice that his wife is having some difficulty. Her shoelaces are not tied and when you mention it, she looks down and pushes them into the inside of her shoes instead of tying them. Her emotions seem blunted, she has been neglecting her personal hygiene, and her husband is worried about her decreased energy and motivation and lack of initiative. This, in combination with her problem understanding some of your conversation with her about her husband's bandages, leads you to believe she may be having some cognitive problems. Under these circumstances, an assessment of the wife is warranted.

TABLE 14-1 ■ Comparing Delirium, Dementia, and Depression

	Delirium	Dementia	Depression
Diagnostic Features	Disturbance of consciousness accompanied by a change in cognition unaccounted for by a pre-existing or evolving dementia. Reduced clarity of awareness of the environment. Impaired ability to focus, sustain, or shift attention. Change in cognition may include memory impairment, disorientation to time and/or place, or language disturbance such as rambling, irrelevant, or pressured and incoherent speech. Simple or complex perceptual disturbances may include misinterpretations, illusions, or hallucinations.	Multiple cognitive deficits, including memory impairment and either aphasia, apraxia, or agnosia; or a disturbance in executive functioning (the ability to think abstractly, to organize, plan, initiate, sequence, monitor, and stop complex behavior). Impairment in occupational or social functioning that represents a decline from earlier level of functioning.	Dysphoric mood, loss of interest or pleasure in usual activities and pastimes, appetite disturbance, change in weight, sleep disturbance, psychomotor agitation or retardation, decreased energy, feelings of worthlessness or guilt, difficulty concentrating or thinking, thoughts of death or suicide or suicide attempts.
Associated Features	Emotional disturbance: fear, anxiety, irritability, anger, euphoria, apathy. Disturbance in sleep–wake cycle with daytime sleepiness or nighttime agitation and difficulty falling asleep. Disturbed psychomotor behavior including groping or picking at bedclothes, sudden movements, or sluggishness and lethargy. Possible extremes of psychomotor activity during the day.	Spatial disorientation, poor judgment, poor insight, violence, suicidal behavior, disinhibited behavior, slurred speech, anxiety, mood and sleep disturbances, delusions, hallucinations, vulnerability to physical and psychosocial stressors. Progressive disease that slowly but steadily destroys the neurons of the brain and reduces, among other neurotransmitters, the concentration level of acetylcholine.	Depressed appearance, tearfulness, feelings of anxiety, irritability, fear, brooding, irrational guilt, excessive concern with physical health, panic attacks, phobias. Delusions or hallucinations may be present. In older adults, symptoms suggesting dementia (i.e., disorientation, memory loss, distractibility, apathy, difficulty in concentration, inattentiveness).
Onset	May begin abruptly. Relatively rapid: over hours. Short period of time: a few days. Especially common in children and after the age of 60.	Depends on underlying etiology. May be rather sudden (e.g., head trauma) or insidious in onset and slow, but progress is relentless over several years (i.e., primary degenerative dementia).	Usually able to date onset with some precision. Onset is variable; symptoms usually develop over a period of days to weeks but may be sudden. In some instances, prodromal symptoms may occur over several months.
Course	Fluctuates; symptoms usually worse at night; lucid intervals usually in the morning.	Depends on underlying etiology. May be progressive, stable, or (less likely) remitting.	Often not recognized or misdiagnosed in older adults. Need to differentiate from dementia.
Duration	Transient. May resolve in a few hours or a few weeks.	May progress to death over several years. May be slowed.	Can be self-limiting. Median time period is 8 months; may last up to 2 years.
Outcome	Depends on severity. Poorer prognosis with severe delirium. Recovery possible if underlying disease is corrected or self-limiting. If disorder persists, delirium would shift to another more stable organic brain syndrome. May cause death.	Generally irreversible. Slowing of deterioration depends on underlying pathology, timely diagnosis, and treatment. The more widespread the structural damage to the brain, the less likely the clinical improvement.	Can be successfully treated if identified and treated. Recurrent depression common in the elderly. Severe depression may end in suicide.
Etiologic Factors	Multifactorial. Systemic infections. Metabolic disorders (hepatic or renal disease, hypoxia, hypercapnia, hypoglycemia, ionic imbalances, thiamine deficiency). Postoperative states. Substance intoxication and withdrawal. Head trauma. Lesions of the right parietal lobe and occipital lobe. Toxin exposure. Anticholinergic effects of medication.	Primary degenerative dementia, Alzheimer's type. Infections of central nervous system. Brain trauma. Virus (i.e., AIDS). Prion (i.e., Creutzfeldt–Jakob disease). Toxic metabolic disturbance. Vascular disease (i.e., vascular dementia). Normal pressure hydrocephalus. Neurologic conditions such as Huntington's disease, multiple sclerosis, Parkinson's disease. Postanoxic or posthypoglycemic states.	Situational: bereavement, loss of health, major catastrophic event in person's life, trauma. There is a cardiac link to depression that is still being explored.

Source: Adapted from Voyer, P., Richard, S., Doucet, L., & Carmichael, P.-H. (2011). Factors associated with delirium severity among older persons with dementia. *Journal of Neuroscience Nursing, 43*(2), 62–69 and Blazer, D., Hughes, D. C., & George, L. K. (1987). The epidemiology of depression in an elderly community population. *The Gerontologist, 27,* 281–287.

Dementia is a mental disorder involving functional declines in multiple cognitive areas, including memory, along with behavioral and psychological symptoms. Symptoms related to specific areas of brain damage are shown in FIGURE 14-1 ■. The DSM further differentiates dementia as "sufficiently severe to cause impairment in occupational or social functioning" (American Psychiatric Association [APA], 2000, p. 148).

Dementias are classified according to either the cause or the area of neurologic damage (such as cortical or subcortical). Dementia of the Alzheimer's type (DAT) is the classic cortical dementia, whereas Huntington's disease and Parkinson's disease are common subcortical types. The cortical and subcortical types are quite similar. People with subcortical dementias, however, have a higher order of functioning.

Some sources suggest that as many as 5% of dementias evaluated in clinical settings may be attributable to reversible causes. Some of these causes include metabolic abnormalities (e.g., hypothyroidism), dementia syndrome due to depression, paraneoplastic disease, or Hashimoto encephalitis (Rosenbloom & Atri, 2011). How dementia affects function depends on the area of the brain involved in the disease. There will be different behavioral, neurologic, psychiatric, and cognitive symptoms depending on the type of dementia. An added frequent complication is the presence of mixed dementias. With such a broad array of dementias, establishing a clear diagnosis is complex, difficult, and time consuming but worth the effort in order to determine appropriate psychiatric treatment.

Sleep apnea increases with age and is significantly associated with cognitive impairment and dementia (Kim, Lee, Lee, Jhoo, & Woo, 2011). It is important to assess nocturnal breathing patterns in clients with dementia. Do not assume that their sleep pattern disturbance is the phenomenon called sundowning—increased restlessness and agitation during the evening and night hours. Sleep deprivation can lead to restlessness, reduced concentration, and, if prolonged, hallucinations and delusions. Poor sleep quality and greater severity of sleep apnea were associated with impaired language function in clients with mild cognitive impairment. This suggests that vulnerability to specific brain damage associated with sleep apnea could increase the risk for dementia. Likewise, chronic sleep deprivation may exacerbate dementia behaviors, as in this clinical example.

Clinical Example

Ellen, an older adult, was recently hospitalized for management of a medical condition. She was known to have early dementia of the Alzheimer's type (DAT) but had been managing alone in her apartment up to this point. Over a period of several days, she became increasingly agitated, demanding cigarettes from nursing staff, other clients, and visitors. Attempts at distraction or providing unsolicited attention were unsuccessful.

A nursing student began questioning how much sleep this client had been getting. At that point the nurse's only cue was the lack of success

FRONTAL LOBE
Perseveration, concrete thinking, reduced problem-solving capacity, lack of foresight and insight, loss of social and moral sense, impulsiveness, indifference, aggressiveness, insistence, regression

TEMPORAL LOBE
Amnesia, dementia

Lateral view of brain

PARIETAL LOBE
Disorientation, body agnosia

BRAIN STEM, THALAMUS, HYPOTHALAMUS
Apathy, dysphoria, lability of affect, polydypsia, hyperphagia, anorexia, altered libido, impaired consciousness, sleep disturbance

RIGHT CEREBRAL HEMISPHERE
Difficulty copying designs and doing jigsaw puzzles, spatial disorientation

RIGHT TEMPORAL LOBE
Spatial sequencing problems, musical atonality

Frontal view of brain

LEFT CEREBRAL HEMISPHERE
Thought blocking, inability to initiate action

LEFT TEMPORAL LOBE
Memory difficulties, aphasias, atypical psychoses, personality deterioration

FIGURE 14-1 ■ Behavioral changes related to specific areas of brain damage. Damage to each part of the brain results in specific alterations and deficits in client behaviors and skills.

with other interventions, but the nurse also knew that sundowning is common in clients with dementia. The brief chart notes made by the night staff offered little information. From a neighbor who came to visit, the nurse found out that prior to the hospitalization Ellen had been phoning the neighbor during the night in an agitated state. The night staff agreed to observe and record the amount of time that Ellen spent sleeping, and the day staff did the same. With this additional data it was soon apparent that Ellen was averaging no more than 4 hours of sleep per 24-hour period. Meanwhile, her agitated behavior was increasing.

After a client conference in which the nursing student offered her nursing diagnosis hypothesis of Sleep Deprivation, the nurse practitioner agreed to try a mild short-acting hypnotic for the next three nights. Nursing staff continued to monitor Ellen's sleep patterns and behavior. By the end of the three nights, during which she did appear to sleep for longer periods, the agitated behavior and demands for cigarettes subsided considerably.

The use of hypnotics was not a long-term solution for the client in the above example, but it broke the escalating cycle of increasing agitation and decreasing sleep. Recognizing the role of sleep deprivation in contributing to a daytime behavior problem can facilitate effective short-term intervention and create a context for more comprehensive assessment of possible contributing factors such as fear, relocation stress, powerlessness, or sensory and/or perceptual alterations.

Another feature to be aware of is how culture and ethnicity play a significant role in the health care practices of clients with dementia and their families. How individuals view their body and their functioning has an effect on diagnosis and treatment of dementias as well (Chin et al., 2011). See

Developing Cultural Competence for ways to consider incorporating culture into your practice with these clients.

Dementia of the Alzheimer's Type (DAT)

Dementia of the Alzheimer's type (DAT), also known as *Alzheimer's disease* or *Alzheimer's dementia (AD)*, a chronic progressive disorder, is the most common form of dementia among older adults. (See the summary of diagnostic criteria for cognitive disorders.) Reference to this disease with either abbreviation—DAT or AD—is accepted; however, to keep the distinction clear that this is one of many different types of dementia, and to prevent confusion with the abbreviation AD used to refer to anxiety disorder, it will be referred to as DAT throughout this chapter.

DAT cannot yet be prevented or cured. In addition to the quality-of-life issues for the clients involved, there are financial realities that affect the individual, the family, the community, and our health care system in general. Care for those with DAT costs the U.S. economy over $180 billion a year. You can access additional data through links to DAT resources through the Online Student Resources for this book.

Alois Alzheimer first recognized the features of what would come to be called DAT in 1907 while conducting an autopsy on a 51-year-old woman with a 4-year history of dementia. He discovered senile plaques in the brain and other pathologic lesions that he called *neurofibrillary tangles* (Alzheimer, 1907). Neurofibrillary tangles are illustrated in FIGURE 14-2 ■. These are now called *Alzheimer-type changes.*

DEVELOPING CULTURAL COMPETENCE

Culture and Dementia

Because dementia is a product of biologic and cultural factors, be aware of the following points in developing your cultural competence with dementia clients and their families. Evidence suggests that the prevalence of DAT may be lower in non-Hispanic whites. Cultural factors influence perceptions about what is normal aging. Minority groups can have delayed dementia diagnoses. Look for cultural bias (language, expected response, speed, etc.) in cognitive screening tools and discuss these biases with colleagues.

Nurses who are involved with ethnoracial minority groups promote effective health practices in the community setting; for example, taking blood pressure, discussing healthy diet, and noticing early symptoms of dementia. Education and outreach to diverse populations can provide support for clients and their families.

CRITICAL THINKING QUESTIONS

1. What are some possible explanations for why the prevalence of DAT is lower in non-Hispanic whites?
2. What are some possible reasons for delayed dementia diagnoses in minority groups?
3. How do ideas of normal aging vary among cultures?

FIGURE 14-2 ■ Neurofibrillary tangles. This photomicrograph of a brain tissue specimen from an Alzheimer's client shows the characteristic plaques (dark patches) and neurofibrillary tangles (irregular pattern of strandlike fibers).
Photo courtesy of SIU/PHOTOLIBRARY PETER ARNOLD INC

This disease may also destroy the neurons that secrete the neurotransmitter acetylcholine, which plays a role in memory and learning.

Signs of Dementia of the Alzheimer's Type (DAT)

Signs of this disease include the following:

- *Aphasia:* The loss of language ability.
- *Anomia:* Over time, the person experiences difficulty remembering words.
- *Agraphia:* An inability to express thoughts in writing.
- *Alexia:* An inability to understand written language (eventually, the condition progresses to a loss of all verbal ability).
- *Apraxia:* The loss of purposeful movement without loss of muscle power or coordination in general. The ability to conceptualize or perform motor tasks deteriorates. People with apraxia may have difficulty carrying out complex tasks.
- *Agnosia:* The loss of sensory ability to recognize objects. Initially, the person has difficulty recognizing everyday objects. In the later stages, people with agnosia recognize neither loved ones nor their own body parts.
- *Mnemonic disturbances:* Memory loss. The inability to remember recent events, especially in new or changing environments, extends to profound memory loss of both recent and past events (American Psychological Association [APA], 2011).

Frequently, symptoms of DAT occur insidiously. Family members may notice that routine tasks cannot be completed or items are placed in unusual places. The movie *Away From Her* (see Mental Health in the Movies) demonstrates some of the small and odd changes that take place in the beginning stages of DAT.

Hallucinations, more often visual than auditory, can be quite disturbing to the unsuspecting client. Behaviors can become agitated and will run counter to the client's usual personality and interactional style. Spending time in a health care facility for physical reasons such as rehabilitation or surgery can bring some of the symptoms to the attention of health care providers. See Box 14-1 for Behavioral Changes of DAT. The following is a clinical example of dementia.

Clinical Example

Therese Thomas, an 81-year-old retired piano teacher, is recuperating from knee replacement surgery at a rehabilitation center. Nursing staff noticed slight changes in her interactions over the past 2 weeks, including refusing to use silverware during meals, a significant difference from her typically fastidious habits. During an assessment interview, Ms. Thomas was asked how her vision and hearing have been lately, because seeing well and hearing well frequently become issues with older adults. She replied that she has been seeing and hearing just fine. These questions can be asked or stated in such a way as to seem more a physical set of questions than an emotional or psychiatric-focused set of questions (e.g., "Sometimes people may not hear as well as others and words are missed."). Then the question was asked, "Sometimes your hearing may be such that you are hearing things that other people don't hear. Does that ever happen to you?" Ms. Thomas admitted she did hear things to which other people were not reacting. When asked to elaborate, Ms. Thomas stated that her silverware had begun speaking to her. When the nurse asked what was being said, Ms. Thomas replied, "Nothing good."

Progression of Dementia of the Alzheimer's Type (DAT)

There are three clinically distinct global stages of DAT based on functional and cognitive capacity: Stages 1, 2, and 3. One assessment tool useful in assessing the cognitive capacity in DAT is the Mini-Mental State Exam (MMSE, see Chapter 11∞). Usually, a score of 18 or higher is seen in the early stages of DAT, between 12 and 18 in moderate DAT, and lower than 12 in severe DAT. The average decline in MMSE scores is approximately 3 points per year.

Functional disability can be assessed grossly through determining competence with activities of daily living (ADLs). When you assess a client for DAT, observe for functional disabilities. There is a correspondence between the stages of central nervous system (CNS) aging and DAT. Note cognitive decline and the corresponding functional disability when you formulate your assessments. In as many as 20% of clients with DAT, you can expect mild rigidity and a slowing of movement, called *bradykinesia* (Scarmeas et al., 2011). This will affect how quickly and how well they will be able to function. Mental Health in the News lists the many famous people who were diagnosed with dementia.

MENTAL HEALTH IN THE MOVIES
Away From Her

The movie *Away From Her* is the story of a man coping with the institutionalization of his wife because of DAT. Their wonderful life full of love and adventure is reduced to infrequent and brief glimpses of its former glory as he watches the progression of her disease from putting a frying pan away in the refrigerator to not knowing who he is. The movie brings us along on the waves of his gut-wrenching feelings of loneliness as he leaves her at a specialty facility, sleeping without her for the first time. He faces the unimaginable changes in their relationship as he watches her transfer her affections to another man who also lives at the long-term care facility. Her fear and confusion from DAT are palpable as she tells him she doesn't want to be near him because she doesn't know how to feel.

Both sides of the DAT story are told with frankness and candor while being true to presenting the symptoms of the disease and the practical side of lives changed by DAT.

Photo courtesy © Lions Gate/courtesy Everett Collection.

Box 14-1 Behavioral Changes of Dementia of the Alzheimer's Type (DAT)

DAT has an average course of 5 to 10 years, with a range of 2 to 20 years. Early onset often leads to very rapid deterioration.

Stage 1 (2–4 Years): Early

Changes in behaviors include the following:

- Complex tasks become more difficult, related to a recent decline in memory.
- Concentration decreases while distractibility increases.
- Making accurate judgments becomes difficult.
- Disorientation about time occurs, but memory about people and places remains.
- Personal appearance may decline and the person needs help in selecting appropriate clothing.
- Planning in general is seriously limited, so incomplete verbal or written reports are common at work sites.
- Verbal skills decline and word finding and object naming become difficult. Speech in noisy, distracting environments is too difficult.
- Client may accuse others of wrongdoing because of transitory delusions of persecution ("You hid my keys"). People recognize their own confusion and are frightened by it. They cover up and rationalize symptoms.
- Poor driving skills because of misperceptions and errors in judgment can lead to accidents.
- *Hypertonia* (an increase in muscle tone) can happen with dementia and may result in muscle twitching.
- Anxiety and depression are common, as are frustration, helplessness, apathy, and shame.
- Psychotic symptoms are common.
- Depression worsens the symptoms of dementia and should be treated.

Stage 2 (Several Years): Middle

Changes in behavior include the following:

- Progressive recent and remote memory loss are characteristic.
- New information cannot be retained.
- Failure to recognize family members or past significant events signals loss of remote memory.
- Behavior deteriorates rapidly and is often socially unacceptable.
- Poor impulse control leads to outbursts and tantrums.
- Emotional lability is common—the mood quickly shifts from a flat affect to marked irritability.
- Comprehension of language, interactions, and significance of objects is greatly diminished.
- Disorientation occurs to the three spheres of person, place, and time.
- Wandering occurs.
- The person has difficulty tracking the sequence of events especially for bathing, dressing, and toileting.
- Psychotic symptoms are common.
- *Misidentification syndrome* frequently occurs, in which familiar people are seen as unfamiliar and vice versa.
- Sleep cycle is impaired, with a decrease in total sleep time and frequent awakenings.
- Accidents are common, especially falls and injuries because of difficulty in using sharp objects.

Stage 3 (1–2 Years): Late

Changes in behavior include the following:

- Hyperorality (placing everything within reach into the mouth) and periodic binge eating occur.
- Hypermetamorphosis occurs (the need to compulsively touch and examine every object in the environment).
- Motor skills seriously deteriorate.
- Emotional responses dwindle to nonresponsiveness.

MENTAL HEALTH IN THE NEWS

Famous People With Dementia

A number of people have been in the news for their struggles with dementia. These people all had DAT:

- Ronald Reagan, the 40th president of the United States
- Charlton Heston, an American film actor
- Rita Hayworth, an American film actress
- Sugar Ray Robinson, a professional boxer
- Peter Falk, an American actor
- Otto Preminger, a film director
- Tommy Dorsey, a noted big band leader
- Arlene Francis, American actress
- Burgess Meredith, American actor

These people had unspecified dementias:

- Barry Goldwater, five-term U.S. Senator
- Norman Rockwell, famous painter and illustrator
- Joe Adcock, professional baseball player
- Molly Picon, actress
- Betty Schwartz, Olympic gold medal winner in track
- Joyce Chen, chef
- Louis Feraud, fashion designer

Sources: Adapted from Famous People Who Have and Had Dementia http://www.disabled-world.com/artman/publish/famous-dementia.shtml *and* About Alzheimer's, Famous People with Alzheimer's http://alzheimers.about.com/od/familyandfriends/a/alz_celebs.htm

Photo courtesy of Corbis Images.

Treatment for DAT

The available treatment choices for a person with DAT include pharmacologic interventions. Chapter 7∞ discusses the science of psychopharmacology, Chapter 31∞ addresses the medication treatment issues, and this discussion explains how the brain chemistry affects what symptoms you see in those with DAT. The target symptoms are agitation, aggression, psychosis, and to a lesser extent, memory. Two main groups of medications used in DAT are acetylcholinesterase inhibitors, or cholinesterase inhibitors, and a glutamate pathway modifier. At this time these medications slow progression of the symptoms but do not treat the disease. The important neurotransmitters altered by the disease, and attempted to be corrected by these medications, are acetylcholine and glutamate.

Acetylcholine is useful in storing and retrieving memories. People with DAT need all the help possible in storing and retrieving memory, so working on increasing the amount of acetylcholine helps memory. The enzyme that breaks down the acetylcholine—acetylcholinesterase—is inhibited when an acetylcholinesterase inhibitor is used. The result is a slight increase in the amount of acetylcholine in the brain. This has the chance to improve memory.

Glutamate is a primary excitatory neurotransmitter in the brain and glutamate receptor activity is associated with information processing, storage, and retrieval. There is a glutamate excitotoxicity hypothesis to DAT in that too much glutamate causes an overexcitation that can lead to toxic effects. We see the overexcitation when the client cannot figure out a simple task, do a series of steps to a process such as dressing or hygiene, and has memory difficulties. When the pathway is modified, the client has less toxic effects and can function more competently.

Dementia With Lewy Bodies

Dementia With Lewy bodies (DLB) is the second most common late-onset dementia after DAT, accounting for 15% to 20% of the neurodegenerative dementias. The name of this dementia subtype comes from the pathologic feature of Lewy body inclusions. Lewy bodies are abnormal concentrations of protein that develop inside nerve cells and appear as masses that displace other cell components and their function.

DLB research identifies a distinct presentation of the dementia with parkinsonism (symptoms that resemble Parkinson's disease resulting from effects on the extrapyramidal tracts of the CNS), fluctuating confusion, disturbances of consciousness, falls, and psychiatric symptoms (Higashi et al., 2011).

One of the main concerns regarding DLB is making the diagnosis before pharmacologic treatment is initiated. This is important because people who have DLB are unusually sensitive to many antipsychotic medications given for dementia and can have a severe and even fatal sensitivity to the extrapyramidal side effects. These clients are at much higher risk of developing side effects such as tardive dyskinesia or neuroleptic malignant syndrome in response to traditional antipsychotics (such as haloperidol). Although the newer atypical

antipsychotic agents are generally less likely to provoke side effects in clients overall, DLB clients can be at unacceptably high risk. Quetiapine (Seroquel), however, is an atypical antipsychotic that has a relatively low risk of provoking these side effects and clients with DLB are often better able to tolerate quetiapine than other antipsychotics.

The three core diagnostic features of DLB were defined by McKeith et al. (1996):

1. Spontaneous parkinsonism or extrapyramidal signs
2. Persistent or recurrent visual hallucinations
3. Fluctuating cognition

Clients who have only DLB are much less common than those who have a concomitant DAT. Neuropathologic studies have found that 20% to 30% of older adult clients with degenerative dementia have an overlap of both DAT and DLB. It is also difficult to differentiate DLB that is comorbid with DAT as a unique clinical syndrome from DAT alone. It is challenging to distinguish these clients from those with a Parkinson's disease (PD)–DAT blended syndrome.

An action tremor may precede other parkinsonian features, and dementia is often heralded by myoclonus and hallucinations, and if the client is treated with levadopa you may notice levodopa-induced sedation. Early on, the response to treatment with levodopa can be substantial, making it difficult to differentiate DLB from Parkinson's disease (Murray, 2011). The progression of symptoms of DLB appears to be intermediate, as compared with the progression of symptoms in the PD and PD–DAT subgroups.

In addition to parkinsonian features, dementia, and a frequent tendency to episodic delirium, the syndrome may be clinically indistinguishable from DAT. On autopsy, there will be diffuse involvement of cortical neurons with Lewy body inclusions and an absence of, or inconspicuous number of, neurofibrillary tangles and senile plaques.

Vascular Dementia

Vascular dementia, also known as *ischemic vascular dementia* (IVD) and formerly known in DSM-IV as *multi-infarct dementia,* accounts for about 19% of the dementias. Unlike Alzheimer's disease, vascular dementia is abrupt in onset and episodic, with multiple remissions. The client also demonstrates focal neurologic signs, such as one-sided weakness, emotional outbursts, and a stepwise—rather than progressive—decline in intellectual functioning, and has a history of hypertension, diabetes, or cardiovascular disease affecting other organs.

In vascular dementia, the brain tissue is destroyed by intermittent emboli that can range from a few to over a dozen. Individual infarcts may vary by 1 cm in diameter. Symptoms are commonly absent until 100 to 200 cc of brain tissue have been destroyed.

Parkinson's Disease (PD)

The association between **Parkinson's disease** (PD) and dementia has deepened over the years. A minority of clients with dementia have PD. A subset of clients has both PD and DAT, and this diagnosis may be difficult to determine. There are several varieties of PD, and the cause of classic PD is unknown. Another type, postencephalitic, has been linked to previous viral infection in the brain.

Huntington's Disease

Huntington's disease is a genetic, progressive, degenerative disorder characterized by both motor and cognitive changes, chorea, and dementia. This disease, one of the more frequently observed types of hereditary nervous system diseases, usually begins between the ages of 40 and 50. By the time of diagnosis, the client has usually reproduced, passing this inherited disease to another generation. The movement disorder is thought to be caused by vulnerability to damage and subsequent loss of nerve cells in the brain.

Movement abnormalities slowly increase, ultimately involving all muscle groups. The motor dysfunction is characterized by *chorea*: quick, jerky, purposeless, involuntary movements. The average life span after an initial diagnosis is 15 years. Mood disturbances, particularly depression, are common early in the disease, followed by deterioration of cognitive function.

Supplementing with coenzyme Q10 (CoQ10 or ubiquinone) has been known to replace deficient levels of the enzyme in muscle and decrease cerebellar-based ataxia. The enzyme could have an impact by slowing the disease's progression. Interestingly, CoQ10 has been tolerated very well while other treatments have been associated with several adverse effects (Bank, Kagan, & Madhavi, 2011). Rigorous research is required to explore this issue further. Associated concerns are the cost (from $60 to $150 per month) and the fact that as a nutritional supplement, CoQ10 may not have the quality and control guarantees of a pharmaceutical-grade product. CoQ10 cannot be taken by people who have diabetes or any platelet disorder.

Pick's Disease

Pick's disease is a rare disorder in which cerebral atrophy is present in the frontal and/or temporal lobes. These circumscribed pathologic changes are different from DAT, where the atrophy is mild and diffuse. The two patterns of behavior evident in Pick's disease represent the temporal and frontal types of the disease. People with the temporal type are talkative, lighthearted, joyous, anxious, and hyperattentive. People with the frontal type are locked into inertia, emotional dullness, and lack of initiative. As the disease progresses, the deterioration becomes more global, affecting memory and language. There is profound atrophy of the frontal and/or temporal lobes. Pick's disease worsens rapidly.

Clinical Example

Marlene was a respected member of the faculty at a large state university. Three years after she first stated her concern about forgetting things—where she put her keys, frequently used phone numbers, the occasional word to describe an object or person—she became a resident in a skilled nursing facility. Marlene became unable to feed or bathe herself or to recognize friends and family.

The expected life span after the original diagnosis is 7 years. A higher incidence is seen in some families, suggesting a genetic predisposition. Because language is affected, you will be charged with attending to the behavioral messages of clients with Pick's disease.

Creutzfeldt–Jakob Disease (CJD)

Creutzfeldt–Jakob disease is an infectious, transmissible degenerative dementia affecting the cerebral cortex through cell destruction and overgrowth. It is marked clinically by a very rapid onset and involuntary movements. This profound dementia is evidenced by cerebellar ataxia, diffuse myoclonic jerks, and other visual and neurologic abnormalities. There are distinctive electroencephalographic changes with this disease. The infection is presumed to be caused by a *prion*, a small protein particle that is resistant to treatment and sterilization procedures. There may be a genetic susceptibility to infection; however, the only definitive spreading mechanism is iatrogenic as seen after corneal transplantation and after the injection of human growth hormone derived from the pituitary gland of cadavers with the disease. Elevated levels of brain-derived proteins are detected on lumbar puncture. Levels in the cerebrospinal fluid (CSF) may increase over time; therefore, repeated testing—even when the first test is negative—may be diagnostic.

New Variant Creutzfeldt–Jakob Disease (nvCJD)

Once the disease known as mad cow disease (bovine spongiform encephalopathy [BSE]) became widespread, an unusual presentation of Creutzfeldt–Jakob disease was noted and since 1996 has been identified as **new variant Creutzfeldt–Jakob disease (nvCJD)**. It appears to be caused by the same agent as BSE, although it is unclear how transmission to humans takes place. There is no blood or tissue test for nvCJD. Studies show that nvCJD can be transmitted through blood transfusions. There is evidence suggesting that nvCJD is linked to eating contaminated beef. Usually, CJD occurs in older clients and begins as dementia. This new variation can occur in younger clients and includes unusual spongiform changes in the cerebellum. nvCJD is currently more of a problem in Europe than in North America due to varying health codes and standards.

Binswanger's Disease (BD)

Binswanger's disease (BD) is a subcortical vascular dementia caused by widespread, microscopic areas of damage to the deep layers of the brain's white matter. As the arteries become more and more narrowed by atherosclerosis, less blood is supplied, and the subcortical areas of the brain are not properly nourished and cannot survive. Changes in the person's behavior may be sudden or gradual and then progress. BD often coexists with DAT.

All the behaviors and treatments that slow the progression of disease processes such as high blood pressure, diabetes, and atherosclerosis can lower the likelihood of developing BD. However, there is no specific cure for BD. Consistent use of the proper medication as well as eating a healthy diet and keeping appropriate activity and rest cycles, and not smoking or drinking too much alcohol can also slow the progression of Binswanger's disease.

Pseudodementia

Affective disorders, particularly depression, can be masked by symptoms suggestive of dementia. Clinical symptoms may include impaired attention and memory, apathy, self-neglect, and without complaints of depression. The term **pseudodementia** has been used to describe the reversible cognitive impairments seen in depression. It is essential to detect pseudodementia in clients because, with appropriate treatment, they can recover. Pseudodementia should be suspected when the onset is abrupt, the clinical course is rapid, and the client complains about cognitive failures. Clients with dementia often fail to perceive, or attempt to cover up, their deficits. Evidence of these deficits can be seen, such as in the clinical example that follows.

Clinical Example

Ms. Salerno, a 57-year-old woman, was having problems selecting the words she wanted to use and putting her thoughts on paper. She began to miss appointments and her scheduled workdays, and she could no longer handle her daily responsibilities.

Mr. Jorgensen, a 45-year-old man, was in the hospital. He would forget what day it was and whether or not his family had visited. Occasionally he had visual hallucinations and on one occasion seemed to think he was at summer camp. He was quite upset about these changes in "who I am."

Medical Conditions Affecting Cognition

Studies suggest that physiologically-based clinical neuropsychiatric manifestations or disorders are common among adult persons with AIDS (Gannon, Khan, & Kolson, 2011). A neurologic syndrome or neurocognitive impairment may be the first clinical manifestation of HIV disease. Neurocognitive changes associated with HIV consist of cognitive, behavior, and motor dysfunction. Significant numbers of people with HIV experience neuropsychiatric manifestations for two major reasons:

1. Because the virus is capable of invading CNS tissue, several of the opportunistic infections and neoplasms associated with AIDS also affect the CNS.
2. Prescribed pharmacologic treatment may have neuropsychiatric side effects.

In addition to neurocognitive changes, more ominous changes—delirium, dementia, and coma—can occur.

Focal Brain Processes

The most common focal brain processes are toxoplasmosis (a parasitic opportunistic infection), cryptococcal meningitis (a fungal opportunistic infection), cytomegalovirus (CMV) encephalitis (a viral opportunistic infection), progressive multifocal leukoencephalopathy (PML, a viral opportunistic infection), and CNS lymphoma (a neoplastic process). Signs and symptoms associated with these processes include focal deficits, altered level of consciousness, confusion, memory disturbances, headaches, and seizures.

Medication Side Effects

Several antiretroviral medications and medications used to treat associated symptoms and opportunistic infections cause significant neuropsychiatric side effects. For example, acyclovir, isoniazid, pentamidine, thiabendazole, vincristine, and zidovudine may cause hallucinations. Sleep disturbances—including insomnia, vivid dreams, and nightmares—can be a side effect of most of the medications listed earlier, as well as amphotericin B, cotrimoxazole, didanosine (ddI), interferon, procarbazine, stavudine (d4T), and steroids. Isoniazid can cause memory impairment. Several cause one or more of the following: agitation, anxiety, confusion, delirium, depression, headache, and irritability. Be sure to know which medications your clients receive in order to assess accurately the presence of neurologic and emotional signs and symptoms.

HIV-Associated Dementia

A syndrome caused by direct HIV infection of the CNS, **HIV-associated dementia (HAD)**, is rare—but the milder form, HIV-associated neurocognitive disorders (HAND), persists in this population. The positive impacts of antiretroviral therapy (ART) on neurocognitive functioning is the result of clients following their medication regimen precisely.

HAND pathogenesis includes the following:

- Persistent systemic and CNS inflammation
- Aging in the HIV-infected brain
- HIV subtype (clade) distribution
- Potential neurotoxicity of ART

HAD is characterized as a progressive dementia with the following signs and symptoms:

- Cognitive dysfunction: forgetfulness, loss of concentration, confusion, and slowness of thought
- Declining motor performance: loss of balance, muscle weakness, and deterioration in fine motor skills such as handwriting
- Behavioral changes: apathy, withdrawal, dysphoric mood, and regressed behavior
- Other symptoms such as headaches or seizures

HAD is often initially confused with psychiatric depression but may progress in a period of months to the point at which the affected individual is bedridden. Individuals with HAD may also quickly succumb to opportunistic infections because they are unable to take care of themselves.

AMNESTIC DISORDER

Amnestic disorder, a relatively uncommon cognitive disorder, is characterized by short- and long-term memory deficits, an inability to recall previously learned information or past events, an inability to learn new material, confabulation, apathy, and a bland affect. Impairment ranges from moderate to severe. Possible causes include head trauma, hypoxia, encephalitis, thiamine deficiency, and substance abuse. These causes shape the three main types of amnestic disorder, which are briefly described here: those due to (1) a medical condition, (2) a substance, or (3) other causes.

Traumatic brain injury (TBI) is an acquired brain injury and is frequently associated with amnesia. The cause of the trauma creates a connection between the general medical condition (which includes physical trauma), and the amnestic disorder when this type is diagnosed. The diagnosis of amnestic disorder is supported by the timing of the onset of amnesia (the amnesia is coordinated with physical trauma), an atypical presentation of a memory problem, and the ruling out of other explanations for the disorder. The emotional and behavioral sequelae of a TBI need explicit and intense team efforts for successful treatment (Doering & Exner, 2011).

Substance-induced amnesia persists beyond the immediate effects of the substance and the duration of intoxication or withdrawal from the substance. Deficits can worsen over the years despite abstinence from the substance.

Amnestic disorder not otherwise specified (NOS) is the diagnosis used when the criteria are not met for the two other types described earlier, or when there is not enough supporting evidence to link a cause to the amnesia.

BIOPSYCHOSOCIAL THEORIES

Theories about the causes of cognitive disorders are as varied as the disorders themselves. Genetics, infection, and vascular insufficiency are all believed to be causative factors. Because delirium is usually caused by an underlying systemic illness, a prompt search is essential for treatable conditions such as dehydration, diabetes, hyponatremia, hypercalcemia, thyroid crisis, infection, silent myocardial infarction, drug intoxication, or liver or renal failure (Voyer et al., 2011). If the cause is removed quickly, complete recovery from delirium can be achieved.

The actual cause of DAT remains unknown, but several factors are believed to play a role. DAT has been correlated with the loss of specific groups of nerve cells and the disruption of communication between nerve cells from acetylcholine and serotonin deficits. Researchers are working to identify a

slow-acting, virus-like causative agent. This work has been prompted by the findings of just such an agent in CJD.

To date, advanced age, family history of the illness, Down's syndrome, and a history of head trauma are risk factors for DAT. There are linkages between genetic markers and DAT on a number of chromosomes—namely, chromosomes 1, 14, and 21, and one or both alleles coding for the e4 variant of apolipoprotein on chromosome 19 (referred to as APOE e4). People with DAT have four times the family incidence of dementia. Yet in identical and fraternal twins, in only 40% of cases do both get DAT, suggesting that DAT cannot be due to a single autosomal dominant gene. The disease also appears in twins and in various family members at different times, making it difficult to interpret the markers found in genetic studies.

Other possible risk factors are environmental toxins, stroke, thyroid disorder, lower educational status, and female gender (Alzheimer's Association, 2011). Ongoing research focuses on causes and medication treatment that can either protect or restore neurons, thereby combating memory loss. Additional medication studies focus on ameliorating behavioral symptoms. Vitamin B_{12} deficiency in DAT is explained in Caring for the Spirit.

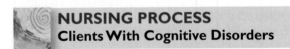

NURSING PROCESS
Clients With Cognitive Disorders

The nursing process with all cognitive disorders revolves around the principles of care used in dementia.

Assessment

Your skills in assessing clients with these disorders are important for developing and delivering competent client care. Use this information in each subsequent step of the nursing process.

Subjective Data

It is often difficult to gather data about clients with delirium, dementia, amnestic disorder, and other cognitive disorders.

CARING FOR THE SPIRIT

Vitamin B_{12} Deficiency

There are numerous dementia-related metabolic dysfunctions such as the imperfect metabolism of vitamin B_{12}. DAT interferes with vitamin B_{12} metabolism. We now know that vitamin B_{12} deficiency is one way in which DAT affects the body.

People who have the variation of the apolipoprotein-E gene (abbreviated as APOE), variation e4, are at increased risk for developing late-onset DAT. Continuing research shows us that people who have the APOE e4 gene are much more likely to be dysfunctional metabolizers of vitamin B_{12}. When a person is deficient in vitamin B_{12} there are numerous behavioral disturbances such as bizarre behaviors and psychotic symptoms, as well as alterations in circadian rhythm patterns and

mood disorders. These problems are slightly more frequent in people who have the APOE e4 variation of the gene.

Vitamin B_{12} depletion can occur outside the occurrence of DAT. It is common among older adults because of age-induced changes in the gastrointestinal tract. A lack of vitamin B_{12} causes anemia, and in time anemia is accompanied by neurologic signs and symptoms, including diminished vibration and position senses and dementia.

Being up to date on information about whole-body effects of DAT such as metabolic dysfunction can prevent a great deal of misery and spiritual distress among older adult clients. Change the stress level for your clients and their families by attending to the spiritual value of food and nutrition.

They are sometimes anxious, defensive, and confused, and give unreliable histories. Often, there is no dependable secondary source of information. To maximize your efforts, gather all data in a setting that is free from distraction and discomfort:

- Decibel levels of ambient (surrounding) noise must be low.
- Light should be sufficient to dispel shadows.
- Room temperature should be comfortable for the client.

When you ask questions, pace the questions slowly to allow the client time to answer comfortably. Aging people can normally process information after receiving it but may have difficulty taking in information. Placing the client in a situation that interferes with an already compromised sensory apparatus only heightens the client's anxiety and seriously compromises your attempts to evaluate.

Health History When completing the client's health history, include all past and present medical conditions, paying special attention to chronic conditions for which the client is being treated and any recent changes in health status. Ask the client: "Are you seeing a health care provider at this time?" "Why did you seek medical help?" "What does your health care provider say is the problem?" Infections may present as confusion and other symptoms of dementia before any change in temperature, pulse, and respirations is noted.

Sensory Impairment Older adults are particularly sensitive to the confusion associated with sensory deprivation. Physiological changes in their sensory apparatus may be directly related to aging or to pathologic processes. Both diminish sensory receptive ability. The changes in sensory apparatus, however, are not clear cut. The older adult may have difficulty hearing high-frequency sounds, such as consonants. Turning up the volume on the radio may help the person hear one range of sounds but may also cause sensory overload because the rest of the sounds are too loud. The overall result is deprivation and distortion.

Try to ascertain any possible sensory problems, especially in hearing and vision. To test hearing, stand so that the client cannot see your face, and ask a question in a normal tone of voice. The question should require more than a yes or no answer. Test vision with pictures that the client will easily recognize. See Chapter 10 ∞ on communicating with a hearing-impaired person.

Dietary History When possible, obtain an estimate of the client's food intake. "What do you usually eat for breakfast? Lunch? Dinner?" Make special note of protein and vitamin intake. Avitaminosis, pellagra, anemia, and hypoglycemia have all been associated with reversible brain syndromes. Hydration is also an important factor, easily noted in the client's physical state (adequate hydration is indicated by a saliva pool below the tongue). Dehydration can also cause confusion. Anticholinergic side effects from any number of typically prescribed medications and over-the-counter (OTC) drugs can cause dehydration and confusion.

Head Trauma Falls are common among older adults. Misjudging distances and not being aware of obstructions also contribute to injuries. Cerebral contusions, midbrain hemorrhage, and subdural hematoma may result from a fall. Confusion may be the result of any of these conditions.

Medication Older adults are prone to adverse drug reactions as a result of age-related bodily changes. These factors are compounded by high consumption of many different medications: More than one third of all drugs are consumed by the 15% of the population who are older clients. Older adults are particularly susceptible to medications with anticholinergic properties (major tranquilizers, antidepressants, barbiturates, adrenal steroids, atropine, antiparkinsonians, antihistamines, antihypertensives, and diuretics). Question the client about both prescription and over-the-counter medications: "Are you now taking any medicines that your doctor prescribed?" "Do you take laxatives, cold pills, or other medicines that you buy at your drugstore without a prescription?" "Have you tried some of the health foods, herbs, supplements, or remedies they have at some of these stores?"

Alcohol Consumption Ask the client about alcohol consumption. Beyond being another source of dehydration, alcohol is a CNS depressant, and intoxication may mimic symptoms of cognitive disorders. Alcohol also compromises nutritional status and may cause withdrawal effects. Ask questions such as "What is your favorite drink?" "How much alcohol do you drink in one day/week?" and "Have you ever had periods of not remembering after you have been drinking?" Beer, wine coolers, and hard lemonade are sold in grocery stores with advertising and packaging that may be perceived as nonalcoholic or not "counting" as alcohol consumption. You could ask questions about these substances separately from alcohol consumption questions, possibly when discussing diet and eating habits.

Family History The families of impaired older adults can be a major source of information and support. In the United States, the majority of older adults have seen one or more relatives the previous week, and many live within 30 minutes of their nearest child. Common living arrangements include living with a spouse, child, or sibling. Family assessment should include the following:

- Living arrangements
- Care arrangements for the client (e.g., shopping assistance, daily visits, telephone calls)
- Family knowledge of the current illness
- Family expectations for the future
- Special family concerns about client care
- Family style of coping with stress (e.g., death of a relative, illness)
- The identified spokesperson for the family
- The family's perception of the client's coping abilities

Throughout the interview, note the interactions between family members and the client. Do family members support the client and respect what the client says? Do people listen to one another? What is the atmosphere in the family group? What is the level of intimacy between family members? Do they relate to each other with warmth and affection? Chapter 29 ∞ includes an expanded family assessment.

Activities of Daily Living Assess the client carefully for level of self-care. This is often called a *functional assessment*. What activities of daily living can the client do without help? For which activities is help required? What type of help is needed? As cognitive deficits increase, the client becomes more dependent on others for assistance. For a study about the ADL needs of clients with DAT, see Evidence-Based Practice.

Community Functioning The Comprehensive Functional Assessment (CFA) tool measures the ability to sustain oneself in the community. It covers the basic skills of living, working, relating to others, and recreating in community settings. Assess not only the ability to live independently in the community but also the degree of social involvement. Does the client belong to any clubs or groups? Do friends visit the client at home? Does the client belong to a particular church or temple? Ask about attendance at senior citizen programs and the level of participation in activities involving others.

Objective Data Evaluating older adults with mental impairment is usually organized into three areas: physical assessment, laboratory assessment, and imaging techniques.

Physical Assessment A thorough assessment, including a complete neurologic exam (evaluation of cranial nerves, motor and sensory systems, and reflexes) and a psychiatric consultation for possible psychiatric illness, is important for all older adults with mental impairment. Because older adults with organic illness frequently manifest confusion and depression, clinicians work from the assumption that reversible illness is present. Chest X-ray films and an electrocardiogram are taken.

Laboratory Assessment The following tests are routinely ordered for older clients:

- Complete blood count, including folic acid and vitamin B_{12} levels to detect anemia
- Erythrocyte sedimentation rate (ESR) to detect infection
- SMA (sequential multiple analyzer) to detect electrolyte imbalances
- Syphilis tests (Venereal Disease Research Laboratory [VDRL])
- Thyroid function studies
- Serum levels of barbiturates, bromides, and digitalis
- Liver function studies
- Human immunodeficiency virus (HIV)
- Serology
- Heavy metals
- Toxicology
- Urinalysis

Imaging Techniques Views of the brain's structure and function can be provided through a computed axial tomographic brain scan (CAT scan) or computed tomographic brain scan (CT scan), positron emission tomography (PET), and single-photon emission computed tomography (SPECT). FIGURE 14-3■ presents PET scan images of a normal brain and the brain of an individual with DAT. These tests can be ordered for clients at high risk, that is, those having acute deterioration in cognitive functioning of recent onset. Acute deterioration is often associated with focal lesions and hydrocephalus.

EVIDENCE-BASED PRACTICE

Developing a Sensitive and Humane Bathing Protocol for a Cognitively Impaired Client

You are a nurse in a treatment setting that combines long-term community care and short-term respite care. Abe, a 76-year-old client with dementia who owned his own business for years, is being treated at the long-term care section of the center. His daughter Esther is his caregiver and has been involved in both her father's care and in some program development at the clinic. Bathing has become an issue with Abe—it seems to frighten and embarrass him. Discussions with his daughter revealed this to be a new problem.

The first difficulty arose when staff members entered Abe's room with bathing equipment and announced it was time to wash up. This time, what had been a usual routine was not received well. Abe grabbed a female staff member and murmured that there was no way she was going to see what he needed to keep private, nor could she squeeze the life out of him with "that stuff." Calm explanations of the staff's intentions did not dissuade Abe. He was determined not to allow bathing.

Abe needs to exercise some control over the situation, and understand that bathing routines can be designed to be pleasant and comfortable for him. Letting Abe have a say in when he bathes ("Not now" is an acceptable response) and what gets cleaned (wash his hair first, last, or not at all) has immediate positive results. Keep in mind that older skin can be dry, bathing can cause further drying (soybean oil–based no-rinse cleansers promote healthier skin), and arthritis and other conditions make movement painful. This also helps make bathing more pleasant, more comfortable, and safer. Embarrassment can be alleviated if Abe is washed under a bath blanket or a towel of sufficient size to adequately cover him.

The interventions for Abe are based on the following research:

Gallagher, M., & Long, C. O. (2011). Advanced dementia care: Demystifying behaviors, addressing pain, and maximizing comfort: Research and practice: Partners in care. *Journal of Hospice & Palliative Nursing, 13*(2), 70–78.

Sheu, E., Versloot, J., Nader, R., Kerr, D., & Craig, K. D. (2011). Pain in the elderly: Validity of facial expression components of observational measures. *Clinical Journal of Pain.* Advance online publication. doi: 10.1097/AJP.0b013e31820f52e1

CRITICAL THINKING QUESTIONS

1. What are the physical and emotional benefits to clients of altering a general routine to meet their specific needs?
2. Staff members derive benefits also. How can altering Abe's bathing routine help the staff?

(a)

(b)

PET/SPECT Dementia Animation

FIGURE 14-3 ■ PET scan brain images in dementia of the Alzheimer's type. Compare a normal brain scan (a) with the brain of a person with Alzheimer's disease (b). (a) The red and yellow areas indicate normal metabolic rates. (b) Note the blue areas indicating abnormally low metabolism in the parietal and temporal lobes. *Photo courtesy of* Dr. Robert Friedland/Photo Researchers, Inc.

A number of other diagnostic procedures may be used. Because of their intrusive nature or their cost, their use should be limited unless indicated. These are as follows:

- Lumbar puncture
- Skull X-ray films
- Electroencephalography (EEG)
- Magnetic resonance imaging (MRI)
- Cerebral angiography
- Isotope cisternography

The amygdala plays a key role in enhancing pleasant and unpleasant memories and it modulates our memory processes. Because the medial aspect of the amygdala is involved in DAT, some imaging such as an MRI could provide insights into behavioral and emotional changes in clients if the nature of the testing would not be problematic for the client (Cavedo et al., 2011).

Cognitive Functioning

Cognitive functioning includes memory, reasoning, abstraction, calculation ability, and judgment. Refer back to Box 14-1 on page 275 for detailed information on cognitive functioning during the various stages of DAT. Clients will not respond effectively unless they feel that the information requested is relevant, they see some purpose in the interview, and they are interested in the material. Choose testing materials carefully, and keep the client's endurance in mind at all times. When assessing cognitive functioning, pay particular attention to the following clinical manifestations.

Appearance Clients who appear disheveled, dirty, or unkempt may be experiencing problems with poor memory or a shortened attention span. This diminished ability to perform self-care may not be apparent if the client has a caregiver who helps with grooming.

Manner and Attitude Some clients may exaggerate mannerisms to compensate for a perceived decline in functioning. For example, clients who have compulsive tendencies may become more set in their ways. An attitude of defensiveness, withdrawal, or paranoia may be a response to increasing anxiety about diminished abilities.

Communication Assess communication in the areas of speech, gestures, facial expression, and writing. Difficulty in finding words and naming objects may suggest **expressive aphasia**. Difficulty grasping complex concepts may suggest **receptive aphasia**. Assess the client's ability to use gestures and facial expressions to compensate for verbal aphasia. Not using facial expressions and gestures and speaking in a monotone may indicate depression. Also test the client's written communication and reading ability and assess language ability. Older individuals whose primary language is not English may revert to their native language; therefore, make arrangements for a translator/translation service.

Perception Perception is the client's ability to recognize and integrate sensory information, including the conscious recognition of oneself in relation to the environment. Clients with asymmetric brain involvement of DAT may neglect one side of their body. These clients may also have difficulty recognizing objects (agnosia). Clients with perceptual difficulty may distort sensory information, with resulting hallucinations and delusions.

Attention and Wakefulness Attention refers to alertness and the ability to attend selectively to stimuli and to direct one's focus. Can the client sustain or pay attention to the interview process, or is he or she easily distracted by the environment? You can assess attention by asking the client to spell a word backwards. Wakeful states range from hyperalertness to stupor. Stupor can be the result of medication intoxication or an acute systemic disease.

Motor Activity Lethargy is often a symptom of depression, but it can also be the result of such medications as tranquilizers, antihypertensives, antidepressants, and antihistamines. Combinations of medications can also cause lethargy even when one of the medications alone may not be sedating. Lethargy can be caused by a number of disease processes, such as urinary tract infection, anemia, and meningitis. A shift between hypermotor and hypomotor activity is a sign of delirium. Agitation and physical striking out are occasionally demonstrated.

Mood and Affect Depression may accompany the earlier stages of dementia. The more serious the dementia, however, the less depressed the client. Clients with organic disease of the cerebral area are emotionally labile. Ask the client about any changes in eating or sleeping habits, and inquire about a recent loss of energy and interest in usual activities. If depression is suspected, evaluate the client for risk of suicide (see Chapter 23 ∞). Explore thoughts about dying, plans regarding self-harm, or self-neglect to the point of harm or death. Ask questions about suicide in a matter-of-fact manner, without hesitation, and record the findings carefully in your assessment notes.

Orientation Measure disorientation to time, place, and person in an environment where the client has easy access to the information. Days in a hospital are all the same to clients housed without calendars and seasonal cues. Acute disorientation in all spheres is commonly found in people having toxic states and traumatic brain disease. Disorientation to place and person usually indicates a degenerative disorder.

Memory People with dementias have difficulty acquiring recent memory or learning; this symptom may be a key to the early detection of dementia. At present, there is no set of tests that can adequately measure the memory capacity of clients with dementia. Most tests measure *episodic memory:* the processing and storage of information, like recalling the events of the day. This type of memory is impaired in most clients with cognitive disorders, depression, and drug or alcohol intoxication. *Semantic memory,* or knowledge memory, is the ability to synthesize and think about events. It is used in language, abstraction, and logical operations. People with DAT have difficulty with semantic memory; however, depressed clients do not.

Test episodic memory by asking the client to repeat a series of words or recall a recent event, such as a meal. Test semantic memory by asking the client to develop a scenario, such as describing the events from dinner until bedtime. Episodic memory is also tested in relation to time and is usually divided into three spheres: recent, remote, and past.

Abstract Reasoning Proverbs are the most common way of testing abstract reasoning. You might ask: "What does it mean when we say, 'People who live in glass houses shouldn't throw stones'?" or "What does 'A stitch in time saves nine' mean to you?" Clients with DAT often interpret these proverbs quite literally or concretely; for example, they may reply to your question about the latter proverb with a statement such as "If you sew a single stitch, you won't have to sew nine."

Calculation Ability The most common test of calculation ability is the serial sevens test: The person subtracts 7 from 100 and continues to subtract 7 from the answer. This is a difficult process for the client with dementia or delirium. The test measures the client's ability to concentrate and focus thought. It may also be a measure of educational level.

Judgment The test for judgment should predict whether a person will behave in a socially accepted manner, including the planning and carrying out of activities that require the client to discriminate reality from unrealistic situations. You might ask the client, "If you needed help during the night, how would you get it?" or "If you lost your wallet while doing errands, what would you do?"

Nursing Diagnoses: NANDA

A discussion of several nursing diagnoses common to clients with cognitive disorders follows.

Impaired Physical Mobility

Gait changes due to neurologic involvement are seen in people with a number of the dementias. These include DAT, Huntington's disease, Parkinson's disease, and Creutzfeldt–Jakob disease. Restlessness in the client with delirium is reflected in hyperactive behavior. The client usually alternates between hyperactivity and hypoactivity.

Self-Care Deficit: Bathing/Hygiene, Dressing/Grooming, Feeding, Toileting

Clients with delirium are unable to perceive, organize, or carry out the activities of daily living (e.g., bathing/hygiene, dressing/grooming, feeding, toileting). They are far too distracted by stimuli and unable to focus. The DAT client has a distinct problem: apraxia, the loss of ability to perform formerly known skills. In the late stages of all the dementias, total care is a necessity as the client moves toward brain failure.

Readiness for Enhanced Sleep

Also called *sundowner syndrome,* **sundowning** is commonly understood as confused behavior when environmental stimulation is low. It can be seen in clients with delirium and dementia. The client catnaps during the day and wanders at night. Poor sensory processing can also occur in clients who wander at night. The client with DAT may not sleep for several days, moving about in a confused state. The client becomes increasingly agitated, disoriented, or even aggressive/paranoid or impulsive and emotional later in the day and at night.

Disturbed Thought Processes

Altered thought processes can occur as a variety of experiences. Clients behave differently depending on their ability to think as a result of these alterations.

Agnosia Agnosia, the failure to recognize familiar objects, is a progressive problem that eventually renders the person unable to recognize or remember loved ones. Overall, in both delirium and dementia, the client's ability to use information in making judgments may be seriously impaired.

Memory Episodic short-term memory is affected by delirium, dementia, and mood disorders. Long-term memory is diminished in the later stages of DAT and acute delirium. See FIGURE 14-4 ■ for a diagram of how short-term and long-term memory is established.

Orientation Disorientation is seen in clients with both dementia and delirium. In the former, it is related to progressive cerebral changes; in the latter, to an acute, usually identifiable, causal agent.

FIGURE 14-4 ■ The path to short-term memory, whether short-term memory is created, and the conversion of short-term to long-term memory.

Impaired Verbal Communication

Confabulation is a common defense used by clients who cannot remember required information and therefore use fantasy to fill in the memory gaps. Confusion and paranoid ideation require that you interact with the client in a nonthreatening manner. Rx Communication: Client With Dementia describes interactions with this in mind.

Aphasia, both receptive and expressive, is one of the hallmarks of DAT. In the late stage of the illness, the client is completely mute. When this occurs, your observations are vital to assess discomfort and pain. The scales providing descriptors that correspond to how people actually display facial expressions of pain are effective at differentiating intensities of pain (Sheu, Versloot, Nader, Kerr, & Craig, 2011).

Risk for Self-Directed Violence and Risk for Other-Directed Violence

In clients with DAT and most of the other dementias, there is a gradual decline in the social acceptability of their behavior. Overstating distress and making threats are common, especially if this was the mode of coping when the client was more intact. See Rx Communication: Client With Dementia

at Risk for Self-Harm for an example of an interaction with a client making threats. High risk for violence is linked with impulsivity and unpredictability in these clients (see also Chapter 35∞). The client may also strike out at others while hallucinating or in a hyperactive phase. These behaviors are also seen in delirious clients, who are similarly unpredictable.

Ineffective Role Performance

As a result of decreasing intellectual competence, the client with dementia moves from the role of spouse, parent, employee, and community member to that of a dependent, regressed family member. The role loss and role change are anxiety provoking and at times overwhelming for the client and family. Characteristically, the family members experience a period of acute grief after receiving the diagnosis. Assess their level of depression. Feelings of isolation and being overwhelmed are also common.

Disturbed Sensory Perception

The inability to attend and focus concentration is a hallmark of delirium. Decreased attention is also seen in the later

---

R_X RX COMMUNICATION

Client With Dementia

CLIENT: "What are you doing here?"

NURSE RESPONSE 1: "Hello, my name is Betty and I would like to talk to you."	**NURSE RESPONSE 2:** "I'd like to talk with you. Can you tell me if anything is hurting you?"
RATIONALE: This response helps you make contact with the client, establish what you are going to do to allay fears, and give an opportunity to interact in a nonthreatening manner.	*RATIONALE:* Many clients find it easier to talk about physical pain than to articulate complex notions such as feelings and desires.

RX COMMUNICATION

Client With Dementia at Risk for Self-Harm

CLIENT: "I'm going to walk outside and get hit by a truck."

NURSE RESPONSE 1: "Tell me about why you are so upset."	**NURSE RESPONSE 2:** "Let's take a walk together."
RATIONALE: Client ventilates feelings in more constructive ways when discussing feeling states with the nurse.	*RATIONALE:* Client has the opportunity to use physical energy constructively by being distracted with empathic and supportive social interaction.

stages of the dementias when the client loses the ability to encode. Delirium alters perception by reducing the client's ability to distinguish and integrate sensory information. As a result, the client has difficulty discriminating reality from hallucinations, dreams, illusions, and imagery. In the later stages of dementia, clients also experience hallucinations and delusions, which complicate delivery of care. The client is prone to hallucinations and delusions as a result of a reduced ability to distinguish and integrate sensory information. Rx Communication: Client With Dementia and Hallucinations shows an interaction with a client who experiences hallucinations.

Risk for Situational Low Self-Esteem

During the first stage of DAT and other dementias, the client is acutely aware of cognitive failure. This awareness and the resulting anxiety can be damaging to the self-esteem of a person living in a culture that does not tolerate or provide for dependence.

Functional Urinary Incontinence, Bowel Incontinence

Incontinence of urine or feces is usually the result of confusion and difficulty finding or using the bathroom facilities. In the later stages of dementia, clients lose cortical control, but physiological function remains. It is essential to ensure proper hygiene for clients; poor hygiene will result in infections and skin breakdown.

Imbalanced Nutrition, Less Than Body Requirements

Poor nutrition and some metabolic disorders can be the direct cause of confusion in older adult clients. The reverse can also be true; confusion and cerebral change can cause nutritional deficits. Without supervision, many older clients are not capable of preparing or ingesting adequate amounts of food.

Clients who are in the later stages of DAT have symptoms of bulimia followed by total loss of appetite.

Outcome Identification: NOC

Clients with these disorders have varying outcomes; delirium in many cases is reversible, while dementia is not. Specific outcomes for clients experiencing cognitive disorders are listed in the nursing care plans. Clients' abilities to return to their previous lifestyles remain somewhat intact when disorders are reversible. However, in the deterioration of dementing conditions, carefully scrutinize the expectations for outcomes. Family members and the client must have information about the illness and how it will change lifestyle. Maximizing the quality of life can be an outcome for clients who have dementia.

Planning and Implementation: NIC

Nursing interventions for clients with cognitive disorders can be divided into two broad groups: interventions for (1) clients with dementia and (2) clients with delirium. A sample nursing care plan for a client with delirium is presented at the end of this chapter. A case study for a DAT client can be accessed on the Online Student Resources for this text.

With few exceptions, the interventions are similar, although the overall goals are different as noted earlier in the Outcome Identification. The goal with the dementia client is to minimize the loss of self-care capacity. Although functional loss is progressive, at every stage of the illness you must assess and support the client's self-care capacity. Family members must also learn how to work with the client. See Partnering With Clients and Families for suggestions for families. With delirious clients, the overall goal for nursing intervention is to support existing sensory perception until their cognitive function can return to previous levels of

Case Study: Needs of the Client With DAT

RX COMMUNICATION

Client With Dementia and Hallucinations

CLIENT: "Get those women out of here!"

NURSE RESPONSE 1: "Come with me. We'll go down the hall."	**NURSE RESPONSE 2:** "You must be very nervous. Let's get you something to help you feel better."
RATIONALE: Distracting the client from the internal stimuli, which may be transient, calms and addresses the emotional component of the client's experience.	*RATIONALE:* Client may need interventions (nonpharmacologic or pharmacologic) to control breakthrough symptomatology.

PARTNERING WITH CLIENTS AND FAMILIES

Suggestions for Families Who Have Just Had a Family Member Diagnosed With DAT

- Have a family meeting and discuss strategies to care for the client at the present time and in the future, based on family responsibilities and resources.
- Contact the Alzheimer's Disease and Related Disorders Association (ADRDA) and request information. View their videotapes and read the available written material.
- Go to a support group for family caregivers.
- Contact an attorney and make decisions about power of attorney and the control and distribution of client/family assets.

- Consider developing a psychiatric advance directive (discussed in Chapter 12∞).
- Familiarize yourself with community resources such as day care treatment centers, nursing homes for your family member with DAT, and respite care for the caregivers.
- Purchase a bracelet for the client identifying her/him as having DAT.

functioning. Of course, in both conditions, keeping the client safe is the first priority.

Promoting Normal Motor Behavior

Because of impaired coordination in dementia, falls become a safety concern. Living areas must be well lit and furniture must remain in the same place. Remove any loose rugs and ensure that clients are wearing properly fitting shoes with a strap. Evaluate the client for visual and balance disturbances. Safety bars should be installed near toilets, showers, and tubs. Teach clients who need assistance the safe use of walkers and wheelchairs. Evaluate all clients using tranquilizers and antidepressants for postural hypotension. A difference in blood pressures (BPs) taken supine and standing, wherein the standing BP is lower than the supine BP, is an indication of postural hypotension. Restlessness and wandering can be dealt with by allowing the client to wander in a safe, enclosed environment. Avoid crowds or large open spaces without boundaries.

Hyperactivity in clients with delirium can be decreased by controlling environmental stimuli. If this does not help, medications can be used judiciously. Take vital signs 1 hour before and after the administration of any medication, and observe the client carefully for signs of stupor. Interrupt prolonged periods of hypoactivity with range-of-motion exercises, frequent turning, and having the client stand up at the bedside, as tolerated. During periods of fluctuating motor behavior, there is always concern for the client's safety. A staff member should be present at all times; keep the bed lowered and the side rails up. In DAT, wandering is a common and troublesome behavioral symptom. See Your Intervention Strategies for guidelines for working with the wandering client.

Maintaining Self-Care

Allow the client to do as much as possible unassisted. The more the client can effectively control the daily routine, the less anxiety the client will experience. Remind the client about daily grooming and personal hygiene, and repeat instructions. If the client resists oral hygiene, use mouth swabs with dilute hydrogen peroxide. If the client resists this as well, having the client eat an apple may help to clean the mouth. If the client resists any routine procedures, wait a few moments and try

YOUR INTERVENTION STRATEGIES
Guidelines for Working With the Wandering Client

Strategy	Rationale
■ Stay with the client, or be sure the client is in a safe, enclosed area.	■ Wandering clients can get hurt. Safety is the first priority.
■ Maintain a calm demeanor.	■ Clients notice the feelings of others.
■ Approach the client slowly and give her or him space. Use touch only if the client responds positively to it.	■ The aim is to prevent aggressiveness, fear, and anxiety. Each client is different in response to touch, and with specific people.
■ Determine why the client is wandering. Is she or he upset? Thirsty? Hungry? Searching for family?	■ When we understand why the client wanders, we can plan client-specific interventions.
■ Meet the client's needs. If the client is searching, be supportive: "You are looking for X. . . ." "You must miss X. . . ."	■ Support decreases anxiety, fear, and hostility.
■ Attempt to engage the client in a repetitive activity such as rolling yarn or folding towels.	■ Repetitive activities use energy and can be diversional.

again. The client often forgets to offer new resistance. Clients who are acutely delirious or in the last stages of dementia need total bed care.

Promoting Adequate Sleep

Clients with dementia and delirium respond poorly to hypnotics, which increase confusion and aggravate the disorientation that may be experienced in lowered light in older adults. A small amount of beer or wine at bedtime may produce enough relaxation without side effects. The most helpful measure may be to allow sleepless clients to wander in a confined area until they are tired. If the client is disoriented at night, make sure the room is light and without shadows. Possibly leave a radio on to provide more stimulation. Low doses of risperidone or an antianxiety agent may be prescribed. (Use antianxiety medications with caution and re-evaluate them regularly if used on a nightly basis.)

In some instances, it may be necessary to use mechanical restraints to protect the client from injury or prevent the client from disrupting necessary medical treatments (e.g., a delirious client repeatedly tries to bear weight on a damaged limb or attempts to remove IV tubing or bandages). Use mechanical restraints only as a last resort and according to established policy. Before using restraints, apply effective and imaginative alternatives. If restraints are deemed unavoidable, remember to evaluate their use and replace them with less restrictive alternatives. Reassure clients who have been restrained that they are safe and that the restraints are there to protect and help them. See Chapter 35∞ for guidelines in the use of restraining techniques.

Supporting Knowledge Processes

The same interventions that are used to support memory and orientation are applied to the support of knowledge processes. Family education is imperative and can take the form of professional help and/or self-help groups. For a listing of professional help and/or self-help groups, refer to the Online Student Resources.

Supporting Optimal Memory Functioning

Gently orient the client. To allay anxiety, do not argue with the client about verbal discrepancies. Rather, direct the client toward areas of interest that are familiar and pleasurable. The environment should support whatever memory functions are still intact. Do not test the client for episodic memory unless it is absolutely necessary. If the client uses confabulation to fill in the memory gap, do not argue; remember that it is an ego-protective mechanism. Other strength-enhancing behavioral and psychotherapeutic treatment reminders are summarized in Your Intervention Strategies.

Because of their episodic memory loss, DAT clients do not respond well to reality orientation classes. However, you can trigger semantic memory by initiating a procedure the client can then complete. In this leading technique, a combination of words and nonverbal cues are used. For instance, while handing the client a toothbrush and pointing toward the mouth with a brushing motion, say, "Brush your teeth." Constant repetition in a kind, firm manner is often necessary. See Your Self-Awareness to evaluate your skills in this area. Music therapy may also trigger past associations, aid the client's long-term memory, and help a normally aphasic client participate in a group.

Promoting Optimal Medication Management

Medication therapy has also been proposed to assist the client in the early stages of DAT to maintain memory and orientation (see Chapter 7∞). Galantamine (Reminyl), donepezil (Aricept), rivastigmine (Exelon), and tacrine (Cognex), all potent acetylcholinesterase inhibitors, are available to treat DAT. Clinical trials and treatment outcome information for these medications have resulted in both positive and negative results. The problems in demonstrating overall efficacy are believed to be due to the heterogeneity in DAT clients and the fact that these medications provide mild to moderate improvement.

YOUR INTERVENTION STRATEGIES   Guidelines for Supporting Optimal Memory Functioning

Behavioral and Psychotherapeutic Reminders

- Use calendars or other concrete reminders of what is going on by day of the week, date, and time.
- Use objects or wall hangings that mirror the current season or holiday events; pictures that reflect seasonal events and people's actions and behaviors around those events (remember to be culturally sensitive).
- Use a photo album and sign-in book for visitors to remind clients of who visited and when.
- If the client is very attached to a family member who visits, prominently display a large photo of that family member in the client's room.
- Discover a client's preferred hobbies and interests to add cues to the environment, which will be positively received (e.g., a team schedule for a sports fan).

Reminiscence

- Clients often need to talk, even repetitively, about important prior experiences, which encourages the process of resolving feelings about these experiences as well as the difficulties the client has in recalling them.

- Encourage discussion of likely social and historical contexts operative during earlier phases of the client's life (e.g., The Great Depression of the 1930s, World War II, and important events of the 1950s).

Adaptive Functioning and Cognitive Preservation

Careful evaluation of remaining cognitive strengths through the following:

- Observation
- Psychological testing
- Diagnostic interviewing

When areas of strength are diagnosed, do the following:

- Provide opportunities for the client to exercise them.
- Give positive reinforcements such as praise, a pleasant experience such as listening to music, or a caring interaction when the client is exercising his or her better preserved abilities.

When areas of deficit are diagnosed, do the following:

- Assist the client in coping with deficits (e.g., training and encouragement to use written reminders to compensate for failing memory).
- Give the client positive reinforcement for using such strategies.

YOUR SELF-AWARENESS
Triggering Semantic Memory

DAT clients experience episodic memory loss; therefore, interactions may not be retained, and repetition is necessary. Answer the following questions about your skill level at triggering semantic memory.

1. In this leading technique, a combination of words and nonverbal cues are used. Are your words and nonverbal cues:

   Precise?   ☐ Yes   ☐ No
   Concise?   ☐ Yes   ☐ No
   Clear?   ☐ Yes   ☐ No

2. Constant repetition in a kind, firm manner is necessary. When you have to repeat yourself a number of times, are the following interaction impacts present?

   Is your tone on the third repetition identical to your tone the first time you said this? ☐ Yes ☐ No

   Is your affect kindly the fourth time you've repeated yourself? ☐ Yes ☐ No

   Do your movements remain the same even though you have to repeat them? ☐ Yes ☐ No

   Are you consistent? ☐ Yes ☐ No

   If you answered "Yes," you are using this technique effectively and your communication with clients who have these disorders is more likely to be successful. If any of these areas has a "No" response, you may need to improve the connection between your verbal and nonverbal cues and evaluate your personal reaction (action, emotion, attitude) to the need to repeat basic instructions.

Memantine (Namenda) is the first DAT medication to work by targeting glutamate rather than acetylcholine. This medication is for moderate to severe disease treatment and expands the choices in the psychopharmacologic management of the disease.

Medication management with this group of disorders has a variety of purposes and options. Examples of these options are included in TABLE 14-2 ∎.

Promoting Optimal Orientation

Structure the client's environment to support cognitive functions. The client should be wearing whatever aids (hearing, vision) are necessary to prevent sensory loss or distortion.

Familiar objects from home, such as sweaters, robe, and photographs, may also help orient the client. Easily read clocks, orientation boards, and a consistent daily routine that includes physical activity and socialization without sensory overload will also help orient the client. Verbally orient the client during conversation. Do not quiz the client about discrepancies.

Supporting Optimal Verbal Expression

As communication skills decrease, the client's nonverbal communication becomes more important. Clients respond physically to the environment, especially if they feel threatened. Call the client by name, approach in clear view, and give simple directions.

Supporting Appropriate Conduct/Impulse Control

The client may strike out in response to hallucinations or delusions. All measures used to support perception and orientation are imperative here because clients function best in an environment where stimulation is controlled and sensory overload prevented. All changes, whether environmental or personal, need to be made slowly wherever possible. Always approach the client in full view, calling his or her name, and refrain from touching the client. Requests should be simple and nondemanding.

Supporting Optimal Role Performance

To promote functioning in the family, the client must be viewed as an active member. Most clients with dementia remain at home until the caregiver can no longer manage the client's needs. The family needs support throughout this time, such as home visits, day care, respite care, and support groups.

If the client is institutionalized, the family can be an integral part of the client's daily routine. Family members need extra emotional support as the rewards for maintaining involvement diminish. For the client with dementia, role maintenance involves supporting the client's need to be oriented.

Maintaining Optimal Attention Span

Repeat requests as needed. Speak in simple phrases, loud enough to be heard, and reinforce meaning with gestures. To decrease distractibility and hyperalertness, keep environmental stimulation at a minimum. Make every effort to lower the client's anxiety level by moving slowly, speaking clearly, and providing new information slowly.

TABLE 14-2 ∎ Common Medications Used to Treat Certain Cognitive Disorders

Cognitive Disorder	Common Medications (generic and trade names)	Use
Dementia of the Alzheimer's type (DAT)	donepezil (Aricept)	Slow the rate of cognitive decline
Dementia with Lewy bodies	escitalopram (Lexipro)	Reduce symptoms of depression when present
Pick's disease	valproic acid (Depakote)	Reduce problematic mood swings and agitated behavior
Vascular dementia with psychosis	quetiapine (Seroquel)	Reduce or eliminate delusions and hallucinations

Promoting Optimal Self-Concept/Self-Esteem

During the early stages of dementia, make every effort to maintain clients' self-esteem as they struggle with the personal awareness of cognitive loss. Encourage clients to express their fears and concerns, and listen attentively. Allow for the verbal expression of anger and sadness.

Manipulate the environment to help the client with a failing memory. Helpful measures include labeling the bathroom and bedroom, posting notes to remind the client to turn off the stove and lock the door, and labeling the contents of drawers. Gently remind the client of forgotten events, and do not confront confabulations. Encourage the family to maintain the client as a productive member of this important group.

Supporting Optimal Perceptual Functioning

A quiet environment with soft music prevents the client from experiencing sensory overload. When speaking with the client, stand or sit so that you are in direct view. Use touch with caution. First give a verbal warning before touching the client's shoulder or forearm, and slowly and clearly explain all procedures. Sometimes even a very soothing touch can overexcite the client, who may respond by striking out. Make sure that the client is wearing hearing aids and eyeglasses if necessary.

In responding to hallucinations, simply state that you understand that these sensations can be very powerful and even disturbing. Do not argue or ask the client to elaborate. Take care of the emotional response (e.g., if the client is frightened, reassure) in your interactions. Give reassurance that these thoughts will go away. Say, "We will help you." Do not leave the client alone or in an isolated room without some stimulation to help the client block out the hallucinations and support reality testing. The room should be well lit and without shadows or glare. If the client becomes combative, briefly intervene to redirect and prevent harm to self or others. Then attempt to distract, reassuring the client, "You are in a safe place."

Promoting Optimal Patterns of Elimination

A regular toileting schedule helps clients with dementia control bowel and urinary incontinence. Clients are often not able to let the nurse know when they have to use the toilet or have soiled themselves. Use clothing that is easy to remove and clean.

During the early stage of dementia, a toileting routine is essential. It helps confused clients to place a large sign on the bathroom door labeled, "Toilet." As the disease progresses, the client no longer recognizes a toilet or its purpose. Such a client may resist sitting on the toilet. Forcing the client will only produce agitation and combativeness. Distract and try again. If all efforts at maintaining a routine fail, use disposable pants or diapers. The use of catheters and external drains is not recommended because of the possibility of infection and their certain removal by a confused client.

Promoting Optimal Nutritional Status

Monitor the client's food and fluid intake. Give hyperactive clients a diet high in protein and carbohydrates in finger-food form. Some clients may need double portions. Clients who chew constantly need to be reminded to swallow. Depending on the client's level of perception and motor activity, supervision and assistance at mealtimes may be necessary. Weigh the client routinely, and increase caloric intake as needed. In the final stages of the disease, the client loses all interest in food and may receive nasogastric, gastrostomy, or intravenous feedings.

Evaluation

Assess both the effectiveness of all interventions and the client's response to them. For guidance on self-assessment, see Your Self-Awareness.

Delirium Evaluation Criteria

The evaluation of nursing care for clients with delirium is based on the premise that clients are capable of returning to their previous level of functioning. During that process, the goal is to help the client maintain optimal levels of sensory perception, participate in activities of daily living, and maintain physiological homeostasis.

Dementia Evaluation Criteria

Dementia entails progressive intellectual, behavioral, and physiological deterioration. The goal of nursing care is not to cure, but rather to sustain the client at the optimal level of self-care. Help the family sustain a personally rewarding relationship with their loved one throughout this terminal process.

CASE MANAGEMENT

Case management of the client with dementia involves developing and organizing a program to address the symptoms present. It must be a flexible system to respond to the changing

---

YOUR SELF-AWARENESS
An Inventory for Nurses Who Care for Clients With Cognitive Disorders

Caring for clients with cognitive disorders can be difficult and frustrating at times. The self-awareness information you gather by thoughtfully considering your responses to the following questions will help you to become more successful in working with cognitively impaired clients and their families.

- How do I feel about working with clients with cognitive disorders?
- What do I like about working with them?
- What frustrates me about working with them?
- What behavioral symptoms (e.g., wandering, agitation, hallucinations, delusions, hostility, eating problems, etc.) do I feel most competent to deal with? Least competent?
- What strategies have I used with clients that have been successful? Unsuccessful?
- Who are my favorite clients? Why? My least favorite clients? Why?
- What can I do to become more knowledgeable and/or skilled in dealing with clients with cognitive disorders?

PARTNERING WITH CLIENTS AND FAMILIES

Nutrition and Feeding

Suggestions for families on effective nutrition and feeding skills with someone with advanced dementia include the following:

- Recognize that eating problems are not unusual in people with late-stage dementia and, in fact, are quite common.
- Extending the quality of life through feeding can be accomplished with involved caregivers.
- Discuss with the treatment team some of the nutritional needs specific for your family member.
- Assist your family member with oral feeding for as long as possible—this promotes comfort and provides basic contact.
- Take the client's food preferences into account; and remember that tasting and smelling senses may be poor.

- Routinely proceeding to tube feedings has not been shown to extend life, improve nutritional status, or reduce aspiration.
- Be aware of the typical problems in feeding at this stage. Your family member may be easily distracted, spit out or cheek food, and have swallowing difficulties or poor coordination.
- Helpful environmental features include lighting sufficient to contrast and illuminate food and utensils and avoid overcrowding.
- Maintain eye contact.

Sources: Chang, C.-C., & Roberts, B. L. (2011). Strategies for feeding patients with dementia. *American Journal of Nursing, 111*(4), 36–44 and Lee, T. J., & Kolasa, K. M. (2011). Feeding the person with late-stage Alzheimer's disease. *Nutrition Today, 46*(2), 75–79.

---

needs of the client as deterioration progresses. There is a great deal of contact with the caregiver(s). Provide regular monitoring and supervise the following:

- Regular physical examinations with a primary care provider
- Prescription medications
- Nutrition
- Over-the-counter medications
- Finances
- Interpersonal relationships

One of the challenges in managing the care of a client with advanced stages of dementia include how to physically intervene in everyday activities. Nutrition concerns are relevant, especially in how to feed someone who has advanced DAT when other problems are likely and contribute to difficulties. Lee & Kolasa (2011) explore some of the options that families and professionals can try in developing the best possible combination of strategies. See Partnering With Clients and Families on the issue of feeding.

COMMUNITY-BASED CARE

Community-based care for the client with dementia could involve appointments in a clinic setting, a day program designed for the current level of difficulties in functioning, medication clinic appointments, a supportive group, or some combination. Frequently, a family member or caregiver is involved, especially due to the need for transportation.

Counseling and face-to-face contacts are a way to decrease the social isolation inherent in a client with dementia. Psychotherapy can be useful to help clients with mild to moderate dementia cope with the loss of cognitive functions. The features of counseling or therapy would include the following:

- Empathic listening
- Support
- Working on coping methods

- Providing the client with outlets for distress that might otherwise exacerbate disturbed behavior (e.g., talking over fears rather than acting out behaviorally)

HOME CARE

The most effective treatment for the client with dementia is a balance between stimulation/environmental demand and whatever internal resources remain for the client. The home would need to be evaluated to determine if it will meet the changing needs of the client. Some revisions are usually necessary so that safe wandering is possible, dangers are minimized through safety devices, and activity can be controlled. A cycle of stimulation and rest is best so the client's abilities are engaged but not overwhelmed.

Supportive counseling is frequently helpful when providing home care for clients with dementia. You must understand the premorbid personality and developmental history of someone with dementia because the dementing process is superimposed on the pre-existing personality. Determine what role anxiety played in clients' lives, their previous self-view, and how conscious they were of themselves and the impact of their actions on others. Once the client's anxiety is reduced, the tendency toward better functioning will ensue.

The focus of treatment for clients with dementia expands to include caregivers. Whether the caregivers are relatives, friends, or health care providers, they may require explanations of symptoms and help in designing behavioral interventions. Caregivers working with severely demented clients may require help in coping with stress, discouragement, and a sense of hopelessness.

The concept of respite care is one where caretakers are able to either have someone come into the environment to care for the client and the caregiver can exit the situation temporarily, or the client is cared for in a facility with skilled and experienced respite services. This allows caregivers the freedom of movement and action. In either case, the caregiver can have a few days to attend to other matters.

NURSING CARE PLAN: CLIENT WITH DELIRIUM

Identifying Information

Mr. Hennessey is a 50-year-old married man who entered the hospital to have colon surgery. He is a physically fit man in a physically demanding job, typically jogging several miles a week for exercise. This is his first serious physical problem. His wife of 25 years is extremely devoted and stayed with him following his surgery. While still in the ICU, Mr. Hennessey became disoriented. Staff members were careful to check his electrolyte balances, which were within normal limits. Within 2 days he began hallucinating. He cried out that the hovering bats he saw in the corners of the room were trying to kill him. He has had other hallucinations and believes that his life is at great risk. When his wife offered him a newspaper, he whispered

that she should give him the bucket of pills he'd been hiding under his bed. He lashed out at his wife following this exchange and ripped out his IV and nasogastric tube.

History

Mr. Hennessey has no prior psychiatric history, nor are there any family members with major psychiatric problems. His wife and two grown children, who live nearby, are concerned about his well-being. All are attentive to Mr. Hennessey, love him, and are willing to help with his care.

Mr. Hennessey is a contractor and owns his own business. He and his wife have many friends and activities. He was diagnosed with a colon tumor 1 month ago and had a colon resection. The pathology

report was positive for cancer. Mr. Hennessey had been healthy all his life until he noticed rectal bleeding a month ago. He has had regular physicals and responded immediately when symptoms of a problem arose.

Current Mental Status

Mr. Hennessey is disoriented the majority of time, and he is often aggressive. He has been having frightening visual hallucinations, especially at night. He is delusional that people are trying to hurt him.

Other Clinical Data

Mr. Hennessey is on morphine for pain management.

Nursing Diagnosis: High Risk for Violence related to confusion and fear inherent in delirium

Expected Outcome: Mr. Hennessey does not attempt to harm self or others.

Short-Term Goals	Interventions	Rationales
Mr. Hennessey will have decreased symptoms of persecutory delusions.	■ Directly address the fear he is feeling (i.e., "I understand how frightening this all is, and we will make sure you are safe"). ■ Prevent overstimulation and understimulation.	Talking about the feelings is more reassuring and shifts interactions from argumentation. ICUs can be overwhelming in certain sensory areas while not providing enough cues to the outside world (such as windows).
Mr. Hennessey displays considerably less agitation and fear.	■ Orient Mr. Hennessey whenever he is confused. ■ Promote relaxation in both active and soothing modes. ■ Move slowly, speak clearly, and explain all procedures. ■ Make sure only one person is speaking to Mr. Hennessy at a time. ■ Following clearance on neurologic examination, medicate Mr. Hennessey with a low-dose antipsychotic. ■ Explain to family about ICU psychosis and the temporary nature of it.	Decrease the stimuli that can exacerbate symptoms or confusion.

Pearson Nursing Student Resources

Find additional review materials at
nursing.pearsonhighered.com

Prepare for success with NCLEX®-style practice questions, interactive assignments and activities, web links, animations and videos, and more!

REFERENCES

Alzheimer, A. (1907). Uber eine eigenartige Erkraukung der Hirwrinde. *Allegmeine Zeitschrift fü r Psychiatrie, 64,* 146–148.

Alzheimer's Association. (2011). *2011 Alzheimer's disease facts and figures.* Retrieved from http://www.alz.org/downloads/Facts_Figures_2011.pdf

American Psychiatric Association. (2000). *Diagnostic and statistical manual of mental disorders* (4th ed., Text Revision) (DSM-IV-TR). Washington, DC: Author.

American Psychological Association, Task Force to Update the Guidelines for the Evaluation of Dementia and Age-Related Cognitive Decline. (2011). Guidelines for the Evaluation of Dementia and Age-Related Cognitive Decline. Adopted by the APA Council of Representatives on February 18, 2011. *www.apa.org/pi/aging/resources/dementia-guidelines.pdf*

Bank, G., Kagan, D., & Madhavi, D. (2011). Coenzyme Q10: Clinical update and bioavailability. *Complementary Health Practice Review, 16*(2), 129–137.

Blazer, D., Hughes, D. C., & George, L. K. (1987). The epidemiology of depression in an elderly community population. *The Gerontologist, 27,* 281–287.

Bowman, G. L., Shannon, J., Ho, E., Traber, M. G., Frei, B., Oken, B. S., . . . Quinn, J. F. (2011). Reliability and validity of food frequency questionnaire and nutrient biomarkers in elders with and without mild cognitive impairment. *Alzheimer Disease & Associated Disorders, 25*(1), 49–57.

Cavedo, E., Boccardi, M., Ganzola, R., Canu, E., Beltramello, A., Caltagirone, C., . . . Frisoni, G. B. (2011). Local amygdala structural differences with 3T MRI in patients with Alzheimer disease. *Neurology, 6*(8), 727–733.

Chang, C.-C., & Roberts, B. L. (2011). Strategies for feeding patients with dementia. *American Journal of Nursing, 111*(4), 36–44.

Chin, A. L., Negash, S., & Hamilton, R. (2011). Diversity and disparity in dementia: The impact of ethnoracial differences in Alzheimer disease. *Alzheimer Disease & Associated Disorders.* Advance online publication. doi: 10.1097/WAD.0b013e318211c6c9

Doering, B., & Exner, C. (2011). Combining neuropsychological and cognitive-behavioral approaches for treating psychological sequelae of acquired brain injury. *Current Opinion in Psychiatry, 24*(2), 156–161.

Gallagher, M., & Long, C. O. (2011). Advanced dementia care: Demystifying behaviors, addressing pain, and maximizing comfort: Research and practice: Partners in care. *Journal of Hospice & Palliative Nursing, 13*(2), 70–78.

Gannon, P., Khan, M. Z., & Kolson, D. L. (2011). Current understanding of HIV-associated neurocognitive disorders pathogenesis. *Current Opinion in Neurology, 24*(3), 275–283.

Higashi, S., Moore, D. J., Minegishi, M., Kasanuki, K., Fujishiro, H., Kabuta, T., . . . Iseki, E. (2011). Localization of MAP1-LC3 in vulnerable neurons and Lewy bodies in brains of patients with dementia with Lewy bodies. *Journal of Neuropathology & Experimental Neurology, 70*(4), 264–280.

Kim, S. J., Lee, J. H., Lee, D. Y., Jhoo, J. H., & Woo, J. I. (2011). Neurocognitive dysfunction associated with sleep quality and sleep apnea in patients with mild cognitive impairment. *American Journal of Geriatric Psychiatry, 19*(4), 374–381.

Lee, T. J., & Kolasa, K. M. (2011). Feeding the person with late-stage Alzheimer's disease. *Nutrition Today, 46*(2), 75–79.

McKeith, I. G., Galasko, D., Kosaka, K., Perry, E. K., Dickson, D. W., Hansen, L. A., . . . Perry, R. H. (1996). Consensus guidelines for the clinical and pathologic diagnosis of dementia with Lewy bodies (DLB): Report of the consortium on DLB international workshop. *Neurology, 47,* 1113–1124.

Murray, K. (2011). Creutzfeldt-Jacob disease mimics, or how to sort out the subacute encephalopathy patient. *Practical Neurology, 11*(1), 19–28.

Rosenbloom, M. H., & Atri, A. (2011). The evaluation of rapidly progressive dementia. *Neurologist, 17*(2), 67–74.

Rudolph, J. L., & Marcantonio, E. R. (2011). Postoperative delirium: Acute change with long-term implications. *Anesthesia & Analgesia, 112*(5), 1202–1211.

Scarmeas, N., Luchsinger, J. A., Brickman, A. M., Cosentino, S., Schupf, N., Xin-Tang, M., . . . Stern, Y. (2011). Physical activity and Alzheimer disease course. *American Journal of Geriatric Psychiatry, 19*(5), 471–481.

Sheu, E., Versloot, J., Nader, R., Kerr, D., & Craig, K. D. (2011). Pain in the elderly: Validity of facial expression components of observational measures. *Clinical Journal of Pain.* Advance online publication. doi: 10.1097/AJP.0b013e31820f52e1

Voyer, P., Richard, S., Doucet, L., & Carmichael, P.-H. (2011). Factors associated with delirium severity among older persons with dementia. *Journal of Neuroscience Nursing, 43*(2), 62–69.

Substance-Related Disorders

15

EILEEN TRIGOBOFF

LEARNING OUTCOMES

After completing this chapter, you will be able to:

1. Discuss the major theoretic explanations for substance-related disorders.
2. Describe the populations at risk for substance-related disorders.
3. Explain how the physical, psychological, and withdrawal effects of the major categories of substances manifest.
4. Identify treatment approaches for the major categories of abused substances.
5. Discuss how the presence of both a substance-related disorder and a major mental disorder (such as schizophrenia) complicates nursing care.
6. Compare and contrast the short-term and long-term nursing intervention strategies for clients with substance-related disorders.
7. Implement the strategies for helping a client avoid relapse.
8. Formulate outcome criteria for clients who have substance-related disorders.
9. Assess your own feelings and attitudes about clients with substance-related disorders and how they may affect your professional practice.

CRITICAL THINKING CHALLENGE

Billie is a 19-year-old homeless African-American woman pregnant with her third child and addicted to crack cocaine. When she appeared at your hospital's Family Practice Clinic for prenatal care 1 month before her delivery, she was referred to your team for assessment and treatment for her addiction. Billie is concerned about losing her children if she enters a drug treatment program, and she is fearful that her unborn baby is already damaged. She shuns Alcoholics Anonymous (AA) and Narcotics Anonymous (NA) because admitting "powerlessness" and "turning her life over to God the Father" is unacceptable to her; as a marginalized poor black woman, she's had it with powerlessness and would rather empower her daughters so that they "don't turn their lives over to men." Others on your treatment team refuse to accept her as an outpatient because she will not promise complete abstinence and is reluctant to commit to attending one NA or AA meeting per day.

1. Under what conditions does the treatment team have the right to refuse outpatient treatment for Billie?
2. What are some other options for Billie's care?
3. Should Billie lose her children? Why, or why not?

Drug and alcohol abuse, already a widespread problem, is rapidly escalating. Substance abuse is a psychosocial and a biologic problem. Television and radio advertisements entice viewers with the hope of relief from pain and problems; they portray life without stress. The values portrayed are clear: Discomfort should be erased; drinking is vital to a stress-free life; drugs are acceptable mediators of emotions. When people do not have the skills to effectively self-soothe, maladaptive coping such as using substances can be put into effect.

Substance abuse is a complex public health issue with grave ramifications. It increases the crime rate, auto accident deaths, number of teenage pregnancies, HIV infection rate, and the suicide rate. Individuals and families are destroyed. Every part of a substance abuser's life—social life, family life, physical health, work productivity and relationships—is affected.

Two critical features—how substances are taken into the body, and how substances are combined with other substances—pose public health dangers. Active injection drug users (IDUs) who are also hazardous alcohol users are thought to be at particularly high risk for HIV and HIV transmission. The transfer of small amounts of blood in shared needles or syringes constitute a bridge to others—their fetuses, newborns, and sex partners—putting them at increased risk. IDUs are likely to minimize their HIV risks as nil or small. Alcohol and cocaine use, both injection and noninjection, substantially increases the risk for HIV infection. A group with persistent drug and sex risk behaviors is adolescents, especially those who have been brought to the attention of the juvenile justice system. Older adults with illicit drug use and at-risk drinking are less likely to be receiving behavioral health care when needed. And in general, drug users are less likely to take antiretroviral medications. Substance abuse in the work environment increases accidents, workers' compensation claims, absenteeism, and theft while decreasing the quality of life for other workers and potentially decreasing the quality of the work performed overall.

This chapter is a biopsychosocial exploration, applying the nursing process to clients who have substance-related disorders. Be aware of the need to keep up-to-date on the trends, fads, and activities related to substance abuse, because they change quickly. The importance of having a knowledge base on this topic, developing caring attitudes, and developing skilled therapeutic interventions are discussed in the standards of addiction nursing, jointly written by the American Nurses Association and the International Nurses Society on Addictions. These standards can be found on http://nursesbooks.org, the website of the publishing arm of the American Nurses Association.

SUBSTANCE-RELATED DISORDERS

According to the DSM-IV-TR (American Psychiatric Association [APA], 2000), substance-related disorders are disorders that are: (1) a consequence of abusing a drug (such as alcohol), (2) the side effects of a medication (such as antihistamines), or (3) related to exposure to a toxin (such as fuel). Substance-related disorders are divided into the following two groups:

1. Substance use disorders that include substance dependence and substance abuse

2. Substance-induced disorders (including substance intoxication and substance withdrawal as well as other substance-induced disorders such as substance-induced cognitive disorders and mood disorders)

This chapter focuses on substance dependence and substance abuse, including the intoxication and withdrawal issues for those classes of substances traditionally called psychoactive drugs.

SUBSTANCE ABUSE

Substance abuse is characterized by a pattern of repeated use of substances that is maladaptive in that significant adverse consequences occur. Examples include recurrent social and relationship problems. Refer back to the summary of the DSM-IV-TR diagnostic criteria for substance abuse.

SUBSTANCE DEPENDENCE

Substance dependence is defined as a maladaptive pattern of substance use leading to clinically significant impairment or distress. (See DSM Essential Features for diagnosing substance dependence, abuse, intoxication, and withdrawal.) The hallmarks of this pattern are as follows:

- **Tolerance**—needing increased amounts of a substance to achieve the desired effect
- **Withdrawal**—the uncomfortable physiological and cognitive behavioral changes that are associated with lowered blood or tissue concentrations of a substance after an individual has been a heavy user

People typically display common characteristics when they depend upon substances—the compulsive use of that substance, and unsuccessful efforts to cut down or schedule their use. You may have noticed when you have been in contact with someone with this problem that he or she spends a great deal of time trying to obtain the substance and either use or recover from the effects of using it. Dependence involves continuing to use the substance despite the recognition that there are costs (physical, financial, and emotionally) and difficulties.

This diagnosis can be made for every class of substance except caffeine. The latest information on substance abuse can be found at the Substance Abuse & Mental Health Services Administration (SAMHSA) website at http://www.samhsa.gov/

SUBSTANCE INTOXICATION

Substance intoxication refers to a reversible syndrome of maladaptive physiological and behavioral changes that are due to the effects of a substance on a person's central nervous system (CNS). The continuum of CNS depression with substance use can be seen in FIGURE 15-1 ■. The syndrome includes disturbances of mood (such as belligerence or mood lability), perception, the sleep–wake cycle, attention, thinking, judgment, and psychomotor as well as interpersonal

DSM ESSENTIAL FEATURES

Substance Abuse, Dependence, Intoxication, and Withdrawal

In order to receive one of these diagnoses, the maladaptive pattern of substance use must cause clinically significant impairment or distress. Several accompanying issues must also have occurred within a 12-month period.

Substance Abuse: At some point, recurrent substance use caused a failure to fulfill major role obligations. This occurred at work, school, or home. There may have been substance-related legal problems, the substance was used in physically hazardous situations, and the individual continued to use the substance despite the problems associated with its use.

Substance Dependence: The client has some combination of tolerance, withdrawal, and taking the substance often in larger amounts or over a longer period than intended. There is

a persistent desire to cut down with unsuccessful efforts to control substance use. The client spends a significant amount of time obtaining the substance, often reducing or stopping important work, social, or recreational activities to do so. Substance use continues despite increasing medical or psychological consequences.

Intoxication: During or shortly after use of a substance, the client develops a reversible pattern of clinically significant maladaptive changes in behavior, thoughts, or feelings caused specifically by the substance.

Withdrawal: During or shortly after decreasing or stopping heavy or prolonged substance use, the client develops distress or impairment in an important area of functioning which can include work or social life.

---

behavior. See the essential aspects of the diagnostic criteria for substance intoxication.

SUBSTANCE WITHDRAWAL

Substance withdrawal refers to the development of maladaptive physiological, behavioral, and cognitive changes that are the result of reducing or stopping the heavy and regular use of a substance. **Substance withdrawal syndrome** is associated with distress and/or impairment in important areas of social functioning. The clinical example that follows describes the difficulties of withdrawing from the long-term

Clinical Example

Paul is a 40-year-old unemployed banker with a history of daily alcohol consumption that has gradually exceeded a quart of vodka per day for 25 years. He is estranged from his ex-wife and their two teenagers. He has tried unsuccessfully to cut back on his drinking on numerous occasions. His attempts to quit were particularly motivated when it became clear he would lose his job because of his declining performance and when he received a second arrest for driving while intoxicated. He is brought into the community crisis unit for medical detoxification and referral to Alcoholics Anonymous (AA) meetings and a mandatory outpatient recovery group program. He smokes at least a pack of cigarettes each day and drinks 6 cups of strong coffee as well. His physical examination reveals hypertension that is not responsive to medication, elevated liver enzymes, and ascites. He complains of dull abdominal pain, dry skin, diarrhea, and indigestion. He is sweaty, shaking, and irritable. He repeatedly asks the nurse practitioner (NP) to write a prescription for pain medications to ease his current discomfort.

use of a substance. See the summarized diagnostic criteria for substance withdrawal earlier in this chapter in DSM Essential Features.

SUBSTANCE-INDUCED SLEEP DISORDERS

Substances of abuse or by prescription (e.g., alcohol, cocaine, opioids, hypnotics, anxiolytics) may cause a severe sleep disorder during intoxication or withdrawal. Even after prolonged abstinence, the abuse of some substances such as alcohol and hallucinogens may affect sleep architecture.

Substance-induced sleep disorder is characterized by sustained use of stimulants for staying awake, or of alcohol to induce sleep. You will probably work with many clients who use stimulants or alcohol periodically for their effect on sleep. For example, the use of stimulants is not uncommon among long-distance truck drivers, and alcohol is and has been one of the most frequently used hypnotics. While a drink at bedtime usually helps a person to fall asleep, it usually induces wakening later in the night.

A wide range of biochemical substances can contribute to this sleep disorder by their presence in sufficient quantities (such as caffeine and prescription drugs), their unaccustomed absence (alcohol), or their abuse (street drugs). Clients with psychiatric disorders, especially schizophrenia or mania, or clients with a history of traumatic brain injury are particularly vulnerable to sleep disorders due to chemical imbalances.

SAMHSA (Substance Abuse & Mental Health Services Administration)

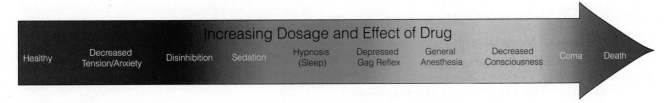

FIGURE 15-1 ■ Continuum of CNS depression when using substances of abuse, showing increasing dosage and effect of drug.

Clinical Example

Judith and Karina participate in a program setting for people with schizophrenia. They often meet for a drink together at the conclusion of a meeting. Although they consume similar amounts of alcohol, Karina, who also has a history of minor brain injury, experiences greater disordered sleep.

The vulnerability may be twofold: direct effects of biochemical imbalance plus the use of alcohol or drugs as an attempt to cope with a psychiatric disorder.

With acute alcohol intoxication, adults have an urge to sleep that is increased for 3 to 4 hours. Sleep may be deep with rapid eye movement (REM) suppression. However, after that, sleep tends to be fragmented, restless, and often accompanied by bizarre dreaming. During alcohol withdrawal, sleep tends to be very fragmented, with REM rebound. The vivid dreaming may be associated with alcohol withdrawal delirium (APA, 2000). Sleep pattern disturbances persist even after a year or more of abstention.

Other abused drugs follow a similar pattern of exacerbation of their usual effect (sedation or stimulation) after excessive intake, along with rebound effects upon withdrawal. The diagnostic criteria for substance-induced sleep disorders are summarized in DSM Essential Features.

BIOPSYCHOSOCIAL THEORIES

The theoretical frameworks for understanding substance problems include biologic/genetic, psychological, sociocultural, and family systems theories.

Biologic/Genetic Theories

The biologic explanation of alcoholism gained a great deal of importance in the last few years. Following are some examples of research that contribute to our evidence-based practices.

- Classic research by Jellinek (1946) during the 1940s to 1960s, described as the Disease Model of Alcoholism, revealed that alcoholics proceed through phases (prealcoholic symptomatic phase, prodromal phase, crucial phase, and chronic phase). He recognized "loss of control" in addictive alcoholics and hypothesized that it may have a biochemical basis. Building on this early work, current research examines biochemical differences in these clients such as lower levels of dopamine (DA) neurotransmission,

increased density of dopaminergic D_2 receptors in the brain, and early relapse in alcohol-dependent clients.
- Pharmacologic management of addictions, as opposed to psychosocial interventions, includes the use of standard and new compounds.

1. Acamprosate (Campral) Delayed-Release Tablets were approved by the U.S. Food and Drug Administration (FDA) in 2004. Acamprosate is indicated for the maintenance of alcohol abstinence in clients with alcohol dependence who are abstinent at treatment initiation. This compound alleviates the physiological and psychological distress during the postacute withdrawal period, making it easier not to drink. Its mechanism of action is not completely understood; the main interaction is believed to be with the glutamate system.
2. Naltrexone (ReVia, Trexan) was developed in 1984 for the treatment of heroin abuse, and was approved in January 1994 for blocking the craving for alcohol and the pleasure derived from drinking it.
3. Disulfiram (Antabuse), inhibits acetaldehyde metabolism. With disulfiram, acetaldehyde, which is highly toxic, accumulates in the bloodstream when alcohol is consumed. This combination of disulfiram and alcohol produces nausea, vomiting, dizziness, and other uncomfortable and potentially dangerous symptoms. It is used to discourage alcohol use.

- Advances in genetics help explain some aspects of vulnerability to substance abuse (Swendsen & Le Moal, 2011; Crabbe, Harris, & Koob, 2011; Hack et al., 2011); however, genetic risk factors for such complex diseases are modest and therefore difficult to detect (Bergen et al., 2011).
- Substance abuse prior to conception and pregnancy has grave consequences for fetuses. In both males and females, it has been validated as damaging to the genetic makeup of the child (Kraft et al., 2011).
- Children growing up in adverse social environments (such as having inebriation and behavioral drama a regular feature of home life) had increased behavioral problems and compromised language development. Conversely, an easy temperament acts as a protective factor for social–emotional development and could be related to resilience (Derauf et al., 2011).

DSM ESSENTIAL FEATURES

Substance-Induced Sleep Disorder

A disturbance in sleep that is prominent and severe enough to need treatment and is related to substance abuse or medication intake. Other potential causes of the sleep disturbance, including delirium, have been ruled out. This sleep disorder causes distress or impairment in social, occupational, or other areas of functioning.

- Drug use affects human development on the genetic level because drug use negatively affects sperm and egg health. Each partner contributes to the negative effect—when a male uses a substance and subsequently impregnates a woman, when a woman uses drugs prior to pregnancy, and when a woman uses substances during pregnancy. Birth defects are more commonly linked with paternal DNA damage than with maternal DNA damage.
- The National Drug Threat Assessment (a survey of drug use in the United States) and other topical information can be found at the National Drug Intelligence Center at http://www.justice.gov or on this text's Online Student Resources.

Psychological Theories

From the psychological perspective, the substance abuser is viewed as regressed and fixated at pregenital, oral levels of psychosexual development. Some writers relate the pattern of drug taking to parental inconsistency, self-centeredness, and inner dishonesty. The following personality traits are often associated with disruptive drug abuse:

- Dominant and critical behavior with underlying self-doubts and passivity
- Overt extroversion
- Tendency to describe one's own parents as self-reliant and efficient but not emotionally warm
- Personal insecurity, with low self-esteem and self-criticism
- Problems with sexual identification
- Rebellious attitudes toward authority
- Tendency to use defense mechanisms that are primarily escapist or sensation seeking
- Difficulty with intimacy
- Absence of a strong and efficient superego
- Marked narcissistic trends
- Difficulty with impulse control and feelings

There is no real agreement about whether certain personality traits are sufficient to account for drug dependence, because the personality traits in question are studied after the diagnosis of substance abuse is made.

Sociocultural Theories

Sociocultural models of substance abuse emphasize social forces, role models, and adaptive responses to stress in the sociocultural environment. Life's harsh realities come in many forms: the hopelessness and defeat of urban poverty, the academic and social pressures generated by upper-middle-class families, the adolescent's feeling of impotence and alienation, the peer group pressure to join in and share experiences, the social vacuum of unloving families in which meaningful attachments are dissolved or dissolving.

All of these social conditions and contexts help create and sustain substance abuse. Another sociocultural aspect is situational—people who become addicts or alcoholics tend to live in environments where access to chemicals is easy and initiation into their use is widespread. Such an environment might include a neighborhood where abandoned houses become places to sell, buy, and use substances. Substance abusers describe in interviews how they learned to drink or use drugs at school, in social circumstances with their peers, or at home by watching their families. They recognized chemicals as a social lubricant, an escape, or a remedy for psychic and physical pain. See Developing Cultural Competence for specific information about culture and drug use.

Family Systems Theories

A family systems explanation for substance abuse has gained increasing acceptance among health care professionals. When assessing substance abuse and the psychological impacts, ask yourself, "Could the substance dependence be serving a purpose in this family?" It may serve to do any or all of the following:

- Shift the family's focus away from other more anxiety-provoking feelings or events
- Give them a purpose or a challenge to distract them from other issues
- Relieve one family member of a burden or provide a needed burden to one or several members
- Provide a cohesive cause in which all family members can involve themselves

The family systems perspective includes the phenomenon of codependence. **Codependency** involves being preoccupied with controlling another person's behavior. Codependency can be seen when a family member both rescues and blames (persecutes) the substance abuser.

Although Alcoholics Anonymous (AA), a support group for alcoholics, does not openly endorse the family systems theory, it does recognize that alcoholism is a family disease. Al-Anon and Ala-Teen are groups for spouses, parents, friends, coworkers, and teenage children of alcoholics. The

DEVELOPING CULTURAL COMPETENCE

Substances of Abuse in Specific Cultures

Studies clearly show that substance abuse is present in all cultures; however, which substance people abuse is often culturally determined. In Western culture, alcohol is the drug of choice. In Muslim countries, marijuana is used because Islam prohibits alcohol use. Opium is used in China and other Eastern countries, while people in India, Africa, and South America use native herbs and chemicals. Native Americans use peyote (a cactus button with hallucinogenic properties) and alcohol more than other drugs. South Americans use ayahuasca (an hallucinogenic herb) in cleansing spiritual hallucinogenic rituals.

CRITICAL THINKING QUESTIONS

1. What use is knowing the specific substances someone may use depending on their culture?
2. What complications could you anticipate when someone uses these substances for a spiritual reason?

focus is on helping these nonalcoholics learn to live and work effectively with alcoholics.

The underlying process, as the clinical example illustrates, is that other people assume an **enabling** role, or co-alcoholic behavior, and this perpetuates the alcoholic's drinking patterns.

Clinical Example

Louise has been drinking for many years. She works full time as a secretary in a financial office setting. Adrienne, Louise's coworker for many years, routinely does Louise's work when Louise is too tired, confused, or otherwise unable to perform her duties. Adrienne believes she is helping Louise keep her job and her self-esteem. In reality, Adrienne is enabling Louise to continue to drink and not suffer the consequences of her drinking.

A cycle begins when people who enable cover for the person dependent on a substance—such as by saying that he or she has a cold, is bruised because of stumbling in the dark, is asleep because of fatigue. Protected by the enabling behavior, there are no consequences of bad behavior and no motivation to stop drinking or using drugs. The person who is enabling, believing that the substance user is coping with family, marital, or work problems "the best way he can," denies the disease of addiction. The addict blames the person who is enabling; the person who is enabling feels guilty and then attempts to control family life and the behaviors of the alcoholic/addict by throwing out liquor or taking the car keys. Enabling behavior was employed to protect, rescue, control, and blame, but none of these behaviors is effective in altering the course of the disease. Those who enable feel worthless and helpless because they are unsuccessful in terminating the addiction. Intervention and confrontation are necessary to break the cycle.

Enabling can also allow someone to stay in a relationship with an addict. This occurs when someone outside the relationship, such as the best friend of the nonaddict, provides a way to continue to ignore or deny the problem. See Box 15-1, How Significant Others Enable, for an example of a relationship involving enabling.

Dysfunctional Family Roles

When a family includes one parent whose role consists of addictive behavior and who is incapable of being emotionally present and adequately fulfilling the parenting role, and one parent whose role involves codependency or enabling, whose attempts to fix addictive behaviors prevail, children may be forced into dysfunctional family roles. Such children are consumed with meeting family needs and miss out on nurturing. Children's roles may consist of the following:

- The Hero or Martyr
- The Troublemaker or Scapegoat
- The Lost Child
- The Mascot

These defensive personalities represent survival strategies for children living in what they perceive to be a frightening family environment. Behaviors associated with each of these dysfunctional family roles appear in FIGURE 15-2 ■.

Box 15-1 How Significant Others Enable

Enabling can allow the addict to continue using the drug without immediate consequences; however, enabling can also allow a relationship with an addict to continue. Best friends being supportive in their relationship can have enabling occur when a 3rd party is an addict.

Nell's friend Tish married an alcoholic. Following the honeymoon, Tish called Nell every day to describe how stressed she felt, to talk about her feelings, and to receive support. Allowing Tish to vent daily gave Tish the energy to stay in her marriage. Because this took the lid off her stress, she did not have to acknowledge the negative aspects of her marriage. Eventually, Nell realized she was enabling Tish and actually helping her to avoid recognizing that she needed help to deal with her husband's addiction.

Nell explained this process to Tish along with her decision to refuse to talk with Tish about her husband and his addiction. This decision needed to be reinforced every time Tish brought up the topic. Eventually Tish got "fed up" with her predicament, sought therapy, and made changes so she could take better care of herself.

Adult personalities are partially imprinted during childhood, and the roles that children take in order to cope in a family burdened by addiction can continue into adulthood if appropriate treatment is not provided.

ALCOHOL

Alcohol is a common, accessible substance that has just as much destructive power as any other substance of abuse. According to the World Health Organization, alcohol is one of the most widely used and abused substances in the world and causes as much, if not more, death and disability as measles, malaria, tobacco, or illegal drugs. It is a liquid recreational drug that happens to be legal. Characteristic features of abuse of this drug are seen in the clinical example that follows.

Clinical Example

Colleen, a 48-year-old woman, arrived at the hospital to be admitted for the fifth time. Her gait was unsteady and her speech slurred. She avoided eye contact, appeared embarrassed, and apologized profusely for "getting into this mess again." She said, "I really don't need to be here. I can handle this." Then Colleen burst into tears, began to say something, got distracted, and argued repetitively with staff. Blackouts were evident; Colleen had no memory of how she got to the hospital (she had, in fact, driven herself and parked her car on the front lawn of the hospital).

Interacting with someone who is intoxicated from alcohol requires implementing a set of guidelines and understanding the processes at work.

Because of the increasing incidence of alcoholism and the highway carnage attributed to alcohol use, alcoholism is now the focus of magazine articles and radio and television programs. Media attention heightens awareness of the devastating effects of chronic alcoholism: depression; loss of self-respect; alienation from family, friends, and coworkers;

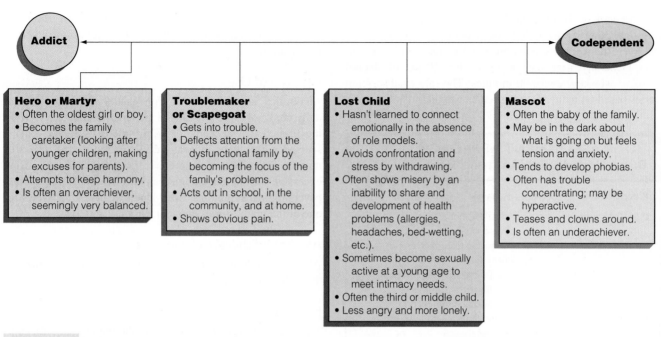

FIGURE 15-2 ■ Dysfunctional family roles in the presence of addiction–codependency.

malnutrition; infections; and damaging physiological effects to most body systems. The effects of chronic alcoholism can be found in your medical–surgical nursing textbooks.

Although alcoholism was historically viewed as a moral problem, increased awareness played a part in redefining alcoholism as a disease. As research about its biochemical aspects became known, earlier beliefs were challenged. The social stigma attached to alcoholism is decreasing, and more people are seeking help. Professionals, laypeople, alcoholics, and nonalcoholics are attending workshops and seminars on alcoholism; college courses at the undergraduate and graduate levels are offered. Recovery programs are reported widely in the media. The latest research related to the treatment of alcoholism and other drug abuse can be accessed at the website for the National Institute on Drug Abuse (NIDA) at http://www.nida.nih.gov/

The Effects of Alcohol

Alcohol is a sedative anesthetic and a central nervous system (CNS) depressant. It depresses physiological (gag, heart rate, breathing rate) and psychological functions. If taken in high doses, alcohol can depress respiration and cause death. Intoxication occurs when a person's blood alcohol level (BAL) is 0.10% or more. This blood alcohol level is the legal definition of inebriation in most states, although 0.08% is the drunk driving limit in all 50 states and represents definite impairment in coordination and judgment. FIGURE 15-3 ■ illustrates the amount of alcohol that results in a BAL of 0.10%.

National Institute on Drug Abuse

6 shot glasses
of liquor
(1.3 oz. each/80 proof)

24 oz.
of table wine

15 oz.
of fortified
wine

6 beers
(12 oz. each)

FIGURE 15-3 ■ Intoxication. These amounts of alcoholic beverages, when consumed within a 2-hour period, will give a 160-lb person a BAL of 0.10.

Alcohol is absorbed in the mouth, stomach, and small intestine. Approximately 95% of alcohol is broken down by the liver; the rest is excreted through the lungs, kidneys, and skin. Generally, a person can metabolize 10 mL of alcohol (1 oz of whiskey) every 90 minutes. The rate of absorption varies based on many factors, such as weight, intake of food,

and liver function. Your Assessment Approach compares BALs and the behaviors you will observe at various levels of intoxication.

Patterns of Use

Alcoholics manifest one of three patterns of use: regular daily intake of large amounts of alcohol, regular heavy drinking limited to weekends, or long periods of sobriety interspersed with binges of heavy drinking lasting for weeks or months. Regardless of the preferred pattern, people who drink excessively experience numerous negative physiological and psychological symptoms. See Mental Health in the News for one of the many stories about alcohol use and abuse.

Alcohol Withdrawal Syndrome

Alcohol withdrawal often includes the symptoms described in the following section.

Hangover

The term *hangover* is used to describe the unpleasant symptoms of mild alcohol withdrawal occurring approximately 4 to 6 hours after alcohol ingestion. These symptoms include the following:

- Nausea and vomiting
- Gastritis
- Headache
- Fatigue
- Sweating and thirst
- Restlessness
- Irritability
- The "shakes"
- Vasomotor instability

The cause of the symptoms is unclear, but they are attributed to dehydration, hypoglycemia, and the accumulation of lactic acid and acetaldehyde in the blood.

Alcoholic Hallucinosis

Alcoholic hallucinosis refers to auditory hallucinations reported by clients with alcohol dependence. The hallucinations occur approximately 24 to 48 hours after heavy drinking and may be vivid and frightening.

YOUR ASSESSMENT APPROACH
Blood Alcohol Level (BAL) and Behaviors

Blood Alcohol Level (BAL)	Behavior
0.05–0.15 g/dL	Initial euphoria
	Mood lability
	Cognitive disturbances, including:
	■ Decreased concentration
	■ Impaired judgment
	■ Sexual disinhibition
0.15–0.25 g/dL	Mood lability with outbursts
	Slurred speech
	Staggered gait or ataxia
	Drowsiness
	Diplopia
0.3 g/dL	Aggressive behavior
	Incoherent speech
	Labored breathing
	Vomiting
	Stupor
0.4 g/dL	Coma
0.5 g/dL	Severe respiratory depression
	Death

Adolescents do not have the same behaviors in response to BALs as adults. Their neurologic and physiological responses vary, so their behaviors vary significantly as a result. We need to know three important differences:

No slurred speech

No ataxia

No drowsiness

As a result, the adolescent will not know they are intoxicated, neither will adults. Because they do not get drowsy nothing stops them from drinking, so their levels will become toxic.

MENTAL HEALTH IN THE NEWS

David Hasselhoff

The media exposes us to a variety of situations concerning alcohol. Some are fictional, some are partially autobiographical, and some are real. The fully-fictional or partially fictional depictions often glamorize the situation and minimize the damage and embarrassment. When actor David Hasselhoff was so intoxicated he was crawling around eating a cheeseburger off the floor, he was videotaped. The 2007 home video clip surfaced of Hasselhoff apparently in a drunken stupor. The video showed

him shirtless, lying on the floor, drunkenly trying to consume a cheeseburger in a hotel room. His 17-year-old daughter, who shot the video, can be heard saying, "Tell me you are going to stop, tell me you are going to stop." The video brought the undeniable reality of alcoholic intoxication to light. In 2009, David Hasselhoff was hospitalized with a BAL of 0.39. He has publicly admitted past treatment for alcoholism. As of 2010, he has been hospitalized for an alcohol-related seizure and continued drinking.

Photo courtesy © Everett Collection Inc/Alamy.

Generalized Seizures

Generalized seizures (also known colloquially as "rum fits") may occur 2 to 3 days after the person stops drinking. They can be prevented in a well-monitored medical withdrawal program.

Delirium Tremens

Delirium tremens (DTs), one symptom of withdrawal, is a condition of severe memory disturbance, agitation, anorexia, and hallucinations. The symptoms are described more thoroughly in the section on withdrawal that follows.

Generally, DTs begin a few days after drinking stops and end within 1 to 5 days. They may, however, appear as late as the second week, especially when there is cross-addiction to other drugs. Additional medical illnesses may be present, such as pneumonia, pancreatitis, and hepatic decompensation.

Withdrawal from Alcohol and Medical Treatment

Alcohol withdrawal occurs after the dependent individual stops drinking. This syndrome is composed of a constellation of physiological and behavioral symptoms that occur when the alcohol level drops. Medical treatment of alcoholism involves the management of withdrawal symptoms.

Minor Withdrawal

A *minor withdrawal* from alcohol can occur within 6 to 12 hours after the alcoholic's last drink. These symptoms may last 48 to 72 hours. The appearance of hallucinations (visual, auditory, olfactory, or tactile) and seizures marks the onset of a *major withdrawal*. See the stages of withdrawal from alcohol in Your Assessment Approach.

Major Withdrawal

A major withdrawal is the most advanced, potentially life-threatening stage of alcohol withdrawal. Symptoms appear within 2 to 3 days following the last drink and may last 3 to 5 days. Symptoms associated with DTs usually develop 72 hours after the last drink.

Clinical Example

Sindi and Bert were married for 2 years when Sindi left Bert because of his abusive behavior when drunk. Several weeks later, Bert called and asked Sindi to go on a 3-day cruise with him in a couple of days so he could show her he was sober and to mend their relationship. While on the cruise Sindi noticed how Bert, who was sober, was making special efforts. On the last day of the cruise Bert became very sweaty and feverish during dinner and told Sindi that he thought he caught the flu. On returning to their stateroom, Bert became disoriented, had a seizure, and collapsed. The ship's doctor told Sindi that Bert was going through major withdrawal. He had stopped drinking just before they went on the cruise and was now in the 5th day of abstinence from alcohol.

Treatment of Withdrawal

The best treatment for major alcohol withdrawal involves early detection. Medical treatment for withdrawal includes the following:

1. Monitoring the client's fluid status. If the client is unable to take fluids by mouth, fluids may be administered intravenously.

YOUR ASSESSMENT APPROACH   Stages of Alcohol Withdrawal

State	Peak Time of Onset After Last Drink	Symptoms	Potential Duration of Symptoms
Tremulousness	24 hours	At rest: slight tremors; during activities: gross and irregular tremors	1 week
		Diaphoresis	3–4 days
		Anorexia, nausea, vomiting	3–4 days
		Increased vital signs	3–4 days
		Sense of agitation and inner shakiness	2 weeks
		Insomnia with nightmares of seemingly real events	2 weeks or longer
Tremors and transitory hallucinosis	24 hours	Tremors plus visual hallucinations of events (e.g., having an accident while driving drunk)	3 days
Alcoholic hallucinosis	24 hours	Cues of tremulousness state plus vivid persecutory and auditory hallucinations, agitation, increased suicide, preassaultive potential	3 days–2 weeks
Delirium tremens	24–48 hours	Cues of tremulousness state plus delirium, generalized seizures, disorientation for time and place, visual hallucinations, agitation, panic level of anxiety	3–5 days
Rum fits	24–48 hours	2–6 generalized seizures; cues of delirium tremens	3–5 days

2. Administering magnesium sulfate to decrease the irritability caused by low magnesium levels and to prevent seizures.

3. Administering vitamins, especially thiamine (vitamin B_1) because alcohol interferes with the absorption of B vitamins.

4. Prescribing benzodiazepines, such as diazepam (Valium) or chlordiazepoxide (Librium), to help prevent DTs. Seizures may be treated with IV diazepam, and the client may be placed on phenytoin (Dilantin).

Withdrawal from alcohol, or any chemical substance, should include: controlling the dangerous symptoms of withdrawal and reducing the extreme discomfort. A separate pathway of intoxication, from the agents such as benzodiazepines used to support the withdrawal, needs to be minimized.

Blackouts

Having **blackouts** is frequently confused with passing out. In fact, passing out refers to unconsciousness, whereas a blackout is anterograde amnesia: loss of short-term memories with retention of remote memories. A person can function effectively for several days—talking on the telephone, working, and shopping—yet have absolutely no memory of doing so. To others, the alcoholic may appear normal or "high." This is because the cognitive impairment occurs before motor impairment. Interestingly, alcoholics appear unconcerned about the blackouts and eventually learn to cover them up. This appearance of unconcern may, in part, be due to euphoric recall: The alcoholic recalls feeling good but does not recall his or her behavior. Reality is distorted. Some clients find blackouts very disturbing and seek treatment at that point.

There are two types of blackout, *en bloc* or complete inability to recall a time period and *fragmentary* where the memory loss is not complete. The faster the client's BAL increases, the more likely there will be a blackout. Women are more susceptible to blackouts due to pharmacokinetics and female body composition (Rose & Grant, 2010). When assessing an alcoholic client, determine whether blackouts are part of the symptoms. See the Nursing Care Plan for chronic alcoholism at the end of this chapter.

Alcohol-Induced Persisting Amnestic Disorder

Alcohol-induced persisting amnestic disorder (Korsakoff's syndrome) is a disturbance of short-term memory that occurs in people who have been drinking alcohol heavily for many years and have a thiamine deficiency. Korsakoff's syndrome is the result of damage to the hippocampus and surrounding tissue from heavy alcohol ingestion. If treated early, Korsakoff's syndrome may be avoided. Once this disorder is established, however, it has a chronic irreversible course, and impairment can become severe. It often follows an acute episode of alcoholic encephalopathy.

Alcoholic Encephalopathy

Alcoholic encephalopathy (Wernicke's encephalopathy) is a neurologic disease associated with chronic alcoholism and is characterized by ataxia, sixth cranial nerve palsy, nystagmus, and confusion. Wernicke's encephalopathy may clear spontaneously in a few days or weeks and responds rapidly to large doses of parenteral thiamine in its acute, early stage.

Fetal Alcohol Syndrome

Nurses need to be aware of the harmful effects of alcohol on pregnant women and unborn children. **Fetal alcohol syndrome (FAS)** occurs in children of women who engage in heavy alcohol ingestion during pregnancy. Approximately 1% to 3.5% of babies are born with FAS (Watson, Finkelstein, Gurewich, & Morse, 2011). It is considered the most common nonhereditary form of intellectual disorders.

Physical and mental defects of FAS include severe growth deficiency, heart defects, malformed facial features, intellectual disorder, low birth weight, learning problems, and hyperactivity. The characteristic physical features of a child with FAS are seen in FIGURE 15-4 ■. If a child has one or two of these characteristics, the condition is called fetal alcohol effects (FAE). A baby born to an alcoholic mother may need to be withdrawn gradually from alcohol immediately after birth. Even brief exposure to very small amounts of alcohol may kill fetal brain cells and cause peripheral nerve damage as well.

There is hope as a result of ongoing FAS research at the National Institute of Child Health and Human Development. For up-to-date information about FAS, see the link to the National Organization on Fetal Alcohol Syndrome on the Online Student Resources for this text.

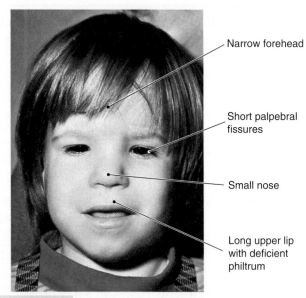

Narrow forehead

Short palpebral fissures

Small nose

Long upper lip with deficient philtrum

FIGURE 15-4 ■ Fetal alcohol syndrome is the result of alcohol consumption during pregnancy, and it can have many severe effects on the child, including physical malformations such as those shown here: narrow forehead, short palpebral fissures, small nose, and long upper lip with deficient philtrum.
Photo courtesy of Streissguth, A. P., Landesman-Swyer, S., Martin, J. C., & Smith, D. W. (1980). Teratogenic effects of alcohol in humans and laboratory animals. "Science, 209," 353–361.

Suicide and Alcoholism

Be alert to the possibility of suicide attempts by alcoholics. Watch for other self-destructive behavior and for events in a client's life that represent a loss such as work, family, health, or legal problems. Such behavior and events put people in a high-risk category. Suicide is thoroughly discussed in Chapter 23 ∞.

BARBITURATES OR SIMILARLY ACTING SEDATIVES OR HYPNOTICS

Barbiturates can be overprescribed for anxiety, stress, and sleep difficulties when health care practitioners treat the symptoms of anxiety, stress, or insomnia without first determining the cause, as in the clinical example that follows.

Clinical Example

Elizabeth, a 45-year-old housewife, has been depressed and irritable over an impending divorce. Her physician prescribed diazepam (Valium) 5 mg for sleep and for anxiety (every 6 hours as needed). Because this dosage was not helping decrease her anxiety as much as she wanted, she increased her dosage and began taking 50 to 100 mg a day over a period of a few weeks. This evening, Elizabeth's estranged husband found her mumbling incoherently. Her speech was slurred, she was bumping into furniture, and she was quite drowsy.

The Effects of Barbiturates, Sedatives, or Hypnotics

Barbiturates are highly addictive drugs that cause people to feel euphoric, yet relaxed. They are frequently prescribed to relieve pain, reduce anxiety (sedative effects), and induce sleep (hypnotic effects). Barbiturates were the first drugs used to treat anxiety and insomnia. They were considered dangerous because of their ability to cause significant CNS depression and their lethality upon overdose.

Anxiolytic drugs, the benzodiazepines (BZDs), began to be widely used because of their ability to reduce anxiety without causing significant CNS depression. However, they also have the drawbacks of producing dependence and withdrawal syndromes. BZDs include many widely prescribed drugs, including diazepam (Valium), clorazepate (Tranxene), lorazepam (Ativan), and alprazolam (Xanax). These drugs are thought to modify anxiety by altering the balance of neurotransmitters, especially norepinephrine (NE) and gamma-aminobutyric acid (GABA) in the brain's limbic system. The limbic system is involved in the regulation of emotion (see Chapter 6∞). These drugs have a high risk for abuse and physical dependence. When the drug stops working and tolerance builds up, people tend to increase the dosage just "to cope." Even the nonbenzodiazepines such as zolpidem (Ambien) and zaleplon (Sonata) can be used to excess and have dependence issues associated with their use (see Chapter 7∞).

Patterns of Use

In party situations, some teenagers and young adults take high doses of barbiturates, often in combination with alcohol, to get "high." The resultant CNS depression makes this practice especially dangerous. "Speed freaks" (amphetamine abusers) use barbiturates to "come down" from a high. Dependence, tolerance, and cross-tolerance to other depressant drugs develop rapidly.

Action

Barbiturates are metabolized in phases by the liver. When taken orally, they are initially absorbed and partially metabolized. However, the unmetabolized parts become active metabolites that are stored in the fatty tissues. Consequently, taking these drugs over a period of time results in a cumulative effect, unsuspected dependence, and possible overdose. Nurses in every area need to be aware of the frequency of substance abuse among their clients and its impact. See What Every Nurse Should Know for further information.

More Americans die from barbiturate overdose than from opioid dependence. Many take alcohol and barbiturates together. While judgment is impaired they take more pills, thereby unintentionally overdosing. Because alcohol and barbiturates are synergistic, an overdose can occur quickly. Barbiturates are often used in suicide attempts (see Chapter 23 ∞).

Withdrawal

Barbiturate withdrawal is unpleasant and life threatening. A deep sleep is followed by decreased respiration, coma, and sometimes death. Babies born to mothers addicted to barbiturates are physically dependent and need to be helped through withdrawal.

Withdrawal from BZDs may produce symptoms similar to those of barbiturate withdrawal. Symptoms include autonomic hyperactivity (alterations in vital signs and diaphoresis), marked anxiety, agitation, insomnia, depression, and seizures. Medically supervised detoxification treatment can prevent a potentially serious emergency during withdrawal.

WHAT EVERY NURSE SHOULD KNOW

Substance-Abusing Client

Imagine that you are an emergency department nurse. When a client comes in, the complaint may be physical or psychiatric in nature and either could be the result of substance use or abuse. Look for the hallmark signs of substance use. In an emergency situation, you would be able to detect substance-abusing clients because they may not be able to answer key questions like these:

- Have you had any medications or drugs today?
- What did you take?
- How much did you take?
- When did you take it?
- What have you taken in the last 24 hours? In the last week?

When clients are not able to provide necessary information, you must rely on family or friends as data sources, and then corroborate what you learn with the client once he or she is alert.

Case Study: Prescription Substance Abuse

OPIOIDS

The opioids include heroin and morphine, derived from the poppy plant, and synthetic drugs, such as oxycodone (OxyContin), meperidine (Demerol), codeine, methadone, and others.

The Effects of Opioids

Opioids have analgesic qualities and are prescribed after surgery. They are quite potent and have the ability to remove painful stimuli. Depending on the person, the drugs may produce a euphoric high, as in drug addicts, but they generally cause people to feel drowsy and out of touch with the world. Postoperative nurses, for example, need to be knowledgeable about the use of opioids as a substance of abuse. See What Every Nurse Should Know for information on this topic.

Heroin addiction by itself is not inherently dangerous. Unless there is an accidental overdose, heroin alone as a substance will not harm the individual. The ancillary issues of possibly contaminated diluting agents, needle cleanliness, and exposure to transmissible diseases such as hepatitis C, tuberculosis, and HIV, along with typically criminal behaviors necessary to support the addiction, put the individual at great risk and make the addicted individual of concern to others. Methadone as a treatment option for these clients has been successful to a certain extent, but is controversial ethically and economically and is viewed as a public health concern.

Patterns of Use

In 1898, heroin became widely available and initially was not believed to be addictive. Within a short time, its addictive properties became known, and the government intervened (Harrison Narcotics Act of 1914). Because most opioid abusers take the drugs intravenously, they are at high risk for HIV/AIDS and hepatitis C. Addiction to opiates has increased recently. Overdose, malnutrition, and infections spread by dirty drugs and needles are dangers. The potency of the drug can vary. Dealers often add impurities to "cut" the heroin, thus increasing the quantity and their own profit. The impurities may cause poisoning and other problems. The varied potency can also cause accidental overdoses as the client may use more than intended because of a delay in effect or a suboptimal intoxication.

Overdose

Constricted pupils, euphoria, psychomotor retardation, slurred speech, and/or drowsiness indicate opioid intoxication.

> ### Clinical Example
>
> Steven, a 20-year-old male, arrived at the hospital in an ambulance. He was unconscious. His respirations were slow, and his pupils were pinpoints. "Tracks" were visible on his arms and behind his knees. A source said Steven had just "shot up" heroin.

If a client overdoses, naloxone (Narcan) is given intravenously (IV). It is a fast-acting narcotic antagonist that counteracts respiratory depression. Abdominal cramps, rhinorrhea, and lacrimation may be treated with belladonna alkaloids or with phenobarbital.

Withdrawal

Because opioids are physically addictive, withdrawal is a threat. People who use high doses of a drug and who "shoot up" or "mainline" (IV drug use) are at high risk for severe withdrawal symptoms. Withdrawal symptoms are usually evident within 12 hours after the last dose. The person experiences the most severe withdrawal within 36 to 48 hours, with the symptoms decreasing gradually over 2 weeks. During this stressful time, the person craves the drug and may terminate treatment against advice of health professionals.

Babies born to addicted mothers must be treated for opioid withdrawal. These babies are irritable and have high-pitched crying, increased respirations, fever, sneezing, yawning, and tremors.

Treatment

In 1964, methadone was introduced to treat opiate addiction. By the late 1960s and early 1970s, when federal governments allocated money for treatment, methadone maintenance programs mushroomed all over North America. Methadone, a synthetic narcotic, was dispensed daily at clinics to narcotic addicts.

Although addictive, methadone does not produce the ecstatic feeling (rush) associated with heroin. Methadone alleviates the addict's craving for narcotics and, therefore, was expected to decrease the illicit drug trafficking, theft, prostitution, and crime necessary to obtain money for the drugs, thereby allowing addicts to lead productive lives. Also, methadone therapy is far less expensive than residential programs or jail. Methadone maintenance programs are only one treatment option for opioid addicts.

WHAT EVERY NURSE SHOULD KNOW

Pain Medication Use and Overuse

Imagine you are a postoperative nurse. Following a surgical procedure, it is important to instruct your clients on the proper use of pain medications to prevent establishing chronic pain pathways. At the same time, you have to be vigilant not to instruct your clients in such a way that promotes inadvertent or deliberate overuse of pain medications. There will be times when people electively choose repeated surgeries so they have access to pain medications. Under these circumstances, it is important to evaluate the client's intent for surgical interventions and also attend to the client's follow-up behaviors after each surgery. Assess for substance dependence in the form of prescription pain medication overuse or dependence. Use the assessment skills described in this chapter to ensure healthy recoveries and intervene appropriately.

EVIDENCE-BASED PRACTICE

Office-Based Treatments for Substance Abuse

Craven is a 33-year-old native of Britain who has been in the United States since high school. Although bright and active in sports in high school, he began socializing with a group using alcohol and marijuana regularly and cocaine and heroin on occasion. After high school his activities dwindled and his opportunities shrank as he spent more and more time with these friends. Within a few years he was marginally functional and lived solely to obtain heroin. Five years ago, Craven agreed to enter a treatment program on the insistence and with the help of his large extended family.

A significant barrier to Craven's treatment and subsequent recovery has been the lack of available treatment slots at methadone clinics. You are involved as the nurse in an office-based buprenorphine treatment program that incorporates psychosocial treatments and education. Research shows that selected clients do well in this type of program in an office setting.

As part of your role, you present information about access to these types of office-based programs at various community centers. It was at one of these presentations that you met Craven and his mother. As a result, you were able to assess his circumstances, noting that best practices and guidelines at your site outline treatment options for Craven's problems. You provided Craven with the access to treatment that may allow his recovery to proceed unimpeded.

Action should be based on more than one review of treatment modalities, but the following may be helpful in this situation.

Nicholls, L., Bragaw, L., & Ruetsch, C. (2010). Opioid dependence treatment and guidelines. *Journal of Managed Care Pharmacology, 16*(1–b), S14–S21.

CRITICAL THINKING QUESTIONS

1. What factors do you believe will increase the likelihood that Craven will benefit from an office-based treatment program?
2. What factors do you believe will decrease this likelihood?
3. How can Craven's mother be helpful to him?

Another option is buprenorphine (Buprenex), a partial opioid agonist that relieves opioid withdrawal symptoms and cravings for 24 hours or longer. Buprenorphine has a much lower risk of overdose than methadone and is preferred for people at high risk for methadone toxicity, those who might need shorter-term maintenance therapy, and those with limited access to methadone treatment. The initial dose should be given only after the client is in withdrawal. The therapeutic dose range for most clients is 8 to 16 mg daily. People at higher risk for abuse and diversion (selling or bartering) such as IV drug users are given fewer tablets of buprenorphine at each appointment. This means the client must return more frequently to receive the medication. People who fail buprenorphine treatment should be referred for methadone- or abstinence-based treatment. Office-based treatment of opiate addictions is discussed in Evidence-Based Practice.

AMPHETAMINES OR SIMILARLY ACTING SYMPATHOMIMETICS

Amphetamines belong to a group of compounds called *sympathomimetics;* amphetamines are also referred to colloquially as "speed." This group of compounds contains synthetic drugs derived from ephedrine that stimulate the release of adrenaline and speed up the user's system—hence the common name. There are growing problems with chemicals being used as substances of abuse. See TABLE 15-1 ■ for a list of the many versions and effects of these drugs, as well as the original purpose of some of them. The following clinical example shows how the best intentions can lead to dire and unexpected consequences.

Clinical Example

Laura, a 16-year-old high school girl, was on a diet so she could get into her favorite bathing suit. Her friend's brother, a pharmacist, gave her some Dexedrine "just until you lose the weight." Laura's mother initially noticed her rather unusual hyperactivity, her euphoria, and the fact that she refused dinner. Over a period of a few weeks, Laura's behavior changed. She appeared suspicious and irritable and continued to speak and move rapidly, and her grades dropped significantly. Laura was rushed to the hospital after being found unconscious in the girls' locker room at school.

The Effects of Amphetamines

In small doses, amphetamines cause a person to feel energetic and euphoric. A growing number of people take amphetamines (uppers) to counteract the effects of barbiturates (downers) in a cyclic fashion. Amphetamines are dangerous because they alter judgment and obscure feelings. Taken in high doses or intravenously, amphetamines can have dangerous side effects. Tolerance develops rapidly, and chronic abusers may suffer a toxic, paranoid psychosis. Argumentativeness, delusions, hallucinations, stereotypic compulsive behavior, increased libido, interpersonal sensitivity, panic, and violence may occur (APA, 2000).

Amphetamines act by mimicking two of the brain's most important neurotransmitters, dopamine (DA) and norepinephrine (NE). A drug must be able to act on a receptor site or on a number of receptor sites to have an impact. The body may not have a specific amphetamine or cocaine receptor site, so amphetamine and cocaine will take what is called *illegal control* at the existing receptor sites. Dopamine and dopamine

TABLE 15-1 ■ Chemicals Used as Substances of Abuse

Chemical/Herb	Street Name	Used/Abused for	Physical Effects	Chemical Use
Combined methedrone and methylenedioxypy-rovalerone	Bath Salts Ivory Bliss Wave Bliss White Lightening Hurricane Charlie Vanilla Sky	Stimulant	Increase blood pressure Increase heart rate Agitation Hallucinations Extreme paranoia Delusions Death	Insecticide Plant food Pond scum cleaner
Salvia divinorum	Salvia Shepherdess's Herb Maria Pastora Magic Mint Sally-D	Hallucinogenic plant Feeling apart from the body (dissociated)	Hallucinations	
Ayahuasca	Ayahuasca	Hallucinogenic plant	Purging Cleansing Hallucinations	
Inhalants	Laughing Gas Poppers Snappers Whippets	Loss of inhibitions Feeling high	Headache Nausea or vomiting Slurred speech Loss of motor coordination Wheezing/cramps Muscle weakness Depression Memory impairment Damage to cardiovascular and nervous systems Unconsciousness Sudden death	Aerosol propellants Paint thinner Gasoline or fuel Adhesives or glues

receptor sites are intricately involved in the effects substances of abuse have on the nervous systems of clients. (The specific ways in which morphine, amphetamine, and cocaine are involved in this process are shown in FIGURE 15-5 ■.) Chronic use of methamphetamines changes the way a person thinks and behaves because the brain's cortex is no longer activated during decision making. This change in the ability of the brain to transport dopamine, to any significant degree, creates the clinical characteristics you see as severe psychiatric symptoms.

Patterns of Use

Amphetamine was first synthesized in 1887, and experimental medical use began in the 1920s (McGuinness, 2006). In the 1950s and 1960s, amphetamines were heralded as wonder drugs for depression, management of obesity, and exhaustion. By the 1970s their dangers became known and today they are prescribed less frequently because alternative compounds are available to safely and effectively treat those symptoms. Amphetamines are still used to control appetite and treat depression, narcolepsy, minimal brain dysfunctions, and attention deficit disorders in children. Amphetamine abusers are usually teenagers or young adults who are looking for a good time. The uninformed—truck drivers on long road trips, students studying for exams, and athletes—hoping for alertness and improved performance can be lured into the "speed trap."

Amphetamine abusers crave these drugs and require higher and higher dosages. Abusers are rowdy, paranoid, and irritable. A depression (crash), often with suicidal symptoms, may last for several weeks. It is so uncomfortable that the user ingests more amphetamines in an attempt to feel better and develops a cyclical pattern of using and crashing.

Physiologically, the overuse of speed has been tied to stroke and death. Diazepam given intravenously (IV) decreases tachycardia and the chance of convulsions. Depression, anxiety, and increased stress symptoms are the most common psychological pitfalls in recovering from the use of speed. Changes in neurotransmitter activity increase the client's sensitivity to stress and may contribute to the spontaneous recurrence of amphetamine and methamphetamine psychosis, called *flashbacks* (Akiyama, Saito, & Shimoda, 2011). Recurrent flashbacks contribute to recurrent major mood disorders.

Methamphetamine

The most hypercharged form of speed is methamphetamine (MA). It is less expensive than cocaine and has similar CNS stimulant characteristics. MA use has become an enormous public health/substance abuse issue. Recipes for manufacturing MA in home drug labs using everyday ingredients (over-the-counter pseudoephedrine, starter fluids, and drain cleaner) are widely available and have influenced how these products

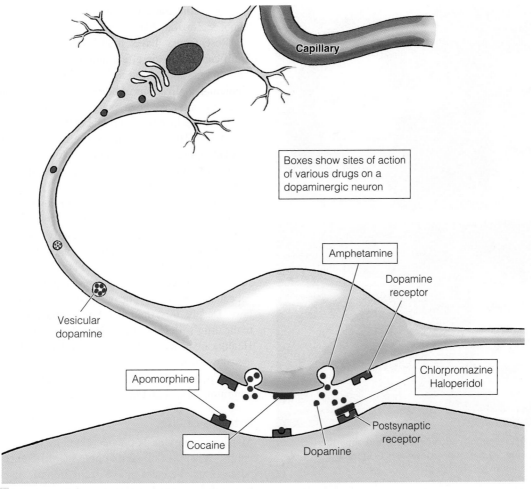

FIGURE 15-5 ■ Action of drugs on dopaminergic neurons. Note how apomorphine can take the place of dopamine in the receptor, and cocaine can perform the blocked reception of a neurotransmitter instead of an antipsychotic.
Source: Smock, T. K. (1999). *Physiological psychology: A neuroscience approach.* Upper Saddle River, NJ: Prentice Hall.

are sold. For example, as a result of the Combat Methamphetamine Epidemic Act of 2005, pseudoephedrine is now stocked behind the pharmacist's counter and buyers, especially those who purchase pseudoephedrine frequently or in large quantities, can be tracked and reported. Lower-quality MA is called "speed" or "crank"; higher-quality MA is sold in small chunks as "glass" or "ice" because of its crystalline appearance. It is a maximum stimulant with maximum risks.

Exposure to MA is neurotoxic, and long-term use leads to extensive neural damage. Physiological changes include cognitive impairments, MA-induced psychosis, inadequate perfusion, and ischemic lesions of the brain. MA morphologically changes the corpus callosum and causes skin lesions, perinatal complications, and hypertension (Nakama et al., 2011). Each of these impacts has consequences that are far reaching for a person's health and functioning. See FIGURE 15-6 ■ for before and after pictures of methamphetamine users. The changes in appearance demonstrate the severity of the physiological effects.

The National Survey on Drug Use and Health (NSDUH) Report (2009) on Methamphetamine Use is available online at http://www.oas.samhsa.gov/nhsda.htm and on the Online Student Resources for this text. Methamphetamine use is an enormous public health problem; young adults 18 to 25 years old were more likely than adolescents (12 to 17 years old) to use methamphetamine in the past year and more likely than adults older than 26 years to use MA.

Treatment for MA addiction continues to be a combination of behavioral and psychosocial approaches. Cognitive–behavioral therapy (CBT) and contingency management where the client has a backup plan for each stage of recovery have been the most successful versions of behavioral and psychosocial treatment (Roll, Rawson, Ling, & Shoptaw, 2009). CBT and other behavioral therapies are discussed further in Chapter 30 ∞. There is reason to be hopeful and optimistic about the recovery of MA addicts.

Withdrawal

Chlorpromazine (Thorazine) combats the physiological effects of amphetamines. Diazepam (Valium), given intravenously, decreases tachycardia and the chance of convulsions. Depression and anxiety are the most common psychological

FIGURE 15-6 ■ Weight loss, apparent stress, and opportunistic infections are some of the visible consequences of using methamphetamine.
Photo courtesy of Faces of Meth Program.

pitfalls in recovering from the use of speed. Physiologically, the overuse of speed has been tied to stroke and even death.

CANNABIS

Marijuana arrived in North America in the early 1900s. Although it has been illegal in the United States since 1937 and remains so even with individual states making exceptions under certain circumstances, marijuana is used more than any other chemical except tobacco, alcohol, and caffeine.

The Effects of Cannabis

Derived from an Indian hemp plant (*Cannabis sativa*), marijuana contains the psychoactive substance delta 6-3,4-tetrahydrocannabinol (THC). THC is found in the sticky yellow resin secreted by the tops and leaves of the ripe plants. Unlike alcohol, which is water-soluble and leaves the body through urine, breath, and perspiration, THC is stored in the fatty tissues (especially the brain and reproductive system). Consequently, it can be detected in the body for up to 6 weeks. The potency of marijuana has steadily increased over the years. Although marijuana contains over 400 chemicals, the THC content determines the potency. With an increase in potency comes an increase in health problems. There is compelling evidence that underlying neurochemical mechanisms reinforce the reward and dependence features of this

drug and contribute to continued use and relapse (Logrip, Koob, & Zorrilla, 2011).

Researchers have found that marijuana produces a significant analgesic effect and is modestly effective against the nausea and vomiting associated with chemotherapy. Medicinal applications of both THC and cannabidiol (a derivative) on pain have been examined, showing significant pain relief. Dronabinol is a synthetic delta 9-tetrahydrocannabinol or delta-9-THC that contains standardized THC content in an FDA-approved pharmaceutical. It is mainly used to treat weight loss, nausea, and vomiting associated with a number of medical conditions.

The medical use of marijuana for the treatment of nausea, glaucoma, cachexia, pain, and spasticity has been consistently supported by the medical community, but there are legal and ethical risks for us as professionals that are not new and remain problematic (Nelson, 2011). The U.S. Department of Justice announced in 2009 that users and distributors of medical cannabis would not be pursued as long as they follow state laws. Despite this, the federal government resists any change to the drug's illegal status at the national level (Nelson, 2011). Health care providers in 14 states and the District of Columbia are allowed to treat with medical marijuana without risking loss of license. The use of medical marijuana is a subject of continuing social and medical debate.

Patterns of Use

Marijuana smoking is prevalent among teenagers and young adults. Schepis et al. (2011) note the differences in use with adolescents. Females move from initially using marijuana to regular use much faster than males. Long-term marijuana use has been associated with both physical and emotional changes, as seen in the clinical example.

Clinical Example

Joe, a 35-year-old captain of a rescue squad, was having trouble at his job. He paid less and less attention to the accuracy of his client reports; he was often late for work; he forgot to repair and replace his equipment, causing his unit to be unsafe and ill-equipped. Joe told an emergency department nurse that he felt all the marijuana he was smoking was beginning to affect him. He revealed that he'd been a daily smoker for 5 years. At first, he felt there were no long-term effects, but lately he was concerned because "I never feel like doing anything." He has trouble concentrating, forgets what he is talking about in midsentence, and is unmotivated to make any positive changes in his life.

Because marijuana smoking is so prevalent among teenagers and because its dangers are becoming increasingly known (see Box 15-2), some health care professionals advocate urine screening when teenagers have a checkup by a family doctor. Chemical dependence takes 10 to 15 years to develop in adults and only a few years to develop in a child. Children are less successful in drug rehabilitation than adults. Because of this danger, pediatric clinicians should initiate educational and treatment programs on drug and alcohol abuse. Likewise, psychiatric–mental health nurses need to respond to this vital

---

Box 15-2 Dangers of Marijuana

Marijuana

- Appears to lower testosterone levels in males.
- Chemicals may accumulate in ovaries, although hormone levels remain normal.
- Affects brain wave test results; teenagers who get high twice a week or more often have evidence of diffuse brain impairment for up to 2 months after the last time they use the drug. They experience disruptions in learning, short-term memory loss, problems concentrating, and amotivation syndrome (confusion, declining performance, and difficulty finishing tasks).
- Causes neurocognitive deficits in attention, learning, memory, and intellectual functioning.

- After effects are durable; THC can be found in the blood and urine for up to 2 weeks after smoking; if the THC is radioactively labeled, it can be detected for up to a month.

Marijuana Smoke

- Has 50% more tar than regular cigarette smoke
- Produces greater cellular damage in the lungs than cigarette smoke.
- Contains 70% more benzopyrene, a major cancer-causing chemical.
- Can cause emphysema 20 times faster than tobacco.
- Increases airway resistance 25% under laboratory conditions in which a similar amount of tobacco smoke produces no significant increase in airway resistance.

---

public health issue. For information on efforts to prevent and treat youth drug abuse, see the Center for Treatment Research on Adolescent Drug Abuse (CTRADA) website via the Online Student Resources for this book.

Marijuana use is endemic in the teenage culture. Therefore, nurses who work with teenagers must be knowledgeable about marijuana and its effects. When admitting a teenager to a psychiatric unit or interviewing a teenager as an outpatient, be aware of a variety of indicators of marijuana use. Parents need to be knowledgeable about marijuana use and alert to the following indications that it is being used:

- Marijuana smells like hemp or burning rope.
- Teenagers often burn incense or use perfumed sprays to mask its pungent odor.
- Teenagers may use eyedrops (Murine) so that their eyes will not be red, and they may cough a lot. Conjunctival redness and coughing can occur with marijuana use.
- A teenager who uses marijuana may have smoking paraphernalia—plastic baggies filled with dried leaves, rolling papers, and "roach" clips (clips that hold the marijuana cigarette once it becomes too small to handle).

COCAINE

Since cocaine abuse has been recognized as a widespread problem, government agencies have spent significant amounts of money trying to block cocaine shipments from South America. Planes, boats, and "mules" (people who transport cocaine) have been seized, and tons of cocaine have been confiscated and destroyed. Yet, it remains plentiful and is purer today than ever before. The cocaine industry is a multibillion-dollar enterprise involving bribery, corruption, and murder.

The Effects of Cocaine

Cocaine is a stimulant extracted from the leaves of the coca plant that has long been known and used. For hundreds of years, South American Indians chewed coca leaves, enjoying the effects of decreased appetite and increased ability to

work at high altitudes. Slaves became more productive when given cocaine. Freud experimented with cocaine. It was an ingredient in Coca-Cola before federal regulations prohibited it in 1903. Today, cocaine is used as a local anesthetic in ear, nose, and throat surgery. When inhaled or injected, cocaine produces alertness and energy and makes users feel sociable, confident, and "in control." The drug blocks appetite and erases fatigue, which makes it appear to be an ideal performance booster.

Although cocaine is not believed to be physically addicting, it is psychologically addicting. Those who use cocaine heavily or regularly frequently encounter great difficulty in discontinuing its use. Cocaine addicts develop a tolerance to the drug, using amounts that would previously have been lethal to them. Euphoria diminishes with tolerance. The development of new dendrites (branches of the nerve cells) to aid the uptake of the increased amount of DA accounts for the tolerance. Ultimately, the cocaine no longer produces pleasure, but not taking it feels even worse. Dopamine is eventually depleted, and the user becomes chronically fatigued, irritable, and anxious, even mentally confused and paranoid, as in the clinical example that follows.

Clinical Example

Will, a 32-year-old male, was brought to the hospital by his father. He was talkative and jumpy, and his eyes darted around the exam room. He repeatedly wiped his nose with his finger and rubbed the bottom of his face. He acted suspicious and kept saying someone was after him. His family stated he had a $400-a-day cocaine habit. He began casually snorting a few lines once in a while when he needed a sense of control over his full load of graduate school courses and full-time job. His cocaine use increased to every day, then every few hours.

Suicide attempts, accidents, and overdoses are common. The only effect of cocaine that is increased as tolerance develops is its ability to induce a convulsion or seizure. Be sure to carefully assess clients to differentiate the symptoms of cocaine use from the symptoms of bipolar disorder and chronic anxiety. Figure 15-7 ■ illustrates the cocaine use cycle.

CTRADA

Animation: Cocaine Drug Mechanism in Action

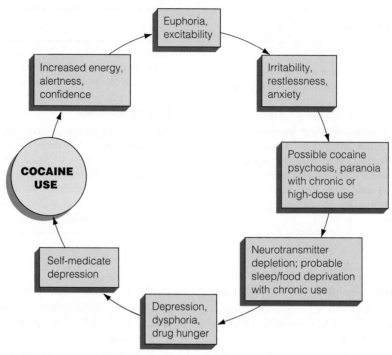

FIGURE 15-7 ■ The cycle of cocaine use.
Source: Reprinted with permission from Mim Landry, Danya International, Silver Spring, MD.

Cocaine Intoxication

Interestingly, the symptoms of low-level cocaine intoxication are similar to those of alcohol withdrawal: sweating, dilated pupils, psychomotor agitation, and increased blood pressure/heart rate. With higher doses of cocaine, a person becomes increasingly intoxicated. Symptoms include high fever, cardiac arrhythmia, seizures, hallucinations, and a paranoid schizophrenic syndrome. Hallucinations typically involve "cocaine bugs," which feel like bugs under the skin. The client may scratch furiously in an attempt to get rid of them. Haloperidol (Haldol) is used to combat the psychotic symptoms; phenothiazines should not be used because they may decrease the seizure threshold.

The strength of the physiological effects of cocaine is revealed in animal research. Monkeys work harder at pressing a bar to receive cocaine intravenously than to get any other drug. Even when starving to death or when confronted with a sexually receptive female, monkeys continue pressing the bar. Receiving an electric shock every time they touch the bar does not alter their behavior. Research with cocaine users indicates that the medication bromocriptine mesylate (Parlodel), a DA receptor agonist, eliminates the craving that users feel after they stop using cocaine. Cocaine initially increases DA neurotransmission. Over time, however, cocaine abuse depletes DA in the brain, and this depletion may be the basis for craving.

The "Post-Coke" Blues

It has not been proven that cocaine is physically addictive, but its ability to cause psychological dependence is clear (recall that cocaine users crave the drug). After a brief post-use euphoria (lasting approximately 5 to 10 minutes), they experience a strong desire to repeat the high. This high is followed by a crash—a terrible letdown called the "post-coke blues," or *cocaine abstinence syndrome*. Anxiety, depression, and fatigue are part of this syndrome. The cocaine crash, lasting approximately 30 to 60 minutes, results from depletion of DA, the neurotransmitter responsible for feelings of pleasure and well-being. The addict responds to the crash by feeling irritable, depressed, and tired. Although the brain needs to synthesize more DA (because of chemical misprogramming resulting from the addiction) it craves more cocaine, which offers immediate relief. The crash intensity appears to be related to the amount of cocaine used. In an attempt to feel better and reduce these uncomfortable symptoms, addicts often use other drugs, such as alcohol, marijuana, or sleeping pills, during the crash.

One addict described the post-coke blues as "pure hell, the most painful depression I have ever felt. I wanted to die from the pain." This painful depression, along with the memory of the cocaine high, causes people to want to use cocaine again and again to recapture the momentary ecstasy. The period of agitation, anxiety, and insomnia usually ceases within 2 weeks.

Patterns of Use

Smokable forms of cocaine that have an effect similar to that of the injectable drug are in great demand. With the advent of cheaper rock cocaine, cocaine is now available to people in all cultural and socioeconomic groups. Intranasal cocaine users place themselves at risk for hepatitis C. Those who inject cocaine place themselves at risk for HIV/AIDS as well as hepatitis C.

Treatment

Detoxification for cocaine abusers depends on the client's symptoms. In some treatment centers, the procedure is detoxification by going "cold turkey"; no medications are used to ease withdrawal symptoms. Options using medications include diazepam administered intravenously at a slow rate, oral diazepam, or PRN diazepam protocols. Phenobarbital in decreasing doses and imipramine hydrochloride (Tofranil) are other options.

Because the depression is so great, Tofranil or other tricyclic antidepressants (TCAs) may be given for several weeks after detoxification. TCAs build up existing levels of neurotransmitters and make them available for transmission. Beta-adrenergic blockers such as propranolol (Inderal) may be used to counteract the tachycardia and hypertension that accompany acute cocaine intoxication, but their use may result in paroxysmal hypertension due to unopposed alpha-adrenergic stimulation. Therefore, they should be used cautiously and with constant blood pressure monitoring.

Using TCAs to increase the number of neurotransmitters in the synapse is called *synaptic treatment*. Postsynaptic treatment for cocaine withdrawal and dependence includes the use of medications such as bromocriptine (Parlodel) or amantadine (Symmetrel), which increase dopaminergic activity in the synapse and enhance the effects of DA on the postsynaptic receptors.

Crack

Crack, or "rock" cocaine, is a potent form of hydrochloride cocaine that is mixed with baking soda and water, heated, allowed to harden, and then broken or "cracked" into little pieces and smoked. Crack is more insidious, addictive, and toxic than cocaine. One user said, "I am worse in 3 weeks of using crack than in 6 years of using cocaine."

Crack is cheap and fairly easily acquired. A crack high has a rapid onset and is intensely euphoric, followed by a dramatic crash. Within seconds after "coming down," users feel compelled to smoke more crack. Because addiction is so rapid, many people are "hooked" and seek help when they can no longer support their habit. Crack users are flooding treatment centers, many of which have long waiting lists. Recidivism is estimated at over 90%. See Your Self-Awareness for guidance in dealing with the frustration and discouragement common in work with substance-abusing clients.

Symptoms of Crack Use

Symptoms of crack use include irritability, paranoia, depression, and physical symptoms that accompany the smoking of a toxic chemical, such as wheezing and coughing blood and black phlegm. Cardiac dysrhythmias caused by crack use may lead to death.

The number of babies being born to mothers who use crack is growing. These babies are more likely to be premature or have low birth weights and microcephaly. They are irritable and exhibit tremors and muscle rigidity.

YOUR SELF-AWARENESS
Maintaining Therapeutic Optimism

- *Realize that both mental illness and substance disorders are chronic, relapsing conditions.* Understand that progress may be slow and setbacks inevitable despite your best efforts and those of the client. Appreciate small steps forward and reframe setbacks as learning opportunities.
- *Understand that even if a client is not currently making much effort toward better management of his or her disorders, the development of a trusting relationship with you is helping to set the stage for movement toward recovery in the future.* A positive, valued relationship with a mental health professional is one of the factors that prompt mental health clients to move toward sobriety.
- *Talk to people who are in recovery.* Hearing about how these individuals overcame challenges to become happier and more stable will give you more confidence that clients who are currently struggling with similar obstacles can also overcome them.
- *Don't be afraid to talk to clients about spirituality.* Mental health providers often underestimate how important spiritual concerns are in the lives of clients with substance disorders. Ask clients about their spiritual beliefs and practices, and be flexible in helping clients find support for their spirituality. Access to these inner resources is especially important when clients lack external support.
- *Find mentors who are successful in working with clients with substance disorders.* Seek their help in dealing with situations you find difficult or frustrating.
- *Take good care of your own physical, mental, and spiritual health.* You can role-model healthy behavior for clients (never underestimate the power of a good example!), and renewing your own energy means you have more to give in your relationships with clients.

Freebase

Freebase is a purified form of cocaine made by applying solvents to ordinary cocaine. Melting the cocaine with small butane torches helps in the purifying and delivery process. This action alone is dangerous due to the hazard of the solvent exploding. The effects of freebase are brief but intense, and the short euphoria (3 to 5 minutes) immediately becomes a restless desire for more "base."

PHENCYCLIDINE (PCP)

PCP was originally used as an anesthetic for humans and as a tranquilizer for animals. Because of its dangerous side effects, it was removed from the market except for veterinary use. However, by the mid-1960s PCP was readily available as a street drug. PCP is inexpensive and easily synthesized by home chemists, making a ready supply always available.

The Effects of PCP

People who use PCP frequently arrive at the emergency department in a psychotic, violent, and agitated state. The agitation and sensations generate incredible power and strength in the user so that even a small, slight person is capable of breaking heavy glass or fighting several people.

Clinical Example

Pete, an 18-year-old college student, was offered marijuana at a fraternity party. After smoking several joints, he was driving home with a friend when he became severely agitated. He insisted his friend stop the car near a pay phone; he jumped out and attempted to call the police, believing someone was trying to kill him. When the police arrived because of the disturbance he was causing (by then he was shouting and hallucinating), he rushed them, kicking at a passerby and shooting at them as if he had a gun. During an assessment interview, the friend confessed to putting PCP in the marijuana.

Some users fluctuate between coma and violence. Hallucinations are common. A differential diagnosis is important but difficult because the symptoms are similar to those of schizophrenia. It is believed that schizophrenics are particularly sensitive to PCP and that PCP may aggravate symptoms of schizophrenia.

A PCP high appears about 5 minutes after a person takes the drug and lasts 4 to 6 hours. Effects may last up to 48 hours. PCP may be recovered from the blood and urine for 7 to 10 days. While using PCP, a person experiences an unpredictable and wide variety of feelings ranging from euphoria and utter peace to violence, confusion, and disorganization. Distorted sensory perceptions are common. During a bad "trip," anxiety, fear, and paranoia predominate. The dramatic physical and emotional effects of PCP may last for several weeks. Users may suffer from depression, fatigue, memory loss, concentration difficulty, and poor impulse control.

A substance very similar to PCP is ketamine, also known as Special K, K, Vitamin K, and Cat Valium, among other names. Distorted perceptions of sight and sound and feelings of detachment—dissociation—from the environment and self are mind altering but not hallucinations. PCP and ketamine are therefore more properly known as "dissociative anesthetics." Dextromethorphan, a widely available cough suppressant, when taken in high doses can produce effects similar to those of PCP and ketamine. Dissociative drugs act by altering distribution of the neurotransmitter glutamate throughout the brain. Glutamate is involved in perception of pain, responses to the environment, and memory. PCP is considered the typical dissociative drug, and the description of PCP's actions and effects largely applies to ketamine and dextromethorphan as well.

Ketamine has a much shorter duration of action than PCP and is used recreationally because of its sedative and hallucinogenic properties. It can cause delirium, amnesia, tachycardia, anxiety, and high blood pressure. Ketamine use increases every year, as does the use of the club drug GHB and Rohypnol (the date rape drug, discussed later in this chapter and in Chapter 24 ∞).

A vital problem with PCP is the question of its purity and concentration. Because it is generally manufactured illegally, users never really know what they are buying.

Adulterants used in street drugs are often toxic to humans, causing a wide variety of responses, including death. Originally called the "peace pill," PCP is now recognized for its potential to cause violence, especially when the drug is taken in high dosages.

Treatment

Treatment of acute PCP intoxication may include the use of diazepam (Valium) for muscle spasms, seizures, and agitation. Risperidone (Risperdal) or haloperidol (Haldol) may be used for severe psychotic behavior, but phenothiazines should not be used because PCP is anticholinergic. The combined anticholinergia of phenothiazines and PCP creates a number of severe side effects, including hallucinations. Calcium channel blockers such as verapamil may be given. These drugs are thought to prevent or reverse PCP-induced vasospasm, thereby decreasing the hallucinogenic effects of PCP. This treatment is controversial, however, because some clinicians believe that the use of verapamil may potentiate the effects of PCP.

Treatment during the acute phase of PCP intoxication should focus also on protecting the client and others from injury and reorienting the client to reality. Providing a quiet, safe environment and addressing the client calmly in a reassuring manner are important.

HALLUCINOGENS

Hallucinogens are synthetic and natural drugs that cause hallucinations and unusual sensory experiences. Developed in 1938 for scientific research, LSD (lysergic acid diethylamide) became popular in the 1960s when Timothy Leary, a Harvard psychologist, described how it stimulated great insight and increased awareness. In the 1960s and 1970s, the U.S. Army experimented with LSD by giving it without informed consent to unsuspecting army employees. One dramatic and much-publicized event concerned an army officer who leapt to his death from a window after unknowingly ingesting LSD. Once the danger of LSD use was publicized, the unethical research became public knowledge. Physician researchers also were interested in experimenting with the uses of LSD in the treatment of a variety of diseases; however, in 1966 LSD became illegal and could no longer be used in human research.

Peyote, the active hallucinogen in cactus buttons, is still an integral part of religious rituals of Native Americans in the southwestern United States and Mexico. Psilocybin is the active hallucinogen in certain mushrooms, sometimes called "magic mushrooms." Ayahuasca is an herb used in South America and Canada that also causes hallucinations as well as the physical symptoms of extreme gastrointestinal distress.

The Effects of Hallucinogens

After a lull in use, LSD ("acid") is again being used by teenagers because it is cheap ($2 to $5 a "hit") and causes an intense high that lasts 6 to 12 hours. It is typically delivered orally, usually on absorbent blotter paper (FIGURE 15-8 ■), a sugar cube, or gelatin. Teenagers today are unacquainted with the LSD horror stories of the 1960s. Today, people use LSD

FIGURE 15-8 ▧ Blotter LSD. Both LSD and the psilocybin in "magic mushrooms" induce psychedelic effects; however, LSD is much more potent than psilocybin (a product of various kinds of mushrooms).
Photo courtesy of Martin/Custom Medical Stock Photo.

predominantly to get high rather than to expand consciousness. Psychological and physical dependence are unlikely because each experience with a hallucinogen is different. Increased creativity and brilliant personality revelations, presumed effects of the drugs, are short-lived at best.

Clinical Example

Two high school seniors decided to take LSD. After 8 hours, one student was enjoying music, describing the varied colors he saw as the music changed in tempo. The other student was sweating profusely. His pupils were dilated, and he was trembling. He saw brightly colored dogs with huge teeth and claws changing into cats, snakes, and lions. He said he felt his gallbladder working with his liver and stomach. He eventually became so out of control that the other student took him to the emergency department.

Treatment

The dangers of hallucinogens include "bad trips" and flashbacks.

Bad Trips

Users who experience *bad trips* may appear psychotic and extremely fearful. Reassuring the person and pointing out reality are helpful; occasionally, tranquilizers or antipsychotics are given. The symptoms usually disappear within 12 hours but may persist for months. People who are mentally ill or emotionally conflicted are more likely to have bad trips and flashbacks and to require hospitalization than are ordinary users.

Flashbacks

Flashbacks are a spontaneous reliving of the experiences the person felt while under the influence of the drug, although the person is drug free. The experience may involve perceptual distortions, a variety of physical feelings, and strong emotions

such as fear and pleasure. Flashbacks are generally brief, and they occur less frequently over time. Flashbacks may be induced by stress, fatigue, and drug or alcohol ingestion.

Some authorities believe hallucinogens pose a particular danger to adolescents in that they may precipitate a psychosis. Because teenagers' egos and defenses are weak, they may be especially susceptible to the effects of hallucinogens.

INHALANTS

Inhalants—glue, fuels, paints, aerosols, air fresheners, the substance used to resole shoes, hairspray, and the propellants in canned whipped cream—are popular among school-age children because they are cheap and easy to obtain. An unusual new development in preferences for inhalants has recently been noted: embalming fluid.

The Effects of Inhalants

The abuse of inhalants is increasing at a frightening rate. Inhalants are inexpensive, easily available, and often legal. Their use causes euphoria, light-headedness, and excitement. Children are the most frequent users. Adult users often have a long history of polydrug abuse.

Clinical Example

Carlos is an 11-year-old homeless child from Brazil living on the streets in Miami, Florida. He came to the attention of the clinic because he had been arrested for purse snatching. On clinical examination, Carlos appears giddy, dirty, disheveled, confused, and belligerent. His speech is slurred, he has an unsteady gait, and he smells like glue. His eyes are red and tearing, he is coughing, and he is nauseated. He has avoided attending school and has received no health care.

Patterns of Use

Inhalants are sniffed or inhaled (called "huffing") in a variety of ways, such as from a rag soaked with the inhalant and placed in a plastic bag. Gas is frequently inhaled directly from a tank. Amyl and butyl nitrate (called "poppers") can be easily concealed and passed around a classroom, and paint thinner can be concealed in a soft drink can. Metallic colored spray paints are popular choices as the propellant—the substance being inhaled—must be more powerful to push out the heavy metal flakes. You will know this is occurring when you see a paper bag concealing the spray paint and tell-tale gold or silver flecks around the mouth. Use of these inhalants and solvents can cause ventricular fibrillation, decreased cardiac output, serious brain damage, and sudden death.

Treatment

Although withdrawal must be managed as with the other substances covered in this chapter, careful assessment, early identification, detoxification, education, and prevention are particularly critical because so many inhalant abusers are children under the age of 12. Be aware of the programs and resources available and support legislation to make it more difficult for minors to obtain glue and paint products.

NICOTINE

Nicotine is the psychoactive stimulating substance found in tobacco. The behavioral and physiological effects of nicotine frequently lead to addiction. Access to this legal drug for adults endangers those under the legal smoking age. Populations with psychiatric conditions and substance abuse problems have higher rates of smoking and show a lack of responsiveness to smoking cessation treatments.

The Effects of Nicotine

Nicotine is a stimulant that acts in the central and peripheral nervous systems at cells that are normally acted upon by the neurotransmitter acetylcholine. In the CNS, nicotine occupies the receptors for acetylcholine in both dopamine and serotonin neural pathways. This causes the release of both dopamine and norepinephrine. The stimulant nicotine initially increases alertness and cognitive ability, and then has a depressant effect.

Research suggests that dopaminergic processes have a role in regulating the reinforcing effects of nicotine, making cessation of use more difficult. Dopamine blockers can alter smoking behavior for a limited time, but people compensate for this by smoking more. The usual effect of increased dopamine turnover in the system is the reduction of hunger impulses. Once someone tries to quit smoking and dopamine is reduced, hunger impulses return and the person may gain weight.

Although the amount of cigarettes consumed by smokers in the general population has fallen somewhat over the past 25 years, smoking is still of concern as the numbers of smokers increases (U.S. Department of Health and Human Services, Substance Abuse and Mental Health Services Administration [SAMHSA] Office of Applied Studies, 2009). Nicotine is associated with cancer, heart disease, emphysema, hypertension, and death. Given its negative physiological impact, nicotine consumption in the United States remains a major public health issue.

Patterns of Use

Smoking cigarettes is an extremely common addiction and is seen routinely despite smoke-free environments and restrictions on cigarette access. Approximately 59 million adults and adolescents in the United States smoke. There are also socioeconomic differences in smoking rates; the highest rates are among those living below the poverty line. Cigarette and cigar smoking is more common among unemployed adults aged 18 or older than among adults who are working full time or part time. This is especially true with psychiatric–mental health clients. Their work activities may be dictated by their symptom level, and they frequently experience unemployment.

Typically, people begin smoking at a young age, because of peer pressure, or during times of stress. Use of tobacco products can be interrupted briefly during respiratory illnesses, hospitalizations, pregnancy, and following health care providers' advice on smoking cessation. Return to tobacco use after a brief time is all too common; smokers find it very difficult to quit smoking successfully. Only 10% to 25% of people maintain their smoking abstinence over a long period of time even if they received pharmacologic cessation support, such as nicotine replacement systems and psychopharmacology (Raupach & van Schayck, 2011). Evidence indicates that smoke-free environments only protect people from the force of secondhand smoke but do not reduce actual smoking. Smokers practice anticipatory smoking (that is, they smoke more before they are going into a smoke-free environment) to ensure their desired level of nicotine is maintained. Smokers also continue to smoke to avoid the symptoms of nicotine withdrawal.

Treatment

The most commonly used approach for treating nicotine dependence is nicotine replacement therapy (patch, inhaler, lozenge, gum), which reduces craving by maintaining the blood level of nicotine. Bupropion (Zyban), an antidepressant, has demonstrated effectiveness in shorter-term abstinence. Support in a variety of forms is also useful in assisting clients with this difficult addiction. Office-based nursing and centralized telephone counseling services with an emphasis on relapse prevention have demonstrated long-term abstinence effectiveness. Understanding the mechanisms of behavior change identified in Table 32-1 ∞ on page 700 will enhance your ability to help clients transition to healthier behaviors.

CAFFEINE

Caffeine is available in a number of products: coffee, tea, chocolate, and some pain relievers. It is a common substance totally integrated into our social and occupational lives. In the United States, more than half the population over the age of 10 drinks coffee. As with most other foodstuffs, an excessive intake of caffeine is not recommended; around 300 mg per day is safe for most people. Over 600 mg per day is considered excessive.

Coffee has variable amounts of caffeine, depending on its preparation method; there are 64 mg of caffeine in a cup of instant coffee and 150 mg in a cup of filter coffee. A cup of coffee contains two or three times more caffeine than a cup of tea or chocolate. The amount of caffeine in tea varies according to the plant variety and how long the tea is brewed—the longer it is brewed, the higher the caffeine level—but on average a 6-ounce cup of tea contains 40 mg of caffeine. The average amount of caffeine ingested by a coffee-drinking adult each day is around 360 to 450 mg. TABLE 15-2 ■ lists the caffeine content of selected beverages and drugs.

The Effects of Caffeine

Caffeine acts as a stimulant, increasing the heart rate and stimulating the CNS. It is also a diuretic. There is evidence that a relationship exists between the amount of coffee consumption, total cholesterol, and low-density lipoprotein (LDL) cholesterol levels (Lopez-Garcia et al., 2006). The greater the amount of caffeine ingested, the higher the total cholesterol and LDL cholesterol levels. Peak concentrations of caffeine are achieved 30 to 60 minutes after ingestion, and it takes around 3 hours to clear the system.

TABLE 15-2 ■ Caffeine Content of Certain Beverages and Drugs

Source Beverages	Approximate Caffeine Content per 5 oz/dose
Drip coffee	56–176 mg (average 112)
Percolated coffee	39–168 mg (average 74)
Instant coffee	29–117 mg (average 66)
Decaffeinated coffee	1–8 mg (average 3)
Tea (bag or leaf)	30–91 mg (average 37)
Cocoa	2–7 mg (average 4)
Cola drinks (12 oz)	30–46 mg
Jolt (12 oz)	71.2 mg
Red Bull (8.2 oz)	80 mg
Over-the-Counter Drugs	
Analgesics	
Aspirin (plain)	0 mg
Anacin, Bromo Seltzer, Cope, Empirin Compound, Midol	32 mg
Excedrin Migraine	65 mg
Vanquish	33 mg
Diuretics	
Aqua-Ban	100 mg
Stimulants	
NoDoz	100 mg
Vivarin	200 mg
Caffedrine	250 mg
Weight Control Aids	
Dexatrim	200 mg
Dietac	200 mg

If coffee is withdrawn suddenly from people who drink large quantities of filtered coffee (6 or more cups a day), they may become irritable and can even suffer from headaches. Strong coffee is capable of causing palpitations. Given the stimulant effect of caffeine, it makes sense to advise those who complain of insomnia to switch to decaffeinated coffee or to have their last cup of coffee at least 3 hours before going to bed. Because tea has much less caffeine per cup than coffee, it does not have such a strong stimulating effect. However, if there is a complaint of insomnia, it is worth not drinking large quantities of tea just before going to bed to address that problem. Because of its stimulant properties, very young children should not drink coffee.

The negative physiological effects of caffeine, especially those related to cardiac risks, are of grave concern. There have been variable research outcomes in this regard; however, it has become clear that some of the difficulty results from the use of coffee and nicotine together.

Patterns of Use

People who use caffeine use it for its stimulant properties. It is typically taken upon awakening, during times of low energy or fatigue, and when an external source of comfort is required. Once a pattern of use has been established, individuals continue to use caffeine in order to avoid withdrawal symptoms.

Treatment

Reduction-of-harm modes of caffeine ingestion have been successful. The individual decreases the overall intake of the substance vehicle (such as coffee or tea), begins using decaffeinated mixtures in increasing proportions, then completes the effort by ceasing to ingest caffeine. This process weans the individual from the substance without causing, or by at least minimizing, jarring and uncomfortable withdrawal symptoms. Treatment facilities frequently limit or restrict access to caffeinated beverages so that interference from their stimulating effects does not complicate psychiatric treatment. Advance planning for alternatives to caffeine in social and occupational situations is helpful.

POLYDRUG USE

Most substance abusers today are polydrug users, that is, they abuse more than one drug. This fact complicates diagnosis and treatment and increases the hazards associated with abuse. The impact of these multiple drugs on each other and on our clients occurs in a variety of ways, as follows:

- *Synergistic or potentiating effects* are possible where the effects of two or more drugs taken together are greater than the singular effects of each drug.
- *Addictive effects* occur when two drugs that have similar effects are used together.
- *Paradoxical effects* occur if a drug causes a reaction opposite to that expected. Paradoxical effects may occur when only one drug is taken or when several drugs are taken.
- A *pathologic reaction* may also result from the ingestion of only one or several drugs; it is an unexpected and dramatic response to the drug. For example, the combination of alcohol and marijuana is especially dangerous because THC suppresses the nausea that results from an overdose of alcohol. Consequently, the person may continue to drink, risking respiratory depression, coma, and death.

Cocaine and alcohol are frequently used together; the cocaine gives the user a brief high, and the alcohol masks the ensuing depression. When the cocaine wears off, the person is intoxicated and unable to drive safely. Prescription drugs and alcohol are also a common combination. For up-to-date information on drugs of abuse, prevention, and treatment, see the resources and links listed in the Online Student Resources for this text.

As illustrated in the clinical example on PCP, polydrug use can be inadvertent. Marijuana is often laced with PCP. In recent years, dealers have also been putting heroin in marijuana. When heroin is smoked, it becomes a hidden addiction. The individual smokes more marijuana, increasing the amount of heroin needed to get the same high. The move from marijuana use to heroin use is then completed.

DESIGNER DRUGS

According to the Controlled Substance Act of 1970, controlled substances (federally regulated substances) are classified from I (most regulated) through V, according to the potential for abuse and the current accepted medical use. As new information is made available, drugs may be reclassified. Designer drugs, also called "club drugs," are chemical derivatives of controlled drugs. They are called *analog drugs* because they retain properties of controlled drugs but one molecule is changed, making them initially not classifiable as controlled.

Produced by underground and cottage industry chemists, analog drugs are initially legal until the government has them analyzed and researched by chemists. Once a dangerous pattern of use is determined (often 3 to 6 months after police discover the drug), the drug may be classified as a controlled substance.

Fentanyl citrate (Sublimaze), a synthetic anesthetic agent, is similar chemically to some designer drugs. Fentanyl is 100 times as strong as morphine and 20 to 40 times as strong as heroin. It provides a fast rush and an extraordinary high. A person can become addicted after one shot of fentanyl. MTPT (China white), an analog of meperidine (Demerol), has an adverse reaction similar to the rigidity caused by Parkinson's disease.

Methylenedioxymethamphetamine, also called Ecstasy, X, MDMA, Adam, XTC, Clarity, and Lover's Speed, has recently been classified as a Schedule I narcotic because research demonstrates that it causes structural damage to the brain. It is an amphetamine with hallucinogenic properties with effects lasting 3 to 6 hours. Currently, Ecstasy is the drug of choice for adolescents. It is easily and readily accessible. In high doses, MDMA has been associated with malignant hyperthermia and rhabdomyolysis.

Flunitrazepam, also known as Rohypnol, Roofies, Rophies, the Date-Rape Pill, and the Forget-Me Pill, is a fast-acting benzodiazepine that causes anterograde amnesia (memory loss of events occurring while under the influence of the drug) and is tasteless, colorless, and odorless. Because it can be used to sexually victimize women when mixed into drinks, it is the modern-day version of a Mickey Finn (alcohol and chloral hydrate). Another date-rape substance is gamma-hydroxybutyrate (called GHB, G, Liquid Ecstasy, Grievous Bodily Harm, and Georgia Home Boy). It produces euphoria and disinhibition, is used by body builders because of its anabolic properties, and is available on the Internet and in health food stores.

GROUPS AT RISK FOR SUBSTANCE ABUSE

People in a number of different circumstances can use and abuse a substance. However, there are those who are at greater risk for substance problems than others.

Teenagers

Drug abuse among teenagers is pervasive in our society. Although many adolescents experiment with drugs for only a brief time, many more who do so become addicted.

Susceptibility to addiction seems to depend on the following variables:

- Form and potency of the drug
- Dosage
- Frequency of use
- Pattern of use
- Stress
- Personality and genetic makeup of the user
- Family culture

People use drugs that initially produce good feelings to escape from the stress and strain of life. A teenager who relies on a quick "fix" (a drug) to ease mental pain does not learn healthy coping skills. If teenagers do not learn healthy coping skills or work through the pains and mood swings associated with living, they fail to complete a necessary developmental stage. Consequently, they remain fixated at a dependent level of development. They enter a dangerous cycle that is unlikely to be interrupted without professional intervention. Drug use, regardless of what drug is used, inevitably affects all areas of a teenager's life: school, work, social and family relationships, and sense of self-worth. (See Chapter 26 ∞ for an assessment of teenage drug use.)

Adolescent drug users manifest more psychopathologic conditions than nonusing adolescents do. Symptoms include feelings of depression, inadequacy, frustration, helplessness, and self-alienation. These teenagers also have ego structure deficiencies and poor impulse control. As you can imagine, once a client starts using a substance instead of doing the personal work to learn how to self-soothe and cope, it predicts continued substance use. The earlier a child begins using a dependence-producing drug, the more likely the child is to use other dependence-producing drugs. Teenagers who use alcohol and drugs are likely to continue to use them in adulthood.

Psychiatric Clients With Coexisting Substance Abuse Disorders

You need to be alert to possible, and very likely, substance abuse by psychiatric clients. Problems may occur if clients take a combination of substances, and treatment is hindered if clients are under the influence of drugs or alcohol. There are a number of different ways to refer to psychiatric clients who use substances. *Mentally ill chemical abusers (MICAs), chemically abusing mentally ill (CAMI), co-occurring mental and substance use disorders,* and *dual diagnosis* (referring to both a mental illness and substance abuse diagnosis), among others, are terms that try to explain the coexistence of two or more demanding and divergent disorders. The numerous problems facing psychiatric–mental health clients make them susceptible to both substance use and targeting by drug dealers. Poor coping mechanisms, heightened stress, economic factors, and challenging and demoralizing illnesses influence a client's ability to steer clear of the escapism drugs offer. The characteristics of clients who have coexisting disorders are discussed in FIGURE 15-9 ■.

It is estimated that between 16% and 60% of psychiatric clients have a substance use or abuse issue. In the United States, integrated substance abuse/mental health treatment is

FIGURE 15-9 ■ Characteristics of clients with coexisting disorders.

infrequently available (Dugmore, 2011). Both types of disorders are chronic, and clients tend to relapse. You should ask clients directly if they are taking drugs. In most psychiatric hospitals, urine is routinely tested for the presence of drugs if there is suspicion of use. Drug screening is usually carried out on admission and when the client returns from a pass. Close observation of teenagers and their visitors is also useful.

Treatment programs for clients with psychiatric and substance use/abuse problems are best constructed with a reduction-of-harm perspective and built-in extensive psychosocial supports. Because this combination creates consequences (see Box 15-3) of which people may not be aware, it is important to educate yourself and your clients. Staff members with credentials in psychiatry and substance treatment and rehabilitation work collaboratively with the client to manage the numerous chaotic upheavals characteristic of either one of the disorders at any time. When a client with

Box 15-3 Consequences of Using Substances When Having a Serious Mental Illness

- Increased psychiatric symptoms
- Poor treatment adherence
- Increased need for, and use of, emergency health care services
- Poor response to psychiatric medications
- Unstable clinical course
- Increased frequency and length of hospitalization
- Chronic threats to health
- Increased risk of tardive dyskinesia
- Behavioral problems
- Suicide
- Homelessness
- Violence

these problems is treated in a setting designed for one or the other disorder, not both, the client is not likely to receive the specialized care for his or her condition.

The same demographic factors that are associated with substance use disorders in the general population affect people with mental illness. Being male, unmarried, young adult, and poor are associated with a higher risk of substance abuse.

Clinical Example

Ian is a 25-year-old man who was diagnosed with schizophrenia 6 years ago, when he was a student at a local junior college. After becoming ill, Ian lost most of his friends because he was preoccupied with a delusional relationship with a radio talk-show host and spent most of his time alone in his room. He dropped out of college because his mental disorganization and frequent psychiatric hospitalizations interfered with his ability to attend classes. He has tried several times to work, but has not been able to keep a job.

After Ian's most recent hospitalization, he moved into a supervised residence for psychiatric clients and began receiving biweekly injections of a long-acting neuroleptic medication. He became much less delusional and started making friends. Several months ago, Ian and two of his male friends from the halfway house moved into an apartment in a neighborhood known for its high incidence of crack cocaine use.

Ian's case manager believes Ian is using crack. He has lost weight, become aggressive and paranoid, and has been threatened with eviction for failing to pay his rent. Ian was brought to psychiatric emergency services by the police after becoming agitated and threatening the cashier in a convenience store. Ian's urine toxicology screening was positive for cocaine.

People with coexisting disorders display a wide range of clinical characteristics and service needs, depending on the nature and severity of their psychiatric and substance-related problems (Dickerson & Johnson, 2010).

Gender Differences

Because men and women have different rates of substance use disorders and different rates of some psychiatric disorders, gender differences in the range of coexisting psychiatric and substance use disorders also exist. Women have a lower prevalence of all types of substance use disorders when compared to men; however, women—across ethnic groups—often have more serious and disabling medical complications from alcohol dependence.

Women are more likely to have pre-existing mood and/or anxiety disorders than men. They are also reported to link their substance abuse with specific past traumas such as physical or sexual abuse much more often than men do. Women are much less likely to have antisocial personality disorder, which is a significant risk factor for substance use disorders.

Women tend to undergo treatment earlier, possibly due to their increased comfort with socialization and accessing help systems, or perhaps because of more rapid escalation of medical and social consequences. Women often have different motivations for entering treatment, such as child custody concerns. Research on women and alcohol makes it clear that treatment programs should be geared to women's needs. Such programs might include women-only groups, lesbian-only groups, female therapists, meetings with recovered women alcoholics/addicts, and help for the client families.

Biologic Aspects

Biologic, as well as psychological, factors are thought to contribute to the person's use of drugs and alcohol to **self-medicate** (use substances such as drugs and alcohol to address symptoms of mental illness). Some substances of abuse may stimulate neurotransmitter systems in the brain that have been altered both by the disease and by some of the agents used to treat schizophrenia. Animal studies indicate that addictive agents increase activity in brain systems dependent on dopamine (DA), a neurotransmitter whose functioning is altered in schizophrenia. The use of stimulants by people with schizophrenia may be seen as an attempt to "normalize" certain brain functions that have been impaired by the disease. In addition, nicotine relieves problems with sensory processing caused by schizophrenia and counteracts side effects of psychotropic medication, which may help to explain the extremely high frequency of smoking in this group (Gandhi, Williams, Menza, Galazyn, & Benowitz, 2010).

Although substance use may produce symptom relief, it is often true that this decrease in symptoms is short lived and likely to be followed by an exacerbation of symptoms. It is also true that the same substance may relieve some psychiatric symptoms and worsen others—for example, stimulants may briefly elevate depressed mood and increase energy, but exacerbate anxiety and psychotic symptoms.

General Hospital Clients

When you work in general hospitals, be alert to the possibility that clients with physical illnesses may be substance abusers and may be in danger of withdrawal. If you see symptoms that do not mesh with the condition under treatment, you may want to keep in mind that you may be seeing symptoms of substance withdrawal. Be alert and sensitive if physical assessment reveals any of the following:

- Debilitation out of proportion to the presenting health problem
- Physical findings that do not correlate to the chief complaint
- Unsteady gait, slurring of speech, dilated pupils, night sweats, chills, blackouts, tremors, skin tracks, abscesses, nasal septum perforation, or jaundice
- Weight loss, poor hygiene, and poor nutrition
- Symptoms of substance withdrawal
- Failure to attain pain relief with the usual and customary dosage of medication

Alert the primary health care provider and suggest appropriate laboratory studies (such as liver function tests). A nursing assessment may include questions about a client's drinking habits. If alcoholism is suspected, a helpful, matter-of-fact, but nonjudgmental stance will facilitate the client's acceptance of treatment for possible withdrawal symptoms. Even among obviously intoxicated clients, however, responses to such direct questions may be angry and defensive.

Older Adults

Older clients who are being treated for several chronic illnesses by different health care providers are at risk for drug problems from drug interactions and/or for drug dependence. For this reason, you should obtain a good history from the client, including a list of all the drugs taken, frequency of use, dosage, and duration of use. It is often useful to ask the family of an older client to bring all drugs to the hospital for review rather than relying on memory. Frequently, the confusion seen in older clients is a direct consequence of drug interactions or malabsorption.

In addition, substance abuse (especially alcoholism) is less likely to be detected and treated in older adults than in younger clients. It often goes unrecognized because the signs of substance abuse are difficult to distinguish from the changes associated with normal aging or degenerative brain disease. The overall health burden predicts subsequent problematic substance abuse behavior (Ruiz & Cefalu, 2011). Therefore, it is likely that problematic drinking behaviors are likely to increase with the future graying of America. Early- and late-onset older adult alcoholics have reported loneliness, losses, depression, and meager social support networks as antecedents of their alcohol abuse.

Adult Children of Alcoholics

Adult children of alcoholics (ACOA) are at great risk for becoming alcoholics. This type of alcoholism has been labeled *familial*. Research on familial alcoholism has shown the following:

- A family history of alcoholism is present.
- Alcoholism develops early, usually by the time the person is in his or her late twenties.
- The alcoholism is generally severe and usually requires treatment.

■ The risk of alcoholism is increased, but not the risk of other psychiatric disorders.

However, research also indicates that resiliency (the power to rebound, resist, or recover readily) typically overtakes the expression of genetic predisposition with alcoholism. ACOAs' resiliency levels are similar to those of non-ACOAs. Self-help exposure increases resiliency when compared to ACOAs who have not had self-help exposure. There are no universal ACOA personality traits.

Health Care Providers

Many factors place health care providers at risk for developing chemical dependence. Health care providers in general tend to work under a great deal of stress and have easy access to drugs. Every day, they give people medication to relieve pain. It is an easy leap to self-medication. However, such behavior is a violation of state practice acts and ethical standards of practice and, depending on the drug and method of obtaining it, may be a criminal offense.

Colleagues of chemically dependent health care workers need to be alert to behavior that suggests a problem. They should attempt to talk with the professional who is having difficulty before documenting and reporting such behavior to a supervisor. It is very common for colleagues to cover up for one another. Shielding a chemically dependent health care provider—whatever the professional discipline—puts clients, the health care provider, and the profession at risk and violates professional practice, the code of ethics, and the law in many states. Nurses, however, need to understand that their chemically dependent colleagues suffer from a disease, not a moral problem. This understanding empowers us to work together to help one another. Warning signs of behavior by health care providers that suggest chemical dependency are in Your Assessment Approach.

YOUR ASSESSMENT APPROACH
Warning Signs of Chemically Dependent Health Care Providers

Be alert for the following behaviors that suggest a colleague may have a problem with chemical dependency:

■ Frequent absenteeism before and after days off; always working (in order to obtain a supply)
■ Irritability
■ Abrupt mood changes; inappropriate affect
■ Sloppy charting and client care
■ Problems with record keeping of drugs or drug inventory (missing drugs, frequent "wasting" of drugs, inaccurate records)
■ Frequent errors in judgment
■ Alcohol (stale or fresh) on breath
■ Frequent disappearance from the assigned area
■ Offering to give medication to clients who do not request or do not seem to need it
■ Frequent night shift work
■ Having clients who complain of little or no pain relief after the health care provider has administered the medication

---

NURSING PROCESS
Clients With Substance-Related Disorders

As substance abuse becomes a greater problem in society, more clients will be admitted to hospitals and clinics for help with intoxication and withdrawal. Substance abuse is a disease and not a weakness or flaw. It may be true that some health care providers have negative biases regarding addicts, labeling their behaviors as selfish and self-destructive. Some may question whether the substance abuse client has a right to health care resources. A moralistic attitude always alienates the client and is not scientifically sound.

It is always important for the health care provider to maintain an objective, clinical perspective that does not lapse into personal bias or prejudice, particularly in ways that sabotage the delivery of quality health care to the recipient. Recognizing and accepting that the disease is chronic, often with remissions and exacerbations, should keep you from succumbing to the frustration felt by many who treat substance abusers who relapse. At stressful times in life, anyone may develop a dependence on drugs or alcohol; however, certain people seem to be predisposed to the illness. Your expertise in the stages of the nursing process is vital to the care of clients with substance abuse problems. Your focus should be on helping clients work toward self-awareness, good health, and good interpersonal relationships so that they can lead productive, fulfilling, happy lives.

Drugs change rapidly, and nurses must keep up with the "drug scene" to assess and treat clients. Along with the knowledge acquired from reading, continuing education programs, and seminars, nurses need self-knowledge to be good therapists with substance abusers. Ongoing critical self-analysis of your own susceptibility to substance use is useful. See Your Self-Awareness for a list of questions to guide this self-analysis.

Assessment

Carry out an accurate assessment of the substances used and abused to anticipate potential toxic and withdrawal effects and to make nursing care plans as specific and relevant as possible. For example, a methamphetamine user who is malnourished, exhausted, and depressed needs immediate diet regulation, rest, and gradual involvement in a treatment program. See the Nursing Care Plan for the Client With Methamphetamine Intoxication at the end of this chapter. Cocaine or crack abusers are likely to be resistant to treatment and need active staff intervention and a structured program to involve them in treatment. They should not be left alone or purposefully isolated, as might be done with an alcoholic.

Subjective Data

As part of the mental status exam and the psychiatric history, conduct a thorough, nonjudgmental substance use assessment. Include the following interview questions:

1. How many packs of cigarettes do you smoke?
2. Do you take any prescription drugs now?
3. Do you drink alcohol each day? If yes, do you drink a pint or about a quart? (Let the client correct you

YOUR SELF-AWARENESS
Your Stress Response and Susceptibility to Substance Use

Examine who you are when you are stressed by answering the following questions. Attend to what your answers suggest about your coping mechanisms and your susceptibility to substance use.

Check the substances you choose to use when you seek comfort from stress:

- ❏ Food (carbohydrates)
- ❏ Food (noncarbohydrates)
- ❏ Cigarettes
- ❏ Coffee
- ❏ Wine
- ❏ Beer
- ❏ Liquor
- ❏ Chocolate
- ❏ Tea
- ❏ Pain relievers (ASA, acetaminophen, ibuprofen, other)
- ❏ Marijuana
- ❏ Recreational drugs

At what rate do you use any of the above?

- ❏ More than five times a day
- ❏ More than two times a day
- ❏ Daily
- ❏ Only at work/school
- ❏ Only on the weekends
- ❏ Only at dinner
- ❏ Only at parties
- ❏ Monthly
- ❏ Occasionally

At what rate would you use these substances if you had the money, time off, no weight concerns, or other release from responsibility?

- ❏ More than five times a day
- ❏ More than two times a day
- ❏ Daily
- ❏ Only at work/school
- ❏ Only on the weekends
- ❏ Only at dinner
- ❏ Only at parties
- ❏ Monthly
- ❏ Occasionally

YOUR ASSESSMENT APPROACH
Interview Questions for Substance Use

Your assessment of individuals who may have difficulty with a substance can include general types of questions about their substance use and what kind of feedback they have received from others, if any. The following questions help explore those possibilities:

1. What have you thought about your drinking or substance use?
2. Do you think it is contributing in a negative or a positive way to your life?
3. How would you describe it?
4. What have those who are important to you said to you about your drinking or substance use?
5. Do you agree or disagree with their input?
6. Tell me what happens the next day after you drink or use a substance.
7. Do you notice when you are drinking or using a substance whether you must do certain actions or cannot do others?

lifestyle inquiries about cigarette smoking, coffee consumption, and exercise habits. Experts agree that skillful assessment interviewing of clients and their family members remains the best source of data.

Common Defense Mechanisms in Client Responses Denial, rationalization, and projection are three defense mechanisms common to substance abusers. These defense mechanisms, along with other behaviors—conning, bargaining, feigning illness or an injury—complicate the assessment. Chapter 8 ∞ has details of these defense mechanisms.

Alcoholics and other drug abusers tend to deny that they have a problem or minimize the problem: "I drink/use drugs every day, but it rarely interferes with my work." Rationalization is common: "I know I shouldn't drink, and I'll stop as soon as I get through this problem. Drinking keeps me calm enough to function." Projecting the problem onto others is also common: "You are so uptight that perfectly normal social drinking bothers you for no good reason. It's your issue, not mine."

A detailed assessment, along with family/coworker interviews, reveals that the problem is generally worse than the client says. Cocaine users tend to project and blame their difficulties on others, often a spouse. For instance, a man may bring up the issue of his wife's drinking and give a dozen reasons why he does not need treatment.

Substance abusers sometimes manipulate ("con") people to get drugs. Drug-seeking behaviors (DSB), a term used in some treatment centers, refers to feigning illness or an injury to get a drug. Clients also bargain with themselves and staff members to get what they want. An alcoholic/drug abuser is likely to think, "I know I shouldn't hang out with Benny and Paul since we all get loaded together, but I like them. I'll just be with them, I won't drink/use." Later on, the person may think, "I'll only use a gram of cocaine"; later, "I'll just do an eight-ball." This client might tell the nurse, "I'll be glad to go to group therapy next week; just let me rest for a few days." Of course, substance abusers always con themselves first.

Motivation for Treatment Nurses need to consider some important psychosocial issues when clients come for treatment.

on your overstatement rather than fear shocking you with the truth.)

4. How often do you drink a pint or quart of alcohol or more? When was your last drink?
5. When did you last drink more than you wanted to?
6. Do you have a drug habit?
7. What drugs do you use, and what is your daily cost?

Simply asking, "How many drinks do you have at a time?" can be misleading and can minimize the problem if each drink exceeds standard bar amounts of about 2 ounces. The questions in Your Assessment Approach can be helpful to assess any substance use.

Accurate responses to these questions are most likely when they are part of an interview that includes general

Clients may enter a treatment program voluntarily. This situation is best, because they are internally motivated and therefore have a better chance of success. However, they may be coerced by family, friends, physicians, or the police to undergo treatment. See the website for the National Center on Addiction and Substance Abuse at Columbia University, http://www.casacolumbia.org, for information on every form of substance abuse.

Coerced treatment inevitably causes anger and resentment. These clients may lash out at people, blame them (including you, the nurse), and demonstrate resistant or arrogant behavior. In these difficult situations, you must remain detached and nonjudgmental to avoid both power struggles and taking the role of persecutor or rescuer. At this time, you function as a data gatherer: "I know you are [uncomfortable, anxious, afraid, angry] now. To help you feel better, I need to ask you some questions about your drug use." A judgmental question is, "Don't you know that if you don't get help now you will only get worse?" Such questions prevent rapport and alienate the client.

The Importance of Language Knowing the language of the drug world is important in obtaining an accurate nursing assessment of a substance abuser. Drug users have a language all their own; to understand them and the extent and nature of their habit, you need to be familiar with this language. For example, "basing and balling" refer to freebasing (using ether to purify cocaine and make it more potent) and speed-balling (combining heroin and cocaine); "copping an eight-ball" means acquiring one-eighth ounce of cocaine; a "mission" is several days' use of crack; "drug of choice" is the client's favorite drug. Often, the clients themselves or a recovering addict can teach you this language.

Mental Status Abnormal mental status findings are seen in substance-induced disorders but are not specific to them.

- Confusion, disorientation, and agitation are often seen in intoxicated individuals, but can also indicate other problems, such as dementia, head injury, or metabolic abnormalities.
- Paranoia is common in stimulant abuse but can also indicate paranoid schizophrenia.
- Hallucinations can be caused by hallucinogens, withdrawal from alcohol, or psychotic illnesses.
- Signs of impaired thinking, such as loose associations, are unlikely to be caused by substance use and are more likely to be due to schizophrenia.

Objective Data

In addition to assessing subjective data, you should include a thorough consideration of relevant objective data. An assessment of behavioral changes can cue you to drug use.

Physical Findings Less dramatic physical findings may include dry skin, hangnails, malnutrition, ascites, elevated blood pressure, and the smell of alcohol or an inhalant on the client's breath. As alcoholism progresses, be alert to signs and symptoms of liver cirrhosis. Your medical–surgical nursing textbooks will have these physical signs and symptoms.

Laboratory Tests For years, researchers and clinicians have been searching for an objective biologic marker that will reflect problem drinking and make assessment less challenging. Following are common laboratory tests in which elevated values are associated with excessive alcohol intake:

- Blood alcohol concentration
- Gamma-glutamyl transferase (GGT)
- Alanine aminotransferase (ALT, formerly SGPT)
- Aspartate aminotransferase (AST, formerly SGOT)
- Lactate dehydrogenase
- Alkaline phosphatase
- Total bilirubin
- Cholesterol
- Triglycerides
- Uric acid
- Mean corpuscular volume (MCV)

Elevated laboratory test values are only one of the alerting factors for problem drinking. No single test or combination of tests alone is appropriate for clinical screening. Confirmation of the excessive use of alcohol in a sensitively conducted assessment interview remains the preferred assessment approach and is considered a prerequisite for successful intervention.

Nursing Diagnoses: NANDA

Because substance-related disorders are associated with biologic, psychosocial, and even spiritual distress, a wide variety of nursing diagnoses is likely to be fundamental to planning comprehensive care. Nursing diagnoses for clients with substance-related disorders may include, among others:

- Ineffective Coping
- Dysfunctional Family Processes
- Fear
- Imbalanced Nutrition: Less Than Body Requirements
- Decisional Conflict
- Chronic Pain
- Disturbed Sensory Perception
- Impaired Social Interaction
- Disturbed Thought Processes

Outcome Identification: NOC

When designing care for clients who have substance abuse disorders, specifically delineate desired outcomes. While the outcome of total and permanent abstinence may be achievable for some clients, for others it may be an unattainable goal. Reducing the harm of substance use may be an intermediate step that is attainable for some. This is referred to as **harm reduction**. The harm reduction approach is used with those who are not ready for abstention and must be counseled on how to reduce the risk to themselves and to others. As a concept, harm reduction respects work on any positive change as a person defines it for himself or herself and focuses on minimizing the personal and social harms and costs associated with the substance use. Assess each situation individually. Make sure your outcomes are measurable so both you and your client are aware of progress and relapse. Outcome

Casa Columbia

criteria for substance abusers that relate to sobriety, abstinence from drugs and alcohol, and "being clean" include coping, decision making, and impulse control.

Further outcomes include risk reduction; improvement of work, family, and social relationships; and lifestyle changes that may include a growing sense of spirituality. Clients become more effective in using new attitudes and behaviors. As a result, clients feel better about themselves. Although the fear of relapse is always present, over time the craving for chemicals diminishes, and the client establishes a new, healthy lifestyle.

Ask yourself, "Is the outcome one this client can relate to and invest energy into?" None of the addictions or abuse situations discussed in this chapter is easy for a client to abandon as a lifestyle. Imagine a habit you have that is not in your best interests (we all have such habits to one extent or another). Then, imagine how you would best be able to work with a nurse to change that habit or eradicate it completely.

Planning and Implementation: NIC

Your role may be slightly different in each of the following settings, depending on the client's stage of illness and presenting symptoms. Remember, when you work with clients with substance-related disorders in any of these settings that addiction is a chronic, progressive disease. Each treatment setting calls for different skills. For example, in general or specialty hospitals, nurses need psychosocial skills along with technical skills to assess and monitor the physiological components of abuse and withdrawal. In residential rehabilitation and extended residential care centers, nurses may educate clients about the disease, help clients re-enter the community as much as possible, and facilitate or lead support groups. At a student counseling center in a university or college, nurses are involved in treating the college student who has difficulty with drugs or alcohol.

General Hospital Care

Substance abusers who are suicidal or acutely ill with DTs, hepatic coma, respiratory depression, or cardiac dysrhythmias are often treated in the medical–surgical unit of a general hospital. See Rx Communication on interacting with an alcohol-intoxicated individual.

Attend to life-threatening physiological symptoms first. In this setting, nurses perform the following tasks:

- Monitor vital signs and respiratory and cardiovascular support.
- Administer prescribed medications.

- Apply ice packs for fever, such as fever caused by amphetamine intoxication or following cocaine use.
- Decrease stimulation; provide a darkened, quiet room.
- Point out reality: "I know you are seeing things, and I know you are frightened. You are in the hospital, and we are caring for you. There are no bugs or monsters here. You are safe and will feel better soon."
- Make sure that clients receive adequate nutrition and fluids (they are disoriented and generally forget to eat and drink).
- Assess changes in level of consciousness.
- Monitor fluid intake and output.
- Protect skin integrity.
- Offer emotional support and encouragement to the client and family.
- Refer clients to community resources for recovery programs.

When the client is out of danger, then the alcoholism or drug addiction issues are addressed.

Specialty Hospital Care

Specialty hospital care is given in inpatient hospital units that are geared specifically for the treatment of substance abuse. If the hospital is equipped with trained personnel and appropriate resources, acutely ill clients, including those who are intoxicated, may be admitted. The physical environment is modified to handle problems with substance abusers. For example, rooms devoid of furniture and potentially harmful materials offer a quiet, unstimulating environment that prevents convulsions and decreases anxiety.

A primary nurse may be assigned to decrease confusion and stimulation. Members of the staff are experts in detoxification, education, and treatment. Clients also receive treatment for coexisting medical and psychiatric problems. Staff efforts are geared toward stabilization.

Residential Rehabilitation

Residential rehabilitation facilities offer inpatients expert care for substance abuse. These residential centers have a variety of lengths of stay (21 days to months duration) that is sometimes dictated by insurance or 3rd-party payer and not a clinical determination of effective length of stay. Note that in some cases many staff members are not nurses and therefore may not be skilled in treating medical or psychiatric problems.

℞ COMMUNICATION

Client With Alcoholism Who Is Intoxicated

CLIENT: "I'm so sorry I'm such a burden to you. You're such a good nurse, and I never want to be the type of person who. . . ."

NURSE RESPONSE 1: "I'm going to take your vital signs and then you will have some time to yourself."

RATIONALE: This interaction treats the event as an illness in which there are physical consequences to the behavior as well as set limits on the interaction.

NURSE RESPONSE 2: "We will talk later when you are able to concentrate."

RATIONALE: An intoxicated client is not able to benefit from a detailed discussion.

Extended Residential Care

Extended-care facilities provide services for people with physical impairments and a home for recovering alcoholics or drug addicts who have been rejected by their families. Apartments for independent living, a relatively new concept, are useful for these clients.

Outpatient Care

Outpatient care may consist of daily, weekly, or monthly individual, group, or family therapy in a variety of treatment centers. Daily care is usually given only in intensive programs of limited duration, usually 3 to 4 weeks. Employee assistance programs (EAPs) are now common in many industries and are one example of outpatient care given not in a clinic but in the workplace. Substance abuse outreach counselors work with chemically dependent employees.

Self-Help Groups

In self-help groups, also called *mutual help groups*, people with similar problems help one another. Groups composed of peers share experiences and knowledge of the problem to support and educate one another.

Twelve-Step Programs In contrast to the previously described treatment programs, twelve-step programs such as Alcoholics Anonymous (AA) and Narcotics Anonymous (NA) are not specifically treatment programs. They are spiritual programs based on the fellowship among its members. Both are successful self-help groups that meet daily or more often in different parts of large cities and weekly in smaller towns. Meetings are held in places of worship, schools, town halls, and various mental health treatment facilities. Anyone with a desire to stop drinking or taking drugs is welcome. This belief pervades both organizations: "Once an alcoholic/addict, always an alcoholic/addict." Members admit they are powerless over chemicals, live "one day at a time," recite the serenity prayer, and believe in "a power greater than man." Members learn to turn their problems over to "the God of my understanding." Their philosophy is revealed in part through their key slogans, "First things first," "Easy does it," and "Let go and let God." Members of both organizations learn the "twelve steps." The twelve steps of AA are reproduced in Box 15-4. Jellinek's work is thought to be the basis for the contemporary view of alcohol addiction as a disease and the foundation upon which twelve-step programs are based (1946).

Through AA/NA, people learn to change negative attitudes and behaviors into positive ones. A key concept of AA/NA is that total abstinence is essential to recovery. As members become sober or drug free, they begin "sponsoring" (helping) other substance abusers. This offering of support is believed to be vital to recovery, as is regular attendance at AA/NA meetings. Twelve-step recovery programs also emphasize spirituality through meditation and prayer rather than willpower as the means to recovery.

Recognize that AA's twelve steps were written in the 1930s by and for white Christian males and may not be culturally relevant for all people. Adapting the language to a less

---

Box 15-4 The Twelve Steps of Alcoholics Anonymous

1. We admitted we were powerless over alcohol—that our lives had become unmanageable.
2. We came to believe that a Power greater than ourselves could restore us to sanity.
3. We made a decision to turn our will and our lives over to the care of God, as we understood Him.
4. We made a searching and fearless moral inventory of ourselves.
5. We admitted to God, to ourselves, and to another human being the exact nature of our wrongs.
6. We were entirely ready to have God remove all these defects of character.
7. We humbly asked Him to remove our shortcomings.
8. We made a list of all people we had harmed, and became willing to make amends to them all.
9. We made direct amends to such people wherever possible, except when to do so would injure them or others.
10. We continued to take personal inventory and when we were wrong, promptly admitted it.
11. We sought through prayer and meditation to improve our conscious contact with God, as we understood Him, praying only for knowledge of His will for us and the power to carry that out.
12. Having had a spiritual awakening as the result of these steps, we tried to carry this message to alcoholics, and to practice these principles in all our affairs.

Source: The Twelve Steps are reprinted with permission of Alcoholics Anonymous World Services, Inc. (AAWS). Permission to reprint the Twelve Steps does not mean that AAWS has reviewed or approved the contents of this publication, or that AAWS necessarily agrees with the views expressed herein. AA is a program of recovery from alcoholism *only*—use of the Twelve Steps in connection with programs and activities which are patterned after AA, but which address other problems, or in any other non–AA context, does not imply otherwise.

---

patriarchal, less traditionally Christian, approach that is spiritual yet culturally relevant to diverse groups of people makes the twelve-step principles available to people who might otherwise discount them. Caring for the Spirit includes adaptations that are spiritually focused and culturally relevant.

AA and NA, while excellent for clients with substance abuse problems, may cause some difficulties for the psychiatric client with a coexisting abuse or use problem. The AA/NA philosophy of complete abstinence from substances has been said to include psychiatric medications. This requirement causes a rift between what clients are told by their psychiatric–mental health nurses and the path toward wellness according to AA/NA. Programs designed to provide the most effective treatment for the psychobiologic underpinnings of psychiatric disorders and accommodate the added stress of substances of abuse work best.

Women for Sobriety Women for Sobriety (WFS) is another self-help group. Unlike AA/NA, WFS is not based on a spiritual philosophy; instead, the program is based on abstinence. WFS's 13 acceptance statements focus members on new ways of thinking. The women learn to cope and, over time, to change their daily lives. The group recognizes the differences of alcoholism in males and females. For example, women become inebriated faster than men.

CARING FOR THE SPIRIT

A Culturally Broadened Twelve-Step Recovery

The twelve steps are grouped here into four categories: Surrender, Acceptance, Fellowship, and Bliss of Living. Each step is given a one-word description to indicate how the step works in the recovery process.

Surrender Steps

Step One: Honesty
Step Two: Hope
Step Three: Faith

Because many view surrender as a negative activity, using the words *honesty*, *hope*, and *faith* to describe each of the steps in the first category gives new meaning to the purpose of these steps. When seen from a patriarchal hierarchical view, the first step may appear to be a command. However, when it is a call to "get honest" with oneself, the step takes on new meaning without rewriting it or discounting the value it has had in helping others find recovery.

When seen as a way to expand one's spirituality through meditation and contemplation, the second step takes on new meaning as well. Hope comes from observing others who have given up the need to control and be self-centered and have found peace as a result of that action. The "came to believe" part of this step occurs over time as the client hears similar stories from multiple sources who share at twelve-step meetings. This is in part why a new member is urged to "Keep coming back so more can be revealed."

The faith that results from taking the third step allows the client to move from ego-centered thinking to belief in a power greater than self, permitting that power to work on his or her behalf.

Acceptance Steps

Step Four: Courage
Step Five: Integrity
Step Six: Willingness

The next three steps follow from the change of attitude in the first three steps. These are action steps.

In the fourth step, clients use newly discovered courage to examine the specific aspects of their character that they need to nurture and develop, as well as those character aspects that need to be eliminated because they are responsible for the client's current discomfort and distress.

The fifth step works to restore integrity to the client's life and may be responsible for the euphoria reported by many during early recovery. The client may feel a growing spiritual connection, and the nurse may be in a position to support the client's awareness of how the steps have contributed to his or her improved condition.

The sixth step is a willingness activity in which clients must decide how to convert their growing spirituality into a change of behavior.

Fellowship Steps

Step Seven: Humility
Step Eight: Forgiveness
Step Nine: Discipline

The fellowship steps help clients progress in their spiritual awareness and recovery by developing qualities of humility, forgiveness, and discipline in their personal relationships and public lives.

Bliss of Living Steps

Step Ten: Perseverance
Step Eleven: Love of self
Step Twelve: Gratitude

The bliss of living steps bring clients back to a life with meaning. By developing perseverance, clients gain a freedom from worry about when the accumulation of undesirable behavior will be discovered and how it will lead back to the pain of the past. In the eleventh step, clients learn through prayer and meditation the love of self, love of others, and love of life. They come to feel that they are not in charge of the world and that trusting in a higher power who is in charge is "OK." In the twelfth step, recovering addicts and alcoholics express their gratitude for what they have achieved and learn to value reaching out to other sufferers to share the hope of step two, the courage of step four, and the love of step eleven.

Nurses have the opportunity to assist with the unfolding of the process of twelve-step recovery. Clients do the work supported by their spiritual beliefs. Nurses can nourish the process of learning to live life in a new way.

Rational Recovery (RR) Alcoholics Anonymous is the most popular mutual-help recovery organization in the world, but it is not the only one. Alcoholics and addicts who failed to find a comfortable home in AA but were nevertheless determined to become sober have founded at least one other major organization to help others become clean and sober. This group, Rational Recovery (RR), rejects the spiritual approach of AA.

In addition, RR rejects the notion that alcoholics and addicts are powerless to stop their addictions, suggesting instead that until now they simply have not chosen to do so. Instead of reliance on a higher power (which RR considers another form of dependence), RR members are urged to build on strengths within themselves; the movement inspires independence whenever humanly possible. A constant theme is "Think yourself sober."

In RR, there are no steps, sponsors, moral inventories, making amends to others, or even caring about what others think of you. According to rational emotive therapy, on which RR is based, human beings should love themselves because they are human beings and not because others think well of them. The concept of staying sober one day at a time is rejected in favor of a decision to never drink or use again, period. Sobriety is not supposed to become the cornerstone of one's life. The goal is for members to wean themselves from dependence on alcohol, then from dependence on people, and finally from dependence on the group.

Meetings take place only twice a week, and most people attend for only 1 year, after which they may be considered "recovered." They can, however, return to meetings whenever the need arises. Discussions at meetings focus on the here and now rather than past history, and interactive discussion is encouraged.

Whereas AA relies totally on nonprofessionals helping one another, professional coordinators lead RR, and each group has volunteer professional advisors available for advice and input. This is necessary because, unlike AA, there are no old-timers around to help newcomers. Advisors attend meetings only occasionally. RR, like AA, offers written materials, the core of which is *Rational Recovery From Alcoholism: The Small Book* (meant to contrast with the *Big Book* of AA).

Looking within oneself for strength and direction is a major focus in RR. We all have within us an inner voice, RR believes, that challenges us to go wrong. It is this voice, nicknamed "Beast," that urges one to drink or use drugs, takes over during blackouts, encourages one to do terrible things, and speaks louder than one's rational self. It is the voice that tells one "You can stop anytime (but not now)" or "You're not really addicted (you just like the taste)" and that tears angrily into those who criticize or try to help. BEAST is an acronym used to help RR members avoid taking another drink or drug. The BEAST acronym is outlined in Box 15-5.

Relapse

Relapse is common among substance abusers, and it seriously complicates treatment. Authorities in the field of alcoholism estimate that 60% to 75% of those who complete treatment programs drink again within the first 90 days. Data suggest that only 10% to 20% of alcoholics remain abstinent for 1 year following treatment, and that only 35% of these are abstinent 5 years later. In fact, recidivism rates are notoriously high across the spectrum of addictive behaviors.

Stages of Recovery Several common stages of the recovery process are as follows:

1. Commitment to recovery and motivation for abstinence
2. Initiating change
3. Maintaining change

As a result of a successful initial change, the person experiences perceived control while remaining abstinent.

Box 15-5 BEAST Acronym

- **B** is for Boozing Opportunities (weddings, parties, trips, etc.). Rational Recovery (RR) cautions to be aware of the pitfalls but not necessarily avoid them. You are not powerless in the face of temptations, and you can choose not to succumb.
- **E** is for Enemy Recognition. Recognize as the Enemy (Beast) those thoughts that are positive about booze or drugs.
- **A** is for Accuse the Beast of Malice. You can be angry at the Beast for its evil deeds (trying to tempt you), or you can laugh at it. Either way, make clear to the Beast that you have the upper hand and you won't relinquish it.
- **S** is for Self-Control and Self-Worth Reminders. Find ways of showing the Beast that you have self-control (like moving your hands in front of your face and holding them there, totally in your control, until the Beast backs down). Find ways of telling yourself that you are a worthwhile person. Choose not to drink for the same reason you drank: to feel good about yourself.
- **T** is for Treasuring Your Sobriety. Focus on the pleasures of life that are attainable only in sobriety (a concept similar to that in AA).

Stages of Relapse The feeling of perceived control continues until the person encounters a high-risk situation involving negative emotional states, interpersonal conflict, or social pressure. Partnering With Clients and Families includes a checklist of symptoms leading to relapse. The person can avoid relapse by using effective coping responses in the high-risk situation. (See Rx Communication for an example of how you might discuss these issues with a client dependent on substances but not currently using them.)

If, however, the individual cannot cope successfully, an initial "lapse" occurs in which he or she resorts to the use of a chemical to control stress. The person then feels less able to exert control and develops a tendency to "give in" to the situation ("It's no use, I can't handle this"). In subsequent high-risk situations, the individual again resorts to the use of chemicals to relieve stress. Repeated lapses set the stage for a return to uncontrolled use (relapse).

Relapse Prevention Many treatment centers incorporate the concept of relapse prevention into their treatment programs. This concept is designed to teach clients how to anticipate relapse. By learning skills to use in high-risk situations, clients

Care Plan: Potential for Relapse

R℞ COMMUNICATION

Client Dependent on Substances but Not Currently Using Them

CLIENT: "I don't need to spend a lot of time talking to you about this stuff. I'm not going to take it anymore and you can bet on that."

NURSE RESPONSE 1: "I hear that you have no intention to use again, and that's good. I also want to make sure you have every support available to you when that time comes when your resolve gets shaky."	**NURSE RESPONSE 2:** "We don't have to do a lot of talking, but you have to make the changes in what you do and who you do it with."
RATIONALE: This interaction provides direction around the eventual difficulties that face everyone dependent on a substance—temptation and relapse.	*RATIONALE:* Clear statements about how the client is responsible for his or her behavior and for making necessary changes interfere with urges to shift blame.

PARTNERING WITH CLIENTS AND FAMILIES

Teaching About Relapse

A Checklist of Symptoms Leading to Relapse

1. *Exhaustion.* Don't allow yourself to become overly tired or to have poor health. Many chemically dependent people are also prone to work addictions. Perhaps they are in a hurry to make up for lost time or are overworking to compensate for feelings of guilt or personal inadequacy. Good health and enough rest are essential to recovery. Good feelings of physical well-being are associated with a healthy, optimistic mental outlook. Fatigue and feelings of physical illness often induce negative thinking and a pessimistic attitude. You may begin to think a drug or drink would help you return to a positive frame of mind.

2. *Dishonesty.* This symptom begins with a pattern of unnecessary little lies and deceits with fellow workers, friends, and family. Then come important lies to yourself. This is called *rationalizing*—making excuses for not doing what you do not want to do, or for doing what you know you should not do.

3. *Impatience.* Things are not happening fast enough; others are not doing what they should or what you want them to.

4. *Argumentativeness.* Arguing about small and ridiculous points of view indicates a need to always be right. Chemically dependent people need to learn an attitude of acceptance of their disease and the value of the tools of recovery.

5. *Depression.* Unreasonable and unaccountable melancholy and despair may occur from time to time as a *natural part of recovering* from chemical dependence. Periods of depression are times when the risk of relapse is very high. Deal with your negative feelings; talk about them.

6. *Frustration.* Remember, not everything is going to be just the way you want it.

7. *Self-pity.* "Why do these things happen to me?" "Why must I be chemically dependent?" "Nobody appreciates what I'm doing for them."

8. *Cockiness.* "I've got this problem licked; I have nothing to fear from drugs or booze." This dangerous attitude may lead to going into situations where friends are drinking and using drugs to prove to others that you don't have a problem.

Do this often enough and your defenses against relapse will wear down. Don't *test* your recovery. You may lose!

9. *Complacency.* It is dangerous to let up on discipline because everything seems to be going so well. Always having a little fear is a good thing when it comes to maintaining abstinence. *More relapses occur when things are going well than when things are going badly.*

10. *Expecting too much from others.* "I've changed—why hasn't everybody else?" It's a plus if they do, but be prepared to deal with disappointment in your expectations of others. They may not trust you yet or they may be looking for more evidence of your improved physical and mental health. You may be setting yourself up for a lot of frustration and other negative feelings if you expect others to change their lifestyle just because you have.

11. *Letting up on discipline.* Continue with prayer, meditation, daily inventory, and twelve-step meeting attendance. This attitude may stem from complacency or from boredom. No chemically dependent person can afford to be bored with his or her recovery. The cost of relapse is too great.

12. *Wanting too much.* Do not set goals you cannot reach with normal efforts.

13. *Forgetting gratitude.* You may be looking negatively on your life, concentrating on problems that still are not totally corrected. It is important to remember where you started from and how much better life is now.

14. *"It can't happen to me."* This kind of thinking is very dangerous. Almost anything can happen to you and is all the more likely to happen if you become careless with your recovery. Remember that you have a progressive disease and will be in even worse shape if you relapse.

15. *Omnipotence.* This is a feeling that results from a combination of many of the attitudes listed here. You may come to believe you have all the answers for yourself and for others. No one can tell you anything new. You may begin to ignore suggestions or advice from others. Relapse is probably imminent unless drastic change takes place.

Source: Anonymous.

---

gain confidence and the expectation of being able to cope successfully, thus decreasing the probability of relapse. Research indicates that participation in a twelve-step program with a focus on the individual being "in recovery" and maintaining sobriety, as opposed to having recovered or being cured, can prevent relapse. See Partnering With Clients and Families for suggestions on discussing the realities of relapse.

General Treatment Approaches

A number of general interventions for substance abuse that have been found to be useful are discussed next.

Using Confrontation Strategies For many years, it was believed that alcoholics and drug abusers needed to "hit bottom" before they could accept their problem and request help. Today, most people believe that intervention can occur as soon

as the problem is identified. Group intervention/confrontation is one strategy that aims to break down the substance abuser's denial. Nurses are often "intervention specialists" and leaders in the process.

Several family members, friends, employers, coworkers, and an alcohol/drug intervention specialist confront the substance abuser in a private meeting. They list the evidence by going around the group, one by one. The family/friends/ employer, following the leader's cues, speak calmly and slowly with minimal emotion, presenting the facts, the objective evidence, to the alcoholic/drug abuser. Shouting, blaming, and haranguing are avoided because the alcoholic/drug abuser inevitably responds by denying the behavior or making excuses for it. However, confrontation by several people who really care and who persistently present the facts can break

PARTNERING WITH CLIENTS AND FAMILIES

How to Interact During a Group Intervention

Use this series of steps to educate family or friends on how to interact with the substance-abusing client during a group intervention. Encourage family members to integrate the tone and style cues described in the chapter text.

Presentation of Facts

"You had slurred speech and didn't even respond when I told you I had to be hospitalized for surgery."

"You have not made your daughter's dinner all week. And you forgot to pick her up from school."

"You missed work for 3 days, and you have been late 8 days in the past month."

"You have alcohol on your breath (or needle marks on your arms)."

"I found two bottles (a syringe and empty vial) hidden in the bathroom."

Consequences

"Either you get help now or you will have to leave your job."

"Either you enter a treatment program now or I will move out with the kids."

---

through the denial. Examples of confrontation strategies are given in the Partnering With Clients and Families feature.

The next step in group intervention/confrontation requires the family/friends/employer to make clear and direct statements to the alcoholic/drug abuser about the consequences of his or her behavior:

- "Either you get help now or you will have to leave your job."
- "Either you enter a treatment program now or I will move out with the kids."

If the client agrees to treatment, the caring people agree to remain involved.

Educating Videotapes and talks by recovered substance abusers or experts in the effects of substance abuse are helpful. A videotape of the substance abuser recorded when the client was doing well can be motivating and instructive. The person would say, for example, "This is how well I am doing. I feel good and my relationships are going well. It is all because I am not using right now and it proves I can do it."

Education may take place in or out of the hospital, in one comprehensive session or several sessions over time. Nurse educators focus on the types of abused substances and their physical, psychological, and social effects. Families are often involved in these sessions because substance abuse is a family problem. The belief underlying such education is that knowledge and awareness may be useful in decreasing self-destructive behavior. But knowledge alone is never enough. Culturally sensitive and relevant educational resources should be used.

Referral and Self-Help Groups Support and self-help groups are extremely useful in helping clients feel better about themselves and acquire new attitudes and behaviors. Merely being with many people who are suffering in similar ways is beneficial. By observing people who have been sober or drug free for long periods, clients can begin to learn similar behaviors. They can see that there is hope and that recovery is possible. Self-help groups also provide new friends, generally with healthy lifestyles. Clients may choose to attend support groups for the rest of their lives. Some clients who experiment with drugs or alcohol during one period of their lives

(for example, during a crisis) may choose to attend only during the crisis once they succeed in discontinuing their drug or alcohol use.

Lifestyle Change An emphasis on the requirement for a total lifestyle change is necessary. You can help clients discuss ways to alter their destructive habits by suggesting different coping strategies and by encouraging clients to discover new interests and capabilities within themselves. You and your clients can role-play new responses to old situations. Recognizing that relapse is always a threat, you may set up contracts with clients. For example, clients may agree to contact the nurse or an AA/NA sponsor if and when they feel the urge to drink or do drugs. This agreement represents new behaviors that are necessary for a lifestyle change.

Clients must realize that spending time with friends who are substance abusers or hanging out at places where they used to take drugs or alcohol is not helpful. The mere sight or smell of paraphernalia or the desired substance is often enough to trigger a relapse. The client must break old ties and pursue new friends and activities.

Helping the Family

Substance abuse affects not only the client but also the entire family system. Family members often engage in behaviors that enable clients to continue their substance abuse by protecting them from its consequences. Helping family members includes clarifying the problem and presenting possible solutions (treatment) and creating a support system for family members. See Mental Health in the Movies for a compelling example of a family dealing with this problem. Referring family members to Al-Anon or Ala-Teen can be a very useful strategy.

In dysfunctional families, the substance abuser often becomes the "identified patient," focusing attention on that individual and away from the other problems in the family. Treatment for the substance abuser may require some type of family therapy. Family members may need treatment for codependence through group or individual therapy or involvement in a twelve-step program such as Al-Anon or Codependents Anonymous (CODA). The Adult Children of Alcoholics (ACOA) support groups are also helpful.

MENTAL HEALTH IN THE MOVIES
When a Man Loves a Woman

The movie *When a Man Loves a Woman* brings us along on the developing story of an alcoholic wife (Meg Ryan) and her loving husband (Andy Garcia). Their family begins to disintegrate when the wife and mother of two young girls starts to have blackouts and irritable, and then violent, responses to stressors. The stages of controlling behavior bring to light the enabling behavior the husband has been participating in throughout the problem of alcoholism. How they manage to put their lives back together after ultimately forcing his wife into a rehabilitation program provides hope without hiding the truth of the illness' devastation of lives.

Photo courtesy © Buena Vista/courtesy Everett Collection.

Evaluation

Evaluating the recovery process requires an evaluation of the client's ability to change. Is there evidence that the client is being honest, open, and willing to take responsibility for his or her own actions? Regardless of the substance of abuse, once a client stops blaming others for his or her use/abuse, treatment has made a positive impact. Another criterion is the amount of substance the client is placing in his or her body. Has it decreased? Other indications of positive treatment outcome are increased job stability, improvement in interpersonal relationships, and improved problem-solving techniques. Evaluating clients for emotional maturity and the ability to make lifestyle changes that include people, places, and things are critical for victory over substance dependence. Improvement in these areas is a good indication that the client is well on the road to recovery.

CASE MANAGEMENT

Case management services for clients with addictions have the potential to cover many areas. At any time, for any client, you would be involved in the following:

- Arranging for services at clinics
- Responding to emergent and chronic health care needs
- Designing access to educational resources
- Monitoring the client's living situation and residential movements
- Revamping recreational options

In fact, there are as many different case management needs as there are different substance abuse clients. See the Nursing Care Plan for the Client With Methamphetamine Intoxication at the end of this chapter for examples of the variety of case management needs a client may have.

Perhaps the most important task of the nurse case manager for a substance abuse client is availability and flexibility in response to client needs. These clients can experience a plethora of difficulties in their social, occupational, living, and familial/relationship arrangements. Any one of these has the potential to serve as a trigger for relapse into substance abuse or dependence. Assist the client in managing difficulties in these areas to lower the risk of a relapse. This must be done in a manner that does not breach interpersonal boundaries and maintains the client's responsibility for self-care.

COMMUNITY-BASED CARE

In an outpatient treatment center, where the nurse functions in a community-based care environment, you may take the role of a counselor or a therapist. In all cases, the nurse must have psychosocial, physiological, and spiritual skills. Such skills include interviewing, teaching clients about the disease process and alternative coping strategies, referring clients to appropriate sources and community support systems, and knowing how to conduct individual, group, or family therapy (for advanced practice nurses). You cannot give quality care without an in-depth understanding of the disease process—from the varying theoretic explanations to the varying methods of treatment at different stages.

Another feature of community-based care for substance abuse is that of court-mandated treatment. Addicts often exhibit poor judgment. For example, alcoholic clients may continue to drive while intoxicated. In most states, driving under the influence of alcohol or drugs is considered a crime for which the driver will face legal penalties. The law enforcement system may interact with the mental health system to force treatment on those found guilty of driving while intoxicated. A psychiatric–mental health nurse may care for those clients who have been mandated for treatment.

Clients with poor judgment mandated to treatment may initially respond with minimal or superficial cooperation, although many clients do make positive changes as a result of mandated therapy. All clients mandated for treatment must be informed in writing of all policies related to the treatment process and the court mandate. Often, this mandate will include written evidence of participation in one–to–one therapy, family therapy, educational programming, and attendance at twelve-step meetings. At times, random drug testing may be court ordered.

Clients may attempt to manipulate you into withholding information from the court. Allowing the client to manipulate you will jeopardize the treatment process. Successful manipulation may decrease the client's feeling of responsibility for recovery. At no time can you consider violating the court mandate. The law enforcement system has the right to file charges against a nurse who fails to cooperate fully with court mandates.

When state laws clearly mandate a treatment course, you must work within legal mandates. It is much more difficult to decide what to do when public opinion and legal mandate are less clear, or when the mandates seem to interfere with prudent treatment. For example, pregnant women who suffer from substance addiction potentially face conflict between the legal system and basic prenatal care. States vary in their approach to the pregnant addict. Some states seek to incarcerate pregnant women who continue to use illegal drugs, and others mandate that health care workers report all women who have tested positive for drugs, determining such behavior to be child abuse.

At times you may need to interact with the legal system during mandated treatment. You may serve as an advocate who will facilitate treatment for the addict and her baby. This process of intervention can be complex. For example, it is difficult to identify active addiction, secondary use, and recreational use. While any drug use is potentially hazardous, regular use seen in addiction may be more damaging to mother and baby.

HOME CARE

Home care can revolve around a physiological event resulting from substance use or abuse. Cerebral vascular accident from crack use, injury from driving while intoxicated, or brain damage from inhalant abuse are all likely scenarios requiring nursing home care services. In these circumstances, recovery from the physiological threat is coupled with treatment for substance abuse.

One aspect of treatment for substance abuse that can be accomplished in the home is helping the client to develop drink- or drug-refusal skills. In many cases, substance abuse clients who are sober relapse into using substances when they encounter stressful events in their home lives with which they are poorly equipped to cope. Often, these events can lead to situations that include the offer of alcohol or drugs for personal use. A home-based training component can help clients develop the interactional and social skills needed to successfully negotiate refusals of these offers. You can play an instrumental role in designing and implementing this training.

NURSING CARE PLAN: CLIENT WITH CHRONIC ALCOHOLISM

Identifying Information
John Mills is a 54-year-old married civil servant. He is Catholic, has a high school education, and was referred from the Care Unit (a specialty hospital) where he has been for the last 28 days.

John states, "I've had a drinking problem for 35 years. My wife and boss told me if I don't shape up they'll kick me out of my home and my job. I want to feel better. It's been a living hell. But, I'm not sure I can stop drinking; I've tried before." He describes his drinking as a way "to cope with my problems for most of my life." He "wants to stay dry." Fifteen years ago, his social drinking escalated and he began binge-drinking on the weekends. Then he began drinking throughout the week. He has been drinking daily for most of the last 3 years. He drank "enough to keep a buzz on" and occasionally "enough to pass out." John's problems with work include tardiness, absenteeism, and errors on the job. Marital problems are described as "she either yells at me or takes care of me." He gives as examples his wife

pouring out his hidden liquor and calling his boss to say John had the flu when he was really "hung over."

History
John has been in and out of AA groups and has seen three psychiatrists. He has been hospitalized three times for car accidents and injuries due to drinking (broken leg and ribs, contusions, concussion). After the last general hospital admission, he was admitted to the Care Unit for a 28-day alcohol treatment program.

Both of John's parents are deceased and both were alcoholics. His sister, age 58, is a recovering alcoholic (has been "dry" for 10 years). The family has never been close. John feels he was "never allowed to be a normal, active kid." His sister cared for him when he was young and functioned as a surrogate mother.

John developed normally but always "felt different." He worked every summer and took a full-time job after high school graduation. He enjoyed being with his

"drinking buddies" from work, but has never had a close friend on whom he could depend. He smokes one pack of cigarettes daily and uses no other drugs. He spends his leisure time watching TV and at bars with friends.

John has cirrhosis of the liver. He is malnourished from chronic alcoholism and has a long history of insomnia.

Current Mental Status
John is well groomed, clean, and alert. His sensorium is within normal limits; affect appropriate yet apathetic. He appears depressed and expresses feelings of self-reproach and guilt for his years of drinking and its effect on others. Speech is slow and spontaneous. Motor behavior, thought content, and thought processes are within normal limits. Insight is questionable.

Other Clinical Data
Multivitamins qd; no indications of suicide or violence potential.

(Continued)

NURSING CARE PLAN: CLIENT WITH CHRONIC ALCOHOLISM (*Continued*)

Nursing Diagnosis: Ineffective Coping related to alcohol abuse

Expected Outcome: John will reduce ineffective and self-destructive coping through alcohol abuse and regular use of more effective coping styles

Short-Term Goal	Interventions	Rationale
Identification of two effective coping mechanisms	■ John inventories those situations that challenge his ability to cope. ■ John recognizes the automatic mechanisms involved in habitually responding to stress with alcohol. ■ John rehearses various coping strategies to prepare to select two for regular use. ■ John begins to substitute effective coping for alcohol use when stressed.	Revision of coping styles requires identification of the situations that place him at risk, typical problematic responses, and acknowledgment of the need to learn new coping styles. Rehearsing new behaviors and thoughts incorporates them into a repertoire.

Nursing Diagnosis: Insomnia related to alcohol abuse

Expected Outcome: John will use sleep-inducing strategies nightly and report satisfaction with his quality of sleep.

Short-Term Goal	Interventions	Rationale
John will sleep a total of 6 hours per night.	■ Assess current pattern and effective strategies. ■ Respond to awakening with sleep hygiene: warm milk, reading, relaxation strategies. ■ Employ effective strategies regularly.	Re-establish a consistently healthy sleep routine.

Nursing Diagnosis: Imbalanced Nutrition: Less Than Body Requirements, related to alcohol abuse

Expected Outcome: John eats three meals every day plus snacks and takes a multivitamin as recommended.

Short-Term Goal	Interventions	Rationale
John identifies the relationship between alcoholism and malnutrition. John gains weight through a balanced diet.	■ Monitor intake of meals and snacks. ■ Initiate dietary consult. ■ Investigate dietary preferences to maximize John's abilities to expand his intake appropriately. ■ Educate regarding the impact of chronic alcohol ingestion on the digestive tract, metabolism, and overall health. ■ Offer frequent food and fluids throughout contacts.	Malnutrition from chronic alcoholism can be addressed with a comprehensive nutrition program. John is more likely to eat food he prefers, as part of a balanced diet. Alcohol impairs the ability of the digestive tract to absorb nutrients.

NURSING CARE PLAN: CLIENT WITH METHAMPHETAMINE INTOXICATION

Identifying Information

Brianna is a 29-year-old married woman. Her husband brought her to the hospital. Brianna was an advertising executive with a large local firm prior to being recently fired. She has an MBA in marketing. She is not now, and has never been, in treatment or therapy.

Brianna does not believe she needs to be hospitalized, especially because she needs to find work. She asserts she is extremely creative and productive and needs "to get my ideas down on paper before someone steals them as their own." She is agitated, aggressive, elated, loud, and occasionally incoherent during the interview. Her only complaint is increased libido "that my husband can't keep up with." Brianna admits to "working very hard at working very hard," but does not believe she needs treatment right now. She feels she can handle this herself.

She has been using methamphetamine for 1 year, spending most of her salary on it. For the last 5 days she has used methamphetamine two to three times a day. Prior to that, her use was once or twice weekly. Brianna explains her recent increase in use as "helping me work harder and faster to find a job somewhere in this town. I feel more productive." She is having trouble sitting still and she is perspiring visibly. Brianna states she has been feeling nauseous for several days. Brianna's husband and one female friend are her main support system.

History

Brianna has no prior psychiatric history. Her parents are both living and work together in their own business (retail shoe store). Her younger brother is a college senior. Although close and loving, Brianna's family is 2,000 miles away and they seldom see each other. Brianna's father is an alcoholic who has not been actively drinking for 5 years.

Brianna is a competitive woman who has always excelled at academics and at work. She "likes being number one." Brianna has few close friends and socialized with acquaintances from work who have not been accessible to her since her firing. Smoking cigarettes since age 17, Brianna admits to "moderate" drinking with occasional weekend alcohol bingeing. She has experimented with a variety of recreational drugs but states "meth really works for me." Brianna describes herself as "the best kind of hard-driving, career-focused woman" but enjoys reading and tennis when time permits.

Brianna has no current or past medical problems. She states she is in good health despite "feeling horrible now." Her blood pressure is 140/90, and her apical pulse is 110.

Current Mental Status

Brianna is attractive, disheveled, agitated, hyperalert, alternatively compliant and hostile, and occasionally incoherent. Sensorium is impaired. She is oriented to time, place, and person. Her judgment is impaired. Her affect is labile, and mood swings are evident. Her motor behavior is notable for rapid and frequent movements. Her thought content is grandiose. Delusions are present. Brianna reports seeing "signs" on billboards that are messages to her that she should "move onward and upward to take over a company." Thought processes are occasionally incoherent, tangential, with difficulty concentrating and easy distraction. There is limited insight: "I can take care of myself. I have a great deal of innate skill and knowledge. I know what I'm doing."

Other Clinical Data

Brianna is not taking any medications; suicide/violence potential is minimal.

Nursing Diagnosis: Ineffective Coping related to methamphetamine abuse

Expected Outcome: Brianna will complete detox program and will remain free of methamphetamine.

Short-Term Goals	Interventions	Rationale
Meets with staff and attends group meetings according to schedule without prompting.	▪ Hold individual meetings with Brianna regarding consequences of drug use in work, home, social, and physical arena.	Improve Brianna's awareness of her behaviors, reduce denial, and educate about the addictions process.
"Clean" urine 72 hours after last use.	▪ Convey agreement to work with Brianna on her problem areas.	Monitor drug-seeking behavior as an inevitable aspect of her problem.
Brianna discusses problems created by methamphetamine use.	▪ Assign Brianna to daily individual and group therapy.	
Replaces destructive coping with two effective individual coping options.	▪ Observe every half hour. When drug-seeking behavior commences, encourage Brianna to express feelings, educate about cravings and timeframes for resolution.	
	▪ Assist Brianna in recognizing the automatic mechanisms involved in turning to methamphetamine.	Revision of coping styles requires learning and practice.
	▪ Encourage Brianna to rehearse various coping strategies and select two for regular use.	
	▪ Explore with Brianna how to substitute effective coping for methamphetamine use.	

Pearson Nursing Student Resources

Find additional review materials at
nursing.pearsonhighered.com

Prepare for success with NCLEX®-style practice questions,
interactive assignments and activities, web links, animations
and videos, and more!

REFERENCES

Akiyama, K., Saito, A., & Shimoda, K. (2011). Chronic methamphetamine psychosis after long-term abstinence in Japanese incarcerated patients. *American Journal of Addictions, 20*(3), 240–249.

American Psychiatric Association. (2000). *Diagnostic and statistical manual of mental disorders* (4th ed., Text Revision). Washington, DC: Author.

Bergen, S. E., Balhara, Y. P. S., Christoforou, A., Cole, J., Degenhardt, F., Dempster, E., . . . DeLisi, L. E. (2011). Summaries from the XVIII World Congress of Psychiatric Genetics. *Psychiatric Genetics, 21,* 136–172.

Crabbe, J. C., Harris, R. A., & Koob, G. F. (2011). Preclinical studies of alcohol binge drinking. *Annals of the New York Academy of Sciences, 1216*(1), 24–40.

Derauf, C., LaGasse, L., Smith, L., Newman, E., Shah, R., Arria, A., . . . Lester, B. (2011). Infant temperament and high-risk environment relate to behavior problems and language in toddlers. *Journal of Development and Behavior in Pediatrics, 32,* 125–135.

Dickerson, D. L., & Johnson, C. L. (2010). Mental health and substance abuse characteristics among a clinical sample of urban American Indian/Alaska Native youths in a large California metropolitan area: A descriptive study. *Community Mental Health Journal.* Advance online publication. doi: 10.1007/s10597-010-9368-3

Dugmore, L. (2011). Partnership working in dual diagnosis. *Nursing Times, 107*(7), 20–1.

Ewing, J. A. (1999). Screening for alcoholism using CAGE. *Journal of the American Medical Association, 281*(7), 611.

Gandhi, K. K., Williams, J. M., Menza, M., Galazyn, M., & Benowitz, N. L. (2010). Higher serum caffeine in smokers with schizophrenia compared to smoking controls. *Drug and Alcohol Dependence, 110*(1–2), 151–155.

Hack, L. M., Kalsi, G., Aliev, F., Kuo, P., Prescott, C. A., Patterson, D. G., . . . Kendler, K. S. (2011). Limited associations of dopamine system genes with alcohol dependence and related traits in the Irish affected Sib pair study of alcohol dependence (IASPSAD). *Alcoholism: Clinical & Experimental Research, 35*(2), 376–385.

Jellinek, E. (1946). *Phases in the drinking history of alcoholics.* New Haven, CT: Hillhouse Press.

Kraft, W. K., Dysart, K., Greenspan, J. S., Gibson, E., Kaltenbach, K., & Ehrlich, M. E. (2011). Revised dose schema of sublingual buprenorphine in the treatment of the neonatal opioid abstinence syndrome. *Addiction, 106*(3), 574–580.

Logrip, M. L., Koob, G. F., & Zorrilla, E. P. (2011). Role of corticotropin-releasing factor in drug addiction. *CNS Drugs, 25*(4), 271–287.

Lopez-Garcia, E., van Dam, R. M., Willett, W. C., Rimm, E. B., Manson, J. E., Stampfer, M. J., . . . Hu, F. B. (2006). Coffee consumption and coronary heart disease in men and women: A prospective cohort study. *Circulation, 113*(17), 2045–2053.

McGuinness, T. (2006). Methamphetamine abuse. *American Journal of Nursing, 106*(12), 54–59.

Nakama, H., Chang, L., Fein, G., Shimotsu, R., Jiang, C. S., & Ernst, T. (2011). Methamphetamine users show greater than normal age-related cortical grey matter loss. *Addictions, 106*(8), 1474–1483. doi: 10.1111/j.1360-0443.2011 .03433.x

Nelson, R. (2011). Cannabis use in long-term care: An emerging issue for nurses. *American Journal of Nursing, 111*(4), 19–20.

Nicholls, L., Bragaw, L., & Ruetsch, C. (2010). Opioid dependence treatment and guidelines. *Supplement to Journal of Managed Care Pharmacy, 16*(1–b), S14–21.

Raupach, T. & van Schayck, C. P. (2011). Pharmacotherapy for smoking cessation: current advances and research topics. *CNS Drugs, 25*(5):371-82.

Roll, J. M., Rawson, R. A., Ling, W., & Shoptaw, S. (2009). *Methamphetamine addiction: From basic science to treatment.* New York, NY: Guilford Press.

Rose, M. E., & Grant, J. E. (2010). Alcohol-induced blackout: Phenomenology, biological basis, and gender differences. *Journal of Addictions Medicine, 4,* 61–73.

Ruiz, M., & Cefalu, C. (2011). Palliative care program for human immunodeficiency virus-infected patients: Rebuilding of an academic urban program. *American Journal of Hospital Palliative Care, 28*(1), 16–21.

Schepis, T. S., Desai, R. A., Cavallo, D. A., Smith, A. E., McFetridge, A., Liss, T. B., . . . Krishnan-Sarin, S. (2011). Gender differences in adolescent marijuana use and associated psychosocial characteristics. *J Addict Med, 5*(1):65–73.

Swendsen, J., & Le Moal, M. (2011). Individual vulnerability to addiction. *Annals of the New York Academy of Sciences, 1216*(1), 73–85.

U.S. Department of Health and Human Services, Substance Abuse and Mental Health Services Administration Office of Applied Studies. (2009). National survey on drug use and health. Retrieved from https://nsduhweb .rti.org/

Watson, E., Finkelstein, N., Gurewich, D., & Morse, B. (2011). The feasibility of screening for fetal alcohol spectrum disorders risk in early intervention settings: A pilot study of systems change. *Infants & Young Children, 24*(2), 193–206.

Schizophrenia

EILEEN TRIGOBOFF

16

LEARNING OUTCOMES

After completing this chapter, you will be able to:

1. Describe the central features of schizophrenia.
2. Distinguish among the subtypes of schizophrenia.
3. Compare and contrast the various biopsychosocial theories that address the possible causes of schizophrenia.
4. Explain how psychological and social pressures can influence the course of schizophrenia.
5. Implement the major nursing implications in caring for clients with difficult and chronic illnesses such as schizophrenia.
6. Partner with and provide support to the families of persons with schizophrenia.
7. Incorporate methods to prevent or minimize relapses in schizophrenia.
8. Analyze the personal characteristics you bring to the care of clients with schizophrenia that might cause you to distance yourself or fail to understand their experience and difficulties.

CRITICAL THINKING CHALLENGE

Like most individuals with schizophrenia, Alicia is extremely sensitive to her environment. When stressed, she often runs the risk that her symptoms will worsen. In the course of living in usual ways, everyone experiences stress related to conducting day-to-day activities. Alicia's nurse at the mental health clinic has been preparing her to cope with working at a local store. Specific environmental features, such as noise and visual distractions, are particularly difficult for Alicia to deal with.

1. Why do mental health care providers advocate that people with schizophrenia interact with the larger community in treatment programs, jobs, and living in the community?
2. Would people with schizophrenia be better off in protected environments such as semistructured group homes or structured and sheltered workshops? Why, or why not?
3. How would you help Alicia deal with noise and visual distractions?
4. How do most working people create an environment that suits their strengths and weaknesses? Can these methods be useful for Alicia?

Schizophrenia is a complex disorder with an extremely varied presentation of symptoms. It affects cognitive, emotional, and behavioral areas of functioning. According to the National Institute of Mental Health (2011), the prevalence rate for schizophrenia is approximately 1.2% of the population over the age of 18. The age of onset is typically between the late teens and midthirties, although there are cases outside that range. For example, there is a rarely seen childhood schizophrenia (1/10,000) as well as a late-onset schizophrenia (referred to as LOS) that is diagnosed after age 45 and seen more often in women. The illness is diagnosed most frequently in the early twenties for men and late twenties for women. The progression of the disease is as variable as its presentation. In some cases, the disease progresses through exacerbations (an increase in the seriousness of the disease marked by greater intensity in symptoms) and remissions; in other cases, it takes a chronic, stable course; while in still others, a chronic, progressively deteriorating course evolves. The National Institutes of Health website on schizophrenia (http://www.nlm.nih.gov/medlineplus/schizophrenia.html), which can be accessed through a direct link on the Online Student Resources for this book, will also serve as a resource on schizophrenia for you, your clients, and their families.

SYMPTOMS OF SCHIZOPHRENIA

The diagnosis of schizophrenia requires not only the presence of distinct symptoms but also the persistence of those symptoms over time. Symptoms must be present for at least 6 months, and some symptoms (called *active-phase symptoms*) must be present for at least 1 month during that time, before schizophrenia can be diagnosed. See DSM Essential Features about schizophrenia.

The symptoms of schizophrenia are conceptually separated into **positive symptoms**, which represent an excess or distortion of normal functioning, or an aberrant response; and **negative symptoms**, which represent a deficit in functioning.

Positive Symptoms

Positive symptoms include the three most pronounced outward signs of the disorder: hallucinations, delusions, and disorganization in speech and behavior. They are called *positive* symptoms because if the person has these symptoms it is because they are ill. It is similar to when you have a positive tissue biopsy—it means there is evidence of a problem.

FIGURE 16-1 ■ Distorted perceptions. The distorted visual perceptions indicated by this figure exemplify what is experienced by someone during visual hallucinations.
Photo courtesy of Dennis Potokar/Photo Researchers, Inc.

Hallucinations

Hallucinations are the most common perceptual disturbance in schizophrenia. **Hallucinations** are subjective sensory experiences that are not actually caused by external sensory stimuli. One or more of the five senses are involved in hallucinations. Hallucinations may be auditory (heard), visual (seen), olfactory (smelled), gustatory (tasted), or tactile (touched). FIGURE 16-1 ■ represents how someone with visual hallucinations may distort a scene.

The most common form of hallucination in schizophrenia, at least in the western hemisphere, is hearing voices or sounds that are distinct from the person's own thoughts. If a voice is heard, it (or they) may be friendly or hostile and threatening. It is particularly characteristic of schizophrenia if the person hears two or more voices conversing with each

DSM ESSENTIAL FEATURES

Schizophrenia

The client presents with some combination of symptoms including delusions, hallucinations, disorganized speech/behavior, reduced range of emotion, little speech, or low motivation and has not received treatment for at least a month. Work, social life, or self-care are poorly conducted. There is evidence these symptoms have been present for months. Also, no sustained symptoms of mania or depression are noted and substance ingestion, a medical problem, or developmental disability do not explain the symptoms.

other, or hears a voice that provides continuous comments on the train of thought.

Having auditory hallucinations does not necessarily mean that the individual hears human speech. As you will see later in Table 16-3, several other sounds may be hallucinated. Do not confuse hallucinatory experiences with *synesthesia,* which is the experience of having multiple senses involved in a single event. Synesthesia is not a disease or disorder. Distinguishing between synesthesia and hallucinations can be accomplished by ensuring that there is no external stimulation to the sensations. Examples of synesthesia include seeing sounds, seeing colors when in pain, and hearing smells.

Hallucinations also occur in several other illnesses besides schizophrenia. Dementia (Chapter 14∞), substance abuse (Chapter 15∞), and depression (Chapter 17∞) are some of them. TABLE 16-1■ links hallucinations with commonly associated disease processes. Hallucinations can also be experienced under extreme physiological stress or as a side effect of medications.

Delusions

Delusions are mistaken or false beliefs about the self or the environment that are firmly held even in the face of disconfirming evidence. Delusions may take many forms. In *delusions of persecution,* the person may think that others are following him, spying on him, trying to damage or take something of value like a reputation, or trying to torment him (e.g., "They have misters in my apartment that spray LSD onto me when I walk around."). In another common form, delusions of reference, the person thinks that public expressions, like a story on the television or a newspaper article, are specifically addressed to him or her or that the event occurred because of his or her thoughts or actions (e.g., "When the newscaster wears navy blue, she is speaking my thoughts to the world."). **Folie à deux** is a delusion shared by two people, who are usually emotionally close to each other. Specific delusions are discussed in TABLE 16-2 ■.

Disordered Speech and Behavior

Other positive symptoms represent excesses of language or behavior. Disorganized speech is the outward sign of disordered thoughts and may range from less severe forms (the person moves rapidly from one topic to another), to severe forms (the person's speech cannot be logically understood). Positive symptoms include low-level behavioral responses to the environment characterized by such disorganized behavior as agitated, nonpurposeful, or random movements, and waxy flexibility (discussed and defined later in this chapter). The positive symptoms of schizophrenia are discussed in TABLE 16-3 ■.

TABLE 16-1 ■ Types of Hallucinations

Perceptual Disturbance	Commonly Associated Disease Process
Auditory	Schizophrenia
Visual	Dementia
Tactile*	Acute alcohol withdrawal
Somatic*	Schizophrenia
Olfactory*	Seizure disorders
Gustatory*	Seizure disorders

*Also called *proprioceptive hallucinations,* associated with infections, heavy metal poisoning or vitamin and mineral toxicities, and tumors.

TABLE 16-2 ■ Types of Delusions

Disturbances in Thinking	Definition	Example
Delusions of persecution	Belief that others are hostile or trying to harm the individual	A woman notices a man looking at her and believes that he is trying to follow her.
Delusions of reference	False belief that public events or people are directly related to the individual	A man hears a story on the evening news and believes it is about him.
Somatic delusions	Belief that one's body is altered from normal structure or function	An elderly woman believes that her bowel is filled with cement and refuses to eat.
Thought broadcasting	Belief that one's unspoken thoughts can be heard	A young client believes that everyone around him knows he's attracted to a nurse although he has said nothing.
Delusions of control	Belief that one's actions or thoughts are controlled by an external person or force	A woman believes that her neighbor controls her thoughts by means of his home computer.
Nihilistic delusions	Belief that reality and existence are gone or were never there	A young man states that nothing exists. Makes statements such as "Everything is lost," "I have no head, no stomach," "I cannot die," or "I will live to eternity."
Delusions of self-deprecation	Belief that one is not worthy of routine or usual aspects of life	A young mother believes she is ugly and smells like garbage. Severe depression can cause feelings of being unworthy, sinful, ugly, or foul smelling.
Delusions of grandeur	Inflated sense of self-worth and abilities	A woman with mania believes she is "extraordinarily wealthy and intelligent with a fully evolved value system."

TABLE 16-3 ■ Positive Symptoms

Positive Symptom	Examples	
Hallucinations		
Auditory	Human speech (speaking clearly, mumbling, whispering, singing, yelling, screaming, one voice, several voices, voice speaking to client, voices speaking to each other, male, female, both, indistinguishable, imitating nonhuman sounds)	
	Mechanical sounds (clocks, metal clanging, clicking)	
	Music	
	Animal sounds	
	Insect sounds	
	Wind through the trees	
	Grating sounds made by walking on sand	
	Crinkling sound from plastic or aluminum wraps	
	The sound of the earth moving or heaving as during an earthquake	
Visual	Blood	People
	Animals	Movement of large objects
	Distortions of everyday sights	Auras
Olfactory	Green peppers	Blood
	Fumes	Burning materials
	Garlic	Urine or feces
	Semen	Rotting meat
	Sulfur	
Gustatory	Metallic flavor	Blood
	Urine or feces	Semen
Tactile	Being pregnant	Giving birth
	Being beaten	Electrocution
	Being raped	Band around head
	Grease on hands	Moving tumors
	Internal movements	
Delusions		
Persecutory	"I cannot leave my apartment more than once a month. I have to have this cardboard in my pockets when I go out so the CIA can't take pictures of me."	
Referential	"I didn't mean to do it. I was just thinking what would happen if the train derailed. I'm sorry I killed all those people."	
Somatic	"I am going to be hemorrhaging, bleeding to death through my mouth." Or: "I have an alien gestating in my belly. When he is mature he'll drip from my palms like sweat."	
Religious	"My daughter is the devil, saturated with evil, because her age of ascendancy is 666 (June 6, 2006)."	
Substitution	"It looks just like my wife but it's really a robot."	
Thought insertion	"These thoughts are being put in my head by the alien conspiracy." Or: "When I get angry it's because the NSA is altering my brain waves."	
Nihilistic	"Everything is falling apart. My insides are rotting away and so is everything else."	
Grandiose	"I made $7 million from a software program I developed and they're keeping it from me until I tell them my secret programming wizardry." Or: "I am not who you think I am. I work midnights at all the top law firms so I can get all their work done for them."	

TABLE 16-3 ■ Positive Symptoms *(Continued)*

Positive Symptom	Examples	
Disorganized Speech		
Loose associations	"I take a shot of Haldol every 4 weeks, it's not weak, it's strong and so is the pill twice a day. I don't care if it does me wonders or not, wonder bread, soviet. I'm taking it for the hell of it. Bread and comrad. Who cares if it helps me or not. I'm doing phenomenal."	
Word salad	"Wimple sitting purple which the twilighted cheshire, for then frames of silver ticking bubble and."	
Clanging	"I want to eat neat treat seat beat."	
	"I'm fine it's a sign fine whine wine pine dine."	
Echolalia	Client repeats pieces of what is said or entire phrases: Nurse asks, "How are you today?" and the client states, "You today." Or client states, "I love smelling roses. I love smelling roses."	
Behavior		
Disorganized	Client walks around aimlessly picking up everything available to him and touching all objects and surfaces.	
Catatonic	Excited catatonia: A client in the emergency department is repeatedly assaultive, hyperactive, or cannot sit still.	
	Waxy flexibility: Client maintains a rigid position, allows another to move him or her into new positions and maintains the new position.	
Thinking		
Lack of planning skills	Indecisiveness	Lack of problem-solving skills
Concrete thinking	Blocking	Difficulty initiating tasks

Negative Symptoms

Negative symptoms of schizophrenia are less dramatic but just as debilitating as positive symptoms. They are called *negative* symptoms because people are missing something they would normally have if they were not ill. They lost the ability to do or feel because of their illness. Negative symptoms are also predictors of a poor outcome to treatment (Stanford et al., 2011). TABLE 16-4 ■ gives examples of negative symptoms of schizophrenia.

Flat Affect

People with schizophrenia often appear to have unemotional or very restricted emotional responses to their experiences. **Flat affect** "is the absence or near absence of any signs of affective expression" as well as poor eye contact (American Psychiatric Association [APA], 2000). To see how flat affect differs from a normal range of affect, imagine someone responding to winning a prize ("This is great! I'm so happy!"). Now imagine that same person with much less emotion in her response and no emotion showing on her face ("Oh."). The difference between the two responses is the flattening of affect.

Alogia

Brief, empty verbal responses are known as *alogia*. Rather than saying a few sentences in response to a question, clients with alogia reply with a single word or a very limited number of words. This **poverty of speech** is thought to be symptomatic of diminished thoughts and is different from a refusal

TABLE 16-4 ■ Negative Symptoms

Negative Symptom	Examples
Flat Affect	The client maintains the same emotional tone when told his mother has died as when told it is time to attend programs. "OK."
Apathy	The client has feelings of indifference toward people, events, activities, and learning.
Avolition	The client does not get to the job he really wanted because he couldn't get up and take the bus.
Anhedonia	The client apparently derives no pleasure from bowling when, prior to getting sick, he used to enjoy it.
Alogia	Rather than using a series of sentences or several words, the client, when asked about his day, speaks sparsely in a limited, stilted manner: "Fine."

to speak. With alogia, the client does not use many words to express experiences or thoughts.

Avolition

A symptom that is frequently misunderstood by families and the community is **avolition**, an inability to pursue and persist in goal-directed activities. Another name for it is *amotivational syndrome*, or not being motivated. You may see

MENTAL HEALTH IN THE MOVIES
A Beautiful Mind

The movie *A Beautiful Mind* is based on the true story of Nobel Prize-winning mathematician and economist John Nash and his life with schizophrenia. The movie begins with his college years at an ivy league school and moves through the beginning of his career and the formation of his relationship with his wife. His brilliance and unique perspectives, as well as his quirky behaviors and strongly held views, bring you to the realization that something else may be shaping his experiences. You find out about his illness when he finds out about his illness. John's best friend and roommate from college and his friend's young niece turn out to be visual hallucinations. Delusions of being involved in special government work greatly influence his behavior. Antipsychotic medication had not yet been developed when he was diagnosed, so his journey included insulin shock therapy and then, later, the traditional or conventional antipsychotics.

In one scene, John sits and stares while his wife tells him, "Meaning is all around you, all you have to do is look for it." Her exasperation is evident. The side effects of the medications interfere with his relationship with his wife in other ways as well. After he stops taking them, he is once again plunged into symptoms. This movie shines a light on the illness of schizophrenia, how an individual and his family cope, provides hope about the power of caring relationships, and demonstrates how people can propel their own recovery.

Photo courtesy of Everett Collection.

evidence of this negative symptom when a client fails to go for a job interview or fails to become involved in an easily available activity. The person with schizophrenia who has avolition is often misinterpreted as being lazy or unwilling to support him- or herself, rather than as a symptom of the illness. This misunderstanding often affects the ability of family members and friends to stay involved in relationships with the client. They may feel frustrated, as if their efforts have been wasted, or personally rejected because their suggestions have gone unheeded.

Anhedonia

Anhedonia, the inability to experience pleasure, may challenge you as you work with clients who have schizophrenia. It is difficult to imagine, and even more arduous to empathize with, someone who cannot seem to enjoy even small aspects of life. It is important to remember that people who have schizophrenia cannot enjoy experiences because of a physiological reason over which they have no control.

Recognizing the Presence of Negative Symptoms

Negative symptoms of schizophrenia are difficult to assess because they are part of our everyday experiences, just more intense and durable. While few of us have experienced true hallucinations, many of us know what it is like to have a day without the energy to pursue goal-directed activities. Another difficulty in recognizing the presence of negative symptoms stems from the fact that people with schizophrenia often live in difficult situations that may lead to restricted emotional expression and disturbed goal-directed activities. Living in poverty or in unsettled circumstances—homelessness, for example—can induce feelings of desperation or despair, which may mimic the negative symptoms of schizophrenia. It is important to try to separate environmental influences on experience from the disease

process, and to note the persistence of the symptoms over time across a variety of circumstances. For example, if a client is living in a rooming house where others around him are likely to steal, that client will not be safe talking excitedly about having received a gift from his parents. If, however, the client is not excited when in his own home in front of his parents and trusted others, the presence of his limited verbalizations is likely a negative symptom of schizophrenia.

While the media is not typically a reliable source of accurate information about schizophrenia, the movie *A Beautiful Mind* is a wonderful exception. See Mental Health in the Movies for details about the plot. You see exactly what families struggle with in the depiction of negative symptoms in the movie.

Another important criterion for recognizing schizophrenia is detecting an impaired ability to perform and complete social and work obligations. It is diagnostic of schizophrenia when the person has difficulty performing in one or more areas of life including work, school, social relationships, and the maintenance of everyday activities such as dressing and providing food for oneself.

SUBTYPES OF SCHIZOPHRENIA

Subtypes of schizophrenia are used to designate which symptoms are prominent. The subtypes are discussed in this section.

Paranoid Type

Prominent hallucinations and delusions are present in the **paranoid type** of schizophrenia. Delusions are often persecutory or grandiose, and they often connect into a somewhat organized story. Delusions may also be varied and include somatic or religious delusions. Hallucinations often link with the delusions, although this is not necessary. For example, a person who believes he is being monitored by the FBI may hear the voices of people he identifies as FBI agents laughing at him or talking about him.

Disorganized Type

The central features present in the **disorganized type** of schizophrenia are disorganized speech and behavior and flat or inappropriate affect. The client appears disorganized and unkempt because the client cannot accomplish basic everyday tasks like dressing oneself. The client may have all the necessary clothing on, but the order of putting on each item of clothing or the steps required to accomplish dressing (e.g., buttoning, zipping, tying) may be too much to handle. Emotional expression may be either inappropriate to the content of what the client is saying (e.g., laughing when discussing being thrown out of the house by roommates) or restricted and flat. Hallucinations and delusions are typically more fragmented and disorganized than in the paranoid type. This subtype has been referred to as potentially being the most severe form of the disease.

Catatonic Type

Although not seen frequently in the United States, the **catatonic type** of schizophrenia is a distinctive type characterized by extreme psychomotor disruption. The client may display substantially reduced movement to the point of stupor, accompanied by negativism and resistance to any intervention. A client could display a type of posturing known as **waxy flexibility**, a feature of catatonic motor behavior in which, when clients are placed in peculiar positions, they remain almost completely immobile in the same position for long stretches of time. Alternatively, extremely active and purposeless movement (excitement) that is not influenced by what is going on around the person may be present. Additional signs of the catatonic type of schizophrenia are repeating what others say or mimicking their movements.

Undifferentiated Type

When a client is in an active psychotic state and does not have prominent symptoms that match any of the prior subtypes, then **undifferentiated type** is diagnosed. Remember that a client's diagnosis may also change over the years as symptoms form and re-form. The particular subtype diagnosed at one point in time may not match what is currently happening to a client. The subtype of schizophrenia may have shifted, with the undifferentiated subtype now most representative of the course of the disease.

Residual Type

The **residual type** of schizophrenia is a subtype diagnosis reserved for a client who has had at least one documented episode of schizophrenia but now has no prominent positive symptoms of the illness. Negative symptoms such as flat affect and inability to work are present, but prominent hallucinations, delusions, and disorganized thoughts and behavior are not. When a client has these characteristics, the client is considered to have residual features of the illness and receives this subtype diagnosis.

SOMATIC TREATMENTS

Prior to the 1950s—which is called the *pre-neuroleptic age*—insulin coma, drug or electrically induced shock treatments, and psychosurgery, including prefrontal lobotomies, were used to treat schizophrenia. The impact of these extreme somatic treatments did make a difference, for a time, in symptomatology but were not durable or beneficial and often not ethical. Many hoped these treatments were the long-sought-after cure for schizophrenia because they were relatively quick and inexpensive compared to lengthy and costly analytic therapies. This hope was not realized.

Contemporary psychosurgery has been refined from a gross assault on cranial tissue (the lobotomy of decades past) to procedures in which specific involved areas of the brain are delicately shaped to reduce repetitive and destructive behaviors (amygdalotomy, cingulotomy). Electroconvulsive therapy (ECT) has been improved upon and crafted to an impressive degree in the last 30 years. Effective treatment with minimal risks has been offered mostly for mood-disordered clients.

The introduction of psychoactive drugs in the 1950s provided new alternatives for the treatment of schizophrenia. Psychotropic medications, which influence the thoughts, mood, and behavior of clients, made previously uncontrolled symptoms manageable. In the period following the introduction of psychotropic medications, the use of seclusion and restraints declined dramatically, as did the duration of hospital stays and numbers of clients in state mental hospitals.

A new optimism arose regarding the possible outcomes of mental illness. Because they controlled the most difficult symptoms of psychosis, psychotropic medications made psychosocial or behavioral treatments possible for a much greater percentage of psychiatric clients. There is no cure yet for schizophrenia; however, these drugs relieve the most debilitating symptoms for many clients and are the first step toward recovery or a higher level of functioning. Refer to Chapters 5, 6, 7, and 31∞ for more details on the history and the science behind somatic treatments. Ethical and legal aspects of somatic treatments are discussed in Chapter 12∞.

RELAPSE

A client with schizophrenia is vulnerable after a period of stability, however brief or extended, partial or complete, to a return of symptoms. This is called a **relapse**, and the disease itself has a pattern of relapse and recovery. As a chronic disorder, schizophrenia is characterized by relapses alternating with periods of full or partial remission.

Although antipsychotic medication is effective in reducing relapse rates, 10% to 30% of clients relapse within 1 year after hospital discharge even if they are receiving maintenance medication (Emsley, Chiliza, Asmal, & Lehloenya, 2011). Acknowledge the sense of demoralization likely with such a recurrent and debilitating course and the need to improve methods for relapse prevention. The following two clinical examples detail how relapses can occur under certain circumstances.

Clinical Example

Daryl, a 26-year-old man with a diagnosis of paranoid schizophrenia, decided to stop taking his quetiapine (Seroquel) because he didn't think he needed it anymore. Within a few days of stopping the medication, he was unable to leave the house for fear of someone harming him. Although he liked his job at the local cannery and knew that he had the chance to earn more money in the near future, he refused to go to work for fear that he would be hit by a bus on his way there. He was eventually fired because of poor attendance. The loss of a structured schedule furthered his deterioration and Daryl relapsed, requiring hospitalization.

In this instance, a decrease in medication increased Daryl's biologic vulnerability, with marked behavioral, and eventually environmental, consequences. His relapse began with a medication issue and could have been prevented.

Clinical Example

Jeanne, 22, lived with her divorced mother and younger sister Maura since her release from the hospital after her second psychotic episode. She found living alone too frightening and was more comfortable staying in her old room at home. When Maura began preparing to leave home for college, Jeanne became increasingly anxious, demanding to sleep in Maura's room at night and hiding Maura's belongings. As Maura's departure grew near, Jeanne began actively hallucinating and withdrew to her room, refusing to talk to her mother or sister.

In this case, the client did not have sufficient coping skills to deal with her sister's departure from the household, and her psychosis re-emerged. Jeanne's relapse may have

been averted had she been taught coping skills and had the opportunity to practice them. However, learning is unfavorably affected by schizophrenia, motivation and energy are problems, and even a competent program of teaching cannot remove all the negative consequences in response to life stress.

OTHER PSYCHOTIC DISORDERS

Psychosis occurs in a number of disorders in addition to schizophrenia. The problems with symptoms can be short lived or may extend into significant periods of time with disability.

Schizophreniform Disorder

Schizophreniform disorder is very similar to schizophrenia except the person has not been ill for very long. The main difference is that the client has experienced the symptoms for at least 1 month and either recovered from the symptoms before 6 months, or 6 months have not yet elapsed since the original symptoms began. Under the latter set of circumstances, the diagnosis of schizophreniform disorder is provisional until the 6 months have elapsed and then a diagnosis is set. A second difference, besides duration, is that the client may show no impairment in social and work functioning.

Schizophreniform disorder may occur just prior to the onset of schizophrenia (i.e., be prodromal to [precede] schizophrenia), yet approximately one third of clients diagnosed with this disorder recover. The other two thirds go on to have either schizophrenia or schizoaffective disorder.

Schizoaffective Disorder

In **schizoaffective disorder**, two sets of symptoms—psychotic and mood symptoms—are present concurrently in the same period of illness episode: positive symptoms of schizophrenia and symptoms of a mood disorder (either a major depressive or manic disorder; see Chapter 17∞). Schizoaffective disorder is less common, and has a slightly better prognosis, than schizophrenia, but it has a substantially worse prognosis than mood disorders. Interacting with a client who has schizoaffective disorder may require the same skills you would employ with a client who has schizophrenia. Disorganized speech may be an expression of this client's psychosis. Rx Communication

R_X COMMUNICATION

Client With Clang Associations

CLIENT: "The dining room lining trying to eat forever."

NURSE RESPONSE 1: "Jack, are you having a problem getting your food?" *RATIONALE:* A direct question allows the client with clang associations to answer with a "yes" or "no" response, models how the communication can be stated, and labels the situation as a problem.
NURSE RESPONSE 2: "Come with me and let's get you set up." *RATIONALE:* This response reinforces the appropriateness of the client's coming to the nurse with a problem and concretely shows the client how to resolve the problem.

provides examples of therapeutic communication with a client with the clang association form of disorganized speech.

One of the defining characteristics of schizoaffective disorder is when the hallucination or delusion occurs. A person who has schizoaffective disorder is likely to have hallucinations or delusions regardless of mood state. In other words, if the person were delusional only when he or she had extreme problems with mood (mania or depression), it is likely the diagnosis would be mood disorder with psychotic features rather than schizoaffective disorder.

Delusional Disorder

Delusional disorder is diagnosed when the client holds one or more nonbizarre delusions for a period of at least 1 month. Although it is sometimes difficult to differentiate bizarre from nonbizarre delusions, the key is that the nonbizarre delusions could conceivably arise in everyday life. A nonbizarre delusion is the focus of the clinical example that follows.

Clinical Example

Martin holds the delusional belief that the police are trying to entrap him. He goes to extremes to protect his home with surveillance and security equipment. At the same time, he believes that the police won't bother him at work because his boss, with whom he gets along well, is the son of a policeman.

People with delusional disorders may function quite well in areas of their life not affected by the delusion, yet behave oddly in activities touched by the delusion. Delusional disorders are not common and arise predominantly during middle and late adulthood.

A subtype of delusional disorder, the erotomanic type, occurs when clients believe that another person is in love with them. Typically this other person has no relationship whatsoever to the client, or the relationship is superficial at best. Contacting the person, stalking the person, and displays to impress the imagined lover have involved celebrities, politicians, and the man or woman next door.

Brief Psychotic Disorder

In a brief psychotic disorder, at least one of the positive symptoms for schizophrenia is present (hallucinations, delusions, disorganized speech or behavior) for at least 1 day, but for less than 1 month. Upon remission of these symptoms, clients return to their level of functioning prior to the onset of the illness. This disorder may be brought on by a particular stressful event in the person's life, including childbirth. In other instances, a stressful life event cannot be specifically identified. Brief psychotic disorder is an unusual and seldom-seen phenomenon.

Additional Psychotic Disorders

Several additional psychotic disorders are specified in the DSM, as follows:

- Shared psychotic disorder
- Psychotic disorder due to a general medical condition
- Substance-induced psychotic disorder
- Psychotic disorder, not otherwise specified (NOS)

Consult the DSM-IV-TR for diagnostic criteria for these disorders. However, in diagnosing any psychotic disorder, the diagnostician must explore the alternative explanation that symptoms may be caused by an underlying medical disorder or by substance use.

BIOPSYCHOSOCIAL THEORIES

Beliefs about the causes of schizophrenia have changed over the centuries since schizophrenia was equated with early senility. Theories about the treatment for schizophrenia have also undergone change. For example, at one point it was erroneously believed (based on the writings of Sigmund Freud) that people with schizophrenia could not be treated because they were unable to form a therapeutic relationship with a psychoanalyst. At another point, a now discredited theory pointed to the behavior of parents, especially mothers, causing schizophrenia in their offspring. It is likely that several factors inter-relate to cause schizophrenia and several forces influence the effectiveness of treatment. A multifactorial cause and a varied approach to treatment, responsive to the individual's needs, seem to be most accurate and effective.

Biologic Theories

It is unlikely that schizophrenia is caused by one specific biologic abnormality. Scientists have searched unsuccessfully for a unique biologic marker consistently present in people with schizophrenia but absent in healthy people. At the same time, evidence suggests that the disorder is not merely psychological and that biologic alterations are present. Particularly convincing is the fact that the symptoms associated with schizophrenia, such as delusions or hallucinations, are found in healthy people only when they are in a state of metabolic imbalance or suffer from organic diseases. Individuals who have brain tumors, have infections, or have ingested certain drugs, for example, may experience hallucinations.

Genetic Theories

People with schizophrenia inherit a genetic predisposition to the disease rather than inheriting the disease itself. What supports this theory is the fact that relatives of people with schizophrenia have a greater chance of developing the disease than do members of the general population. While 1.2% of the population develops schizophrenia, 10% of the first-degree relatives (parents, siblings, children) of persons with schizophrenia are diagnosed with the disease during their lifetimes. The risk of developing schizophrenia increases with the closeness of one's relationship to a diagnosed person. Siblings have a greater risk of developing the disease than do half-siblings or grandchildren, and these have a greater risk than more distant relatives, such as cousins.

There is no clear genetic marker for schizophrenia at this time, although several research projects are involved in the search for susceptibility genes. The most promising development has been research looking at the large number of genes involved in developing our nervous systems and the smaller number of genes called *epigenetic regulators,* or genes that can moderate genetic expression (Zahir & Brown, 2011). Because schizophrenia is complex and there are so many forms of the disorder, a single gene is not responsible for causing schizophrenia. It has been suggested that schizophrenia may be a collection of disorders rather than a single disease entity.

Research examining the occurrence of schizophrenia in twins indicates that both environmental and genetic factors are important. Rates of concordance (in which both twins either express or do not express the trait) for schizophrenia are consistently higher for monozygotic twins than for dizygotic twins. Interestingly, monozygotic, or identical, twins need not both have schizophrenia, but the chance of both twins having schizophrenia is 25% to 40%. This finding supports the hypothesis of some level of genetic transmission. The fact that both twins are not always affected when they are genetically identical, however, indicates that environment plays a large part in the expression of the illness. If the disease were solely genetically determined, the concordance rates in this group would be close to 100%. (See also pages 95 and 97 in Chapter 6 ∞ for another discussion of genetics in schizophrenia.)

Brain Structure Abnormalities

As a group, people with schizophrenia differ in their brain structure from people who do not have schizophrenia. People with chronic schizophrenia show changes to their frontotemporal cortical gray matter, among other areas. Magnetic resonance imaging (MRI) studies show

hippocampal structural differences between people who have schizophrenia and those who do not. When the hippocampus is formed, brain-derived neurotrophic factor (BDNF) is involved. Checking for abnormalities in BDNF may be able to tell us who is at risk for developing schizophrenia. Also, the BDNF increases when clients are on antipsychotic medication (Lee, Lange, Ricken, Hellweg, & Lang, 2011).

Altered brain structures may be genetically based and could represent a marker of vulnerability to schizophrenia that precedes any other symptomatology. How the brain structure abnormalities influence the progress of the disease is not well understood and requires further study. An example of PET scan differences between someone who has schizophrenia and someone who does not is seen in FIGURE 16-2 ■.

Biochemical Theories

The biochemical basis of schizophrenia is captured in the **dopamine hypothesis**, which states that schizophrenic symptoms may be related to overactive neuronal activity that is dependent on dopamine (DA). In other words, positive psychotic symptoms are associated with excessive DA transmission.

The hypothesis was supported by numerous studies demonstrating the alleviation of symptoms from treatment with DA blockers, which are medications that decrease DA activity. The traditional antipsychotic medications were shown to be effective because of their ability to antagonize DA receptors; however, this causes undesirable side effects such as extrapyramidal symptoms. The relief of positive symptoms with these traditional agents was not complete,

FIGURE 16-2 ■ PET scans measuring regional cerebral blood flow. (a) Areas of lower blood flow and brain activity are seen in the individual with schizophrenia. (b) Areas of normal blood flow and brain activity are visible in the unaffected individual.
Photo courtesy of R. Haier/Photolibrary.

PET/SPECT Schizophrenia Animation

Extrapyramidal Side Effects Videos

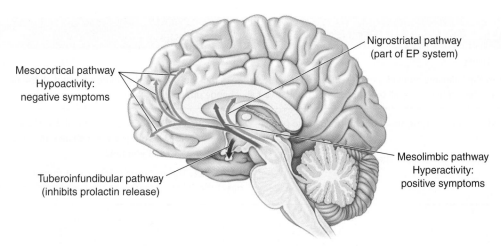

Mesocortical pathway
Hypoactivity:
negative symptoms

Nigrostriatal pathway
(part of EP system)

Tuberoinfundibular pathway
(inhibits prolactin release)

Mesolimbic pathway
Hyperactivity:
positive symptoms

FIGURE 16-3 ■ The dopamine hypothesis of schizophrenia holds that the amount of dopamine in various areas of the brain creates the various symptoms of the disease. Note how too much dopamine in the mesolimbic area (the middle of the limbic system) is thought to cause positive symptoms, while too little dopamine in the mesocortical area (the middle of the cortex of the brain) is thought to cause the negative symptoms of schizophrenia. Antipsychotic medications are designed to address this problem and attempt to stabilize these excesses and deficits.

and the negative symptoms of the disorder were much less responsive to DA blockers. See FIGURE 16-3 ■ for a graphic representation of this concept.

Research suggests that the relationships between DA activity and schizophrenic symptoms are much more complex than originally hypothesized. It is now known that there are multiple types of DA receptors, and different types of receptors are concentrated in different regions of the brain. The regulation of DA activity continues to be thoroughly studied, because DA dysregulation is recognized as being inherently involved in the pathology of schizophrenia.

Psychological Theories

Most psychological theories focus on the processing of information as well as attention and arousal states in schizophrenia.

Information Processing

Many clients with schizophrenia have information-processing deficits. Two central types of information processing have been identified, as follows:

1. Automatic processing
2. Controlled or effortful processing

Automatic processing occurs when you take in information unintentionally. Automatic processing can occur without your being aware of it and does not interfere with conscious thought processes that occur at the same time. An example of automatic information processing is being aware of the physical features of a new environment, such as a room being large and spacious as opposed to small and confined.

People with schizophrenia have difficulty in the skill called *controlled information processing*. Their ability to perform directed, conscious, sequential thinking—for example,

making comparisons between two stimuli or organizing a set of stimuli—is consistently inferior to that of people who do not have schizophrenia. Someone with schizophrenia would not be easily able to perform the series of steps necessary to organize a classroom debate. Any level of cognitive dysfunction creates ripple effects in treatment and quality of life. See Rx Communication for an example of an interaction with a client who is unfocused and having a problem processing information.

We do not know whether the inability of a person with schizophrenia to sustain conscious, directed thought is the primary problem or the result of a primary deficit in automatic thinking. If the primary deficit is in automatic processes, then the person is forced to complete automatic tasks at the conscious level, inhibiting and slowing controlled information processing. Sufficient evidence to resolve this question is not yet available.

Attention and Arousal

Attention and arousal are measured by physiological states and alterations, such as galvanic skin response, heart rate, blood pressure, skin temperature, and pupillary response. Physiological studies of attention and arousal in clients with schizophrenia show promise in identifying clinically significant subgroups.

One subgroup of clients exhibits abnormally low response levels to novel, or different, stimuli. This finding suggests that these clients are less adept than healthy people at attending to and responding to novel situations. An example of this state can be seen when a client with schizophrenia does not register that a ball is being thrown at him during a game of catch. The ball may even strike him, drop to the ground, and roll away before the client looks at it.

R$_X$ COMMUNICATION

Unfocused Client

CLIENT: "I went to the ballgame and I had great seats and I saw the whole game and I saw all the home runs and all the hits and all the strikeouts and I saw the pitcher throw all the pitches, fast ball, curve ball, change up, and. . . . "

NURSE RESPONSE 1: "Keith, tell me about this more slowly so I can keep up with you." *RATIONALE:* This response defines the special skills required for a conversation.	**NURSE RESPONSE 2:** "How about if I ask you some questions about the game? If you give me a chance to ask questions I'll have a better idea of what you saw." *RATIONALE:* This response is structured to be brief, focused, and to direct the client's attention to the speed with which he speaks.

A second group of clients with schizophrenia demonstrates a state of hyperarousal evidenced by elevated electrodermal activity, heart rate, and blood pressure. Hyperarousal has been noted during both symptomatic and nonsymptomatic periods. These clients demonstrate symptoms of irritability, excitement, and anxiety rather than apathy and withdrawal. An example of this state occurs when a client with schizophrenia angrily and loudly criticizes someone for using incorrect grammar in a sentence.

Family Theories

Numerous theories implicating family interaction alone as a cause of schizophrenia have been proposed and unsupported. Research has failed to support the theory that dysfunctional family interaction alone causes the illness.

Suggestions have been supported that disordered family communication (the inability to focus on and clearly share an observation or thought) causes schizophrenia only in the presence of a genetic predisposition to the disease. For example, the communication taking place at the dinner table may be chaotic and constant. No one finishes a sentence and nothing is discussed to its logical conclusion. Living with this pattern of family communication during early development is thought to impair the ability of the person with schizophrenia to perceive the environment and communicate with others about it. People with schizophrenia are more likely to show symptoms of thought disorder when they are raised by people who have dysfunctional communication.

Individuals with schizophrenia who are raised by adoptive parents, who themselves showed elevated levels of communication deviance, demonstrate as much thought disorder as those raised in birth families. In contrast, adoptees who were raised by adoptive parents with more functional communication were less likely to show thought disorder. This means there is not a "schizophrenogenic" environment for individuals who do not have a pre-existing genetic liability. These examples support the view that genetic factors alone do not explain the development of schizophrenia, and that interactions with the environment are important. Individuals who live in aversive environments tend to have higher rates of schizophrenia, suggesting there may be a neighborhood and social context to development of the disease.

The family or the environment's emotional tone can influence the course of schizophrenia over time. Researchers found that individuals with schizophrenia from families who are highly critical, hostile, overprotective, or overinvolved tend to relapse more often. Families exhibiting such characteristics have been described as having high **expressed emotion (EE)**. There is some evidence that family expressed emotion, life events, and biologic factors combine with the individual's genetic liability to the disorder to cause schizophrenia. In other words, the disorder is responsive to psychosocial attributes such as the emotional climate of the interpersonal environment (Rylands, McKie, Elliot, Deakin, & Tarrier, 2011). Recent research on schizophrenia can be found on the website for NARSAD at http://www.narsad.org and through a direct link on the Online Student Resources for this book.

Humanistic–Interactional Theories

An interactional model of schizophrenia integrates many of the biologic and psychosocial theories already discussed. In this view, schizophrenia is due to the interaction of a genetic predisposition or biologic vulnerability, stress or change in the environment, and the individual's social skills and supports. In an interactional model, the influences are multidimensional. A biologic vulnerability may inhibit the individual's capacity to cope with even minor stressors such as the loss of a primary source of support. Similarly, the symptoms of schizophrenia may worsen upon entering an environment that demands coping skills the person with schizophrenia may not have developed.

A precursor to present-day interactional theories is the enduring interpersonal–psychiatric theory of Harry Stack Sullivan (discussed in detail in Chapter 5 ∞). Sullivan, a psychiatrist, emphasized modes of interaction and the role of anxiety as the real focus of psychiatric inquiry in his work with people with schizophrenia. Hildegard Peplau (known as the "mother" of psychiatric nursing) based her interpersonal psychiatric nursing approach on the work of Sullivan. However, Peplau had more to say than Sullivan about the social and cultural conditions that influence behavior. The ideas of Sullivan and Peplau continue to influence our practice with clients who are schizophrenic.

Stress–Vulnerability Model

An interactional model for understanding schizophrenia that has received wide acceptance is the stress–vulnerability model, which suggests that people with schizophrenia have a genetically based, biologically mediated vulnerability to personal, family, and environmental stress. In this model, risk factors and protective factors interact in any of the following three ways:

1. Stressors, risk, and vulnerability factors combine and potentiate each other.
2. As long as stress is not excessive, it enhances competence.
3. Protective factors modulate or buffer the impact of stressors by improving coping and adaptation.

People with schizophrenia have a potentially increased vulnerability to stress. High-EE relatives or environments may cause them great stress, resulting in an exacerbation of symptoms and/or a relapse. It is now almost standard practice to aim to reduce high EE and criticism in the environment and relationships of people who have schizophrenia.

As we know, the stressors a client with schizophrenia experiences can overwhelm the resources available, and symptoms result. Psychobiologic stressors include the stress of living with schizophrenia itself. Altered attention and perception, as well as problems with motivation and energy, create stresses for people with schizophrenia. Environmental and interpersonal stressors include those we all encounter; however, a person with schizophrenia is particularly sensitive to them. These include stressful life events, environments that are highly demanding or stimulating, and family or living environments that are highly negative.

It is not unusual for clients to make statements that point to the validity of the stress–vulnerability concept, especially the protective qualities. One client said, "I'm not saying it [referring to an antipsychotic medication] is a perfect solution. It's not. There are painful side effects. But I know I can count on it when the going gets rough. If things get stressful it will help me through it." A second client said: "I feel raw inside and out when I'm off it [referring to an antipsychotic medication]. Everything bothers me. So it cushions the blows that are my life."

Resources That Moderate Stress

Resources that can moderate stress (and are thought to affect the development of symptoms in schizophrenia) include having someone who will recognize symptoms and help manage them, having social support, and taking antipsychotic medication. Social support has proven helpful in moderating stress for general populations and for people with schizophrenia in particular. Supportive others who provide empathy, interpersonal contact, financial aid, problem solving, and other forms of support help to mitigate the difficulties of schizophrenia. Finally, antipsychotic medications moderate some, and sometimes most, symptoms of the disease, and thus some of the stressors induced by the disease.

The capacities to self-monitor the waxing and waning of schizophrenia and to develop coping strategies to influence symptoms at the first sign of trouble show promise in influencing the longer-term course of the illness. Help your client learn how to self-monitor symptoms and develop effective coping strategies. This capacity to detect prodromal symptoms and acute symptoms and institute self-care before completely decompensating (having symptoms interfere significantly with functioning) is a resource that may work to mediate the stress that occurs in the person, family, or environment. Evidence-Based Practice shows how some coping mechanisms are better than others.

EVIDENCE-BASED PRACTICE

Assessing the Coping Skills of an Adolescent Client With Schizophrenia

Marvin is a 16-year-old male who has paranoid schizophrenia. He is one of the people with whom you work in an outpatient clinic for moderately ill people who have schizophrenia. Your education and experience have taught you that schizophrenia is a complex illness that requires more than medications to address it adequately.

As a teenager, Marvin has difficulties with interactions, problem solving, and coping that an older client may not have to the same extent. Older clients would have developed those skills prior to getting ill, or had access to psychoeducation and treatment from nurses and other professionals. You note that Marvin becomes stressed very easily and typically retreats into sleeping or wishful thinking to cope. He often feels anxious, fearful, and irritable. You notice that, although he will feel better for a brief time after he withdraws to bed or to daydreaming, over time Marvin is not learning how to cope nor is he developing problem-solving approaches.

This situation suggests the need to be active in helping Marvin learn new skills. Coping based on problem solving instead of emotions can lower Marvin's stress levels. Base your plan to teach Marvin on more than one study, but the following is a study that would be helpful in this situation.

Lee, H., & Schepp, K. G. (2011). Ways of coping in adolescents with schizophrenia. *Journal of Psychiatric & Mental Health Nursing, 18*(2), 158–165.

CRITICAL THINKING QUESTIONS

1. Is it possible for Marvin to learn new coping skills? Why, or why not?
2. How will you know if Marvin is using a problem-solving coping mechanism?

NURSING PROCESS
Clients With Schizophrenia

Schizophrenia is a difficult and chronic illness requiring understanding and competent care in every facet of the client's life. In addition to the discussion that follows, a nursing care plan for the client with schizophrenia is presented at the end of the chapter.

Assessment

Assessing clients who have schizophrenia occurs at individual, family, and environmental levels. Be aware of the client's status and of changes in the client's personal life, family situation, and environment in order to plan care and intervene effectively. In addition, care that addresses multiple levels of the client's life is consistent with the interactional theory of schizophrenia because it is assumed that changes in any aspect of the client's environment influence all other aspects of the personal environmental balance.

Subjective Data

These data describe the client's inner experience of schizophrenia.

Perceptual Changes The perceptions of clients with schizophrenia may be either heightened or blunted. These changes may occur in all the senses or in just one or two. For example, a client may see colors as brighter than normal or may be acutely sensitive to sounds. Another may have a heightened sense of touch and therefore be extremely sensitive to any physical contact. **Illusions** occur when the client misperceives or exaggerates stimuli in the external environment. A client with schizophrenia may mistake a chair for a person or perceive that the walls of a hallway are closing in. The perceptual changes are sufficient to cause the client to mistake the stimulus for something else (see the example of an illusion in Figure 10-1 on page 185∞). Hallucinations are the most extreme and yet the most common perceptual disturbance in schizophrenia. Auditory hallucinations are the most common form of hallucination. Although hallucinations are a hallmark of schizophrenia, their presence alone does not establish the presence of the disorder. Refer back to Table 16-1 on page 335, which lists various types of hallucinations.

Assess perceptual disturbances by asking the client about the experience and by observing for behaviors that indicate the client is frightened or attending to internal stimuli. Ask the client, "What are you seeing and hearing?" Note the degree to which this description differs from your perceptions of the environment. Clients may be reluctant to discuss the extreme perceptual disturbance of hallucinations. One of the ways you can introduce the topic is to discuss physical symptoms such as pain or discomfort. Then ask about hearing and vision skills. From there it is a smooth transition to asking about unusual experiences with hearing and seeing.

A classic sign of auditory hallucinations is placing the hands over the ears when clients are frightened by the voices and attempt to block them out. Less obvious signs of hallucinations are inappropriate laughing or smiling, difficulty following a conversation, and difficulty attending to what is happening at the moment. Fleeting, rapid changes of expression that are not precipitated by events in the real world can be another sign. The degree to which clients believe the hallucinatory experience is real and their ability to verify the reality of the experience by checking with others have important implications for interventions. Note the client's emotional response to hallucinations. Some clients experience depression or despair about the continued presence of voices; others may be comforted or kept company by their voices. Client coping strategies, and their effectiveness or ineffectiveness, are also an important aspect of assessment. Finally, clients may talk to themselves, presumably in answer to the voices they hear. Specific guidelines for assessing hallucinations are given in Your Assessment Approach.

Sleep Disturbances Significant sleep disruption occurs with an exacerbation of the symptoms of schizophrenia. Great difficulty getting to sleep (called *extended sleep latency*) may accompany extreme anxiety and concern about delusional and hallucinatory phenomena. The overall circadian cycle may also be disrupted. Clients with schizophrenia have a deficit of deeper sleep in stage 4, and reduced rapid eye movement (REM) sleep. A careful sleep history looks for other contributing factors—such as obesity-hypoventilation syndrome. In that case, the sleep problem can be minimized by continuous positive air pressure (CPAP).

Objective Data

These data are the observable symptoms and manifestations of schizophrenia that you, as a nurse, will assess.

YOUR ASSESSMENT APPROACH
Hallucinating Client

A complete assessment of hallucinations should identify the following:

- Whether the hallucinations are solely auditory or include other senses
- How long the client has experienced the hallucinations, what the initial hallucinations were like, and whether they have changed
- Which situations are most likely to trigger hallucinations, and which times of day they occur most frequently
- What the hallucinations are about (Are they just sounds, or voices? If the client hears voices, what do they say?)
- How strongly the client believes in the reality of the hallucinations
- Whether the hallucinations command the client to do something, and if so, how potentially destructive the commands are
- Whether the client hears other voices contradicting commands received in hallucinations
- How the client feels about the hallucinations
- Which strategies the client has used to cope with the hallucinations and how effective the strategies were

Disturbances in Thought and Expression Clients with schizophrenia find that their thinking is muddled or unclear. Their thoughts are disconnected or disjointed, and the connections between one thought and another are vague. The clarity of the client's communication often reflects the level of thought disorganization. Client responses may be simply inappropriate to the situation or conversation. They may have difficulty responding or stop in midsentence, as if they are stuck, a sign of **thought blocking**.

Note the rate and quality of the client's speech. Is it unusually loud, insistent, and continuous? Does the client wander from topic to topic or have *tangential communication* (communication with only a slight or tenuous connection to the topic)? An example is, "You want to know how I came here? I came here by bus, but bussing is kissing, I wasn't kissing but if you keep it simple that is a business tenet for KISS. That was a great group that played on and on but I'm not playing with you." Does the client bring up minute details that are irrelevant or unimportant to the topic at hand (*circumstantial communication*)? An example is, "You want to know how I came here? I came here on a blue and yellow bus with a lady bus driver. There were three teenage kids and a blind man with a seeing-eye dog on the bus. It didn't have to make a stop at the corner of Main and 9th." Are the client's responses slow and hesitant, reflecting difficulty in taking in stimuli and responding to them?

Clients with schizophrenia also have difficulty thinking abstractly. Their responses may be inappropriate because they interpret words literally rather than abstractly. For example, when told to prepare to have his blood drawn, a young man readied some paper and marking pens. You can assess abstract thinking by asking clients the meaning of proverbs, a test requiring the client to abstract a general meaning from a specific or metaphysical statement, for example, "People who live in glass houses shouldn't throw stones." Clients with schizophrenia are more likely to give concrete ("If you throw a stone the glass will break") rather than abstract ("Don't criticize someone else if you behave the same way") responses.

Disruptions in Emotional Responses Tone of voice, rate of speech, content of speech, expressions, postures, and body movements indicate emotional tone. Many individuals with schizophrenia demonstrate inappropriate affect—emotional responses that are inappropriate to the situation. For example, a client may smile or laugh while relating a history of having been abused as a child. Or, a client may become angry or anxious when asked to join a group of other clients for dinner. The degree to which a client's emotions are inappropriate is a prognostic indicator. Clients whose emotional response is preserved and generally appropriate have a more favorable prognosis than clients who demonstrate inappropriate affect.

A marked decrease in the variation or intensity of emotional expression is called **blunted affect** and is discussed earlier in this chapter with negative symptoms. The client may express joy, sorrow, or anger, but with little intensity.

Motor Behavior Changes Disruptions seen in schizophrenia include disorganized behavior and catatonia. Disorganized behavior lacks a coherent goal, is aimless, or is disruptive. Catatonic behavior is manifested by unusual body movement or lack of movement. This activity disturbance includes *catatonic excitement* (the client moves excitedly but not in response to environmental influences), *catatonic posturing* (the client holds bizarre postures for periods of time), and *stupor* (the client holds the body still and is unresponsive to the environment). Another motor concern is body posture and falls. People who have schizophrenia—especially those who are older—are more likely to be overweight, have extrapyramidal side effects (from their medication), and have some postural instability. Recognize these risk factors for falling (Koreki et al., 2011).

Neurologic Signs Schizophrenia involves neurologic deficits in many cases. Assessing for soft and hard neurologic signs can help you design appropriate interventions, given the individual client's needs. See Box 16-1 for specifics on these neurologic signs.

Changes in Role Functioning An important factor in predicting the course of schizophrenia is the client's level of functioning before the symptoms of the disease became pronounced. Assessment should therefore include a complete history of the client's success at completing developmental tasks. The prognosis is best if the client functioned at a high level prior to the onset of schizophrenic disturbance. Assess how well the client fulfilled role responsibilities in the family, in school, in relation to peers, and at work. Obtain a history of the rate of decline in these various roles. The onset of schizophrenia may be relatively acute, or degeneration may be slow.

Box 16-1 Neurologic Soft and Hard Signs

Neurologic soft signs are as follows:

- Increased frequency of eye blinking
- Difficulty following moving objects (abnormal smooth-pursuit eye movements called SPEMs)
- Impaired fine motor skills
- Abnormal motor tone
- Mild muscle twitches, choreiform movements (rapid, jerky movements that can cause leaping, jumping, or dancing motions), ticlike movements, facial grimaces not related to emotional responses
- Not able to recognize objects simply by touch (astereognosis). Clients have to look at the object.
- Cannot identify letters or numbers traced out on their skin (agraphesthesia)
- Impaired in ability to smoothly alternate and sequence movements such as alternating palm up and palm down (dysdiadochokinesia)

Neurologic hard signs are as follows:

- Loss of physical function
- Loss of strength
- Slowing of reflexes
- Impairment in motor and sensory behaviors

Drug Use Clients with drug toxicity, intoxication, or withdrawal may have behavior disturbances similar to those seen in clients with schizophrenia. They may have auditory or visual hallucinations and may be confused, illogical, and highly anxious. For this reason, it is essential to obtain a detailed drug history. Assess both long-term and recent use of chemical substances. If the client is not a reliable historian, you may try to interview the client's family or friends. In addition, both blood and urine should be tested for drugs if you cannot obtain reliable information.

Family Health History Part of a thorough and complete assessment is noting any history of mental disorder in the client's family. Of particular interest is a history of schizophrenia or any thought disorder, mood disorders (such as cyclical highs or depressions), or alcoholism in any family member. Note any report that family members had "nervous breakdowns" or any other colloquial descriptions of mental or emotional disorders.

Family Cohesion and Emotion In families of people with schizophrenia, enmeshment (see Chapter 29 ∞), combined with a negative emotional tone, is thought to be detrimental to the ill member's well-being. However, the presence of acquaintances and family members showing emotional warmth in low expressed emotion (EE) situations can have a protective function.

Much of the nursing assessment of family cohesion and emotion can be carried out unobtrusively. Chapter 29 ∞ has specific guidelines for assessment of these and other family dynamics. The nursing staff, in conjunction with the interdisciplinary team, can also arrange formal family assessment interviews (also discussed in Chapter 29 ∞). When you are observing interactions, note signs of dysfunction.

Family Overinvolvement and Negativity At present there are no clear-cut clinical determinants of exactly how much overinvolvement and negative emotion in families is problematic. Note families who seem excessively bonded emotionally. The inability of family members to maintain emotional, social, or physical separateness is a clear sign of this problem. Also assess for the presence of a high level of criticism among family members. Discuss families that seem seriously enmeshed or hypercritical with the treatment team.

Family Communication Problems Unclear or incomplete communication is frequent in families of people with schizophrenia. This area requires nursing assessment. Unclear communication may result from continual interaction with the ill member or may contribute to the disorder. Clinicians must evaluate how effectively the family communicates to determine the potential need for intervention.

Assess the following aspects of family communication:

- Ability to focus on a topic
- Ability to discuss a topic in a meaningful way with other family members
- Ability to maintain the discussion without wandering from the subject or becoming distracted
- Use of language and explanations that are generally understandable (not peculiar to that family alone)

Also note who in the family seems to do the talking, who talks to whom, and whether members talk for, or interrupt, one another. Box 16-2 shows communication problems that commonly occur with the diagnosis of schizophrenia and interfere with interpersonal relationships.

Family Burden Most families of individuals with schizophrenia report that caring for the ill member places a burden on the family unit. Ask about the challenges the family is facing so that you can determine the information and support needs to be met. See Chapter 29 ∞ for examples of common family burdens.

Environment Assess the availability of support and services beyond the bounds of the family, including extended family and friends, as well as community groups and organizations that support people with schizophrenia. Assess also the availability of mental health programs that address the specific mental health needs of people with schizophrenia.

Nursing Diagnosis: NANDA

Nursing diagnoses with clients with schizophrenia focus on alterations in the patterns of activity, cognition, emotional processes, interpersonal processes, and perception. Alterations in ecologic, physiological, and valuation processes are assessed as well; however, the central nursing problems relate to the former five processes.

Impaired Communication

Schizophrenia interferes with the ability to communicate, a complex and demanding function.

Box 16-2 Problematic Communication Patterns Common in Schizophrenia

Blocking

The client has trouble expressing a response or stops in midsentence, as if stranded without a thought.

Clang Associations

Words that rhyme or sound alike are distributed throughout conversations without necessarily making sense.

Echolalia

Phrases, sentences, or entire conversations said to the client are repeated back by the client.

Neologisms

Words or meanings are invented by the client. This can include multisyllabic, pseudo-scientific words or simple words.

Perseveration

The client maintains a particular idea regardless of the topic being discussed or attempts to change the subject.

Word Salad

An incoherent medley of words is emitted in conversation as if it was a sensible and articulate phrase.

Verbal Clients with schizophrenia may communicate in a disorganized, sometimes incomprehensible fashion. Some clients, because their thinking is disorganized, speak very little (alogia, or poverty of speech). Also note there may be a poverty of content in speech, in that the client converses but actually says very little. Often, clients with schizophrenia communicate in ways that are overly concrete (a sign of an inability to think and communicate abstractly) or overly symbolic (a sign of preoccupation with unreal or delusional material). The symbols are usually difficult to decipher because their meanings are idiosyncratic to that particular individual.

Nonverbal The facial and bodily expressions that accompany the verbal communication of people with schizophrenia frequently do not match the content of the verbal message. This lack of congruence is primarily due to the blunting of emotions found in schizophrenia. Expected facial expressions—smiles, looks of concern or disgust—may not accompany the client's statements. In addition, clients with motor or behavioral abnormalities—posturing, unusual movements, or grimacing—convey a confusing mix of verbal and nonverbal messages.

Self-Care Deficits

People with schizophrenia frequently appear indifferent to their personal appearance. They may neglect to bathe, change clothes, or attend to minor grooming tasks such as combing their hair. Some show little awareness of current fashion styles, and many wear clothing that makes them look out of place. Of greater concern are those who wear clothing that is inappropriate to the current season and weather conditions.

Although lack of attention to grooming might be a simple annoyance to those who must live in close proximity to the person with schizophrenia, health risks related to prolonged poor hygiene can arise. Assess immediate problems, such as inadequate nutrition, fluid intake, and elimination, as well as long-term problems, such as dental caries and increased susceptibility to infections.

Disregard for appearance and hygiene may extend to the client's environment. The client may fail to maintain a clean and safe living space. He or she may not take good care of personal belongings and may misplace them. Self-care deficiencies may result from consistently disturbed thought and perceptual processes. For example, a client whose chronic hallucinations are only partly relieved by medication may have difficulty concentrating for long periods and paying attention to grooming.

Activity Intolerance

The emotional disturbances of ambivalence and apathy, common in schizophrenic disorders, can result in lack of interest and inactivity. Inactivity induced by ambivalence is associated with higher levels of emotion. Anxious about choosing one course of action and rejecting another, the client is immobilized. The following clinical examples describe the experience of intolerance to activity.

Clinical Example

Jim is ambivalent about taking a pass to go out alone from the inpatient unit for the first time. He is undecided about taking the risk of leaving the hospital setting without a staff member, yet yearns for the freedom of walking the streets alone. Indecision leaves him standing, immobilized, by the doorway to the unit.

Extreme ambivalence can manifest itself in even the most automatic of behaviors.

Clinical Example

Melissa cannot eat because of ambivalence about where to sit or what to eat. She stands in the center of the dining room, turning first to one chair and then another, unable to choose where to sit so that she can begin eating.

Clients who are inactive because of apathy demonstrate little emotional tone. Such clients may spend long hours lying in bed staring into space or listening to music. Often, but not always, apathetic individuals prefer isolation. You might find several clients sitting in the same room, engaged in no apparent activities, and interacting with one another only when absolutely necessary.

Social Isolation

Extreme anxiety about relating to others often leads clients with schizophrenia to withdraw from interaction and to isolate themselves. Some clients tolerate only a few moments of direct communication, whereas others can manage extended periods of contact. Assess the client's tolerance of brief periods of contact with staff and other clients. Document patterns of relating and withdrawal, also noting in which activities the client engages when in contact with others and which activities the client undertakes when alone. Nurses who work in skilled nursing facilities also need to be able to diagnose social isolation as a symptom of schizophrenia (see What Every Nurse Should Know).

Decisional Conflict

Decisional conflict in schizophrenia is probably due to biochemical alterations in the brain that make it difficult for clients to take in, synthesize, and respond to information. Decisional conflict may be evident both in the mundane activities of daily life (e.g., selecting one's diet) and in major life decisions. This can be frustrating for caregivers and for clients. The following clinical example shows how decisional conflict can remove what is a pleasant aspect of life from the client.

Clinical Example

Murray refuses to take medications, even though not taking them means that he will be evicted from the residential treatment program he likes.

Disturbed Sensory Perception

Alterations in the five senses (sound, sight, smell, taste, touch) create an altered perception of the world.

WHAT EVERY NURSE SHOULD KNOW

Primary Symptoms of Schizophrenia

Imagine you are a skilled nursing facility (SNF) nurse. You need to be familiar with the primary symptoms of schizophrenia—delusions, hallucinations, agitation, and general decompensation in order to competently assess your clients. There are two reasons SNF nurses should be familiar with these symptoms:

1. These symptoms are part of a disease process that require treatment.
2. The presence of these symptoms can distort or mask the presentation of symptoms of physical illnesses, and severe psychiatric distress can impair healing from medical and surgical procedures and injuries.

When an SNF resident has symptoms that appear to include behavioral and psychiatric features, the SNF nurse should be prepared and able to document, classify, and report these symptoms correctly, and to help ensure the resident receives necessary treatment. Knowing the interventions, pharmacologic and nonpharmacologic, can speed stabilization and improve the quality of life the residents experience.

Hallucinations Hallucinations are both a clinical diagnostic sign of schizophrenia and a focus for nursing care. You need to know the extent and nature of clients' hallucinations so that you can document the hallucinatory experience. Discuss with the client, if the client is able to, the details of his or her symptoms. Look for major themes in the content of the hallucinations, particularly whether the hallucinations command the client to take action. *Command hallucinations* such as "Jump up and down. Jump up and down. Don't look at her, she has cancer and you'll catch it," can be difficult for the client to cope with and can affect the client's behavior. The client may not be able to withstand pressured commands to say things or perform acts that could include a refusal to remain in

a housing situation (which could lead to homelessness), violence, or suicide (Kasckow, Felmet, & Zisook, 2011).

Illusions Illusions (mistaken perceptions) make the client vulnerable to emotional and physical injury. We all have these experiences from time to time and they are not part of a pathologic process. For example, you may see what you think is a palm tree, but another look tells you it is an evergreen. But for someone with schizophrenia, the level of misperception may vary from day to day and even throughout the day. Misperceptions of the social environment make the client vulnerable to inappropriate responses that may be ridiculed by others. Misperceptions of the physical environment, such as misjudging the speed of an oncoming car, may lead to physical harm.

Disturbed Body Image

A body image disturbance is common in people with schizophrenia. Clients may lose the sense of where their bodies leave off and where inanimate objects begin. They may become dissociated from various body parts and believe, for example, that their arms and legs belong to someone else. They may worry about the normalcy of their sexual organs. Clients often verbalize this altered sense of self directly, saying "I don't feel like myself" or "I feel like I am looking at my body from somewhere else in the room."

Excess Fluid Volume

Excess fluid intake, or water intoxication, is a problem that is observed primarily in clients who reside in institutions such as state mental hospitals. This physiological state is brought on by excessive drinking, characterized by hyponatremia, confusion, and disorientation, and progresses to apathy and lethargy. In severe cases, seizures and death may result. This behavior can lead to irreversible brain damage. Polydipsia appears to be significantly associated with male gender, smoking, celibacy, and psychiatric chronicity. Polydipsia in schizophrenia is a difficult problem to treat in that behavioral interventions struggle to balance protecting the client while maintaining the client's independence. Acetazolamide (Diamox) and clozapine (Clozaril) are included as effective

MENTAL HEALTH IN THE NEWS

Henry Cockburn

Patrick Cockburn is a foreign correspondent for the British press who recently found out his son, Henry, is schizophrenic. While on assignment in Afghanistan in the winter of 2002, his 20-year-old son Henry was fished fully clothed from an icy river back home. Henry's mother had noted "sinister changes" in his behavior for months, but this latest episode included hallucinatory voices and visions so threatening to Henry that the river seemed the best place to hide. Henry was taken to a mental hospital and since then, like many people with unremitting schizophrenia, has never lived unsupervised or entirely free from his disease.

This father and son tell their story in the book *Henry's Demons: Living with Schizophrenia, A Father and Son's Story*. Patrick tells

of his first naïve assumptions that Henry would recover and resume his previous life, and how this moved to his final stark, resigned descriptions of Henry at age 27. Living in a halfway house in London, Henry is a person who "spent a lot of his waking life thinking about where he could get his next cigarette and where he could smoke it."

Henry contributes his own version of the story by highlighting his obsessive need to be outdoors (he has escaped from even top-security facilities dozens of times) and his profound reluctance to medicate all his vivid hallucinations away. "The forest would come alive and speak to me," he writes. "The tree roots would move at the touch of my finger."

Photo courtesy © Rosie Hallam/eyevine/Rudux.

pharmacologic treatments for this population (Takagi, Watanabe, Takefumi, Sakata, & Watanabe, 2011). For clients suspected to be at risk because of frequent drinking, preventive measures include regular measures of urine specific gravity, and regular weights designed to screen for increases in the body's fluid volume.

Disturbed Thought Processes

Schizophrenia changes the way thoughts are processed by distorting logic and organization.

Delusions Clients express delusional thinking in direct interactions and, to a lesser extent, through behaviors. When asked, many clients willingly describe their delusional beliefs in detail. They seldom withhold this information because they believe firmly in the validity of the delusion, no matter how bizarre it seems to others. Clients' actions reflect the fixedness of their beliefs.

Clinical Example

Gerry has the somatic delusion that her body is riddled with holes. She flatly refuses to drink, convinced that the fluid will flow directly out of the holes and soil her dress.

The content of delusions varies: delusions of persecution, reference, and so on (see Table 16-3). Reality-based delusions may seem plausible because they could, under some circumstances, actually occur. Bizarre delusions, more common among clients with schizophrenia, have no possible basis in reality. On the other hand, the false belief that one's husband is having an affair with a neighbor has a possible basis in reality, and is called a *reality-based delusion*. In contrast, the belief that one's thoughts are directed by a television announcer, or that one's unspoken thoughts can be heard by others, are known as *bizarre delusions*.

Delusions often reflect the client's fears, particularly about personal inadequacies. For example, a man's grandiose delusion that he is the mayor of New York City could be a defense against feelings of inferiority. Similarly, persecutory delusions defend against the person's own feelings of aggression. Aggressive feelings are projected onto a person or organization—for example, the police, whom the client then fears.

Magical Thinking Magical thinking is the belief that events can happen simply because one wishes them to. Some people with schizophrenia claim they can exert their will to make people take certain actions or make specific events occur, like winning the lottery.

Thought Insertion, Withdrawal, and Broadcasting Hallmarks of schizophrenic thought are the beliefs that others can put ideas into one's head (*thought insertion*) or take thoughts out of one's head (*thought withdrawal*). In addition, some clients believe that their thoughts are transmitted to others via radio, television, or other means but not directly by the client. This belief is known as *thought broadcasting*.

Dysfunctional Family Processes

When a family has a member with a significant illness, regardless of whether it is a mental or physical illness, that family's functioning and dynamics change. The operations of the family must change to accommodate the ill family member as well as how the rest of the family deals with the illness. The symptoms of the illness may be alien to family members, and they may not know how they should respond. See Partnering With Clients and Families for guidelines on how to teach families about the negative symptoms of schizophrenia.

Interrupted Family Processes

Families burdened with the long-term responsibility of caring for a relative with schizophrenia may suffer disruptions in their household routine, work, social interactions, and

PARTNERING WITH CLIENTS AND FAMILIES

Teaching About the Negative Symptoms of Schizophrenia

Families and caregivers have a difficult time understanding that symptoms of an illness include not just those experiences that are unusual and extra, such as hallucinations and delusions, but also those aspects of being human that are missing, such as enjoyment and motivation. You need to evaluate the family's current level of awareness of negative symptoms and provide important information.

Suggestions	Rationale
Discuss how not having motivation and not seeming to care about surroundings are part of the illness.	Families may be comforted to know that their loved one is not choosing to behave in this way.
Inform the family members about how these symptoms look and feel to the client.	Frequently, family members may blame medication for causing the client to be "zoned out" or "just sitting and staring."
Help families identify their responses to the negative symptoms.	Families often misinterpret negative symptoms as laziness or refusing to cooperate, and communicate this to the client. This increases the negativity to which the client is exposed.
Talk about when and how negative symptoms respond to medications.	The time frame of 18–24 months before negative symptoms respond to atypical antipsychotics may seem a long time to family members, and they will need support so their expectations are realistic.

physical well-being. The household may be disrupted by the client's insistence that the family act on and accommodate delusional beliefs. The family may bend to the client's wish, fearing an increase in the client's anxiety and possible fighting or shouting if they do not comply.

Clinical Example

The Walker family built an extra bathroom rather than fight with Tim, their son with schizophrenia, who spends hours in the bath completing elaborate washing rituals.

The Sherman family must eat out several times a week because Suzanne, their daughter with schizophrenia, refuses to allow anyone in the room when she eats.

The family social life may be disrupted. For instance, the family may fear leaving the ill person alone, or they may fear that the ill person will embarrass visitors if friends are invited in. Some families are willing to be open about the adjustments they make in living with a loved one with schizophrenia, whereas others choose to live isolated lives.

Family members' work can suffer because of the emotional strain of living with an ill member. They must take time off to accompany the schizophrenic person to doctors' appointments, make hospital visits, and help during interviews with social agencies or the police. Family health may suffer because of general inattention or because of prolonged stresses within the home.

Outcome Identification: NOC

The outcome criteria established for a client with schizophrenia need to be flexible and include the option to acknowledge a partial behavior change as success. For example, the outcome for Body Image Distortion may include (a) recognizes symptom regularly, (b) speaks often with important other person regarding body feelings, and (c) manages to function despite symptomatology much of the time. Setting realistic goals and continually re-evaluating expectations based on

your client's current desires and status is imperative with outcomes development. Other issues for outcomes with this population are an awareness of the client's multiple functional deficits, your personal response to working with this population, cultural differences, and lethality factors. See Caring for the Spirit for cultural awareness contributions to outcomes.

Outcomes for other psychotic disorders, such as delusional disorder or brief psychotic disorder, have similar features. However, as the underlying process is less debilitating, your goals will likely be at a higher level of functioning. Someone with a delusional disorder will learn how to live with the symptom while remaining functional at work and in social and home life situations.

Planning and Implementation: NIC

Nursing interventions are most effective when they focus on the needs and wants of the client to maximize functioning. In order to accomplish this, you must attend to the issues that are important to the client. The client's perspective is the most valuable tool you have to create competent and meaningful treatment interventions. Box 16-3 discusses the issues most important to the client with schizophrenia, from the unique perspective of the client.

When planning care for any client with a chronic illness, nurses must be careful to set realistic goals for client change. Take particular care with clients who are schizophrenic because they are extremely sensitive to change and failure. Deterioration in all aspects of functioning is characteristic of the disease. Focus on the most troublesome areas of client functioning and set incremental, short-term goals that pave the way for successes in achieving long-term goals. Answering the questions in Your Self-Awareness: Working With Clients Who Have Schizophrenia will increase your effectiveness in working with a psychotic client.

Preventing Relapse

Programs for relapse prevention with schizophrenia typically combine standard doses of maintenance antipsychotic medication

CARING FOR THE SPIRIT

Can Culturally Adapted Interventions Make a Difference in Outcome?

Schizophrenia is a difficult illness with many presentations. The distress people experience during symptom exacerbation motivates the search for treatments that are effective and useful in fulfilling the needs of the client. The search for answers has taken a variety of pathways, including the realm of spirituality and cultural sensitivity.

The quality of mental health services available to people who have schizophrenia are greatly enhanced when the relevant content of both psychoeducational and mental health interventions are culturally linked. Think about the last time you spoke with somebody about a problem you were having. If that person had an understanding of both your culture and your value system, such as spirituality, you probably had

an easier time explaining your problem. Now think about a time when you spoke with somebody about a problem you were having and that person had no idea what you were talking about. How would you describe that experience? As you can imagine, this happens quite often with people who have schizophrenia when their symptoms are unusual or they are not able to articulate them clearly.

Culture, spirituality, and a value system are intricately interwoven. They form the fabric for a system of meaning. Symptom expression, stressors, coping mechanisms, and interactions with others arise from this system. Keeping the cultural and spiritual context of a client's experience in mind while interacting around psychiatric symptoms and treatment reduces the client's frustrations and increases the effectiveness of your communication.

Box 16-3 Important Issues for the Client With Schizophrenia

People who have schizophrenia have to deal with an illness different from any other disease. The symptoms are unlike anything else, and anosognia (unawareness of the illness) can further complicate their lives. Imagine not knowing you have an illness and not, therefore, needing help. It makes accepting treatment and staying in treatment particularly challenging. Developing meaningful treatment and conducting effective interventions incorporate the following vital aspects into effective nursing care:

- Personal power and efficacy
- Interpersonal relationships
- Social expectations
- Differences between what one hoped for oneself and what one has now
- Connecting with people
- Personal growth
- Stability
- Coping with relapses
- Expression of spirituality
- Understanding the symptoms of the illness

with psychosocial treatment. Early clinical intervention when low-level symptom worsening occurs is effective in preventing a full relapse in clients with schizophrenia. And for clients residing with their families, educational and supportive family interventions have an important effect on relapse prevention. A further discussion can be found in Chapter 32 ∞.

YOUR SELF-AWARENESS
Working With Clients Who Have Schizophrenia

To increase self-awareness about working with a person with active psychosis, ask yourself the following questions:

- How do I feel about approaching a person who is having hallucinations?
- How do I feel about talking to someone who has delusions that frighten him?
- Have I ever encountered someone in public who was psychotic?
- Do I fear that I might do something that might make the person's illness worse?
- What kinds of understanding and knowledge do I need to feel comfortable working with clients with psychosis?

To increase self-awareness about working with clients with disrupted ability to care for themselves, ask yourself the following questions:

- Do I react negatively when I think about someone my age who has never worked?
- What goes through my mind when I see someone who is disheveled, unclean, or oddly dressed?
- How can I find a point of connection between myself and someone whose life is so dramatically different from my own?

Promoting Adequate Communication

Clients with schizophrenia try to communicate, even though their statements may be difficult to understand. Close attention to what the client is saying and honest attempts to understand the real and symbolic aspects of the message are important. The client will perceive nuances of your behavior. Therefore, one of the most direct and successful ways to demonstrate caring and respect is to attend seriously to the client (this is discussed in depth in Chapter 10 ∞).

Clients make valid observations about their environment, needs, and concerns. Some, if not all, of their observations and sensations exist in reality and are not to be treated as if they are all totally psychotic symptoms. The sensitivity to the environment that can overwhelm someone with schizophrenia also clues him or her into aspects to which others may not have access. A client may make observations about events or situations that are beyond your awareness. For example, take seriously a client's statement about another client's drug use or suicidal threats. If a client complains of a physical symptom such as stomach distress, consider the symptom as real until there is evidence otherwise. It is easy to dismiss a client's statements, particularly those of a delusional client. Doing so, however, shows lack of respect for the client's intact capacities to see and respond to what is happening in the environment.

Promoting Adherence With Medication Regimen

Psychotropic medications play an important part in the treatment of schizophrenic disorders. Drugs that diminish focal symptoms (hallucinations and delusions) and yet produce relatively few untoward effects are now available. Adherence to treatment, which for schizophrenia means medications, is a complex demand. You will need to be creative and ever-mindful of your client's specific barriers to learning and maintaining specific behaviors. The disease itself causes difficulty in adhering to a treatment regimen when a client lacks the ability to recognize the illness. This is called poor insight and can be compared to the unawareness or lack of insight into neurologic deficits following a stroke. Recognize that individuals respond to their illness, their circumstances, and their medications in different ways.

The idea of adherence can be expressed through a number of terms such as treatment adherence, role reliability, collaboration for health behaviors, and cooperation. Interviews and clinical contacts tell us that clients are able to participate in the treatment if they are included and made an integral part of the design of their care. See Box 16-4 for a description of the barriers and challenges to treatment adherence. Consistent adherence in taking medications as prescribed is not common among this client population, although psychiatric clients are not unique in that regard. People in endocrine, pediatric, antiretroviral, and antibiotic situations also struggle with adherence to medications. Nonadherence is especially problematic for psychiatric clients because nonadherence often leads to an exacerbation of illness, violence, and suicide.

Clients who do not take their medications are more vulnerable to stressors and risk more frequent relapse of

---

Box 16-4   Challenges to Adherence

Clients may stop taking their medications for these reasons:

- Difficulties with prescribed psychotropic medications
- Severe level of symptomatology
- Cognitive difficulties secondary to thought disorder
- Motivational problems secondary to negative symptoms
- Motivational problems secondary to flight into health (wanting to be "normal")
- Unpleasant side effects
- Persistence of positive symptoms (delusions) mitigating against adherence
- Financial issues
- Misperceptions and misunderstanding of the information presented in medication teaching
- Cursory or minimal medication teaching that lacks relevance to all areas of the client's life
- Unresolved issues with treatment providers
- Cultural impacts
- Misunderstanding the administration instructions
- Disorganization that prevents the client from following the instructions
- Uncomfortable side effects of major tranquilizers
- Rejecting treatment in order to avoid being stigmatized as having schizophrenia
- Feeling better and believing the medication is no longer necessary
- Having difficulty in easy access to pharmacies because of transportation, financial, or interpersonal difficulties

---

symptoms. Efforts to educate clients about their medications and to have them practice self-medication prior to discharge have increased the rate of adherence marginally. Client attitudes toward the medications prescribed also influence their willingness to adhere to the regimen. You must be an active participant in assessing adherence and fostering a positive attitude toward medications. Commonly used antipsychotic medications and side effects are presented in Chapter 31 ∞.

Clients are often ambivalent about taking medications. Maintaining adequate blood levels of therapeutic medications is important for clients with schizophrenia. To help them overcome ambivalence, give them time to think about taking the medications. Set a time limit. For an inpatient who fails to take the medication, come back later and try again. Two useful strategies are reminding clients of the positive effects of the medication and framing the action as a way for them to help themselves get better. Your Intervention Strategies is a compendium for increasing treatment adherence for clients with schizophrenia.

Assisting With Grooming and Hygiene

Helping clients establish and maintain personal care habits is a complex process. If the client clearly lacks the skills, then teach the skills. If, however, the client has learned grooming skills but does not practice them, focus on ways to motivate the client. Intervention begins by establishing clear expectations about essential grooming habits. The frequency and timing

of all aspects of grooming—including bathing, dressing, hair care, oral hygiene, and room care—can be specified in writing if that would be a useful learning device for your client.

Formal training programs for helping chronically mentally ill clients improve their grooming skills can be applied in inpatient as well as outpatient settings. These programs are well developed and tested. They systematically help clients in all steps of personal grooming, including collecting grooming supplies, moving to the grooming area (a bathroom or bedroom with sink and mirror), completing each grooming step, completing appropriate dressing, and storing grooming materials. Nursing interventions at each step can progress from simple verbal coaching, to modeling, to gentle physical guidance. Acknowledge client efforts during each phase with realistic encouragement and praise. The success of these programs probably depends on daily staff attention to the client's training, along with consistent, meaningful rewards. Avoid power struggles regarding the completion of tasks. If initial prompts don't work, leave the client alone for a short period.

Promoting Organized Behavior

Clients whose behavior is disorganized require direction and limits to make their actions more effective and goal directed. In working with a disorganized client, proceed slowly and remain calm. The client's perception of the environment may be distorted, but your calmness can help calm the client. Try to direct the client in simple, safe activities. Nursing goals and interventions for a disorganized client must focus on manageable steps. A clinical example of one such intervention follows.

Clinical Example

George is moving quickly yet aimlessly from the refrigerator to the cupboard. He pulls a box of cereal from the cupboard, opens it, and then wanders away. Next he goes to the refrigerator, opens the door, peers in, and closes the door. Rummaging through all his pockets, he locates a comb, combs through his hair, sets the comb on the counter, and wanders back to the cupboard. This effortful yet unproductive behavior continues for several minutes when the nurse enters.

Nurse: "George, are you trying to get some cereal for yourself?"

George: "Sort of. I was going to . . . brush . . . no . . . comb . . . no . . . eat something. Yeah, I wanted something to eat."

Nurse: "Try to concentrate on one thing. First, put the comb back in your pocket." (He does so.) "Now, come over here and get the cereal box. Here's a bowl. Here's a spoon." (She hands him the utensils.) "Why don't you sit right here?" (She seats him so that he has his back to the rest of the activity in the room.) "Can you sit still for a bit?"

George: "I think so."

Nurse: "Pour yourself some cereal. I'll get the milk for you." (She does so.)

George begins to eat his cereal quietly. The nurse stays with him for a few minutes and directs him to continue eating each time he becomes distracted by others who come into the room.

YOUR INTERVENTION STRATEGIES Increasing Medication Adherence
for Clients With Schizophrenia

- Involve the client as a partner in medication-based treatment planning decisions.
- Change to another medication with a different neurotransmitter action with lower or different side effects that may be more tolerable. Atypical antipsychotic medications have a lower side-effect profile and can increase adherence because they're not so hard to take.
- Teach the client how to report side effects, such as dry mouth, priapism (persistent, usually painful, erection of the penis). This may require role-playing or assertiveness training.
- Teach the client how to manage the side effects he does get (sugar-free hard candy or sugar-free gum helps with dry mouth, and a rubber pillow case liner helps with nighttime drooling). It may make it tolerable to continue on the medication.
- Instruct, educate, and arrange for reminders well before discharge (especially with geriatric recipients) to maximize both knowledge and adherence (knowledge can be the number-one factor determining adherence).
- Simplify the medication regimen.
- Match the medication dosing strategy to the client's schedule, preferences, work situation, and recreational pursuits.
- Discuss the client's expectations of the medication—are they realistic?
- Take cultural impacts into account during comprehensive treatment planning.
- Use concrete educators. The tried-and-true cognition enhancers are: pamphlets, booklets, handbooks, workbooks, sheets, cards, videos, audiotapes, posters, magnets, logs, journals, and so on.
- Assess the client's perception of control over the treatment regimen.
- Assess the client's self-administration of medications.
- Help the client take action to prevent untoward effects, such as maintaining fluid intake to avoid postural hypotension.

- Teach coping efforts that involve problem solving, which increases adherence.
- Encourage peer support. Hearing from *peers* how a new medication could help with symptoms, and asking the prescriber to consider it, improves adherence.
- Give hope—it pays to be well. It takes all the small steps to recovery in addition to medications to get better.
- Use repetition—say the same thing over and over, with patience, especially if clients have schizophrenia or depression.
- Develop reminders, cues to remembering (visual cues—when I see this I need to take my pills, when I eat lunch I take my pills, rubber band on wrist, calendars, to-do lists; auditory cues—alarm clocks or watches).
- Recommend the use of depot medications, which are given weekly, biweekly, or monthly; these can contribute to adherence because the client does not have to remember to take pills. The marketing of an atypical antipsychotic in depot form (risperidone, olanzapine) adds to the choices.
- Teach the client to use pill boxes—come in many shapes, sizes, and organizational styles (multiple daily doses, layers for time of day, Braille markings, timer with small alarm clock feature that opens compartment). If the medication cannot be taken out of its original container without affecting the potency, place a small button or candy in the pill box to serve as a reminder.
- Keep all medications and information about them in one dry, cool place. Use plastic products such as containers and bags—*not* in the bathroom or by a dishwasher in the kitchen.
- Involve the family.
- Match the degree of client autonomy in treatment to the needs of the individual client.
- Inform the client that financial assistance might be available.
- Have clients teach other recipients or their significant others about their medications (after they have learned sufficiently). Nothing speeds learning as much as teaching others.

Care Plan: Social Isolation and Schizophrenia

Promoting Social Interaction and Activity

The client's efforts to withdraw from social contact stem from past relationship failures and fear of rejection. Clients often find their internal world less risky and therefore more attractive than a world that requires interpersonal relating. When making efforts to help the client become less withdrawn, respect the client's sometimes overwhelming anxiety about human contact.

After establishing a basic level of trust, encourage the client to try out new behaviors within the relationship. The goal is to have the client experience success; therefore, encourage even small increments of change. If, for example, the client has difficulty initiating conversation, encourage the client to practice this skill once a day. Similarly, if the client avoids any activity in the environment because of fear of relating to groups, structure an activity involving the client, yourself, and one other client. Encourage client to communicate, even if that communication contains

problematic patterns (refer back to Rx Communication on pages 340 and 344).

Promoting Social Skills and Activities

Address social skills that are essential to functioning in the environment: introducing oneself, starting a conversation, ending a conversation, saying no, asking for assistance, and listening. Staff members can model these skills and help clients role-play each skill. Focus discussion on situations in which clients might need the skill. If they see its applicability to dilemmas in their personal lives, they will be motivated to learn the skill. Praise and, if available, material rewards can also motivate clients. Social skills training can also be done in small groups (see Chapter 28 ∞).

Schizophrenia can disturb a person's will and capacity to accomplish meaningful activity. Clients with distorted perceptions and thinking expend considerable energy merely taking in and interpreting their immediate worlds. In addition, major tranquilizers, which control the positive symptoms of the disease, can further inhibit a client's active involvement and interest in activities. Be aware of how much work it takes to cope with schizophrenic symptoms. Do not assume that periods of quiet or inactivity are due to laziness or lack of interest. Rather, assess each individual's need for quiet periods in which to organize perceptions and thoughts. At the same time, clients with schizophrenia live in a culture in which action and accomplishment are highly prized and rewarded. They are not immune to the pressure for personal productivity as a measure of personal worth. For this reason, they feel better about themselves when they are involved in meaningful activities. Your task is to help clients find activities that are intrinsically rewarding or that bring some social or tangible reward, yet are within their capacities. See Developing Cultural Competence for ideas about this aspect of psychiatric–mental health nursing.

Learning clients' personal interests is a first step. Providing opportunities for the client to actively engage in an activity of interest (by providing records, books, craft materials, or access to newspapers and television) is the next intervention.

DEVELOPING CULTURAL COMPETENCE

Culture, Religion, and Schizophrenia

In developing your cultural competence with clients who have schizophrenia and their families, keep in mind the potent influences culture has on the perception of illness. In a very religious family, a young man who hears an ancestral spirit speaking to him and sees its movement around him may be considered blessed or chosen, as opposed to ill or disordered. Therefore, there would be no reason to seek treatment for an experience thought to be special and advantageous. This could continue for a significant period of time, deepening problematic neurochemical processes.

In order to determine whether intervention is necessary, you would need to know the elements of the cultural environment and obtain additional information. An assessment of the young man would include his spiritual and cultural beliefs. You would also consider his overall functioning, because the concept of schizophrenia encompasses more than sensory experiences. If you found him to have poor interaction skills—he does not make sense when speaking—and he has been poorly groomed over a long period of time, you may consider these to be clues to a disorder, and not necessarily related to religiosity.

If the family continued to see their son's experience as religious despite evidence of cognitive and emotional dysfunction, education and outreach could provide support. You might discuss with his family how it would be possible to explore the need for diagnosis and treatment while maintaining the possibility of this being a unique religious experience.

CRITICAL THINKING QUESTIONS

1. Why is it important to know the client and family's interpretation of unusual experiences?
2. How does the client's religious and cultural background shape your plan for therapeutic interventions?

In addition, activities within the therapeutic milieu, such as attending groups and completing unit "jobs," can provide the external rewards of praise from staff and peers. These activities give clients confidence and develop and promote their work habits. Success in these activities can lead to success in volunteer or paid work in the community after discharge.

Intervening With Hallucinations and Delusions

Delusions or hallucinations often frighten clients. You can intervene by doing the following:

- Reassure clients that they are safe.
- Protect them from physical harm as they respond to their altered perceptions.
- Validate the feelings they are having in response to their experience.
- Validate reality.
- Help them distinguish what is real from what is a hallucination or a delusion.

Hallucinations are especially frightening if the client has never experienced them before or if their content is threatening or angry. Attempt to alleviate this anxiety by describing your perception of the frightened behavior and asking clients to discuss what they are experiencing. Make simple reassuring remarks, such as "I hear what you are telling me. This sounds very frightening. No one means to harm you." See Your Intervention Strategies for intervention strategies that help a client manage hallucinations.

Protect clients from harm and reassure them about safety. A client may take impulsive action to escape the frightening experience or to obey voices in the hallucination. Prevent this by doing the following:

- Closely observe client behavior during active hallucinations.
- Use calming techniques and one–to–one interactions to shape and guide the situation.

YOUR INTERVENTION STRATEGIES
Helping a Client Manage Hallucinations

- Determine the kind of hallucinations (auditory, visual, etc.).
- Can the symptom be managed with current coping?
- Access resources (advocacy groups, peers, staff, literature) for fresh ideas or better management techniques.
- Discuss options and success rate with professionals.
- Select options for coping with the stimuli:
  Distraction
  Resisting
  Calming
  Treatment (such as medication)
- Practice using an option to cope.
- Use a technique based on the success you have with it.
- Address the emotions evoked by the hallucinations (so that even if the hallucinations are not eradicated by medications, they can be managed).
- Be ready to replace coping styles when they do not work anymore.

YOUR INTERVENTION STRATEGIES
Helping a Client Manage Delusions

- Determine if the client can tell the difference between the delusion ("I don't drink the water because it's poisoned") and a personal preference ("I'm not drinking water because I prefer orange juice").
- Work with advocacy groups, peers, and professional staff to clearly demarcate what constitutes delusional thinking.
- Suggest options to cope with delusional thoughts:
  Support from others
  Concrete tasks
  Caretaking activities
  Refocusing thoughts
  Determined efforts to steer thinking in another direction
- Make sure client understands how important it is to be surrounded by people who reinforce the client's efforts.
- Encourage clients to self-validate the struggle they are in and any level of effectiveness they achieve at coping.

- Reduce excess noise and distractions. One person speaks to the client at a time.
- Intervene quickly by giving additional doses of psychotropic medications or placing the client in a quiet room.
- If necessary, secure the unit so that the client cannot leave and take self-destructive or impulsive action.

Make every effort to help the client attend to real rather than internal stimuli, orient the client to the real situation, and encourage the client to focus on you rather than on the hallucination. "George, listen to me rather than to the sounds you hear. Remember, you are in the hospital and I am your nurse. I will help you find your shoes. Come with me." Active involvement in some activity, such as finding shoes, will help the client maintain a focus on real events and perceptions.

General guidelines for working with delusional individuals are to avoid arguing with their false beliefs, to focus on the reality-based aspects of their communication, and to protect them from acting on their delusions in a way that might harm themselves or others. It may also be important to teach clients that sharing their delusional content directly with others in community settings such as the workplace or the social club may frighten others and lead to stigmatization. Keeping delusional content to oneself in these situations can improve interpersonal relationships. See Your Intervention Strategies for suggested nursing interventions that contain or manage delusions.

Promoting Congruent Emotional Responses

Working with clients who display blunted or flat affect can be confusing for nurses who are accustomed to reading emotional responses that fall within a more normal range. Be aware that these clients have feelings about events around them, including their interaction with you and other staff members, yet may have difficulty expressing those feelings.

Note any lack of congruence between the person's affect and the content of the message. If your relationship with the client is well established, you might comment on the incongruity and explore it with the client. ("Malcolm, what you are telling me is sad but you are laughing. What shall I pay attention to?") Modeling clear, congruent communication is helpful. Little can be done to change the client's anhedonia, yet empathic listening might comfort the client.

Ambivalence, the simultaneous experience of contradictory feelings about a person, object, or action, can trouble clients with schizophrenia. Ambivalence can become great enough to immobilize a client. Such clients cannot express one emotion or the other, or choose one action over the other. You may be able to partially alleviate the client's unease by identifying aloud the emotions the client may be experiencing. ("Lily, I think you might be feeling both very happy to see your father and at the same time very angry.") Naming the conflicting emotions gives the client the opportunity to talk about them, although many times he or she may not be able to do so.

Immobility due to ambivalence is extremely uncomfortable. One way of intervening is to limit the number of choices the indecisive client has to make. For example, a man may be immobilized by his inability to decide whether to go out alone for the first time. You can help by telling him that it seems too soon for him to go out alone and that, for today, he must be accompanied. Another example is a young woman who is undecided about where to sit. You can remove extra chairs at the table in the dining room so that she has only one choice.

Promoting Family Understanding and Involvement

When a person with schizophrenia is hospitalized, encourage the family and help them remain involved in the client's care. Except for unusual circumstances, share information on the client's status, treatment program, and future treatment plans, including discharge plans. Nurses may need to be active advocates for families' rights to information about, and involvement in, the care of their loved one with schizophrenia. Of course, nurses need to comply with the client's wishes and with the laws governing disclosure of information, which vary by state and by institution.

Referral to Psychoeducation Programs If assessment suggests that family members need information about the disease and treatment, refer the family to education programs, if they are available. Family psychoeducation programs are preferable to direct teaching because they often combine education with mutual support. In such groups, families can meet others who share their life difficulties. These peers can provide informal support and information to help the family deal with the tasks that lie ahead. You can reinforce the formal teaching that occurs in such programs when you meet with individual families.

Referral to NAMI Without exception, families should know about a national family support group with many local and state affiliates. The National Alliance on Mental Illness (NAMI) serves families through educational programs, local support groups, and political activism. Most local organizations are listed in telephone directories or can be reached through the local community mental health agency responsible for information and referral. For a resource link to NAMI, go to the Online Student Resources for this book.

Clinical Example

The Oldstads were worried about their daughter's failing grades at college for the last semester and were surprised to learn that she had ended a relationship with her boyfriend. When she came home for spring break, she seemed disinterested and uncommunicative and wouldn't eat or socialize with the family. Her parents found her burning incense and chanting to herself in the mirror at 3:00 a.m. In a panic, they took her to the local emergency department. After a complete workup, they were shocked to learn that the probable diagnosis was schizophrenia. Furthermore, the physician wanted their daughter to begin taking medication.

The rapidity of the decline in their daughter's functioning, and the fact that she had hidden many of her symptoms from them, left the Oldstads feeling guilty, sad, and disbelieving. They could not fathom how this had happened to their beautiful daughter. A nurse at the emergency department had given them the number of a local NAMI support group and hotline. In their anguish, they called and were able to speak with other parents, who helped them begin to deal with their emotions and directed them to helpful books that explained schizophrenia and its treatment.

The importance of NAMI to families and the NAMI education program are discussed in detail in Chapter 29 ∞.

Promoting Community Contacts

An awareness of a client's community supports and potential treatment programs can guide nurses in preparing clients for discharge. For example, the client's most important peer support group might be the clientele at a local day treatment program or social club. If so, several visits prior to discharge will help the client make the transition back to the community.

Preparing clients for the residence they will enter after hospital discharge is a central nursing task. Often, placement depends on how the client functions in the hospital. If the client is able to manage medications, participate in a variety of groups, and live cooperatively with other clients, then placement in a residential care facility that supports independent functioning is appropriate. In contrast, clients who need assistance with structuring free time, resist taking medications, or cannot be responsible for self-care require a more structured and supervised environment. Nurses work with clients to help them achieve their highest level of functioning. They document clients' abilities to perform various tasks and make recommendations to the treatment team about appropriate placements.

Evaluation

To complete the nursing process, nurses evaluate changes in client status and behavior in response to nursing interventions. Evaluation criteria are linked to nursing goals and reflect an understanding of the limitations of clients with schizophrenia. However, you must keep the concept of recovery in mind, because every client can improve and recover to a certain extent. The National Library of Medicine MEDLINEplus website offers search options on schizophrenia and other topics and can be accessed via the Online Student Resources for this text.

Communication

Clients will, with greater regularity, express their thoughts clearly and congruently. They will feel sufficient trust to talk to the nurse about troublesome symptoms or experiences. Because clients will probably continue to experience some symptoms even after medications have taken effect, this trust allows them to express what has changed and what is still troublesome.

Self-Care

Clients will consistently appear clean and well groomed and will independently manage personal grooming and hygiene. Clients will have clean and reasonably appropriate clothes, in terms of both fashion and season. Individual styles of dress, which are the client's way of expressing or presenting the self, will be supported by nurses. The means for maintaining self-care after discharge from acute care are identified.

Activity Intolerance

Clients will participate in goal-directed activities with minimal intervention. Clients will complete the activities they begin. Clients will demonstrate a broader range of interest and activities than they did on admission.

Social Isolation

Clients will demonstrate the capacity to interact, at least for brief periods, with nursing staff, with other clients, and in small groups. They will consistently demonstrate socially required interactions, such as greeting and starting a conversation with a stranger, asking for assistance, saying no, and listening to another's conversation. Clients will be inactive for shorter periods and spend more time engaged in interesting or meaningful activity. They will demonstrate the capacity to function outside the protective environment of acute or sheltered care.

Sensory/Perceptual Alterations

Clients will have fewer episodes of attending to internal stimuli. If hallucinations or delusions persist, clients will begin to identify stressors or situations that precipitate them. Clients will identify and practice personal coping strategies that decrease the hallucinations, delusions, or their effects, such as going to a quiet room, engaging in social activities, and performing activities that demand concentration.

Thought Processes

Clients will engage in reality-based discussions. If delusions persist, clients will not act on delusions in ways that are harmful or detrimental to themselves or others. They will also identify significant others in their current living environment who can help them limit their hallucinations via distraction or social contact.

Emotional Responses

Clients will have increased awareness that their emotional expressions at times do not match their verbal communications. They will monitor others' responses to them to learn cues about how they are varying their emotional expressions. Clients will experience fewer episodes of extreme discomfort due to ambivalence about people, events, or actions.

Family Functioning

If appropriate, families will be involved in all aspects of client care, including assessment, planning and carrying out interventions, inpatient treatment choices, and planning for discharge. Family understanding of the illness trajectory and the client's capacities and limits will improve. Family difficulties in caring for clients will be considered in treatment and discharge planning, and adequate resources will be identified to support family needs. Families will report that their questions about the schizophrenic disease process, and about varying modes of treatment for the disorder, have been answered.

CASE MANAGEMENT

Knowledge of the impact schizophrenia has on the way an individual thinks and functions is the underpinning of a competent case management program. In order to carry out any particular task, an individual with this illness must have specific duties coupled with realistic expectations. The case management strategies that work best with schizophrenia and other psychotic disorders include the following:

1. Tasks broken into manageable steps
2. Concrete actions
3. Structured environment
4. Routines and schedules
5. Dependable professionals
6. Flexibility to accommodate the shifts of the illness

Intensive Case Management (ICM) assists people with schizophrenia in outpatient settings (discussed in Chapter 13∞). With a smaller caseload, you have greater involvement with clients who require more supervision and care. You would orchestrate appointments and daily functioning issues to enhance the client's abilities to remain in the community and to foster a more independent lifestyle. Whether your assignment involves case management or intensive case management, the difficulties with thought processing and communication mentioned earlier in the chapter will shape your management of the case.

COMMUNITY-BASED CARE

People who have schizophrenia can have repetitive inpatient hospitalizations. The transition from an inpatient unit back to the community setting must begin prior to the client's discharge from the inpatient setting, forming a bridge from inpatient to outpatient care.

There are a number of services necessary and available in the community to maximize both quality of life and more independent functioning for people with schizophrenia and other psychotic disorders. Following are some examples.

1. Continuing day treatment programs
2. Independent living centers
3. Day hospitals
4. Community mental health centers
5. Social clubs
6. Wellness centers

These various settings are described in Chapter 13∞.

Counseling, psychotherapy, medication management, and other treatments are part of the care delivered in the community. In addition, remember that recreation is a quality-of-life issue. Community-based care can be instrumental in providing the guidance needed for clients to integrate into community living with an illness that can be debilitating and difficult.

HOME CARE

You may conduct different roles in delivering clinical services and care to clients with schizophrenia in a home setting. For example, you may function as a case manager and make home visits. This can be particularly important for clients with schizophrenia who often have great difficulty successfully meeting daily responsibilities and maintaining independence in a healthy home environment.

An important function of the nurse, whether or not you are a case manager, is to assist clients who have schizophrenia with medication adherence. Clients with schizophrenia are at high risk for relapse because they may stop taking their antipsychotic medications. This can happen because of side effects (those reported and not reported to the prescriber), confusion about medication administration schedules, environmental factors that do not encourage adherence to a medication regimen, or any number of other factors. You can play an important role in reducing the likelihood of relapse during home care visits. The home will shape adherence practices because the home is the environment in which most doses of their medications are taken.

Home interventions by nurses, however, are not limited to case management or medication adherence issues. Some people with schizophrenia can benefit from supportive psychotherapeutic interventions delivered by you in the client's home. These interventions can help generalize what they have learned beyond the confines of the nurse's office or the clinic. When people who have schizophrenia live with significant others, it is sometimes possible for you to deliver psychoeducational interventions for everyone living together as a unit. This allows the significant others and the client the opportunity to increase their skills in living together and coping with this serious illness in a way that lowers the probability of client relapse.

NURSING CARE PLAN: CLIENT WITH SCHIZOPHRENIA

Identifying Information

Jack May is a 24-year-old single male who lives with his mother and supports himself with Social Security Insurance (SSI). He is brought to the psychiatric emergency service by his mother. He currently attends a structured work program 5 days a week, but stopped attending 8 days ago.

Jack says that he does not need to be hospitalized and that his mother is the one with the problem. He wants to be left alone to work on his computer projects. He admits that he has been hearing multiple voices in his head for the past week. For the past 2 weeks, Jack has been increasingly isolated, working on his personal computer in his room. He will not tell anyone what the work is about, but his mother has seen printouts that suggest it is a plan to soundproof and secure his room. Jack stopped attending his work program a week ago, saying that he had "more important work" to do at home. He refuses to eat or talk with his mother. His mother believes he stopped taking his medications. An identifiable stressor is that 2 weeks ago his father announced plans to remarry in the near future.

History

Two years ago, Jack had a serious psychosis precipitated by his move to a college out of state. He was diagnosed with schizophrenia, paranoid type. He was hospitalized for 2 weeks, stabilized on Haldol, and discharged home. Persecutory delusions that shift with news events are always present at a low level. He has lived with his mother since diagnosis, attending day treatment and, for the last 8 months, a structured work program. He occasionally attends client support network meetings. His work attendance has been sporadic, and he has been on and off probation for nonattendance in this structured work environment. He receives medications and follow-up treatment at the community mental health center.

The Mays are both living and well. They were separated 3 years ago and divorced 2 years ago. Jack's father is an attorney, and Jack sees him approximately once a month. Their relationship is pleasant but not close. His mother runs her own crafts store and is agreeable to having Jack live with her. There are no other children.

Jack has completed high school and a few courses at the local community college. He was an above-average student and was always involved in school and extracurricular activities, until about 9 months before his first psychotic episode. Since that time, he has socialized primarily with his mother and rarely with a few acquaintances from the client support group. He smokes a pack of cigarettes a day and drinks beer occasionally. He denies any illicit drug use. Jack has a keen interest in computers. He took extensive coursework in computers in school and has collected considerable equipment and software, primarily gifts from his father. Other pastimes are listening to rock music and watching television.

No notable medical problems.

Current Mental Status

Jack is a healthy-looking 24-year-old man who is anxious, somewhat guarded, but cooperative in the interview. He is oriented to person, time, and place, and demonstrates good memory and recall. Judgment is impaired. His affect is anxious. Speech is rapid, pressured, tangential. He is hyperalert to his environment and is notably startled by a siren outside. Persecutory delusions about people trying to take over his home and work are present, and he has hallucinations of unrecognizable voices and the voice of his father. He has no command hallucinations. Some loosening of associations is present. Abstractions are concrete and self-referential. His insight is poor; he believes that his mother is "sick" and that she should not impede him in his important projects.

Other Clinical Data

There is evidence that Jack may have stopped taking medications approximately 2 weeks ago. Suicide/violence potential is minimal.

Nursing Diagnosis: Disturbed Thought Processes

Expected Outcome: Jack will demonstrate the ability to cope competently with delusions.

Short-Term Goals	Interventions	Rationales
Jack is able to function in a variety of settings without intrusive delusional thought content.	■ Allow description of delusional thoughts and acknowledge emotional impact of same. ■ Focus discussions on Jack's feeling level concerning the delusions, and not the content. ■ Teach Jack how to cope with delusional thinking through engagement in activities for distraction, active self-talk promoting his efforts, support from others, treatment. ■ Reinforce adaptive efforts.	Some contacts can be overwhelming for a client with schizophrenia and need to be of a manageable length. Jack must be taught how to cope with the symptoms of the illness in an effective manner.

NURSING CARE PLAN: CLIENT WITH SCHIZOPHRENIA (*Continued*)

Nursing Diagnosis: Anxiety related to delusions

Expected Outcome: Jack will demonstrate decreased anxiety.

Short-Term Goals	Interventions	Rationales
Jack is able to describe a reduction in his anxiety. Jack participates in his treatment.	■ Make frequent, supportive, and brief contacts.	Some contacts can be overwhelming for a client with schizophrenia and need to be of a manageable length.
	■ Reassure Jack verbally, with a structured routine, and by giving explanations congruent with Jack's ability to understand.	People with schizophrenia often do not have their feelings acknowledged. Reassurance validates their feelings.
	■ Prompt Jack to interact with others when able to reduce feelings of isolation and alienation.	
	■ Provide an array of coping skills Jack may use when anxious.	You must teach a variety of coping skills to suit various situations.

Pearson Nursing Student Resources

Find additional review materials at
nursing.pearsonhighered.com

Prepare for success with NCLEX®-style practice questions, interactive assignments and activities, web links, animations and videos, and more!

REFERENCES

American Psychiatric Association. (2000). *Diagnostic and statistical manual of mental disorders* (4th ed., Text Revision). Washington, DC: Author.

Emsley, R., Chiliza, B., Asmal, L., & Lehloenya, K. (2011). The concepts of remission and recovery in schizophrenia. *Current Opinion in Psychiatry, 24,* 114–121.

Kasckow, J., Felmet, K., & Zisook, S. (2011). Managing suicide risk in patients with schizophrenia. *CNS Drugs, 25*(2), 129–143.

Koreki, A., Tsunoda, K., Suzuki, T., Hirano, J., Watanabe, K., Kashima, H., & Uchida, H. (2011). Clinical and demographic characteristics associated with postural instability in patients with schizophrenia. *Journal of Clinical Psychopharmacology, 31,* 16–21.

Lee, A. H., Lange, C., Ricken, R., Hellweg, R., & Lang, U. E. (2011). Reduced brain-derived neurotrophic factor serum concentrations in acute schizophrenic patients increase during antipsychotic treatment. *Journal of Clinical Psychopharmacology, 31,* 334–336.

Lee, H., & Schepp, K. G. (2011). Ways of coping in adolescents with schizophrenia. *Journal of Psychiatric & Mental Health Nursing, 18*(2), 158–165.

National Institutes of Mental Health (2011). Statistics on Serious Mental Illness. http://www.nimh.nih.gov/statistics/index.shtml

Rylands, A. J., McKie, S., Elliott, R., Deakin, J. F., & Tarrier, N. (2011). A functional magnetic resonance imaging paradigm of expressed emotion in schizophrenia. *Journal of Nervous and Mental Disorders, 199,* 25–29.

Stanford, A. D., Corcoran, C., Bulow, P., Bellovin-Weiss, S., Malaspina, D., & Lisanby, S. H. (2011). High-frequency prefrontal repetitive transcranial magnetic stimulation for the negative symptoms of schizophrenia: A case series. *Journal of ECT, 27,* 11–17.

Takagi, S., Watanabe, Y., Takefumi, I., Sakata, M., & Watanabe, M. (2011). Treatment of psychogenic polydipsia with acetazolamide: A report of 5 cases. *Clinical Neuropharmacology, 34*(1), 5–7.

Zahir, F. R., & Brown, C. J. (2011). Epigenetic impacts on neurodevelopment: Pathophysiological mechanisms and genetic modes of action. *Pediatric Research, 69*(5), 92R–100R.

17

Mood Disorders

EILEEN TRIGOBOFF

LEARNING OUTCOMES

After completing this chapter, you will be able to:

1. Compare and contrast the similarities and differences between major depressive disorder and bipolar disorder and between bereavement and dysfunctional grieving.
2. Describe the elements of the biopsychosocial theories discussed here that contribute most to the current understanding of mood disorders.
3. Explain the principles upon which the various biologic therapies for clients with mood disorders are based.
4. Systematically conduct a nursing assessment of a client with a mood disorder.
5. Implement an understanding of suicide prevention and safety promotion in the plan of care for clients with mood disorders.
6. Design a plan of care to reduce negative thinking and promote improved self-esteem.
7. Educate clients and their families about biologic treatment for mood disorders such as antidepressant medications and electroconvulsive therapy.
8. Assess personal feelings, values, and attitudes toward clients with mood disorders that may provide challenges to professional practice.

CRITICAL THINKING CHALLENGE

Consuela is a 38-year-old woman with severe mania who has not responded to psychopharmacologic interventions. The treatment team on her inpatient psychiatric unit has recommended electroconvulsive therapy (ECT) to Consuela and her family. Consuela is quite fearful of this procedure and believes that it will enable others to control her mind. She is adamantly opposed to it.

1. What are the rights of severely ill psychiatric clients in determining their own treatment? Do they differ from those of other clients with physiological disorders who now enjoy almost complete self-determination if they choose to exercise it?
2. At what point does a client's right to autonomy and self-determination end?
3. How might a treatment facility's philosophy on this issue be implemented to ensure consistency of care?

Approximately 12% of Americans suffer from the wide spectrum of mood disorders. Mood disorders are a group of psychiatric diagnoses characterized by disturbances in physical, emotional, and behavioral response patterns. These patterns of **affect** (mood) range from extreme elation and agitation to extreme depression with a serious potential for suicide. They are the most common of all mental disorders, largely due to the prevalence of depression. Other mood disorders that occur less frequently than depression, but can be severely incapacitating, include dysthymic disorder and the bipolar disorders. The spectrum of bipolarity in the community, estimated at more than 6%, is of great public health significance. Mental Health in the News lists just some of the people who have these disorders.

The symptoms of mood disorders—poor memory and concentration, fatigue, apathy, indecisiveness, and loss of self-confidence in depressed clients and grandiosity and unrealistic overconfidence in those with mania—reduce the capacity to work and maintain the activities of daily living. Some mental health authorities believe that major depression is more disabling than many medical disorders, such as chronic lung disease, arthritis, and diabetes. It is the leading cause of lost workdays and diminished productivity on the job.

Many people with mood disorders are never seen for treatment in psychiatric settings because of the following:

1. Some people may not realize they have a problem.
2. Other people do not realize they have a treatable illness.
3. Physical complaints brought to primary health care providers may be determined to require medical, or surgical, treatment instead of mental health care.
4. Health care policy and insurance coverage for mental disorders may be nonexistent or meager.

Nearly two thirds of depressed people in this country go undiagnosed and untreated. As a nurse and a citizen, you are in an excellent position to identify early signs of mood disorders and initiate action leading to early treatment.

MAJOR DEPRESSIVE EPISODE/DISORDER

A **major depressive episode** is characterized by a change in several aspects of a person's life and emotional state consistently throughout at least 14 days. Of prime importance is the client's mood state. Be aware that clients do not always describe their mood as "depressed." Instead, they may say they are sad, discouraged, "down in the dumps," or say that they feel helpless. Or, they may complain of having no feelings at all or of feeling "blah." In other cases, vague somatic complaints such as aches and pains are reported, while other clients report increased anger, frustration, and irritability, with uncharacteristic outbursts over minor matters. It is not difficult to imagine that someone who looks and feels sad or empty is depressed. A diagnosis of depression is more likely to be missed when a person simply seems anxious or irritable. The description of the diagnostic criteria for single-episode and recurrent major depression is found in DSM Essential Features.

Major depressive disorder may consist of a single episode or may recur as recurrent major depression at various points in life. Key facts about major depression are in Box 17-1. When a person experiences a major depressive disorder, activities that previously gave pleasure, such as socializing, hobbies, sports, and sexual activities, often are no longer enjoyed. This condition is known as **anhedonia**. Changes in physiological functioning during depression are called **vegetative symptoms**. Changes in appetite, usually experienced as a reduction or loss of interest in food, are often seen, although increased appetite and cravings are also reported.

MENTAL HEALTH IN THE NEWS

Famous People With Mood Disorders

- Drew Carey, comedian and star of the ABC sitcom "The Drew Carey Show"; depression
- Sheryl Crow, singer and musician; depression
- Richard Dreyfus, comedian and actor (Jaws, Down and Out in Beverly Hills); depression
- F. Scott Fitzgerald, writer (The Great Gatsby); depression
- Sigmund Freud, "father of psychoanalysis"; depression
- Billy Joel, musician; depression
- Margot Kidder, actress ("Lois Lane" in Superman); bipolar disorder
- Joey Kramer, drummer ("Aerosmith"); depression
- Vivian Leigh, actress (Gone With the Wind, A Streetcar Named Desire); bipolar disorder
- Abraham Lincoln, President of the United States; depression
- Greg Louganis, winner of five Olympic medals for diving; depression

- Marilyn Monroe, actress (Some Like It Hot) and immortal vixen; depression
- Alanis Morissette, platinum album singer and musician (Jagged Little Pill); depression
- Jimmy Piersall, baseball player for the Boston Red Sox; bipolar disorder
- Axl Rose, singer, musician, member of "Guns n' Roses"; bipolar disorder
- Charles Schulz, cartoonist, creator of Peanuts; depression
- Brooke Shields, actress and model; postpartum depression
- Sting (Gordon Sumner), musician, singer; depression
- Mike Wallace, award-winning journalist (the CBS newsmagazine, 60 Minutes); depression
- Robin Williams, comedian, actor (Good Morning Vietnam, Dead Poets Society); depression
- Bert Yancey, professional golfer; bipolar disorder

Photo courtesy of Helga Esteb/Shutterstock.com.

DSM ESSENTIAL FEATURES

Depressive Disorders

Types of depressive disorders include major depressive disorder—single event or recurrent episodes—and dysthymic disorder. These problems cause significant distress in social, occupational, or other important areas of function. The individual can never have had a manic episode or symptoms of mania. Any of these depressive disorders can vary in relation to the seasons or to the time of year, and cannot be due to ingesting a substance or from a medical problem or another psychiatric problem.

Major Depressive Disorder: The various symptoms of a major depressive disorder include a depressed mood and loss of interest or pleasure, changes in appetite and weight, sleep problems, observable restlessness or underactivity, and low energy. Additionally, depressed individuals may have trouble concentrating and have feelings of worthlessness and/or excessive guilt that are inappropriate for the behaviors. Thoughts of suicide or death occur. Symptoms also have to be more than would be expected after the loss of a loved one.

Dysthymic Disorder: Symptoms of a dysthymic disorder include depressed mood for most of the day for more than 2 years, accompanied by some of these symptoms: changes in appetite and eating, sleep problems, low energy, low self-esteem, and hopelessness.

Sleep disturbances are also common, particularly **insomnia** (the inability to fall asleep or stay asleep, or awakening early in the morning) with depression. An association between depression and the chronic inability to get to sleep or to remain asleep during the usual sleep period was observed as long ago as the time of Hippocrates. Two types of insomnia are most often experienced by people having a major depressive episode. *Middle insomnia* refers to waking up during the night and having difficulty falling asleep again. *Terminal insomnia* refers to waking at the end of the night and being unable to return to sleep. The sleep pattern disturbance may actually precede other symptoms of depression and likewise may respond to antidepressant medication more rapidly than the depression. Also reported is **hypersomnia**, in which the person sleeps for prolonged nighttime periods as well as during the day, but still wakes up tired or fatigued.

Fatigue and decreased energy are characteristic symptoms of depression, a condition known as **anergy or anergia**. Individuals report being tired upon awakening, regardless of how long they have slept. Even the smallest task seems insurmountable, and routine activities require substantial effort and take longer to accomplish. Decreased energy may be manifested in **psychomotor retardation**, in which thinking and body movements are noticeably slowed and speech is slowed or absent. Psychomotor agitation also may occur, in which the person cannot sit still, paces, wrings the hands, and picks at the fingernails, skin, clothing, bedclothes, or other objects. Psychomotor retardation is a prominent symptom in the clinical example that follows.

Clinical Example

Becky is a 26-year-old insurance underwriter who visited a local Planned Parenthood clinic for a yearly checkup and Pap test. During the examination by the family planning nurse, Becky asked whether she might be anemic because she was "just exhausted all the time." Becky revealed that for the past month she had had difficulty getting out of bed in the morning. Getting dressed and ready for work left her drained. She described standing in front of her closet for long periods, unable to decide what to wear. Becky was also having extreme difficulty calling potential clients. Whereas she was normally an assertive salesperson who called on perfect strangers with ease, she now described sitting at her desk for hours, trying to work up the motivation to pick up the phone. Coworkers, including her boss, had commented on her 15-pound weight gain, and these comments precipitated several uncharacteristic angry and tearful outbursts at work. Other common symptoms in significantly depressed individuals include guilt or a sense of worthlessness, self-blame, impaired concentration and decision-making ability, even about trivial things, and suicidal ideation.

Sleep disturbances secondary to psychiatric disorders are generally related to mood disorders and anxiety disorders. While recognizing that a cyclical relationship is usually

---

Box 17-1 Key Facts About Major Depression

- The average age of onset is the midtwenties, although major depressive disorder can begin at any age and seems to be occurring in younger and younger people.
- The risk of developing major depressive disorder during one's lifetime ranges from 15% to 25% for females and from 8% to 15% for males, making depression twice as likely for women as for men.
- First-degree biologic relatives (parents or siblings) of people with major depressive disorder are up to three times as likely to develop depression as are members of the general population (APA, 2000).

- Symptoms usually develop over a period of time. The person may experience anxiety and mild depression for several days, weeks, or months before the onset of a full major depressive episode.
- If untreated, major depression lasts 6 or more months. In about 20% to 30% of cases, some depressive symptoms persist for longer periods, ranging from months to years. This is considered a partial remission and thought to be predictive of later depressive episodes and the development of chronic depression.

involved, it is helpful to try to differentiate primary sleep disorders from those that are secondary to a psychiatric disorder. Such differentiation can be particularly important for clients with depression.

Differentiating sleep disorder secondary to psychiatric disorder from primary sleep disorder is a complex process that requires collaboration among clients, families, and health professionals. The sequence of onset may provide a clue. Many persons with unipolar depressive disorder initially see primary care practitioners or sleep clinics because of insomnia. It may take trying an intervention known to be effective for one or the other type of disorder to assess the circumstances and help clarify the primary diagnosis.

You need to be vigilant for the potential effects of a mismatched primary diagnosis and intervention. A depressed client misdiagnosed as having a primary sleep disorder of insomnia may be at risk of suicide if given a usual supply of hypnotic medication; likewise, obstructive sleep apnea with modest ingestion of alcohol can be mislabeled as alcohol abuse. As in any area of nursing practice, all components of the nursing process must be carefully and critically used.

The characteristics of a major depressive episode are illustrated in FIGURE 17-1 ■. Individuals with a history of a manic or hypomanic episode (discussed later in this chapter) are considered to have a bipolar disorder and are not classified under these categories.

A fairly recent association has been made between depression and cardiac health issues. Because this is a new area of research, it is still unclear if cardiac difficulties result from depressive states, coexist with depression, or whether a depressive state results from a cardiac condition. Stress hormones and mortality concerns following a cardiac event such as a myocardial infarction (MI) could increase an individual's vulnerability to depression. Psychopharmacologic treatments for depression need to be cardiac-safe (do not challenge a client's cardiac

functioning) so that people with depression can adhere to treatment. It had been a concern at one point that some antidepressants may somehow precipitate MIs, and that led to cardiac clients not being treated for depressive symptoms. This concern has been dispelled by Scherrer et al. (2011) who found significantly reduced rates of MI with all classes of antidepressants.

DYSTHYMIC DISORDER

The term **dysthymic disorder** describes chronic depression for the majority of most days for at least 2 years (1 year for children and adolescents). Throughout those 2 years, no more than 2 months can be described as symptom free. In general the symptoms of dysthymic disorder, while distressing, tend to be less severe than those in major depressive disorder, with fewer physiological symptoms. The diagnostic criteria for dysthymic disorder were given in DSM Essential Features. Dysthymic disorder tends to predispose people to the development of major depressive disorder. According to the DSM-IV-TR, 10% to 25% of individuals diagnosed with dysthymic disorder will develop major depressive disorder within the next year (American Psychiatric Association [APA], 2000). The lifetime risk of developing dysthymic disorder is approximately 6% in the general population. Dysthymic disorder often occurs in childhood, adolescence, or early adulthood and tends to be chronic. While both females and males are equally affected as children, there are two to three times as many adult females as males with dysthymic disorder.

The symptoms of dysthymic disorder are similar to those of chronic major depressive disorder. This similarity makes it difficult, even for experienced clinicians, to make an accurate differential diagnosis. In clinical practice, nursing care of the dysthymic client is similar to that of depressed clients. The clinical example included here describes such a case.

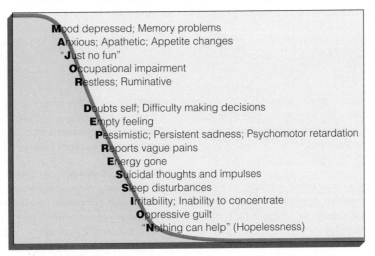

Mood depressed; Memory problems
Anxious; Apathetic; Appetite changes
"**J**ust no fun"
Occupational impairment
Restless; Ruminative

Doubts self; Difficulty making decisions
Empty feeling
Pessimistic; Persistent sadness; Psychomotor retardation
Reports vague pains
Energy gone
Suicidal thoughts and impulses
Sleep disturbances
Irritability; Inability to concentrate
Oppressive guilt
"**N**othing can help" (Hopelessness)

FIGURE 17-1 ■ Characteristics of major depression.

Clinical Example

Gregory is a 14-year-old boy who was brought to a nurse psychotherapist by his mother on the suggestion of the guidance counselor in his private school. In the letter of referral, the counselor stated that she was concerned because of Gregory's "persistent pessimistic outlook on life."

According to Gregory's mother, who was interviewed alone, Gregory has always been a cranky and irritable child. Since starting kindergarten, he has had difficulty relating to other children and is often left out of activities and social invitations. At home, he stays in his room much of the time where he plays computer games and writes poetry. He does not do well in school, although testing has shown him to have far above average intelligence. Despite their best efforts, his parents have never been able to interest him in scouting, sports, or other activities they deem appropriate for a boy his age. His parents reported that Gregory's weight, eating habits, and sleeping patterns were unchanged.

When Gregory was interviewed, he responded in monosyllables, made poor eye contact with the therapist, and sat slumped in his chair with no facial expression. He stated that he knew his parents were "disappointed" in him.

SEASONAL AFFECTIVE DISORDER

Natural light is frequently taken for granted, and most people may be unaware of how it influences the human experience. As early as the days of Hippocrates, observers of human behavior noticed that some people suffer mood changes as the seasons change.

The relationships between light, biologic rhythms, and mood are the subject of robust and thorough scientific study. This research focuses on the use of light in the treatment of **seasonal affective disorder (SAD)**, a depressive disorder that occurs in relation to the seasons, usually during winter months. Natural light may help modulate daily rhythms that influence sleep and activity patterns, neuroendocrine functions, and brain chemical systems.

Many antidepressants are typically used to treat the depressive features of SAD, but only one currently is indicated for this diagnosis by the Food and Drug Administration (FDA). Bupropion extended release (Wellbutrin ER) may prevent major depressive episodes in people with SAD. Treatment for SAD has entered areas well beyond therapy and medication. Researchers are exploring the application of different forms of light to the skin and eyes at different times of day, and the results indicate a reduction of fatigue and depression as well as improved alertness (Joseph, 2006). The exact relationship between SAD and light, biologic rhythms, and events at the cellular level has not yet been determined. Information on SAD and the clinical application of light therapy is available through the Society for Light Treatment and Biological Rhythms http://www.sltbr.org) and the Seasonal Affective Disorder Association http://www.sada.org.uk) and can be accessed through the Online Student Resources for this book.

BIPOLAR DISORDERS

The **bipolar disorders** are a group of mood disorders that include manic episodes, hypomanic episodes, mixed episodes, depressed episodes, and cyclothymic disorder. A *bipolar I disorder* consists of one or more manic or mixed episodes, and the course of illness can be accompanied by major depressive episodes. A *bipolar II disorder* consists of one or more major depressive episodes accompanied by at least one hypomanic episode. See the components necessary to diagnose these disorders in DSM Essential Features.

Bipolar disorders tend to be recurrent, and have the unusual tendency to increase in frequency as the individual ages. The majority of bipolar I disorder clients do not have the chance to experience a baseline mood—called euthymic mood—because a major depressive episode may quickly follow. Many clients return to normal functioning during remissions, but approximately 20% to 30% have residual mood symptoms and as many as 60% have continuing interpersonal and occupational difficulties. Of clients with bipolar II disorder, 5% to 10% have four or more mood episodes in a given year, and approximately 15% experience continuing mood lability and interpersonal and occupational difficulties (APA, 2000).

Manic and Hypomanic Episodes

Mania is characterized by an abnormal and persistently elevated, expansive, or irritable mood lasting at least 1 week, significantly impairing social or occupational functioning,

---

DSM ESSENTIAL FEATURES

Bipolar Disorders

Types of bipolar disorder can include manic, hypomanic, or mixed episodes, and cyclothymic disorder. The symptoms cause significant distress in social, occupational, or other important areas of function, and are not caused by ingesting a substance, from a medical or another psychiatric problem.

Bipolar Disorder: The manic or hypomanic episodes of bipolar disorder include an elevated, expansive, or irritable mood for at least 1 week for a manic episode, and 4 weeks for a hypomanic episode. The individual has a specific combination of the following symptoms: inflated self-esteem, reduced sleep, is talkative and hard to interrupt, has racing thoughts, has quick and unusual series of ideas, is distractible, is overactive, and takes risks that are not typical for the individual. Mixed episodes include almost daily symptoms of mania and depression for at least 1 week.

Cyclothymic Disorder: A diagnosis of cyclothymia disorder requires 2 or more years of numerous periods with both hypomanic and depressive symptoms (less severe than depressive disorder), with no history of major depressive disorder or manic or mixed episodes for the initial 2 years of the cyclothymia.

and generally requiring hospitalization. This disturbance in mood must be accompanied by at least three additional symptoms such as "inflated self-esteem or **grandiosity**, decreased need for sleep, pressure of speech, **flight of ideas** (rapidly changing, fragmentary thoughts), distractibility, increased involvement in goal-directed activities or psychomotor agitation, and excessive involvement in pleasurable activities with a high potential for painful consequences" (APA, 2000, p. 362). Psychotic symptoms, such as delusions or hallucinations, may be a feature of severe mania.

Hypomania is a less extreme form of mania that is not severe enough to markedly impair functioning or require hospitalization. Individuals experiencing hypomania feel wonderful, "on top of the world," and do not recognize changes in themselves. Those who know them well, however, are aware of the changes in mood and behavior. There are no psychotic features in hypomania.

The onset of manic episodes is usually in the early twenties but may begin at any time. It often follows a severe disappointment, embarrassment, or other psychic stressor. The mood of clients experiencing a manic episode is euphoric or "high." Their behavior is excessive and out of bounds. It is characterized by overly enthusiastic involvement in projects of an interpersonal, political, religious, or occupational nature. When someone or something gets in the way or appears to put a snag in their way, they become irritable. Moods alternate between euphoria and irritability. Increased sexual behaviors are often seen, including flirting, making sexual overtures, having inappropriate sexual relationships, and feeling compelled to seduce and be seduced. Women may dress in an uncharacteristically flashy or seductive manner and wear garish makeup. Speech is pressured, and racing thoughts or flight of ideas are often present. Grandiosity can reach delusional proportions. Clients with mania rarely believe they are sick, even when they are in financial or legal trouble, and may vehemently protest the need for treatment. The characteristics of a manic episode are described in the clinical example and illustrated in FIGURE 17-2 ■.

Clinical Example

Mr. Gery, a 52-year-old engineer, was brought to the emergency psychiatric clinic by two adult sons at 2:00 a.m. Their mother had called them to come help with their father, who had not slept in 3 days. When they arrived at their parents' home, they found their father working in the backyard on a large landscaping project involving stonework, a waterfall, a fish pond, and extensive plantings of trees, shrubs, and flowers.

According to the sons, Mr. Gery had three prior episodes of manic behavior, beginning when he was in the Army many years earlier. He was stabilized on lithium carbonate for years, but stopped taking it about a year ago because he felt so good. The current episode began about 1 week ago after he was passed over for a promotion at work. He then took a leave of absence from his job to create what he called "the world's first home-based theme park." Any attempt by his wife to talk him out of the project was met with anger and renewed resolve. Mr. Gery angrily told the admitting nurse, "I don't know why these boys brought me here. I need to get back to work! I'm going to get millions for this franchise."

Depressed Episodes

A diagnosis of bipolar disorder does not always mean that manic or hypomanic behaviors will be manifested in the current illness. There are several types of bipolar disorders in which manic or hypomanic episodes have occurred in the past, but the features of the current episode are purely depressive. This is termed a *depressed episode*. Treatment of depressed bipolar disorders is similar to treatment of depression, with the exception that pharmacologic treatment adds a mood stabilizer to antidepressant treatment.

Recent studies explain what many clinicians have been struggling with when treating people who are not responsive to antidepressant pharmacotherapy. People who have already been diagnosed with major depression may very well have bipolar disorder as opposed to depression. Nearly half of all people who have bipolar disorder are first diagnosed with major depression. Many clients with bipolar disorder are not correctly diagnosed in a timely manner. This can mean that an individual loses years of his or her life to an illness that could have been successfully managed if correctly diagnosed and treated.

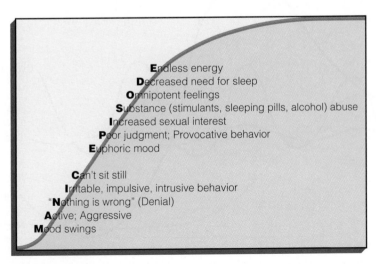

FIGURE 17-2 ■ Characteristics of a manic episode.

Mixed Episodes

In a *mixed episode,* symptoms of both mania and depression are present nearly every day in rapidly alternating succession over a period of at least a week. These clients are often agitated, are suffering from insomnia and appetite disturbances, and may exhibit suicidal and psychotic thinking. The presentation also can resemble depression, with a great deal of energy and animation behind the sadness. Clients may have recently had a manic episode or a major depressive episode, although this is not always the case. Because depressive symptoms are part of the clinical picture, clients suffer more psychic pain than do individuals who are in a state of mania, and they may seek help more readily. The clinical example that follows illustrates one type of presentation of a mixed episode.

Clinical Example

Mrs. Kent is a 32-year-old high school teacher who was readmitted to the psychiatric unit 2 weeks after she was discharged following treatment for a major depressive episode. Her husband described her recent behavior as extremely unstable, with a strange mix of moods. "She is driving herself and me crazy, crying and talking about killing herself because her life is so sad and she is so depressed, but every action is so full of energy. She tried to go back to work right after she got out of the hospital the first time, but the principal put her on a leave of absence until the end of the year. He said she made wildly gesticulating movements while describing how miserable she was to some of her students."

Cyclothymic Disorder

When clients have suffered for at least 2 years from "chronic, fluctuating mood disturbances involving numerous periods of hypomanic symptoms and numerous periods of depressive symptoms," they are diagnosed with **cyclothymic disorder** (APA, 2000, p. 398). They must be free of severe symptoms that qualify for the diagnosis of manic disorder or major depressive disorder. These individuals are often considered to be moody, unpredictable, or temperamental, and they may go on to develop an overlay of symptoms that are of major depressive or manic intensity. FIGURE 17-3 ■ compares mood in major depressive disorder, bipolar disorders, dysthymia, and cyclothymia.

Cyclothymic disorder begins early, usually in adolescence or early adulthood. Although not common, with a lifetime risk of only 0.4% to 1% of the general population, it is thought to predispose the person to other mood disorders. The incidence is approximately equal between males and females.

MOOD DISORDERS DUE TO OTHER CONDITIONS

It is widely recognized that mood disorders may be manifestations of physiological conditions such as hepatitis or thyrotoxicosis. Mood disorders may also be induced by substance abuse, such as cocaine or amphetamines; prescribed medications, such as antihypertensives or oral contraceptives; or toxins, such as lead or carbon monoxide. Mood disorders may also be precipitated by withdrawal from substance intoxication or abuse. Chapter 15∞ has details on this phenomenon. The general medical condition of clients should be carefully evaluated before making a diagnosis of mood disorder.

POSTPARTUM MOOD EPISODES

The majority of women experience the "baby blues"—transient mood changes, usually depression, that do not impair functioning—in the 2-week period after the birth of a baby. However, when the symptoms meet the criteria for any of the mood disorder categories discussed earlier in this chapter, the client is diagnosed as having a mood disorder with postpartum onset or **postpartum mood episode**. This rate is set conservatively at 13% to 19%. The onset of a mood disorder

FIGURE 17-3 ■ Comparison of affect (mood) in major depressive disorder, bipolar disorder, dysthymia, and cyclothymia.

with postpartum onset occurs within 4 weeks of giving birth but may occur anytime in the first year following childbirth (McCoy, 2011).

The symptoms the client experiences are no different from the symptoms of other mood disorders except for a major one—preoccupation with infant well-being. This preoccupation can range from overconcern for the safety of the infant to severe ruminations about the infant's safety. Sometimes, but not always, psychotic features are evident. For example, the woman may have delusional thoughts about her infant (the infant is possessed by an evil presence) or command hallucinations (to kill or injure the infant). The following clinical example describes the illness.

Clinical Example

A woman drowned her six children, ages 2 months through 7 years old, believing that they were evil and that she was saving them from hell. Each of the six births, all within a period of 7 years, was characterized by a postpartum mood episode, some with psychotic features that required hospitalization and psychotropic medications. She had attempted suicide at least twice during a mood episode. Despite the severity of her postpartum mood episodes, which occurred after each pregnancy, the couple did not modify their dream to have a large family.

The risk for a postpartum mood episode with psychotic features is increased in women who have had a prior mood disorder (especially bipolar I disorder) or a previous postpartum episode with psychotic features, or in women with no history of a prior mood disorder but with a family history of bipolar disorders. The risk for recurrence with a subsequent delivery is between 30% and 50% (APA, 2000). You can refer depressed postpartum women to Postpartum Support International for a postpartum self-assessment test and help in locating a support group. You can access their website, http://www.postpartum.net, through the Online Student Resources for this book.

BEREAVEMENT

Bereavement is a term that refers to the state of loss. We all have losses that have to be dealt with, and how we cope affects not only us but our loved ones. Bereavement is a natural process and not a mental illness. Certainly, people may have significant difficulties at some point; however, this is a transient state. Overall, bereavement is a process that everyone handles in a slightly different manner. Although we might wish for a logical and firm set of rules, there is no lock-step progression of bereavement or grieving through routinized categories, but rather an ebb and flow.

You will notice in your work with depressed clients that many episodes of major depressive disorder are preceded by a major loss of some kind. **Grief** (the feeling of sadness for a loss) is a multifaceted reaction to loss. It has emotional components as well as physical, cognitive, behavioral, social, spiritual, and philosophical dimensions. Caring about someone or something and having a real relationship means putting yourself at risk for intense feelings of grief when the

relationship changes or ends. People do not grieve for losses that are unimportant to them. The term "grief struck" is an apt one, for many people are shocked by the jarring impact of the loss. Grieving is a personal process that is best supported by others who understand and care.

Dysfunctional Grieving

Dysfunctional grieving is a term that describes the failure of an individual to follow the course of normal grieving to a point of resolution. When normal grieving deviates from the norm, the individual becomes overwhelmed and resorts to maladaptive coping. Nursing care can focus on lowering the risk for spiritual distress, anxiety, depression, and dysfunctional grief in situations where trauma and grief are issues (O'Baire-Kark & Klevay, 2011). The following clinical example is of a dysfunctional grief reaction.

Clinical Example

Jacki was particularly close to her father all of her life. As she matured into adulthood, she developed healthy relationships with others, including friendships, marriage, and motherhood. Through it all she maintained a very close relationship with her father. When he died suddenly when she was 50, Jacki reacted strongly, as everyone expected she would. She accused other family members of not caring and was estranged from some for months following his death. As the months, then years, went by, Jacki exhibited tearful and grief-stricken reactions especially on her father's birthday and the anniversary of his death.

In telephone conversations with her siblings she would ask, sobbing, "Do you know what today is?" When her siblings did not recognize the date as being significant, Jacki would yell and accuse them of never loving their father because they failed to note that this was the day he usually held the first barbecue of the year (or some other fairly insignificant activity). Ten years following her father's death Jacki is still highly emotional, erratic, and not functioning well interpersonally. She is having a dysfunctional grief reaction.

Treatment for dysfunctional grieving can resemble treatment for depression, including cognitive–behavioral therapy, other talk therapies, and antidepressants. Group therapy can consist of groups composed of people all of whom are experiencing complicated or dysfunctional grief reactions. Focusing on competent relationships and receiving support from capable others can prevent problems.

BIOPSYCHOSOCIAL THEORIES

People with certain personality types or temperaments are more prone than others to develop depressive and elated behaviors. Significant efforts have been devoted to identifying a single psychological factor, trait, or mechanism that is unique to the development of mood disorders.

Research exploring the causative factors of mood disorders has focused on reactions to early separation from parents or parental loss, early mother–child relationships, errors in thinking, inherited tendencies, biologic factors, and other aspects of human development and experience. To date, no single personality type, biologic or psychological trait, or constellation of experiences has been established to account for all forms of mood disorders. Multiple complex factors contribute to the development of mood disorders.

Psychoanalytic Theory

The psychoanalytic theory of depression was originally formulated by Freud and later refined by others. It focuses on an unsatisfactory early mother–infant relationship as the primary factor predisposing individuals to later depression. If an infant's needs go unmet, a sense of loss occurs. Unresolved grief over the loss results in anger turned inward and the development of self-hate. The child's ego development is thereby adversely affected, resulting in a weak ego and an overdeveloped, punitive superego.

The psychoanalytic school of thought suggests a different etiology for bipolar disorder. This theory holds that the mother/primary caregiver derives pleasure from the infant's early dependence but feels threatened by increasing autonomy as the child develops. Independent behaviors are considered "bad," and the child must suppress his or her needs in order to sustain parental affection. Ambivalence resulting from the coexisting desires to please the parents and become more autonomous causes resentment and leads to a love–hate relationship with the parenting figures. Again, a weak ego and punitive superego create depression. Mania is seen as the denial of depression taken to the extreme. Contemporary theorists and researchers criticize psychoanalytic theory for its tendency to blame mothers while ignoring biologic factors.

Cognitive Theory

Cognitive theorists such as Clark and Beck (1999) believe that depression results from impaired cognition, or distorted thinking processes. People who think negative thoughts evaluate themselves critically and interpret stressful events as having a powerful, global impact on them. They feel guilty, inadequate, and hopeless about the future. Recent models of cognitive vulnerability to depression theorize that negative thoughts alone are not sufficient to cause depression unless the individual already suffers from a mildly depressed mood. In these instances, the combination of adverse life events (or the perception of adverse life events) and mildly depressed mood combine to create a downward spiral into depression. The Beck Depression Inventory is a clinical assessment tool. It asks clients to rate themselves on 21 groups of questions designed to detect negative thinking. Cognitive therapy seeks to teach individuals how to stop negative thinking and replace it with more positive self-appraisals. Cognitive therapies are discussed in detail in Chapter 30 ∞.

The theory of **learned helplessness** is a cognitive theory that proposes that learning plays an instrumental role in the development of depression. This theory holds that depression is based on the person's belief that he or she has no control over life situations. This conclusion is drawn from repeated failures, either real or perceived, to control life events and environmental influences. The result is that the individual gives up, stops trying to control, becomes dependent on others, and is thereby predisposed to depression (Lazenby, 2011).

Biologic Theories

Promising findings are emerging from studies of biologic factors that alter brain function. Research on the physiological basis for depression has been under way for more than 60 years and has generated a variety of hypotheses. Because mood disorders vary widely, it is unlikely that any single biologic causative factor can be isolated. This has led to research on how the various biologic factors already identified relate to one another, how they affect behavior, and how they respond to different therapies. In searching for biologic changes in mood disorders, it is important to remember that although a biologic abnormality may coexist with a mood disorder, it is not necessarily a causative factor. It could be a cause, a coexisting factor, or a consequence. Your Assessment Approach lists some abnormal findings on laboratory tests that may indicate the presence of a mood disorder.

Gender and Age

Women are more prone to major depression and dysthymia than are men. This is true across cultures. Endocrine and reproductive cycles may play a role, although menopause alone, contrary to popular belief, does not appear to be a risk factor for depression in women. It is also unclear whether prenatal and postpartum depressions are hormonal in nature, result from the increased stress of motherhood, or represent an interaction of these and other factors. Gender is important given the propensity of women to succumb to depression

---

YOUR ASSESSMENT APPROACH
Abnormal Biologic Findings in Mood Disorders

While there are no laboratory studies that definitively diagnose mood disorders, some abnormal findings are noted more often in mood-disordered individuals when symptoms are present than in control subjects. These are as follows:

- Sleep abnormalities in 40% to 60% of outpatients and up to 90% of inpatients with major depressive episode and in 25% to 50% of adults with dysthymic disorder; decreased need for sleep and abnormal polysomnographic findings in people with manic episode (sleep abnormalities may precede the onset of a mood disorder and may persist in the absence of other symptoms)
- Neurotransmitter and neuropeptide dysregulation in major depressive episode and manic episode
- Hormonal disturbances (blunted growth hormone and thyroid-stimulating hormone); elevated urinary free cortisol; dexamethasone nonsuppression of prolactin; elevated plasma cortisol
- Brain imaging studies may show increased blood flow in limbic and paralimbic regions and decreased blood flow in the lateral prefrontal cortex in depression; increased rates of right hemispheric lesions, or bilateral subcortical or preventricular lesions in persons with bipolar I disorder
- Preventricular vascular changes when depression begins in late life
- Urine and blood drug screens may indicate a substance-induced mood disorder

more than men. However, environment and life experiences play a major role in the development of depression in both men and women. It is clear, however, that of all population groups, those at greatest risk for depression are the elderly, especially those with physical illness (Mark et al., 2011).

Genetic Theories

Numerous studies have concentrated on the role heredity plays in depressive illness. Interest in this field of research was stimulated by the observation that the incidence of depression is higher among relatives of depressed individuals than in the general population. Studies of illness rates within and between generations of families, of monozygotic and dizygotic twins, and of the general population, and those using known genetic markers such as blood type or color blindness all validate the increased incidence of depression in relatives of depressed individuals.

Studies have demonstrated that bipolar disorder is also increased among first-degree relatives of individuals with that disorder. Studies of identical twins report an 80% concordance rate in bipolar disorder. This means that if one twin has the disorder, there is an 80% chance that the other twin will also develop it.

The role of genetics in the development of major mood disorders is complicated by the familiar question: Which plays the more important role, genes or environment? People who are biologically related tend to spend time together and influence one another's thinking. They share similar values and beliefs and are subjected to similar stressors, such as poverty or death of loved ones. It is therefore difficult to determine the relative weight of genetics, thinking patterns, family relationships, and learning in the development of mood disorders.

Depression and the most effective treatments for it can now be tested. Following the recent FDA approval of a test to predict differences in the cytochrome P_{450} (CYP450) gene, clinicians and clients must decide whether using genetic tests to select a specific antidepressant medication from the class known as selective serotonin reuptake inhibitors (SSRIs) might improve the response to treatment for depression. New research on gene-based tests intended to personalize the dose of SSRIs to improve outcomes, or aid in treatment decisions in the clinical setting, is still a challenge at this writing (Teutsch et al., 2009).

Biochemical Theories

Early biochemical studies established that an error in metabolism results in an electrolyte imbalance that seems to play a role in depression. The studies demonstrated that sodium and potassium were transposed in the neurons of depressed individuals. This transposition alters the sensitivity of the neuronal cell membranes. Alterations in sensitivity of neuronal receptors are likely to lead to alterations in behavior. This may account for the efficacy of medications, such as lithium carbonate and antidepressants, in the treatment of mood disorders.

Since then, scientific research has focused on the role of certain chemicals, the neurotransmitters, in the central nervous system. These are chemicals that transmit nervous impulses along neuronal pathways in the limbic area of the brain. Levels of certain monoamine neurotransmitters— norepinephrine, serotonin, epinephrine, and dopamine—were found to be deficient in many depressed people. Until the 1980s scientists believed that major depression resulted from norepinephrine or serotonin deficiencies, and the early antidepressants were formulated accordingly.

The monoamine hypothesis prevailed for years until it was found insufficient to explain fully the etiology of a complex disorder such as depression. Deficient levels of monoamine neurotransmitters have not been consistently found in depressed people and have not been able to relieve symptoms reliably. It is now believed that monoamine deficiencies are only one manifestation of depression. Many pharmacologic agents successfully used to treat depression and mania, however, do enhance monoamine activity. For example, study of the metabolism of serotonin and the discovery of the dysfunction of certain serotonergic neurons in depressed individuals led to the development of the SSRIs and subsequent generations of these useful antidepressants.

Much current biochemical research focuses on the role of psychosocial stress in the pathophysiology of depression. The damaging effects of chronic stress, including its impact on limbic activity, are under extensive study. Current research indicates that the underlying biochemical process involves the neurotransmitters dopamine, gamma-aminobutyric acid (GABA), serotonin, and norepinephrine (Lin et al., 2011). Interferences with the smooth transmission of impulses from one neuron to another, associated with depressive and manic phases of bipolar disorder, can be explained by inadequate release of neurotransmitters or faulty storage mechanisms. It is expected that interactive hypotheses of depression—that is, those that take into consideration a variety of biologic and psychosocial factors—are likely to be most useful in the future understanding of these complex disorders.

Biologic Rhythms

It is widely recognized that we have self-sustained internal physiological cycles that occur every 24 hours. These circadian rhythms, which include body temperature, sleep, and appetite, are activated, controlled, and integrated by the hypothalamus in the brain. The central controlling pacemaker is commonly known as the biologic clock. You can access a biologic clock cell animation through the Online Student Resources for this book.

Diurnal variations in mood, rest and activity cycles, EEG patterns, and neuroendocrine secretions have been clinically demonstrated, and you have no doubt seen the impact of many of these variations yourself. Circadian rhythm dysfunction can explain a number of mood disorder symptoms, such as insomnia, hypersomnia, early morning awakening, and variations in appetite, rest, and activity cycles. Animal studies have demonstrated that alcohol and antimanic medications, such as lithium, slow the biologic clock, while estrogen and tricyclic antidepressants accelerate it or restore normal rhythms. The precise role biologic rhythms play in mood disorders is yet to be determined.

The presence of physical problems has also been thought to play a role in mood disorders. There may be a common factor at work with certain illnesses in which both depression and another physical problem are present, as referred to earlier in this chapter regarding cardiac dysfunction. It is interesting to note that in order to make a diagnosis of mood disorder, the diagnostician must rule out infections, chemical imbalances, environmental toxins, alcohol abuse, and other biologic processes. All of these physical problems may present in such a way as to look like depression.

Psychological Factors

Regardless of temperament and personality patterns, people can and do become depressed. Mild depression is widely acknowledged as a part of the human experience. Although most of us have had "the blues" from time to time, it has been established that certain people are more prone to developing true depression than others. Individuals who exhibit certain attitudes and beliefs—such as low self-esteem; lack of personal goals and direction; the tendency to avoid difficult situations rather than facing them directly; dependence and passivity in interpersonal relationships; acting and reacting impulsively; a limited ability to form enduring, mature relationships; and internalization of blame—are thought to be at risk for the development of depressive disorders.

Sociocultural Factors

Most clinical investigators believe that life events and environmental stress play a role in mood disorders. There is less agreement, however, as to whether life events play a primary role or merely contribute to the onset of an inevitable episode of a mood disorder. Certain events, such as the death of a loved one, divorce, and other losses, are widely recognized by both mental health professionals and the general public as precipitating events for depression. The impact of stress reactions and stress hormones on mood has been established. The unremitting stresses of living in poverty, and society's devaluation of the disadvantaged, also seem to predispose people to developing depression.

Predictors of bipolar mood disorder episodes, for the most part, include stressful life events, increased number of previous bipolar episodes, decreased interval between bipolar episodes, and persistence of the effect of symptoms on functioning. The stressors of pregnancy are excellent examples of life events that can create a psychological vulnerability (Abdel-Hay, El-Sawy, & Badawy, 2011). Their study found that, in addition to the previously listed risk factors, discontinuation of medications and more prior episodes during pregnancy resulted in a recurrence of bipolar disorder during or following pregnancies.

Having longer periods between episodes is typically associated with active involvement in psychotherapy, adhering to a medication regimen, and having a strong support system. Unfortunately, the presence of substance abuse interferes with any semblance of stability, and the prevalence of substance abuse in this population is notably high.

Culture exerts a powerful influence on how individuals experience and communicate psychic distress. Spiritual or religious concerns such as guilt may predominate and mask the underlying mood disorders. Some cultures experience depression largely in somatic terms. Be alert to complaints of headaches or "nerves" in Hispanic clients, of weakness or "imbalance" in Asian clients, and of body metaphors involving the heart in Middle Eastern and certain Native American clients (see Chapter 9 ∞ for a discussion of culture-bound syndromes). These may be culturally determined ways of expressing depression.

Be aware of the unique needs of clients who are likely to perceive the meaning and severity of psychiatric symptoms in relation to the norms of their cultural reference group. They include new immigrants to this country, individuals who are still heavily involved in the culture of origin, those who do not speak English, and those whose entire network of social and religious support remains embedded in the culture of origin.

Differences in culture and social status of clients and caregivers can create problems in diagnosis and treatment. Language differences, for example, create barriers in forming therapeutic relationships in talk therapies and in other treatment settings such as clinics. Cultural differences in the expression of symptoms make it difficult to determine whether a behavior is normal or pathologic, and the culture itself may dictate or affect clients' attitudes toward and adherence to treatment (Buckner-Brown, Tucker, & Rivera, 2011). The influence of culture on clients' attitudes toward treatment and beliefs about healing are discussed in Chapter 9 ∞.

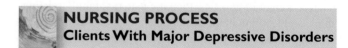

NURSING PROCESS
Clients With Major Depressive Disorders

Nursing care of clients with mood disorders follows a problem-solving model you are already accustomed to using, the nursing process.

Assessment

As already discussed, depression is characterized by low mood, often related to a loss. The loss may be concrete, such as the loss of a loved one or a job, or perceived, such as the loss of a cherished wish or disillusionment with a respected role model.

Subjective Data

Clients with depressive disorders may express some of the following:

- Feelings of sadness
- Fatigue
- Lack of interest in relationships and activities that were previously pleasurable
- Feelings of worthlessness
- Impaired concentration
- Impaired decision-making ability
- Sleep disturbances
- Appetite changes; weight loss or weight gain
- Excessive sleep

Clients will often describe how long it takes them to complete activities that formerly were easily accomplished, such as preparing a simple meal. Tearfulness and emotional outbursts may also be a part of their description of the problem. They may or may not mention a loss or disappointment that they relate to the feelings.

Somatic Concerns Somatic concerns are often the presenting complaint. Depressed clients may complain of abdominal pains, headaches, and vague bodily aches. A problem with sexual functioning or lack of desire may also be a presenting complaint. Constipation is a common result of the general slowing of metabolism due to inactivity. Some cultures more easily express symptoms of depression through complaints about body function and discomfort. See What Every Nurse Should Know for information on how you can detect depression evidenced by somatic concerns in other settings.

Suicide Assessment Assess all clients who describe depressive symptoms for suicide risk. This is best accomplished through direct questioning. Ask about suicidal thinking, history of suicide attempts, and whether the client has a specific suicide plan. This aspect of assessment is reassuring, not alarming, to clients. Ask these questions in a direct fashion. You might ask, for example, "Tell me how you plan to kill yourself. Do you have or can you get the gun/pills/poison?" It is important to know whether the client has actually planned the suicide or if it is a vaguely formed thought. The more organized the plan is, the more concern it generates, particularly if the client has access to a lethal weapon, chemical, or other means of self-injury. Further discussion of other aspects of

WHAT EVERY NURSE SHOULD KNOW

Physical Complaints and Depression

Imagine you are a medical office nurse. Frequently, you would note that people feel aches and pains more acutely when they are depressed. The natural reaction to pain is to seek help from one's primary medical health care provider. One out of every six people going to a medical office is depressed. Only one out of every six of those people are diagnosed and treated for depression. It is important for people who are suffering from depression to talk to their health care providers about other experiences and symptoms over their lifetime. Be aware that in some cultures, people express depression through body systems—headaches, stomachaches, muscle spasms, and visual problems, among others. When you assess people from these cultures, consider the possibility that they may be depressed. A discussion of culture and depression is integrated throughout Chapter 9∞.

People seldom self-diagnose depression. They are much more likely to assume that not enjoying their usual activities, experiencing changes in eating or sleeping habits, and feeling bad in one way or another are caused by a medical problem. Ferreting out the real cause of distress will ensure effective responses to treatment.

suicide will be discussed under the heading "Preventing Suicide and Promoting Safety." Suicide lethality assessment is thoroughly discussed in Chapter 23∞.

Objective Data

Depression is a common disorder in the general population. Depressed clients are more likely to be female than male; however, the lifetime rate of depression is approximately 1 out of 4 women and 1 out of 6 men. Both genders are at significant risk for a depressive event. Clients with depression often have had prior episodes of depression and a family history of depression or bipolar disorder. A history of a recent stressful event and the lack of social support are also common features.

Objective Signs Objective signs and symptoms of depression are few. Psychomotor agitation or retardation may be observable if it is profound or if the nurse is familiar with the client's usual level of functioning. Family members may report observations of the client's agitation or apathy and lack of pleasure in usual activities. They may describe a pattern of social withdrawal and lack of social participation, combined with an intense preoccupation with the client's own feelings. Be alert to a change in behavior.

Checklist Depression Inventories During assessment, many clinicians find it useful to provide a list of symptoms and ask clients to check the ones they are experiencing. A widely used and highly regarded self-reporting instrument designed to assess mood state is the Beck Depression Inventory, mentioned earlier in the chapter. It has been in use for over 35 years and has been revised several times based on clinical research. This inventory is useful for detecting depression, anxiety, apathy, and irritability. Several different types of Beck inventories are now available (Beck, Steer, & Brown, 1996).

Medical Illnesses Other objective information to obtain during the nursing assessment includes concurrent general medical illnesses. Autoimmune, neurologic, metabolic, oncologic, and endocrine disorders often trigger depression. For example, hypothyroidism may be accompanied by depressive symptoms due to the underlying medical disease, while a client with AIDS or cancer may become depressed as a result of the diagnosis, prognosis, or disability connected with the disease.

Substance Use and Abuse Alcohol, which is a CNS depressant, and certain legal and illegal drugs can cause or complicate depression. Obtain a complete list of all substances and medications used by the client through matter-of-fact questioning. A few prescription medications have depression as a side effect; do not overlook these in the complete assessment. Birth control pills, sedatives, reserpine, glucocorticoids, and anabolic steroids have all been associated with the development of depression.

Laboratory Tests There are currently no laboratory tests specific for depression, but abnormal findings on several tests were discussed earlier in this chapter in Your Assessment Approach on page 370.

Nursing Diagnosis: NANDA

The following sections discuss the implications of several nursing diagnoses commonly seen in depressed clients.

Risk for Self-Directed Violence

Thoughts about and impulses toward self-harm are related to feelings of worthlessness, feelings of guilt, repeated failure experiences, feelings of helplessness and hopelessness, or psychotic thinking. Suicidal clients should be hospitalized on either a general or a specialized hospital unit. Regardless of setting, whenever a client is at high risk for self-harm, that becomes *the* priority nursing diagnosis, and client safety becomes the most important aspect of nursing care.

Situational Low Self-Esteem or Chronic Low Self-Esteem

Depressed clients often express, either directly or indirectly, negative feelings about themselves and their abilities. Reduced self-esteem may be related to a variety of factors, including feeling abandoned by loved ones, experiencing repeated failures or losses, lacking positive feedback from others, thinking negative thoughts, engaging in negative "self-talk," or feeling guilty over real or perceived transgressions.

Evidence of low self-esteem is seen in clients who withdraw from social interaction; have difficulty accepting compliments or positive feedback; are harshly critical of themselves or others; are reluctant to try new activities because of fear of failure; express feelings of inferiority, worthlessness, and pessimism about the future; are overly sensitive to criticism; see social slights where none are intended; or set unrealistic goals and engage in grandiose thinking (denial of low self-esteem).

Hopelessness

Individuals who lead lives characterized by hopelessness believe that their own actions cannot significantly influence an outcome. They believe there is no solution to their problems. They come to doubt their own abilities and are passive in response to others.

Evidence of hopelessness is seen in the behavior of clients who lack energy and initiative, refuse to engage in self-care, do not participate in decision making, verbally express a lack of control and doubts about their abilities, are reluctant to express feelings, avoid eye contact, generally lack involvement, and exhibit decreased affect.

Social Isolation

Low self-esteem and doubts about abilities lead many depressed clients to withdraw socially. Because inadequate social skills and self-absorption create impediments to positive interpersonal relationships, clients with low self-esteem frequently *are* avoided by others. This further reinforces their fears of undesirability and increases their social isolation. Evidence of social isolation and impaired social interaction is seen in behaviors such as spending inordinate amounts of time in bed, lack of verbalization, lack of eye contact, dull or monosyllabic responses to others' attempts at conversation, a preference for being alone, turning away or closing the eyes, and exhibiting discomfort in the presence of others.

Outcome Identification: NOC

Suggested outcomes for each NANDA diagnosis presented in the previous section are discussed in the following section.

Risk for Self-Directed Violence

NOC outcomes have not yet been identified for this nursing diagnosis. Appropriate potential choices for depressed clients include Impulse Control: Ability to restrain compulsive or impulsive behavior, and Suicide Self-Restraint: Ability to refrain from gestures and attempts at killing self.

Situational Low Self-Esteem or Chronic Low Self-Esteem

The suggested NOC outcome for depressed clients with this nursing diagnosis is Self-Esteem: Personal judgment of self-worth.

Hopelessness

Several NOC outcomes are relevant to depressed clients with this nursing diagnosis. They include Decision Making: Ability to choose between two or more alternatives; Hope: Presence of internal state of optimism that is personally satisfying and life supporting; Mood Equilibrium: Appropriate adjustment of prevailing emotional tone in response to circumstances; and Quality of Life: Expressed satisfaction with current life circumstances.

Social Isolation

The depressed client with this nursing diagnosis has several potentially appropriate NOC outcomes. These outcomes include Loneliness: The extent of emotional, social, or existential isolation response; Social Interaction Skills: Use of effective interaction behaviors; Social Involvement: Frequency of social interactions with persons, groups, or organizations; and Social Support: Perceived availability and actual provision of reliable assistance from other persons.

Planning and Implementation: NIC

When planning and implementing interventions designed to help depressed clients, keep the following two general principles in mind:

1. It is impossible to make depressed people feel better by being cheerful. In fact, an overly cheerful attitude tends to make them feel even worse because it trivializes or minimizes the impact of their feelings. Try to adopt a more emotionally neutral attitude while maintaining confidence that they will feel better.
2. Recognize that working with depressed people may eventually lower your mood and make you feel "down" yourself. This is called *emotional contagion*. Stay in touch with your own feelings. If you find yourself feeling down, assert yourself by asking to be assigned to a different type of client for a time.

Examine and learn from your interventions by processing your interactions with depressed clients. The process recording method will help you to structure your examination. A process recording usually consists of three columns—one for the nurse's statements, one for the client's, and one that identifies the process or action taking place. A sample process recording of an interaction between a nurse and a depressed client is in Box 17-2.

Box 17-2 A Sample Process Recording With a Client Who Is Depressed

Client	Nurse	Process
"I don't think I can take this anymore—it's too much for me."	"You sound so overwhelmed. How long have you felt this way?"	Validating Exploring
"It's been like this for as long as I can remember. It just never ends."	"How have you handled these feelings over the long time you've had them?"	Opening the topic of client's successes in managing
"I just put one foot in front of the other. It doesn't make it better, though."	"It does seem to work to some extent. You've made it through this long."	Reframing the effort as a success
"I guess. I just don't know how I can keep doing it."	"It can be tiring. Keep in mind you're not alone in this effort. You have people who support you and care about you."	Validation Reinforcing the social supports in place
"As long as I have some help."	"There is help you can depend on."	Reassurance

Preventing Suicide and Promoting Safety

There are few times when "always" and "never" are applicable. Client safety, however, *always* takes priority over other nursing care concerns. When the risk for self-directed violence is high, a number of actions call for immediate intervention. These actions are discussed in Your Intervention Strategies. *Be aware that the risk of suicide increases as the severest stage of depression is alleviated, because clients then have sufficient energy and cognitive ability to plan and successfully implement a suicide plan, even though they are still deeply depressed.*

Encourage discussing all feelings. Clients need to know that all feelings are valid and that it benefits them to express their emotions, particularly anger and hopelessness, rather than act them out through maladaptive behaviors. Having the feeling is always accepted. Acting on the feeling, however, may be problematic. What counts in the long run is what one decides to do about the feeling. Assist in the transition from hospital to home by helping clients identify people in their usual environments to whom they can express feelings candidly without being judged.

Use a calm, reassuring approach and teach calming measures, such as time-outs and controlled breathing. Provide safe physical outlets for expression of anger or increasing tension. Specific nursing interventions for anger are discussed in Chapter 22 and Chapter 35∞.

Collaborate with clients to identify community resources to which they can turn if suicidal thoughts recur outside the treatment setting. Almost all communities have access to hotlines that are staffed around the clock with trained volunteers or professionals who are available to discuss feelings before they reach crisis proportions. Refer to Chapter 23∞ for specific information on suicide and suicide prevention.

Promoting Self-Esteem

While low self-esteem is a chronic problem, there are a number of actions you can take to reduce negative thinking, thereby promoting improved self-esteem.

- Provide distraction from self-absorption by involving the client in recreational activities and pleasant pastimes. Simple conversation with a staff member or another client helps interrupt the pattern of negative thoughts. Use care to select activities that are not too complex for the client's current level of functioning. Experiences of success, not more failures, are needed. Increase the complexity of activities as the client progresses.
- Dispel the notion clients often have, that *when* they feel better, they will want to engage in activities. Explain that they must begin doing things *in order* to feel better. Being active promotes a more balanced feeling state. Be sure to acknowledge that it takes

YOUR INTERVENTION STRATEGIES   Preventing Inpatient Suicide and Promoting Safety

Be sure to check the policy and procedures of the individual inpatient treatment facility and implement those guidelines as well.

- Evaluate the level of suicide intent regularly, and institute the appropriate level of staff supervision following unit protocol.
- Suicidal clients need to know that the environment is safe for them. Reassure them by removing sharp objects, razors, breakable glass items, mirrors, matches, and straps or belts, and explain why these objects are being removed. Monitor the use of scissors, razors, and other potential weapons.
- Place suicidal clients in a centrally located room near the nurses' station to facilitate ease of observation.

- Avoid establishing a predictable pattern of observation during the day and especially at night.
- Be particularly alert during change of shifts and on holidays or other times when staffing is limited, and during times of distraction, such as mealtimes and visiting hours.
- Examine items brought by visitors and monitor for safety.
- The no-suicide contract, discussed in detail in Chapter 23∞, is a useful intervention.

Encourage clients to seek you or another staff member when bothered by suicidal thoughts or impulses. Discussing these thoughts and impulses may be sufficient to diminish them and prevent a suicidal crisis from occurring. Avoid discussing suicidal ruminations in repetitious detail, because this may reinforce maladaptive behavior.

self-discipline and energy to do something when one does not really feel like it.

- Recognize accomplishment; do not use flattery or excessive praise. Give positive, matter-of-fact reinforcement, such as "I notice that you combed your hair," rather than overly enthusiastic compliments, such as "What a great hairstyle!" Appropriate recognition will increase the likelihood that the client will continue the positive behavior, while insincerity can be perceived as ridicule or infantilizing.
- Help clients identify their personal strengths. It may be useful to write these down. Recognize that it often takes some time for clients with low self-esteem to realize that they have any strengths. Avoid the temptation to point out the characteristics you have noticed. It is far more useful to support their ability to recognize their own positive qualities.
- Be accepting of clients' negative feelings, but set limits on the amount of time you will listen to accounts of past failures. Be alert for opportunities to interrupt the negative conversational patterns with more neutral ones.
- Teach assertiveness techniques, such as the ability to say "no" to protect one's own rights while respecting the rights of others. Clients with low self-esteem often allow others to take advantage of them. Defining passive, aggressive, and assertive behavior and giving examples of each are also helpful when teaching assertiveness (Partnering With Clients and Families has a description). Encourage clients

and their family members to practice the new techniques in their relationship with you, so that you can give feedback on how it feels to the recipient of an assertive communication or action.

Instilling Hope

Assisting depressed clients to develop a positive outlook is a priority nursing intervention. Clients who feel hopeless tend to form dependent relationships. Be aware of this tendency, and work from the first contact to minimize the likelihood that maladaptive dependence occurs in your nurse–client relationship. The list in Your Self-Awareness will give you direction on minimizing maladaptive dependence. Provide clients choices in the planning of their own care and encourage them to assume some responsibility for that care. For example, allow a client to choose whether to bathe in the morning or at night, or to choose from a short list of activities to attend. Encouraging clients to set their own goals that identify what they hope to achieve during hospitalization or outpatient therapy reinforces the message of self-determination. Remember that unrealistically optimistic goals will ensure another failure experience and reinforce the client's sense of powerlessness. Make sure that goals are attainable.

Clients who feel hopeless also need help in identifying how they can gain a sense of control in their relationships and lives outside the hospital. Collaborate with clients to identify changes they wish to make and action steps toward achieving them. Make the steps small and manageable. Accomplishing even small steps leads to a sense of mastery and optimism.

PARTNERING WITH CLIENTS AND FAMILIES

Teaching About Aggressive, Passive, and Assertive Behaviors

Assertiveness is a learned behavior. Everyone has assertiveness potential, but we are not born knowing how to be assertive. Children learn patterns of communicating from the adults around them. However, you can unlearn communication patterns if they are not working and learn new ones. The goal is to help people express themselves without fear of disapproval from others. Being assertive does not guarantee that others will always agree with you, but you do have the satisfaction of giving your opinion.

Definitions

Aggressive behavior is directed toward getting what one wants without considering the feelings of others. Aggressive communicators want to get their own way at any cost. They want others to "back off" and use intimidation to convey this message. An example of aggressive behavior is insisting on going to a certain movie even though you know your companion does not enjoy that type of movie. The outcome of aggressive behavior is that although you may get what you want in the short run, others feel discredited and tend to avoid you.

Passive behavior consists of avoiding conflict at any cost, even at the expense of one's own happiness. An example of passive behavior is agreeing to go to a movie you do not want to see because your friend pressures you to go. Passive communicators

hold their feelings in and allow anger to build up. Anger can come out suddenly in an explosion or can be expressed in what is known as passive–aggressive behavior. An example of passive–aggressive behavior is taking a long time to get ready to go out while your friend is waiting because you are angry at him for insisting on seeing a movie you do not want to see. The outcome is that the passive person gives up control and is left with resentment, which usually emerges in other ways that damage relationships.

Assertive behavior consists of expressing one's wishes and opinions, or taking care of oneself, but not at the expense of others. An example of assertive communication is saying, "I really don't care for violent movies. Let's look at the movie listings and see if there is something playing that we can both enjoy." The outcome of assertive behavior is self-confidence and self-esteem. Clients and family members can learn about assertiveness in other ways as well. Share with them the helpful hints in Partnering With Clients and Families: Teaching About Assertiveness on page 766 of Chapter 35 ∞. Also refer them to books that can be obtained through your local library or bookseller: *My Answer is No... If That's OK With You,* by Nanette Gartrell, 2009; *Peace at Any Price: How to Overcome the Please Disease,* by Deborah Day Poor, 2005; and *Civilized Assertiveness for Women: Communication With Backbone...Not Bite,* by Judith Selee McClure, 2007.

YOUR SELF-AWARENESS
Minimizing Maladaptive Dependence

Be aware of the tendency of hopeless clients to form dependent relationships and work from the first contact to minimize the likelihood that maladaptive dependence occurs in the nurse–client relationship.

- Emphasizing the short-term nature of the relationship is essential.
- If the client singles out one staff member exclusively and refuses to relate to others, this is a clue that undue dependence is developing.
- Avoid giving dependent clients the hope that the nurse–client relationship can continue after the end of the therapy.
- Kindly, but firmly, refuse requests for your address or telephone number.
- Remind clients that social contact will not be allowed.
- If you find yourself wanting to continue relationships with certain clients, discuss these feelings with your instructor (if you are a student), or your supervisor or a respected professional peer (if you are a practicing nurse). It is essential that you separate your professional life from your social life.

Teach clients coping measures such as problem-solving techniques, and encourage them to use them when confronting life situations. For example, if a client has difficulty paying the rent, help him or her identify options, such as moving to a less expensive apartment or taking in a roommate. Explore the pros and cons of each option and their possible consequences. Emphasize confidence in the client's ability to identify, select, and carry out problem-solving activities that will result in a greater sense of involvement in his or her life. Equally important is to help clients identify the aspects of their lives that are not within their control. The ability to accept what *cannot* be changed is just as essential as developing the ability to bring about positive change.

Planning for discharge should begin with the first client contact and is particularly important with hopeless, dependent clients. Help them and their families and significant others to identify resources in the community and to build support systems. Support groups, therapy groups, and social groups can all help clients separate from caregivers more readily when the time comes to end therapy.

Enhancing Socialization

When designing interventions for promoting social interactions, realize that both the quality and the quantity of a client's social behavior may be impaired. Early in the nurse–client relationship, make brief but frequent contacts with withdrawn clients, without making any demands. Your interest can increase a client's self-worth.

With extremely uncommunicative clients, simply spending time sitting quietly without any demand for interaction may be helpful. This approach communicates your belief that they are worth the investment of time. If you find it difficult to be comfortable with silence, you may communicate that discomfort to clients. Remember that silence conveys acceptance and is a useful therapeutic communication technique. Using silence therapeutically is discussed in Chapter 10 ∞.

When clients express feelings or cry, remember to be nonjudgmental. Avoid showing surprise or disapproval. Two examples of how you can do this are in Rx Communication. Recognize that ventilating feelings may provide temporary relief, particularly if anger is expressed. If clients are unable to verbalize feelings, they sometimes can act them out in safe and appropriate ways, such as tearing up an old magazine or beating on a pillow or bed. Provide privacy during these times.

Encourage both verbal and nonverbal expressions of feelings by teaching clients that these are healthy behaviors. This intervention reinforces your acceptance of clients as unique and valuable individuals. Avoid disagreeing with, or otherwise belittling, a client's feelings by using overly cheerful reassurances like, "Now, now, Mrs. Hamilton. You're feeling down right now but you'll feel better after a good night's sleep."

Once clients are comfortable interacting with one person, encourage group activities. Although this step may be difficult and frightening for clients, you can minimize their discomfort by attending activities with them at first. If their anxiety becomes too uncomfortable, let them know that they can leave the situation without losing your approval. Give recognition for even small steps, gradually removing yourself and allowing them to stay in groups on their own.

℞ COMMUNICATION

Client With Major Depression

CLIENT: "I am upset and irritated all the time. All I do is yell at my kids and snap at my husband."

NURSE RESPONSE 1: "What can you tell me about feeling so upset?"	**NURSE RESPONSE 2:** "It sounds like you are feeling out of control right now."
RATIONALE: Open-ended questions elicit the client's perception of the problem and allow her to begin to explore her feelings where she can. Accepts the client where she is now without judging her.	*RATIONALE:* This response shows empathy and acceptance. By reflecting her expression of feelings, you validate the accuracy of your understanding and lay the groundwork for further exploration.

Sometimes clients avoid social situations because they lack social skills and self-confidence. Create opportunities for clients to learn social skills and practice them in a protected environment. For example, teach them to read the newspaper or see a movie and select several items of interest to use in making "small talk." Demonstrate making small talk, and encourage them to practice with you. Give feedback on their progress. Make sure this is an enjoyable and nonthreatening activity.

Individuals who are either extremely passive or too aggressive in their social interactions are often avoided by others. Teaching such clients how to use assertive behavior can improve their interpersonal relationships. Use role-playing to help them become comfortable with new skills. (Refer again to Partnering With Clients and Families on page 766 in Chapter 35∞.)

Administering Medications

The main types of antidepressants nurses will administer to depressed clients are tricyclic antidepressants (TCAs), monoamine oxidase inhibitors (MAOIs), selective serotonin reuptake inhibitors (SSRIs), serotonin and norepinephrine reuptake inhibitors (SNRIs), and atypical antidepressants such as bupropion. See Chapter 7∞ for detailed discussions of these medications. The intended action of all antidepressants is to exert positive effects on mood and behavior. Because some are sedating and others are energizing, the individual client's symptoms guide the choice of medication. The use of antidepressants during pregnancy may be necessary and is weighed against both the dangers to the fetus of an untreated, unstable mother and the risk of birth defects. Current clinical practice is to treat the mood disorder to protect both the mother and the baby.

Antidepressants are generally effective in alleviating most clients' symptoms and are helpful adjuncts to treatment. Because they do nothing to affect underlying psychosocial conflicts, they should not be used as the single treatment modality for depressed clients but should be used in conjunction with individual, family, and/or group therapy. Responsibility for correct administration, monitoring for effects, and client education rests with nurses. Specific information such as maintaining a low-tyramine diet (**tyramine** is an amino acid) while on MAOIs is an educational point that must be discussed with clients and families. People taking MAOIs cannot consume anything (food, drink, medications) containing tyramine because this can cause a dangerous rise in blood pressure called *hypertensive crisis*. Chapter 31∞ has additional information about antidepressant therapy and related nursing responsibilities.

Monitoring Electroconvulsive Therapy

Electroconvulsive therapy (ECT), a treatment procedure during which a small electric current is passed through particular areas of the brain, is extremely useful to clients with severe depression, acute mania, some psychotic conditions, and those who are acutely suicidal. It is usually given several times a week until a course of 12 treatments

is completed. Exactly how ECT works is not well understood. Evidence suggests that it may resynchronize circadian rhythms, like a "brain defibrillator"; it may act as an anticonvulsant like carbamazepine; it may restore the equilibrium between cerebral hemispheres; or it may help prioritize function over depressive thoughts. Historically, ECT caused some controversy, probably due to its crude beginnings. Current use, known as modified ECT, is not the intense physiological event it used to be because of the use of muscle relaxants and short-acting anesthetic agents.

Contrary to popular belief, ECT causes no tissue damage or neuronal cell loss (structural brain damage). Most ECT clients report positive associations with the treatment and general improvement in cognition, in addition to relief from depression for several weeks following ECT. The vast majority of ECT clients would recommend ECT as a treatment for their loved ones. There are very few cautions or contraindications for ECT use. Guidelines for working with clients receiving ECT are discussed in Your Intervention Strategies.

During a course of ECT, a transient short-term memory loss is expected. This is distressing to some clients, and they need to be reassured that memory is usually completely restored. Because ECT is not curative, ongoing psychotherapy and pharmacotherapy are often continued to prevent *relapse*. This treatment modality is considered the treatment of choice for treatment-resistant depression. The practical issues of ECT treatment and how the treatment is conducted are described in the following clinical example.

Clinical Example

Barry has been depressed for a number of months after having been accused of unfair practices at work. His feelings of guilt and worthlessness are far out of proportion to reality. Although he believes he has a successful defense against these charges, many people at work see it differently. His prescriber has tried several different antidepressants with him, but his symptoms of depression continue to worsen. Barry developed severe depressive symptoms such as suicidal thinking, psychomotor retardation, and weight loss because he believes that he does not deserve to eat.

Barry's psychiatrist has recommended a course of ECT for his treatment-resistant depression. Barry is concerned because he has heard many rumors about the negative effects of ECT. The prescriber has explained that it is a safe and effective treatment about which there are several negative and inaccurate myths. After several discussions, Barry agreed to try ECT. He was given a course of six ECT treatments over 2 weeks and experienced a significant improvement in his mood. He is no longer suicidal or delusional, and no longer has psychomotor retardation. It has become possible for him to function more effectively at work, including defending himself against what he declares are unfounded charges. Due to advances in ECT techniques Barry had no discomfort during or after any of the ECT treatments. He is relieved that ECT has been an effective treatment for his depression.

Evaluation

Specific client behaviors indicate that nursing interventions have been successful. Evaluation criteria answer the question, "How do we know that the depressed client's condition has improved?"

YOUR INTERVENTION STRATEGIES   Working With Clients Receiving ECT

- Prepare the client by explaining the procedure and answering all questions as fully as possible.
- A separate consent for treatment must be signed because ECT requires the administration of anesthesia. While informing clients and obtaining consent forms is legally a medical responsibility, in practice it is often shared by nurses.
- Clients are kept NPO for at least 4 hours before treatment.
- Just prior to treatment, request that the client void and remove contact lenses, jewelry, hairpins, and dentures.
- Assess vital signs.
- The anesthetic preparation usually consists of the following:
    1. Generally, an atropine-like medication, such as glycopyrrolate (Robinul), is given to decrease secretions and block cardiac vagal reflexes during the seizure.
    2. A short-acting anesthetic, such as methohexital sodium (Brevital), is administered intravenously.
    3. Following induction, a skeletal muscle relaxant, such as succinylcholine chloride (Anectine), is administered to prevent injuries during the seizure.
    4. The client must be artificially ventilated until the muscle relaxant is fully metabolized, usually in 2 to 3 minutes. Oxygen is

administered with a rubber bite block in place. If necessary, oxygen may be administered by positive pressure.

- An electrical current is passed through the brain by means of unilateral or bilateral electrodes placed on the temples. This causes a generalized (or tonic–clonic) seizure, the effects of which are masked by the muscle relaxant. Often the only observable signs of seizure are a fluttering of the eyelids and carpopedal spasms.
- Clients are recovered in the lateral recumbent position to facilitate drainage and prevent aspiration. Upon awakening, they will be confused and somewhat disoriented. After they are fully recovered and have been reoriented by the nurse, they may eat breakfast.

Photo courtesy of Will McIntyre/Photo Researchers, Inc.

Impulse Control and Suicide Self-Restraint

The risk for self-directed violence is lessened when the client reports a decrease in suicidal thoughts and impulses and commits no acts of self-violence. Clients who are not suicidal can vent negative feelings appropriately and avoid high-risk environments or situations. They become more adept at identifying alternative ways of coping with problems and no longer depend on suicide as their primary coping skill.

Self-Esteem

Clients who have improved self-esteem can verbalize self-acceptance and identify positive characteristics of themselves. They can speak about increased feelings of self-worth. Their behaviors are consistent with increased self-esteem; for example, their posture is erect, and they groom and dress themselves with some care. They are able to accept a compliment, to express feelings directly and openly, and to communicate assertively with others, including maintaining eye contact. They express some optimism and hope for the future. Clients demonstrate self-esteem when they evaluate their own strengths realistically; set realistic, attainable goals for themselves; and work toward reaching them.

Hopelessness

Depressed clients demonstrate progress toward eliminating hopelessness by consistently weighing and choosing among alternatives and by expressing faith, the will to live, reasons to live, meaning in life, optimism, and belief in self or others. They can identify their own personal strengths, show interest in achieving life goals, and demonstrate satisfaction with life conditions or work to change them.

Social Involvement

Improved social involvement is apparent when clients communicate and socialize with others. Voluntarily attending group activities is a measure of success. They can initiate interaction with another person appropriately and assume responsibility for dealing with feelings, including finding others with whom to talk. Clients can identify their own personal characteristics or behaviors that contribute to social isolation and accept responsibility for them. They report fewer experiences of feeling excluded. For additional information about working with depressed clients, see the Nursing Care Plan at the end of this chapter. Clients plan for discharge by establishing or maintaining relationships, a social life, and a support system outside the hospital, and by participating in leisure activities.

CASE MANAGEMENT

Case management with depressed clients attempts to ensure that they receive needed services in a timely, flexible, cost-effective manner. This requires that the case manager understands risk factors and possible complicating factors of major depression, recognizes prodromal/recurrence/relapse symptoms early, anticipates possible complications, and understands effective case management outcomes. Depending on his or her educational preparation and experience, the case manager may or may not deliver direct psychotherapeutic care to depressed clients.

Risk factors for recurrence or *relapse* (a return of symptoms after a period of time with no or very few symptoms)

WHY I BECAME A PSYCHIATRIC–MENTAL HEALTH NURSE

Kay K. Chitty, RN, EdD

My first psychiatric nursing course when I was a junior in college included a practicum in the locked psychiatric ward of a huge public hospital in Atlanta. I was petrified! My only previous exposure to psychiatric clients took place when my Girl Scout troop toured the back wards of the state hospital in my hometown. Although I never lost my initial anxiety about stepping off the elevator onto "the unit," I emerged from that semester with the realization that I had found my niche in nursing, and I have never looked back.

Psychiatric nursing has been good to me. I have had a wonderfully varied career, ranging from staff nurse in a New York City psychiatric hospital to independent practice in North Carolina. I have practiced, written about, and taught psychiatric nursing for 40 years in several states and never once considered changing to another field. Every day is different and no day is predictable. Working with people who have emotional problems is, to me, the most challenging field in nursing. There have been many times when I felt inadequate—it goes with the territory. But additional study, further experience, and supervision by more experienced nurses gradually molded me into a competent (I'd like to think excellent) psychiatric nurse. I love sharing my knowledge with students and I never forget how they feel when they embark on their first course in psychiatric nursing!

of depression include female gender, family history of depression, previous depression, lack of family/social support, stressful life events or losses, and substance abuse. Suicide attempts, substance abuse continuance or increase, having a personality disorder, having a coexisting medical or psychiatric condition, resistance to treatment, and/or failure to respond to treatment complicate the course of a depressive episode. While recurrence of depressive symptoms is of concern, the length of time it takes to recover from depressive symptoms affects longer-term planning and case management services. Symptoms of depression must resolve to a certain extent before the person can experience healthier functioning (Sheehan, Harnett-Sheehan, Spann, Thompson, & Prakash, 2011). And as treatment continues, symptom relief and then functionality proceed hand-in-hand. Recognizing depressive symptoms, and treating them, earlier in the process can be an effective tool in reducing the long-term impacts of the illness.

Symptoms that would alert the case manager to evaluate a client's need for treatment for major depression have been discussed in DSM Essential Features on page 364. Case management interventions would respond to suicidal thoughts, suicide plans, or suicide attempts, prior self-destructive violence, concurrent chronic or severe acute medical problems, prior medication-resistant depression, social withdrawal, and decline in work productivity. Teach clients and family members to also be alert for symptoms that indicate the need for treatment.

Clients and families may find the following websites helpful:

- National Institute for Mental Health: http://www.nimh.nih.gov/health/publications/depression/complete-index.shtml (information presented in both English and Spanish)
- International Foundation for Research and Education on Depression (iFRED): http://www.ifred.org/

These sites can be accessed through the Online Student Resources for this book.

Desired case management outcomes include symptom remission; improvement in social, family, and occupational functioning; reduced risk of self-harm; and either avoidance of hospitalization or shortened hospital stay. Clients who lack financial resources and family, social, and employer support, and who resist or respond poorly to treatment, represent greater challenges for the case manager. The ultimate case management goal is the earliest possible detection of symptoms, effective symptom reduction, and a rapid return to maximal premorbid functioning.

COMMUNITY-BASED CARE

A number of depressed clients can be effectively treated in community-based settings such as mental health centers, schools, occupational health settings, doctors' offices, hospices, skilled nursing facilities, and rehabilitation centers, among others. Nurses in community settings play a major role in recognizing symptoms of depression, providing screening and assessment, providing emotional support and information, monitoring antidepressant therapy, and educating family members and significant others about depression. Severely depressed and/or suicidal clients, however, should be referred to inpatient treatment to ensure their safety. What Every Nurse Should Know presents information on depression for nurses in this specialty area as well as for nurses in skilled nursing facilities and rehabilitation centers.

Nurses working in community health settings may not be educationally prepared as psychiatric–mental health nurses. However, with minimal continuing education focused on the detection and treatment of depression, they can play a valuable role in the recovery of depressed clients while enabling them to remain in the community while in treatment.

HOME CARE

Nurses functioning in the home serve as bridges between hospital, home, and community. Home care may substitute for inpatient care in carefully selected cases, or it may precede or follow the client's inpatient treatment. Home care aims to maximize the client's ability to stay in the family context and overlaps somewhat with the case management model discussed earlier. The APRN psychiatric–mental health nurse, however, is prepared to provide psychotherapeutic interventions directly to depressed clients and their families.

WHAT EVERY NURSE SHOULD KNOW

Grief and Depression

Imagine you are a hospice nurse helping people live the last months of their lives. Depression is thought to be the natural reaction when people have been diagnosed with a terminal illness. When people know that their life is coming to an end, there is sadness and grieving. However, depression is much more than that. Symptoms of depression that last for 14 days or more are not a necessary emotional state. The final months of someone's life, while sad, can be made more comfortable, functional, and potentially satisfying when depression is treated. Nurses working in hospice settings interact with people whose lives will end in a few short months. Spending those months in an emotionally healthy setting is the priority.

Differentiating between normal sadness and grieving and the state called depression is done in clinical interviews and through observations. Statements such as, "I never should have sold the house. That house is where my children grew up and I took all their memories away when I sold it," represent irrational guilt more than legitimate regret. Similarly, taking more responsibility than is reasonable, interpreting interactions in morbid ways, not being able to enjoy any aspect of their current life, and drastic changes in appetite and sleeping pattern that are not related to their medical condition are all signs of depression. Make arrangements for a psychological consult when you detect depressive symptoms as a hospice nurse. Consultations of this nature are performed by advanced practice psychiatric–mental health nurses, psychologists, or psychiatrists.

Effective treatment of depressive symptoms, even during the final stages of life, is not only a possibility but a responsibility. Talk therapy and/or medications can have an impact within a matter of days or weeks, allowing clients to say goodbye and face this transition positively and peacefully.

Working with depressed clients in the home and family contexts allows the nurse to observe the family dynamics and their impact on the family members, including the depressed client. These nurses provide education to client and family about medications, side effects, desired effects, adverse effects, and possible medication and/or food interactions. In addition, home care nurses educate clients and families about the nature of depression, the usual course of depression, what to expect, and when to seek help. They assist clients and families in establishing realistic goals, both short and long term. They collaborate with other professionals such as physicians, psychologists, psychiatrists, social workers, and others to improve communication and prevent gaps and overlaps in services. They also serve as client advocates, ensuring that depressed clients receive comprehensive, cost-effective care in the home setting.

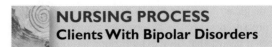

NURSING PROCESS
Clients With Bipolar Disorders

Because the nursing care of clients experiencing depressive symptoms is the same whether the diagnosis is major depressive disorder, dysthymic disorder, or depressed episode bipolar disorder, this section will focus on hypomania and mania, which constitute the other half of the bipolar continuum of behaviors.

Assessment

The onset of a hypomanic or manic episode may be gradual or dramatic. Affect is euphoric or elated, but can change quickly to irritability or hostility if the person is confronted with limits or is otherwise frustrated. The signs and symptoms range in severity from mild (in hypomania) to extreme (in a frank manic episode).

Subjective Data

Clients who experience mania have changes in their thought processes, sometimes stating that their "thoughts are racing." They often experience inflated self-esteem, sometimes to the extent of having delusions of grandeur. Delusions of persecution also may be a feature. They ignore fatigue and hunger, being too involved in activity to focus on physiological sensations. Suffering from an inability to concentrate, they are easily distracted by the slightest stimulus in the environment. They may experience hallucinations. Hypomanic individuals and those early in manic episodes feel wonderful and do not understand why people are upset with their behavior. See Box 17-3 for all the main symptoms seen in mania.

Objective Data

Clients who are experiencing mania for the first time are most likely to be young people in their twenties, although adolescents are sometimes affected. Although bipolar disorder appears to have little gender specificity, the initial episode is likely to be manic in males and depressive in females (APA, 2000). To date, there is no documented evidence of the effect of race or ethnicity on bipolar disorder.

The hallmark of mania is constant motor activity. During a manic episode, clients will not stop to eat. They do not rest, have disordered sleep patterns, and may go for days without sleep. Bruises and other injuries sometimes result from the constantly agitated behavior.

Box 17-3 Mania Symptoms—DIGFAST

Distractable
Insomnia
Grandiose
Flight of ideas
Agitation
Speech
Thoughtlessness (impulsivity)

Flight of ideas is manifested in the manic communications, and pressured speech is an obvious symptom. Family members often report that they exhibit poor judgment, such as going on spending sprees and committing sexual and other indiscretions that are completely out of character with their usual behavior. Appearance may be unusual, such as inappropriate dress and garish makeup or being disheveled and unkempt. Just as they fail to settle down long enough to eat and sleep, they also neglect bathing. In time, the absence of personal hygiene alienates them from other people.

Impairment in occupational functioning may result in work layoff or being placed on a leave of absence because the behavior is disruptive in the workplace. People who have mania cause interpersonal chaos with their manipulative behavior, testing of limits, and playing off one person against another. If their manipulation attempts fail, they become irritable or hostile, and such behavior further alienates others. The movie *Michael Clayton* depicts a bipolar character and the occupational sequelae in Mental Health in the Movies.

There are no laboratory findings specific for the diagnosis of mania. Abnormal biologic findings were discussed earlier in this chapter in Your Assessment Approach. Individuals experiencing manic episodes have been noted to have abnormal cortisol levels as well as abnormalities in neurotransmitter systems, but it is not known whether these abnormalities are a cause of or result from the disorder.

Clients who have mania are not usually able to cooperate fully in the assessment process. In many cases, you will find it necessary to rely on your own assessment skills and secondary sources, such as family members, to obtain essential assessment data. Family members can often provide detailed information about the onset and progression of symptoms, as well as information about previous episodes, if any.

Nursing Diagnosis: NANDA

Several nursing diagnoses are common in the care of clients who have mania.

Risk for Injury

Individuals with mania are at risk for injury because their usual adaptive and defensive abilities are impaired. Because of their hyperactivity and agitation, they often lose control of their movements and bump into objects, fall, and otherwise injure themselves.

Their impulsivity, poor judgment, and propensity toward hostile outbursts also place them at risk for injury. Other clients are often extremely annoyed by inappropriate or unacceptable social behavior and may attack clients who are manic. As with self-directed violence, preventing injury becomes the nursing priority.

Disturbed Thought Processes

Clients with mania experience disruption of their usual cognitive processes. This may be related to a variety of factors, including the following:

- Biochemical alteration
- Genetic predisposition
- Sleep deprivation
- A severe blow to self-esteem
- Massive denial of depression

Evidence of altered thought processes is seen in clients who cannot concentrate, have short attention spans, are easily distracted, and have impaired problem-solving abilities. They exhibit unwarranted optimism and poor judgment due to inaccurate interpretations of the environment. Delusional belief systems held by clients indicate a severe impairment of thought processes, as do hallucinations. Pressured speech, tangentiality, and flight of ideas are ample evidence of disrupted cognitive operations.

Impaired Social Interaction

Unlike depressed clients who may isolate themselves and avoid social interaction, most clients with mania are extremely gregarious and excessively social. But their social interactions are highly dysfunctional. Manipulating other people to meet

---

MENTAL HEALTH IN THE MOVIES
Michael Clayton

Michael Clayton is a movie about an attorney, Michael Clayton (played by George Clooney), who fixes problems in law firms caused by the idiosyncratic behaviors of various attorneys. Crimes, sexual misconduct and ethics issues, along with behaviors related to mental disorders, are his usual assignments. One of the attorneys he is asked to extract from an embarrassing situation is a brilliant man who happens to have bipolar disorder. Arthur Edens (played by Tom Wilkinson), has had a bizarre outburst in the middle of a deposition in a class action lawsuit against a conglomerate. Michael arrives to fix the situation for his good friend and colleague. He convinces the authorities to let Arthur out of jail and brings him back to their hotel where he is successfully sedated. However, Arthur escapes from the hotel in the middle of the night.

The general counsel for the conglomerate obtains Arthur's briefcase and discovers that Arthur has documentation detailing the conglomerate's decision to manufacture a chemical they know to be carcinogenic. Public knowledge of this decision would severely disrupt the finances of the conglomerate. In addition, the general counsel knows about Arthur's bipolar disorder, his failure to take his medications, and his outbursts. They follow Arthur, tap his phone, and bug his apartment. The conglomerate's general counsel has Arthur assassinated in a manner designed to resemble suicide, a common occurrence with people who are bipolar and unmedicated.

Michael, saddened by his friend and colleague's death, is suspicious about the circumstances. He cannot reconcile his friend's beliefs and energies with suicidal intent. Because he searches for and finds Arthur's evidence and plans to publicize it, he is also targeted for assassination. However, the attempt is botched. The movie resolves with Michael recording the general counsel's admission of murder and attempted murder.

Photo courtesy of CAP/FB Supplied by Capital Pictures/Newscom.

their own wishes and needs is a major impediment to positive social interactions. Egocentrism, impulsiveness, lack of interest in the needs and concerns of others, and an unwillingness to accept responsibility for the effect of their behavior on others all make clients with mania difficult to tolerate. Poor personal hygiene aggravates the situation.

Nurses often have difficulty dealing with the challenging and unreasonable behavior of clients with mania. Your Self-Awareness will help you determine how you may be affected by these behaviors.

Self-Care Deficit

Clients experiencing a manic episode have an impaired ability to perform the self-care activities of feeding, bathing, toileting, dressing, and grooming. This is related to hyperactivity, the inability to make accurate judgments about personal needs, alterations in thought processes, lack of awareness of personal needs, and fatigue. Self-care deficit is evidenced by inadequate food and fluid intake, an inability or refusal to bathe, a lack of interest in grooming and appropriateness of appearance, and an inability or unwillingness to toilet without assistance.

Sleep Deprivation

The sleep pattern of clients in a manic episode is so disrupted that exhaustion and even death can result. Disrupted sleep is related to hyperactivity, agitation, and possibly to biochemical

alterations. Sleep pattern disturbance includes the inability to fall asleep, roaming or pacing the halls during the night, awakening frequently during the night, and sleeping only for short naps with long periods of hyperactive, restless behavior in between.

Outcome Identification: NOC

Outcomes for mood disorders include the expectation of a return to premorbid functioning. Suggested outcomes for each NANDA diagnosis presented in the previous section are discussed in this section.

Risk for Injury

NOC outcomes appropriate for the client with mania include Risk Control: Actions to reduce or eliminate actual, potential, and modifiable health threats; and Safety Behavior: Fall prevention: Individual or caregiver actions to minimize risk factors that might precipitate falls.

Disturbed Thought Processes

Outcomes that address the client's altered thought processes include Cognitive Orientation: Ability to identify person, place, and time; Concentration: Ability to focus on a specific stimulus; Decision Making: Ability to choose between two or more alternatives; and Distorted Thought Control: Ability to self-restrain disruptions in perception, thought processes, and thought content.

Impaired Social Interaction

Nursing outcomes relevant to the client's impaired social interaction include Social Interaction Skills: An individual's use of effective interaction behaviors; and Social Involvement: Frequency of an individual's social interactions with persons, groups, or organizations.

Self-Care Deficit

Clients' self-care deficits are addressed in the outcomes related to Self-Care: Feeding, bathing, toileting, dressing, and grooming. Some or all of these outcomes may be appropriate for a particular client.

Sleep Deprivation

Outcomes that address the client's tendency to physical and mental exhaustion include Rest: Extent and pattern of diminished activity for mental and physical rejuvenation; and Sleep: Extent and pattern of sleep for mental and physical rejuvenation.

Planning and Implementation: NIC

With clients who are manic, your demeanor should be calm and relaxed but firm and matter of fact, particularly when communicating limits. Your own behavior serves as a model and is reassuring to out-of-control clients. As with all clients, building a trusting relationship is important. Therefore, make promises only when you are certain you can keep them.

Promoting Client Safety

Taking steps to ensure the safety of clients and others in the environment is a priority.

Providing a Safe Environment Provide a safe environment for clients in a manic episode by reducing environmental stimuli. For inpatients, this means providing a simply furnished private room that has had all unnecessary items removed. It should be in a quiet location to reduce noise stimulation. Low lighting can also be calming to the hyperactive client. Some hospitals have "quiet units." From there, clients can be transferred to milieu units when they are better able to deal with the distractions of community living.

Because clients experiencing mania have difficulty interacting appropriately with others, their participation in group activities should be limited until they are less agitated. Group settings tend to overstimulate these clients, and their behavior may antagonize others.

Smoking materials are particularly hazardous in the hands of agitated clients. They may burn themselves or leave burning cigarettes lying around when they become distracted by other stimuli. While not an issue in most institutions, allow the client who is experiencing mania to smoke only under supervision.

Monitoring Activities Scheduling a program of appropriate activity, interspersed with rest periods, helps provide an outlet for tension while protecting clients from exhaustion. Appropriate activities include walks, exercising or dancing with the supervision of an activity therapist, and supervised vacuuming or sweeping chores. Avoid highly competitive activities that bring out hostility and overtly aggressive behaviors.

Setting and Enforcing Limits Set and enforce limits on unsafe or socially inappropriate behavior when clients are unable to control their impulses. Matter-of-fact intervention rather than angry scolding is the most effective approach.

Clients may respond to verbal reminders, or you can use their distractibility to redirect them into safer and more appropriate activities. Remember to reward appropriate behavior with positive reinforcement such as, "I enjoyed our walk today because you were able to walk with me rather than running ahead." See Evidence-Based Practice for more information on setting limits and other interventions, and Your Intervention Strategies for options in communicating limits.

Administering Medications

Mood stabilizers form the basis of medication treatment for bipolar disorders. Lithium is still the optimum choice, with antiepileptic drugs (AEDs) that have mood stabilizing features chosen according to their effectiveness in addressing specific symptoms. Antipsychotic medications also contribute to helping clients think more clearly and help manage psychotic thinking (grandiose delusions).

Nursing interventions include monitoring clients for adverse side effects of mood stabilizing and antipsychotic medications. Side effects include sedation, agitation, postural hypotension, dizziness, dry mouth, and blurry vision (see Chapter 31∞).

Lithium Carbonate Lithium carbonate has been used in the treatment and prevention of acute manic episodes since the 1960s. It is now used in preventing the recurrence of bipolar disorder as well. Toxic symptoms begin appearing at blood levels above 1.5 mEq/L. Because there is such a narrow margin of safety, serum concentrations must be closely monitored until stabilized. The need for close monitoring means that clients are often hospitalized when lithium therapy

---

EVIDENCE-BASED PRACTICE

MANIA AND SUBSTANCE ABUSE

Brent is a large, muscular 22-year-old man diagnosed with bipolar disorder 2 years ago. He was admitted to the crisis unit in your community after his parents called the police. He stopped taking lithium last month and had been up and screaming for 3 days and nights. Today he shouted obscenities at his mother, pushed his father to the floor, and broke the windows of neighbors' cars parked along the street as he ran from his home. Brent's parents also reported that he abuses a variety of substances, although they did not know specifics.

Within an hour of his arrival on the unit, he began breaking light fixtures in the hall and in other clients' rooms with a broom he found in a closet. Other clients were visibly distressed and frightened by his behavior. Your plan for intervention options for the immediate situation and Brent's long-term care are based on current research results. For example, in your review of studies of psychosocial approaches for improving treatment adherence in people with bipolar disorder who are substance abusers, you

consider the possibility that Brent will more quickly and effectively gain self-control of his behavior if you work with him on specific techniques in private. Decreasing stimulation and setting limits on his free activity both contribute to Brent being able to focus. Less stimuli and brief interactions allow a therapeutic relationship to develop. Once Brent is more stable, psychoeducation about his diagnosis and treatment can proceed. The success rate of treatment for his disorder can be discussed at that time. Involving his family would be an integral part of this approach.

You should base your action on more than one study, but the following research was helpful in developing this set of multiple intervention strategies:

Gaudiano, B. A., Weinstock, L. M., & Miller, I. W. (2011). Improving treatment adherence in patients with bipolar disorder and substance abuse: Rationale and initial development of a novel psychosocial approach. *Journal of Psychiatric Practice, 17,* 5–20.

CRITICAL THINKING QUESTIONS

1. What elements would you take into consideration when planning to interact with Brent?
2. How can Brent and his family benefit from psychoeducation?
3. What topics would be considered priorities for this family?

YOUR INTERVENTION STRATEGIES Setting and Enforcing Limits

Effective limit setting requires that all members of the mental health team participate in establishing limits and determining and enforcing the consequences of exceeding them.

1. Establish limits only when and where there is a clear need. Limits must help client growth.
2. Establish reasonable and enforceable consequences for exceeding limits.
3. Explain the limits and consequences to clients in language they can understand. Explain why the limits are necessary, and allow clients to express their feelings about them.
4. Enforce the limits consistently. Written care plans help ensure consistency.
5. Evaluate the continued need for limits frequently. Turn control over to clients as soon as the client's behavior indicates the ability to exercise self-control.
6. Keep the client's dignity in mind at all times. Limit setting is not a punishment but a part of therapy.

is initiated. Before discharge, both clients and families must learn how to continue lithium therapy safely at home. Look at Chapter 31∞ for nursing considerations for clients on lithium carbonate.

Anticonvulsant Drugs (AED) as Mood Stabilizers Agents used in therapy for those with bipolar disorder include the anticonvulsants or AED medications. Individuals may have good responses to any of the mood-stabilizing AEDs; however, lamotrigine (Lamictal) or topamirate (Topamax) are generally better for depressive symptoms of bipolar disorder, while valproic acid (Depakote) or oxcarbazepine (Trileptal) are effective for mania. These medications cannot be discontinued abruptly because this may precipitate a seizure. Additional information about the pharmacotherapy of mood disorders is found in Chapter 7∞ and the practical issues of psychopharmacology are found in Chapter 31∞.

Antipsychotic Medications For many years haloperidol (Haldol) has been added to lithium as part of the treatment of bipolar disorder. Psychotic symptoms, such as grandiose delusions, usually respond fairly rapidly to antipsychotic medications. Hyperactive and agitated behavior also can be managed well with these medications. The atypical antipsychotics such as risperidone (Risperdal) and olanzapine (Zyprexa) have proven effective as mood-stabilizing medications, are often given in conjunction with anticonvulsive mood stabilizers. Atypical antipsychotics are used to help manage the symptoms of mania when individuals have started on lithium carbonate therapy, because lithium takes 1 to 3 weeks to become effective.

Intervening With Delusions and Hallucinations

Present reality by spending time with clients. Identify yourself, the time and day, location, and other orienting information as needed. Engage clients in reality-based, somewhat concrete activities, such as discussing a current event. Consistency is reassuring to clients with altered thought processes. Establish consistency by having a schedule so clients understand what is expected of them. Consistency is also enhanced by assigning the same caregivers to work with the client whenever possible.

When dealing with delusional or hallucinating clients, communicate your acceptance of their need for false beliefs, while clearly stating that you do not share their perceptions. A statement such as, "I understand that you believe you are the owner of this facility, but I see it differently," conveys acceptance without supporting delusional thinking.

It is nontherapeutic to argue or try to reason with delusional clients. This often serves to harden the belief system and can impair the development of trust. Instead, use statements such as, "I find that hard to believe" or "That is extremely unusual," to instill reasonable doubt as a therapeutic intervention.

When clients communicate altered reality perceptions, reflect their statements back to them for validation. For example, "Are you saying that your husband is trying to poison you with monosodium glutamate?" can help a client understand how her perceptions sound to others. You will recognize that clients are becoming less delusional when they make statements such as, "I know this sounds bizarre, but. . . ." Remember to give positive reinforcement when clients begin to focus on reality.

Enhancing Socialization

Nursing activities are designed to facilitate the client's ability to interact with others by identifying specific needed behavior changes and assigning tasks that will improve the client's interactions with others. This may require mediating between the client and others when the client exhibits negative behavior. Nursing actions should encourage and demonstrate honesty and respect for others' rights.

A maladaptive behavior of clients who are manic that significantly impairs social interactions is manipulation, an indirect way of getting their needs met. This may take a simple form, such as borrowing money from other clients rather than using their own. Or it may be highly complex, such as pitting staff members against one another, as in Rx Communication, by giving them false information about each other.

Manipulation meets a need for the client. It serves the purpose of increasing a client's sense of control and interpersonal power (the mania can be frightening as it spins out of control). Nursing interventions, such as setting limits, promote client security and often enable clients to curb their manipulative behavior or give it up entirely. Be aware of your own control needs, and provide opportunities for clients to be in control when appropriate.

℞ COMMUNICATION

Client With Bipolar Disorder

CLIENT: "I can't go to community group today! I'm expecting some top-level government officials to visit. The other nurse told me I didn't have to go."

NURSE RESPONSE 1: "I understand, Francis, but it is time for community group now and we expect everyone to attend. Let's walk over together." *RATIONALE:* This response acknowledges his need for the false belief without reinforcing or arguing with it. This response also maintains a consistent, routine schedule wherein this delusional client can feel safe, clearly articulates what is expected of the client, and offers self.	**NURSE RESPONSE 2:** "All clients and staff members attend these meetings, Francis. You made some constructive comments last week. Let's go so we can get a good seat." *RATIONALE:* This response sets limits on manipulative behavior. Matter-of-fact enforcement of rules and expectations without allowing the client to involve you in a dispute with another staff member defuses the manipulative behavior and provides positive reinforcement of adaptive behavior.

Setting Limits on Manipulative and Out-of-Control Behavior Out-of-control and manipulative behaviors require setting limits. All staff members must agree upon the established limits and must enforce them consistently. Violations of limits must have established consequences, also agreed upon by all staff. Clients must know what behaviors are expected and what consequences will result if they exceed limits. Inconsistent application of consequences will cause failure in the efforts to decrease manipulative behavior.

You can expect clients to give charming explanations of why they had to exceed this or that limit, but do not be disarmed by these explanations. They are another form of manipulative behavior. Matter-of-fact limit enforcement and the consistent application of consequences are essential in promoting adaptive behaviors. Your Intervention Strategies provides an overview of how to effectively set and enforce limits. (See also Chapter 22∞.)

Monitoring Intake and Output and Promoting Nutrition

Well-being is compromised when clients do not receive sufficient nourishment and fluids for extended periods of time, particularly during periods of hyperactivity. Monitoring intake and output is an important nursing activity. Frequent small snacks that can be eaten "on the go" are most likely to be consumed by the hyperactive client who is unable to sit down to eat. Work with a dietitian to ensure that high-calorie finger foods and nutritious liquids are available on the nursing unit until the client is able to attend regular meals.

Promoting Improved Self-Care

A minimal level of personal hygiene is needed to ensure health, self-esteem, and healthy social interactions. Assist hyperactive clients who are unwilling or unable to bathe, brush their teeth, shave, wash their hair, change clothes, or use the toilet. Autonomy is desirable, so allow clients to do as much for themselves as possible with verbal encouragement. Reinforce any attempts at self-care with recognition, for example, "I see you shaved today, Mr. Adams."

Incontinence of urine or feces is occasionally seen in severely regressed clients during mania. This can be very disturbing to other clients and staff and insults the dignity of the client who is experiencing incontinence. Nursing activities include establishing a schedule of frequent, regular toileting. Accompany the client to the bathroom every hour or half hour until "accidents" no longer occur.

A more common elimination problem is constipation. Hyperactive clients suppress the urge to defecate and may become severely constipated. The anticholinergic effect of some medications may also exacerbate constipation. Frequent fluid intake and a high-fiber diet can reduce constipation.

Enhancing Rest and Sleep

Clients in the manic phase of bipolar disorder appear deceptively energetic when they may actually be nearing the point of exhaustion. Design nursing activities to facilitate regular sleep–wake cycles. Monitor clients closely for signs of fatigue, and make provisions for rest periods. Promote nighttime sleeping by limiting extended daytime naps. Sleep may promote the rapid resolution of first episodes of mania. Prior to bedtime, decrease light and noise and encourage quiet activities and presleep routines, such as listening to soothing music. A warm bath and snack may aid relaxation, as may a backrub. Administer medications that do not suppress REM sleep, such as zolpidem tartrate (Ambien) as prescribed.

If clients experience extended nighttime wakefulness, avoid engaging them in long conversations or otherwise stimulating or giving extra attention during the night. Firmly encourage clients to stay in their darkened rooms with the expectation that they will fall asleep. If they will not stay in their rooms, assign a monotonous, repetitive task, such as folding towels or sorting papers to encourage drowsiness. When clients are able to sleep, avoid waking them for nonessential care or activities. Allow for sleep cycles of at least 90 minutes.

Evaluation

Specific client behaviors indicate that nursing interventions have been successful. Evaluation and outcome criteria answer the question, "How do we know that the client's condition has improved?"

Risk for Injury

If nursing interventions have been successful in promoting safety, clients will be free of accidental injuries. They will not engage in agitated or impulsive behaviors that can endanger them. Their social behaviors will no longer irritate or enrage other people, so they will no longer risk attacks from others. Clients will be able to enumerate safe ways of relieving excess tension when it occurs, such as verbal expression of feelings, writing feelings down in a diary or journal, or other adaptive methods. Clients will name their medications, understand the proper dosages, describe adverse effects, and explain lab monitoring needed, if any.

Cognitive Orientation and Reality-Based Thinking

Clients who base their thinking on reality will be oriented to time, place, and person. They will no longer experience delusional thinking or hallucinations. They will be able to establish trust relationships. Their attention spans will increase. Their speech will be less pressured and will reflect diminished flight of ideas and tangentiality. Clients will recognize and verbalize errors in perception when they occur. Their thought processes and perceptions of environmental stimuli will be accurate and can be validated by others. They will demonstrate logical, organized thought processes.

Social Interaction Skills

Improvements in social interaction skills will be demonstrated when clients can recognize and describe which of their interactions is successful and which is unsuccessful, and acknowledge the effect of their own behavior on social interactions. They demonstrate behaviors that may increase or improve social interactions. Clients put significant effort into treatment in order to prevent relapse, and having more appropriate social contacts and interactions is an enduring signal of emotional health (Delmas, Proudfoot, Parker, & Manicavasagar, 2011). Clients acquire or improve skills such as cooperation, sensitivity, genuineness, and compromise. The absence of, or dramatic decrease in, the use of manipulation as a method of meeting their own needs also will signal improvement in social interaction. They now accept responsibility for their own behavior.

Other signs of improved social interaction include nondisruptive participation in activities, re-establishment of a social life, and identification of individuals with whom they can develop a social and support network.

Intake, Output, and Nutrition

Clients will demonstrate the ability to establish and main adequate nutrition and fluid intake.

Self-Care

Clients who have re-established self-care will demonstrate this ability by performing the activities of daily living autonomously and willingly. This includes adequately bathing and grooming themselves, selecting appropriate clothing and makeup, establishing and maintaining adequate nutrition and fluid intake, and establishing and maintaining patterns of elimination without reminders or assistance.

Rest and Sleep

The need for uninterrupted sleep varies from person to person depending on age, activity level, and usual pattern of sleep. Generally, clients who are able to sleep 6 or more hours per night without sleeping medication and awaken feeling refreshed will have demonstrated healthy sleep patterns. Being able to fall asleep within 30 minutes or less is another indicator. Recognizing fatigue and voluntarily resting or napping appropriately also indicates that clients are attending to their bodily sensations once again.

CASE MANAGEMENT, COMMUNITY-BASED CARE, AND HOME CARE

Case management and community-based care for clients with depressed phase bipolar disorders were described earlier in the nursing process section discussing the care of depressed clients. Clients in the manic phase of bipolar disorders, however, often require hospitalization until stabilized on medication or through ECT.

Following discharge, goals for clients who have mania are the same as for others—high-quality, cost-effective treatment aimed at returning the client to full functioning as soon as feasible. Communication with family members, mental health professionals, employers, social workers, and others involved in the client's case is essential.

Monitoring the client's lithium level is an important aspect of the community-based nurse's role for the treatment of mania. Additional client and family teaching are often required to reinforce the information they received in the inpatient setting. ECT is increasingly used as an outpatient procedure, again calling on the community- and home-based nurse's teaching skills and sensitivity to concerns about safety, memory loss, and effectiveness.

Nurses in case management, community settings, and home care must be alert for "red flags" that signal exacerbation of the client's manic symptoms. These include nonadherence with treatment, including refusal to take medications as ordered, escalating activity level that may include psychomotor excitement/agitation, spending sprees, shortened attention span, impaired occupational functioning, and grandiosity. Early recognition of red flags and mobilization of the treatment team can ward off rehospitalization and enable the client to stay at home while being treated and maintained in a community setting. Be sure that family members are also aware of behaviors that signal exacerbation of the client's symptoms.

Clients and their family members will find help from Continuing Medical Education http://www.cmellc.com/topics/bdfaq.html). A self-help resource for bipolar disorder and other mood disorders can be located at http://www.mentalhealthrecovery.com. Both websites can be accessed through the Online Student Resources for this book.

NURSING CARE PLAN: CLIENT WITH DEPRESSION

Identifying Information

Margaret M. is a 59-year-old, unmarried legal assistant who was admitted to the psychiatric unit following a gastric lavage in the emergency department. She had ingested 30 antidepressant tablets in a suicide attempt. Margaret stated that she had been home alone for 2 days, became increasingly depressed and hopeless, and took the antidepressants that her family doctor had prescribed for depression a few weeks ago. She became frightened almost immediately thereafter, was unable to make herself vomit, and called 911. Margaret stated, "I just don't have anything to look forward to anymore. No one would care if I died."

History

Margaret is the eldest of seven children from a small rural community. She had to leave school after the seventh grade to stay home and help with the younger children. At the age of 22, she returned to school and became a legal assistant. She moved to a large city over 100 miles from her home and built her life around her work. She never married. Because she works long hours in a large metropolitan law firm, she has virtually no social life and, except for a few coworkers, no friends. She stopped going to church recently, stating, "I just don't fit in anywhere and I never have."

Margaret reports that she has been concerned about her impending retirement at age 65 and her elderly mother's declining health. About a month ago, the health of her 86-year-old mother, who still lives in their small town, began to deteriorate. Margaret now fears that she will have to go care for her mother, with whom she has never gotten along. Her siblings are pressuring her to move back home, live with their mother, and serve as her caregiver. She fears that because she has no family of her own and no family ties in the city, she will eventually have to give in to their pressure.

She has no prior psychiatric history and no significant health problems. Vital signs are: temperature, 98.4°F; pulse, 88; respirations, 18; height, 5'3"; weight 157 pounds; blood pressure, 138/78.

Current Mental Status

Margaret is somewhat disheveled and weeps occasionally during the interview. She is cooperative with the interviewer, even eager to talk. She reports being "exhausted" for the past 3 weeks. She has not slept well, has lost weight, had crying spells, has been irritable with coworkers, and had difficulty concentrating at work. She reports having had suicidal thoughts but did not have a specific plan until the weekend after the firm's senior partner told her to take a few days off to "get yourself together." She fears being fired, in which case she will have no reason to resist her siblings' pleas to "come take care of Mama."

Margaret is alert, responsive, and well oriented. There is no sign of a thought disorder, confusion, or impairment. She weeps as she discusses her situation, stating, "I have always been unattractive and nobody has ever loved me. If I died, all my family would lose is a nursemaid for Mama."

Other Clinical Data

Margaret reports being in good health, although she is somewhat overweight. She has mild arthritis in her knees, which she treats symptomatically with aspirin. Until she began taking antidepressants, she took no other medicine.

Nursing Diagnosis: Risk for Self-Directed Violence related to recent suicide attempt

Expected Outcome: Impulse Control: Ability to restrain compulsive or impulsive behavior
Suicide Self-Restraint: Ability to refrain from gestures and attempts at killing self

---

Short-Term Goals	Interventions	Rationales
Margaret will not harm herself during hospitalization.	■ Remove all dangerous articles from Margaret's environment.	Margaret's safety is ensured.
	■ Observe Margaret closely, using irregular schedule.	Irregular schedule prevents her from predicting when she will be alone.
	■ Adopt a neutral, matter-of-fact attitude.	A neutral attitude prevents client dependency.
	■ Evaluate suicidal intention at every shift and institute appropriate level of supervision.	Suicidal thoughts and impulses may change rapidly.
	■ Establish a no-suicide contract.	Nurse–client collaboration promotes self-responsibility.
	■ Encourage Margaret to seek nurse out when bothered by suicidal thoughts or impulses.	Margaret learns to substitute talking it out for acting it out.
	■ Limit repetitive discussion of suicidal ruminations.	Repetition reinforces preoccupation with self-directed violence.
Margaret will demonstrate alternative ways of dealing with stress, such as talking, exercise, and relaxation techniques.	■ Assist Margaret to verbalize at least one reason for living.	Identifying reasons for living counteracts negative thinking.
	■ Encourage the expression of feelings in one–to–one and group activities.	Self-expression decreases isolation and elicits peer support.
	■ Assist Margaret to identify and practice alternative ways of dealing with stress.	Margaret's coping behaviors are expanded.

NURSING CARE PLAN: CLIENT WITH DEPRESSION (*Continued*)

Short-Term Goals	Interventions	Rationales
Margaret will identify resources where she can seek help if suicidal thoughts recur following discharge, such as a crisis line, or a minister.	■ Help Margaret identify community resources and supports.	Margaret becomes more aware of social supports available to her.
Margaret will verbalize safe uses of antidepressant medication and describe potential drug/food interactions.	■ Teach Margaret safe use of antidepressant medication.	This is information every client should know.

Nursing Diagnosis: Self-Esteem Disturbance related to impaired cognition, fostering negative view of self

Expected Outcome: Self-Esteem: Personal judgment of self-worth

Short-Term Goals	Interventions	Rationales
Margaret will sit and walk erectly; comb hair neatly; wear clean, matching clothes.	■ Help Margaret with hygiene and grooming as needed.	Competent self-care increases feelings of self-worth.
Margaret will participate in unit activities.	■ Teach Margaret that activity helps decrease depression. ■ Involve Margaret in simple, noncompetitive recreational activities. ■ Increase the complexity of activities as Margaret progresses.	This is information all depressed clients should know. Cooperative recreation allows Margaret to experience success. Margaret's growth and self-regard are enhanced by appropriate challenges.
Margaret will verbalize positive aspects of self and increased feelings of self-worth.	■ Set limits on time spent reviewing past failures. ■ Help Margaret enumerate her own personal strengths.	Focusing on personal strengths counteracts negative self-view and increases self-worth.
Margaret will communicate assertively with others; will explain to siblings that she will not give up her career to come home to care for mother.	■ Teach Margaret assertiveness techniques. ■ Practice (role-play) Margaret's direct expression of feelings. ■ Stay with Margaret during difficult interactions, if desired. ■ Give positive recognition when progress is shown.	Learning assertiveness validates Margaret's right to take care of herself. Role-playing promotes confidence in asserting herself. Encouragement and recognition support healthy behaviors.

Nursing Diagnosis: Hopelessness related to inability to make and carry out decisions on her own behalf

Expected Outcome: Decision Making: Ability to choose between two or more alternatives
Hope: Presence of internal state of optimism that is personally satisfying and life supporting
Mood Equilibrium: Appropriate adjustment of prevailing emotional tone in response to circumstances
Quality of Life: Expresses satisfaction with current life circumstances

Short-Term Goals	Interventions	Rationales
Margaret will verbalize feelings about situations over which she has no control; will realize that siblings' expectations do not control her responses.	■ Assist Margaret to identify situations over which she has no control. ■ Assist Margaret to identify situations over which she can attain control.	A realistic appraisal of her situation allows Margaret to focus on areas in which she can effect change.

NURSING CARE PLAN: CLIENT WITH DEPRESSION (*Continued*)

Short-Term Goals	Interventions	Rationales
Margaret will set realistic goals for herself and work toward them.	■ Engage Margaret in goal setting for herself. ■ Provide options when possible.	Setting goals is a crucial step toward self-determination. Options help Margaret understand the concept of choice.
Margaret will demonstrate a problem-solving system that she has used successfully.	■ Explore problem-solving models with Margaret and encourage her to select one. ■ Practice problem-solving with small daily problems.	Information and practice help build Margaret's confidence.
Margaret will verbalize plans to attain control over life situations; works with siblings to find appropriate caretaker for mother.	■ Role-play possible situations with siblings. ■ Assist Margaret to prepare for siblings' potential untoward responses. ■ Assist Margaret to plan for retirement.	Role-playing increases Margaret's confidence and resourcefulness.
Magaret expresses some hope for the future.	■ Identify community resources that assist individuals toward fulfilling retirement (e.g., AARP). ■ Involve Margaret in identifying enjoyable leisure pastimes.	Planning for the future decreases fears of the unknown and introduces new sources of support. Positive use of leisure time is promoted.

Nursing Diagnosis: Social Isolation related to fear of rejection

Expected Outcome: Social Interaction Skills: Use of effective interaction behavior

Social Involvement: Social interactions with persons, groups, or organizations

Social Support: Perception of availability of reliable assistance from other persons

Short-Term Goals	Interventions	Rationales
Margaret will communicate with nursing staff and socialize with other clients on the unit.	■ Make brief, frequent contacts with Margaret. ■ Spend time with Margaret with no demands. ■ Use a nonjudgmental attitude. ■ Encourage Margaret to ventilate verbally or through activity.	Frequent contact demonstrates your availability and interest. A nonjudgmental approach demonstrates acceptance. Appropriate self-expression decreases internal tension and increases sociability.
Margaret voluntarily attends group activities.	■ Accompany Margaret to group activities initially, withdrawing as tolerated. ■ Teach social skills and assist Margaret to practice them.	Providing support as needed fosters gradual independence. Practice increases Margaret's self-confidence in social situations.
Margaret assumes responsibility for dealing with feelings, including seeking others out; identifies key individuals outside hospital and initiates contact to renew relationships; makes concrete plans to go to church again.	■ Teach assertive communication. ■ Encourage role-playing of phone calls, other contacts, anticipating others' possible responses. ■ Give positive feedback for all signs of progress.	Learning assertiveness helps Margaret take care of herself. Role-playing decreases social anxiety and builds resourcefulness and flexibility. Positive feedback validates Margaret's efforts and reinforces growth.

Pearson Nursing Student Resources
Find additional review materials at
nursing.pearsonhighered.com
Prepare for success with NCLEX®-style practice questions,
interactive assignments and activities, web links, animations
and videos, and more!

REFERENCES

Abdel-Hay, M., El-Sawy, H., & Badawy, A. (2011). Predictors of recurrence of bipolar disorder during pregnancy and postpartum periods in a sample of Egyptian women. *Middle East Current Psychiatry, 18*(1), 45–50.

American Psychiatric Association. (2000). *Diagnostic and statistical manual of mental disorders* (4th ed., Text Revision). Washington, DC: Author.

Beck, A. T., Steer, R. A., & Brown, G. K. (1996). *Manual for the Beck depression inventory-II.* San Antonio, TX: Psychological Corporation.

Buckner-Brown, J., Tucker, P., & Rivera, M. (2011). Racial and ethnic approaches to community health. *Family & Community Health, 34*(1S), S12–S22.

Clark, D. A., & Beck, A. T. (1999). *Scientific foundations of cognitive theory and therapy of depression.* New York, NY: John Wiley & Sons.

Delmas, K., Proudfoot, J., Parker, G., & Manicavasagar, V. (2011). Recoding past experiences: A qualitative study of how patients and family members adjust to the diagnosis of bipolar disorder. *Journal of Nervous and Mental Disorders, 199,* 136–139.

Gaudiano, B. A., Weinstock, L. M., & Miller, I. W. (2011). Improving treatment adherence in patients with bipolar disorder and substance abuse: Rationale and initial development of a novel psychosocial approach. *Journal of Psychiatric Practice, 17,* 5–20.

Joseph, A. (2006). *The impact of light on outcomes in healthcare settings.* Concord California Center for Health Design, Issue Paper #2.

Lazenby, R. B. (2011). Depression in the college population: An E-S-A approach to primary prevention. *Nurse Practitioner, 36*(2), 33–39.

Lin, K.-M., Chiu, Y.-F., Tsai, I.-J., Chen, C.-H., Shen, W. W., Liu, S. C., . . . Liu, Y.-L. (2011). *Pharmacogenetics and Genomics, 21,* 163–170.

Mark, T. L., Joish, V. N., Hay, J. W., Sheehan, D. V., Johnston, S. S., & Zbun Cao, M. A. (2011). Antidepressant use in geriatric populations: The burden of side effects and interactions and their impact on adherence and costs. *American Journal of Geriatric Psychiatry, 19*(3), 211–221.

McCoy, S. J. B. (2011). Postpartum depression: An essential overview for the practitioner. *Southern Medical Journal, 104*(2), 128–132.

O'Baire-Kark, M., & Klevay, A. (2011). Another perspective on finger replantation surgery: Nursing support for the psychological levels of recovery. *Journal of Trauma Nursing, 18*(1), 34–42.

Scherrer, J. F., Garfield, L. D., Lustman, P, J., Hauptman, P. J., Chrusciel, T., Zeringue, A., . . . True, W. R. (2011). Antidepressant drug compliance: Reduced risk of MI and mortality in depressed patients. *American Journal of Medicine, 124*(4), 318–324.

Sheehan, D. V., Harnett-Sheehan, K., Spann, M. E., Thompson, H. F., & Prakash, A. (2011). Assessing remission in major depressive disorder and generalized anxiety disorder clinical trials with the Discan Metric of the Sheehan Disability Scale. *International Clinical Psychopharmacology, 26,* 75–83.

Teutsch, S. M., Bradley, L. A., Palomaki, G. E., Haddow, J. E., Piper, M., Calonge, N., . . . Berg, A. O. (2009). The Evaluation of Genomic Applications in Practice and Prevention (EGAPP) Initiative: Methods of the EGAPP Working Group. *Genetic Medicine, 11*(1), 3–14.

18

Anxiety Disorders

SUE C. DELAUNE

LEARNING OUTCOMES

After completing this chapter, you will be able to:

1. Discuss the theories that are helpful in understanding anxiety disorders.
2. Explain how the concept of anxiety relates to anxiety disorders.
3. Incorporate a knowledge of the common themes and distinctive characteristics of anxiety disorders into the care of clients with anxiety disorders.
4. Conduct a thorough and comprehensive assessment in the care of clients with anxiety disorders.
5. Design a plan of care for intervening into mild, moderate, severe, and panic levels of anxiety.
6. Educate clients and their families about pharmacologic and nonpharmacologic measures for anxiety disorders.
7. Analyze personal feelings and possible challenges in caring for clients with anxiety disorders.

CRITICAL THINKING CHALLENGE

JoAnn, a 35-year-old single parent of two small children and the owner of a beauty salon, went to the emergency department stating, "I can't breathe! Help me! I feel like I'm smothering and going to die." JoAnn has been treated for similar symptoms in this emergency department three times over the past year. You, the RN, overhear another staff member say that JoAnn is a "frequent flyer who is making up her symptoms. She just wants attention."

1. Do you think this staff member's comments are valid? Why, or why not?
2. How do you respond to the staff member?
3. Why is it important that a complete physical assessment be done on JoAnn, even if health care providers believe her symptoms are of psychogenic origin?

Although anxiety is a universal experience, people vary in their ability to tolerate anxiety and anxiety-producing situations. Anxiety, a subjective feeling experienced in response to stressors, is a normal response that usually helps people cope with threatening situations. There are four levels of anxiety: mild, moderate, severe, and panic. Mild anxiety serves as a catalyst for change and is an ideal time for learning to occur. In the moderate level of anxiety, the perceptual field is narrowed and the individual is able to attend to selected stimuli. People experiencing the severe and panic levels of anxiety have varying levels of functional impairments. It is essential that a person experiencing the panic level be closely monitored for safety reasons. Common coping behaviors of individuals experiencing anxiety include withdrawal, acting out, avoidance, somatization, and problem solving. See Chapter 8∞ for a thorough discussion of the levels of anxiety and effects of anxiety on individuals.

This chapter examines the experience of individuals with anxiety disorders. People with these disorders have one thing in common: anxiety so disabling that their functioning is adversely affected. The functional disabilities they have may affect all dimensions of life, including physical, emotional, cognitive, sociocultural, and spiritual, as well as social, work, and family relationships (see Figure 18-1 ■).

Anxiety disorders are the most common of all mental illnesses. According to the National Institute of Mental Health (NIMH), there is a 28.8% lifetime prevalence of anxiety disorders (see Box 18-1) in the U.S. adult population (NIMH, 2010). You will encounter clients with anxiety disorders in every clinical practice setting including primary care and general hospital settings, not just mental health facilities, and in your own community. Anxiety disorders affect people of every socioeconomic status. It is also relatively common for a person to have one anxiety disorder coexist with another. Anxiety disorders can also coexist with other mental disorders, such as depression. You can readily apply what you learn about anxiety disorders in this chapter to any area in which you choose to work.

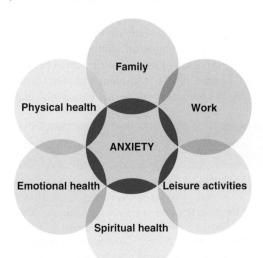

FIGURE 18-1 ■ The holistic impact of anxiety.

Box 18-1 Anxiety Disorder

Prevalence of Anxiety Disorders in U.S. Adult Population

Acute stress disorder	No long-term statistics available
Agoraphobia	0.8%
Generalized anxiety disorder	3.1%
Obsessive–compulsive disorder	1%
Panic disorder	2.7%
Post-traumatic stress disorder	3.5%
Specific phobia	8.7%
Social phobia	6.8%

Note: Percentages and numbers refer to the estimated incidence of occurrences in American adults within a given year.

Source: National Institute of Mental Health. (2010). Statistics. Retrieved from http://www.nimh.nih.gov/statictics/index.shtml

ANXIETY DISORDERS

Anxiety disorders are characterized by a mixture of physiological, psychological, behavioral, and cognitive symptoms. Anxiety disorders affect individuals across the entire lifespan. Even though each anxiety disorder has its own distinct characteristics, they all have the common theme of excessive, irrational fear and dread. Worry is a major component of anxiety disorders.

In anxiety disorders, anxiety is either the predominant disturbance (as in generalized anxiety disorder) or anxiety is experienced as avoidance behavior when the person attempts to master the symptoms (as in confronting the dreaded object or situation in a phobic disorder). When anxiety is not related to a specific stimulus, it may be called **free-floating anxiety**.

People in anxiety states experience anxiety both as a subjective emotion and as a variety of physical symptoms resulting from muscular tension and autonomic nervous system activity. When acute, the anxiety drives the individual to seek help. When chronic, anxiety can lead to a number of somatic discomforts or disabilities (e.g., heartburn, epigastric distress, diarrhea, and constipation). Chronic muscular tension can lead to a variety of musculoskeletal aches and pains.

The onset of anxiety may be sudden or gradual. Some people experience an unexpected, incapacitating outbreak of acute anxiety, as in panic disorder. In other people (especially those with generalized anxiety disorder), anxiety may express itself through relatively mild somatic symptoms in which the existence of underlying anxiety is overlooked. Therefore, it is necessary to specifically assess the client's level of anxiety. There are several types of anxiety disorders. They are discussed in the following sections and their essential diagnostic criteria are presented in DSM Essential Features.

Panic Disorder

A common disorder, **panic disorder**, is characterized by recurrent attacks of severe anxiety lasting a few moments to an hour. These attacks are not a response to a specific stimulus but

DSM ESSENTIAL FEATURES

Anxiety Disorders

Acute Stress Disorder: Dissociative symptoms that include numbing, detachment, and amnesia. Anxiety symptoms including exaggerated startle response, motor restlessness, and ANS hyperarousal. The symptoms occur within 1 month after exposure to an extreme traumatic stressor.

Agoraphobia: Intense fear and avoidance of any situation in which escape might be difficult or help is unavailable.

Generalized Anxiety Disorder (GAD): Persistent, pervasive, and exaggerated sense of worry and anxiety.

Obsessive–Compulsive Disorder (OCD): A combination of intrusive, irrational thoughts and stereotypical behavioral rituals performed to dispel the unwanted thoughts that cause the person marked distress. The thoughts, impulses, and ritualized behaviors are recurrent and persistent.

Panic Disorder: Recurrent and unexpected feelings of extreme fear that occur for no apparent reason and are accompanied by intense physical symptoms or cognitive symptoms. Fears of losing control, having a heart attack, or dying are common.

Post-Traumatic Stress Disorder (PTSD): A reaction to, and re-experiencing of, a traumatic event that involved intense fear, helplessness, or horror. The person has persistent symptoms of avoidance/numbing and hyperarousal.

Social Phobia: Fear of extreme embarrassment of social or performance situations. The fear is persistent and the feared situation is avoided when possible or is endured with marked anxiety upon exposure to the feared situation. The individual recognizes the unreasonable nature of the fear.

Specific Phobia: Marked and persistent fear of an object or situation combined with the compulsion to avoid the feared object or situation. The individual recognizes the unreasonable nature of the fear.

---

instead seem to occur suddenly and spontaneously. They may, however, become associated with certain situations, such as going to a shopping mall or driving a car. The person usually experiences physical symptoms such as palpitations, nausea, diarrhea, dyspnea, rapid pulse, and a feeling of choking or suffocation. The pupils are dilated, and the face is flushed. The person may feel dizzy or faint and often has a sense of impending doom or death. Restlessness is acute, and the person may make pleading, apprehensive appeals for help. Mental Health in the Movies describes, in amusing terms, one person's plea for help.

In its most advanced state, panic may create a group of symptoms that mimic myocardial infarction and mitral valve prolapse. Thus, the diagnosis of panic disorder is often not made until expensive medical procedures fail to provide a correct diagnosis. The following clinical example describes Loretta, who is experiencing a panic disorder.

Clinical Example

Loretta has been to her primary care physician on two different occasions convinced that she was having a heart attack. Both times, she was told that she was healthy. However, Loretta continued to experience palpitations, rapid pulse, and dizziness. Fearful that she would be labeled a hypochondriac, Loretta was reluctant to visit her physician again.

When panic attacks occur frequently and interfere with the person's functional abilities at work, school, or in the family, the condition is called *panic disorder*. People who have repeated attacks, or persistently worry about having another attack, are diagnosed with panic disorder. Anticipatory fear of helplessness or of losing control during a panic attack is a common occurrence. The individual frequently avoids situations that induce the fear, sometimes developing a phobic avoidance reaction. The next clinical example shows the impact of panic attacks on a person's functional abilities.

Clinical Example

Loretta's panic attacks persisted, gradually increasing in frequency and severity. She noticed that her symptoms seemed to begin every time she entered the elevator in her office building. Loretta began to take frequent sick days rather than report for work and avoided all social activities with friends whenever a ride in an elevator was required.

Agoraphobia, the marked fear of being in public places from which escape might be difficult or in which help might not be available (which often leads to the fear of being alone), is secondary to panic attacks. A diagnosis of panic disorder with agoraphobia is appropriate for an individual who experiences

---

MENTAL HEALTH IN THE MOVIES
As Good As It Gets

In this romantic comedy, a waitress, a misanthropic author, and a gay artist form an unlikely interdependent relationship. Melvin Udall (Jack Nicholson) is cranky, bigoted, and controlled by his obsessive–compulsive behavior and a germ phobia. When Carol, the only waitress at his favorite diner who will tolerate him, must leave the restaurant to care for her asthmatic son, Melvin finds it impossible to eat breakfast. His trials and tribulations

with obsessive–compulsive behavior and his germ phobia steer the film until its ending when Melvin comes to understand Carol's son's need for medical care, respect his gay neighbor, Simon, and make a start, with Carol's help, toward managing his behavior. While *As Good As It Gets* is a great deal of fun, it underestimates the seriousness and the complexities involved in dealing with obsessions, compulsions, and phobias on a day-to-day basis.

Photo courtesy of SONY PICTURES/Album/Newscom.

panic attacks and has phobic avoidance. In the absence of phobic avoidance, the condition is called *panic disorder without agoraphobia*. Agoraphobia without panic attacks is uncommon. Agoraphobia with symptoms of panic attack is now treatable with some medications (e.g., antidepressants, anxiolytic agents).

Panic disorder is usually first noted in late adolescence or early adulthood. It may be limited to a single brief period lasting several weeks or months, recur several times, or become chronic. Physical disorders such as hypoglycemia, hyperthyroidism, and amphetamine or caffeine intoxication must be ruled out before a diagnosis of panic disorder can be made. The ways in which hypoglycemia mimics a panic attack are discussed in Caring for the Spirit.

Phobic Disorders

A **phobia** is a persistent and irrational fear of a specific object, activity, or situation that results in a compelling desire to avoid the dreaded object or situation. Nearly all phobic individuals experience panic when in contact with the phobic situation. The fear is recognized by adults or adolescents as unreasonable in proportion to the actual danger. However, children do not always identify their fears as unrealistic.

In the development of phobia, fear arises through a process of displacing an unconscious conflict onto an external object symbolically related to the conflict. Thus, in becoming phobic, the individual fears a specific external object rather than an unknown internal source of distress. The phobic person can then control the intensity of the anxiety by avoiding the object with which the anxiety is associated.

A diagnosis of phobic disorder is generally made when the avoidance behavior becomes extreme or the problem so pervasive that it interferes with the person's normal functional ability. Phobic disorders are classified into three main types: agoraphobia, social phobia, and specific phobia. They are described next.

Agoraphobia

Individuals with agoraphobia often fear leaving the safety of home, worrying that they might develop an incapacitating symptom, such as dizziness, loss of bowel or bladder control,

or cardiac distress. Normal activities are increasingly curtailed as the fears dominate the person's life. Agoraphobic people often limit travel and need a companion when away from home. Those who endure the phobic situation experience intense anxiety.

Agoraphobia without panic attacks is relatively rare. More commonly, people with agoraphobia have spontaneous panic attacks. Most people with agoraphobia have a history of generalized anxiety or anxiety attacks at the onset of the phobic behavior. Onset of this disorder usually occurs in the middle to late twenties. Agoraphobia is more frequently diagnosed in women than in men. Separation anxiety in childhood and sudden object loss appear to be predisposing factors. Depression, anxiety, rituals, minor checking compulsions, and rumination are frequently associated features of agoraphobia.

The prognosis for people with agoraphobia is variable. Some less severely disturbed individuals experience intermittent symptoms and may have periods of remission. Those who are more severely impaired may experience lifelong disability.

Social Phobia

Social phobia (also called *social anxiety disorder*) is characterized by persistent fear and avoidance of situations in which the person may be exposed to scrutiny by others. The person especially fears being humiliated or embarrassed. Examples of social phobias are extreme fear of performing or speaking in public, making complaints, or writing or eating in front of others. Other common phobias include fear of interacting with members of the opposite sex, superiors, or aggressive individuals. Usually, a person has only one social phobia. This disorder is characterized by overwhelming anxiety and excessive self-consciousness in everyday situations.

According to the DSM-IV-TR (American Psychiatric Association [APA], 2000), 10% to 20% of people who have anxiety disorders are also affected by social phobias. Generalized anxiety, agoraphobia, or specific phobia may also coexist with social phobia. Often appearing in late childhood or early adolescence, social phobia usually progresses to a chronic course. Although symptoms may decrease in middle age, the

CARING FOR THE SPIRIT

Can Hypoglycemia Mimic an Anxiety Attack?

Much has been written in the lay press about the dangers of low blood sugar. Some popular authors claim it is a major scourge that afflicts millions of Americans, causing severe psychological harm.

Postprandial hypoglycemia is a drop in plasma glucose following a carbohydrate load. It can occur after gastric surgery or in the very early stages of diabetes. However, when it has no clear-cut organic cause, it is called *functional hypoglycemia*.

Functional low blood sugar occurs in two major ways. Epinephrine-like signs and symptoms include nervousness,

faintness, weakness, tremulousness, palpitations, sweating, and hunger. Central nervous system signs and symptoms include headache, confusion, visual disturbances, muscle weakness, ataxia, and marked personality changes.

Although there is little controlled clinical research to support the popular media view, psychiatric–mental health nurses should not dismiss hypoglycemia as a hypochondriac's invention. Negating a client's symptoms is akin to accusing the client of lying. Such insults wound the soul by dehumanizing the person. As holistic healers, nurses tend to the spirit by actively listening to the client and demonstrating support in all domains—physical, emotional, cognitive, and spiritual.

disorder is usually lifelong with only occasional remissions. Familial pattern and predisposing factors are unknown and the incidence is evenly distributed between men and women.

Specific Phobia

More common than any other type of phobic disorder, a **specific phobia** is an isolated fear focused on one situation or object, such as darkness, heights, or animals. This category of phobic disorders encompasses all phobias not included in agoraphobia or social phobia. Many specific phobias begin in childhood and subsequently disappear as the person ages. Phobias that persist into adulthood rarely go away without treatment. Specific phobia is more often diagnosed in females than in males. School phobia, which affects some children, may result in academic failure, impaired social relationships, and self-esteem problems.

Specific phobias generally cause minimal impairment if the phobic object is rarely encountered and easily avoided; for example, a fear of snakes does not seriously impair an individual living in a high-rise condominium. The phobia can, however, be incapacitating if the phobic situation is frequently encountered and not easily avoided. A fear of heights or elevators would seriously incapacitate a person living or working in a high-rise building. A specific phobia may lead to lifestyle restrictions that vary in severity according to the degree of anxiety. A list of common, uncommon, and curious specific phobias appears in TABLE 18-1 ■.

The object or situation avoided determines the subtype of specific phobia. The DSM (APA, 2000) identifies these subtypes as follows:

- Animal type: Fear related to animals, birds, or insects.
- Natural environment type: Fear triggered by elements of nature, such as water or weather.
- Blood–injection–injury type: Fear caused by the sight of blood or injury, or by receiving invasive medical procedures, such as an injection. The vasovagal response often occurs with this type of phobic reaction. There is a strong familial pattern with this subtype.
- Situational type: Fear resulting from contact with enclosed places, bridges, and/or public transportation.

TABLE 18-1 ■ Common, Uncommon, and Curious Phobias

Name of Phobia	Specific Fear
Acrophobia	Heights
Agoraphobia	Open spaces or crowds
Algophobia	Pain
Androphobia	Men
Arachnophobia	Spiders
Astraphobia	Thunder and lightning
Astrophobia	Stars and celestial space
Aviophobia	Flying
Claustrophobia	Enclosed places
Coprophobia	Excrement
Cynophobia	Dogs
Entomophobia	Insects
Erythrophobia	Blushing
Hematophobia	Blood
Hydrophobia	Water
Iatrophobia	Doctors
Lalophobia	Speaking
Necrophobia	Dead bodies
Nyctophobia	Darkness, night
Odynophobia	Pain
Ophidiophobia	Snakes
Pathophobia	Disease
Peccatophobia	Committing a sin
Phonophobia	Speaking aloud
Pyrophobia	Fire
Sitophobia	Food, eating
Taphophobia	Being buried alive
Thanatophobia	Death
Toxophobia	Being poisoned
Xenophobia	Strangers
Zoophobia	Animals

Generalized Anxiety Disorder

Generalized anxiety disorder (GAD) is considered less specific and less debilitating than panic disorder and phobic disorder. GAD is characterized by pervasive, persistent anxiety of at least 6 months' duration but without phobias, panic attacks, or obsessions and compulsions. The person experiences chronic feelings of nervousness and apprehension for no apparent reason and is unable to control the worry. The worry is greatly exaggerated in relation to the probability that the event will actually occur.

People with GAD are unable to stop worrying, even though they realize that their anxiety is more intense than the situation warrants. Overall, those with GAD are unable to relax. The excessive worries usually lead to insomnia and/or impaired quality of sleep and are associated with physical symptoms such as muscle tension, headaches, sweating, hot flashes, headaches, shortness of breath, and dizziness. Irritability is a common psychological manifestation of GAD. Autonomic symptoms may be less frequent or less severe than in panic attacks. In order to accurately diagnose GAD, a thorough physical examination must be done to determine the presence of any medical conditions that lead to anxiety. Some medical conditions that may contribute to the development of anxiety are thyroid imbalances, endocrine problems, and cardiovascular disease.

There is little generally accepted information about age of onset, predisposing factors, cause of illness, prevalence, familial pattern, or sex ratio, although there appears to be a more equal sex ratio than in panic disorder. Associated mild depressive symptoms are not uncommon in individuals with GAD. Although impairment in social or occupational functioning is rarely more than mild, the abuse of alcohol or other drugs may be a serious complication that interferes with effective motivation for treatment.

Obsessive–Compulsive Disorder

Obsessive–compulsive disorder (OCD) is classified as an anxiety disorder because of the anxiety symptoms that develop when an individual tries to resist an obsession or compulsion. OCD is more common in males than it is in females.

An **obsession** is a recurring thought that cannot be dismissed from consciousness. These intrusive thoughts are sometimes trivial or ridiculous, often morbid or fearful, and always distressing and anxiety provoking. Other common obsessive thoughts have to do with violence or contamination. The following clinical example compares an innocuous obsession to a serious one.

Clinical Example

Ernesto's inability to get the nursery rhyme "snips and snails and puppy dog tails" out of his mind is an example of a strange but trivial obsession. Even though Ernesto tried to distract himself with activities, he found the rhyme running through his mind at work and at home, especially when he was trying to sleep at night.

Melinda's obsession was much more ominous. She could not stop thinking that she must kill her children in order to prevent a worldwide race war.

A **compulsion** is an uncontrollable, persistent urge to perform certain acts or behaviors in order to relieve an otherwise unbearable tension. Most compulsive acts are attempts to control or modify obsessions because the person either fears the consequences or is afraid he or she will not be able to control the primary impulse. Although compulsions are attempts to reduce tension, they eventually increase tension because the individual becomes increasingly agitated, unable to decide whether to stop or continue the compulsive actions.

Typical compulsive acts are endless handwashing, checking and rechecking doors to see if they have been locked, and elaborate dressing rituals. Such compulsive acts are defenses used to contain, neutralize, or ward off the anxiety related to the primary impulse. Compulsive acts such as counting and elaborately checking routine duties are frequently associated with the fear of failing or making a mistake, or with the need to be perfect. The following clinical example describes the progression of obsessive thoughts to compulsive behaviors.

Clinical Example

Ernesto, the young man who could not dismiss the rhyme from his mind, developed a compulsion that involved ritualistic washing of his genitals to ward off the anxiety generated by his apparently silly obsession.

Melinda, obsessed with thoughts about killing her children, engaged in symbolic rituals of touching religious objects to repel evil influences through magical interventions by the saints.

People with OCD usually fear that they will harm someone or something. They rely heavily on avoidance and are best understood in terms of their control needs. Individuals who develop obsessive–compulsive symptoms have a great need to control themselves, others, and their environment. Obsessions and compulsions have the following features in common:

- An idea or impulse persistently intrudes into the person's awareness.
- A feeling of anxious dread accompanies the primary manifestation and often leads the person to take countermeasures against the forbidden thought or impulse.
- Both the obsessions and the compulsion are ego alien—that is, they are foreign to one's self-perception.
- No matter how compelling the obsession or compulsion, the person has enough insight to recognize it as irrational and experience it as a significant source of distress.

TABLE 18-2 ■ lists some common obsessions and compulsions.

Many of the personality traits associated with obsession and compulsion are highly valued in American culture. Success in several professions and occupations demands cautiousness, deliberateness, and rationality. These traits are usually associated with the tendency toward obsession or compulsion. When these personality traits are carried to an extreme, or when the balance between control and impulse expression leads to paralysis, they become a liability.

Pediatric Autoimmune Neuropsychiatric Disorders Associated With Streptococci (PANDAS)

Although OCD is usually diagnosed in older adolescents or young adults, children may also be affected by the disorder. Some children are at risk for developing **pediatric autoimmune neuropsychiatric disorders associated with**

TABLE 18-2 ■ Common Obsessions and Compulsions

Behavior	Related Compulsion	Related Obsession
Repetitious handwashing	Urge to wash, scrub, or clean	Fear of disease or contamination
Returning home often to make sure appliances are turned off	Need to recheck related to self-doubt	Fear of disaster
Hoarding junk mail, receipts, and all types of papers	Need to keep everything	Fear of losing things
Ritualistic counting of number of stairs climbed	Urge to count repeatedly	Belief that counting will yield control and thus prevent making mistakes
Avoiding stepping on seams of tiles, carpets, sidewalks	Need for order and routine	Belief that order and routine will negate all anxiety

Videos: Obsessive–Compulsive Disorder

Care Plan: Obsessive–Compulsive Behavior

streptococci (PANDAS). The term *PANDAS* is used to describe a subset of children who have OCD and/or tic disorders, such as Tourette's syndrome, and in whom symptoms have exacerbated following streptococcal infections, such as strep throat. (Tic disorders are discussed in Chapter 25∞.) It is theorized that an antibody against strep throat bacteria mistakenly acts on a brain enzyme and disrupts communication between neurons.

Children with PANDAS seem to have dramatic fluctuations in OCD and/or tic severity; that is, the children have "good days" and "bad days." OCD does occur in children without PANDAS. However, when a child has a very episodic course of OCD/tic symptoms and has had strep throat prior to or during a dramatic worsening of the symptoms, the possibility of PANDAS should be considered. Also, the symptoms due to PANDAS have a sudden onset as compared to the gradual development that occurs with OCD (Children's Center for OCD and Anxiety, 2009).

Post-Traumatic Stress Disorder

Post-traumatic stress disorder (PTSD) is the experience of a significant stressor or trauma, outside the range of usual experience, which is followed by recurrent subjective re-experiencing of the trauma. The types of trauma that precipitate PTSD are varied, including military combat, criminal attack (i.e., assault, rape), child abuse (especially incest), terrorist attack (i.e., bombing, skyjacking), and natural catastrophes (i.e., earthquakes, tornadoes, hurricanes). Children who have witnessed violence in their families, schools, or communities are also vulnerable to developing PTSD. First responders (e.g., paramedics) and other health care providers, especially those who work in critical care areas and trauma centers, are at risk of developing PTSD as a result of witnessing extreme suffering. The trauma that precipitates the development of PTSD has to be extreme; therefore, the client's cultural context must be considered in the diagnostic

DEVELOPING CULTURAL COMPETENCE

War and Mental Disorders

Several cultures associate the effects of war with the origins of mental disorder. Bosnians and Serbs seem familiar with post-traumatic stress disorder (PTSD) as a result of the devastating impact of events related to war in their country. Cambodians believe that emotional problems resulted from the Khmer Rouge brutalities, and that evil spirits or ancestors may cause mental disorder. Jewish Holocaust survivors may have experienced psychiatric effects because of war atrocities. The Hmong appear to accept those who have depression and PTSD because these conditions are common among those who experienced war.

CRITICAL THINKING QUESTIONS

1. What advantages can you identify for knowing the origins of a mental disorder?
2. How would experiences such as war provide a platform for structuring therapeutic interventions?

process. An example of an extreme trauma is war (see Developing Cultural Competence).

The psychological effects of trauma affect individuals throughout their lifetimes. For example, a child who observes domestic violence (especially repeated episodes) is at risk for developing PTSD as an adult. The violence associated with rape, whether experienced or witnessed, is severe enough to precipitate the onset of PTSD. For further discussion of PTSD as it relates to the experience of rape or incest, see Chapter 24 ∞ to. The following clinical example provides a description of combat-related PTSD.

Clinical Example

Bill and Joe, who are veterans of military action in Afghanistan and Iraq, are enrolled in a PTSD program at a veterans' hospital outpatient clinic. Upon returning home from combat, they essentially relived their experiences through recurrent nightmares about intermittent explosive devices. They both experienced insomnia and a loss of pleasure in previously enjoyed activities. Both men had trouble concentrating. Bill felt guilty about surviving when other men in his unit did not. Joe felt guilty about the actions he had to take in order to survive.

A common manifestation in individuals with PTSD is hyperarousal while re-experiencing the traumatic event. As a result, the person is unable to relax; hypervigilance occurs and the person is always "on edge." Another common feature of PTSD is dissociation, in which emotions about the traumatic event are blocked. The individual becomes emotionally numb and experiences impaired social relationships. People with PTSD may also avoid the stimuli associated with the traumatic event. For example, a woman who is raped in an elevator may avoid using any elevator—an example of how PTSD can restrict daily functioning. A significant complicating problem is the person's use of alcohol or other substances in an attempt to maintain control and soothe emotions.

The course of PTSD is variable. Most people who have suffered a significant stressor tend to have an acute reaction from which they recover spontaneously. In others, however, the reaction may be delayed or prolonged and eventually become chronic. PTSD is characterized by high rates of chronicity and comorbidity. PTSD is divided into categories according to onset and duration of symptoms:

- Acute: Symptoms occur within 1 month of trauma and last less than 3 months.
- Chronic: Symptoms last 3 months or more.
- Delayed onset: At least 6 months have elapsed between the trauma and the occurrence of symptoms.

PTSD can occur in people of any age, including children and elders. Following a traumatic event, it is important to thoroughly assess everyone, including children and older adults. To be complete, the assessment should include physical, psychological, sociocultural, and spiritual domains. Across the lifespan, associated symptoms of depression, anxiety, and increased irritability are common, sometimes leading to unpredictable explosions of hostility with little or no provocation.

Acute Stress Disorder

Acute stress disorder (ASD) is the development of anxiety and dissociative symptoms that occur within 1 month of an extremely traumatic event. The precipitating stressors of ASD are similar to those of PTSD. They include exposure to a trauma in which the individual experienced or witnessed event(s) that involved actual or threatened injury or death and were accompanied by feelings of intense helplessness, fear, or horror. As in PTSD, the precipitating event must be a trauma that is outside the usual human experience. The traumatic event may be a natural disaster or human-induced event (e.g., rape, terrorist bombing). One type of trauma that often triggers ASD is disasters that affect entire communities. Individuals feel overwhelmed as a result of the trauma and are unable to cope effectively.

Although it is similar to PTSD, ASD can be differentiated in the following ways:

- The duration is shorter.
- The interval from the trauma to the development of symptoms is shorter.
- The person has at least three of these dissociative manifestations: sense of detachment or numbing, depersonalization, derealization, dissociative amnesia, decreased awareness of surroundings (being in a daze).
- The dissociative symptoms interfere with effective coping.

Individuals with ASD may experience depression accompanied by despair and helplessness. Thus, there is a very real danger of suicide (refer to the thorough discussion of suicide in Chapter 23 ∞). The individuals may feel they are responsible for the outcome of the trauma. For example, if another person was killed in the traumatic event, survival guilt frequently occurs. People affected by ASD often neglect safety precautions and basic needs for daily living. First responders and other emergency personnel are at high risk for developing ASD. The next clinical example describes the onset of ASD as a response to a natural disaster.

Clinical Example

William was a member of a team of firemen from California who volunteered to help with rescue efforts in Japan following a massive earthquake and tsunami. William and his fellow volunteers worked through rubble, at first looking for survivors, then removing bodies. William's symptoms of acute stress disorder began 1 week after returning home from the traumatic event.

BIOPSYCHOSOCIAL THEORIES

There are several schools of thought regarding the causes of anxiety disorders. These theories include biologic, genetic, psychosocial, behavioral, and humanistic, which are discussed in the next section.

Biologic Factors

Refresh your understanding of the biologic basis of anxiety disorders by referring to FIGURE 18-2 ■, which illustrates the

FIGURE 18-2 ■ Physiological responses in anxiety disorders.

physiological responses in anxiety disorders in relationship to the sympathetic and parasympathetic divisions of the central nervous system. Notice that they are the same as the fight–or–flight response described in Chapter 8 ∞. A major research question that remains unanswered is: Are the physiological imbalances a *cause* or a *result* of the anxiety disorder?

Recent research findings point to biologic changes in the brains of individuals experiencing anxiety disorders. Some of those findings are as follows:

- The noradrenergic system in the brain is especially sensitive to the neurotransmitter norepinephrine (NE). One section of the noradrenergic system, called the *locus ceruleus* (located in the brain stem), appears to be involved in precipitating panic attacks. Drugs that increase the activity of the locus ceruleus have been found to cause panic attacks; drugs that inhibit the activity of the locus ceruleus block panic attacks (see Figure 18-2). Tricyclic antidepressant medications stabilize the locus ceruleus and noradrenergic system; thus, they are sometimes useful in alleviating the symptoms associated with panic attack (Sadock & Sadock, 2010).
- Functional MRIs showed that individuals with generalized anxiety disorder experienced irregular activity in the medial prefrontal and anterior cingulated regions of the brain (Paulesu et al., 2010). Another study indicates that the medial prefrontal cortex is activated in people with excessive anxiety levels (Etkin, Prater, Hoeft, Menon, & Schatzberg, 2010).
- The brain's benzodiazepine (BZD) receptor system is especially sensitive to BZDs. The BZDs enhance the action of gamma-aminobutyric acid (GABA), an inhibitory neurotransmitter. With the administration

of GABA, or medications that potentiate GABA, anxiety is reduced. On the other hand, medications that inhibit the activity of GABA increase anxiety (Sadock & Sadock, 2010). GABA may have a slight tranquilizing effect (Bourne, 2011).

- Hormonal changes experienced during pregnancy may affect the onset, duration, and intensity of certain anxiety disorders. A recent poll conducted by the Anxiety Disorders Association of America (2010–2011) shows that 52% of women who had been pregnant reported increased anxiety or depression during pregnancy.
- Lactic acid levels are higher in some individuals experiencing panic attack. Lactic acid may actually precipitate anxiety in some people (Bourne, 2011).
- Many substances increase anxiety levels. Caffeine stimulates the central nervous system (CNS) and increases NE production. In fact, caffeine produces the same physiological arousal response experienced with exposure to stress. The result is increased sympathetic nervous system activity and a release of adrenalin. Caffeine causes some people to remain in a chronically tense, aroused condition and may trigger panic attacks.
- Nicotine is another substance that is a suspected trigger for panic attacks. Nicotine, which is a strong stimulant, results in increased physiological arousal, vasoconstriction, and increased blood pressure. Nicotine consumers tend to sleep less well than tobacco product users.

Genetic Theories

Research evidence indicates that a familial predisposition for anxiety disorders may exist. According to twin studies, there is a genetic factor in OCD and panic disorder (APA, 2000). First-degree relatives of people with panic disorder are four to seven times more likely to develop panic disorder (APA, 2000). In approximately 25% of individuals with GAD, there is a family history of the disorder (Sadock & Sadock, 2010). Transmission of certain genes may contribute to the development of OCD; early-onset OCD has been shown to be familial (Walitza et al., 2010).

Psychosocial Theories

Psychoanalytic theory views anxiety as a sign of psychological conflict resulting from the threatened emergence into consciousness of forbidden or repressed ideas and/ or emotions. The individual fears expressing the forbidden impulses; anxiety is an outcome of repressing such impulses. Other analytic views sometimes called *neo-Freudian,* evolved from the work of Freud and differ on the nature of anxiety. Rank (1952) believed that anxiety can be traced back to birth trauma. According to the psychoanalytic model, the unconscious conflict must be brought into conscious awareness through psychoanalysis so that the real source of anxiety can be discovered and resolved.

Social-interpersonal theorists such as Sullivan (1953) stressed the importance of the early relationship between the mother and the child and the transmission of the mother's anxiety to the child. In the interpersonal model, treatment takes the form of the less time-consuming psychodynamic psychotherapy.

Behavioral Theories

Behavioral learning theorists view anxiety as a learned response that can be unlearned. For example, behaviorists believe that the cause of phobias is traumatic exposure to the avoided object, situation, or activity. According to this theory, during the development of obsessions, an original neutral obsessive thought evokes anxiety because it becomes associated with an anxiety-provoking stimulus. In compulsions, a person discovers that a certain action relieves anxiety associated with the obsessive thought. The person repeats the action to achieve relief until eventually the act becomes a learned pattern of behavior. Compulsive behavior is viewed as a maladaptive attempt to alleviate anxiety.

Behavior modification (discussed in Chapter 30 ∞) is a treatment approach that teaches clients new ways to behave. Conditioning techniques—using positive and negative reinforcements—are examples of modification techniques. One behavior modification technique is systematic desensitization, a process in which a client builds up tolerance to anxiety through gradual exposure to a series of anxiety-provoking stimuli. The client is taught relaxation techniques that are to be used whenever the anxiety increases.

Behavioral approaches are often effective in the treatment of anxiety and are widely used for modifying symptoms in phobic disorder and obsessive–compulsive disorder. Behavioral therapists believe it is unnecessary to use insight-oriented psychotherapy to help clients cope with the anxiety. Instead, clients need only face the anxiety repeatedly until it becomes manageable. Behavioral treatment approaches are often used in treating phobias because the methods are more efficient, less costly, and less time consuming than insight-oriented psychotherapy. Like some psychodynamically and psychoanalytically oriented therapists, behavioral therapists tend to avoid the use of medication because they believe it may interfere with the client's ability to learn more appropriate behaviors.

Humanistic Theories

The humanistic perspective is particularly important in understanding anxiety disorders. Environmental stressors, biologic factors, and intrapsychic fears or conflicts cannot be adequately dealt with separately but only as they interact with one another. For example, clients suffering from a phobic disorder experience shame and helplessness as they attempt to cope with fears of annihilation in the presence of the dreaded object or situation. The result may be interpersonal withdrawal and functional impairment, which create long-lasting disability.

This perspective has given rise to a multifaceted approach to the care of clients with anxiety disorders. Humanistic treatment approaches are integrative and may include a range of psychotherapeutic interventions, including psychotherapy (cognitive, behavioral, and/or dynamic), measures to develop effective social support systems, measures to reduce environmental stress, and psychopharmacologic treatment.

THE NURSING PROCESS
Clients With Anxiety Disorders

Chapter 8 ∞ covers concepts of anxiety, stress, and coping that are relevant to the care of clients with anxiety disorders; it also covers the general anxiety continuum and the need to identify the client's level of anxiety. The subject of this section is the nurse's role with clients whose anxiety is severe enough to be classified as an anxiety disorder. A nursing care plan for a client experiencing panic disorder with agoraphobia is at the end of this chapter.

Assessment

Clients with anxiety disorders have impaired psychosocial and physiological function. The emotional disturbances and physical and intellectual changes that take place as a result of extreme or chronic anxiety affect the client's work, school, and social functioning and frequently impair or threaten previously meaningful interpersonal relationships. The clinical manifestations are listed in Your Assessment Approach: Anxiety Disorder. Clients can also review a variety of self-tests for GAD, OCD, PTSD, and other anxiety disorders on http://www.adaa.org. You can also access these self-tests through the Online Student Resources for this book.

The occurrence of acute anxiety and its related symptoms is common to a number of physical conditions and acute medical emergencies. Therefore, a careful evaluation should always be conducted to initiate appropriate treatment quickly.

YOUR ASSESSMENT APPROACH
Client With an Anxiety Disorder

Use the questions that follow as guidelines for assessing clients with anxiety disorders.

Physiological Assessment

- How often do you experience palpitations (heart pounding)?
- Do you have difficulty breathing?
- Do you experience muscle tightness? If so, where, and how long does it last?
- How often do you experience changes in bladder or bowel function?
- How do your symptoms affect your sleep?

Psychological Assessment

- Do you feel sad and/or hopeless?
- How often do you lose your temper?
- Do you enjoy being with other people?
- How often do you criticize yourself?

Cognitive Assessment

- Do you think about the same things over and over?
- Do you frequently have trouble concentrating on important activities?
- How often do you worry about the past or the future?
- Do you still enjoy activities that were pleasurable for you in the past?

A history and physical examination should rule out such conditions as hyperthyroidism and other endocrine problems, Ménière's syndrome, brain disorders, caffeine intoxication, mitral valve prolapse, and medical emergencies (such as myocardial infarction).

Differentiation from other psychiatric diagnoses is difficult when anxiety and depression are mixed. The question of which one predominates can puzzle many practitioners and necessitates ongoing thorough assessment. Some ways to differentiate anxiety and depression are listed in TABLE 18-3 ■. Anxiety is part of many other clinical syndromes, such as schizophrenia and mood disorders. The medical diagnosis may be made on the basis of the dominant, most debilitating symptom.

During assessment, determine not only whether the client is anxious (and, if so, to what extent) but also the possible source of the anxiety. Knowing the source will help you plan and implement effective care. It is important to assess the client's perception of threat; the greater the perceived threat, the more intense the anxiety. For extremely anxious clients, suspend formal data gathering in favor of immediate, direct action to reduce anxiety. Common features of panic attack are listed in Your Assessment Approach: Panic Attack.

Subjective Data

Clients with an anxiety disorder may report a variety of physical and emotional symptoms. It is important to encourage clients to describe symptoms in their own words and to explain how the symptoms affect their daily activities. They may report emotional distress, cognitive and perceptual changes, somatic discomforts, and/or role impairments.

Emotional Distress Clients with anxiety disorders may reveal a number of distressing emotional feelings, such as the following examples:

- "I feel like something terrible is going to happen."
- "I feel helpless for no reason at all!"
- "I just can't seem to enjoy life—everything bothers me."

Anger, guilt, feelings of worthlessness, and anguish frequently accompany anxiety. When the anxiety is acute

TABLE 18-3 ■ Comparison of Anxiety and Depression		
Clinical Manifestations	**Anxiety**	**Depression**
Affect	Fear and/or dread	Sadness, despair, helplessness, and/or hopelessness
Insomnia	Initial difficulty in falling asleep	Early morning awakening followed by difficulty returning to sleep
Motor activity	Agitation	Retardation (slowing)
Negativism	Limited to specific areas	Global

YOUR ASSESSMENT APPROACH
Client With Panic Attack

To determine the psychological effects of panic on your client, ask:

- How do you feel right now?
- When did you start feeling this way?
- Did this feeling start gradually or all at once?
- How well are you able to concentrate?
- How do you feel about the future?
- Do you sometimes feel out of control?

To determine the somatic effects of panic on your client, ask:

- Are you having chest pains or shortness of breath?
- Have you felt dizzy or faint?
- Can you hold your hands steady, or do they shake?

or extreme, as in panic disorder or PTSD, the client feels in immediate danger and may seek protection and reassurance from others. If the anxiety is too severe, however, clients may become immobilized and unable to report their terrifying feelings at all, or they may refuse assistance and run away or become physically aggressive.

Sometimes clients with anxiety disorders may deny the existence of anxious feelings. They try to protect themselves by dissociating these feelings. It is important to recognize clients' anxiety despite their denials. In such instances, assessment requires an especially careful observation of objective data.

Cognitive and Perceptual Changes Anxious clients frequently have difficulty concentrating and making decisions. Some clients report feeling as if they are "going in circles," unable to think through a problem in order to make an effective decision. They may worry about their effectiveness at work and fear job loss as a result of attention and judgment problems. In the clinical situation, clients may ask staff members to make decisions for them. At the same time, however, they may express difficulty following through with suggestions, finding many loopholes or possible problems with the plan of action. Other clients become forgetful or misinterpret what they hear.

In extreme anxiety, as in a panic attack, the client is unable to assess a situation accurately and realistically. The client may later report having had a frightening feeling of personality disintegration. The client needs immediate attention from, and orientation by, you.

Somatic Discomfort Clients with anxiety disorders may complain of nausea, indigestion, headache, decreased appetite, a constant feeling of fatigue, or other somatic problems. They may relate these somatic disturbances to having "bad nerves," or they may be unaware of any psychological component of their discomfort.

Clients with OCD who engage in repetitive activity, such as compulsive handwashing or hair pulling, may report special health problems (tissue breakdown or hair loss)

as a result. You must compare the psychological benefits to the physical consequences of the client's compulsive rituals when determining appropriate interventions for these clients.

Clients with PTSD may report fitful sleep, terrifying nightmares, and a fear of returning to sleep. The subsequent sleep loss becomes an additional physiological stressor. Be sure to assess the sleep pattern of clients with PTSD. Common features of PTSD are listed in Your Assessment Approach: Client With PTSD.

Role Impairment Clients may be aware of the impact that emotional, cognitive/perceptual, and somatic changes have on their social, family, and work roles. They report worry about losing their jobs or being unable to continue caring for their families. This worry only exacerbates the underlying anxiety and sets up a vicious cycle of worry compounding anxiety, which adds to the worry. The next clinical example describes two people who are experiencing interpersonal difficulties as a result of anxiety.

Clinical Example

Gisela despairs that she is unable to take her daughter to the playground because her phobias prevent her from leaving the house.

Abe, a middle-aged accountant, obsessed about tallying his firm's financial data, is unable to put his job aside for the weekend, and misses his son's football game. He experiences anger, guilt, and self-recrimination as a result.

Objective Data

In addition to noting general signs and symptoms of anxiety as discussed in Chapter 8 ∞, other specific physical, emotional, cognitive, and role performance changes may be observed in very anxious clients. Look for indicators of hypervigilance, such as guarding and suspiciousness; these are common occurrences in people experiencing PTSD.

YOUR ASSESSMENT APPROACH
Client With PTSD

The questions that follow will help you to assess PTSD.

- When was the last time you struck out in anger?
- Are you able to laugh and cry at appropriate times/situations?
- How would you describe your mood right now? Happy? Sad? Depressed?
- How much time do you spend thinking the same thing over and over?
- Are you able to relax?
- When was the last time you lost your temper? Or said something without thinking first?
- How do you sleep at night? Any nightmares or repetitive dreams?
- How is your memory?
- Are you able to finish tasks?

Physical Findings Clients with acute or extreme anxiety—clients with PTSD or panic disorder, and clients with phobic disorder who cannot avoid the phobic situation—may experience a panic reaction and show extreme discomfort. Look for acute physical changes, such as breathing difficulty, sweating, trembling, and/or vomiting, during these incidents. The client may be unable to verbalize, or verbalizations may be confused and incoherent. During a panic episode, clients may be so frightened that they refuse help at the moment and may require firm reassurance and protection until the episode subsides.

The client with an anxiety disorder may develop long-term physiological effects, such as susceptibility to viral infections or the development of ulcers, hypertension, or asthma. Substance abuse may develop when clients try to alleviate anxiety through chemical means and can become a serious complicating problem. Substance abuse (discussed in Chapter 15∞), which frequently occurs in individuals experiencing PTSD, may be the client's attempt to avoid traumatic memories by self-medicating. Other physical findings may be the effects of ritualistic or compulsive activity—skin lesions in a client who obsessively picks at the skin, for example.

Emotional Changes Family and friends of a client with PTSD may report personality changes in the client, including increased irritability, suspiciousness, angry outbursts, and a tendency to blame others and to withdraw emotionally. Remember to pay attention to your own feelings when interacting with highly anxious clients. Because anxiety can be transmitted interpersonally, use self-awareness to determine the source of your own anxiety when interacting with anxious clients.

Individuals with phobic disorder and obsessive–compulsive disorder show a lack of emotional distress as long as the phobic object or situation is avoided or alleviated with activity. There may be little spontaneity or active involvement by the client during assessment, because rigid, stereotyped behavior patterns are common.

Cognitive Deficits Unrealistic or distorted perception of a situation is common in anxiety states. During panic attacks, clients may distort or exaggerate details. They may complain about some seemingly insignificant detail. Clients may lose their ability to take in other pertinent data, and thus make errors in judgment. In assessment interviews, clients with anxiety disorders are often forgetful and unable to concentrate or attend to details. Errors in calculation and grammar are also common. Eyewitness accounts to stressful events, such as crimes, are notoriously inaccurate for these same reasons.

Clinical Example

Nine people witness a hit-and-run automobile accident. It becomes clear to the police officers interviewing the witnesses that there are major discrepancies in the description of the car that caused the accident. Three people say it was blue, two people say it was green, three people say it was black, and one person says it was white. At the conclusion of the investigation, it was determined that a green car caused the accident.

Impact on Role Function The symptoms of anxiety disorder affect social, work, and family relationships. It is important to understand the possible effects of anxiety symptoms on interpersonal relationships. Obsessive–compulsive acts, for instance, may become so pervasive that they take the place of relating to other people. Sometimes, clients may use obsessions and compulsions to negotiate social interactions and social roles. Nurses who plan intervention strategies for clients with anxiety disorders should first assess the impact of the symptoms on the family system. In the following clinical example, the client knows that her compulsive cleaning is irrational but is unable to stop the behavior. Vanessa does not connect the excessive need for cleaning to an attempt to negate her sense of decreased control over her family members.

Clinical Example

Vanessa's house is so clean and orderly that you could literally "eat off the floor." Vanessa spends a large amount of her time after work and on weekends making sure that the house is sparkling clean. She prepares to-do cleaning lists for her young adult children to follow when they visit. When Vanessa's husband comes home after traveling on business, he is often met with his own to-do list. Family social activities are put on hold until Vanessa's lists have been accomplished. Vanessa's husband and children complain about having to clean an already clean house. Vanessa is upset that her children are visiting less often and that her husband seems to be spending more and more time traveling on business.

Reports from the client and/or family that the client is having trouble at work are additional evidence of role impairment. The client may be in jeopardy of losing a job because of poor performance. A person with PTSD, for example, may be fired for absences, drug or alcohol abuse, or outbursts of temper.

Nursing Diagnosis: NANDA

It is impractical to try to identify all the nursing diagnoses that apply to clients experiencing anxiety disorders. However, there are three fundamental nursing diagnoses pertinent to clients with these disorders:

1. Fear—a response to a threat that is recognized as a danger
2. Anxiety—a vague feeling of dread accompanied by an autonomic response; a feeling of apprehension in anticipation of danger
3. Ineffective coping—an inability to form a reality-based appraisal of the stressors, inadequate selection of responses, and/or inability to use available adaptive resources

Following is a discussion of the three primary nursing diagnoses and other diagnoses that may apply to clients with anxiety disorders.

Fear

Fearful responses to anxiety can occur on a continuum ranging from slight apprehension to paralyzing terror. One anxious person may state, "I'm scared," whereas another may be filled with alarm and unable to verbalize feelings of panic.

In extreme cases of anxiety, panic is communicated through behavioral responses rather than verbalizations. Behaviors such as being immobilized with fear or striking out at others are often exhibited by individuals experiencing panic.

Anxiety

Apprehension and tension are emotional experiences common to clients with anxiety disorders. Clients may worry excessively, ruminating about what might go wrong in the future. They may express anxiety through worry about their physical well-being; somatic preoccupation or hypochondriasis may develop. Sexual drive or behavior may also be inhibited by anxiety. The potential for substance abuse is high, and suicidal potential is increased.

Ineffective Coping

Excessive anxiety can cause alterations in conduct and impulse control. Some clients, such as those with PTSD or panic disorder, manifest unpredictable behaviors in an attempt to cope with their overwhelming fears. Individuals with OCD are unable to alter behaviors, even though they may recognize the behaviors as harmful or irrational. In an attempt to cope, some clients with anxiety begin to self-medicate with alcohol or other drugs, which results in disordered conduct and impaired impulse control.

Ineffective Role Performance

Anxiety disorders impair performance in the family, at school, and at work. Anxious clients may become less efficient and accurate at work or school because of distractibility or other perceptual and cognitive difficulties. Clients may withdraw emotionally from formerly important and meaningful relationships, or they may become overly dependent on others for help. They may isolate themselves and avoid previously enjoyed activities and recreation. Excessive need for reassurance, decreased productivity, reduced creativity, impaired hygiene, and impaired home maintenance are all possible outcomes for the client with anxiety disorder.

Impaired Verbal Communication

Clients with anxiety disorders often have difficulty communicating. They may speak too quickly or too loudly, may overelaborate, or may talk about too many subjects at once. Easily distracted, anxious people may have trouble understanding explanations or retaining information. A client with severe anxiety may be incoherent, making verbal communication impossible. Written communication may also be impaired.

Risk for Trauma

Impairments in motor behavior are often related to hyperactivity and restlessness, which may place the client at risk for accidental injury. Wringing of the hands, poor coordination, and startle reaction are motor behaviors associated with anxiety disorders. Clients with OCD may perform bizarre repetitive acts, such as repeatedly washing the hands; these ritualistic acts often result in self-injury.

Disturbed Thought Processes and Disturbed Sensory Perception

Anxiety disorders affect perception and cognition and reduce the client's ability to solve problems. Judgment, concentration, abstract thinking, and attention are impaired. The client is indecisive but at the same time may make decisions impulsively in an attempt to relieve tension. In panic disorder, the client may become disoriented, misinterpret reality, and distort the meaning of situations or events. Loss of self-esteem and a lowered self-concept often result because the client is unable to use skills that were previously helpful in coping.

Ineffective Tissue Perfusion

Alterations in circulation and elimination may occur as a result of stimulation of the autonomic nervous system. The client may experience increased blood pressure, rapid heart rate, dizziness, and palpitations as well as dry mouth, cold or clammy hands, sweating, shortness of breath, and a bad taste in the mouth. Diarrhea, enuresis, and slowed digestion may occur.

With extreme anxiety or panic, these symptoms are intensified, and the client may faint or vomit. A medical emergency may arise if the client has a coexisting physical problem, such as cardiovascular disease.

Insomnia

Insomnia, which is difficulty falling asleep or maintaining sleep, is a major public health problem affecting over half of the adult population in the U.S. (Hale et al., 2009). Up to 15% of adults report severe or frequent insomnia, and another 15% report occasional episodes (APA, 2000). **Primary insomnia** is the term used in the DSM-IV-TR to describe difficulty initiating or maintaining sleep, or nonrestorative sleep that lasts for at least a month and does not occur exclusively in association with another sleep disorder or mental disorder. Insomnia is a frequent response to anxiety; a majority of clients with anxiety disorders have trouble sleeping. Sleep may be further disturbed by nightmares or night terrors, as experienced by people with PTSD.

Outcome Identification: NOC

When developing client outcomes, specifically state the outcomes in behavioral terms. For example, the statement "Mr. Atkins will be less anxious" is ambiguous and not easily measured. However, the statement "Mr. Atkins will participate in one relaxation session per day" is observable and measurable. Outcome identification is individualized according to the client's clinical manifestations and needs. The following list provides some outcomes that generally apply to clients experiencing anxiety disorders:

- Client will demonstrate absence of physical manifestations of anxiety.
- Client will identify indicators of own anxiety.
- Client will verbalize feelings of anxiety appropriately.
- Client will demonstrate the use of new coping skills.

Planning and Implementation: NIC

When planning and implementing care for anxious clients, remember that anxiety is communicated interpersonally and often affects the client's family and friends, other clients, and staff members as well. Refer to Your Self-Awareness for help in reading your own bodily cues of anxiety.

Most mental health care professionals believe that clients who cope with the stress of anxiety disorders can grow and change with therapeutic intervention. Nursing interventions for clients with anxiety disorders should be geared toward effective coping. Refer to the Nursing Care Plan on panic disorder with agoraphobia at the end of this chapter.

Reducing Fear

Fear and anxiety usually coexist in that a person who is fearful is generally anxious as well. The clinical manifestations of fear and anxiety are very similar. Thus, when dealing with a client who is afraid, nursing interventions for reducing anxiety are appropriate (see the following).

Reducing Anxiety

Because anxiety is such an uncomfortable feeling, we learn early in life to reduce it or diminish its effects as soon as possible. Although individuals use a variety of behaviors, the most common automatic responses to anxiety are anger, withdrawal, and somatization. Automatic responses are limiting, rigid, and inflexible and, therefore, prevent a creative response to the stressor.

Intervening With Clients Experiencing Panic Clients who are extremely anxious or in a panic state require immediate, direct, and structured intervention. During an acute panic attack, perception and personality are disrupted to such a degree that the client cannot solve problems or discuss the source of anxiety. The first priority is to reduce the anxiety to more tolerable

---

YOUR INTERVENTION STRATEGIES
Client in Panic

Strategy	Rationale
Stay with the client.	Being left alone may further increase the anxiety.
Maintain a calm, serene manner.	Prevents transmission of anxiety from nurse to client.
Use short, simple sentences.	Disruption of the perceptual field causes difficulty in focusing.
Use a firm and authoritative voice.	Conveys your ability to provide external controls.
Place client in a quieter, smaller, less stimulating environment.	Prevents further disruption of the perceptual field by sensory stimuli.
Focus the client's diffuse energy on a repetitive or physically tiring task.	Repetitive tasks or physical exercise help reduce excess energy.
Administer antianxiety medications if ordered.	Antianxiety medications may help reduce anxiety by altering brain chemistry.

---

levels. The interventions listed in Your Intervention Strategies can help alleviate the client's panic.

Your goal is to reduce the client's immediate anxiety to more moderate and manageable levels. The family of the anxious person needs counseling about how to respond therapeutically because they are often present during a panic episode.

Intervening in Less Severe Anxiety You can frequently detect subtle indications of increasing anxiety and intervene early to prevent escalation. Some clients are adept at covering up their anxiety, even though their behavior usually transmits cues to the sensitive observer. Often, your own feeling of increased tension is a useful cue that the source of anxiety is in the client. Anxiety may make people excessively demanding. Your response to the client's demands should always consider the possible effects of your response on the client's anxiety. In some cases, it may be reassuring to set limits and deny the request. In other cases, such a response may place further stress on the client.

The intervention strategies for clients who suffer from prolonged anxiety are intended to help clients use their anxiety to learn about themselves and their coping strategies. This requires the client to endure the anxiety while searching out its causes. The client must then develop more effective and satisfying coping strategies to replace the maladaptive ones. To help clients learn to cope more effectively with anxiety, first detect the anxiety and then make thoughtful observations and responses that facilitate learning. Refer to Your Intervention Strategies on page 406 for the client experiencing anxiety.

It is important that you avoid reinforcing clients' justifications for their usual coping patterns. Often, clients try to give plausible explanations for their ineffective anger, withdrawal, or somatization. However, these rationalizations do not explain the relief in terms of the factors that caused the anxiety.

YOUR SELF-AWARENESS
Cues to Anxiety

Because anxiety is communicated interpersonally, it is imperative that you are able to read your own somatic clues that indicate increasing anxiety. Read the list below and identify the cues that you commonly experience when anxious.

Physical Cues	Emotional Cues	Cognitive–Behavioral Cues
Dry mouth	Irritability	Forgetfulness
Profuse sweating	Fearfulness	Short attention span
Urinary frequency	Suspiciousness	Pacing and fidgeting
Nausea ("butterflies" in stomach)	Sadness	Withdrawal

Take a few minutes and reflect on a time when you were very anxious. How did you feel both physically and emotionally? What were your behaviors? If you feel comfortable doing so, share your responses with others and ask for feedback. Are their perceptions of your responses to anxiety-provoking situations similar to yours?

YOUR INTERVENTION STRATEGIES
Client With Anxiety

Strategy	Rationale
Use a quiet, calm approach.	Minimizes the interpersonal transmission of anxiety.
	Role-models expected behavior.
Observe the client's verbal and nonverbal behavior.	Anxiety is manifested verbally and nonverbally. Early detection of cues promotes prompt intervention to prevent escalation of anxiety.
Encourage the client to verbalize feelings.	The act of talking is cathartic and therefore reduces anxiety level.
	Identification of a problem is the first step in the problem-solving process.
Teach relaxation techniques when the client's anxiety is at a mild level.	Clients with moderate, severe, or panic-level anxiety are unable to process new information. Maximum learning is possible at the mild anxiety level.
Encourage the client to use relaxation techniques as needed.	The relaxation response counters hyperarousal of anxiety states.

YOUR INTERVENTION STRATEGIES
Activities That Promote Relaxation

Passive Behaviors	Active Behaviors
■ Soak in a warm bath.	■ Take a long walk.
■ Listen to soothing music.	■ Ride a bicycle.
■ Have a back rub or massage.	■ Phone someone and discuss your feelings.
■ Perform progressive muscle relaxation.	■ Organize your desk, pantry, or closet.
■ Take slow deep breaths, to counter the effects of hyperventilation.	■ Garden or mow the lawn.
	■ Paint a picture, or a house.

The relief afforded by the usual coping patterns does not last long because the needs or expectations that originally caused the symptoms still exist. The underlying needs may become even more intense. Clients can begin to change disturbed coping patterns only when they understand what their unmet needs are, what they did instead of fulfilling these needs, and their subsequent feelings.

Anxious clients have two alternatives. They can change their hopes and expectations, or they can try new tactics or resources to get their needs met. Discuss these options with the client, and negotiate a contract to work on one or both goals. Acting on either option involves problem solving. Simple physical activities often help reduce anxiety to more tolerable levels. Encourage adaptive mechanisms that work, such as the activities that promote relaxation discussed in Your Intervention Strategies: Activities That Promote Relaxation.

You can use a variety of techniques and skills in intervening with clients who experience anxiety. Cognitive–behavioral therapy helps individuals face their fears in order to cope. Progressive muscle relaxation, meditation to activate the relaxation response, thought-stopping techniques, autogenic training, and guided imagery may help clients learn new ways to reduce the disturbing affect. (Chapter 33 ∞ discusses several of these approaches.) Other methods include helping clients test reality, because their sense of danger is often out of proportion to actual danger. Developing goal-oriented contracts such as those suggested in Chapter 30 ∞ may help reduce a client's

sense of inner chaos by providing structure and direction. The use of contracts also actively involves clients in their own healing process. This involvement increases their sense of control, thereby alleviating feelings of powerlessness.

Teaching Clients About Medications

Teach clients about the major medications used to manage acute anxiety and their limitations and possible side effects. Anxiety that is secondary to major medical illness or acute trauma (such as the death of a child) requires a different dosage than that prescribed for the treatment of primary anxiety. A guide to medications for anxiety is offered by the Anxiety Disorders Association of America (http://www.adaa.org) and can be accessed through the Online Student Resources for this book.

Antianxiety medications (also known as *anxiolytics*) should be used cautiously and sparingly. Antianxiety medications (e.g., diazepam) are among the most overprescribed and abused drugs in the United States and Canada. Older adults are particularly sensitive to the effects of CNS depression associated with diazepam. If a benzodiazepine (BZD) is necessary for an older person, lorazepam (Ativan) or oxazepam (Serax) are safer because the risk of toxicity is lower than with longer-acting BZDs such as diazepam (Valium). The toxicity risk is lower due to the short elimination half-life and also because they are not active metabolites and are not metabolized actively in the liver. One study indicates that sertraline (Zoloft) and buspirone (BuSpar) seem to be effective in treating generalized anxiety disorder in older adults (Brown University, 2010).

BZDs have been shown to be effective and relatively safe in controlling situational anxiety for periods of 4 to 8 weeks. Antianxiety agents such as diazepam and alprazolam (Xanax), or adrenergic blocking agents such as propranolol (Inderal) are sometimes used. Some individuals have responded well to a combination of escitalopram (Lexapro) and cognitive–behavioral therapy (Schneier, Belzer, Kishon, Amsel, & Simpson, 2010).

Selective serotonin reuptake inhibitors (SSRIs) are generally first medications of choice for treating anxiety disorders because they exert fewer side effects than other medications. Other types of medications that can be used effectively in treating anxiety disorders include tricyclic antidepressants (TCAs), BZDs, beta blockers, atypical antipsychotic agents, and buspirone, which often helps clients cope with a moderate level of anxiety. Note that some antipsychotic medications may have a paradoxical effect and trigger the development of anxiety disorders. This is especially true of clozapine (Clozaril) as a precipitant to OCD in some individuals. When used to treat anxiety disorders, medications are started at a low dosage level and gradually increased until a therapeutic level is achieved. Inform clients that it may take up to 2 to 4 weeks before they begin to feel better. This information is crucial in helping clients continue to take the medication. These medications are discussed more fully in Chapters 7 and 31 ∞.

Although medications may alleviate the symptoms of anxiety, they do nothing to help clients understand the source of their anxiety. Ideally, these medications should be used for the short-term treatment of anxiety—days, weeks, or months instead of years. However, some clients may require longer-term treatment, depending on the degree of anxiety relief. Thus, it is necessary to closely monitor each client's anxiety level to determine the efficacy of medication. You will provide medication education to all clients; see Partnering With Clients and Families for some specific teaching guidelines for anxiolytic and antidepressant medications.

Promoting Effective Coping

Coping skills can be taught to clients with every type of anxiety disorder. In addition to anxiety alleviation, there are other therapeutic benefits to using previously learned coping skills, such as increased self-esteem, improved self-efficacy, and more effective problem solving. You need to demonstrate patience in order to project a sense of calm when working with anxious clients.

Interventions for Clients Experiencing Obsessive–Compulsive Disorder

Clients with OCD avoid anxiety by engaging in compulsive acts and rigid thinking. Regardless of your practice setting, you will likely encounter an obsessive–compulsive client whose problem is severe enough to require hospitalization such as in What Every Nurse Should Know. It is essential that you establish a therapeutic alliance with your clients. One way to foster a therapeutic bond is to let clients know that although their thoughts are irrational, they are individuals worthy of respect.

Clients with OCD use compulsive rituals to control anxiety. Therefore, schedule your intervention to avoid increasing the client's anxiety. It is usually countertherapeutic to interfere prematurely with a ritual unless it is life

WHAT EVERY NURSE SHOULD KNOW

Anxious Client in an Emergency Department

Imagine that you are a nurse in an emergency department:

- When clients enter your emergency department, it is important to assess their level of anxiety, just as you assess every client's vital signs and pain level.
- Knowing your client's level of anxiety will help determine your next action.
- Approach each client with a calm, reassuring manner; this will help the client feel less threatened and more secure.
- Involve clients in their own care as much as possible. This will increase their sense of control, which helps keep anxiety in check.
- Protect the safety of the client whose anxiety is escalating, as well as the safety of other clients and yourself.
- Call for help from team members immediately if your interventions have not de-escalated the client's anxiety.

threatening. Generally, the client needs plenty of time to complete the ritual. When the client is interrupted during or prohibited from performing the compulsive behavior, anxiety escalates. It is best to time therapeutic activities to occur immediately following the ritual because the client's anxiety level is temporarily decreased by the compulsive behavior.

Clients with OCD often have a strong tendency toward negativism, which may cause them to become more firmly entrenched in their defenses if modifications are introduced prematurely or hurriedly. Attempt to develop an affirming, dependable relationship before suggesting that clients change their behavior patterns, gradually introducing a substitute behavior. Balance the value of intervening in behavior that protects clients from mental anguish against the need to prevent physical deterioration caused by the behavior.

Interventions for Clients Experiencing Post-Traumatic Stress Disorder

Clients with PTSD frequently experience behavioral disturbances as a result of the intense anxiety triggered by re-experiencing the trauma. Alcohol or other drugs, when used to relieve anxiety, may contribute to destructive and

PARTNERING WITH CLIENTS AND FAMILIES

Teaching About Medications for Anxiety Disorder

- Drowsiness is a common side effect. Avoid activities requiring mental alertness, such as driving, until you know how the medication will affect you.
- Do not consume alcohol while taking this medication. Check labels on over-the-counter drugs and toiletries (e.g., mouthwash) because many contain alcohol.
- Because drinking caffeine decreases the effect of your medication, use decaffeinated beverages.
- Do not take other medications without first discussing it with your health care provider. Many drugs interact negatively with others.
- Do not increase the dosage or stop taking the medication without checking with your health care provider.

impulsive acts. Clients often experience disordered family relationships, physical disability, social and recreational disruptions, and impaired ability to work or attend school. They may experience symptoms and attitudes of demoralization that further hamper their functional abilities. In the acute stage, crisis counseling is essential. Because of the chronic course of PTSD and the many psychosocial problems associated with it, a comprehensive treatment approach is needed.

When planning care for the client with PTSD, determine the type and duration of trauma experienced. Was the trauma a single, brief incident? Several ongoing incidents? A human-induced trauma (combat or rape)? A natural trauma (hurricane or earthquake)? Natural disasters and human-induced traumatic events can have very different effects on an individual. For example, a survivor of human-induced trauma (such as rape) frequently experiences guilt and humiliation. After a natural disaster, a person may experience feelings of survivor guilt. The effects of trauma-included crises are discussed in chapter 34 ∞.

Clients with PTSD verbalize feelings of no longer being safe and will often exhibit passive–dependent behaviors. The goal of therapy in treating clients with PTSD is to desensitize them to the memories of the traumatic event so that they are able to cope with the anxiety. The techniques listed in Box 18-2 may be used singly or in combination to help alleviate anxiety.

Recent advances in psychopharmacology have led to the use of medication as an adjunct to the psychological treatment of PTSD. As is true for the other anxiety disorders, however, you must be aware of the heightened potential for chemical abuse among extremely anxious clients. The desire for immediate, total relief is powerful and may foster chemical abuse and dependence.

BZDs, TCAs, SSRIs, lithium, beta blockers, alpha-adrenergic antagonists, and neuroleptics have all been reported to relieve PTSD symptoms. During the initial stage (4 to 8 weeks) of PTSD, the use of BZDs may be helpful in the treatment of anxiety, insomnia, and nightmares.

Sleeplessness, another common feature of PTSD, is best treated with a behavioral approach such as relaxation techniques, guided imagery, muscle relaxation, and exclusion of daytime naps. Use of sedatives is discouraged except for a very brief time. Your goal is to help the client re-establish the ability to sleep naturally and cope more effectively without relying on the use of drugs. See TABLE 18-4 ■ for a partial list of medications that affect sleep.

Interventions for Clients Experiencing Phobic Disorders

Clients with phobic disorders attempt to avoid anxiety by symbolically binding it to a specific object or situation. It is essential to recognize that forcing clients to come into contact with the feared object or the basic source of their anxiety can create an intense, disorganizing flood of panic.

Many clinicians agree that clients with phobic coping patterns are highly resistant to most insight-oriented therapies. Such therapies require clients to confront and, at least temporarily, experience some of their originating anxiety. It is not surprising that insight-oriented therapists are ineffective with phobic clients, because avoidance is a major dynamic in phobias. Some symptomatic improvements have been made using techniques derived from behaviorist theory. The most commonly used interventions are desensitization, reciprocal inhibition, and cognitive restructuring. They are discussed in TABLE 18-5 ■ and in Chapter 30 ∞. Read Evidence-Based Practice on page 410 for an example of planning care for a client with social phobia.

Promoting Effective Communication

Nursing interventions that reduce anxiety are important measures to promote more effective communication and behavior. Often, simply offering the opportunity to acknowledge and discuss feelings of anxiety helps the client regain control. At this point, clients are more likely to share their concerns because you have already taken the first steps in demonstrating genuine interest and concern. See Rx Communication for the client with social phobia on page 410.

While encouraging the client to express feelings, be sure to listen attentively. Clients may express fear, anger, sadness, disappointment, or alienation, and it may be difficult for you to hear about the client's pain. Some nurses feel helpless in the face of their client's catharsis and think they should be able to provide ready answers. Instead, ready answers are more likely to interfere with and thwart the client's communication. Genuine, concerned listening without judgment or giving advice is an effective intervention in itself.

Explanations should be simple, clear, and concise. Be careful not to overload severely anxious people with more information than they can handle. If anxiety has contributed to knowledge deficit, reduce the anxiety before trying to teach

---

Box 18-2   Therapeutic Techniques for Clients with PTSD

- **Abreaction:** Focuses on exploring and reliving painful repressed experiences.
- **Cognitive restructuring:** Provides new, less threatening interpretations of events. Includes techniques such as thought stopping and thought substitution (see Chapter 30 ∞ for specific cognitive therapies).
- **Education:** Provides an explanation of the dynamics of the disability and of treatment modalities.
- **Exercise and nutrition:** Strengthens the body's adaptive resources.
- **Family conference/counseling:** Provides support to the client by encouraging the family to work on resolving the many psychosocial effects evoked by the trauma.
- **Group therapy:** Provides support and reinforces new coping skills.
- **Hypnosis:** Brings repressed material to conscious awareness so it can be integrated into the ego structure.
- **Individual therapy:** Provides important ego-supportive and/or cathartic benefits.
- **Relaxation training:** Focuses on developing new skills that the client may use when faced with memories of the traumatic event.

Note: You must have extra training such as graduate education or certification in order to practice hypnosis and abreaction.

TABLE 18-4 ■ Medications That Affect Sleep

Type	Examples	Comments
Antidepressants	Tricyclic antidepressants such as amitriptyline (Elavil)	Induce drowsiness to varying degrees; effect on insomnia associated with depression usually occurs earlier than antidepressant effect. Suppress REM.
	Selective serotonin reuptake inhibitors such as fluoxetine (Prozac)	Generally decrease total sleep time, increase wakefulness, may induce vivid dreaming.
Anticonvulsants	Phenytoin (Dilantin) and phenobarbital	Sedation common, less so with newer seizure control medications.
Antihistamines	Chlorpheniramine (Chlor-Trimeton) and pseudo-ephedrine compounds (Benylin cold capsules)	Induce drowsiness to varying degrees. Sometimes used as sleep-promoting agents because of their availability over the counter.
Antiparkinson medications	Levodopa–carbidopa combinations (Sinemet)	Low doses may improve sleep, but generally persons on medication for Parkinson's have poor sleep with insomnia, vivid dreaming.
Antipsychotics	Traditional antipsychotics such as chlorpromazine (Thorazine) and haloperidol (Haldol)	Chlorpromazine very sedating, haloperidol less so.
	Atypical antipsychotics such as clozapine (Clozaril), quetiapine (Seroquel), risperidone (Risperdal)	High incidence of sedation with clozapine and quetiapine, less so with risperidone.
Anxiolytics	Benzodiazepines such as temazepam (Restoril)	May be used as hypnotics to induce and sustain sleep (note differences between short- and long-acting types).
	Buspirone (BuSpar)	Little effect on sleep and alertness.
Caffeine	Additive to some pain and headache remedies, coffee, tea, colas	Increases wakefulness, effects may last 8–14 hours.
Cardiovascular medications	Antihypertensives such as propranolol (Inderal), clonidine (Catapres), captopril (Capoten)	Insomnia, sedation, and nightmares, less so with captopril and other angiotensin-converting enzyme inhibitors.
Corticosteroids	Prednisone	Generally disturb sleep, especially if taken late in the day; suppress REM sleep.
Hypnotics	Zopiclone (Imovane)	Effective for sleep-onset insomnia because of rapid absorption.
	Zolpidem (Ambien), zaleplon (Sonata), eszopiclone (Lunesta)	Indicated for treatment of insomnia by U.S. Food and Drug Administration.
	Flurazepam (Dalmane)	Longer half-life, useful for sleep onset and maintenance insomnia.
Mood stabilixers	Lithium (Lithane)	Improves sleep but may cause daytime sleepiness initially.

TABLE 18-5 ■ Cognitive–Behavioral Techniques for Treating Phobias

Technique	Description	Example
Systematic desensitization (exposure therapy)	A client is exposed to a series of increasingly anxiety-provoking situations, beginning with the least threatening. The client gradually becomes desensitized to each stimulus in the series until the stimulus that induced the most anxiety is no longer threatening.	A man who is terrified of earthworms might first talk about earthworms until the topic no longer evokes the same level of anxiety. Then he might be shown pictures of earthworms until he masters that level of closeness. Over time, he will progress to holding a live earthworm in his hand without experiencing severe or panic-level anxiety.
Reciprocal inhibition	The anxiety-provoking stimulus is paired with another stimulus associated with an opposite feeling strong enough to suppress the anxiety.	Through the use of meditation, yoga, biofeedback training, hypnosis, or antianxiety medications, clients learn how to induce a calm state.
Cognitive restructuring	This intervention is based on the belief that anxiety stems from erroneous interpretations of situations. The client learns to reframe (or relabel) a frightening situation, object, activity, or event so that it becomes less threatening.	A woman who fears she is going to die if she leaves her apartment learns to change her perception to one that is more reality based by saying, "I may feel uncomfortable but I will not die. I can do this."

EVIDENCE-BASED PRACTICE

Integrative Therapy for Anxiety

Charlene is a 19-year-old female client at a community mental health center. During her initial session, she tells you, the admitting nurse, her story: "I couldn't go on dates or to parties. For a while, I couldn't even go to class. My freshman year of college, I had to come home for a semester. My fear would happen in any social situation. I would be anxious before I even left the house, and it would escalate as I got closer to class, a party, or whatever. I would feel sick to my stomach—it almost felt like I had the flu. My heart would pound, my palms would get sweaty, and I would get this feeling of being removed from myself and from everybody else. When I would walk into a room full of people, I'd turn red and it would feel like everybody's eyes were on me. I was too embarrassed to stand off in a corner by myself, but I couldn't think of anything to say to anybody. I felt so clumsy, I couldn't wait to get out."

Your plan for intervention options is based on current research results. For example, in your review of cognitive–behavioral therapy (CBT) and social phobia, you understand that Charlene will likely experience positive long-lasting effects by participating in CBT groups.

After further sessions with Charlene, you determine that she has negative perceptions of her ability to interact with groups of peers at her college. Because of your understanding of current research findings, you decide to use the technique of cognitive restructuring with Charlene.

The multidisciplinary treatment team working with Charlene understands that current research shows the efficacy of BZDs and antidepressants in the treatment of social phobia. Therefore, Charlene is prescribed paroxetine (Paxil), an SSRI antidepressant, as an adjunct to the CBT group sessions and cognitive restructuring techniques.

This set of multiple intervention strategies is based on the following research:

Harvard Medical School. (2010). Treating social anxiety disorder. *Harvard Mental Health Letter, 26*(9), 1–4.

Jorstad-Stein, E. C., & Heimburg, R. G. (2009). Social phobia: An update on treatment. *Psychiatric Clinics of North America, 32*(3), 641–663.

CRITICAL THINKING QUESTIONS

1. Why would cognitive restructuring be helpful to Charlene?
2. How do SSRIs help individuals with anxiety disorders?
3. Is it realistic for Charlene to expect total remission?

about health or provide information. If the client's perceptual field (see Chapter 8 ∞) is narrow or disrupted, the client will be unable to assimilate information.

Clients with OCD require patience and an unhurried attitude, especially in regard to details and ruminations. If you use the techniques of paraphrasing and reflecting, these clients will say you did not get the details right. They will then go on to correct, qualify, and clarify. This striving for accuracy produces greater vagueness and confusion. It is as if parallel conversations are going on simultaneously. Clients hear only themselves repeating and correcting insignificant details and completely lose the overall meaning of the message. Developing patience in listening and skill in providing well-timed, simple direction is crucial to working effectively with clients with OCD.

Promoting Safety

Lack of coordination, tremors, and impaired concentration make anxious clients prone to accidents. Counsel clients not to perform potentially dangerous activities, such as driving a car, when anxiety is high. Advise them to move more slowly or to repeat instructions carefully when they undertake new tasks or use tools and/or equipment that are potentially dangerous. Provide this same instruction to clients receiving anxiolytics which can also affect their ability to perform potentially dangerous activities.

Promoting Optimal Tissue Perfusion

Tissue perfusion improves when anxiety is reduced. Focus on proper nutrition and adequate activity, because clients

R℟ COMMUNICATION

Client With Social Phobia

CLIENT: "I just had to get out of that room. I couldn't stand it with all those people looking at me. I thought I was going to die!"

NURSE RESPONSE 1: "That sounds very frightening. Tell me more about it."	**NURSE RESPONSE 2:** "Think of other times when you've felt that way. What helped you feel less frightened?"
RATIONALE: This response demonstrates reflection of the client's affect and encourages the client to continue to verbalize feelings.	*RATIONALE:* This response asks the client to identify specific coping methods that were helpful in a similar situation. Such methods can then be used in anticipatory planning for future anxiety-provoking situations.

with anxiety frequently overlook self-care and their health needs. Encourage clients to engage in activities that improve circulation. For example, walking and participating in sports promote healthy physiological functioning and should be part of a comprehensive treatment plan for anxious clients.

Promoting Effective Sensory Perception and Thought Processes

To function more effectively and independently, the client needs to know about normal anxiety and anxiety disorders. Providing accurate information at the right time and in an appropriate manner is an essential nursing responsibility. Other nursing strategies to promote effective perception and cognition include the following:

- Use adjuncts to verbal communication, such as visual aids or role-playing, to enhance the retention of information.
- Practice problem-solving vignettes to improve judgment and insight.
- Identify misperceptions that clients hold as a result of a narrowed perceptual field. Begin with comments such as "I wonder if you've considered this possibility?" or "Perhaps if we tried. . . ."
- Help clients perform a reality test, that is, explore their opinions in the light of validated experience rather than emotional needs that block accurate perception.

Promoting Sleep

Nonpharmacologic nursing measures to promote sleep should be used before medications. Such measures may include a variety of relaxation techniques. One effective method is the use of music that promotes a relaxing atmosphere; listening to the sounds of nature is soothing and induces sleep in some people.

Suggest that the client read a boring book in bed, drink warm decaffeinated liquids, or take a warm bath before retiring. A client with PTSD may fear going to sleep because of nightmares. Having another member of the family nearby and aware of the client's fear may be reassuring. Other suggestions for helping anxious clients sleep are listed in Partnering With Clients and Families.

Evaluation

Evaluation is used to determine the client's response to interventions. In other words, is the client demonstrating progress? Are the anxiety-related symptoms decreasing? Does the client use coping skills effectively? In addition to these questions, it is also important to evaluate clients in the following areas: anxiety, coping ability, role performance, communication, safety, thought processes, perception, tissue perfusion, and sleep.

Anxiety

Specific client outcomes indicative of decreased anxiety levels are described in this section. Clients will show no evidence of acute or intense anxiety and be able to perform activities of daily living independently when appropriate. Clients will verbalize feeling less anxious, they will have fewer somatic complaints, and they will state they feel more comfortable.

Clients will have fewer symptoms of physiological distress, such as racing pulse, diaphoresis, and/or hyperventilation. Clients will be without signs of increased psychomotor activity. They will no longer complain of tearfulness, feelings of rage, or impatience. When appropriate, they will more readily engage in interactions with others. Although they may feel some anxiety, phobic clients will tolerate the presence of the feared object, activity, or situation without experiencing panic or the need to flee.

Individual Coping

Clients will demonstrate the ability to continue with necessary activities even though some anxiety is present. They will be

---

PARTNERING WITH CLIENTS AND FAMILIES

Teaching About Improving Sleep Quality

1. Think about the kind of sleep schedule that seems to fit you best.
2. Make a list of things that help you get to sleep (how dark you like it to be, what temperature, how you get ready for bed).
3. Jot down all the "rules" and "suggestions" you have heard about how to get better sleep. Cross out the ones that don't seem to fit. (Some people sleep better by not having a bedtime snack; other people sleep better after having a snack. Do what feels best for you. If you aren't sure, try an experiment doing it one way for a week and then the other way for the next week.) Put a question mark by the rules and suggestions you have never really tried, and underline the ones you think are important for you.

4. Consider what you could change to get an extra half-hour of sleep each night.
5. Keep a sleep diary for 2 weeks. For the first week, just keep track of your usual pattern (time you went to bed and got up, number of hours of actual sleep, how you felt in the morning, etc.). At the end of the first week, review the diary and your responses to items 1 through 4. In the second week, experiment with one change you think would be helpful to you.
6. Carry on the process a bit longer if you like, but remember:
   - You can manage on very little sleep if you have to.
   - You know better than anyone else what works for you.
   - Your needs and preferences regarding sleep may change as you get older or take on different roles and activities.

less likely to panic or flee. Family members will report that clients are "more like their old selves" and appear less agitated, driven, or explosive in conduct. The client with OCD will limit or cease performing compulsive rituals; for example, a client with a handwashing compulsion will wash hands no more than six times a day.

Role Performance

The client will attend work or school on a regular basis. Family members will report that relationships at home have improved and that the client is once again participating in family activities. Clients will report engaging in recreational or social activities and independently performing self-care. They will express feeling more comfortable about their performance at home, work, or school. Phobic clients will perform daily activities with less restriction or interference from any feared object, activity, event, or situation.

Communication and Safety

Clients will state satisfaction with their communication; they feel heard and understood. There will be open lines of communication between client and nurse and client and family. Clients will report no tremors and will experience no accidents due to poor motor coordination or concentration difficulties. They will report being able to perform the usual small motor tasks, such as writing, in a competent manner.

Thought Processes and Sensory Perception

Clients will be able to recall information you teach them. They will begin to make decisions about their health care and ask questions about anxiety. Clients will describe what led to their anxiety and what happened after they felt anxious. They will verbalize techniques to reduce anxiety. Clients will correctly verbalize the use, side effects, and results of taking

their medications. They will verbalize increased awareness of their environment.

Tissue Perfusion

Clients will report feeling energetic. Somatic complaints will decrease, and clients will report engaging in daily physical activity. Vital signs will be normal, and weight will be stable. When testing the client's capillary refill, you will find it to be normal as a result of the improved perfusion.

Sleep

Clients will sleep through the night without medication or with appropriately prescribed medication. They will have fewer nightmares and waken less frequently during the night. Clients will demonstrate energy during the day as a result of restful sleep during the previous night.

CASE MANAGEMENT

The case manager plays an essential role in collaborating with clients, families, and significant others by providing information about when and where to seek help. The case manager also monitors clients for adherence to the aftercare plan, including the client's medication usage. Issues to be considered during outpatient therapy include: identifying personal strengths, establishing realistic time frames for outcomes, identifying and strengthening support systems, and locating and using community support services.

COMMUNITY-BASED CARE

Individuals with anxiety disorders are usually aware that their behaviors are problematic to themselves and others. However, insight alone does not necessarily result in behavioral changes. Or, when change does occur, it is a very gradual process. As a result, people with anxiety disorders are often treated in the community—in mental health clinics, crisis centers, and therapists' offices.

HOME CARE

Nurses who provide psychiatric–mental health care in the home fulfill a significant role in helping clients with anxiety disorders improve their social interactions and shape behavior. The following interventions are especially helpful for homebound clients experiencing anxiety disorders:

- Meet with the client and family member or significant other to discuss realistic expectations for the client.
- Teach the client home management skills necessary for independent living.
- Determine with the client if testing, placement services, or job skill retraining are desired.
- Refer the client and family to community agencies as needed.

WHY I PLAN TO BECOME A PSYCHIATRIC–MENTAL HEALTH NURSE

Roydella's Story: My clients in the medical–surgical setting are the reason I am going to be a psychiatric–mental health nurse. The things that struck me so often are how their mental attitude either helped or hindered their recovery and how their illnesses caused them to feel stressed and anxious. I found it impossible to try and separate body from mind. They are really interwoven. You can tell someone what to expect after surgery, how to care for their colostomy, how to administer their own insulin, when it's OK to have sex after a heart attack, but if you don't take their level of anxiety into account, they're not likely to hear you. And, if they don't hear you, they aren't likely to do what they need to do to get better. I'm going to work in a state hospital after I graduate. Then, after 1 or 2 years, I plan to go to graduate school and get a master's degree in psychiatric–mental health nursing. I'd like to eventually be in private practice for myself.

NURSING CARE PLAN: A CLIENT WITH PANIC DISORDER WITH AGORAPHOBIA

Identifying Information

Mrs. Randolph is 43 years old, married, and the mother of four daughters in their late teens and early twenties. She was referred to the psychiatric outpatient clinic for follow-up counseling by the emergency department of the local general hospital, where she had been seen on the previous day with symptoms of a panic attack.

History

At the time of the panic attack, Mrs. Randolph believed she was having a heart attack and feared she was dying. She reported racing heartbeat, sweating, and feeling faint. She could not identify any events, thoughts, or feelings that precipitated the incident; it seemed to her to occur "out of the blue." She felt unable to cope with the severity of the symptoms of the attack: "I tried to talk myself out of it; to tell myself it would go away, but it only got worse."

Mrs. Randolph reported she had had similar attacks over the years and that she had always been reassured of her medical and cardiac health, but when these attacks occurred, she "feared the worst" and "lost all perspective." The previous attacks had lasted from 2 minutes to 2 hours. Her daily routine had become quite restricted, because she now sought to have one of her daughters or her husband with her when she went out of the home due to fear of an attack. She did not feel comfortable when alone in her home and could not go to sleep if the other family members were not home. She felt ashamed and angry about her growing disability and often tried to cover up her fears to friends and family.

By interviewing the family, the nurse was able to gather information about a number of significant recent life events preceding the panic episode:

- Recent major surgery: She had a hysterectomy 4 weeks earlier.
- Loss of employment due to her hospitalization: She was abruptly terminated

from her position at a new job because of too many absences.
- There is an upcoming anniversary of her father's sudden death from a heart attack.

Mrs. Randolph had never been hospitalized for a psychiatric condition, although she had been to the emergency department on three prior occasions with symptoms of panic attack. She had seen a therapist years ago when the attacks first occurred, "about the time I left home to marry." She did not follow up with the therapist, however, saying she felt ashamed ("I've always been a strong and effective person!"), that the episodes were not so severe at that time, and that she found relief from panic attacks after she had the children.

Both Mrs. Randolph's parents died within the past 6 years. She was especially close to her father, and the second anniversary of his death was approaching. Mrs. Randolph's mother was considered a "homebody"; she rarely left the house and took part in social activities only if they occurred at the family home. Mrs. Randolph wondered if her mother had "these fears" too. She reported she had begun to curtail social and recreational activities, preferring to stay at home where she was most comfortable.

She described her relationship with her husband as emotionally warm and supportive. Although she sometimes resented his being away from her, she recognized this as part of her "problem" with being alone. Her primary relationships had been with her husband and children. She talked of facing the "empty nest" as her daughters, one by one, left for work or college.

With the exception of chronic gynecologic problems leading to the recent hysterectomy, Mrs. Randolph reported a history of good health. She had no allergies or other chronic illnesses. Her only other hospitalizations were to have her children. The recent hospitalization had been more physically taxing than she

expected, and the fact that she was not allowed to return to work after her recovery came as a blow.

Current Mental Status

Mrs. Randolph is an attractive, carefully groomed woman who looks her stated age. She sits erect in the office chair, appearing somewhat tense. She answers questions cooperatively, but at times with some hesitation as if expecting criticism or judgment from the interviewer.

She is oriented to time, place, and person. Her memory is intact and her recall good. She has no difficulty with calculations. Her judgment is unimpaired. During times of panic, however, sensory and perceptive awareness are greatly impaired.

Affect appears normal, with occasional evidence of anger in the form of irritability and light sarcasm. Mood is within normal limits.

Speech is normal in flow and volume. It appears pressured at times when she attempts to correct an impression she believes the interviewer holds. Posture is at times rigid, but she relaxes as she becomes more comfortable during the interview.

There are no delusions, ideas of reference, or hallucinations. Obsessive worry about the occurrence of panic episodes and her safety is present. Embarrassment and shame over her symptoms are apparent. Suicidal or homicidal thoughts are denied. Associations and abstractions are appropriate, and there is no evidence of thought process disorder or difficulty in concentration, except during acute panic, at which times concentration is impaired and thought processes are disorganized. Some guardedness toward the interviewer is noted. Insight into the meaning of the current situation is minimal.

Other Clinical Data

Mrs. Randolph is considering the use of antianxiety medication, despite "hating the idea" of medication.

Nursing Diagnosis: Ineffective Role Performance related to fear and anxiety level

Expected Outcome: Mrs. Randolph will demonstrate role performance as evidenced by: ability to meet role expectations, knowledge of role transition periods, and reported strategies for role changes.

(Continued)

NURSING CARE PLAN: A CLIENT WITH PANIC DISORDER WITH AGORAPHOBIA (*Continued*)

Short-Term Goals	Interventions	Rationales
Describe specific changes in role function.	▪ Maintain a calm manner.	A calm approach prevents escalation of anxiety.
	▪ Stay with Mrs. Randolph.	Mrs. Randolph's panic is alleviated.
	▪ Use short, simple sentences.	Simple language facilitates anxious clients' ability to concentrate and follow direction.
	▪ Direct Mrs. Randolph's attention to repetitive or physical task.	Distraction serves as an outlet for anxious energy.
	▪ Administer antianxiety medication.	Medication reduces anxiety by altering brain chemistry.

Nursing Diagnosis: Disturbed Thought Processes related to high level of anxiety

Expected Outcome: Mrs. Randolph will demonstrate ability to choose between two or more alternatives.

Short-Term Goals	Interventions	Rationales
Demonstrate appropriate decision making.	▪ Teach relaxation exercises.	Anxiety impairs the ability to concentrate and solve problems.
	▪ Encourage Mrs. Randolph to identify previous coping skills.	Use of previously learned skills can reduce anxiety level.
	▪ Limit number of available options.	Avoids overwhelming the client.

Nursing Diagnosis: Ineffective Coping related to overwhelming fears

Expected Outcome: Mrs. Randolph uses actions to manage stressors that tax personal resources.

Short-Term Goals	Interventions	Rationales
Demonstrate effective coping as evidenced by employing behaviors to reduce stress and reporting decreased negative feelings.	▪ Help Mrs. Randolph identify coping resources (including social supports).	Mrs. Randolph becomes aware of existing resources.
	▪ Teach Mrs. Randolph relaxation techniques.	Relaxation counters the stress response.
	▪ Encourage Mrs. Randolph to verbalize feelings.	Verbalization reduces stress through process of catharsis.

Pearson Nursing Student Resources
Find additional review materials at nursing.pearsonhighered.com

Prepare for success with NCLEX®-style practice questions, interactive assignments and activities, web links, animations and videos, and more!

REFERENCES

American Psychiatric Association. (2000). *Diagnostic and statistical manual of mental disorders* (4th ed., Text Revision). Washington, DC: Author.

Anxiety Disorders Association of America. (2010–2011). *Pregnancy and medication.* Retrieved from http://www.adaa.org/living-with-anxiety/women/pregnancy-and-medication

Bourne, E. J. (2011). *The anxiety and phobia workbook* (5th ed.). Oakland, CA: New Harbinger Publications.

Brown University. (2010). Geriatric psychopharmacy update. *Brown University Geriatric Psychopharmacology Update, 14*(5), 1, 607.

Children's Center for OCD and Anxiety. (2009). *Pediatric autoimmune neuropsychiatric disorders associated with strep (PANDAS): A subtype of OCD.* Retrieved from http://www.worrywisekids.org/anxiety/pandas.html

Etkin, A., Prater, K. E., Hoeft, F., Menon, V., & Schatzberg, A. F. (2010). Failure of anterior cingulate activation and connectivity with the amygdala during implicit regulation of emotional processing in generalized anxiety disorder. *American Journal of Psychiatry, 167*(5), 454–554.

Hale, L., Do, D. P., Basurto-Davila, R., Heron, M., Finch, B., Dubowitz, T., ... Bird, C. E. (2009). Does mental health history explain gender disparities in insomnia symptoms among young adults? *Sleep Medicine, 10*(10), 1118–1123. doi: 10.1016/i.sleep.2008.12.011

Harvard Medical School. (March 2010). Treating social anxiety disorder. *Harvard Mental Health Letter, 26*(9), 1–4.

Jorstad-Stein, E. C., & Heimburg, R. G. (2009). Social phobia: An update on treatment. *Psychiatric Clinics of North America, 32*(3), 641–663.

National Institute of Mental Health. (2010). *Statistics.* Retrieved from http://www.nimh.nih.gov/statistics.index/shtml

Paulesu, E., Sambugaro, E., Torti, T., Daneli, L., Ferri, F., Scialfa, G., ... Sassaroli, S. (2010). Neural correlates of worry in generalized anxiety disorder and in normal controls: A functional MRI study. *Psychological Medicine, 40*(1), 117–124.

Rank, O. (1952). *The trauma of birth.* Philadelphia, PA: Robert Brunner.

Sadock, B. J., & Sadock, V. A. (2010). *Kaplan & Sadock's pocket handbook of clinical psychiatry* (5th ed.). Philadelphia, PA: Lippincott Williams & Wilkins.

Schneier, F. R., Belzer, K. D., Kishon, R., Amsel, L., & Simpson, H. B. (2010). Escitalopram for persistent symptoms of generalized anxiety disorder after CBT: A pilot study. *Journal of Nervous & Mental Diseases, 198*(6), 458–461.

Sullivan, H. S. (1953). *The interpersonal theory of psychiatry.* New York, NY: Norton.

Walitza, S., Wendland, J. R., Gruenblatt, E., Warnke, A., Sontag, R. A., Tucha, O., ... Lange, K. W. (2010). Genetics of early-onset obsessive-compulsive disorder. *European Child and Adolescent Psychiatry, 19*(3), 227–235.

19

Dissociative, Somatoform, and Factitious Disorders

SUE C. DELAUNE

LEARNING OUTCOMES

After completing this chapter, you will be able to:

1. Describe theories that aid in the understanding of dissociative, somatoform, and factitious disorders.
2. Compare and contrast the biopsychosocial characteristics of various dissociative, somatoform, and factitious disorders.
3. Differentiate among somatoform disorders, factitious disorders, and malingering.
4. Perform a thorough and comprehensive assessment of clients with dissociative, somatoform, and factitious disorders.
5. Incorporate an understanding of therapeutic interventions for clients experiencing selected dissociative, somatoform, and factitious disorders into their plan of care.
6. Analyze possible personal challenges to professional practice when caring for clients with dissociative, somatoform, and factitious disorders.

CRITICAL THINKING CHALLENGE

Barbara, a 32-year-old female diagnosed with dissociative identity disorder, has been admitted to the emergency department for attempting suicide by slashing her wrists. This is Barbara's fourth admission for self-inflicted wounds. You, the RN on duty, overhear another staff member refer to Barbara as someone who is "faking" her illness in order to gain attention. This staff person says that he does not believe in the existence of dissociative disorders; that "people who say they have multiple personalities are making up their symptoms just to get some sympathy, just like people who claim to suddenly remember sexual abuse from childhood."

1. Is this staff member's assessment an accurate one? Why, or why not?
2. What elements would you consider in formulating a response to the staff member?
3. Should recovered memories of childhood sexual abuse be taken seriously?

As you know, individuals respond to stress in a variety of ways. Some experience *dissociative disorders*—alterations of consciousness, memory, perception, or identity. Feelings of being unreal, forgetting one's name and past personal history, and splitting into various personalities are characteristic of dissociative disorders. Some individuals have a maladaptive response to stress in which they unconsciously (not deliberately or with intention) transform their emotions into physical symptoms—called a *somatoform disorder,* in which the pain of psychogenic origin is as hurtful as pain with a biologic basis. Occasionally, an individual will pretend to be ill in order to receive a benefit. This process is called a *factitious disorder.* Another disorder in which a client feigns an illness is called *malingering,* which is classified by the American Psychiatric Association (APA) as a condition that may require clinical attention (APA, 2000). Individuals experiencing dissociative or somatoform disorders are sometimes mistakenly considered to be malingering. This chapter emphasizes the differences between dissociative disorder, somatoform disorder, factitious disorder, and malingering. Most clients with these disorders are treated in community settings.

DISSOCIATIVE DISORDERS

Dissociative disorders have, as their common denominator, the defense mechanism of dissociation, in which the client strips an idea, object, or situation of its emotional significance and affective content. (Dissociation and other defense mechanisms are explored in Chapter 8 ∞). Dissociation is a defense against trauma that separates emotions from behaviors. Consciousness, memory, identity, or perception of the environment are impaired in these disorders.

Dissociative disorders are complex and are usually difficult to distinguish from one another; see DSM Essential Features for a comparison of the disorders. In every dissociative disorder, a cluster of related mental events is beyond the client's power of recall but can return spontaneously to conscious awareness. Dissociative disorders are not attributable to mental disorders that have an organic basis, such as dementia. Dissociation is a possible response to extreme trauma, especially trauma experienced during childhood. See Chapter 24 for a discussion of childhood sexual abuse as well as Caring for the Spirit: Repressed Memories or False Memories? in Chapter 8 ∞ on page 154 for a discussion of recovered memory of childhood sexual abuse.

Dissociative Amnesia

Amnesia is a loss of or failure of memory caused by problems in the functioning of the memory areas of the brain. Amnesia can result from concussions, traumatic brain injury, alcoholism (Korsakoff's syndrome; see Chapter 15 ∞), or disorders of the aging brain. *Retrograde amnesia* is a loss of memory for events that occurred prior to the onset of the problem. For example, a hockey player who sustains a head trauma in a game might find that the prior year has been erased. *Anterograde amnesia* is a loss of memory for events that occurred after the onset of the problem. In this instance, the hockey player may find himself unable to remember people he has met after the injury, or where he has parked his car. Dissociative amnesia differs in its cause; its cause is psychological rather than physical.

People with **dissociative amnesia** have one or more episodes of memory loss of important personal information. They suddenly become aware that they have a total loss of memory for events that occurred during a period that may range from a few hours to a whole lifetime. In *localized amnesia,* the most common form, a person forgets only specific and related past times, usually surrounding a disturbing event. *Selective amnesia* for some, but not all, of the events is less common. Least common are *generalized amnesia,* which encompasses the person's entire life, and *continuous amnesia,* in which the person cannot recall events up to a specific time, including the present. *Systematized amnesia* is the loss of memory for certain categories of information, such as all memories related to one's occupation, or all memories related to one's family. Mental Health in the News showcases a current unsolved mystery about a person with dissociative amnesia.

Dissociative Fugue

A person with **dissociative fugue** wanders, usually far from home and for days, perhaps even weeks or months, at a time. During this period, clients completely forget their past life and associations; but unlike people with amnesia, they are unaware of having forgotten anything. When they return to their former consciousness, they do not remember the period of fugue. Clients experiencing dissociative fugue are generally reclusive and quiet, so their behavior rarely attracts attention. During this period, they appear to function unremarkably,

---

DSM ESSENTIAL FEATURES

Dissociative Disorders

Dissociative Amnesia: Inability to recall important personal information, usually of a psychologically traumatic nature; memory loss is too extensive to be caused by simple forgetfulness.

Dissociative Fugue: Sudden, unexpected travel away from home or workplace accompanied by inability to remember one's past, confusion about personal identity, or the assumption of a new identity.

Dissociative Identity Disorder: Presence of two or more distinct personality states or identities; the personality states take control of the person's behavior; accompanied by inability to remember personal information; characterized by identity fragmentation.

Depersonalization Disorder: Persistent or recurrent feeling of being detached from one's thoughts or body; accompanied by intact reality testing.

MENTAL HEALTH IN THE NEWS

Benjaman Kyle

Known now as Benjaman Kyle, the man in the photo has been diagnosed as having dissociative amnesia. Benjaman was discovered badly sunburned near a Burger King dumpster in Richmond Hill, Georgia on August 31, 2004. He has some memories—of living in Indianapolis as a child as well as memories of the area around the University of Colorado at Boulder, and recalls having brothers and attending a Catholic school. In late 2004 and 2005, Kyle was diagnosed with schizophrenia and treated in a

psychiatric facility. Major efforts to identify Kyle have been unsuccessful thus far. An appearance on the *Dr Phil* show in 2008 failed to turn up any useful leads despite 17 million viewers and the efforts of a well-known investigator with more than a decade of experience as an FBI case manager hired by the show. The efforts of Colleen Fitzpatrick, a well-known forensic genealogist have also failed to determine Kyle's identity. A documentary about him, with the working title *Who is Benjaman Kyle*, is scheduled for release in 2011.

Photo courtesy of n03/ZUMA Press/Newscom.

but may behave in a manner inconsistent with their usual pattern of functioning. They may assume a completely new and apparently well-integrated identity during the fugue state. Dissociative fugue has been blamed for the 11-day disappearance of the mystery writer, Agatha Christie.

Dissociative Identity Disorder

Formerly known as multiple personality disorder, **dissociative identity disorder (DID)** is the presence of two or more distinct identities within one individual. Each identity, called an **alter**, at some time takes full control of the person's behavior. Each alter has a unique identity, holds different feelings and memories, and performs different functions. Alters may differ in other ways as well. One alter may have Type II diabetes or asthma while the others may not. Some may be right-handed; others left-handed. Allergies and vision may differ. The voice may differ depending on which alter is in control. Usually, the person's main identity state is unaware of the others' existence.

There is much controversy about dissociative identity disorder. Many professionals are skeptical that such a phenomenon exists. Initially, DID was thought to be a rare condition. Once the popular books and movies *Sybil* and *Three Faces of Eve* brought DID to public attention, the incidence of DID increased dramatically. Controversy exists over whether bringing the condition to public attention encouraged more people to share their symptoms and mental health professionals to make more accurate diagnoses, or encouraged people to fake their symptoms for other more devious purposes. The Mental Health in the Movies feature in Chapter 12 ∞ on page 220 explores the case of Sybil and the therapist's possible role in "creating" her client's multiple personalities. However, clinical evidence of the existence of DID abounds. Refer to the website for the International Society for the Study of Trauma and Dissociation (http://www.isstd.org), which can be accessed through the Online Student Resources for this book.

Depersonalization Disorder

The central feature of **depersonalization disorder** is one or more episodes of feeling detached from oneself so that the usual sense of personal reality is temporarily lost or changed. The individual feels mechanical. Clyde's experience with depersonalization disorder is recounted in the following clinical example.

Clinical Example

Clyde feels as if he is living in a dream or a movie. It seems to him as if he can observe his own life. He explains his experiences by saying, "I don't feel real anymore. It's like I can watch my life as if it's a TV show. I'm afraid I'm going crazy."

The feelings experienced by people with depersonalization disorder are **ego-dystonic**, meaning that they are unacceptable to the person's sense of self as opposed to **ego-syntonic**, meaning in concert with the person's sense of self. The client has intact reality testing; in other words, the client is not experiencing hallucinations or delusions.

BIOPSYCHOSOCIAL THEORIES

Although biologic and genetic factors are being studied as potential etiologic factors, psychosocial theories are used most often to explain dissociative disorders.

Biologic and Genetic Factors

Physiological and neurobiologic functions play a significant role in the development of amnesia and dissociative disorders. For example, the neurotransmitter serotonin affects recall of information. The formation and retrieval of memories relies on intact function of the hippocampus and the limbic system.

- Research suggests that the limbic system may be impaired in individuals who have experienced traumatic experiences in childhood (Sadock & Sadock, 2010).
- One study implicates trauma as an inhibiting factor on the person's ability to process information; there is a disturbance in the cortical visual system (Manning & Manning, 2009).
- Physical illnesses (such as brain tumors, epilepsy, and migraine headaches) may lead to symptoms indicative of depersonalization disorder. Certain drugs (e.g., alcohol, barbiturates, benzodiazepines, and hallucinogens) may cause some people to experience depersonalization symptoms (Sadock & Sadock, 2010).
- One study describes the onset of dissociative disorder after electroconvulsive therapy (ECT) and suggests that ECT may be a risk factor for the occurrence of dissociative episodes (Zaidner et al., 2010).

International Society for the Study of Trauma and Dissociation

According to the DSM-IV-TR, dissociative identity disorder occurs more often in first-degree biologic relatives of people with the disorder (APA, 2000).

Psychosocial Theories

Pierre Janet (1859–1947) was the first to develop the concept of the "splitting off," or dissociation, of a part of consciousness. He believed that the individual needed a normal amount of "mental energy" to maintain integrative mental processes. When the level of energy was high, integration was maintained. When it became low, however, the personality might cease to function as a unit and split or dissociate.

Freud, in contrast, proposed the concept of repression to explain the loss of conscious awareness in dissociation. He then introduced the notion of the dynamic unconscious, a part of the mind in which emotions or ideas that were unacceptable to a person were pushed from awareness. Freud and other early analytic theorists accepted the basic concept of psychological dissociation.

Current explanations of dissociation are based on Freud's dynamic concepts. The repression of ideas that leads to amnesia and other forms of dissociation is conceived of as a way of protecting the individual from emotional pain. External circumstances or internal psychological conflicts are viewed as precipitating factors. A dissociative reaction may be viewed as a flight from crisis or danger—a major psychological route of escape from anxiety. Sometimes, as in states of dissociative fugue and dissociative identity disorder, the dissociated area temporarily assumes direction and control of the entire personality. During such times, the person may appear to be functioning well.

Dissociative identity disorder originates in childhood as a result of chronic trauma, usually child abuse. The trauma may be physical, psychological, or both. The major form of child abuse that contributes to the development of DID is sexual abuse. In attempts to cope with the horror of reality, the child's ego splits through the dissociative process. Each trauma-induced dissociative experience shapes the development of alternate personalities (alters). Chronic abuse leads to a fixation of the dissociated ego splits. Through dissociation, the child may see the abuse as if it were occurring to someone else, as in a movie. This ability to remove the self from the abuse is a mechanism that allows the individual to survive. The development of dissociative identity disorder is illustrated in FIGURE 19-1 ■.

Additional dynamic considerations relevant to dissociative disorders include the following ideas. In dissociative amnesia, the pattern is similar to conversion disorder (discussed later in this chapter in the Somatoform Disorders section) except that the individual does not avoid some unpleasant situation by getting sick. Instead, the person does so by forgetting (repressing) certain traumatic events or stresses. In DID, there appears to be a deep-seated conflict between contradictory impulses and beliefs. A resolution is achieved by separating the conflicting parts and developing each into an autonomous personality or alter.

Behavioral Theories

Behavioral theorists explain the development of dissociative disorders as learned behaviors. An individual learns that avoidance behavior provides protection from a painful experience. After repeated experiences, this avoidance pattern is reinforced. Behavioral theory is the framework for many behavioral and cognitive–behavioral methods currently used in treating symptoms associated with dissociative disorders.

Humanistic Theories

Individuals with dissociative disorders have experienced intense psychological trauma during early childhood. As nurses, we take a holistic approach in dealing with these clients by accepting the fact that the dissociation was used as a defense mechanism that kept the abused child intact. Humanistic theories view the individual as a composite of life experiences, psychobiologic factors, and interpersonal interactions. Individuals are also viewed within the context of their culture. See Developing Cultural Competence for a listing of culture-bound syndromes that may be misdiagnosed as dissociative disorders (APA, 2000).

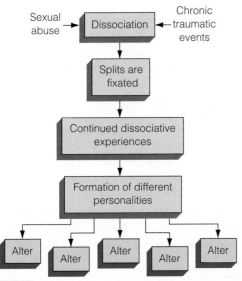

FIGURE 19-1 ■ The development of dissociative identify disorder.

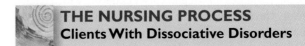

THE NURSING PROCESS
Clients With Dissociative Disorders

When caring for clients with dissociative symptoms, you must use a systematic approach in order to provide holistic, compassionate care. Most clients with dissociative disorders are treated in community rather than inpatient settings.

Assessment

It can become extremely challenging when you begin to gather data on a client with dissociative symptoms. For example, the client's amnesia will likely be problematic when you are collecting a health history. The major areas to focus on

DEVELOPING CULTURAL COMPETENCE

Culture-Bound Syndromes That Can Be Misdiagnosed as Dissociative Disorders

Amok A dissociative episode; characterized by a period of brooding followed by a violent outburst; precipitated by a perceived insult; occurs only in males in Malaysia, Laos, Philippines, Papua New Guinea, Polynesia (*cafard* or *cathard*), Puerto Rico (*mal de pelea*), and among the Navajo (*iich'aa*).

Ataque de Nervios An episode of distress, usually a result of a stressful event involving the family; common symptoms include uncontrollable shouting, crying, heat in the chest rising to the head, and verbal or physical aggression. Dissociative experiences, such as amnesia about the symptoms, may be experienced. Occurs primarily among Latinos from the Caribbean, but also recognized among many Latin American and Latin Mediterranean groups.

Latah Hypersensitivity to sudden fright, often with dissociative or trancelike behavior. Other symptoms include echolalia and echopraxia. Primarily occurs in Malaysia and Indonesia; in Malaysia it is more frequent in middle-aged women.

Spell A trance state in which individuals "communicate" with deceased relatives or spirits; associated with brief periods of personality change. Seen among African Americans and European Americans from the southern United States.

CRITICAL THINKING QUESTIONS

1. Why is it important to know a client's cultural background?
2. How does knowledge of a client's cultural background help you develop therapeutic interventions?

during assessment are identity, memory, and consciousness. Some other areas to assess are awareness of time, amount of unfinished tasks, goal setting, and inconsistent work attendance (Precin & Precin, 2011).

Subjective Data

Clients with dissociative disorders often report a sudden loss of memory of events. Clients may report, for example, that they cannot recall certain important personal events or information. They may not recall important aspects of their own identity, such as their age and where they reside. As you interview clients, listen to their pronoun usage. If the client uses "we" when speaking, this may indicate the presence of alters.

Sometimes amnesia is only partial, and clients remain conscious of what happened, although they report that they feel no control over it. In cases of complete amnesia, the "lost" memories can be recovered under certain therapeutic circumstances (e.g., hypnosis), or they may return spontaneously. Clients who have sustained a loss of their own reality may have adopted a new identity.

If motor behavior is affected in dissociative disorders, clients or their families may report episodes during which clients physically traveled away from home. In clients with DID, the original personality typically is not aware of the existence of the secondary personalities. However, the secondary personalities may be aware of the original personality as well as of each other and may report this awareness to the staff. Clients with depersonalization disorder may report fears that they are going crazy and experience resulting anxiety. See Your Assessment Approach for assessment guidelines for clients with depersonalization disorder.

Objective Data

Conduct a careful assessment of the client's physical condition to rule out the possibility of organic causes, such as a brain tumor. Many of the behaviors of clients with dissociative disorders resemble behaviors associated with organic conditions, including postconcussional amnesia and temporal lobe epilepsy. Your observations of the character, duration, frequency, and context of the dissociative disorder are crucial data. Physical examinations are not continued as part of the long-term intervention program, however, because they

---

YOUR ASSESSMENT APPROACH
Client With Depersonalization Disorder

To determine feelings of unreality, listen for the following client statements:

- "I just feel weird."
- "I'm not myself."
- "I feel like I'm floating away."

To determine altered bodily perceptions, listen for the following client statements:

- "My body doesn't feel real."
- "I looked at my arm and saw that it looked like a piece of wood."
- "When I was looking in the mirror, it was like the image was looking back at me."

To determine impaired behavioral perceptions, listen for the following client statements:

- "I feel like I'm on automatic pilot."
- "I'm walking through life like a zombie."
- "I feel like I'm a machine or a robot."

To determine altered external perceptions, listen for the following client statements:

- "Everything feels different . . . like I'm in a dream while I'm awake."
- "Everyone seems unreal."

reinforce the symptoms and provide secondary gain (defined and discussed later in this chapter in the section on somatoform disorders). Therefore, the completeness and accuracy of the initial physical assessment are of the utmost importance.

A psychosocial assessment is conducted to discover the fundamental source of the anxiety as early as possible. Although many episodes of dissociation appear to occur spontaneously, there may be a history of a specific emotional trauma or a situation charged with painful emotions and psychological conflict. Family or friends may provide clues to the client's conflict; include them in the psychosocial data gathering. When assessing for the presence of DID, consider the clinical manifestations listed in the next Your Assessment Approach.

Events associated with the trauma can trigger memories that have been repressed; these stimuli can precipitate a switch of alters. When interacting with the client, be alert for evidence of forgetfulness and fluctuations of voice tone, speech, and mannerisms. Notice from session to session if there are uncharacteristic changes in behavior. Are there differences in hairstyles, adornment, mannerisms, or dress?

To assess for amnesia, ask if the client has ever had blackouts, blank spells, memory gaps, or has lost time. To assess for dissociation, question whether the client ever "spaces out" or is unable to remember periods of time or events. Ask others who know the client about episodes of uncharacteristic behavior that the client does not recall.

Nursing Diagnosis: NANDA

Several nursing diagnoses may be applicable to clients with dissociative disorders, depending on the client's specific needs. Dissociation is manifested by disturbances in sensory and thought processes. Dissociative disorders markedly interfere with the client's ability to perform role expectations.

Disturbed Sensory Perception and Disturbed Thought Processes

Clients with dissociative disorders may experience sudden memory loss, disorientation, loss of personal identity, and alteration in state of consciousness. Clients with dissociative amnesia have a partial or total inability to recall or identify past experiences. In clients with depersonalization disorder, feelings of unreality and estrangement can affect their perception of the physical and psychological self and of the world around them. Parts of the body or the entire body may seem foreign, and dizziness, anxiety, and distortion of time and space are common.

Ineffective Role Performance

Unexplained disappearances, absences from work, unreliability, and unpredictability are common manifestations of dissociative disorders. Thus, the social or occupational functioning of the client is adversely affected. Symptoms of depersonalization lead to limited or superficial involvement with others and to withdrawal or disengagement in work or social pursuits. As expected, relationships become highly complicated and disorganized when a client has multiple personalities.

Ineffective Coping

In addition to amnesia, a fugue state may occur in clients with dissociative disorders. In this state, clients defend against perceived danger by active flight. They may wander away from home and community. Days, weeks, or sometimes even years later they may suddenly find themselves in a strange place, not knowing how they got there. There is complete amnesia for the period of the fugue. Clients experiencing dissociative fugue may adopt a new identity and life pattern.

Outcome Identification: NOC

When developing expected outcomes, it is important to individualize plans for each client. For example, a client experiencing a dissociative identity disorder will probably need assistance in resolving issues related to self-concept. When planning outcomes, remember that they should be realistic and achievable. Some appropriate expected outcomes would include the following:

- The client will engage in a therapeutic alliance.
- The client will verbalize awareness of personality alters.

Following are some outcomes—written in NOC terminology (Johnson et al., 2012)—for clients experiencing ineffective coping. The client will:

- Seek information about illness and treatment.
- Use stress-reduction behaviors.
- Report decrease in negative feelings.
- Demonstrate impulse control by consistently maintaining self-control without supervision.

Planning and Implementation: NIC

In choosing intervention strategies for clients with dissociative disorders, the treatment team must decide whether to alleviate the troublesome symptoms or reintegrate the anxiety-producing conflict. Some teams emphasize the disruptions in day-to-day functioning precipitated by dissociative disorders. These include unexplained disappearances, absences from work, unreliability, and unpredictability. The

---

YOUR ASSESSMENT APPROACH
Client With Dissociative Identity Disorder

To assess for the presence of DID, ask the following questions:

- Are there blocks of time you are unable to remember?
- Have you ever awakened not knowing your name or where you were at that time?
- Do other people accuse you of being untruthful?
- Have you ever discovered unfamiliar objects, like clothing, in your home and not known how they got there?
- Do you have headaches? If so, how often? How intense are they?
- How often do you have sleeping problems?
- Do you ever have nightmares?
- As a child, were you hurt or abused by others?

dread associated with them justifies intervention strategies designed to change the disruptive behavior pattern. Others believe that new problems are created by removing the dissociative symptoms without considering how they help the client control internal anxiety and maintain some balance in external social life.

Keep in mind that although clients may complain about the difficulties associated with their symptoms, the symptoms often form the basis of relationships with other significant people in their lives. Clients' roles in social groups are likewise built around their coping styles. Anyone who tries to change these coping styles must offer clients more effective and satisfying ways to handle anxiety and obtain support in their social network. Such a task usually requires long-term psychotherapy. However, behavior modification strategies can alleviate some of the problematic behaviors. When planning care for a client with DID, remember that trust is a major issue. The basic building blocks of therapy with the dissociative individual are trust, safety, and acceptance.

For many individuals, receiving a diagnosis of DID actually provides a sense of relief. For years, they have been misdiagnosed and treated incorrectly. However, other individuals may be distressed by the diagnosis; learning the diagnosis may trigger the switching of alters. Thus, a safe, supportive environment is essential when informing the client of the diagnosis. The focus of treatment is to form a therapeutic alliance and work through the issues of each alternate identity.

The goal of integrating the alternate identities into one fused identity is difficult to achieve—but it is feasible. Integration occurs when there is no further need for separateness between identities. The integration process can be very painful for the client, as memories of previous trauma

surface. However, it is important for the client to recall painful memories in order to work through unresolved conflicts. When planning care for clients with DID, you must trust them to express their needs. You also need to actively listen to each identity state and provide support, especially when the client is struggling to accept the realization that he or she has DID.

Promoting Improved Sensory Perception and Thought Processes

Strategies for identifying the underlying source of anxiety include those for recovering unconscious content, such as free association or dream description. At times, more active strategies are used. These may include projective psychometric tests (e.g., Rorschach, Thematic Apperception Test) and hypnosis, with or without intravenous administration of thiopental sodium (Pentothal). These strategies require advanced and specialized training. Strategies that you can use for a client with DID are discussed in Evidence-Based Practice.

Supportive insight therapy may be used by the psychotherapist with the goal of surfacing and integrating traumatic experiences in order to learn new ways of coping with future anxiety. This is especially relevant for clients in whom dissociation arises primarily against a background of intrapsychic conflict.

Promoting Effective Role Performance

It is important to work with the client's family in order to help everyone in the family unit to adjust to role performance alterations. Including family members in a therapeutic counseling relationship helps them learn new ways of dealing with the client. As stated earlier, considerable secondary gain is often associated with dissociative behavior: Some clients may use the illness to escape responsibility

---

EVIDENCE-BASED PRACTICE

An Eclectic Approach to Dissociative Identity Disorder

Jolene is a 34-year-old single female with a history of episodes of which she has no recollection. Family members report that during her blackouts, Jolene would spend money uncontrollably, shoplift, frequent bars, and engage in sexually promiscuous behavior. All of these behaviors are out of character for Jolene. During the past 5 years, Jolene was involved in six motor vehicle accidents during the blackouts. The family reported that during the blackout episodes, Jolene would dress in a provocative manner and speak in a hostile tone of voice. Jolene has a history of being sexually abused between the ages of 8 and 14 by an uncle. She was also physically abused by her mother for several years.

Your plan for intervention options is based on current research results. The primary treatment modality for Jolene is talk therapy. Psychotherapy sessions will focus on desensitizing

traumatic memories. You have also learned that music therapy may be beneficial in promoting relaxation. Other therapies that will be implemented for Jolene include Gestalt therapy to help give voice to opposing feelings and hypnosis to assist in reintegrating the alter personalities.

This set of interventions is based on the following literature findings:

Gleadhill, L., & Ferris, K. (2010). A theoretical music therapy framework for working with people with dissociative identity disorder. *Australian Journal of Music Therapy, 21*, 42–55.

Weber, S. (2009). Treatment of trauma- and abuse-related dissociative symptom disorders in children and adolescents. *Journal of Child and Adolescent Psychiatric Nursing, 22*(1), 2–6.

CRITICAL THINKING QUESTIONS

1. How would you approach a client whose alter personality is in control of behavior?
2. Why would it be useful to determine the underlying meaning of the client's symptoms?
3. What type of environment should be established for a client exhibiting dissociation?

and obtain special treatment. Families often need support in learning to avoid reinforcing dissociative behavior by acting as the source of secondary gain.

Environmental manipulation may be an indicated intervention. For example, it may be necessary to assist the client in problem solving with the goal of minimizing other stressful aspects of the environment. In learning to confront and become desensitized to the underlying conflict, the client will experience some anxiety and discomfort. This anxiety must be kept within manageable limits. Therefore, obvious stressors should be minimized.

Promoting Effective Coping

Psychotherapy, environmental manipulation, and behavior modification help the client cope more effectively with impairments of conduct and impulse, as evidenced by unpredictable and bizarre behavior. Treatment may prove to be long term, and progress may be slow. Establishing a supportive therapeutic alliance with the client and the family is crucial in helping the family and client understand the periodic occurrence of symptoms and in supporting improved behaviors. See Rx Communication for clients with depersonalization disorder.

Evaluation

Evaluating the effectiveness of nursing interventions is essential, although it may be difficult with clients who are experiencing episodes of amnesia. Therefore, you must pay special attention to the client's nonverbal clues and to data obtained from secondary sources.

Sensory Perception and Thought Processes

Clients will no longer experience sudden memory loss, disorientation, loss of identity, or alteration in state of consciousness, or they will experience it less frequently. They will correctly recall and identify past experiences.

Role Performance

Clients will experience increased satisfaction with family and work relationships. Involvement with others will occur more often and will be more fulfilling. Clients will attend work or school regularly, without unexplained absences due to dissociative episodes.

Individual Coping

Clients will no longer exhibit bizarre or unpredictable behaviors, or they will experience them less frequently. For example, incidents of being missing from home without explanation will occur less frequently or not at all.

CASE MANAGEMENT

Case management services for clients experiencing dissociative disorders usually involve extensive tracking of records for previous hospitalizations, especially for clients with DID. Clients with DID may often be disabled as a result of the seriousness of the disorder. The case manager must maintain ongoing communication with the client, family members, mental health professionals, other health care providers, and third-party reimbursers. Medication management is a major issue for many clients with dissociative disorders.

COMMUNITY-BASED CARE

Clients with dissociative disorders are not psychotic and, therefore, are often treated in the community instead of the hospital setting. The community setting includes mental health clinics, crisis centers, and therapists' offices. However, for those clients who are hospitalized, discharge goals seem straightforward but present a challenge: to provide quality, cost-effective care that allows the client to return to full functioning as soon as possible. Community care must focus on the client's safety in light of possible continued memory impairments.

HOME CARE

Some individuals with dissociative disorders are able to live independently. Others, however, may need to live in group homes or halfway houses in order to promote safety and functional ability. The client's ability to live at home is, after all, based on his or her functional abilities. Some individuals with DID need very close supervision, especially if they rapidly switch alters.

SOMATOFORM DISORDERS

The essential features of **somatoform disorders** are physical symptoms suggesting physical disorders for which there is no evidence of organic or physiological causes.

℞ COMMUNICATION

Client With Depersonalization Disorder

CLIENT: "I don't feel like myself. In fact, I don't even feel real."

NURSE RESPONSE 1: "You sound as if you're afraid when those unreal episodes occur."	**NURSE RESPONSE 2:** "When you are feeling this way, you look more anxious. We're here to help you learn to cope better with the anxiety."
RATIONALE: This response demonstrates empathy and reassures the client that it is appropriate to discuss her feelings.	*RATIONALE:* This response provides feedback on the congruence between the client's feelings and behavior. It also reassures the client that she or he can learn methods to decrease the anxiety associated with depersonalization.

DSM ESSENTIAL FEATURES

Somatoform Disorders

Somatization Disorder: Physical complaints that include pain, gastrointestinal symptoms, sexual symptoms, or a symptom or deficit suggesting a neurologic condition that begins before age 30; occurs over a period of several years, and results in significant impairment in social, occupational, or other important areas of functioning.

Conversion Disorder: One or more symptoms or deficits of voluntary motor or sensory function suggesting a medical condition; preceded by conflicts or stressors, not intentionally produced, causing significant distress or impairment in social, occupational, or other important areas of functioning.

Pain Disorder: Pain that is severe enough to cause clinically significant distress or impairment in social, occupational, or other important areas of functioning for which psychological factors

are thought to have an important role, and is not intentionally produced.

Hypochondriasis: A misinterpretation of bodily symptoms that results in preoccupation with the fear of having a serious disease despite appropriate medical evaluation with negative results; minimum duration of 6 months.

Body Dysmorphic Disorder: Excessive preoccupation with an imagined defect in appearance that causes significant distress or impairment in social, occupational, or other important areas of functioning.

Undifferentiated Somatoform Disorder: Physical complaints of at least 6 months that cannot be fully explained following appropriate investigation; not intentionally produced; resulting in social or occupational impairment.

Somatoform disorders, formerly called *psychosomatic disorders,* are sometimes confused with physical disorders because the predominant symptoms are physical. These commonly experienced symptoms include fatigue, pain, and sensory changes such as those described in DSM Essential Features. Client and family educational information about somatoform disorders is available on http://www.psyweb .com and can be accessed through the Online Student Resources for this book.

Somatization Disorder

The diagnosis of **somatization disorder** applies to clients who, like Sonya in the clinical example that follows, have sought medical attention for recurrent and multiple somatic complaints over a duration of several years.

Clinical Example

Sonya has appointments with a gastroenterologist, a gynecologist, a cardiologist, and her primary care physician, all in the same month. Now 54 years old, Sonya has had multiple somatic complaints of nausea, bloating, constipation, heart palpitations, and dizziness for almost 30 years. Although several gastrointestinal X-rays, heart studies, and physical examinations have not indicated the presence of disease, Sonya is convinced her disorders are real. She changes physicians regularly.

Historically, somatization disorder has been referred to as "hysteria," "hysterical reaction," and "Briquet's syndrome." This problem usually begins before the age of 30, has a chronic course, and is often accompanied by anxiety and depressed mood. Clients believe they have been ill for a good part of their lives and report lengthy lists of symptoms, including blindness, paralysis, convulsions, nausea, and other gastrointestinal difficulties. These symptoms are not caused intentionally, nor are they feigned (faked). The pain experienced by individuals with somatization disorder is real.

Even though somatization is common in children, somatization disorder is rarely diagnosed in children and adolescents.

Children who are diagnosed with somatization disorder tend to have caregivers who consistently over-react to the child's somatic complaints, thus reinforcing the complaints.

Conversion Disorder

In **conversion disorder**, clients report impaired physical function that is related to the expression of a psychological conflict. The loss of functional ability is due to psychological, not biologic, problems. However, the symptoms in conversion disorder are not consciously produced. The following clinical example illustrates what occurs in conversion disorder.

Clinical Example

Ronald is the 17-year-old eldest son of a Baptist minister in a rural community. His father expects his family to be pillars of the community and to serve as wholesome examples for the congregation. Ronald has recently developed a paralysis of his right hand, for which no physical basis has been found. Unknown to others, Ronald has been masturbating almost daily since he was 13 years old. He finds masturbation pleasurable, but feels anxiety and guilt at the same time.

Two mechanisms are thought to explain what a person "gets" from having a conversion disorder. The first, **primary gain**, helps the person keep the psychological need or conflict out of conscious awareness. For example, a woman may become blind to avoid acknowledging a traumatic event she has seen. In this instance, the symptom is a partial solution to the underlying conflict (not having to acknowledge witnessing the traumatic event because she has suddenly become sightless). The second mechanism, **secondary gain**, helps the person avoid a distressing, uncomfortable, or repugnant activity while at the same time receiving support from others. For example, a soldier with a paralyzed arm could hardly be expected to fire a gun and is also likely to receive sympathy because of his paralysis. Unlike malingering and factitious disorder, discussed later in the chapter, the symptoms are not deliberately produced to obtain benefits.

Another frequent symptom characteristic of clients with conversion disorder, although not necessarily present in all instances, is **la belle indifférence**, an inappropriate lack of concern about a disability. Tom, in the clinical example that follows, demonstrates la belle indifférence.

Clinical Example

Tom is experiencing a conversion disorder that has led to his inability to walk. Although Tom stated, "I woke up this morning with no feeling in my legs; for some reason they won't move," he seems totally unconcerned about his problem despite its severity.

The person is actually calmer as a result of the somatic symptom. This problem usually begins in adolescence or early adulthood, although a conversion disorder may appear at any time of life. Regardless of the time of onset, a conversion disorder can seriously impede normal life activities. Functional impairments may affect the individual's ability to function at work, at home, or in social situations.

Pain Disorder

In **pain disorder**, clients experience pain for which there is no physiological basis and often have accompanying psychological factors. The pain is usually severe enough to disrupt several functional areas. As a result of this dysfunction, the client often experiences unemployment, disability, and/or family problems. A person with pain disorder is often convinced that somewhere there is a health care provider who can "cure" the pain. Thus, the person may spend much time, money, and energy needlessly in pursuit of a "cure." The pain becomes the central issue of one's life; pain takes control of one's ability to function.

Hypochondriasis

Clients with **hypochondriasis** are preoccupied with the fear or belief that they have a serious disease, which, on physical evaluation, is not present. The preoccupation may be built around any of the following:

- Bodily functions (peristalsis, heartbeat)
- Minor physical problems (an occasional headache, a slight cough)
- Ambiguous, vague physical feelings ("tired ovaries" or "aching veins")

The unrealistic fear or belief persists for a period of at least 6 months despite medical reassurance that no illness is present. This fear impairs the client's social and/or occupational functioning.

Clinical Example

Reading the newspaper and watching the news on television have become anxiety-provoking experiences for Lena. Lena has been worried about AIDS, avian flu, contaminated spinach and bean sprouts, and even head lice. She attributes any symptom she has—an itch, a runny nose, a loose bowel movement—to any one of a number of possible medical conditions. If her worries have not been relieved by her research on the Internet, Lena calls in sick to work and makes an appointment to see her primary care physician or nurse practitioner.

Body Dysmorphic Disorder

Clients with **body dysmorphic disorder (BDD)** are preoccupied with some imagined defect in their physical appearance. The preoccupation is out of proportion to any actual abnormality, as illustrated in the following clinical examples.

Clinical Example

Joanna is very worried about the size of her nose despite reassurances that her nose is normal. She spends an inordinate amount of time in front of the mirror using cosmetics designed to shadow or minimize her nose. Joanna recently turned down a job promotion that would have put her in charge of the entire human resources department at the company at which she works. The job involves training human resources staff at locations in ten other cities. Joanna cannot bear the thought that trainees will have to look at her nose all day.

Fred, a 28-year-old man, has always been shy and very self-conscious about his body. He has a slender stature and perceives himself as being "skinny and weak." Over the past 2 years, Fred has spent a significant amount of time working out at the local gym. As a result he has built muscle and, thus, gained several pounds. However, Fred still sees himself as "a weakling." He is also concerned about the appearance of his nose, which he said "sticks out too much." He sought the opinion of two plastic surgeons. Neither believed that surgery was indicated.

Their beliefs, even though they may be extreme, are not of delusional proportion. The majority of people with BDD have very little insight into the origins of their symptoms.

People with BDD often use avoidance to cope with their perceived defect(s). Such avoidance may result in extreme social isolation. For example, a man who tries to camouflage his "defect" of imaginary hair loss may leave his home only at night, and then only with a hat covering the "defective" part. The preoccupation with one's appearance is very time consuming; thus, it restricts activities. In some cases, clients seek out cosmetic surgery to "cure" the imagined defect. This is a major reason plastic and cosmetic surgeons should do careful screenings before performing cosmetic or reconstructive surgery.

Undifferentiated Somatoform Disorder

In **undifferentiated somatoform disorder**, clients have multiple physical complaints of at least 6 months' duration; extensive evaluation reveals no organic problem. When the client does have an organic disease, the complaints or impairments are grossly excessive. Remember that the symptoms experienced by an individual with this disorder are not intentionally produced. The pain, which is psychogenic in nature, is real to the client.

MALINGERING

Malingering occurs when a person deliberately fakes symptoms in order to benefit. The American Psychiatric Association (2000) categorizes malingering as a condition that may be a focus of clinical attention. In other words, malingering is not considered a psychiatric disorder because it involves deliberate falsification of illness. However, malingering is discussed here because clients with somatoform disorders are sometimes misdiagnosed as faking their conditions. Malingering is consciously motivated and usually results in secondary gain, which may be in the form of extra attention, relief from responsibilities, or financial rewards, as shown in the following clinical example.

Clinical Example

Joyce is a police officer. She fakes episodes of back pain in order to avoid street patrol. Whenever she is assigned to this duty, Joyce claims to be in too much pain to work.

The prevalence of malingering may vary from 20% to 50% in clients with chronic pain who have a financial incentive (Greve, Ord, Bianchini, & Curtis, 2009). It often occurs in the following situations: personal injury and workers' compensation litigation; military service; and criminal cases. Mental Health in the Movies discusses a clever episode of malingering a mental disorder to avoid criminal prosecution. As Chapter 12 ∞ discusses, malingering is fairly often linked with legal pleas of guilty by reason of insanity.

FACTITIOUS DISORDER

Malingering and somatoform disorders are sometimes mistakenly confused with **factitious disorder**, in which clients intentionally produce or feign physical or psychological symptoms (American Psychiatric Association, 2000). The major difference between factitious disorder and malingering is that a person with a factitious disorder has a psychological need to assume the sick role. Unlike malingering, external incentives for the behavior are absent. Several studies (Kradin, 2011; Pasic, Combs, & Romm, 2009; Hagglund, 2009) describe numerous difficulties in diagnosing and treating clients with factitious disorders. It is also costly when medically unnecessary diagnostic procedures are performed. The course of factitious disorder usually consists of intermittent episodes. If undiagnosed or treated ineffectively, the

factitious disorder may become chronic, thereby increasing the risk of danger.

Factitious disorder may occur on a continuum of mild (giving a verbal list of symptoms) to moderate (simulating physical symptoms) to severe (inflicting injury). Dermatologic manifestations are very common; however, physical symptoms can be intentionally induced for many medical conditions. Thelma, in the clinical example that follows, exemplifies factitious disorder.

Clinical Example

Thelma has been admitted to the hospital after being seen in an acute care walk-in clinic with blood in her urine. The admitting physician has ordered several invasive procedures—catheterization, blood work, and cystoscopy, among others. The physician does not know that Thelma has been taking anticoagulants to produce blood in her urine.

Clients with factitious disorders deliberately give false medical histories that can be quite elaborate. It can be difficult to detect a factitious disorder because clients may use several different names and often seek treatment in several agencies to avoid detection or recognition by someone who has encountered the client during a previous hospitalization or clinic visit.

The fabricated symptoms—e.g., fever, anemia, hematuria—are indeed symptoms of "real" diseases; however, there is no organic reason for the appearance of the symptoms. The client provides an untruthful account of symptoms and fakes signs of illness in an attempt to receive medical treatment. Uncontrollable lying is the hallmark characteristic of individuals with factitious disorder; stories are fabricated in order to capture the attention of others. Clients typically describe their symptoms in dramatic terms, yet are vague about the onset and duration of the problems. Individuals with factitious disorder are usually very knowledgeable about medicine. Being knowledgeable, imaginative, and sophisticated about medical systems, medical terminology, and the routines of treatment facilities allows them to convincingly fake a constellation of symptoms.

MENTAL HEALTH IN THE MOVIES
Primal Fear

A young, stuttering, timid altar boy, Aaron Stampler (Edward Norton), is accused of the brutal murder of a Catholic priest. A prominent, spotlight-loving defense attorney, Martin Vail (Richard Gere), interested in the publicity the case will bring, volunteers to represent the young man. Despite the considerable evidence against him (Aaron was found running from the archbishop's home covered in blood), he claims not to remember anything about the murder. When Vail discovers more evidence in the archbishop's home, he confronts Aaron and accuses him of lying. In an emotional scene, Aaron breaks down crying and transforms into the persona of Roy, a violent sociopath. Later, Aaron has no recollection of this event.

In court, Vail arranges a courtroom scene designed to showcase Aaron's vicious alter, Roy. On the basis of his apparent dissociative identity disorder, the judge dismisses the jury and finds Aaron not guilty by reason of insanity. When Vail returns to Aaron's jail cell to tell him the good news, the no-longer stuttering and no-longer timid Aaron reveals that he has been pretending to have a mental disorder the entire time. As a stunned and disillusioned Vail leaves the jail cell, Aaron taunts him. This film raises the controversial issues of both malingering and dissociative identity disorder.

Photo courtesy of Everett Collection, Inc.

When the disorder is severe, chronic, and unremitting—involving repeated hospitalizations, traveling between health care providers and health care facilities, and pathologic lying of an intriguing and fantastic nature (called *pseudologica fantastica*)—it is often called **Munchausen syndrome** or adult factitious disorder (AFD). Ron, in the following clinical example, is an example of such a person.

Clinical Example

Ron is lying on a treatment table in the emergency department. He is in acute pain with a dislocated shoulder. This hospital is located 20 miles from the city in which Ron lives. What the emergency physician does not know is that Ron has been to several different physicians in his city and has had multiple prior hospitalizations for factitious symptoms—pain, fevers of undetermined origin, rashes, and dizziness. All physical assessments proved negative. Ron usually berates the physician, the nurse, or the X-ray technician for being unable to find the cause of his problem and signs himself out against medical advice. The emergency physician also does not know that Ron has dislocated his own shoulder.

As this clinical example demonstrates, Munchausen syndrome can become a lifelong pattern.

Factitious Disorder by Proxy

Factitious disorder by proxy, sometimes called **Munchausen by proxy syndrome** (**MBPS**), occurs when parents or caregivers deliberately induce signs of an illness in another person, usually their own child. MBPS, also called *pediatric condition falsification (PCF)* or *medical child abuse,* is a relatively rare type of child abuse (Kucker, Demir, & Resmiye, 2010). It is difficult for health care providers to deal with situations in which a caregiver (usually a parent) deliberately injures the person under their care. In these situations, health care providers should seek clinical supervision or a consultant to help them to cope with their personal responses.

In factitious disorder by proxy, caregivers deliberately injure their victims in order to gain sympathy or attention for themselves. The victim is usually a preschool child, but could be of any age including adulthood through old age. The individual with this syndrome has an insatiable need for attention, even though the person's behavior is harmful to others. Intentionally producing symptoms in the child (or other victim) is a way to gain attention. The following clinical example discusses a woman with factitious disorder by proxy.

Clinical Example

A mother has been regularly and deliberately administering large doses of laxatives to her 15-month-old toddler over a period of several months. When the child has episodes of cramping, flatulence, and bloody diarrhea, the mother, appearing to be very concerned, takes her to the emergency department of a local hospital. Diagnostic studies show no medical reason for the toddler's symptoms.

It is wise to suspect the presence of factitious disorder by proxy if certain indicators are present. These indicators are identified in What Every Nurse Should Know.

WHAT EVERY NURSE SHOULD KNOW

Factitious Disorder by Proxy and Child Abuse

Imagine that you are a pediatric nurse or a school nurse. Factitious disorder by proxy is a potentially fatal form of child abuse. Not only is the child's life disrupted, the child is usually subjected to frequent hospitalizations and invasive medical procedures. Therefore, the child's safety is of the utmost concern.

An evaluation by an interdisciplinary team that includes health experts is called for whenever this syndrome is suspected. It requires the collection of evidence and the development of a plan to provide appropriate care for the hospitalized child, involve the appropriate authorities (such as child protective services), and obtain help for the child's parent or caretaker. Health care providers should be suspicious of situations in which:

- A child has unexplained, recurrent, or rare symptoms.
- The parent denies knowing the cause of the illness.
- When the caretaker is present, so are the symptoms; however, when the child is separated from the caretaker, the symptoms resolve.
- The illness is unresponsive to treatment.
- The clinical findings are inconsistent.
- There is a history of several hospital visits for treatment.

Unlike factitious disorder, factitious disorder by proxy is not yet recognized in the DSM multiaxial coding system because of insufficient information to warrant inclusion. It warrants further study for possible inclusion in a future edition of the DSM.

BIOPSYCHOSOCIAL THEORIES

Biologic, genetic, and psychosocial theories help us to understand somatoform disorders. The following section presents current research findings about the etiology of somatoform disorders.

Biologic Factors

In somatoform disorders, physical symptoms are present but evidence of physiological disease is not. The symptoms are thought to be linked to psychological factors or emotional conflict. However, there is some evidence that brain abnormalities may lead to altered pain perception (Bourne, 2011; Sadock & Sadock, 2010). Evidence indicates that somatoform disorders are associated with increased activity of limbic regions in response to painful stimuli (Browning, Fletcher, & Sharpe, 2011). Biochemical imbalances, such as decreased amounts of endorphins and serotonin, may cause some people to experience pain more intensely than those with normal brain chemistry. Tocchio (2009) reports some brain imaging studies indicating that, if the circuits that process sensory stimuli receive false information, the voluntary muscles may malfunction.

Genetic Theories

Somatization disorder occurs in 10% to 20% of female first-degree biologic relatives of women with somatization disorder (APA, 2000). The results of adoption studies indicate that both genetic and environmental factors contribute to the risk for somatization disorder (APA, 2000). There may be a possible genetic predisposition because there is an increased incidence of somatization disorder and hypochondriasis in first-degree relatives (Sadock & Sadock, 2010). Other studies with identical twins have shown an increased occurrence of hypochondriasis (Sadock & Sadock, 2010). There is some evidence to support that some children have a genetic predisposition to somatization disorders, especially children who exhibit sensitivity to anxiety and trait anxiety (Silber, 2011).

Psychosocial Theories

Communication theorists believe that manifestations of somatization are nonverbal body language intended to communicate a message to significant others. Sometimes the message is as general as "pay attention to me" or "take care of me." At other times the *conversion of anxiety* actually symbolizes the nature of the specific underlying conflict. For example, a woman who wants to strike her children may develop a paralysis of her arm. A girl who feels guilty about reading erotic books may become blind. Both experience the primary gain of protection from the anxiety-provoking impulses, and both get secondary gains of attention and sympathy. Such behavior patterns are most likely to occur among clients who lack appropriate coping skills.

Many individuals who engage in somatization were reared in chaotic families. The family dysfunction was usually marital discord, substance abuse, and/or personality disorders. For whatever reason, the child received inadequate nurturing. Many adults with somatoform disorders experienced physical or sexual abuse as children. Clients who deal with anxiety by converting it to physical symptoms usually show no other psychological symptoms, such as disturbed thoughts or depressed moods.

Pain is associated with a great many disease processes, including some of the organ-specific somatoform disorders. Pain can be adaptive or maladaptive in that it often indicates real danger but sometimes it interferes with functioning. Consciousness, attention, perception, and cognition are all necessary for the experience of pain. According to modern theories of pain perception, humans have a control system over pain that operates as a "gate." Pain stimuli can be "allowed in" or "shut out" from the cerebral cortex, depending essentially on the meaning the person attaches to the stimulus. This underscores the importance of meaning, symbol, and affect in the experience

DEVELOPING CULTURAL COMPETENCE

Culture-Bound Syndromes That Can Be Misdiagnosed as Somatoform Disorders

Bilis and Colera (also called *munia*) Occurs in Latino groups. Episodes of extreme anger which can exacerbate existing physical symptoms, including headache, stomach upsets, trembling, and loss of consciousness. Chronic fatigue may be a result of these episodes.

Brain Fog Term initially used in West Africa for a condition experienced by students; symptoms include impairments in concentration, memory, and thinking. Somatic symptoms are headache, blurring of vision, burning in the head and eyes.

Falling-Out or Blacking Out A sudden collapse, which may occur without warning but is sometimes preceded by feelings of dizziness. Eyes are open but the individual denies the ability to see; feels powerless to move. Occurs primarily in southern United States and Caribbean groups.

Shenjing Shuairua Characterized by physical and mental fatigue, dizziness, headaches, gastrointestinal problems, sexual dysfunction, other pains, sleep disturbance, and memory loss. Occurs in China.

CRITICAL THINKING QUESTIONS

1. Why is it important to know a client's cultural background?
2. How does knowledge of a client's cultural background help you develop therapeutic interventions?

of pain sensation. Figure 19-2 ■ shows the basic mechanism for so-called idiopathic pain (pain of unknown origin).

In psychoanalytic concepts, the unconscious conflicts are a result of traumatic or frustrating childhood experiences that are reawakened in adult life by a similar stress or frustration. According to this theory, the person cannot express the affect because of feelings of guilt, fear of loss of love, or fear of retribution. The affect is therefore repressed and transformed into physiological correlates, such as pain.

Humanistic Theories

It is important to consider clients with somatoform disorders in the context of what is happening in their lives. Stress related to relationships and work may be the precipitants for somatic symptoms. Tocchio (2009) notes that people with conversion disorder may experience difficulty in dealing with a large amount of stress. Stressful situations encountered by

FIGURE 19-2 ■ The mechanism of idiopathic pain.

some children, such as bullying and abuse (either physical or sexual), may be contributory factors (Silber, 2011). Environmental factors may contribute to the development of somatization in that there is ". . . a preponderance of these conditions among children of families living in lower socio-economic strata" (Silber, 2011, p. 63). Research evidence supports the idea that complicated or unusual medical illness during childhood may also play a role in the development of future somatization disorders (Sansone, Buckner, Tahir, & Wiederman, 2009).

You must view an individual's behavior within the context of the cultural experience. See Developing Cultural Competence for a listing of culture-bound syndromes that may be misdiagnosed as somatoform disorders (APA, 2000).

NURSING PROCESS
Clients With Somatoform Disorders

When you work with clients experiencing somatoform or factitious disorders, you will be challenged by multiple complex problems, not the least of which stem from your values and beliefs. Your values and beliefs will influence how well you implement the nursing process. If you are unaware of your values and beliefs, you are likely to express them nonverbally to clients and family members. Therefore, it is imperative that you increase your self-awareness in order to be more effective when working with clients with somatoform or factitious disorders. Your Self-Awareness is designed to help you examine your feelings.

Assessment

Assessment of clients with somatoform disorders is often difficult because of the many psychobiologic factors involved. Careful and thorough assessment—subjective as well as objective—to rule out the possibility of a physical problem is crucial, as shown in the following clinical example.

YOUR SELF-AWARENESS
Exploring Your Feelings Toward Clients With Somatoform Disorders

Focus on your feelings when you are caring for clients with somatoform disorders. Ask yourself the following questions and then evaluate the relationship between your answers and your reactions to clients with somatoform disorders.

- How well do you handle frustration?
- How do you respond to the expression of anger, either passive or aggressive, by others?
- How patient are you? Are you able to be satisfied with small successes?
- Can you tell when you are becoming defensive?
- How can you tell if another person is experiencing "real" pain?

Clinical Example

Magda was referred for treatment to a local mental health clinic by her primary care physician. She had weakness and numbness of her right arm. When her primary care physician could find no physiological reason for Magda's symptoms, he diagnosed her problem as a conversion disorder and referred her to the mental health clinic. The nurse who admitted Magda to the clinic performed a thorough physical assessment and history. The medical history revealed that Magda had surgery on her left kidney 3 months ago. The nurse made the connection between the surgical position (right lateral) necessary to perform Magda's surgery and Magda's symptoms. The numbness and weakness were actually caused by pressure on the brachial plexus in her right arm during surgery. Magda was discharged from the mental health clinic and referred for physical rehabilitation.

In this clinical example, a complete and accurate assessment of all factors identified the appropriate course of action for Magda and spared her from a stigmatizing psychiatric diagnosis. Some sample questions useful in determining the presence of somatoform disorders are listed in Your Assessment Approach.

Subjective Data

Clients with somatoform disorders report physical symptoms for which there is no positive evidence of organic or physiological cause. For example, clients with hypochondriasis may return many times to the outpatient clinic or emergency department demanding to be re-examined or retested. They believe they are suffering from some major illness that has been undetected. They are not reassured by the lack of physical findings and may go from physician to physician in an attempt to find someone who will validate their fears. This "doctor shopping" may lead to fragmented care and misuse of medication. Because the person is usually a poor historian, a complete medical history (including medications taken) is not always obtained. Although individuals with somatoform disorder usually describe their condition with colorful, exaggerated language, you may find it is difficult to obtain specific facts about previous medical and surgical treatments. In conversion disorder, the individual has loss of or an alteration in function.

YOUR ASSESSMENT APPROACH
Client With Somatoform Disorder

The following list provides some sample questions to help determine the presence of somatoform disorder:

- Have you ever felt as if you were smothering, or couldn't breathe easily?
- Have you ever had problems swallowing or felt as if you were choking? If so, how long did the episode(s) last?
- Have you ever had burning sensations in your mouth or throat?
- Do you ever experience painful menstrual periods?
- Do you have pain in your joints? If so, how often?
- Have you seen many doctors who have told you that nothing is wrong with you?

A nonchalant attitude toward physical problems (*la belle indifférence*) indicates that the symptom is providing primary gain; that is, the anxiety is alleviated through the conversion process. In contrast, clients with somatization disorder or hypochondriasis are overly dramatic and emotional when talking about their symptoms and pain. They report the history in vivid detail and colorful language but often pay more attention to how the symptoms have affected relationships in their lives than to giving a careful description of the nature, character, location, onset, and duration of the symptoms.

Clients with body dysmorphic disorder (BDD) may request unnecessary operations—for example, demanding cosmetic surgery for an imagined or greatly magnified defect in appearance. Societal expectations may pressure women with BDD into seeking unnecessary surgical procedures.

Careful interviewing frequently reveals a stressful life situation with which the client is failing to cope, suggesting that the preoccupation with somatic disorder is a way of avoiding underlying conflict. Helping the client identify and express feelings is a crucial beginning to psychotherapeutic intervention.

Objective Data

Physical examination reveals no organic evidence for the client's symptoms. Likewise, laboratory findings do not substantiate organic or physiological disorder. Despite this, the client may have undergone many exploratory diagnostic and/or surgical procedures without diagnosis or relief. Family members often report that the client is moody, self-centered, or demanding. They feel alienated from the client and are frustrated with the client's chronic preoccupation with physical symptoms.

In a health care setting, these clients often create scenes that bring them attention without regard for the needs of either fellow clients or staff. You may find it difficult to be kind, understanding, and nonjudgmental with such clients. If you do not cope with your reactions, you will be unable to effectively work with them. Recognizing the client's somatization as part of the illness will help you to avoid personalizing the behavior. It may help to remind yourself that these clients do not intentionally produce their symptoms, nor do they understand the effects of their behavior on others. When you understand the psychopathology of the disorder, you are more likely to have empathy for the client's coping style. What Every Nurse Should Know will help you apply these understandings in nonpsychiatric settings.

Nursing Diagnosis: NANDA

Clients with somatoform and factitious disorders experience a multitude of problems; therefore, several nursing diagnoses are likely to be appropriate. The following section discusses five major applicable nursing diagnoses.

Impaired Verbal Communication

Clients with somatoform disorders have an impaired ability to communicate their needs. Although they may be highly verbal, you need to listen carefully for gaps, oversimplifications,

WHAT EVERY NURSE SHOULD KNOW

Somatoform Disorders

Imagine that you are a nurse on a medical-surgical unit.

- Be careful not to rush to judge that "it's all in his/her head" when a client with a somatoform disorder is admitted to your unit. Even individuals with somatoform disorders can be ill or in pain.
- Pain and illness of psychogenic origin is as hurtful as pain of biologic origin.
- Be aware that hypochondriasis, conversion disorder, and other somatoform disorders are maladaptive responses to stress.
- Remember that unconscious (not deliberate) processes are at work, except for instances of malingering or factitious disorder.
- Be alert for signs of secondary gain and avoid reinforcing.
- Use a matter-of-fact approach when the client discusses somatic symptoms.
- Use a calm, patient approach in order to decrease the client's anxiety level.
- Decrease stimuli to promote relaxation.
- Anticipate the client's needs before somatization increases.
- Reward appropriate behavior.

overdramatizations, and overgeneralizations in the clients' stories. Somatoform symptoms are considered to be nonverbal substitutes for the expression of underlying conflicts.

Ineffective Role Performance and Compromised Family Coping

The manipulative and dependent behaviors of the client with a somatoform disorder lead to impairments in social, work, and family relationships and to diminished performance in these roles. Friends and relatives eventually tire of the demands and become less available for support. Clients become emotionally isolated because their self-absorption makes them unable to respond appropriately to the needs of others.

Work performance may suffer from frequent absences due to imagined illness. Preoccupation with health status uses up creative energy that could otherwise be directed toward work-related activities. When this occurs, the individual usually experiences negative consequences in the workplace.

Ineffective Coping

Clients with somatoform disorders generally experience anxiety, anger, and feelings of helplessness. They may feel these emotions acutely and demonstrate these feelings excessively, as in somatization disorder and hypochondriasis. Paradoxically, they may show an uncanny lack of feeling, as in the nonchalant reaction to loss of physical function that often occurs in conversion disorder.

The client's emotions become increasingly restricted. The focus of emotional experience becomes somatic concerns, and clients no longer experience meaningful emotional connections with other people, activities, and events. The range of emotional expression may be limited to making demands, manipulation, and symbolic manifestations of anxiety.

Disturbed Thought Processes and Disturbed Sensory Perception

Clients with somatoform disorders show selective inattention; that is, they filter out stimuli in response to anxiety. In a further effort to prove their ideas, they distort reality and tend to ramble. Judgment is often impaired and it is evident that conclusions are not logical. Clients may also distort memory and show selective memory.

Clients with somatoform disorders have body image disturbances and often sense that they are weak or vulnerable physically. They perceive sensory data incorrectly; for example, they may perceive abdominal discomfort as cancer rather than indigestion.

Outcome Identification: NOC

Expected outcomes are individualized for each client according to personal needs and the situation. However, some expected outcomes that are fairly common to those experiencing somatoform disorders are as follows:

- Demonstrate the ability to cope with anxiety through the use of a new stress management skill (i.e., deep breathing).
- Verbalize feelings instead of expressing them symbolically through physical symptoms.
- Express an increased degree of comfort regarding each physical symptom.

It is essential that you and the client work together in establishing expected outcomes. Include significant others in the planning process in order to help the client achieve the goals.

Planning and Implementation: NIC

In order to intervene effectively, you need to recognize and understand the life problem or adjustment the client is facing. It is also important that you do the following:

- Recognize and understand the client's self-perception as an inability to cope.
- Help the client identify and learn more effective ways of adapting.

These goals may be accomplished by insight-oriented or supportive psychotherapy, behavior modification, hypnosis,

---

YOUR INTERVENTION STRATEGIES
Client With Somatoform Disorder

Intervention	Rationale
Establish a trusting relationship.	Promotes client's psychological safety.
Establish a daily routine.	Decreases client's anxiety.
Encourage verbalization of feelings.	Verbalization is healthier than somatization.
Assist client to relate stress to onset of physical symptoms.	Pointing out a cause-and-effect relationship helps eliminate triggers.
Encourage client to write in a journal.	Increases personal insight.
Limit time for discussing physical symptoms.	Frees up time for problem-solving activities; decreases reinforcement of secondary gain(s).

---

or any of several other psychological, as well as some physical, therapies. No one therapeutic modality can claim superior effectiveness, and new approaches and techniques are indicated when traditional ones prove inadequate. It is important to recognize that many clients with somatoform disorders are highly resistant to change. Thus, progress may be slow and recovery partial. Specific interventions and rationales are discussed in Your Intervention Strategies.

Recall that you may also meet clients with somatoform disorders in general medical–surgical settings. Refer to What Every Nurse Should Know for specific interventions for medical–surgical settings.

Promoting Effective Communication

After assessing the meaning behind the client's communication patterns, plan intervention strategies such as encouraging exploration and demonstrating empathy that enhance the client's verbal communication and self-esteem to the point where the client feels ready to face problems. Rx Communication gives examples of verbal communication strategies.

Establishing a trusting relationship is the key to effective therapy with a somatizing client. It is usually necessary to help clients tone down their characteristic extravagances. Express respectful skepticism regarding oversimplifications and

---

Rx COMMUNICATION

Client With Somatoform Disorder

CLIENT: "How can they help me get better if they can't even figure out what's wrong with me? I know I'm really sick."

NURSE RESPONSE 1: "It sounds as if you are feeling hopeless."	**NURSE RESPONSE 2:** "It must be very frustrating for you. All the exams and tests show no physical cause for your symptoms."
RATIONALE: This response focuses on the client's feelings and encourages further exploration. It also is a way to determine suicidal ideation that may be related to the client's hopelessness.	*RATIONALE:* This response demonstrates empathy while at the same time presenting reality. Reassurance that no organic pathology has been found helps dispute the client's unrealistic belief.

PARTNERING WITH CLIENTS AND FAMILIES

Teaching About Somatoform Disorders

- Provide information about the specific disorder.
- Teach about the relationship between stress and physical symptoms.
- Teach relaxation techniques (e.g., progressive muscle relaxation, guided imagery).
- Provide health promotion education (e.g., healthy diet, balance between exercise and rest, healthy sleep patterns).

- Teach the proper use of medications, including: target symptoms, side effects and adverse drug reactions, contraindications, and when to call for help.
- Teach the indicators for emergency treatment.
- Emphasize the need for continued treatment, including follow-up appointments.

overdramatizations. The group setting provides clients the opportunity to receive feedback about the effect of their behavior on others.

Promoting Improved Role Performance and Family Coping

Working with the family is especially important for clients with somatoform disorders. Partnering With Clients and Families discusses educating the family and the client about the disorder, stressing the importance of avoiding unnecessary surgical or medical procedures.

Encourage independent functioning and reduce the possibility of secondary gain by not focusing on physical symptoms. Assume a matter-of-fact, supportive attitude, with the optimistic expectation that the client will regain functional abilities in work, family, and social roles.

Promoting Effective Coping

The goal of counseling clients with somatoform disorders is to help them express their conflicts verbally rather than acting them out through symptomatic behaviors. The aim of long-term (insight) therapy is to promote effective emotional expression by exploring the sources of anxiety. You will likely be challenged to help clients with somatoform disorders acknowledge the effects of psychosocial stress on symptoms. Supportive therapy seeks to improve self-esteem, perhaps through such measures as expanding clients' interest in their environment.

In general, try to avoid reinforcing the client's symptoms. A well-known psychiatric axiom applies to clients in this general category: *Ignore the symptom but never the client.* Concentrating on the physical symptom by trying to get a paralyzed client to walk or a blind client to see again is giving the symptom more importance than it merits, thus increasing the secondary gain associated with it. Ultimately, this makes it more difficult for the client to relinquish the symptom.

Promoting Improved Perception and Thought Processes

Help clients improve their capacity for perception and thinking by supporting general measures to reduce anxiety such as those discussed in Evidence-Based Practice. Maintain a calm, unhurried attitude toward the client, listen carefully, and maintain an objective, undistorted view of reality. Avoid a premature challenge to the client's symptoms and complaints. As clients gradually relinquish their defenses, propose other ways of understanding the condition, such as by suggesting a psychological explanation for a physical complaint.

EVIDENCE-BASED PRACTICE

Cognitive–Behavioral Techniques for Conversion Disorder

Alfred is a 22-year-old soldier. Even though he voluntarily joined the Army, Alfred never told anyone that he believed that killing under any circumstance is murder. After he finished military basic training, Alfred was deployed to Iraq. When on a routine patrol, Alfred's unit was attacked by enemy forces. While aiming his assault rifle at an Iraqi soldier, Alfred suddenly lost his vision. All medical tests show no physical basis for Alfred's blindness.

Your plan for intervention options is based on current research results. You have learned that Alfred will likely respond to cognitive–behavioral therapy (CBT) techniques such as those discussed in Chapter 30 ∞. Therefore, you teach Alfred the techniques of thought stopping and reframing. Using imagery may also be beneficial to Alfred.

The treatment team also decides to focus on establishing a therapeutic relationship with Alfred that includes an open, honest discussion of his disorder. Knowing that somatization may be triggered by stress, you will also demonstrate empathy and support to Alfred without reinforcing his symptoms.

This set of interventions is based on the following research:

Allan, L. A., & Woolfolk, R. L. (2010). Cognitive behavioral therapy for somatoform disorders. *Psychiatric Clinics of North America,* 33(3), 579–593.

Tocchio, S. L. (2009). Treatment of conversion disorder: A clinical and holistic approach. *Journal of Psychosocial Nursing,* 47(8), 42–49.

CRITICAL THINKING QUESTIONS

1. How would you demonstrate empathy to clients with a conversion disorder without reinforcing the client's symptoms?
2. In what ways would it be useful to determine the underlying meaning of the client's symptoms?
3. How would thought stopping and reframing help someone with conversion disorder?

Evaluation

Consider communication, role performance, coping, perception, and thought processes when evaluating clients with somatoform disorder. When evaluating these areas, it is important that you look for evidence of client progress. Expect that progress will be gradual and encourage the client and family to do the same.

Communication

Clients will express feelings and conflicts verbally and they will have fewer somatic symptoms. Your conversations with the client will "flow," with fewer monologues by the client and more natural dialogue between the client and you. In other words, the client's communication will become more spontaneous.

Role Performance and Family Coping

Clients will attend work regularly without frequent absences due to illness or worry about physical health status. They will be more interested in outside activities and may begin to engage in socialization and recreation. Family members and friends will report being more satisfied with their relationship with the client and will be more willing to interact with the client.

Coping

Clients will be less demanding, manipulative, and attention seeking in interactions with others. They will appear less anxious and will talk about subjects other than their physical status. They will appear less helpless and more able to participate in and make responsible decisions about their health care. For example, they may carry out a plan of treatment without voicing innumerable objections or worries. They will appear more interested and involved in the activities and attitudes of others and be more aware of the impact of their own behavior.

Perception and Thought Processes

The client will distort and misinterpret reality less frequently. Judgment, insight, and memory will improve as a result of reduced defensiveness in perception and cognition. Clients may report feeling more positive about their bodies. They will be more assertive in physical activities because they no longer tend to feel so vulnerable.

CASE MANAGEMENT

Case management for clients with somatoform disorders must focus on occupational functioning, which is usually significantly impaired by the disorder. Provision of job-search skills and communication techniques (e.g., how to listen actively to others) will enhance the client's career opportunities. Rehabilitative agencies can also be called upon to provide specific job-skills training. The case manager will often need to refer significant others to agencies that provide respite care and/or support to family members.

COMMUNITY-BASED CARE

Clients and family members usually need ongoing support for managing in the community setting. One organization that is designed to provide such support is the National Alliance on Mental Illness (NAMI). The website for this organization is http://www.NAMI.org. In addition to informing clients and families about NAMI, you can also encourage the client to adhere to medication therapy through education about the specific medications. Community mental health centers are very useful in helping clients obtain medications and adhere to the prescribed therapies.

HOME CARE

Home health nurses have a unique opportunity to support clients and help them maintain independence in activities of daily living. Home visits are done to provide support and education and to evaluate the client's need for continued treatment. Some tools that are especially useful in the home setting are cognitive–behavioral therapy (discussed in Chapter 30 ∞) and relaxation skills (discussed in Chapter 33 ∞).

National Alliance on Mental Illness

NURSING CARE PLAN: CLIENT WITH DISSOCIATIVE IDENTITY DISORDER

Identifying Information

Sally, a 30-year-old female is brought to the hospital by her friend, who found Sally lying on the floor of her home. Sally had cut her wrist and was bleeding moderately. When admitted to the emergency department, Sally stated her name is Beth and she does not understand why she is in the hospital, unless Sally tried to hurt herself again. Beth says that Sally "is always doing something crazy to herself." When transferred to the psychiatric unit, Beth admits that she tries to protect Sally from "terrible things in the world."

History

Sally experienced sexual abuse from both parents from birth until she was 16 when she ran away from home. She has occasional contact with her younger sister who lives in another state. She states she has never been treated for a mental disorder.

Current Mental Status

Sally is alert and oriented. She answers questions in a vague manner and has several time lapses with no memory. Her speech is slow but coherent. She acknowledges some problems with short-term memory and the ability to concentrate.

Other Clinical Data

A thorough nursing assessment identifies the presence of four alter personalities with specific traits and behaviors. Beth is the host personality. Annie is 4 years old and is looking for "my daddy." Sally is 11 years old and experiences all the pain felt by the others. Bobbie is 17 years old and has the task of protecting the others; Bobbie states she will kill anyone who doesn't do as she wishes.

(Continued)

NURSING CARE PLAN: CLIENT WITH DISSOCIATIVE IDENTITY DISORDER
(*Continued*)

Nursing Diagnosis: Risk for Self-Directed Violence as evidenced by scarring on both wrists

Expected Outcome: Sally will verbalize the lack of suicidal ideation or plans by day 6 of treatment.

Short-Term Goals	Interventions	Rationale
Sally will refrain from harming herself.	■ Place on close observation.	Provides for continuous monitoring of behavior.
	■ Remove all dangerous items from environment.	Reduces risk of harm by ensuring a safe environment.
	■ Ask Sally to sign a no-suicide contract.	Treats Sally as a partner in treatment by increasing her sense of control. Emphasizes seriousness of suicidal thoughts and behaviors.

Nursing Diagnosis: Risk for Violence Directed at Others

Expected Outcome: Sally will exhibit control of aggressive behavior by day 3 of treatment.

Short-Term Goals	Interventions	Rationale
Sally will verbalize feelings of anger.	■ Teach difference between anger and aggression.	Knowledge increases compliance with expectations.
	■ Encourage Sally to list triggers to anger.	Increases self-knowledge.
	■ Encourage Sally to practice relaxation skills and engage in physical activity.	Provides outlets for healthy expression of anger.

Nursing Diagnosis: Disturbed Personal Identity as evidenced by presence of dissociation (alter states)

Expected Outcome: Sally will eventually be able to reintegrate all personality states.

Short-Term Goals	Interventions	Rationale
Sally will identify two triggers of dissociation.	■ Teach relaxation techniques (i.e., focused breathing, progressive muscle relaxation).	Promotes coping with stress due to recognition of current problems.
	■ Have Sally make a list of warning signs of dissociation.	Conscious awareness helps counter dissociation.
	■ Encourage Sally to journal after each dissociative episode.	Increases self-awareness.

Pearson Nursing Student Resources
Find additional review materials at
nursing.pearsonhighered.com

Prepare for success with NCLEX®-style practice questions, interactive assignments and activities, web links, animations and videos, and more!

REFERENCES

Allan, L. A., & Woolfolk, R. L. (2010). Cognitive behavioral therapy for somatoform disorders. *Psychiatric Clinics of North America, 33*(3), 579–593.

American Psychiatric Association. (2000). *Diagnostic and statistical manual of mental disorders* (4th ed., Text Revision). Washington, DC: Author.

Bourne, E. J. (2011). *The anxiety and relaxation workbook* (5th ed.). Oakland, CA: New Harbinger Publications.

Browning, M., Fletcher, P., & Sharpe, M. (2011). Can neuroimaging help us to understand and classify somatoform disorders? A systematic and critical review. *Psychosomatic Medicine, 73*(2), 173–184.

Gleadhill, L., & Ferris, K. (2010). A theoretical music therapy framework for working with people with dissociative identity disorder. *Australian Journal of Music Therapy, 21,* 42–55.

Greve, K. W., Ord, J. S., Bianchini, K. J., & Curtis, K. L. (2009). Prevalence of malingering in patients with chronic pain referred for psychologic evaluation in a medico-legal context. *Archives of Physical Medicine and Rehabilitation, 90*(7), 1117–1126.

Hagglund, L. A. (2009). Challenges in the treatment of factitious disorder: A case study. *Archives of Psychiatric Nursing, 23*(1), 58–64.

Johnson, M., Moorehead, S., Bulechek, G. M., Butcher, H. K., Maas, M. L., & Swanson, E. (2012). *NOC and NIC linkages to NANDA-I and clinical conditions* (3rd ed.). St. Louis, MO: Elsevier.

Kradin, R. L. (2011). Psychosomatic disorders: The canalization of mind into matter. *Journal of Analytical Psychology, 56*(1), 37–55.

Kucker, H., Demir, T., & Resmiye, O. (2010). Pediatric condition falsification (Munchausen syndrome by proxy) as a continuum of maternal factitious disorder (Munchausen syndrome). *Pediatric Diabetes, 11*(8), 572–578.

Manning, M. L., & Manning, R. L. (2009). Convergent paradigms for visual neuroscience and dissociative identity disorder. *Journal of Trauma Dissociation, 10*(4), 405–419.

Pasic, J., Combs, H., & Romm, S. (2009). Factitious disorder in the emergency department. *Primary Psychiatry, 16*(1), 61–66.

Precin, P. K., & Precin, P. (2011). Return to work: A case of PTSD, dissociative identity disorder, and satanic ritual abuse. *Work, 38*(1), 57–66.

Sadock, B. J., & Sadock, V. A. (2010). *Kaplan and Sadock's pocket handbook of clinical psychiatry* (5th ed.). Philadelphia, PA: Lippincott Williams & Wilkins.

Sansone, R. A., Buckner, V. R., Tahir, N. A., & Wiederman, M. W. (2009). Early family environment, borderline personality symptoms, and somatic preoccupation among internal medicine outpatients. *Comprehensive Psychiatry, 50*(3), 221–225.

Silber, T. J. (2011). Somatization disorders: diagnosis, treatment, and prognosis. *Pediatrics in Review, 32*(2), 56–64.

Tocchio, S. L. (2009). Treatment of conversion disorder: A clinical and holistic approach. *Journal of Psychosocial Nursing, 47*(8), 42–49.

Weber, S. (2009). Treatment of trauma- and abuse-related dissociative symptom disorders in children and adolescents. *Journal of Child and Adolescent Psychiatric Nursing, 22*(1), 2–6.

Zaidner, E., Sewell, R. A., Murray, E., Schiller, A., Price, B. H., & Cunningham, M. B. (2010). New-onset dissociative disorder after electroconvulsive therapy. *The Journal of ECT, 26*(3), 238–241.

20

Gender Identity and Sexual Disorders

KAREN LEE FONTAINE

KEY TERMS

LEARNING OUTCOMES

After completing this chapter, you will be able to:

1. Explore the values you hold regarding sexuality.
2. Describe the ranges of transgendered identities and behaviors.
3. Differentiate between adaptive and maladaptive sexual responses.
4. Integrate the various biopsychosocial theories into treatment for people with sexual disorders and gender dysphoria.
5. Construct a sexual history that includes affective, behavioral, cognitive, and sensation components.
6. Develop a more comfortable style when discussing clients' sexuality and sexual problems.

CRITICAL THINKING CHALLENGE

Charles is a 54-year-old man being treated on the inpatient unit for depression. This is his first hospital stay for a psychiatric problem, although he has had difficulties with depression for months. He has been married for 25 years, has no children, and his relationship with his wife Claudia has been strained for some time.

   One of the major problems Charles and Claudia are having is a sexual one. His arousal was based on certain activities in which Claudia no longer wanted to participate. As a couple they decided it would be beneficial to attend therapy focused on this problem. Couples sex therapy provided the opportunity to make some progress on this relationship problem with a specific plan designed for them by a sex therapist. Then Charles's symptoms of depression began affecting their sex life again, and once he began treatment with an antidepressant he experienced significant sexual side effects. The sexual challenge in this relationship was heightened by the problems caused by Charles's antidepressant medication.

1. Do you agree that clients on an inpatient unit should be expected to be celibate? Why, or why not?
2. Are professionals imposing their sexual practice values on clients? Why, or why not?
3. When clients are admitted, do they lose their right to consensual sexual activity with their partner? Why, or why not?

All humans are sexual beings. Regardless of gender, age, race, socioeconomic status, religious beliefs, physical and mental health, or other demographic factors, we express our sexuality in a variety of ways throughout our lives.

Human sexuality is difficult to define. Sexuality is an individually expressed and highly personal phenomenon whose meaning evolves from objective and subjective experiences. Physiological, psychosocial, and cultural factors influence a person's sexuality and lead to the wide range of attitudes and behaviors seen in humans. There are no normal, universal sexual behaviors. Satisfying or "normal" sexual expression can generally be described as whatever behaviors give pleasure and satisfaction to the adults involved, without threat of coercion or injury to others. North America is multicultural and has a sexually diverse population. As nurses, we work toward the goal of acknowledging and appreciating the rich sexual diversity of our clients.

Sexual health is an individual and constantly changing phenomenon falling within the wide range of human sexual thoughts, feelings, needs, and desires. A person's degree of sexual health is best determined by that individual, sometimes with the assistance of a qualified professional. Sexual health includes both *freedoms* and *responsibilities.* Sexually healthy people engage in activities that are freely chosen, including both self-pleasuring and consensually shared-pleasuring activities. Individuals also have freedom of sexual thought, feeling, and fantasy. Sexually healthy people are ethically motivated to exercise behavioral, emotional, economic, and social responsibility for themselves (Crooks & Baur, 2011).

Sexual health care is a relatively new area of involvement for psychiatric–mental health nurses. Until recently, sexuality has not been viewed as falling within their scope of practice. Currently, sexuality is increasingly recognized as an important component of a holistic approach to overall health status. Sexual health care is a legitimate and appropriate nursing concern. The close and often extended relationships that psychiatric–mental health nurses have with clients and families foster the rapport necessary to discuss this private area of clients' health status.

Nursing roles in the area of human sexuality are evolving gradually. Psychiatric–mental health nurses involved in nursing activities related to human sexual functioning need the following:

- Acceptance of, and comfort with, their own sexual values and expressions
- Concrete and comprehensive knowledge about sexual function and dysfunction
- Skill in communication techniques
- A willingness to explore and separate personal values and attitudes from those of clients

The nurse generalist should be proficient in using the nursing process to assess clients' sexual health and sexual concerns, promote optimal sexual health, play a supportive role, and refer clients to advanced practice nurses or other health care professionals with expertise in this area. The advanced practice clinical nurse specialist or nurse practitioner with special training and interest in gender identity and

sexual disorders can diagnose, intervene, and evaluate care to promote optimal sexual health.

Historically, human sexuality has been shrouded in myth and controversy. This history has hindered both the delivery and the receipt of services that promote sexual health and well-being. Although scientific knowledge has expanded immensely during the past several decades, modern North Americans continue to view sex and sexuality with discomfort. Our confusion is complicated by our traditional religious and social values. Basic to nursing is the notion that the nurse's personal beliefs should not influence the quality of care given a client. If nurses hold negative, inappropriate, or stereotyped opinions and ideas, they must confront them before they can meet professional standards of care in helping clients attain optimal sexual health. It is easier for nurses to live up to this standard if they engage in value clarification before providing sexual health care. Giving nonjudgmental nursing care does not mean that the nurse has to agree with others' beliefs and values about sexuality. However, self-awareness can help psychiatric–mental health nurses respect their clients' sexual rights and needs. Use Your Self-Awareness to assess your sexual knowledge and attitudes.

Because *homosexuality* (sexual attraction with same gender) and *bisexuality* (sexual attraction to both genders) are not psychiatric disorders, they are not covered in this chapter. Earlier in the 20th century, homosexuality was viewed as a mental disorder but was removed from the *Diagnostic and Statistical Manual of Mental Disorders* in 1973. Gender and identity issues are separate and distinct from sexual orientation.

GENDER AND TRANSGENDER

Western culture is deeply committed to the idea that there are only two sexes. Biologically speaking, however, there are many gradations running from female to male; these gradations are known collectively as *transgender.* In some cases gender is clear, in some it is unclear, and in other cases there is a blending of both genders within the same individual. This diversity of gender represents normal variations in the human population.

Gender Identity

Gender identity is an individual's personal or private sense of identity as female or male. Gender identity develops from an interaction of biology, identity imposed by others, and self-identity. A newborn is assigned a gender (identity imposed by others) according to the appearance of the external genitals (biology); by 3 years of age, the child says, "I am a girl" or "I am a boy" (self-identity).

Gender identity can be viewed as a continuum. At one end of the continuum are those whose gender identity is congruent with their anatomic sex. In the middle are people who have both male and female gender identities. At the other end of the continuum are those whose gender identity conflicts with their anatomic sex. In addition, sexual identity is fixed for some people, while for others it is more variable and changing.

Videos: Gender Identity Disorder

WebLink Application: Born With Wrong Body

YOUR SELF-AWARENESS
Check Your Knowledge and Attitudes About Sex

Use this checklist periodically to assess changes in your knowledge and attitudes.

Knowledge
Circle True or False for each statement.

Women can and do have orgasms while sleeping. .... **T   F**
It is dangerous to engage in intercourse during menstruation. .... **T   F**
Sex drive usually diminishes after a vasectomy. .... **T   F**
The older male may actually have some advantages over the younger male in sexual activity. .... **T   F**
Masturbation is a relatively common practice of both women and men. .... **T   F**
Females have two kinds of orgasm: clitoral and vaginal. .... **T   F**
Children raised by homosexual couples are very likely to become homosexual. .... **T   F**
An adult male who has been castrated immediately loses his sex drive. .... **T   F**
Intercourse should always be avoided during the last trimester of pregnancy. .... **T   F**
Oral–genital stimulation is unhygienic. .... **T   F**

Attitudes
Circle the letter corresponding to your level of agreement with each statement.

A: Strongly agree;   **B:** Agree;   **C:** Uncertain;   **D:** Disagree;   **E:** Strongly disagree

Sex education has caused a rise in premarital intercourse. .... **A   B   C   D**
Extramarital relations are almost always harmful to a marriage. .... **A   B   C   D**
Relieving tension by masturbation is a healthy practice. .... **A   B   C   D**
Premarital intercourse is morally undesirable. .... **A   B   C   D**
Parents should stop their children from masturbating. .... **A   B   C   D**
Women should have sexual experience before marriage. .... **A   B   C   D**
Homosexual and bisexual behavior should be against the law. .... **A   B   C   D**
Seeing family members nude arouses undue curiosity in children. .... **A   B   C   D**
Promiscuity is widespread on college campuses today. .... **A   B   C   D**
Men should have sexual experience before marriage. .... **A   B   C   D**

Gender Roles

Gender roles are the roles a person is expected to perform as a result of being male or female in a particular culture. The expectation that people will exhibit certain behaviors because they are female or male is referred to as *gender role stereotyping*. Stereotypical images of people do not take into account individual differences. The danger of such stereotypes is that people take them seriously and act on them, turning a blind eye to the qualities and interests of individuals. In North American culture, gender roles are more strictly enforced for males than for females; for example, males are socially punished for female behavior.

Androgyny, or flexibility in gender roles, reflects the belief that most characteristics and behaviors are human qualities that should not be limited to one specific gender or the other. Being androgynous does not mean being sexually neuter, nor does it imply anything about one's sexual orientation. Rather, it describes the degree of flexibility a person has regarding gender-stereotypic behaviors. Adults who can behave flexibly regarding their sexual roles may be able to adapt better than those who adopt rigid, stereotyped gender roles.

Disorders of Sexual Development

Some babies are born with a *disorder of sexual development,* in which there are contradictions among chromosomal gender, gonadal gender, internal organs, and external genital appearance.

WHY I BECAME A PSYCHIATRIC–MENTAL HEALTH NURSE

Karen Lee Fontaine, RN, MSN
Contributor, Chapters 20, 24

I was a young nurse in the 1960s when Masters and Johnson published the first scientific studies of human sexuality. Growing up, my family never discussed sex, and in nursing school we studied all body processes *except* sexual behavior. It was a conspiracy of silence. I was fascinated by this new information and was determined to become a sex therapist. Achieving a master's degree in psychiatric nursing was my route to becoming a sex therapist. One has to be proficient in individual and relationship therapy before specializing in sex therapy.

After earning my MSN in psychiatric nursing, I spent a year interning in sex therapy in one of the few early programs. With the proper preparation, I became certified by the American Association of Sexuality Educators, Counselors, and Therapists. I believe that, as a nurse, I bring a unique perspective to the field with my background in physiology, psychology, and spirituality.

I have always been fascinated by human behavior, thoughts, and feelings—in other words, "what makes people tick." Understanding and empowering people is basic to the practice of psychiatric nursing. Being a part of people's growth is a very satisfying professional experience.

Chaz Bono

Known now as Chaz Bono, the man in the photo was born Chastity Bono, a female, to entertainment artists Cher and Sonny Bono. Chaz is a Female to Male (FtM) transgender man. After being outed as a lesbian by the media years before, Chaz Bono disclosed his preferences and then went on to discuss the process of coming out in two books: *Family Outing: A Guide to the Coming Out Process for Gays, Lesbians, and Their*

Families (1998) and his memoir, *The End of Innocence* (2003). At the age of 39, Chaz underwent gender reassignment surgery and has been an advocate and spokesperson. His recent documentary on his life is an informative tale of how an individual can be empowered to take steps to make sure there is a match between psychological gender and socially recognized and external gender.

Photo courtesy © Allstar Picture Library/Alamy.

The gender of such an infant is ambiguous; he or she has some parts usually associated with males and some parts usually associated with females (Pasterski, Prentice, & Hughes, 2010).

Transsexuals

The medical profession considers *transsexuals* to have a condition called *gender incongruence* (strong and persistent feelings of discomfort with one's assigned sex) or **gender identity disorder**. For the transsexual person, sexual anatomy is not consistent with gender identity. Those who are born physically male but are emotionally and psychologically female are called *Male to Female* or *MtFs*. Those who are born female but are emotionally and psychologically male are called *Female to Male* or *FtMs*. Many consider transsexualism a normal variation and believe that gender identity disorder should be removed from the DSM. Others believe that deleting the diagnosis would lead to the denial of medical and surgical care for these individuals (Cohen-Kettenis & Pfafflin, 2010). A recent FtM in the news is Chaz Bono. See Mental Health in the News.

The practical realities of providing health care to this population have been addressed in a number of treatment centers in the United States. Such centers are designated LGBT, that is, they provide services for the lesbian, gay, bisexual, and transgender (LGBT) individual. Access to treatment is available without stigmatization or discrimination.

Most transsexuals report that they have felt gender *dysphoria* (discomfort) since earliest childhood. They often suffer for many years and try to hide the situation from family and friends for fear of being considered "crazy." Being transgendered puts women and men at extreme risk of being:

- Ridiculed and humiliated
- In constant jeopardy about getting and keeping a job
- Evicted without cause from restaurants and stores

- Denied housing
- Sometimes refused medical treatment, even to save a life

As self-understanding and acceptance increase, many transsexuals live part time or full time as members of the other gender. Cross-dressing (dressing in the clothing of the other gender) not only makes their outward appearance consistent with their inner identity and gender role but also increases their comfort with themselves. A number of individuals elect sex reassignment surgery so that their bodies match their gender identity. The vast majority report a high level of satisfaction with their surgery. Their sexual orientation pre- and postoperatively may be heterosexual, homosexual, or bisexual (Lawrence, 2010). See DSM Essential Features for gender identity disorder.

Cross-Dressers

Cross-dressers are typically males who cross-dress to express the feminine side of their personality. In most instances, people who cross-dress are not interested in permanently altering their bodies through surgical means, especially because the majority of them are comfortable with their original birth gender. Most cross-dressing individuals exhibit stereotypic masculine identity and behavior in their public and professional lives.

Cross-dressing is a conscious choice and may occur at home or in public settings. The frequency of the activity ranges from rarely to often. It is not unusual for cross-dressers to adopt a female name to go with the female personality and wardrobe. Cross-dressing occurs more frequently in cultures in which males are expected to be strong, independent, and unemotional protectors. If the social climate is perceived as one with rigid gender roles, some men may need to express gentleness and dependence by creating a separate world

DSM ESSENTIAL FEATURES

Gender Identity Disorder

Identifying strongly and persistently with the other gender, passing as the other gender, or identifying feelings and reactions of the other gender. There is persistent discomfort with the current gender role and a preoccupation with changing their bodies. In children, four or

more of: wanting to be or stating one is of the other gender, preference for cross-dressing, preference for cross-gender roles, pastimes, and playmates. Children will also feel disgusted with their anatomy and functioning.

and female persona within that social climate (Crooks & Baur, 2011).

Often, cross-dressers do not tell their spouses about the cross-dressing before the marriage. Some are embarrassed and do not know how to bring up the subject. Others view the need to cross-dress as a problem and hope it will disappear after the marriage. Most wives eventually find out. For some women, the discovery raises doubts about their own sexuality and self-worth, and they may decide to terminate the relationship. Some women are not threatened by the cross-dressing but fear it will become public knowledge. Other women move on to full acceptance and understanding of their partner's cross-dressing.

PARAPHILIAS

The DSM classifies **paraphilias** as a group of psychosexual disorders characterized by unconventional sexual behaviors. The person, usually a male, has learned to associate sexual arousal with some environmental stimulus, which triggers the unusual behavior. Paraphilias have a strong obsessive–compulsive component. Affected individuals are often preoccupied with, and feel compelled to engage in, their particular sexual behaviors. One of the distinguishing characteristics of paraphilias is the person's inability to control or stop the behavior. See DSM Essential Features for Paraphilias.

Noncoercive paraphilias are unconventional sexual behaviors engaged in by oneself or with a consenting adult. Many people engage in mild forms of the noncoercive behaviors and consider them simply love play. According to the DSM, the behavior becomes pathologic when it is severe, insistent, coercive, and harmful to self or others. The sexual behaviors known as *coercive* paraphilias are considered criminal acts and are described in the legal code. People with coercive paraphilias become sexually aroused by including nonconsenting persons in their sexual acts. See DSM Essential Features for paraphilias.

Fetishism

Humans respond to a wealth of sexual stimuli. Some people are aroused by the strident beat of rock music, while others are aroused by romantic music. Some people prefer making love in a brightly lit room; others, by candlelight; still others, in the dark. Everyone associates sexual arousal with an individual set of stimuli.

An association or stimulus that is not typical for the culture is called a *fetish*. A fetish is the sexualization of a body part, such as feet or hair, or an inanimate object, such as shoes, leather, or rubber. In **fetishism**, early associations of a particular object or body part with sexual arousal condition the person to respond sexually to that stimulus. Once the initial association is made, repeated viewing or use (fantasized or actual) of the part or object during sexual activity (usually masturbation) reinforces its arousing nature. For instance, a boy may get an erection after trying on his mother's panties. The erection is pleasurable. The next time the boy masturbates, he puts the panties on or fantasizes about them. With repeated experiences, seeing the panties or putting them on becomes a sexual stimulus. The following clinical example illustrates how a fetish can become an obsessive–compulsive behavior.

Clinical Example

LaDarius, a 24-year-old college graduate with a major in accounting, was unable to hold a job because of his foot fetish. LaDarius spent a considerable amount of time fantasizing about women's feet—bare feet, pretty feet, long, narrow feet—and how they looked, felt, tasted, and smelled. He fantasized at work, at the grocery store, and at the library (where he even went under tables to look at women's feet). LaDarius's fantasies made it impossible for him to work effectively or to maintain satisfactory interpersonal relationships with others. LaDarius refused therapy, preferring instead to pray that he would "get over it."

As with all people, fetishists' responses are highly individual. Fetishism is not considered a problem as long as it is not harmful and occurs in the context of consenting adult partners.

Transvestic Fetishism

In contrast with cross-dressers, men who become sexually aroused by dressing in women's clothing are considered **transvestic fetishists**. Almost 3% of men report at least one

DSM ESSENTIAL FEATURES

Paraphilias

Exhibitionism: Recurrent, intense sexually arousing fantasies, sexual urges, or actually exposing genitals to strangers.

Fetishism: Using objects for sexual arousal.

Frotteurism: Sexual arousal from touching and rubbing against people without their consent.

Pedophilia: Fantasizing about or having sex with a prepubescent child when either 16 years old or 5 years older than the child.

Sexual Masochism: Sexual arousal from suffering or being humiliated.

Sexual Sadism: Sexual arousal from causing psychological or physical suffering or humiliation to another.

Transvestic Fetishism: A heterosexual man achieves sexual satisfaction from fantasizing about or cross-dressing.

Voyeurism: Sexual arousal from observing people—without their knowledge—while they are undressing, are undressed, or are having sex.

episode of cross-dressing to obtain sexual excitement. They may wear female underclothes or may cross-dress completely. Like other fetishists, they have often undergone conditioning, and female clothing is an intense sexual stimulus. Many report great emotional stress if they try to resist the urge to cross-dress. Like other fetishes, cross-dressing is not considered a problem among consenting adult partners (Bhugra, Popelyuk, & McMullen, 2010).

Sadism and Masochism (S/M)

Sexual **sadism** (being sexually aroused by *inflicting* emotional or physical pain), and sexual **masochism** (being sexually aroused by *receiving* emotional or physical pain) are highly stigmatized in North American culture. Few people admit to being sexually aroused in this manner. As much as 10% of the population may participate in some form of S/M activity, and all groups—heterosexual, bisexual, homosexual—are represented. Physical behaviors include the following:

- Intense stimulation (scratching, biting, applying ice)
- Discipline (slapping, spanking, whipping)
- Bondage (holding down, tying down)
- Sensory deprivation (using blindfolds, hoods, ear plugs)

Psychological behaviors include humiliation or degradation, such as verbally berating others or requiring them to perform menial acts. S/M behavior varies in intensity and in its significance in the lives of couples. Some couples engage in the behavior only during sex. Some integrate the roles throughout the relationship, but not at all times. Other couples attempt to live out the dominant/submissive roles continuously.

Thus, S/M may be only a part of foreplay, or it may be a significant component of lifestyle. Most sadomasochists do not engage in S/M behavior unless the partner is willing and in that context it is not coercive. Typically, both participants agree to safety "rules," and seldom is the behavior dangerous. Sadomasochists do not see the behavior as a problem and therefore do not wish to change.

A fairly new description, BDSM, has come out of the sexual and gender minority subculture. It combines the behaviors B/D (bondage and discipline), D/S (dominance and submission), and S/M. Thus, BDSM refers to any or all of these behaviors. Participants find these activities highly erotic and emotionally charged. Often, the activities are subtle and sensual and have little resemblance to pornographic material.

A noncoercive but often fatal masochistic sexual behavior is **autoerotic asphyxia**, sometimes called *hypoxyphilia*. It is an example of sexual masochism in the DSM and is a compulsive and unconventional sexual behavior. Called *head-rushing* or *scarfing*, this behavior typically begins in adolescence and is primarily a male affliction. The person fashions a tourniquet-like device that constricts the neck, decreasing the blood and oxygen supply to the brain, masturbates, and, at the point of orgasm, releases the bonds to enhance the sensation or sexual high. Staff in emergency departments may see people who have had an acute event following autoerotic asphyxiation. See What Every Nurse Should Know for an example.

WHAT EVERY NURSE SHOULD KNOW

Autoerotic Asphyxia

Imagine you are an emergency department nurse. Be aware that some adolescents accidentally kill themselves through autoerotic asphyxia. Professionals may mistake the death for a purposeful hanging suicide. Parents are left confused and guilty because they never saw signs of self-harm. The circumstances of the death, such as nudity and the presence of erotic literature or art, often point to autoerotic asphyxia. Helping the parents understand that this was a tragic accident rather than a suicide helps them cope and grieve the loss of their child.

Tragically, this practice causes many deaths. The vagal nerve complex in the carotid artery is stimulated by pressure around the neck, slowing the heart rate and decreasing oxygen flow to the brain even further. The person becomes unconscious, slumps forward, and accidentally hangs himself. Many believe the cause of death is suicide, but family and friends cannot understand the reason for the suicide because these young men are not mentally ill or even troubled. Distinguishing features include evidence of sexual activity or a wide range of sexual paraphernalia such as bondage, hoods, and blindfolds.

Exhibitionism, Voyeurism, and Frotteurism

Exhibitionists and voyeurs, who are almost exclusively men, have powerful urges to display their genitals to strangers (**exhibitionism**) or peep at unsuspecting women involved in intimate behaviors (**voyeurism**). Frotteurs rub up against usually unsuspecting others, often in a crowded train or elevator, to achieve sexual arousal (**frotteurism**). The frotteur does not attempt to engage in sex with the victim and has no desire to form a relationship. Many describe the urge to peep, expose, or rub themselves against others as something that just "happens" to them and thus have difficulty assuming responsibility for their behavior.

Pedophilia

A pedophile is an adult who is sexually aroused by, and engages in sexual activity with, children. All sexual relationships between adults and children are considered coercive and are criminal in North America. The courts consider these acts nonconsensual because minors are presumed to have insufficient knowledge of the consequences of their acts to give meaningful consent. **Pedophilia** activities can include exposure, voyeurism, explicit sex talk, touching, oral sex, intercourse, and anal sex. The child usually knows the pedophile, who may be a family member, neighbor, or friend. Mental Health in the Movies discusses a situation in which a pedophile moves back into a neighborhood after serving jail time. For a thorough discussion of the dynamics and consequences of the sexual abuse of children, see Chapters 24 and 25∞.

MENTAL HEALTH IN THE MOVIES
Little Children

Little Children is a disturbing, complex movie with an uneasy undercurrent running through it. This film takes place in an upper-middle class suburb of Boston, to which Ronnie McGorvey, a registered sex offender, returns. When Ronnie moves in with his mother after serving a 2-year sentence for indecent exposure to a minor, the neighborhood is disrupted. One of the neighbors, Larry, a retired, disgraced cop begins a harassment campaign against Ronnie, handing out posters, vandalizing the house in which he and his mother live, and almost assaulting them. To make matters worse, a blind date for Ronnie goes badly—he masturbates in his date's car outside a children's playground and threatens her with violence if she tells. Definitely not a harmless victim, Ronnie becomes a pariah and a scapegoat for the personal feelings, extramarital affairs, and matrimonial malaise of the adults in the story. The element of danger in the movie surfaces at the end when Ronnie castrates himself. The film views pedophilia from two perspectives—the tortured and dangerous predator himself and the frightened parents and neighbors.

Photo courtesy © New Line Cinema/courtesy Everett Collection.

ALTERED SEXUAL FUNCTION

The ability to engage in sexual behavior is of great importance to most people. Many individuals experience transient problems with their ability to respond to sexual stimulation or to maintain the response. A smaller percentage of people experience problems that are lifelong in duration. FIGURE 20-1 ■ represents the prevalence of various problems for men and women. The problems may be generalized to all sexual interactions and settings, or they may be situational, occurring in a specific setting or with specific types of sexual activity. It is often difficult to sort out the multiple factors contributing to an individual's or couple's sexual problems. Both past factors and situations (lack of sex education, internalizing the belief that sex is dirty) and present (feelings of guilt, anger, or anxiety, fear of failure, spectatoring) contribute to an individual's or couple's sexual problems. For example, *spectatoring* is the detached appraisal of sexual performance of the body during a sexual act: "Am I going to lose my erection?" "Am I going to have an orgasm this time?" "My stomach is too flabby." "When did his thighs get that fat?" DSM Essential Features discusses sexual dysfunctions. For an overview of past and current factors that may contribute to sexual dysfunction, see TABLE 20-1 ■.

Sexual Desire Disorders

Sexual desire disorders are those that include a deficiency or absence of sexual fantasies and a deficiency or absence of desire for sexual behavior, or an aversion to and avoidance of genital sexual contact with a sex partner.

Hypoactive Sexual Desire Disorder

For most people, sexual desire varies from day to day as well as over the years. Some people, however, report a deficiency in or absence of sexual fantasies and persistently low interest or total lack of interest in sexual activity. These clients suffer from **hypoactive sexual desire disorder**. Low desire may be related to relationship problems, other sexual problems, dissatisfaction or boredom with sexual activities, negative messages in childhood, fears, performance anxiety, negative expectations, inaccurate beliefs about sexuality, negative body image, exhaustion, or discordance with sexual orientation. The etiology is most often multifactorial, and treatment focuses on all related factors.

If both individuals in a relationship are similarly uninterested in sex, there really is no problem. More typically, there is a disparity of sexual needs, and the person with the greater desire becomes dissatisfied with the sexual

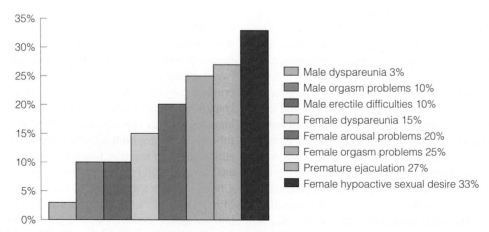

FIGURE 20-1 ■ Male and female prevalence rates of sexual dysfunctions/problems.

TABLE 20-1 ■ Factors Contributing to Sexual Dysfunctions

Type	Past Factors	Current Factors
Physical	■ Trauma: abuse, rape	■ Illness/injuries ■ Organic disorders ■ Medications ■ Substance abuse ■ Failure to engage in effective sexual behavior
Psychological	■ Taught that sex is dirty ■ Childhood sexual abuse	■ Performance anxiety ■ Spectatoring ■ Fear of failure ■ Guilt, anxiety, or anger ■ Negative thoughts
Sociologic	■ Punished as child for normal sex play ■ Lack of sex education	■ Failure to communicate ■ Relationship conflict ■ Not feeling connected to partner
Spiritual	■ Taught that sex is sinful ■ Childhood sexual abuse	■ Lack of intimacy ■ Fear of intimacy

relationship and often initiates seeking help. The key issue in the relationship is not frequency but rather neatly fitting together or combining smoothly and efficiently the different partners' needs.

Physiological factors associated with lack of desire are fatigue, illness, pain, the use of medications, and substance abuse. Maturational factors such as menopause and the effects of surgical procedures that cause menopause can also contribute to decreases in desire. Evidence-Based Practice addresses postmenopausal sexual difficulties.

Sexual Aversion Disorder

Sexual aversion disorder is a severe distaste for sexual activity or the thought of sexual activity, which then leads to a phobic avoidance of sex. It occurs in both women and men. Intense emotional dread of an impending sexual interaction also can trigger the physiological symptoms of anxiety: sweating, increased heart rate, and extreme muscle tension. The client then stops the sexual interaction or prevents it from even beginning. The most common cause of sexual aversion disorder is childhood sexual abuse or adult rape. This severe trauma can lead to a phobic response to sexual activity (Lewis et al., 2010). The following clinical example illustrates how sexual trauma can contribute to sexual aversion.

Clinical Example

Linda and Mike, both 32 years of age, dated all through high school and have been married for 12 years. Linda has a strong aversion to body secretions. She spends hours in the bathtub before she and Mike have sex. Although Mike wears a condom, Linda jumps out of bed before he has finished ejaculating and runs to the bathtub.

Linda can't identify any reasons for her feelings of disgust about body secretions and denies a history of sexual abuse. She does, however, talk about feeling violated by Mike when he "talked me into sex" at age 18. Sometimes she refers to this first sexual experience as date rape.

Despite this problem, Linda and Mike refer to themselves as best friends. Linda has suggested that their marriage be conducted as a platonic relationship. Mike's not sure he wants to live that way the rest of his life. They are in counseling and want to learn how to enjoy one another sexually. Currently, they are learning how to be less genitally focused and to spend more time cuddling, stroking, and touching.

Sexual Arousal Disorders

Sexual arousal refers to the physiological responses and subjective sense of excitement experienced during sexual activity. Lack of lubrication and failure to attain or maintain an erection are the major disorders of the arousal phase. In

DSM ESSENTIAL FEATURES

Sexual Dysfunctions

Dyspareunia: Male or a female genital pain on sexual intercourse.

Female Orgasmic Disorder: Orgasm is less than reasonable for sexual stimulation.

Female Sexual Arousal Disorder: Insufficient excitement leading to lubrication during sex.

Hypoactive Sexual Desire Disorder: Insufficient or absent desire for sexual activity.

Male Erectile Disorder: Inadequate erection.

Male Orgasmic Disorder: Inability, or long delay, in achieving orgasm.

Premature Ejaculation: Ejaculating with minimal sexual stimulation and before preferred.

Sexual Aversion Disorder: Extreme avoidance to sex.

Vaginismus: Involuntary muscle spasms of the outer third of the vagina interfering with sexual intercourse.

EVIDENCE-BASED PRACTICE

Postmenopausal Sexual Difficulties

Peggy is a 57-year-old female who is finding the postmenopausal stage of life a difficult one. Her desire for sexual activity is particularly low, which is affecting her sex life and her relationship with her partner. All physical and psychological sources for the problem have been ruled out. You work in the gynecology clinic where Peggy is being treated. Peggy asked the nurse practitioner about treatment with testosterone.

Following Peggy's appointment, you and the nurse practitioner discussed testosterone's use in postmenopausal hormone replacement therapy. Available data on its use is conflicting and confusing, but the practice is becoming more widespread. One of the problems with this choice of treatment is that women of Peggy's age group are routinely excluded from research examining effectiveness of treatment; therefore, specific information regarding benefits and risks are lacking.

Currently, there is extensive off-label use by women of a variety of testosterone preparations, including implants, creams, and gels. Some men, especially those with muscle-building as well as sexuality concerns, use testosterone regularly. Because the use of this hormone carries risks, there is reason for some concern.

Further research is needed to determine the role of androgen insufficiency as a cause of low desire in premenopausal as well as postmenopausal women. The role androgens can play in female sexuality will become clearer once practitioners attend to the diurnal variation of testosterone in women and examine these impacts on sexual expression. Research that includes women as participants in testosterone treatment studies and androgen correlation studies can shed some light on risk before primary health care providers routinely prescribe testosterone to women experiencing low desire or to postmenopausal women.

Emerson, C. R. (2010). Review of low libido in women. *International Journal of STD & AIDS, 21,* 312–316.

Garcia, F. D., & Thibaut, F. (2010). Sexual addictions. *American Journal of Drug and Alcohol Abuse, 36*(52), 254–260.

Jutel, A. (2010). Framing disease: The example of female hypoactive sexual desire disorder. *Social Science & Medicine, 70,* 1084–1090.

Laughlin, G. A., Goodell, V., & Barrett-Connor, E. (2010). Extremes of endogenous testosterone are associated with increased risk of incident coronary events in older women. *Journal of Clinical Endocrinology & Metabolism, 95,* 740–747.

CRITICAL THINKING QUESTIONS

1. If medications are approved for use in specific conditions or illnesses, should off-label use be allowed? Why, or why not?
2. Is off-label use an ethical and professionally responsible act? Why, or why not?
3. Because menopause is an anticipated maturational transition for women, why not just let the symptoms take their course?
4. If women are not included as research subjects, should study results and recommendations apply to them? Why, or why not?

---

female sexual arousal disorder, the lack of vaginal lubrication causes discomfort or pain during sexual intercourse. The diagnosis of **male erectile disorder** is usually made when the man has erection problems during 25% or more of his sexual interactions.

Some men cannot attain a full erection, and others lose their erection prior to orgasm. The pejorative term commonly applied to this condition, *impotence,* implies that the man is feeble, inadequate, and incompetent. The accurate term is **erectile dysfunction (ED)**, which is objectively descriptive and not judgmental. By the age of 60, 20% to 40% of men complain of at least mild ED. Arousal disorder may also be diagnosed even when lubrication and erection are adequate if individuals report a persistent or recurring lack of subjective sexual excitement or pleasure (Lewis et al., 2010).

There may be other physiological sources for sexual arousal disorders. Medications—especially beta blockers, SSRI antidepressants, SNRI antidepressants, and ADHD medications—can have sexual side effects. In addition, disease processes such as diabetes, hypertension, and cardiovascular disease can cause ED. The side effects of these medications are discussed in Chapters 7 and 31∞.

Oral medications have been the biggest breakthrough for ED. These medications work by relaxing smooth muscles in the penis, thus allowing arteries to expand and increase blood flow into the penis, causing an erection. These medications are sildenafil (Viagra), vardenafil (Levitra), and tadalafil (Cialis). Although research has been conducted using these medications for female sexual problems, the results have been inconclusive. Selective serotonin reuptake inhibitors (SSRIs) may be given for rapid ejaculation, because a common side effect is a slowdown in orgasmic response. The doses are usually lower than those given for depression.

Many prescription medications have side effects that affect sexual functioning. The impact is generally negative, but sometimes there is a positive impact. For example, antidepressants may slow ejaculation. This may be a problem for the man who finds himself suddenly feeling unable to ejaculate. If a man is suffering from rapid ejaculation, however, the antidepressant may "cure" this problem. The two antidepressants with the fewest sexual side effects are bupropion (Wellbutrin) and escitalopram (Lexapro). Some street drugs such as marijuana, amphetamine, and cocaine increase sexual drive and activity. Others, such as opioids and anabolic steroids, interfere with sexual functioning. The following clinical example illustrates how a negative experience with a psychiatric medication can influence the treatment plan.

Clinical Example

Jared is seeing an advanced practice psychiatric nurse for clinical depression. After several weeks with no improvement, the nurse suggested he consider taking an antidepressant to lift his mood and facilitate the psychotherapy. Jared refused outright, saying, "I took Prozac a couple of years ago and it caused me to lose my orgasms. I'm never taking that stuff again. I would rather be depressed than give up my sex life."

Psychological factors may also be a cause of arousal disorders. They include fear of failure, anxiety, anger, poor communication, and relationship conflict. Insufficient vaginal lubrication is less likely than erectile inhibition to create severe distress for couples, because using a water-based lubricant or saliva can correct the immediate problem. An erectile problem may be threatening to a man who feels that his whole sense of masculinity is at stake. Men tend to be dominated by a genital focus more than women. Therefore, difficulty in getting the penis to "perform" results in humiliation and despair. The following clinical example illustrates how thoughts and expectations can become self-fulfilling prophecies.

Clinical Example

Paweena and Morufat, both 45 years of age, sought counseling when Morufat found it impossible to achieve an erection. The first time he was unable to achieve an erection was 6 years ago. This was an emotionally traumatic experience for Morufat, who spent a considerable amount of time worrying that it would happen again. Eventually it did, and Morufat found that he could not attain an erection more and more often. About 6 months ago he consulted an urologist. Nighttime penile tumescence studies showed normal functioning.

The couple was referred to a nurse sex therapist, who discovered that Morufat had believed, from an early age, that sexual functioning stopped once the man reached age 49. In working with the couple, the nurse focused on providing sex education and experiential/sensory awareness training. Once it didn't matter whether Morufat achieved an erection, his performance anxiety was decreased and he was able to do so.

Orgasmic Disorders

Orgasmic disorders are those that occur at, or just before, the peaking of sexual pleasure. There are three types of orgasmic disorders: female orgasmic disorder, male orgasmic disorder, and premature ejaculation.

Female Orgasmic Disorder

The pejorative term commonly applied in the past to women who did not experience orgasm, *frigid,* implies that the woman is totally incapable of responding sexually. The more accurate and objective term is **female orgasmic disorder**, which simply means that the sexual response stops before orgasm occurs. Preorgasmic women have never experienced an orgasm; secondarily nonorgasmic women have had orgasms in the past but do not currently experience them; and situationally nonorgasmic women have orgasms in some situations but not in others. Compounding the orgasmic difficulty is the associated anxiety. In the preoccupation with

orgasm, the real goal of being sexual—mutual pleasuring and intimacy—is lost, and the interchange becomes one of anxiety, frustration, and anger.

Physiological factors related to inhibited female orgasm include fatigue, illness, neurologic or vascular damage, and medications and drugs that interfere with sexual response. In the physically healthy woman, lack of information or negative attitudes about female sexual response often contribute to orgasmic disorder. Women who were taught that masturbation is wrong or sinful may not have explored their own bodies. If so, they cannot teach a partner where, how, and when to touch.

Male Orgasmic Disorder

Some men suffer from **male orgasmic disorder**. Men with this disorder can maintain an erection for long periods (an hour or more) but have extreme difficulty ejaculating, called *retarded ejaculation.* In heterosexual intercourse, the difficulty may be limited to ejaculation in the vagina. Some men ejaculate after self-stimulation or manual or oral stimulation by the partner, whereas others have great difficulty ejaculating with any type of stimulation. This disorder is much less common than rapid ejaculation.

Organic causes inhibiting orgasm include spinal cord injuries, multiple sclerosis, Parkinson's disease, and use of certain medications. Psychogenic factors include fear of pregnancy, performance pressure, fear of losing control, and anxiety and guilt about engaging in sexual activity. As with other dysfunctions, the difficulty can adversely affect the sexual relationship.

Premature Ejaculation

Rapid ejaculation, or **premature ejaculation**, is one of the most common sexual problems among men. There are many definitions, ranging from ejaculating before being touched, ejaculating before penetration, ejaculating with one internal thrust, to ejaculating within a minute or two of penetration. A more helpful description is the absence of voluntary control of ejaculation. The problem is best self-defined: A man is concerned about his ejaculatory control, or the couple agrees that ejaculation is too rapid for mutual satisfaction.

There is very little information about the mechanisms causing rapid ejaculation. Possible influences include the man's:

- Inability to perceive his arousal level accurately
- Lowered sensory threshold due to infrequent sexual activity
- Early conditioning resulting from hurried masturbation or hurried sexual intercourse

Educating about sexual dysfunction can be enhanced with the information in Partnering With Clients and Families.

Sexual Pain Disorder

A **sexual pain disorder** is genital pain that occurs during sexual intercourse. The two types of sexual pain disorders are dyspareunia and vaginismus.

PARTNERING WITH CLIENTS AND FAMILIES

Teaching About Sexual Desire

- Sexual desire varies from day to day as well as over the years.
- Physical factors include low testosterone levels, chronic diseases, and side effects of medications and medical treatments.
- Intrapersonal factors include sexual guilt and anxiety, lack of knowledge, a negative self-concept, and a negative body image.

- Interpersonal factors include conflict, negative communication, fatigue, lack of time, and dislike or fear of the partner.
- Encourage open communication about the situation and each person's feelings about what is or is not happening in their sexual relationship.
- Refer for sex therapy if the issue is not resolved through communication.

Dyspareunia

Both women and men can experience **dyspareunia**, pain during or immediately after intercourse. It is associated with many physiological causes, especially those that inhibit lubrication. Thus, skin irritations, vaginal infections, estrogen deficiencies, and medications that dry vaginal secretions can cause women to experience discomfort with intercourse.

Pelvic disorders, such as infections, small lesions, endometriosis, scar tissue, or tumors, can result in painful intercourse. Engaging in painful intercourse can lead to vaginismus because the body reflexively becomes guarded and tense. Similarly, in males, infection or inflammation of the glans penis or other genitourinary organs can cause pain with coitus (sexual intercourse). Also, some contraceptive foams, creams, or sponges can irritate either the vagina or the penis, causing pain. For both women and men, fear and anxiety in anticipation of pain can undermine the ability to feel pleasurable sexual responses and may lead to an avoidance of sexual activity.

Vulvodynia is constant, unremitting burning that is localized to the vulva with an acute onset. The girl or woman has problems sitting, standing, and sleeping related to the intensity of pain. In contrast, *vestibulitis* causes severe pain only on touch or attempted vaginal entry. Half of women with vestibulitis report lifelong dyspareunia. Women with either of these disorders report a negative impact on their sexual functioning and partner relationship, as well as on their self-esteem and mental health (Goetsch et al., 2010). Vulvodynia and vestibulitis are systemic problems that take some time and a lot of effort to overcome. A low-glycemic diet—no sugar or white foods—is most helpful. It is also important to test for food allergies, because these seem to contribute to the inflammation. When the pain and inflammation are reduced, pelvic floor therapy by specially trained physical therapists is begun. Hands-on techniques include massage therapy and myofascia and pudendal nerve release. Vaginal dilators may be introduced for home use. An individual exercise program is designed to strengthen weak muscles and stretch tight muscles. Pelvic floor biofeedback measures the tension of the pelvic floor muscles and helps clients learn to relax and strengthen them. Other techniques include pelvic floor electrical stimulation and perineal ultrasound.

Vaginismus

An involuntary spasm of the outer one third of the vaginal muscles, making penetration of the vagina painful and sometimes impossible, is called **vaginismus**. The woman often experiences desire, excitement, and orgasm with stimulation of the external sexual structures. Attempts at intercourse, however, elicit the involuntary spasm. She may have similar difficulty undergoing pelvic exams and inserting tampons or a diaphragm.

The vaginismic response may develop initially as a protection against real or anticipated pain. It is often associated with sexual trauma, such as childhood sexual abuse or adult rape. Emotional conflicts, such as extreme fear of pregnancy or intense guilt about engaging in sexual activity, may be additional contributing factors.

The partner of a woman with vaginismus often becomes fearful and anxious about hurting her, or may become resentful, believing that she has spasms on purpose. Partners may develop secondary dysfunctions as a result of these negative feelings and interpretations of rejection.

Increased Sexual Interest

An increased interest in sex and sexual activity is symptomatic of the manic phase of bipolar disorder. Elevated mood is accompanied by a corresponding rise in sexual activity, variety of activity, and, often, number of partners. This behavior occurs despite contrary values, is out of the client's control, and puts the client at risk for HIV and other sexually transmitted infections. The end of the manic episode signals a return to the person's usual level of sexual interest and activity. Because memory is not impaired, the person may feel embarrassed and ashamed about uncontrolled sexual behavior during the manic episode.

Some adult survivors of childhood sexual abuse may go through periods of high sexual activity. This is often a desperate attempt to obtain the nurturance, love, care, and power they were denied in childhood. Having been sexualized at an inappropriately early age, some have learned to survive in a hostile environment by using their sexual availability to make contact with or control others. More information on the impacts of childhood sexual abuse is discussed in Chapter 24 ∞.

Sexual Addiction

Frequency of sexual activity can be viewed on a continuum, with most people falling in the middle range. Some people have sex frequently in a way that enhances their lives; others have sex infrequently and report contentment and satisfaction. A sexual pattern that falls at either extreme of the continuum, however, can signal problems. At the low extreme are individuals who have great difficulty in choosing to be sexual; such people may have a sexual dysfunction. At the high extreme are people who have lost their ability to choose or control their sexual behavior; these people are sexual addicts.

Sexual addiction is a disorder in which the central focus of life is sex. People with this addiction spend 50% or more of all waking hours dealing with sex, from fantasy to acting-out behavior. Acting-out behaviors are often victimless (the partner is consenting), such as having affairs; overindulging in masturbation, fetishism, pornography use, or commercial telephone sex; or visiting prostitutes. Victimizing behaviors (those with a nonconsenting partner) are less frequent. The incidence of sexual addiction is difficult to determine because of secrecy and shame, but it is estimated that 3% to 6% of the population may be affected. It is predominantly a male disorder, with a gender ratio of 3:1 (Garcia & Thibaut, 2010; Cheever, 2008).

It is unethical to label people who do not conform to conventional moral codes as sexual addicts. Sexual addiction is not simply the frequent enjoyment of sexual behaviors. Many people engage in those behaviors without becoming sexual addicts. Rather, sexual addiction is a progressive disorder in which sex is used to numb pain. The payoff is the same as in any other addiction: an intensely pleasurable high, a short-lived release from pain, and an escape from the problems of daily life. The consequences are also the same in that the addict's life eventually becomes unmanageable. The components of sexual addiction are discussed in Box 20-1.

Clients who have a true sexual addiction are usually referred to a twelve-step-based recovery program. As with other twelve-step programs, the initial standard is 90 meetings in 90 days. These programs are generally available in urban settings and have no associated financial cost. There is usually a sense of a "healing community" that includes others with similar hypersexual problems.

BIOPSYCHOSOCIAL THEORIES

Human sexual behavior has been studied from various theoretic perspectives. The most significant are biologic, intrapersonal, behavioral, interpersonal, and sociocultural theories. A review of the various theoretic perspectives shows that human sexuality has been historically characterized by judgments and controversy that have inhibited sexual health care services. It is important for health care professionals to remember that all people to some extent deviate from some physical, social, behavioral, or emotional norm. Some are left handed, some stutter, some are disabled, some are loners, and some are filled with fears. To achieve the highest level of professional practice, nurses must look beyond the characteristics and respond to the whole person.

Only in the past 40 years has human sexuality been scientifically studied from a multidisciplinary approach. With this knowledge came the beginnings of planned interventions for individuals suffering from a variety of sexual problems and disorders. Nursing has been an active participant in the evolution of treatment approaches and programs to provide sexual health care. The current state of nursing involvement—the nursing diagnoses and therapeutic interventions discussed throughout this chapter—indicates nursing's continued dedication to furthering this area of study.

Biologic Theory

Those individuals who take a biologic approach are concerned with the physiological aspects of gender identity and sexual behavior. Some believe there is a neurologic basis for gender differences and look to fetal exposure to sex hormones and adult levels of sex hormones as an explanation of gender dysphoria. They explore sexual dysfunctions to discover factors (e.g., organic disease, injury, medications, pain, and/or depression) that interfere with the physiological reflexes during the sexual response cycle.

It is clear from research over the past several years that the majority of sexual problems are initially physiological in nature. In middle age, for example, normal physiological changes (such as decreased hormone production) may interfere with sexual pleasure and interest. Side effects of many medications or medical treatment may contribute to sexual problems. Arteriosclerosis, diabetes, and other medical problems can interfere with the ability to have an erection. Not understanding the physical basis of the

---

Box 20-1 Components of Sexual Addiction

The components of sexual addiction have the hallmarks of obsessive–compulsive behavior.

1. *Preoccupation.* The person spends hours thinking or obsessing about sex. Preoccupation, in itself, gives a sexual high and is so time consuming that the person cannot fulfill work, school, or family responsibilities.
2. *Ritualization.* The individual engages in specific behaviors done just the "right" way and in the same sequence each time. Ritual behaviors include wearing certain clothing, taking certain steps to get ready, driving certain routes, or looking for partners only in a certain area. The ritual seems to control anxiety; once addicts begin a ritual, they cannot stop until the cycle is completed.
3. *Compulsivity.* The person cannot control sexual behavior, and this behavior becomes the most important aspect of life. Some demonstrate sexually compulsive behavior in a regular pattern; others resist for a time and then have a binge cycle.
4. *Shame and despair.* At the end of the cycle, the person experiences guilt and shame at the loss of control. The pain of despair creates the need to begin the cycle all over again, because the addict seeks to relieve pain by getting high. Like other addicts, these individuals want to stop their behavior, promise to stop, try to stop, and are unable to stop without treatment.

problem, people experience anxiety, shame, or guilt, and the stage is set for the emotional component—distress—related to sexual problems.

At this time, there is no clear understanding of the etiology of transsexualism. Biologic theory is based on animal studies because experimental research cannot be conducted with humans. When exposed prenatally to increased male hormones, experimental animals exhibit increased male behavior. Decreasing the levels of male hormones prenatally increases female behavior in animals. In humans, the male gonads develop and begin secreting androgen during weeks 8 to 12 of gestation. Differentiation of the hypothalamus to a male pattern, which occurs in months 4 to 5 of gestation, requires high androgen levels. Thus, one explanation of transsexualism is that prenatal androgen levels were sufficient for the development of male anatomy but insufficient for differentiation in the brain. In transsexuals who are anatomically female, the androgenic influences may have been high at the critical time of hypothalamic development, although not at the time of genital formation (Crooks & Baur, 2011).

Intrapersonal Theory

Intrapersonal theorists view gender dysphoria, paraphilias, and sexual dysfunctions as problems occurring within the individual. Some view them as expressions of arrested psychosexual development, some seek an explanation in sexual guilt, some see the issue as being one of self-punishment, and others see these as normal variations. People who grew up with rigid family and religious taboos about sex often experience guilt and anxiety about their adult sexual roles and behaviors. Inadequate sex education can lead to ignorance and anxiety about sexuality. Performance anxiety, negative self-concept, and negative body image are all seen as contributing to sexual problems. Problems to be solved during the treatment process include fears of the following:

- Intimacy
- Losing control
- Pain
- Pregnancy
- Sexually transmitted infections

Clients who have difficulties communicating about sexual issues need guidance. You can help clients communicate about sex more clearly and effectively.

Behavioral Theory

Behaviorists believe that gender dysphoria arises from social learning; that is, that the child was rewarded in some way for adopting behaviors of the other sex. They believe paraphilias are learned responses; the person is conditioned to respond erotically to nonsexual objects or particular sexual acts. In the area of sexual dysfunctions, contributing factors include poor communication skills, lack of sexual experience with oneself or a partner, concern with sexual performance, and ineffective stimulation. The dysfunctions, too, are seen as learned responses.

Interpersonal Factors

Relationship difficulties may cause sexual problems. Negative patterns of communication or dislike or fear of one's partner inhibit sexual expression. Conflict over commonplace issues such as money, schedules, or relatives may lead to a loss of sexual interest. An inability to talk about preferences in initiating sex or determining sexual activities creates problems for some people. Fatigue and lack of time due to family and work obligations are other common causes. Likewise, sexual problems can contribute to relationship difficulties, especially when couples do not openly communicate about the situation. Misunderstanding leads to inappropriate guilt or anger and withdrawal from the relationship. Working with clients who have sexual difficulties requires sensitivity and knowledge about how to communicate effectively. See the Nursing Care Plan at the end of this chapter for a full review of a plan of care for a client with sexual difficulties.

Sociocultural Factors

Ideas about sexuality and sexual behavior are based on cultural values and understanding. What is considered normal or abnormal depends on each group's specific viewpoint. The same behavior may be seen as positive in one culture and pathologic in another. Each culture tends to incorporate ethnocentrism in its beliefs; that is, its members believe their particular sexual values and behaviors are superior and preferable to those of any other culture. Ethnocentrism encourages people to view the sexual behavior of other people as eccentric, exotic, and bizarre. See Your Assessment Approach later in this chapter for an example of eliciting a sexuality history that includes cultural factors.

How people communicate about sexuality is culturally determined. In general, North American culture reflects Euro-American values, which include a negative view of public sexual communication, as evidenced by censorship and the attitude that sex is a taboo topic for general discussion. However, there are ethnic differences in communication patterns. African-Americans tend to be very expressive and communicate directly about sexual topics. Latinos from the Caribbean and Central American cultures tend to be restrained in expressing their feelings, while those from Argentina and some other Latin American countries are emotionally expressive. Asian-Americans are often less verbally expressive, so nonverbal communication assumes even more importance. The gay and lesbian subculture has developed private words and expressions in reaction to the homophobia of the dominant culture. Developing Cultural Competence explores attitudes and views of sexual behavior and culture.

Sociocultural theories regarding sexual dysfunctions focus on disturbed relationships between partners, negative early learning, and past or present traumatic events. Women who have had sexual problems related to abuse and pregnancy are seen in a variety of settings. See What Every Nurse Should Know for a perspective on working with survivors of sexual trauma.

DEVELOPING CULTURAL COMPETENCE

Culture and Sexuality

Consider the diversity of sexual values throughout the world. The Mangaia of Polynesia believe that young adolescents of both genders have high sexual drives. However, as they leave young adulthood, they expect their desire to rapidly decline. In contrast, the Dani of New Guinea believe that neither women nor men have high sexual drives and that the primary purpose of sex is reproduction. Following the birth of a child, the husband and wife remain celibate for the next 5 years. Among the Sambrans of New Guinea, young boys around age 7 or 8 have sex with older boys. It is believed that the ingestion of semen is required for physical growth. This pattern of behavior changes to heterosexual interaction as the young men become adults.

Cultures in some parts of Africa and the Middle East practice ritual mutilation of the clitoris, called *female genital mutilation*, as a rite of initiation into womanhood. Because of serious medical complications and psychological trauma, the practice has been outlawed in many countries, although the laws are rarely enforced (Barungi & Twongyeirwe, 2009). Among many cultures throughout the world, there is a third gender. Among the Zuni of New Mexico, this person is called a *berdache*, a male who assumes female dress, gender role, and status. Individuals with this third gender are often considered to have great spiritual power.

The sexual ethics of a culture reflect the culture's assumptions about the purpose of sex. In North American culture, sexual practices have been strongly influenced by the Judeo-Christian tradition, which historically considered procreation to be the primary purpose of sex. As a result, even modern North American culture is fairly sexually intolerant and harshly critical of those whose gender identity or sexual behavior is not in the mainstream. People with little tolerance for cross-gender behavior view transsexuals and cross-dressers as deviants. The sexual acts of noncoercive paraphiliacs conflict with the traditional value of sex for procreation, and they, too, are made to feel like outcasts.

CRITICAL THINKING QUESTIONS

1. What advantages/disadvantages can you identify for the various behavioral patterns concerning sex?
2. How would experiences such as specific acculturation provide dissonance in a sexual relationship?

NURSING PROCESS
Clients With Sexual Problems

The specialized nursing care of clients with gender identity and sexual disorders requires extensive background and experience. While nurses at all levels of practice should aim to develop a trusting relationship and assess clients for sexual concerns, they should refer clients to a health care provider with special expertise in dealing with these complex issues. The actual diagnoses and interventions of these clients are best left to the providers with special expertise.

Assessment

Information about a client's sexual health status should always be an integral part of a nursing assessment. The

WHAT EVERY NURSE SHOULD KNOW

Survivors of Sexual Trauma

Imagine you are an obstetrics nurse. Women who are survivors of sexual trauma may experience difficulty during labor and delivery. There is little sense of privacy during this time, because a variety of people check the progress of labor and are present for the delivery. This may trigger flashbacks to the abusive situation. Some survivors may feel they have little or no control over what is happening to their body, similar to what they felt when they were victimized. It is important for the staff to know when they are working with survivors so they can anticipate what might occur and intervene in a timely fashion.

amount and kind of data collected depend on the context of the assessment, that is, the client's reason for seeking health care and how the client's sexuality interacts with other problems. Including a sexual history as part of the general nursing history is important for some clients and not important for others. It is critical, however, at least to introduce the topic of sexuality to give permission for clients to bring up any concerns or problems.

Subjective Data

The sexual history provides subjective assessment data needed to formulate nursing diagnoses. Elicit sexual information in the same way you elicit a general nursing history. Pay special attention, however, to planning a setting in which privacy and uninterrupted time are available. Such a setting helps clients feel comfortable discussing these private aspects of their lives. It is helpful to begin the interview by explaining why you are asking about sexuality; for example: "Sexuality is a part of people's lives. People often have questions about sexual activity when they have changes in their health. I'd like to take this time to talk with you about your sex life."

Move from general to specific questions. This gradual focus on specific sexual behavior promotes trust and rapport. Initially, questions can relate sexuality to health status. Open-ended questions encourage clients to expand on their sexual experiences and concerns. Reassure clients that it is normal to have sexual concerns and questions, for instance: "It is common for many people to feel concerned about _____. Do you have any questions?" Restate clients' responses to encourage them to expand on their feelings.

All nursing histories should at least include a question such as, "Have there been any changes in your sexual functioning that might be related to your illness or the medications you take?" Nurses might also facilitate communication by saying, "As a nurse, I'm concerned about all aspects of your health. People often have questions about sexual matters, both when they are well and when they are ill. When I take your history, sexual concerns are included to help plan a comprehensive treatment approach." Suggestions for eliciting a sexual history

Affective Assessment

- With whom do you feel most intimate and connected?
- Describe the type of love and affection in this relationship.
- In what way do you experience anxiety about sex?
- In what way do you experience guilt about sex?
- How depressed do you feel?
- In what way does anger interfere with your sexual functioning?
- Do you dislike or feel an aversion toward any parts of your body?

Behavioral Assessment

- Describe your level of satisfaction with the frequency of your sexual activity.
- Describe the positive aspects of your own sexual functioning.
- Describe the negative aspects of your own sexual functioning.
- What concerns do you have about your future sexual functioning?
- What are your partner's concerns about current or future sexual functioning?

Cognitive Assessment

- When you were growing up, how did you learn about sex?
- How has your religion influenced your sexual values and behaviors?
- What "shoulds/should nots," "musts/must nots" do you believe about your sexual behavior/relationships?
- How rigidly were gender roles enforced in your family of origin?
- How are gender roles enacted in your present relationship/family?
- Describe the negative thoughts you have about sex.
- Does the use of fantasy increase or decrease your sexual desire?

Sensation Assessment

- Describe any physical discomfort you feel during sexual activity.
- To what degree do you experience pleasure during sexual activity?

are in Your Assessment Approach. If clients do identify a sexual problem or if they take medications that affect sexual desire or sexual behavior, you can use the information in TABLE 20-2 ■ to formulate additional questions.

Objective Data

Objective data include observed nonverbal behaviors, laboratory data, test results, medical diagnoses, physical examination results, and other documented sources, such as the chart. Objective data may also include results of physiological assessment of sexual function.

Erectile Capacity The nocturnal penile tumescence (NPT) procedure provides a direct measure of erectile capacity. The device measures penile engorgement that occurs during sleep. NPT measurement is considered the best available method to determine if a man's erectile difficulties are physiological. If so, there is minimal penile engorgement during sleep. Men whose erection difficulties appear to be psychological in origin have normal engorgement during sleep.

Female Sexual Function Physiological assessment of female sexual function is accomplished by the use of vaginal plethysmographs or probes. These devices are inserted into the vagina and measure vasocongestion of the vaginal wall tissue.

Laboratory Tests Several sophisticated and expensive laboratory tests are designed to assess sexual function. For instance, testosterone (androgen) and estrogen blood levels may be measured. However, laboratory data must be interpreted with caution because test results are not always reliable indicators of actual sexual behavior. Thus, clients' self-reports of sexual performance, feelings, and values (the subjective data) are of primary importance in assessment.

Androgen levels in women peak in early adulthood and decrease slowly with aging. Women in their 40s have approximately one half the level of women in their 20s. Testosterone has been linked to sexual desire and sexual frequency in menopausal women. At present, it appears that testosterone therapy improves sexual function in women with low levels.

Nursing Diagnosis: NANDA

A number of nursing diagnoses are applicable for clients experiencing gender identity disorders and sexual problems. They are discussed in this section.

Anxiety and Fear

Anxiety and fear inhibit the physiological sexual response as well as the ability to experience pleasure and joy. People who grow up learning that sex is dirty and sinful often experience anxiety in an adult relationship or are so fearful that they develop a phobic avoidance of sex. Adults who have been emotionally, physically, or sexually abused as children often fear intimacy and find they cannot have a trusting relationship with another person. Even individuals with a positive sexual history may at some time feel anxious about their sexual performance and develop a secondary fear of failure as a sex partner.

Spiritual Distress

Lack of fulfillment in a sexual relationship may be related to a temporary feeling of distance from one's partner or an ongoing lack of intimacy in the relationship. Factors relating to lack of intimacy are relationship conflict, multiple fears, adult sexual abuse, or childhood sexual abuse.

Compromised Family Coping

It is difficult to experience sexual fulfillment when the relationship is in trouble in nonsexual spheres. The difficulty may be as straightforward as poor communication or as complex as conflict, anger, and unequal power. Other socioeconomic stressors include underemployment, unemployment, and lack of social network support. When one of the partners cross-dresses, the other partner must come to terms with the behavior if a healthy relationship is to be maintained. Being part of a family with a transsexual involves finding ways to reintegrate the person as a member of the other sex, or else reject the transsexual person and distance the family from this particular member.

TABLE 20-2 ■ Drugs/Medications and Related Sexual Side Effects

	Sexual Side Effects				
Drug/Medication	Increased Sex Drive	Decreased Sex Drive	Decreased Arousal	Retrograde Ejaculation	Inhibited Ejaculation
Alcohol	small amts	large amts	yes		yes
Amphetamines	yes		possible		yes
Antihypertensives		yes	yes		yes
Antipsychotics (atypical)		yes	yes		yes
Antipsychotics (conventional)		yes	yes	possible	possible
Anxiolytics (very few side effects)					
Beta blockers		yes	yes		
Cocaine	yes				yes
Diuretics		yes	yes		
Hallucinogens (unpredictable side effects)		possible	possible		
Heroin		yes	yes		yes
Lithium		yes	yes		
MAO inhibitors		may	may		
Marijuana	small amts	large amts	chronic use		
Mood stabilizers		yes	yes		yes
SSRIs			yes		
Steroids		yes	yes		
Tricyclic antidepressants		yes	yes		yes

Disturbed Personal Identity

In cultures with rigid gender roles, transsexuals and cross-dressers suffer a great deal of pain as they struggle with their gender identity. Transsexuals completely reject their anatomic sex, and cross-dressers alternate between their male and their female personas.

Ineffective Role Performance

Sexual addicts often cannot maintain work, family, and social roles. The addiction is so time consuming that the addict cannot devote time or energy to work or relationships.

Ineffective Sexuality Pattern

Some people cannot achieve sexual arousal and orgasm without the stimulation of an unusual object or situation. These individuals are considered to have one of the paraphilias, which may be coercive or noncoercive. Most often they are preoccupied with, and feel compelled to engage in, their particular sexual behaviors.

Risk for Violence: Self-Directed or Other-Directed

People who engage in autoerotic asphyxia are not suicidal and have no intention of harming themselves but may accidentally kill themselves during sexual activity. People who are coercive paraphiliacs are considered to be violent against others because the victim is nonconsenting and is offended or hurt by the person's sexual behavior.

Pain

A nursing diagnosis of pain applies to women who experience vaginismus. The origin may be past sexual trauma or current emotional conflict. The pain of dyspareunia may occur in both women and men and is typically related to organic factors.

Deficient Knowledge

People who grow up with no or very limited sex education may have difficulties in their adult sexual functioning. For people who do not know what to expect or how to touch themselves or their partners, sexual interactions can be frustrating rather than pleasurable. Lack of knowledge can contribute to ineffective sexual techniques and sexual dysfunctions.

Sexual Dysfunction

Many of the previously discussed nursing diagnoses may be contributing factors to the development of sexual dysfunctions. In addition, illness, injury, surgery, medications, or substance abuse may contribute to sexual dysfunction. Problems with satisfaction may be described under either of these diagnoses: Sexual Dysfunction or Spiritual Distress. Communication about sexual dysfunction can be maximized by using the suggestions in Rx Communication. The impact of aging on sexual expression and satisfaction is explored in Chapter 27∞.

℞ COMMUNICATION

Client With Sexual Dysfunction

CLIENT: "My husband always wants to have sex, and the more he wants, the less I'm interested."

NURSE RESPONSE 1: "Has there ever been a time in your relationship that you enjoyed sexual relations more than you do now?"	**NURSE RESPONSE 2:** "Have you spoken with your medical care provider about this problem?"
RATIONALE: This response explores the history of this problem's development in order to clarify whether the difficulty is interactional, intrapersonal, or perhaps medical in origin.	*RATIONALE:* This response provides an opportunity to gather more assessment data on any contributory medical factors.

Outcome Identification: NOC

The outcomes expected with this group of clients focuses on the specific problem interfering with normal functioning. If the client has been sexually abused or traumatized and sexual functioning has been affected, then the expected outcome is that the client will have sexual abuse recovery. Other issues, such as menopause and aging impacts, are addressed with physical aging status outcomes.

Risk control is important as an outcome for those with sexual addictions or an increase in sexual interest. Actions need to be taken to reduce or eliminate the behaviors associated with risky sexual behavior so that sexually transmitted infections are avoided. Outcomes in this overall area of nursing are related to the likelihood of the disorder.

Planning and Implementation: NIC

Developing the nursing plan of care and putting that plan into action can be structured using a format sensitive to clients with sexuality issues.

Using the PLISSIT Model

You can use the PLISSIT model developed by Annon (1974) to help clients with gender identity issues or sexual problems. The model involves four progressive levels represented by the acronym PLISSIT:

P	Permission giving
LI	Limited information
SS	Specific suggestions
IT	Intensive therapy

At each level, nurses provide additional guidance and information to clients and therefore require more specialized and specific knowledge and skill. All professional nurses should be able to function at the first two levels.

Giving Permission

Clients may feel that they need permission to be sexual beings, to discuss their gender identity, to ask questions, to show affection, and to express themselves sexually. Giving permission means that you, by attitude or word, let clients know that sexual thoughts, fantasies, and behaviors between informed, consenting adults are allowed. Giving permission begins when you acknowledge clients' spoken and unspoken sexual concerns and convey the attitude that these are important to health and healing.

For example, you might ask a client who is diagnosed with major depressive disorder the following question: "Many people who are depressed experience a loss of sexual interest. Has this been a problem for you?"

Supplying Information

Clients need accurate but concise information. You might explain what is usual sexual behavior; how mental disorders and medications affect sexuality; or the impact of cultural expectations on gender role behavior. Continuing with the preceding example, you might say the following: "I notice that you have been on antidepressant medication for 2 months. Although this medication improves mood and general functioning, there are often some sexual side effects, especially related to orgasms."

Suggesting Adaptations

At this level, you will need specialized knowledge and skill about specific interventions. You offer suggestions to help clients adapt sexual activity to promote optimal functioning. If you are working on a cardiac unit, you need specialized knowledge about sexual readjustment during cardiac rehabilitation. If you are working with clients with spinal cord injuries, you need information about the sexual consequences of spinal injuries that occur at various levels. If you are working with a client who has gender identity issues you might say the following: "I'm not sure if you are aware of support groups in the area for people who are transgendered. I can give you a list of these groups, if you would like that information."

Referring for Intensive Therapy

At this level of intervention, nurses must have specialized preparation and knowledge of sexual and gender identity disorders. Nurses who function in the sex therapist role should meet the qualifications for practice as identified by the American Association of Sex Educators, Counselors, and Therapists (AASECT), which differentiate sex counseling from sex therapy. *Sex counseling* helps clients incorporate their sexual knowledge into satisfying lifestyles and socially responsible behavior. *Sex therapy* is a highly specialized, in-depth treatment to help clients resolve serious sexual problems. AASECT publishes a national directory of professionals certified to provide sex education, counseling, or therapy. This directory is an excellent resource for nurses and clients. A resource link to AASECT can be accessed through the Online Student Resources for this book. Some specific sexual counseling strategies are listed in Your Intervention Strategies.

Reducing Violence Against the Self

The most important nursing intervention regarding autoerotic asphyxia is community education. Include warnings about autoerotic asphyxia in adolescent sex-education programs. Encourage teenagers who practice it to seek immediate professional help. Teach parents to look for physical signs of trauma to the neck such as bruising, abrasions, pressure marks, or rope burns. Ropes, knotted sheets, knotted T-shirts, or the like hidden in the bedroom may be warning signs.

Reducing Violence Against Others

Individuals who practice coercive paraphilias typically do not stop their behavior and usually end up in the criminal justice system. The court may or may not mandate therapy. Therapy for sex offenders is a specialized area that should not be undertaken lightly. Although behavior modification techniques, group therapy, and hypnosis are used, they are generally unsuccessful. In severe cases, male sex offenders are treated with the antiandrogen medication medroxyprogesterone

acetate (Provera or Depo-Provera), which induces a reversible chemical castration. The medication reduces the male sex drive, erections, and ejaculation, and decreases the obsessional focus on sex.

Promoting Comfort With Gender Identity

People who experience gender dysphoria have many options for managing the transgendered part of themselves. Physically they may undergo hormonal treatment, genital reassignment surgery, electrolysis, breast surgery, or other cosmetic surgery. They may decide to live in the other gender role part time or full time, prefer to have sex as a woman or as a man with a female, male, both, or neither. They may view themselves as female, male, both, a third gender, or transgendered. Interventions focus on promoting comfort with the chosen gender role.

Transsexuals are usually referred to therapists who specialize in this area or to gender identity disorder clinics. Because gender identity is stable, the goal of treatment with transsexuals is to help them live and function in society in the cross-gender role. Helping people find comfort in their sexual self-esteem is explored in Caring for the Spirit.

If cross-dressing is a newly divulged secret to the partner, offer education and support. If the relationship is to continue, both partners need to agree on where and how cross-dressing will take place. Some couples compromise; for instance, a husband may agree never to cross-dress in front of his wife,

---

YOUR INTERVENTION STRATEGIES Guidelines for Working With Clients With Sexual Difficulties

Some of the intensive therapy interventions in the following list require more specialized and specific knowledge and skills. Refer back to the PLISSIT model to identify which are within your area of expertise and which are level 4 interventions.

Male Orgasmic Disorder
Re-establish a climate of comfort and acceptance for sexual interaction. Encourage the client to masturbate and enjoy touch and body stimulation in general.

Premature Ejaculation
Instruct the client to stimulate the erect penis until the premonitory sensations of impending orgasm are felt. Then the client stops penile stimulation abruptly. This process is repeated to lower the threshold of excitability and make the client more tolerant of the stimuli. Sometimes the client uses the squeeze technique: At the point of orgasm, the client's partner squeezes the head of the penis with thumb and first two fingers for 3 to 4 seconds. This stops the urge to ejaculate.

Female Orgasmic Disorder
Instruct the client to avoid genital sex. Nongenital caressing exercises begin with the partners alternating as the initiator of a session of caressing, thus sharing responsibility for sexual interaction. Next, genital stimulation is added to provide positive sexual experiences without intercourse. When intercourse is attempted, the woman is instructed to assume the superior position and insert the man's penis into her vagina. When setbacks occur, the couple is advised to rely on sexual techniques that do not involve intercourse. The

woman is to place her hand lightly on her partner's to indicate her preference for contact. The emphasis is not on achieving orgasm but on learning erotic preferences. The couple is instructed to use the side-by-side position, which enables both partners to move freely with emphasis on slow, exploratory thrusting. The goal is to develop an ability to enjoy pelvic play with the penis inside the vagina.

Vaginismus
Begin with a physical demonstration to the woman of her involuntary vaginal spasm by inserting an examining finger into her vagina. Then insert Hegar dilators in graduated sizes into the vagina, beginning with the smallest ones. After larger dilators are successfully inserted, instruct the client to retain the dilator for several hours each night. Most involuntary spasms can be relieved in 3 to 5 days with the daily use of dilators. In addition to physical relief from spastic constriction, therapy is directed toward alleviating the fear that led to the onset of symptoms.

Vulvodynia and Vestibulitis
Clients with these disorders need a great deal of empathy and support because they have been living with acute pain for a significant period of time. Instruct them to use nonirritating substances on the vulva such as Lipocream, Aquaphor, or even olive oil or Crisco. Test for food allergies and environmental allergies, because these may be contributing causes. Specially trained physical therapists provide pelvic floor therapy which includes myofascial release, pudendal nerve release, and biofeedback. Yoga and acupuncture may also be helpful.

CARING FOR THE SPIRIT

Experiencing Pleasure and Fulfillment in Sexual Relationships

Sexual problems can create feelings such as guilt, anxiety, or fear that interfere with the ability to experience pleasure and joy. Some people experience guilt when they simply enjoy sex or participate in what they label "unusual" sexual activities, or guilt regarding the choice of partner. Some people internalize negative expectations and beliefs. Those with low self-esteem may not understand how another person could value and love them and also find them sexually attractive. For those who have not yet accepted their sexual orientation or gender identity, this conflict may interfere with sexual relationships.

Help clients identify and label the feelings they are experiencing. Then help them identify one anxiety- or guilt-producing situation within their sexual interactions. Together, review how feelings have been handled in the past and evaluate the range and effectiveness of this past coping behavior. Explore alternative coping behaviors and have clients evaluate their effectiveness after trying them.

Help clients identify the significance of culture, religion, race, gender, and age on their sexual self-esteem. Assist them in setting realistic goals to achieve higher self-esteem. Ask them to formulate positive self-statements and to repeat these aloud several times a day. Help them develop confidence in their ability to experience pleasure and fulfillment in relationships that are best suited for them.

WebLinks: Support Groups

and she may agree to give him privacy. Some agree to limit cross-dressing to the home; others are comfortable going out in public with the partner cross-dressed. The long-term success of the relationship depends on the couple's ability to negotiate these issues.

Reducing Pain

Whenever pain is associated with intercourse, a thorough physical examination is necessary to find and treat the organic cause of the pain. During vaginal examinations, careful attention must be paid to tiny tears in the vaginal wall, which are often overlooked. Even very small tears can cause great pain during intercourse. Vaginismus is treated with education, dilators, and supportive psychotherapy. The initial treatment for vulvodynia and vestibulitis involves decreasing the inflammation, followed by pelvic floor therapy by specially trained physical therapists.

Educating About Noncoercive Sex Patterns

Once paraphilias are a programmed part of arousal, they are very difficult to deprogram. The response to certain sexual or erotic stimuli tends to persist throughout life. A noncoercive, nonharmful paraphilia practiced with a consenting adult partner requires no nursing intervention other than client and partner education and possible couple negotiation about the behavior.

Reinforcing Sexual Health

Clients in a manic episode often exhibit impulsive increases in their sexual activity. Explain to family members that such behavior is a symptom of the manic state, is not within the client's control, and is not an indication of a change in ethics and values. As much as possible, protect clients from sexual acting out until they are able to assume control over this behavior. Set firm limits on inappropriate verbal and physical sexual behaviors. Chapter 17 ∞ discusses details on hypersexuality during mania.

Managing Compulsive Sexual Behavior

Sex addicts, like other people with addictions, respond well to community-based programs. Specific programs are discussed in the section on Community-Based Care.

Addressing Sexual Dysfunctions

Accurate identification of feelings is the first step in the problem-solving process, and clients may need help labeling the feelings they are experiencing. Following this step, help clients identify one anxiety-producing situation within their sexual interactions. At this stage, it is productive to focus diffuse anxiety on a manageable single situation or event. With the client, analyze the situation or event to discover negative anticipatory thoughts that may be the source of the anxiety. Together, review how the client has handled anxiety in the past and evaluate the range and effectiveness of this past coping behavior. It may be appropriate to help the client redefine the sensations of anxiety as sensations of sexual excitement, which is more likely to result in positive expectations. Together, explore alternative coping behaviors, and have the client evaluate their effectiveness after implementing them.

Many adult survivors of childhood sexual abuse are periodically overwhelmed by anxiety, fear, and panic (see Chapter 24 ∞). Refer adult survivors to support groups such as Incest Anonymous or VOICES, as well as individual therapy with a therapist who specializes in this field.

Sexual disorders are explained in comfortable lay terms on the Sexual Disorders website that can be accessed through the Online Student Resources for this book. Because most psychotherapists are not sex therapists, make a referral through AASECT, mentioned earlier in this chapter. The common components of sex therapy programs are listed in Box 20-2.

Enhancing Communication

Good communication is an important part of a sexually fulfilling relationship. Apart from setting specific times to share

Box 20-2 Common Components of Sex Therapy Programs

- **Information and education about sexual functions.** The therapist gives clients specific information about their particular needs. The therapist may discuss the information or assign books to read.
- **Experiential/sensory awareness.** The therapist helps clients recognize feelings of anxiety, anger, and pleasure by tuning into bodily cues. Clients focus on and describe feelings both in therapy sessions and at home. If they believe their genitals are ugly and unclean, the therapist assigns desensitization exercises at home that allow clients to become familiar with their own bodies. Some clients need fantasy training if nonsexual thoughts interfere with sexual arousal.
- **Insight.** The therapist attempts to understand what is causing and perpetuating the sexual problem. The goal is for clients to assume responsibility for their own behavior and recognize that change is possible.
- **Cognitive restructuring.** Clients identify and evaluate their fears about sexual interaction. The therapist encourages them to identify and eliminate negative self-statements and irrational expectations.
- **Behavioral interventions.** Because the focus is on changing nonsexual behavior that contributes to sexual problems, the therapist may assign assertiveness training, communication training, stress-reduction exercises, and problem-solving techniques. Behavioral interventions include assigned pleasuring sessions to discover what is arousing and pleasing to the self and partner.

YOUR INTERVENTION STRATEGIES
Asserting Sexual Needs Tactfully

Couples who communicate about emotionally difficult subjects such as sex convey messages more competently through "I" language than through accusatory "you" language.

"You" Language

- "You only have sex on your mind. You're a pervert."
- "You keep grabbing at me like I'm always ready to go to bed with you."
- "You never pay attention to what turns me on. Are you dumb or hard of hearing?"

"I" Language

- "I'm concerned because we seem to have different expectations of how often we would like to make love."
- "I miss all the hugging and caressing we used to do even when we couldn't make love afterward."
- "I feel frustrated and hurt when it seems like I'm repeating myself. Maybe I'm not communicating my needs very clearly."

feelings and beliefs, some couples need training in more effective communication skills. If they give ambiguous signals to indicate sexual interest, they need to learn how to state their interest clearly. Some people expect their partners to "read their minds" about sexual needs and desires; these people need encouragement to assert their needs tactfully. Teach couples to avoid "you" language, which evokes a defensive response and results in arguments, and to use "I" language, which expresses personal thoughts, feelings, and needs. Some examples of accusatory "you" statements and answerable "I" statements are in Your Intervention Strategies. If couples are able to reduce anxiety and improve communication but still have sexual problems, a referral is appropriate.

Reducing Spiritual Distress

Because the origin of spiritual distress is often a lack of intimacy or connection, the goal of nursing intervention is to help clients achieve and maintain a level of intimacy each partner finds comfortable. In the context of therapy, couples discuss their individual needs for closeness and identify barriers to intimacy. They are instructed to make three or four half-hour "dates" each week, during which they share warmth and intimacy. They spend some of the time discussing specific sexual issues; during other "dates," the couple explores intimate, nonsexual topics, such as hopes and expectations for the future. Couples should give these dates top priority, because a common way of avoiding intimacy is by not setting time aside for each other.

Increasing Knowledge

Providing education for sexual health is important. Many sexual problems exist because of sexual ignorance; many others can be prevented with effective sexual health teaching. You can assist clients to understand their anatomies and how their bodies function. For example, understanding the anatomy of the clitoris may help women learn how their bodies respond to sexual stimulation. Both women and men need to learn what kind of stimulation is pleasing and causes arousal. Encourage open communication between partners. Provide details about physiological changes that occur throughout the life span as part of general health care. For example, you discuss the effects of puberty, pregnancy, menopause, and the male climacteric on sexual function at the appropriate times.

Although there is an increasing awareness today of sexuality and sexual functioning, some people still hold certain myths and misconceptions about sexuality. Many of these are handed down in families and are particular cultural beliefs. It is highly important that you learn about the beliefs clients hold and provide up-to-date information. You are encouraged to visit the website of the Sexuality Information and Education Council of the United States, which has a wealth of information on various aspects of sexuality. The website can be accessed through the Online Student Resources for this book.

Evaluation

Examining your care for effectiveness is especially important where discomfort and bias could interfere with treatment for a client's sexual dysfunction.

AtHealth.com

Care Plan: Sexual Disorder and Communication

Sexuality Information and Education Council

Violence

Community and family education programs addressing the danger of autoerotic asphyxia will be established. Victims of this disorder will be identified and referred for immediate treatment. Clients with this disorder will remain safe. Clients with coercive paraphilias will curb their behavior, or society will set strict limits to protect potential victims.

Gender Identity

Clients will report increasing comfort and satisfaction in their new gender role, which will be congruent with their gender identity. Each will be able to function socially and economically as a person of that gender.

Pain

Individuals will report less pain or no pain during intercourse. Clients suffering from vaginismus will report success in using conscious control to relax vaginal muscles, allowing for pain-free intercourse.

Noncoercive Sexuality Patterns

Clients and partners will verbalize an understanding that noncoercive paraphilias are lifelong patterns. Couples will be able to negotiate the behavior in a way that is mutually satisfying.

Compulsive Sexual Behavior

Clients will attend a twelve-step program for sexual addicts. Partners will attend appropriate self-help groups.

Sexual Dysfunction

Clients will report a satisfying and fulfilling sex life. They will experience minimal difficulty with desire, arousal, or orgasm. They will be able to identify and label feelings and acknowledge responsibility for their own behavior. They will implement a chosen variety of sexual techniques.

Spiritual Distress

Couples will report an acceptable and meaningful level of intimacy in their relationships. They will continue to set aside time for each other and engage in meaningful intimate time.

CASE MANAGEMENT

Case management services tend to revolve around the coercive paraphilias and autoerotic asphyxia. The criminal justice system is involved in the former, and may or may not be involved in the latter case. Case management consists mainly of making arrangements for services for the client, but the majority of effort is focused on protecting others. Treatment for coercive paraphilias has not been successful to any significant extent and recidivism is all too common.

COMMUNITY-BASED CARE

Transsexuals need a great deal of support and assistance as they establish themselves in their new role. If the present job is not gender-role stereotyped, they may be able to remain in the same or similar position. Others may need retraining programs to find acceptable employment. A multidisciplinary approach is most effective in helping transsexuals adjust to their situation. Family and friends need support and counseling to reintegrate this person into their lives as a person of the other sex.

For sex addicts, the cornerstone of recovery is a twelve-step program modeled on the Alcoholics Anonymous program. Partners and codependents are also referred to appropriate self-help groups. A variety of groups, such as Sexaholics Anonymous, Sex Addicts Anonymous, Sex and Love Addicts Anonymous, S-Anon, and Co-Dependents of Sexual Addicts, have been formed throughout the country.

For cross-dressers, a community-based plan of care may include joining a club, such as Tri-Ess, where they can express their female personality in a safe social situation. Counseling for the individual or the couple at a community mental health clinic frequently focuses on the development of compromise within the relationship around cross-dressing issues.

HOME CARE

Sex therapy typically involves 1 hour a week with a sex therapist. The therapist gives clients specific information about their particular needs. The therapist may assign books to read or discuss the information. The therapist attempts to learn and understand what is causing and perpetuating the sexual problem. Clients identify and re-evaluate their fears about sexual interaction. The therapist encourages them to identify and eliminate negative self-statements and irrational expectations.

Clients focus on and describe feelings both in therapy sessions and at home. If they believe their genitals are ugly and unclean, the therapist assigns desensitization exercises at home for clients to explore and become familiar with their own bodies. Some clients need fantasy training if nonsexual thoughts interfere with sexual arousal. Because the focus is on changing nonsexual behavior that contributes to sexual problems, the therapist may assign assertiveness training, communication training, stress-reduction exercises, and problem-solving techniques. Behavioral interventions include assigned pleasuring sessions to discover what is arousing and pleasing to both partners.

NURSING CARE PLAN: CLIENT WITH LOW SEXUAL DESIRE AND ORGASMIC DISORDER

Identifying Information

Susan is a 46-year-old married woman who has come with her 48-year-old husband, Brad, to the local mental health outpatient clinic. Neither of them has received mental health services prior to this time.

History

They both describe their sex life at the beginning of their marriage as fine for the first several years, although Susan states that she was never orgasmic during that time. They never talked about their sex life. Some years ago, after reading a "sex book," Susan experimented with masturbation for the first time and began to experience orgasms. She was never able to share this information with Brad because she felt guilty about touching herself when she was alone. They are verbally and physically affectionate with one another, but, they say, not as much as they used to be. They seldom express their anger to one another, and they manage most relationship conflicts by avoiding the issue.

No prior psychiatric history with either party. Both Susan and Brad are second-generation Americans of Eastern European descent with a common culture. Both describe their parents as very modest and uncommunicative about any sexual issues. No

sex education was given in the family. Susan and Brad have been married 25 years and have two children: a daughter, 19, and a son, 14. They are both pleased with their occupations—Brad in sales, and Susan as a bookkeeper.

The couple describes their routine as Brad initiating sexual activity, primarily nonverbally. Sex typically occurs in the bedroom, after midnight, when they are both tired. Susan determines the length of foreplay, which usually lasts 5 to 10 minutes. The only position they use is man-on-top, but both agree they would like to try other positions. Brad has minimal verbal communication during sex, and Susan says she is too shy to say anything while they are making love. They both have difficulty talking about their sex life with one another. Susan states she is somewhat uncomfortable when Brad touches her body, except for her genitals and breasts. She is comfortable touching Brad's genitals but not touching her own genitals in front of him. She likes to receive oral sex but is uncomfortable giving it because she is afraid Brad will ejaculate in her mouth. Their mutual goals in therapy are to have sex more often, to feel freer to experiment, to discuss sex openly, and to have Susan experience pleasure and orgasms.

Brad has no current or past medical problems. Susan had a hysterectomy 5 years ago for endometriosis and is on hormone replacement therapy.

Current Mental Status

They are both quiet-spoken but articulate individuals. Eye contact is appropriate, mood is stable and appropriate, thought processes are logical, and there are no obvious symptoms of stress. Although they were both uncomfortable discussing sex, it became easier during a 2-hour history-taking time.

Other Clinical Data

Both Susan and Brad agree that there is a disparity of sexual needs. Susan is satisfied to have sex once a month, and Brad wants to have sex several times a week. Susan has never been orgasmic with Brad but does admit to achieving orgasms during masturbation, a fact she has never been able to tell Brad. Susan states that she would probably like to have sex more often if she would enjoy it. Her fear is that she will not become orgasmic. Brad thinks that entering therapy is the first big step, and he is hopeful that their sexual relationship will improve.

Nursing Diagnosis: Ineffective Sexuality Pattern related to disparity of needs.

Expected Outcome: Brad and Susan will demonstrate an understanding of sexual anatomy and physiology, and openly communicate about sex.

Short-Term Goals	Interventions	Rationale
Susan will be able to discuss the frequency of sexual activity with Brad.	■ Explore unspoken expectations and the potential for hurt feelings.	Sexual expectations are seldom similar, and coming to a compromise regarding sex contributes to a healthy relationship.
	■ Discuss and train on the meaning of, and process of, compromising.	
	■ Discuss alternative ways to meet sexual needs besides intercourse.	Masturbation and fantasy may not be readily accessible intercourse alternatives.
The couple will be able to discuss personal preferences for sexual activities.	■ Encourage communication during sex such as what they like and how they like things between them.	Practice establishes behavior.
Susan will be able to achieve orgasm during sexual activity with Brad.	■ Give homework assignments designed to address sexual communication. ■ Discuss physiology of Susan's sexuality related to orgasmic functioning. ■ Encourage Susan to communicate what helps her achieve orgasm. ■ Encourage activities in which Susan has achieved orgasm.	Communication is developed with practice.

Pearson Nursing Student Resources

Find additional review materials at
nursing.pearsonhighered.com

Prepare for success with NCLEX®-style practice questions,
interactive assignments and activities, web links, animations
and videos, and more!

REFERENCES

Annon, J. (1974). *The behavioral treatment of sexual problems: Vol. 1, Brief therapy.* New York, NY: Harper & Row.

Barungi, V., & Twongyeirwe, H. (2009). *Beyond the dance, Voices of women on female genital mutilation.* Kampala, Uganda: Femrite Publications.

Bhugra, D., Popelyuk, D., & McMullen, I. (2010). Paraphilias across cultures: Contexts and controversies. *Journal of Sex Research, 47,* 242–256.

Cheever, S. (2008). *Where sex meets addiction.* New York, NY: Simon & Schuster Paperbacks.

Cohen-Kettenis, P. T., & Pfafflin, F. (2010). The DSM diagnostic criteria for gender identity disorder in adolescents and adults. *Archives of Sexual Behavior, 39,* 499–513.

Crooks, R., & Baur, K. (2011). *Our sexuality* (11th ed.). Belmont, CA: Wadsworth.

Emerson, C. R. (2010). Review of low libido in women. *International Journal of STD & AIDS, 21,* 312–316.

Garcia, F. D., & Thibaut, F. (2010). Sexual addictions. *American Journal of Drug and Alcohol Abuse, 36*(5), 254–260.

Goetsch, M. F., Morgan, T. K., Korcheva, V. B., Li, H., Peters, D., & Leclair, C. M. (2010). Histologic and receptor analysis of primary and secondary vestibulodynia and controls. *American Journal of Obstetrics and Gynecology, 202,* 614–621.

Jutel, A. (2010). Framing disease: The example of female hypoactive sexual desire disorder. *Social Science & Medicine, 70,* 1084–1090.

Laughlin, G. A., Goodell, V., & Barrett-Connor, E. (2010). Extremes of endogenous testosterone are associated with increased risk of incident coronary events in older women. *Journal of Clinical Endocrinology & Metabolism, 95,* 740–747.

Lawrence, A. A. (2010). Sexual orientation versus age of onset as bases for typologies (subtypes) for gender identity disorder in adolescents and adults. *Archives of Sexual Behavior, 39,* 514–545.

Lewis, R. W., Kerstin, S., Fugl-Meyer, S., Corona, G., Hayes, R. D., Laumann, E. O., … Segraves, T. (2010). Definitions/epidemiology/risk factors for sexual dysfunction. *Journal of Sex Medicine, 7,* 1598–1607.

Pasterski, V., Prentice, P., & Hughes, I. A. (2010). Impact of the consensus statement and the new DSD classification system. *Best Practice & Research. Clinical Endocrinology & Metabolism, 24,* 187–195.

Eating Disorders

EILEEN TRIGOBOFF

21

LEARNING OUTCOMES

After completing this chapter, you will be able to:

1. Explain the roles of culture and biology in the development of eating disorders.
2. Compare and contrast the various theories for the causes of eating disorders.
3. Illustrate how psychological and social pressures can influence the course of eating disorders.
4. Assess individual and family problems of clients with eating disorders.
5. Partner with clients and their families in both the prevention and treatment of eating disorders.
6. Formulate intermediate goals in the treatment of clients with eating disorders.
7. Create a nursing plan of care for clients with eating disorders and their families.

CRITICAL THINKING CHALLENGE

A school health nurse in a large public high school is aware that a number of girls diet constantly and several also throw up in the bathroom following lunch period. She learns that boys on the wrestling team use vomiting as a means of "making weight." When the nurse takes her concerns to the principal to ask his support for an eating disorders educational program, he replies: "This is a health problem, not an educational problem. We just don't have time for this kind of thing. It's really up to the parents."

1. In your opinion, what is the responsibility of nurses in educating the public about prevention of eating disorders?
2. What kinds of information do people—particularly parents, teachers, and coaches—need to communicate about eating and health?
3. What messages have you received that have helped or hindered you in developing healthy eating attitudes and behaviors?

For many, eating symbolizes parental nurturing—the love and care that are the prototype of, and basis for, all future intimate relationships. For some, however, eating creates anxiety because of its association with unsatisfactory and unpleasant parent–child interactions. Clearly, food and eating have greater individual and cultural meaning and importance than merely sustaining life. Disturbed eating patterns may develop as a means of coping with stress.

The two major eating disorders discussed in this chapter—anorexia nervosa and bulimia nervosa—create biologic, psychological, and social imbalances that interfere with the individual's normal functioning. Changes in biochemistry, metabolic rate, emotional state, family relationships, and social status brought about by eating disorders can create depression, isolation, and sometimes self-destructive behavior.

Cultural stereotypes contribute to women's preoccupation with their bodies. Attractiveness is determined by how closely a woman's appearance matches the cultural ideal of thinness. Thus, identity and self-esteem are dependent on physical appearance. Being disgusted with one's flesh is the same as having an adversarial relationship with the body—a relationship that often results in eating disorders.

Determining the incidence of anorexia and bulimia is difficult because of the variety of definitions that exist. Certainly, the frequency of these disorders has been increasing, but the increase may be due partly to increased reporting. Ninety percent of women and 25% of men diet at some time in their lives. Over half of teenage girls and one third of teenage boys use unhealthy weight control behaviors such as skipping meals, fasting, vomiting, abusing laxatives, and smoking cigarettes. It is estimated that clinical eating disorders affect 8% to 20% of the population. They are more commonly seen among females, with estimates of the male–female ratio ranging from 1:6 to 1:10, although 19% to 30% of younger people with anorexia are male. The estimate may be low, because primary health care providers tend to be accurate in identifying anorexia and bulimia nervosa, but inaccurate in identifying atypical presentations (e.g., eating disorders not otherwise specified (Allen, Fursland, Watson, & Byrne, 2011).

For those with anorexia or bulimia, the most frequently observed disorder is depression. In some cases, this may be the result of abnormal eating and weight loss. In other cases, the depression is the primary disorder to which the eating disorder is a response. And for yet another group of people, the depression and abnormal eating both are primary disorders.

There is a high prevalence of several anxiety disorders associated with eating disorders. Social phobias may occur in people with eating disorders, possibly in response to others' awareness of their abnormal eating behaviors. Obsessive–compulsive symptoms are common, especially among people with anorexia. Obsessive–compulsive symptoms often continue even after weight is restored in anorexia. Panic attacks are likely when people with anorexia are prohibited from exercising their usual behavior patterns. It is unclear whether these are primary disorders or are secondary to the eating disorders (Swanson, Crow, LeGrange, Swendsen, & Merikangas, 2010). Evidence-Based Practice discusses how constructively expressing distress and emotions helps in recovery from anorexia.

Anorexia nervosa and bulimia nervosa are not single diseases but syndromes with multiple predisposing factors and a variety of characteristics. Although the most obvious symptom is the eating problem, these disorders are not simply a matter of eating too much or too little. It is because of the complex interaction of biologic, psychological, developmental,

EVIDENCE-BASED PRACTICE

Life Roles and Anorexia Nervosa

Suzy is a 45-year-old woman who is extremely thin and jogs several miles every day to maintain her (under) weight. She is 5′7″ and weighs 112 lb. You work with her in an outpatient clinic where she is receiving counseling for marital problems.

Suzy has maintained the same weight since she was 17 years old. Her eating habits have always been tied to her weight. Since she was a teenager, Suzy has added extra miles to her running route, decreased her calorie count, or fasted whenever she was 1 or 2 lb over what she considered her ideal weight. The literature reports that adolescence is the peak time for developing eating disorders. Recovery studies will be most helpful to you in understanding and working with Suzy.

As indicated in the following research, many people, through therapy and close relationships, find nonbodily means to express their distress. Events such as committing to a relationship, forming a family, and settling into an identity and occupation all serve to provide a stable platform for overall functioning. Women's drive to be thin tends to decline as they age (conversely, men's drive to be thin tends to increase as they age), but Suzy does not follow that trend. You will explore her life roles with her (is she a wife, a mother, a daughter, a business executive, a socialite, a student, an athlete, etc.). Identify the ways in which she expresses a range of negative emotions to determine if your work with her needs to focus on problematic feeling expression that may contribute to perpetuating her eating disorder.

You should base action on more than one study, but the following research would be helpful in this situation.

Jenkins, J., & Ogden, J. (2011). Becoming "whole" again: A qualitative study of women's views of recovering from anorexia nervosa. *European Eating Disorders Review*. Advance online publication. doi: 10.1002/erv.1085

CRITICAL THINKING QUESTIONS

1. If Suzy has been maintaining an underweight condition since the age of 17, what are her chances for improvement?
2. What conditions would be necessary for improvement to take place?

MENTAL HEALTH IN THE MOVIES
Superstar: The Karen Carpenter Story

This documentary investigates the story of Karen Carpenter's life with, and death from, anorexia. Karen's visibility as a popular singer only intensified certain difficulties many women experience in relation to their bodies. The short movie re-enacts her life not with actors but with Barbie dolls and gives you a feel for a woman pulled apart at the seams by unrealistic expectations.

Karen Carpenter's anorexia is a debilitating illness brought on by social, not disease, vectors. Clips of Karen and her brother Richard speaking to Herb Alpert, head of A&M Records, are alternated with black-and-white garish shots of food representing Karen's subjective view of the food she denies herself. Her family's attempts to cure her anorexia make matters worse. Unable to comprehend the severity of the psychological disorder, Karen's family simply encourage, then force, Karen to eat, deepening the symbolic power of food in her mind. At one point, Richard callously worries that his sister's gaunt frame will ruin their careers instead of focusing on her withering away. The pace of the film helps us contemplate the sympathetic view of a woman's tragic demise. Although she did not receive psychotherapy, Karen Carpenter began eating normally and was a healthy weight, when she died suddenly of cardiac complications brought on by years of starvation.

Photo courtesy of Michael Ochs Archives/Getty Images.

familial, and sociocultural factors that certain people develop eating disorders. The focus of Mental Health in the Movies, *Superstar: The Karen Carpenter Story,* is on how family dynamics and perception contribute to an eating disorder.

There is no clear-cut distinction between the two disorders, and they have many features in common. The traditional division of anorexia and bulimia is still appropriate until more is known about eating disorders. Body weight may be a significant distinguishing characteristic; people with anorexia are severely underweight and people with bulimia are at normal or near-normal weight. About 30% of people with bulimia have a history of anorexia. As many as 62% of people with anorexia exhibit bulimic behaviors. Conversion from anorexia to bulimia may be a way of moving from a "visible" to an "invisible" eating disorder to deceive family, friends, and health care providers. Thus, the two disorders can occur in the same person, or the person can go from one disorder to the other. Low social support during childhood seems to contribute to vulnerabilities to anorexia and bulimia; there are far more similarities than differences between the two diagnoses (Kim, Lim, & Treasure, 2011). However, to help you understand the differences, the disorders have been separated in this chapter.

ANOREXIA NERVOSA

Anorexia nervosa is a potentially life-threatening disorder characterized by extreme perfectionism, weight fear, significant weight loss, body image disturbances, strenuous exercising, peculiar food-handling patterns, and reductions in heart rate, blood pressure, metabolic rate, and the production of estrogen or testosterone. A well-known pioneer in the treatment of eating-disordered clients, Hilde Bruch (1978), called anorexia nervosa "the relentless pursuit of thinness." DSM Essential Features defines the eating disorders.

Rigidity and over-control are the hallmarks of anorexia. To control themselves and their environment, these individuals develop rigid rules. Such rigidity often develops into *obsessive rituals,* particularly concerning eating and exercise. Cutting all food into a predetermined size or number of pieces, chewing all food a certain number of times, allowing only certain combinations of foods in a meal, accomplishing a fixed number of exercise routines, and having an inflexible pattern of exercises are rituals common to anorexic people. These rules and rituals help keep anxiety beyond conscious awareness. If the rituals are disrupted, the anxiety becomes intolerable. Paradoxically, all these efforts to stay in control lead to out-of-control behaviors (Thornton, Dellava, Root, Lichtenstein, & Bulik, 2011).

Many people with anorexia are hyperactive and discover that exercising excessively is a way to increase their weight loss. Solitary running tends to be the exercise of choice, and there are often obsessional qualities to it. For example, they believe that before they can eat, they have to earn calories by exercising. Conversely, if they overeat, they believe they must punish themselves with excessive exercise. Excessive exercise signifies the triumph of the will over the body and is an indication of psychopathology (Goodwin, Haycraft, Taranis, & Meyer, 2011).

Anorexic young women have a desperate need to please others. Their self-worth depends on responses from others rather than on their own self-approval. Thus, their behavior is often overcompliant; they always try to meet the expectations of others in order to be accepted. They may overachieve in

Videos: Anorexia Nervosa

DSM ESSENTIAL FEATURES

Eating Disorders

Anorexia Nervosa: Refusal to achieve or maintain a healthy body weight with intense fear of becoming fat. Denial of a problem accompanies disturbance in body image. Binge eating and purging may, or may not, be present.

Bulimia Nervosa: Episodes of binge eating accompanied by a sense of lack of control over the binge and by inappropriate compensatory behavior (excessive exercise, vomiting). Purging may, or may not, be present.

academic and extracurricular activities, but these accomplishments are usually an attempt to please parents rather than a source of self-satisfaction.

People with anorexia often feel hopeless, helpless, and ineffective. Because of being overcompliant with their parents, they believe they have always been controlled by others. Their refusal to eat may be an attempt to assert themselves and gain some control within the family. As weight is lost, they are rewarded with praise, admiration, and envy from their peers, which reinforces the restricted eating pattern.

The following clinical example illustrates overcompliant behavior and phobia related to weight gain.

Clinical Example

Simone is a tall, quiet girl who was considered polite, well-liked, and a good student. She was given responsibility beyond her years at both school and home because of her quiet competence and maturity. When she was 15, she entered a beauty contest at a local amusement park as a lark but did not win. She became convinced that she lost because her legs were too large and her abdomen protruded. She decided to diet. To radically control her own intake without arousing the family's suspicions, she began preparing all the family's meals. She herself did not eat, but played with her food during mealtimes.

Simone spent long hours alone in her room studying, dancing, and exercising vigorously. She weighed herself several times daily, and if the scales showed an unacceptable number, she exercised even more frenziedly. As she lost weight, Simone disguised her gauntness with loose, layered clothes. One day, when she and her mother were shopping, her mother saw her disrobed and was dismayed. She insisted that Simone see the family physician, who encouraged her to eat more and prescribed nutritional supplements.

When Simone collapsed at a shopping mall a few weeks later, her parents prevailed on the family doctor to admit her to the psychiatric unit of the community hospital. As an IV was started in the emergency department, Simone asked the nurse, "How many calories are in that bag?"

BULIMIA NERVOSA

There is a cyclic behavioral pattern in **bulimia nervosa**. It begins with skipping meals sporadically and overly strict dieting or fasting. In an effort to refrain from eating, the person may use amphetamines, which can lead to extreme hunger, fatigue, and low blood glucose levels. The next part of the cycle is a period of **binge eating**, in which the person ingests huge amounts of food (about 3,500 kcal) within a short time (about 1 hour). Binges can last up to 8 hours, with consumption of 12,000 kcal. Binge eating usually occurs when the person is alone and at home, and most frequently during the evening. The cycle may occur once or twice a month for some and as often as five or ten times a day for others. The binge part of the cycle may be triggered by the ingestion of certain foods, but this is not consistent for everyone. Although eating binges may involve any kind of food, they usually consist of junk foods, fast foods, and high-calorie foods.

The final part of the cycle is **purging** the body of the ingested food. After excessive eating, people with bulimia force themselves to vomit. They often abuse laxatives and diuretics to further purge their bodies of the food. Some use as many as 50 to 100 laxatives per day. In rare cases, they may resort to syrup of ipecac to induce vomiting. Purging becomes a purification rite and a means of regaining self-control. Some describe it as feeling "completely fresh and clean again." DSM Essential Features on page 461 describes eating disorders.

After the purging, the cycle begins all over again, with a return to strict dieting or fasting. Some people with bulimia eat highly nutritious meals when not binge eating/purging to repair harm done to the body.

Binge eating and purging begin as a way to eat and stay slim. Before long, the behavior becomes a response to stress and a way to cope with negative feelings such as anger, anxiety, and depression. For some, it is poor impulse control; for others, it is an expression of rebellion against family members.

People with bulimia may engage in sporadic excessive exercise, but they usually do not develop compulsive exercise routines. They are more likely to abuse street drugs to decrease their appetite and alcohol to reduce their anxiety. Because their binges are often expensive, costing as much as $100 per day, they may resort to stealing food or money to buy the food. The binge–purge cycle can become so consuming that activities and relationships are disrupted. To keep the behavior secret, the person often resorts to excuses and lies. The following clinical example illustrates the progression of bulimia.

Clinical Example

Beth is a 17-year-old high school student who had been binge eating and purging with vomiting and over-the-counter diuretics and laxatives for about 2 years. She was referred to the mental health center by her school nurse. Beth stated that her school friends became concerned about her increasing preoccupation with purging, even after eating very small amounts of food. She was spending a lot of time in the girls' restroom; after lengthy bouts of self-induced vomiting following lunch period, she was sometimes too exhausted to attend class. Her friends had been "covering" for her but had become frightened and went to the school nurse with their concerns.

Beth is of average weight for her height but admitted that she would be quite heavy if she didn't purge herself of the large amounts of food she consumes in her room at night after her parents have gone to bed. "I'm so embarrassed. My whole life is totally out of control," she told the intake worker.

BIOPSYCHOSOCIAL THEORIES

Although many clinical studies have been published, the literature on eating disorders shows no theoretic consensus on etiology and treatment. Psychoanalytic theory, family systems theory, cognitive–behavioral theories, sociocultural theories, and biologic theories all contribute to an understanding of the development and dynamics of eating disorders. Only by understanding the interrelatedness of the factors in eating disorders can psychiatric nurses take a holistic approach to the care of affected individuals and their families. The interrelationship among these biopsychosocial theories is illustrated in FIGURE 21-1 ■.

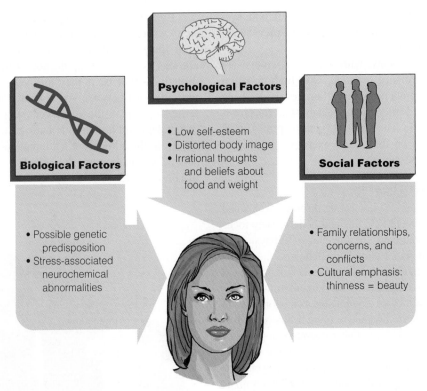

Psychological Factors

- Low self-esteem
- Distorted body image
- Irrational thoughts and beliefs about food and weight

Biological Factors

- Possible genetic predisposition
- Stress-associated neurochemical abnormalities

Social Factors

- Family relationships, concerns, and conflicts
- Cultural emphasis: thinness = beauty

FIGURE 21-1 ▪ Biopsychosocial factors in eating disorders. Nurses who understand the interplay among biopsychosocial factors involved in eating disorders are able to take a holistic approach to client care.

Psychoanalytic Theory

Since Freud first identified it as such, eating has been regarded as a critical aspect of psychological growth and development. An infant at the breast is already beginning to internalize a rudimentary understanding about life through the quality of the feeding experience.

Psychoanalytic theory considers eating disorders to be symptomatic of unconscious conflicts. Little attention is paid to biologic or cultural factors. Psychoanalytic theory relates eating disorders to regression to prepuberty and repudiation of developing sexuality. Anorexics are thought to fear sexual maturity; the anorexia is seen as a rejection of the feminine form and a desperate attempt to regain the contours and dimensions of a prepubertal child.

In psychoanalytic thinking, compulsive overeating represents overcompensation for unmet oral needs during infancy. In other words, people eat to compensate for emptiness in their lives. Obesity is also thought to represent a defense against intimacy with the opposite sex.

The basic treatment modality in the psychoanalytic model is long-term individual psychotherapy, sometimes accompanied by group therapy. The goal of therapy is the development of insight and subsequent "working through" of underlying issues to resolve the unconscious conflicts manifested by the eating disorder. There is little empirical evidence of the effectiveness of psychotherapy in the treatment of eating disorders. Promising new approaches include motivational enhancement therapy and psychotherapies aimed at relapse prevention.

Family Systems Theory

Most family theorists believe family issues are not specific to eating disorders. The family is viewed more as an enabler of the disorder than as a primary causative factor. Some people with eating disorders are survivors of childhood or adolescent sexual abuse, which may or may not have occurred within the family or extended family system.

As the result of anorexia, some families become enmeshed; that is, the boundaries between the members are weak, interactions are intense, dependency on one another is high, and autonomy is minimal. Everybody is involved in each member's concerns, and there is minimal privacy. The enmeshed family system becomes overprotective of the child, and the entire family system becomes preoccupied with food, eating, and rituals involving meals. In contrast, current research indicates that families of people with bulimia are less enmeshed than those of anorexic people. Family members tend to be isolated from one another, and eating behavior may be an attempt to decrease feelings of loneliness and boredom.

Many families of individuals with eating disorders have difficulty with conflict resolution. An ethical or religious value against disagreements within the family supports the avoidance of conflict. When problems are denied for the sake of family harmony, they cannot be resolved, and growth of the family system is inhibited. The anorexic child may protect and maintain the family unit. In some family systems, the parents avoid conflict with each other by uniting in a common concern for the child's welfare. In other family systems, the issues of marital conflict are converted into disagreements over how the anorexic child should be managed. In both systems, the marital problems are camouflaged to prevent the disruption of the family unit.

Many families of clients with eating disorders are achievement and performance oriented, with high ambition for the success of all members. In these families, body shape is related to success, and priorities are established for physical appearance and fitness. The family's focus on professional achievement as well as on food, diet, exercise, and weight control may become obsessional.

Cognitive–Behavioral Theories

Cognitive–behavioral theories view eating disorders as learned behaviors based on irrational thoughts and beliefs. They focus on changing cognitive and behavioral responses to physiological, psychological, and social stimuli. Insight into the nature of the maladaptive behavior (the eating disorder) is integrated with new and healthier responses to emotional stimuli. Education about the psychology of compulsive behavior and the physiological effects of starvation and purging behaviors is usually incorporated into the therapy. Other cognitive approaches include correction of perceptual disturbances of body size and elimination of irrational thoughts and beliefs linking weight to self-esteem, such as, "I've gained a pound; I must run 5 miles today and eat nothing," or "I'd rather be dead than fat."

Cognitive–behavioral therapy has been found to be a successful treatment method for reducing the symptomatology associated with bulimia nervosa and to result in more rapid treatment than with interpersonal psychotherapy. These approaches are also useful in the treatment of binge-eating disorder (Jenkins & Ogden, 2011; Wilfley, Vannucci, & White, 2010).

Sociocultural Theory

In American society, female attractiveness is strongly equated with thinness. Models, actresses, and the media glamorize extreme thinness, which is then equated with success and happiness. The cultural obsession with an extremely thin female body has led to widespread prejudice against overweight people. This prejudice has a significant impact on overall self-esteem and self-acceptance. Self-worth is enhanced for those who are judged attractive and diminished for those deemed unattractive. Mental Health in the News has an excellent example.

Body size and dieting behaviors can determine popularity with peers. Having a heavier body shape is associated with lower popularity for females and adolescent males are less popular if they do not fit the male ideal in either direction—that is, if they are heavier and if they are not muscular or fit. When you consider how important peer relationships are at the adolescent stage of development, you can understand how problematic eating behaviors could result from the adolescent's attempts to cope with these pressures. Current examples of "ideal" body types are presented in FIGURE 21-2 ■.

FIGURE 21-2 ■ Advertisements influence our views of attractiveness. The "ideal" female body is excessively thin. The "ideal" male body is well-toned with a slim waist and hips.
Photo courtesy of Win Initiative/Digital Vision/Getty Images.

MENTAL HEALTH IN THE NEWS

Portia DiRossi

Portia DiRossi is an actress who is lucky to be alive. Her memoir, *Unbearable Lightness: A Story of Loss and Gain*, deftly describes her years with anorexia and bulimia. She starved herself, over-exercised, and felt guilt and distress for eating a 6-ounce yogurt. Portia limited herself to a total of 150 calories in a day and at one point weighed 82 lb as a 5′ 6″ woman. Hiding her true self (as a gay woman), and having distorted views of her body ("I just wanted my legs to be straight"), and needing to fit into smaller wardrobe sizes pushed her to protracted behavioral problems with food. Years of treatment taught her how to eat reasonably and restored her to a normal weight she has since maintained. She is now healthy, has not reverted to bulimic behavior, and is married to talk show host Ellen Degeneres.

Photo courtesy © Reuters/CORBIS.

Magazines marketed for adolescent women often present diet and weight control as the solutions for adolescent crises and contain 90% more articles and advertisements promoting dieting than do magazines read by young men. Frequent exposure to articles about dieting is significantly associated with lower self-esteem, depressed mood, and lower levels of body satisfaction. Thus, the body becomes the central focus of existence, and self-esteem becomes dependent on the ability to control weight and food intake. This preoccupation with body image continues throughout women's lives. In fact, dieting and concerns about weight have become so pervasive that they are now the norm for North American women (Smeets, Jansen, & Roefs, 2011).

The ideal of male attractiveness in American society has been changing and has contributed to an increase in eating disorders among men. The ideal male body is becoming more and more difficult for the average boy or man to attain. Little boys are being taught to base their self-esteem on strength and athleticism. Their action toys have washboard abdominal muscles, and their heroes are members of World Wrestling Entertainment (WWE). Men with eating disorders have an overwhelming fear of fatness and a desire to maintain a masculine appearance or shape. It is not uncommon to see males with eating disorders use anabolic steroids to improve muscle tone and build strength (Neri et al., 2011).

In a sense, anorexia and bulimia could be considered culture-reactive syndromes in the Western world. Developing Cultural Competence discusses this further. Eating disorders are not solely a problem of specific cultural groups, however. Negative body image and body dissatisfaction lead to problematic eating behaviors. It seems that, culture notwithstanding, negative interactions about body size can create stress and challenges that affect eating behaviors (Rivas, Bersabé, Jiméne, & Berrocal, 2010).

Biologic Theory

Family risk studies show that relatives of clients with eating disorders are 5 to 10 times more likely to develop an eating disorder. It appears that in anorexia, the more severe the disorder, the more likely a strong genetic predisposition. Twin studies for eating disorders show that the concordance rate (occurring together) for twins is 55% to 60%. These data suggest that there may be a genetic predisposition (Slane, Burt, & Klump, 2010).

Genetic research focuses on behavioral, neurobiologic, and temperamental variables that may represent core features of these disorders. These features include perfectionism, orderliness, low tolerance for new situations, low self-esteem, and overall high anxiety. Even if an individual has a high genetic risk, however, that person might develop an eating disorder even if he or she did not live in a culture that stresses dieting and thinness (Seal, 2011).

Recently, neurotransmitter dysregulation has been considered to be a contributing factor in eating disorders, particularly serotonin (5-HT). Being full of food to the point of satisfaction is referred to as *satiety*. Normally, a low level of 5-HT decreases a person's satiety and thereby increases food intake. In contrast, a high level of 5-HT increases satiety and

DEVELOPING CULTURAL COMPETENCE

When Thin Is In

What is considered attractive changes over time and from one culture to another. Attractiveness can also be inconsistent within a culture. Centuries ago, a large woman was considered to be the epitome of beauty because it indicated the family had enough money to be well fed, and enough social status to be spared hard labor. The ideal of attractiveness in North American society has been fairly consistent for decades—thin—and has contributed to an increase in eating disorders.

TV, magazines, movies, and advertisements all define beauty. Women tend to be targeted for messages that because thin is good, there is no real lower limit on how thin you should be. This, of course, leads to unhealthy and dangerous levels of calorie deprivation and starvation. Men are targeted for being in shape—not too thin, not too heavy—in messages about body building, weight lifting, or muscle toning. The "ideal" male body is one with well-developed muscles on the chest, arms, and shoulders and a slim waist and hips.

Eating disorders tend to occur predominantly in industrialized, developed countries and less often in traditional societies. For example, Native Canadians (Ojibway-Cree) tend to show a preference for heavier body types than the Euro-Canadian population does. In the Caribbean, the incidence of anorexia among the majority Black population is negligible. African-American women and men in North America are more positive about higher weights in women than are Euro-American women and men. Typically, Asian-American and Latino women were less likely to describe themselves as fat, were less dissatisfied with their body size, and were less likely to diet.

You may see the incidence of eating disorders change, however, as cultures around the world are exposed to each other through media, travel, and social media, and become more Westernized. Recently a cultural shift has been noted. In the shift, Asian, Asian-American, and Latino women are becoming less satisfied with their bodies because their media, similar to the Anglo media. now promotes thin bodies as ideal for women.

CRITICAL THINKING QUESTIONS

1. How would you initiate a conversation about the culture of ideal beauty with a client?
2. How are a person's vocational and recreational activities relevant to culturally influenced eating habits?

thereby decreases food intake. Carbohydrates (CHOs) are involved in the synthesis of 5-HT by increasing tryptophan, the precursor of 5-HT. The neurotransmitter hypothesis of bulimia is that recurrent binge episodes may result from a deficiency in 5-HT and low satiety levels. The tendency of people with bulimia to binge on high-CHO foods may be a reflection of the body's adaptive attempt to increase 5-HT levels.

Other neurotransmitters affect eating behavior. Norepinephrine (NE) and neuropeptide Y (NPY) increase eating behavior, while dopamine (DA) suppresses food intake. DA agonists such as amphetamines and cocaine are appetite suppressants.

Endogenous opioids, such as endorphins, are associated with food intake and mood. Opioids increase food intake and enhance positive mood states; therefore, insufficient levels of endogenous opioids cause decreased food intake and depressed mood. It has been found that underweight people have significantly lower levels of endorphins compared to healthy volunteers. When the person's weight is returned to normal levels, the endorphin level is also within normal limits.

Biologic factors, sociocultural factors, and intrapersonal or interpersonal conflicts cannot—and should not—be dealt with separately. The interaction of these factors is extremely important. For example, clients suffering from severe obesity may experience shame and helplessness as they attempt to cope with fears of rejection and loss of love. These feelings can lead to compensatory overeating, which in turn can create interpersonal conflict with family members. The client may withdraw from others, thus reinforcing the feelings of rejection and increasing social isolation.

NURSING PROCESS
The Client With Anorexia Nervosa

The following section discusses the specific steps of the nursing process for clients with anorexia nervosa. Be aware of your own potential reactions to clients with eating disorders. Self-aware nurses recognize their own emotional reactions to clients and view clients' self-absorption and manipulativeness as symptoms of the disorder. Your Self-Awareness will help you assess your reactions.

> ### YOUR SELF-AWARENESS
> **Possible Reactions to Working With Clients With Eating Disorders**
>
> In order to explore your reactions to clients with eating disorders, determine which, if any, of the following apply to you.
>
> - You feel exhausted and defeated by the structured demands of the client's care plan.
> - You feel resentment at the client's efforts to manipulate and attempts at "staff splitting."
> - You identify with the client because of your own personal body image concerns.
> - You feel overprotective of the client and allow a coalition between yourself and the client to form.
> - You feel annoyance and anger toward the client and are unnecessarily rough during physical care.
> - You have difficulty recognizing that the client's symptoms are as serious as those of a hallucinating or delusional client.
> - You fail to monitor the client's mealtime and after-meal behaviors, allowing the client to continue maladaptive patterns of coping.
> - You allow the client to re-enact power struggles from home, such as those about food, weight, and exercising.
> - You believe that the client is deliberately engaging in maladaptive coping behaviors to upset the staff and family.
> - You feel repelled by the client's eating habits or the appearance of the client's body.
> - You feel hopeless and are affected by the client's despondency.

Assessment

When assessing clients with dramatic weight loss or gain, you must not lose sight of the fact that both can be caused by physical conditions. Certain illnesses must be ruled out before an eating disorder diagnosis can be made. Wasting conditions such as advanced cancer, tuberculosis, AIDS, hyperthyroidism, pyloric obstruction, and drug abuse must be considered when weight loss is a feature. Rapid weight gain can result from a brain tumor, an endocrine disorder, or as a side effect of medications. A good history and physical examination are often needed to provide information to eliminate the possibility of a physical basis for sudden weight loss or gain. After the presence of an eating disorder is established, you will assess the client using the following subjective and objective data.

Subjective Data

Clients with anorexia nervosa perceive themselves as overweight, no matter how thin they may be. However emaciated their bodies, they can always find some body part they believe is fat. They are preoccupied with thoughts of food and simultaneously obsessed with rigidly controlling their own intake. They often collect cookbooks, cook prodigious amounts of food, and insist that others eat while not taking a morsel for themselves. They are fearful of even the slightest weight gain and view with suspicion anyone who encourages them to eat.

Another preoccupation is with exercise. It is not uncommon for anorexics to engage in extremely lengthy sessions of aerobics or calisthenics, or to run, bike, or walk to excess, even when in an emaciated condition. They push themselves to greater and greater levels of endurance and deprive themselves of sleep as a measure of self-control.

Anorexics frequently deny that they have a weight problem. They insist they have never felt better and simply wish to be left alone about food. They report feeling strong, powerful, and good as a result of self-denial. They report feeling guilty, self-indulgent, and weak when they eat. They therefore resist treatment, although they may admit to feeling isolated and lonely and may even describe themselves as exhausted with the effort it takes to achieve the perfection they seek. They tend to have difficulty accepting nurturing behavior from others and therefore have difficulty forming therapeutic alliances. They report a loss of interest in sex but do not perceive this as a problem.

Objective Data

People with anorexia usually experience a weight loss of 25% but a loss as high as 50% is possible. Amenorrhea is extremely common and is thought to be related to the degree of stress the woman is experiencing, the percentage of body fat lost, and altered hypothalamic function. With low estrogen levels, these young women are at higher risk for osteopenia leading to osteoporosis. This is a serious medical complication with no known effective treatment.

The anorexic client is emaciated, with sunken eyes and a skeletal appearance. In very young clients, growth failure may be present. Lanugo growth (babylike, fine hair) on the face, extremities, and trunk may occur. Other physical symptoms include bradycardia, hypotension, arrhythmias, delayed gastric motility, and a hypothyroid-like state manifested by dry skin, listlessness, and dry hair that falls out at a higher-than-normal rate. Peripheral edema may be a feature in advanced starvation. Laboratory tests may reveal leukopenia, anemia, low serum potassium, and elevated blood urea nitrogen (BUN). There may also be low thyroid levels and elevated serum cortisol.

Nursing Diagnosis: NANDA

Once the assessment process is completed, determine appropriate nursing diagnoses.

Imbalanced Nutrition: Less Than Body Requirements

By the time anorexic clients are seen in treatment, their physical condition is often so deteriorated from self-imposed starvation that it becomes the priority for nursing care. Life-threatening malnourishment is seen in 5% to 20% of these clients. Death may occur from malnutrition, infection, or cardiac abnormalities related to electrolyte imbalances. Intravenous therapy, tube feedings, and total parenteral hyperalimentation (TPH) are required in cases of medical emergency.

The client's preoccupation with food, evidenced by reading recipes, discussing food, and preparing food for others, is due to suppression and sublimation of the client's own hunger. Overexercising creates even more extreme nutritional deficits. In those anorexic clients who also purge by vomiting or using laxatives, nutritional status is further endangered.

Clients in a state of starvation experience hormonal, metabolic, and emotional changes. Some of those changes are manifested in amenorrhea or delay of onset of menses, ketosis, severe vitamin deficiencies, depressed immune response, lethargy, weakness, and irritability—conditions that also vitally affect nurse–client relationships.

Ineffective Individual Coping

Clients experiencing anorexia nervosa demonstrate impairment of adaptive behaviors, such as self-care in activities of daily living. They have difficulty meeting daily demands, and role performance may be affected. Their preoccupation with the pursuit of thinness deprives them of the energy necessary for adaptive behavior and distracts them from interest in role fulfillment. The quest for thinness is the entire focus of their lives.

In addition, developmental issues such as the desire for independence and the longing for dependence combine with traditionally adolescent resentment of authority to influence the quality and character of the nurse–client relationship. Family enmeshment and unwillingness to allow the client to separate contribute to self-doubt and the inability to accept responsibility for self.

Disturbed Body Image

Clients with anorexia nervosa are unable to make realistic appraisals of their own body size, although they can accurately evaluate the size of others. They drastically underestimate their own bodily needs, even in the face of overwhelming evidence of malnutrition. Profound disturbances in accurate

perception of size and intense client denial indicate a poor prognosis. The client's body image disturbance is often the source of conflict in family and therapeutic relationships.

Chronic Low Self-Esteem

Anorexic clients' lack of confidence in themselves and feelings of inferiority are main factors in the disorder. Their self-deprivation and self-denial make them feel powerful and superior to others who cannot muster such profound self-control. The quest for perfection is neverending, but they can never achieve a level of thinness that is satisfying; there are always a few more pounds to shed. They often present the picture of "model clients," in contrast to seemingly more disturbed clients. As a result, novice nurses may have difficulty assessing the severity of the illness accurately.

The low self-esteem of anorexic clients stems from unrealistic expectations by self and others, complicated by unmet dependency needs. The clinical picture is further complicated because cultural norms of thinness reinforce maladaptive behavior. The nurse–client relationship is affected by the extreme difficulty these clients have in accepting positive feedback and by their nonparticipation in self-care and therapeutic activities. Their preoccupation with their appearance and with others' perceptions of them may be irritating to other clients. The nurse–client relationship is also affected by the client's need to control, which often leads to manipulative behaviors.

Outcome Identification: NOC

Suggested outcomes for each NANDA diagnosis in the previous section follow.

Imbalanced Nutrition: Less Than Body Requirements

This diagnosis inevitably leads to the desired outcome of improvement of Nutritional Status: Adequate nutrients taken into the body for height, frame, gender, and activity level.

Ineffective Individual Coping

Several NOC outcomes are relevant to anorexic clients with this nursing diagnosis. They include Coping: Actions to manage stressors that tax an individual's resources; Impulse Control: Ability to self-restrain compulsive or impulsive behavior; and Information Processing: Ability to acquire, organize, and use information.

Disturbed Body Image

For the anorexic client, who invariably has a distorted body image, NOC outcomes include Body Image: Positive perception of own appearance; and Distorted Thought Control: Ability to self-restrain altered perceptions.

Chronic Low Self-Esteem

As in many psychiatric disorders, low self-esteem plays a major role in anorexia nervosa, leading to the NOC outcome of Self-Esteem: Personal judgment of self-worth.

Planning and Implementation: NIC

When a client's behavior meets the criteria for a diagnosis of anorexia nervosa, effective nursing intervention is directed toward ensuring that the client will not die and helping the client learn more effective ways of coping with the demands of life. A variety of approaches, including behavioral, insight-oriented, and cognitive therapies, may be useful; pharmacologic therapy may be used also. As a feature of behavioral therapy, a behavioral contract can be very effective. An explanation of how to develop and use behavioral contracts is in Chapter 30∞.

Symptoms can be extreme and dangerous with this disorder. Protection and improvement may require more intensive and constant treatment. In severely debilitated clients, inpatient treatment is indicated. Box 21-1 lists behavioral characteristics identified by Love & Seaton (1991) and White & Litovitz (1998) that indicate the need for hospitalization. The suggestions in these classic references are still used today in clinical settings. Recovery from eating disorders is a long process. Individuals with anorexia are ambivalent about treatment and often terminate treatment early. Symptoms correlated with early termination include higher levels of weight concerns, greater maturity fears, and impulsivity. For those who continue treatment, about 40% recover and the rest experience a chronic course, some with fewer symptoms and some with the same symptoms.

Managing Nutrition

To establish adequate eating patterns and fluid and electrolyte balance, assume a calm, matter-of-fact attitude and a positive expectation of the client. Meeting minimal nutritional goals, with the overall goal of gradual weight restoration, is nonnegotiable. A caloric intake of 1,200 to 1,500 cal/day is the usual range. Changing the eating pattern to a healthier one (called *graded nutritional therapy*) involves timing, education, and reinforcement. Your Intervention Strategies lists guidelines for graded nutritional therapy.

Nursing interventions may include tube feedings or intravenous therapy, which are administered in a nonjudgmental manner. Weighing the client daily, recording intake and output, observing the client during meals, and observing bathroom behavior may be necessary if you suspect the client is discarding food or inducing vomiting. Avoid discussing food, recipes, restaurants, and eating with the client because these conversations

---

YOUR INTERVENTION STRATEGIES
Guidelines for Graded Nutritional Therapy

Strategy	Rationale
■ Acknowledge fears of weight gain.	■ Reassures the client that fears are expected and not unique.
■ Collaborate with the client and dietitian to plan a flexible program for gradual nutrition.	■ Enlists the client as an active participant in treatment.
■ Adopt a matter-of-fact, consistent, and nonjudgmental attitude.	■ Conveys your confidence and acceptance of the client.
■ Collaborate with nutritionists for schedule and nutrition supplement options.	■ Plans the introduction of nutrition because of disruption in normal flora of gastrointestinal (GI) tract.
■ Introduce dietary content slowly.	■ Gives the client a chance to equilibrate to the psychological impact of eating as well as allowing the GI tract to accommodate relatively novel items.
■ Support the client during sensations of fullness and bloating; teach that these are normal and transient feelings.	■ The client's gastrointestinal tract must readjust to unaccustomed intake.
■ Encourage the expression of feelings of loss of control.	■ Upon resuming adequate intake, clients fear "losing control" and "becoming fat."
■ Monitor fluid and electrolyte intake and output, vital signs, body temperature, and mood.	■ Prebiotics and probiotics (see your nursing fundamentals texts) will ease the transition.

Box 21-1 Criteria for Inpatient Admission

Inpatient admission is recommended for eating disordered clients who have the following:

- Suicidal or severely out of control behavior (self-mutilating; abusing large amounts of laxatives, emetics, and diuretics; abusing street drugs)
- Loss of 25–30% of body weight, resulting in severe emaciation
- Cardiac arrhythmias
- Fluid and electrolyte imbalances
- The need for more intensive inpatient contacts and therapy if outpatient treatment has proved insufficient
- The need for extensive diagnostic evaluation to rule out comorbidities

Source: Love, C. C., & Seaton, H. (1991). Eating disorders: Highlights of nursing assessment and therapeutics. *Nursing Clinics of North America, 26*(3), 687; and White, J. H., & Litovitz, G. (1998). A comparison of inpatient and outpatient women with eating disorders. *Archives of Psychiatric Nursing, 12*(4), 181–194. With permission from Elsevier Science.

---

reinforce maladaptive behaviors. Providing a pleasant mealtime environment and adopting realistic expectations of how much the client will eat are critically important aspects of nursing care. Clients find frequent small meals more acceptable than three large meals. Setting a time limit of about a half hour is a good way to forestall mealtime "marathons"—protracted meals during which the client eats little.

Mandatory tube feedings, a controversial intervention, may be the therapeutic regimen in some treatment centers. Although tube feedings will manage a dangerously low weight with perilously disordered electrolytes, tube feedings have a conditioned effect that must be taken into account. (Chapter 30∞ discusses conditioned responses.) Tube feedings do give a message—that is, taking in calories through food is beneficial to overall health. On the other hand, tube feedings can also deliver the message that the problem is too severe for the client to overcome with voluntary action. This message can be demoralizing to the client and may be further amplified by negative associations with treatment providers because of the unpleasant aspects of the experience.

Acknowledge and recognize the efforts of clients who meet weight gain goals, but avoid praise or flattery. Education

YOUR INTERVENTION STRATEGIES Sample Contract for Weight Gain

Name _____ Date _____

Height _____ Weight _____

Goal Weight _____

- I will be weighed _____ daily
  _____ twice weekly _____ weekly
- My weight will be measured upon awakening, after voiding, with bedclothes on
- All exercise, jogging, or calisthenics will only be conducted with treatment team approval
- I will consume all scheduled nutritional supplements as listed below:
  _____ cans of supplement per day if weight is <u>less</u> than ¼ pound over my last highest weight

_____ cans of supplement per day if weight is <u>more</u> than ¼ pound over my last highest weight
- I will consume each can of supplement within 15 minutes

Other issues:
-
-

I agree to abide by the terms of this behavioral contract

Client _____

Nurse _____

Date _____

---

about adequate eating patterns is a necessary part of discharge planning. Consistency and coordination among staff members are essential to avoid manipulation by clients. Interdisciplinary planning conferences and adherence to written care plans promote effective care. Behavior modification programs, which base privileges on weight gain, may be useful for focusing on emotional issues, not just eating behaviors (Wilfley, Kolko, & Kass, 2011). You and the client may engage in a contract for weight gain, such as the sample presented in Your Intervention Strategies.

A target weight is usually chosen by the treatment team in collaboration with a dietitian. Target weight for discharge from treatment is usually 90% of average for age and height. Discharge planning can include referral to self-help groups such as the American Anorexia/Bulimia Association, Anorexia Nervosa and Related Eating Disorders, and National Association of Anorexia Nervosa and Associated Disorders. The websites for these self-help groups are included in Partnering With Clients and Families. These resources can be accessed through links on the Online Student Resources for this book.

PARTNERING WITH CLIENTS AND FAMILIES

Teaching About Eating Disorders

Friends and family members of people with eating disorders are often at a loss as to how to help. Partner with family and friends by introducing the following concepts:

- Food is necessary for life, but moderation (not too much and not too little) must be learned.
- In order for attitudes and behaviors to change, everyone must be willing to do things differently.
- Change takes time.
- The person with the disorder must want to make his or her own change.
- Family and friends must also change to accommodate the person's growth.
- Cooperate fully with the person's therapist.
- Avoid arguments about weight and food.
- Do not force the person to eat, or stop eating, food.
- Learning from others is extremely helpful. Get support and information. (See resource list.)
- Express love, appreciation, and affection both verbally and physically.
- Admit to the normal range of human emotion—your anger, frustration, helplessness, and powerlessness as well as love, appreciation, and affection.
- Feelings are normal; there is no need to fear them.
- Be active with nonfood activities.
- Don't discuss your diet.
- As with any change in behavior, there will be steps forward and steps back.

- Remember, people have the right to make decisions about their health even though you may not approve of the decision.
- If your loved one is engaging in dangerous activities, seek guidance on addressing the situation.

Resources*
National Association of Anorexia Nervosa & Associated Disorders
P.O. Box 640
Naperville, IL 60566
Helpline: (630) 577-1330
http://www.nationaleatingdisorders.org

National Eating Disorders Association
603 Steward St., Suite 803
Seattle, WA 98101
(206) 382-3587
http://www.nationaleatingdisorders.org

Office on Women's Health
200 Independence Avenue SW, Room 730B
Washington, DC 20201
(800) 994-9662 TDD: (888) 220-5446
http://www.womanshealth.gov/bodyimage

Weight-Control Information Network (WIN)
1 Win Way
Bethesda, MD 20892-3665
(877) 946-4627
http://win.niddk.nih.gov/index.htm

*These resources can be found on the Online Student Resources for this book.

Facilitating Coping

The best way to promote individual coping is by involving clients in their own treatment planning. Self-determination fosters adaptive coping mechanisms in clients' day-to-day hospital experiences; this process carries over to daily life outside the hospital setting and helps clients meet its demands.

Although trust is difficult to establish with anorexic clients, it is the basis for all therapeutic relationships. Being honest, available, and matter-of-fact helps establish trust and encourages clients to express their feelings. If necessary, allow clients to assume a dependent role at first, but as trust is developed and physical condition improves, encourage them to take more responsibility for themselves. Participating in the planning of care gives clients opportunities to practice making decisions. Letting clients have input into their treatment plans also fosters adherence. Provide flexibility in activities of daily living, type and timing of exercise, and choice of occupational and recreational therapy activities. This autonomy increases clients' sense of responsibility for themselves.

Giving clients the opportunity to practice problem solving may lead to power struggles if you disagree with clients' choices. Demonstrate positive belief in their ability to regain healthy functioning and a willingness to tolerate "mistakes." The treatment team must set firm and clear limits, however, to provide the secure environment clients need to learn more effective coping behaviors. Also help clients identify ways to feel in control by other than anorexic and manipulative behaviors.

Clients need to explore their extreme fears of gaining weight before they can relinquish maladaptive behaviors. It is helpful to explore with clients their feelings about their family, their role in the family, and their autonomy within the family system.

Enhancing Body Image

To help clients regain an accurate perception of their body size and nutritional needs, first encourage them to express feelings about body size. An example is shown in Rx Communication. Reframe clients' misperceptions by using language that emphasizes health, strength, and evaluation. For example, if the client says "My thighs are huge," reply "Your thighs are becoming stronger now that you're gaining weight. Healthy muscles are rounded and firm, like yours." With practice, clients can replace negative thinking with positive self-talk. Teach and reinforce this skill, and help them practice it. For example, ask clients to make three positive statements (positive affirmations) about their bodies each day.

If clients are unable or unwilling to discuss their feelings about body size, ask them to draw themselves as they are now and as they desire to be. These drawings not only focus the discussion of body size and nutritional needs but also help you understand how clients view their bodies. Because clients with bulimia nervosa and compulsive overeating also have distorted body images, this activity can be incorporated into their plans of care as well. You could also use a more structured tool such as the one illustrated in FIGURE 21-3 ■. In addition, you can access BodyImage, a software program for the assessment of body image disturbance, through a link on the Online Student Resources for this book. Any communication about how clients perceive their bodies is useful in treatment because it removes the hidden, shameful aspects of the perception and allows open discussion.

When clients share feelings honestly, show improvement in accurate perception of body image, or demonstrate healthier eating behaviors, reinforce their efforts through verbal recognition. It is also useful to examine with clients the ways in which the fashion and advertising industries support unrealistic cultural norms of excessive thinness incompatible with healthy functioning.

Improving Self-Esteem

Help clients re-examine negative feelings about themselves and identify their positive attributes. Encourage clients to record in a diary those thoughts that are difficult to share directly. Be nonjudgmental in your acceptance of negative feelings and positively reinforce the honest expression of all feelings. Encouragement is particularly important when clients experiment with independently made decisions, even when outcomes are not entirely positive. The client needs to interpret each experience as worthwhile. Emphasize the feeling of control gained through independent decision making.

Together, you and the client explore the client's attempt to achieve perfection by controlling weight. The idea is for the client to realize that perfection is an unrealistic goal. You are a role model for the person who accepts imperfection yet retains self-esteem. One way to model strong self-esteem is to admit

*(side margin)* Body Image

℞ RX COMMUNICATION

Client With Anorexia Nervosa

CLIENT: [Tearfully] "My doctor says I have to eat and gain weight but I still have this little fat tummy."

NURSE RESPONSE #1: "Tell me what you are feeling right now."	NURSE RESPONSE #2: "It sounds as though you feel caught in the middle of the doctor's expectations and your own."
RATIONALE: Asking the client to focus on her feelings assists her in becoming more self-aware. Obtaining additional subjective data from the client enables you to better understand her.	*RATIONALE:* Nonjudgmental acknowledgement of the client's conflict shows empathy and encourages her to clarify the dilemma from her doctor's point of view as well as her own. Avoids directly challenging the client's distorted perception of her body image.

FIGURE 21-3 ■ Assessing body image. A drawing such as this can be used in several ways: (1) Clients can be asked which image best represents them. This assesses the accuracy of the client's body image. Anorexic clients often believe themselves to be larger than they really are. (2) Clients can be asked which image best represents the ideal for them. This assesses whether a client has a positive (image is similar to the client's own body) or a negative (dissimilar image) body image.

errors willingly. Also model appropriate expressions of anger and teach clients the destructive effects of unexpressed anger.

Evaluation

Evaluation of the effectiveness of nursing interventions with these disorders is an ongoing part of the nursing process.

Nutritional Status

Clients will regain and maintain at least 90% of normal weight for their height and age. Clients will follow eating patterns that demonstrate they recognize the importance of adequate nutrition. They will regain and maintain normal elimination patterns, vital signs, fluid and electrolyte balance, and muscle tone. Female clients will have normal menstrual cycles.

Coping

Clients will demonstrate effective coping when they participate actively in treatment planning and discharge planning using problem-solving skills. They will demonstrate interest and competence in self-care activities such as hygiene, sleep, activity, rest, diversional activities, and nutrition. They will accurately identify both maladaptive coping behaviors and adaptive coping behaviors that they can integrate into daily routines. Clients will express less anxiety about weight gain and will verbalize other means of feeling in control of their lives.

Body Image

Body image disturbance will be alleviated when clients accurately assess their own body size and nutritional needs. They will use criteria such as strength and health, rather than appearance alone, to evaluate body size. They will verbalize less preoccupation with body size. Clients will verbalize positive statements about their own bodies.

Self-Esteem

Clients will demonstrate self-esteem when they verbalize their own positive attributes. They will demonstrate less preoccupation with their own appearance and will focus increasingly on others. They will accept compliments and positive feedback and show greater interest in activities around them. They will verbalize that perfection is an unrealistic life goal. Clients will express anger appropriately without experiencing incapacitating guilt. They will demonstrate interpersonal relationships substantially free of manipulation. Clients will work toward success experiences in work, school, and/or social groups.

CASE MANAGEMENT

Case managers working with clients who have eating disorders must understand the risk factors and possible complications of these disorders. This awareness enables the case manager to recognize symptoms early, mobilize the treatment team and family resources, ensure a smooth transition to inpatient therapy if needed, and ensure adequate follow-up. Failure to respond to treatment occurs in about 50% of cases.

Desired case management outcomes include weight gain/loss, normalization of exercise periods, cessation of binge eating and purging behaviors, and decreased preoccupation with food and body size. Avoidance of hospitalization or the briefest possible hospital stay is a case management priority.

The ultimate case management goal is early detection of symptoms, effective symptom reduction, and rapid return to maximal premorbid function. Despite the best efforts, about half of clients with eating disorders progress from acute to chronic illness, which presents them, their families, and case managers with lifelong challenges.

COMMUNITY-BASED CARE

Although many, if not most, clients with bulimia nervosa and binge-eating disorder can be safely treated in community-based settings, severely anorexic clients usually are admitted to an inpatient program. There are residential treatment facilities for longer-term care of approximately 3 months. Day hospitals are another option. Criteria for hospitalization are found in Box 21-1 on page 468. Nurses in community-based settings, such as school nurses, occupational health nurses, and nurses in doctors' offices, play a major role in recognizing symptoms of eating disorders. They provide screening, information, and support to clients and families; and refer clients for specialized treatment. Eating disorders are not self-limiting and specialized care is required.

Prevention of eating disorders is receiving increased attention as an appropriate and much-needed focus for community-based nurses, particularly those in schools. Due to the early onset of anorexic thinking, education programs as early as grade school should be developed. Eating disorders have become more commonly recognized and, to some extent, normalized. The media have contributed to the idea that the ideal body shape is slimness to the point of extreme thinness. Most recently, the media have called the public's attention to eating-disordered public figures (especially in the entertainment field), thus influencing the public's perception of the illness and the community reaction to treatment and relapse.

Nurses in community-based settings can play a valuable role in the education, support, and referral of clients and their families, often enabling clients to remain in the community while in treatment.

HOME CARE

Historically, clients with eating disorders were isolated from their families during treatment. It was thought that ongoing family conflict would jeopardize their recovery. This approach has been challenged, and attitudes toward home-based care are gradually changing. Having a therapeutic alliance with clients and parents is an important aspect of recovery. Many programs have found that increasing family involvement and integration into the treatment program contributes to improved outcomes.

Just as it is important that families are aware of the helpful websites discussed earlier, it is vital for the family to be aware of Internet websites that are pro-anorexia and promote treatment sabotage. These websites contain information that promote and support anorexia. Content includes lifestyle descriptions, inspirational photos that serve as motivators for weight loss, and "tips and tricks" on being anorexic. Using the information on these websites disrupts the healing process.

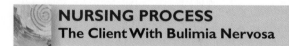

NURSING PROCESS
The Client With Bulimia Nervosa

The following section discusses the nursing process for clients with bulimia nervosa. Some clients with bulimia may also be anorexic. The nursing process in the previous section (on pages 466–471) covers anorexia.

Assessment

Although the two disorders are described separately, the boundary between anorexia and bulimia is blurred. Many bulimics were formerly anorexic, while others may become people with anorexia in the future. It is estimated that as many as half of all people with anorexia binge and purge at some time during their illness. During the assessment phase of the nursing process, keep in mind that these two conditions, although distinctly different, often coexist.

Subjective Data

Clients with bulimia nervosa have feelings of low self-esteem, worthlessness, inadequacy, and guilt. They experience shame and embarrassment over their secret binges (eating several quarts of ice cream, buckets of popcorn, or eight or more candy bars is not unusual) and subsequent purging activities. This shame may be manifested in self-deprecating remarks. Clients report feeling out of control, but at the same time they feel an excessive need to control. Unlike anorexics, clients with bulimia nervosa recognize that their eating behaviors are abnormal and bizarre.

Anxiety and unsatisfactory interpersonal relationships are features of this disorder. Anxiety is intensified when others see the bulimic as successful and in control, and they often appear so to others. They are impulsive and cannot delay gratification. Preoccupation with food, weight, and dieting is a prominent feature. Bulimic clients may report feeling weak and lethargic.

Objective Data

Like anorexic clients, bulimic clients tend to be young females. Bulimia first manifests itself later than anorexia, typically during late adolescence or young adulthood. Clients with bulimia are usually of normal or slightly above-average weight. Appearance does not provide diagnostic clues; hence the term *normal-weight bulimic*. Weight tends to fluctuate but does not become dangerously low unless anorexia occurs concurrently.

Clients with bulimia nervosa are more outgoing than those with anorexia and tend to be more comfortable with sexual relationships. They sometimes manifest impulsive behaviors such as substance abuse, shoplifting, and self-inflicted injury. In inpatient settings, they may steal others' food and hoard food in their rooms.

Physical signs of bulimia nervosa include hoarseness and esophagitis, dental enamel erosion, enlarged parotid glands, abrasions or calluses on knuckles from inducing vomiting, and amenorrhea in about 40% of cases. The client may also have symptoms of fluid volume deficit: concentrated urine, decreased urine output, hypotension, elevated temperature, poor skin turgor, and weakness.

Laboratory tests may reveal electrolyte abnormalities, particularly low serum potassium. Potentially fatal cardiac arrythmias may result. The overuse of syrup of ipecac, an emetic agent, can create cumulative systemic toxicity affecting the gastrointestinal, neuromuscular, and cardiovascular systems, potentially leading to death from cardiotoxicity.

Another concern is the fact that the frequency of bulimia in diabetics is increasing, particularly among young women. This is a potentially deadly combination because binge eating and purging increase the risk for both hypoglycemic episodes and diabetic ketoacidosis (DKA). Closely monitoring blood glucose levels is indicated for these clients.

Nursing Diagnosis: NANDA

Four major nursing diagnoses for clients with bulimia are discussed next.

Anxiety

Clients with bulimia nervosa experience anxiety: vague, uneasy feelings of moderate to intense severity related to preoccupation with body image. A rise in the client's anxiety level is usually a forerunner of binge/purge behaviors and may lead to purchasing or hoarding food in preparation for a binge.

Deficient Fluid Volume

Depletion of body fluids in clients with bulimia nervosa is usually related to self-induced vomiting and the excessive use of laxatives and diuretics, combined with decreased fluid intake. Extreme dehydration may lead to changes in electrolyte balance, causing altered mental status. Lethargy and confusion are symptoms of advanced dehydration. Edema may also be present.

Ineffective Individual Coping

Binge and purge behaviors are ineffective ways to cope with the stresses of life. Other impulse control problems, such as alcohol abuse, drug abuse, and shoplifting, are equally ineffective ways to reduce stress. The bulimic client's ineffective coping is related to issues such as independence/dependence, identity, and self-determination. Ineffective coping is manifested in the bulimic client's preoccupation with body size, poor self-esteem, distorted body image, and excessive overeating followed by purging.

Compromised Family Coping

The families of clients with bulimia nervosa have distorted perceptions of the problems and perceive themselves as unable to deal effectively with the client's eating disorder. Parents may have difficulty allowing the client to grow up and may be overprotective; at the same time, they may have overly high expectations of the client. The bulimic client's behavior may become the family's focus, preventing the fulfillment of essential family roles. If disruption is extreme, the family may not be able to interact effectively with the larger community. Usual problem-solving methods are only partially adequate to deal with the stress of having a bulimic family member.

Outcome Identification: NOC

Suggested outcomes for each NANDA diagnosis in the previous section follow.

Anxiety

Desired outcomes related to anxiety in bulimic clients may involve Coping: Actions to manage stressors that tax an individual's resources; and Impulse Control: Ability to self-restrain compulsive or impulsive behavior.

Deficient Fluid Volume

Two nursing outcomes that are useful with this nursing diagnosis are Electrolyte and Acid–Base Balance: Balance of electrolytes and nonelectrolytes in the intracellular and extracellular compartments of the body; and Hydration: Amount of water in the intracellular and extracellular compartments of the body.

Ineffective Individual Coping

Similar to the anorexic client, several NOC outcomes are relevant to bulimic clients with this nursing diagnosis. They include Coping: Actions to manage stressors that tax an individual's resources; Impulse Control: Ability to self-restrain compulsive or impulsive behavior; and Information Processing: Ability to acquire, organize, and use information.

Compromised Family Coping

NOC outcome statements relevant to the NANDA diagnosis of Compromised Family Coping have not yet been developed. Appropriate outcomes might include those related to improving family communication, reducing family stress, the learning developmental needs of family members, and seeking community resources.

Planning and Implementation: NIC

Several nursing interventions have been somewhat useful in treating bulimia nervosa.

Managing Medication

Medications, primarily antidepressants, are used to reduce the frequency of disturbed eating behaviors such as binge eating and vomiting. In addition, medications are used to ease symptoms that may accompany eating disorders such as depression, anxiety, obsessions, or impulse control problems.

Fluoxetine (Prozac), an SSRI, is effective for clients with bulimia when given at the higher dose of 50 to 60 mg per day. Other SSRIs, paroxetine (Paxil) and sertraline (Zoloft), are useful in that they have antiobsessional and antianxiety effects. Typically, the medication is continued until 6 months following the disappearance of symptoms. In the past, tricyclic antidepressants (TCAs) have been used, but because these individuals already have a risk for cardiac problems, the side effect of cardiotoxicity of TCAs is an unnecessary risk.

Reducing Anxiety

The goal of nursing interventions with anxious bulimic clients is to help them recognize events that create anxiety and to avoid binge eating and purging in response to anxiety. Initially, being available to the anxious client is useful. Project a calm, reassuring attitude, and provide a quiet, nonstimulating environment. After establishing trust, help the client identify anxiety-producing situations. Clients experience anxiety as occurring "out of the blue" and are often unaware that it is related to emotional issues and situations. Help clients identify previously used coping behaviors to determine whether they might be useful in current situations. How did the client handle anxiety before starting to binge and purge? Has positive self-talk or affirmations been beneficial? Box 21-2 shows examples of affirmations. Help bulimic clients identify feelings that precede binge/purge episodes such as those illustrated in FIGURE 21-4 ■ and explore healthier ways of dealing with those feelings.

Teach clients to recognize anxiety early, before it is severe, and to manage increasing anxiety. Energy-consuming activities, such as walking, running, and exercising, are useful but must be used very judiciously if the client's behavior includes overexercising. Clients can benefit from being taught progressive relaxation techniques and meditation (see Chapter 33 ∞). Administer antianxiety medications as ordered, but use caution because of the tendency to habituation. Also review the anxiety sections of Chapters 8 and 18 ∞.

> **Box 21-2 Affirmations for Compulsive Overeaters**
>
> 1. I cherish my mind, body, and spirit every day in every way.
> 2. My actions show that I care for myself and for my loved ones.
> 3. I encourage myself to grow as a kind and loving person.
> 4. I am honest with other people and true to myself.
> 5. My body is nourished and satisfied by moderate meals every day.
> 6. I know that my feelings guide me to my true self—therefore I tolerate them, welcome them, and think about them.
> 7. I am reliable and trustworthy, to myself and to others.
> 8. I am lovable as I am and deserve love and respect.
> 9. A mild level of anxiety stimulates my creativity.
> 10. I am honorable to myself by keeping my word to myself.

Client contracts are useful with bulimic clients. The contract is jointly developed with the client and renegotiated at periodic intervals, depending on the client's goals, severity of symptoms, and compliance with the contract. Such a contract might include agreements about binge eating, vomiting, or hoarding food, such as those in Your Intervention Strategies. Agreeing to a contract encourages clients to assume self-responsibility.

Managing Fluids and Electrolytes

The importance of accurate intake and output records cannot be overstated. Daily consumption of 2,000 to 3,000 mL of liquid promotes rehydration. Accurate daily weights are needed. Always weigh the client at the same time of day (immediately upon arising is preferred) and on the same scale. Assess and document the condition of the skin and

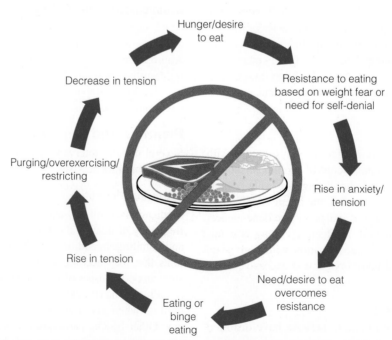

FIGURE 21-4 ■ A disordered eating cycle in bulimia nervosa. A nursing intervention to improve client self-awareness and anxiety reduction involves assisting clients to identify their personal eating cycle, which varies with the individual.

YOUR INTERVENTION STRATEGIES
Sample Contract for a Client With Bulimia

- I will sit with nursing staff for a half hour following each of my meals.
- I will not vomit after my meals.
- I will not take laxatives or diuretics.
- I will not bring any such substances onto the unit.
- I will tell the nursing staff if I feel like binge eating.
- I will stay away from the kitchen if I feel like going on a binge.

Client _____

Nurse _____

Date _____

oral mucous membranes as well as pulses and blood pressure daily, and monitor laboratory values, particularly urine specific gravity, reporting significant alterations to the physician. Observe clients for at least an hour after meals to prevent purging. To promote comfort in the dehydrated client, give frequent mouth care.

Facilitating Coping

Clients with bulimia nervosa can learn adaptive coping mechanisms to replace the out-of-control, binge/purge cycle. Once you have developed trust, help the client plan and practice strategies for dealing effectively with intense feelings and the demands of daily living. It is important for clients to identify situations and patterns of events that precede binge/purge episodes. Rx Communication provides an example of how you might open up the discussion. Clients learn to identify, name, and express feelings that they formerly perceived only as "bad." Once this is accomplished, explore alternative ways for clients to express those feelings.

Help clients identify times when they are at risk for binge eating and lack impulse control, such as when they are bored, frustrated, angry, lonely, or feeling unloved. Teach clients ways to nurture themselves during these times other than eating and purging. Suggest taking a warm bath, calling or visiting an old friend, or a hobby not involving food.

Clients with bulimia nervosa often perceive feelings of guilt and underlying resentment as overwhelming. They need

to learn effective ways of expressing these feelings and assertiveness techniques to diminish guilty interactions in the future. Role-playing with the client helps the client practice assertiveness. The worsening of both mood and bulimic symptoms during the winter has been reported in eating disorder literature with increasing frequency. Bright white light treatment has proven effective in treating bulimics with seasonal mood and symptom patterns. Chapter 17 discusses light treatment.

People who binge may benefit from a behavioral contract around posteating and postpurging behaviors. Refer to the sample contract in Your Intervention Strategies and imagine how this could help instill a sense of control and accomplishment for the client who typically copes by binge eating then purging.

Involve the client in discharge planning. Topics covered in discharge planning include the productive use of time, identification of diversional activities not related to food, and participation in support groups. Coordinate care with other nurses who work in specialty areas such as women's health, school, and pediatric settings that also treat the client.

Mobilizing the Family

Certain family dynamics reinforce maladaptive eating behaviors; therefore, families must also develop effective coping mechanisms to support the client's healthier coping behaviors. Assess the family's feelings and perceptions of the client's bulimia, listening carefully for what is most stressful and threatening to family members. Correct any misperceptions about the disorder. Encourage family members to explore together their usual coping strategies, and determine if any previously used strategies can be useful in the present situation.

Help the family identify their strengths and weaknesses. Encourage family members to share their thoughts and feelings, including feelings of guilt, blame, and resentment, with one another and with the client. Teach family members to use "I" statements, thereby acknowledging their feelings. If the client's disorder impairs family functioning, help the family reorganize roles to reduce stress and ensure that members' needs continue to be met during the client's recovery. Help the family understand that two normal developmental needs of adolescents and young adults are to develop autonomy and to establish identities outside the family. Make appropriate referrals to community resources, such as the American Anorexia/

R℞ COMMUNICATION

Client With Bulimia Nervosa

CLIENT: "Last night I made a pan of brownies and ate the whole thing. Then I had to throw up because I felt so miserable."

NURSE RESPONSE #1: "Let's talk about what was going on yesterday before you ate the brownies."	NURSE RESPONSE #2: "That sounds uncomfortable. What are the miserable feelings about?"
RATIONALE: Shows empathy for the client. Encourages her to focus on her feelings and their influence on her behavior, thereby promoting self-awareness.	RATIONALE: Demonstrates nonjudgmental acceptance. Encourages the client to place events in time sequence. This enables her to connect the cause-and-effect relationship between her experiences, her feelings, and her subsequent behavior.

Bulimia Association, Anorexia Nervosa and Related Eating Disorders, and Anorexia Nervosa and Associated Disorders groups. (Resources are listed in Partnering With Clients and Family on page 469.)

Home visits for an evening or weekend can help both the client and the family learn to use their new coping behaviors. Planning before visits and evaluating the success of visits afterward are essential parts of nurse–client and nurse–family interventions.

Evaluation

The evaluation process determines the effectiveness of the nursing interventions.

Anxiety

Clients will demonstrate anxiety control when they verbally identify situations and events that evoke anxiety. They will communicate needs and negative feelings appropriately. Clients will identify symptoms that indicate their own anxiety. They will identify ways of structuring the environment to prevent stressful situations that result in feeling out of control. Clients will eliminate binge/purge behaviors and demonstrate the use of anxiety-reduction strategies unrelated to eating. They will verbalize their acceptance of normal body weight without intense anxiety or will continue healthy eating patterns even though anxiety persists.

Fluid Volume

Dryness of oral mucosa and skin will not be evident. Skin turgor will be normal. Clients' vital signs and results of laboratory studies will be within normal limits. Input and output are balanced over 24-hour periods. Clients will verbalize their understanding of the relationship between dehydration and self-induced vomiting, laxative abuse, and diuretic abuse. Clients will verbalize understanding the physiological and psychological consequences of dehydration.

Individual Coping

Clients will demonstrate effective coping when they accurately assess maladaptive coping behaviors. They will demonstrate healthier ways to deal with stress and intense feelings. They will identify times of risk and verbalize alternative self-nurturing behaviors. They will demonstrate assertive communication techniques. Clients will demonstrate self-control in eating behaviors, gradually maintaining without supervision. They will verbalize increased self-confidence in the ability to handle the demands of daily life. They will follow through with recommended self-help or support groups and therapy following discharge.

Family Coping

Families will verbalize accurate perceptions of their situation. They will verbalize their feelings about having a family member with an eating disorder. They will acknowledge the needs of both the client and the family unit. They will identify useful strategies for coping with the impact of bulimia nervosa on the family. They will use "I" statements during communication with one another, the client, and the nurse. They will verbalize an understanding of the developmental needs of family members. They will use more flexible problem-solving strategies. The family will reorganize family roles as necessary. They will identify community resources available to them and will follow through on referrals.

For additional information about the nursing process with clients with bulimia nervosa, see the Nursing Care Plan at the end of the chapter.

CASE MANAGEMENT, COMMUNITY-BASED CARE, AND HOME CARE

Community-based care, case management, and home care for clients with eating disorders were discussed earlier in this chapter. Refer to pages 471–472.

NURSING CARE PLAN: CLIENT WITH BULIMIA NERVOSA

Identifying Information

Lauren, a 28-year-old married woman, was admitted to the psychiatric unit from the emergency department where she was taken after collapsing during a marathon. She is a master's-prepared social worker who works in a drug abuse prevention program.

Lauren reports that she has been training for the marathon for about a year, running at least 35 miles a week. She believes that she had to be hospitalized because she did not ingest sufficient carbohydrates and fluids before the race.

Lauren states that she has been binge eating and purging for about 3 years, ever since she read about ballet dancers' and gymnasts' use of purging for weight control. On a typical day, she arises at 5:00 a.m., runs at least 5 miles, then gets ready for work. On the way to work, she buys and consumes a dozen doughnuts. She arrives at work before anyone else and vomits in the employees' bathroom. She eats no lunch unless she can be sure of access to a "good" bathroom, which she describes as one with a single toilet and an outside door that locks. In the evening while preparing dinner, she consumes a can of salted peanuts and four or five glasses of wine. She denies ever getting "high." After a large dinner she showers, vomiting while the

shower is running. Her husband of 4 years is unaware of her "problem" but worries about her drinking and wonders how she can eat so much and never gain weight.

History

No prior psychiatric history. Lauren is the oldest of three children and the only female. Her parents, both retired schoolteachers, live in a nearby town. She sees them infrequently because "they still treat me like I'm a little girl." She rarely sees her younger brothers and feels closer to her husband's family. There is no family history of eating disorders or substance abuse.

NURSING CARE PLAN: CLIENT WITH BULIMIA NERVOSA (*Continued*)

As the daughter of two schoolteachers, Lauren was expected to be the top student in her school. She had few friends because she was "the class geek." In college, she excelled academically but was a "social failure." She states that she can drink an entire bottle of wine, vomit, and "sober up instantly." She has few friends or interests except running. She describes her job as "not fulfilling."

Lauren has no significant health problems. Vital signs are: temperature, 98.2°F; pulse, 68; respirations, 14; height, 5′ 7″; weight, 110 lb; blood pressure, 108/68.

Current Mental Status
Lauren is slim, neatly groomed, and cooperative, but reluctant. She is alert and oriented to time, place, and person. Her judgment is good and her ability to think abstractly is unimpaired. She is articulate; her affect is appropriate to verbal content; she has no delusions, illusions, hallucinations, or other signs of thought disorder. She fidgets in her seat but makes good eye contact. She expresses embarrassment about hospitalization and shame about her behavior. She emphatically does not want her husband or office informed of the extent and details of her "problem." She maintains that she does not need to be hospitalized and can handle this herself.

Other Clinical Data
Lauren reports that she has not had a menstrual period in over 1 year. She takes no medications.

Nursing Diagnosis: Anxiety related to low self-esteem

Expected Outcome: Coping: Actions to manage stressors that tax an individual's resources
Impulse Control: Ability to self-restrain compulsive or impulsive behavior

---

Short-Term Goals	Interventions	Rationales
Lauren will identify at least three sources of anxiety.	■ Adopt a calm, reassuring attitude.	A calm approach conveys safety and confidence.
	■ Provide a quiet, nonstimulating environment.	Reducing stimuli minimizes Lauren's anxiety.
	■ Help Lauren recognize situations and events that create anxiety.	Lauren's self-awareness is enhanced.
	■ Encourage Lauren to identify previously used, successful coping behaviors.	Recognizing successful behaviors promotes self-esteem.
	■ Encourage Lauren to identify alternatives to alcohol abuse, binge eating, and purging in response to anxiety.	Lauren's coping skills are expanded.
	■ Limit overexercising.	Limits counteract unhealthy preoccupations.
	■ Negotiate a contract with Lauren to limit hoarding, vomiting, and other compulsive behaviors.	Contracts promote self-responsibility and self-control.
Lauren will demonstrate the use of relaxation techniques to manage anxiety.	■ Teach progressive relaxation techniques and meditation.	Relaxation techniques improve coping skills.
	■ Assist Lauren to use techniques when feeling tension that would formerly lead to binge eating and purging.	Techniques reinforce and support effective coping.

Nursing Diagnosis: Deficient Fluid Volume related to self-induced vomiting and excessive exercising

Expected Outcome: Electrolyte and Acid–Base Balance: Balance of electrolytes and nonelectrolytes in the intracellular and extracellular compartments of the body
Hydration: Amount of water in the intracellular and extracellular compartments of the body

---

Short-Term Goals	Interventions	Rationales
Lauren will drink a minimum of 2 oz of fluids per hour.	■ Teach Lauren the importance of adequate fluid intake.	This is information every client should know.
	■ Offer Lauren her favorite beverages frequently during the day.	Adequate fluid intake maintains hydration.
	■ Weigh Lauren daily to evaluate rehydration.	Hydration status is monitored.
	■ Keep accurate intake and output records.	

NURSING CARE PLAN: CLIENT WITH BULIMIA NERVOSA (*Continued*)

Short-Term Goals	Interventions	Rationales
	■ Assess skin turgor and condition of mucous membranes daily and record.	
	■ Encourage frequent mouth care to promote comfort.	Comfort measures promote adherence.
	■ Monitor laboratory values, reporting significant alterations to the physician.	Lab values provide information on electrolyte status.
Lauren will not vomit following meals.	■ Establish a no-purging contract with Lauren.	Contracts promote self-responsibility and self-control.
	■ Observe Lauren for at least 1 hour after meals to prevent purging.	Monitoring provides support and reinforcement.
	■ Give positive recognition when progress is shown.	Recognizing progress reinforces healthy behaviors.

Nursing Diagnosis: Ineffective Individual Coping related to feelings of helplessness and lack of control in life situation.

Expected Outcome: Coping: Actions to manage stressors that tax an individual's resources

Impulse Control: Ability to self-restrain compulsive or impulsive behavior.

Short-Term Goals	Interventions	Rationales
Lauren will eat regularly within 1 week.	■ Help Lauren establish a trust relationship with you.	Trust is the basis for a positive nurse–client relationship.
	■ Assist Lauren to plan for and practice dealing with daily demands.	Practice decreases helplessness, promotes self-responsibility and self-control.
	■ Assist Lauren to identify events preceding binge/purge episodes.	Self-awareness is an important step toward self-control.
	■ Encourage Lauren to identify ways of nurturing herself without using food or alcohol.	Concepts of choice, self-determination, and self-control are validated for Lauren.
Lauren will refrain from discussing body image dissatisfactions within 1 week.	■ Engage Lauren in a process of identifying, naming, and expressing negative feelings.	Expressing negative feelings in a responsible manner promotes self-control.
	■ Assist Lauren to identify and practice alternative ways of expressing negative feelings.	Exploring alternative means of expression increases coping skill, improves impulse control, and decreases helplessness.

Pearson Nursing Student Resources

Find additional review materials at
nursing.pearsonhighered.com

Prepare for success with NCLEX®-style practice questions, interactive assignments and activities, web links, animations and videos, and more!

REFERENCES

Allen, K. L., Fursland, A., Watson, H., & Byrne, S. M. (2011). Eating disorder diagnosis in general practice settings: Comparison with structured clinical interview and self-report questionnaires. *Journal of Mental Health, 20*(3), 270–280.

Bruch, H. (1978). *The golden cage: The enigma of anorexia nervosa.* Cambridge, MA: Harvard University Press.

Goodwin, H., Haycraft, E., Taranis, L., & Meyer, C. (2011). Psychometric evaluation of the compulsive exercise test (CET) in an adolescent population: Links with eating psychopathology. *European Eating Disorders Review, 19*(3), 269–279.

Jenkins, J., & Ogden, J. (2011). Becoming "whole" again: A qualitative study of women's views of recovering from anorexia nervosa. *European Eating Disorders Review*. Advance online publication. doi: 10.1002/erv.1085

Kim, Y. R., Lim, S. J., & Treasure, J. (2011). Different patterns of emotional eating and visuospatial deficits whereas shared risk factors related with social support between anorexia nervosa and bulimia nervosa. *Psychiatry Investigation, 8*(1), 9–14.

Love, C. C., & Seaton, H. (1991). Eating disorders: Highlights of nursing assessment and therapeutics. *Nursing Clinics of North America, 26*(3), 687.

Neri, M., Bello, S., Bonsignore, A., Cantatore, S., Riezzo, I., Turillazzi, E., & Fineschi, V. (2011). Anabolic androgenic steroids abuse and liver toxicity. *Mini Reviews in Medicinal Chemistry, 11*(5), 430–437.

Rivas, T., Bersabé, R., Jiméne, M., & Berrocal, C. (2010). The Eating Attitudes Test (EAT-26): Reliability and validity in Spanish female samples. *The Spanish Journal of Psychology, 13*(2), 1044–1056.

Seal, N. (2011). Introduction to genetics and childhood obesity: Relevance to nursing practice. *Biological Research for Nursing, 13*(1), 61–69.

Slane, J. D., Burt, S. A., & Klump, K. L. (2010). Genetic and environmental influences on disordered eating and depressive symptoms. *International Journal of Eating Disorders*. Advance online publication. doi: 10.1002/eat.20867

Smeets, E., Jansen, A., & Roefs, A. (2011). Bias for the (un)attractive self: On the role of attention in causing body (dis)satisfaction. *Health Psychology, 30*(3), 360–367.

Swanson, S. A., Crow, S. J., LeGrange, D., Swendsen, J., & Merikangas, K. R. (2011). Prevalence and correlates of eating disorders in adolescents: Results from the National Comorbidity Survey Replication Adolescent Supplement. *Archives of General Psychiatry, 68*(7), 714–723.

Thornton, L. M., Dellava, J. E., Root, T. L., Lichtenstein, P., & Bulik, C. M. (2011). Anorexia nervosa and generalized anxiety disorder: Further explorations of the relation between anxiety and body mass index. *Journal of Anxiety Disorders, 25*(5), 727–730.

White, J. H., & Litovitz, G. (1998). A comparison of inpatient and outpatient women with eating disorders. *Archives of Psychiatric Nursing, 12*(4), 181–194.

Wilfley, D. E., Kolko, R. P., & Kass, E. A. (2011). Cognitive-behavioral therapy for weight management and eating disorders in children and adolescents. *Child and Adolescent Psychiatry Clinics of North America, 20*(2), 271–285.

Wilfley, D. E., Vannucci, A., & White, E. K. (2010). Early intervention of eating- and weight-related problems. *Journal of Clinical Psychology in Medical Settings, 17*(4), 258–300.

22

Personality Disorders

SUE C. DELAUNE

LEARNING OUTCOMES

After completing this chapter, you will be able to:

1. Differentiate personality traits and styles from personality disorders.
2. Identify the characteristics common to all three clusters of personality disorders.
3. Compare the biopsychosocial characteristics of various personality disorders.
4. Identify the developmental and psychobiologic characteristics that distinguish Odd–Eccentric (Cluster A), Dramatic–Emotional (Cluster B), and Anxious–Fearful (Cluster C) personality disorders from one another.
5. Explain the concepts that enable the psychiatric–mental health nurse to apply the nursing process to the care of clients with personality disorders.
6. Manage the triad of manipulation, narcissism, and impulsiveness when demonstrated by clients with personality disorders.
7. Focus nursing intervention on a client's specific and unique response to the personality disorder.
8. Modify the possible effects of the nurse's positive and negative emotional responses to clients who have personality disorders.

CRITICAL THINKING CHALLENGE

A client requests that you, a newly employed nurse on a crisis inpatient unit, bend the rules for her by extending her therapeutic leave for 2 hours so that she may meet her boyfriend for dinner. When discussing this request with the client, you remind her that decisions about therapeutic leaves are made by the entire treatment team. The client then becomes angry and accuses you of "not being the caring nurse I thought you were." The client states that she will remember this incident and warn her friends about the uncaring nurses at this facility.

1. What would be wrong with bending the rules a little?
2. Should nurses be flexible and autonomous enough not to require approval from the treatment team? Why, or why not?
3. What purpose could the client's accusations serve?
4. How would you handle this situation with the client? What is your rationale?

At times, every individual demonstrates behavior that challenges others. However, working with clients who consistently demonstrate impatient, manipulative, self-centered, or overly suspicious behaviors can be especially challenging. This chapter is designed specifically to help you deal with these difficult behaviors and also asks you to evaluate your responses to interpersonally difficult clients. If you did not familiarize yourself with Chapters 3 and 4 before you began your clinical work in psychiatric–mental health nursing, make sure you do so before you begin this chapter. Chapter 3 emphasizes the need for the nurse's self-awareness and personal integration and Chapter 4∞ emphasizes the therapeutic nurse–client relationship.

What distinguishes an individual is called **personality**, which is defined as the individual qualities, including habitual behavior patterns, that make a person unique. **Personality traits** are persistent behavioral patterns. Even though the behaviors may be annoying or frustrating to others, they do not significantly interfere with the person's life. Both personality and personality traits tend to be stable over time. On the other hand, a **personality disorder (PD)** is a rigid, stereotyped behavioral pattern that deviates markedly from the norm of an individual's culture and persists throughout the person's life. A PD is a lifelong maladaptive pattern of perceiving, thinking, and relating that impairs social or occupational functioning and can be traced back to adolescence or early adulthood.

Individuals with PDs have unique ways of perceiving themselves, other people, and the events in their lives. The range, intensity, and appropriateness of their emotional responses are often exaggerated and their relationships are usually characterized by superficiality. These individuals lack insight; that is, they have no understanding of the impact of their behavior. They fail to accept the consequences of their own behavior and, when feeling threatened, attempt to ease the stress by changing the environment rather than changing their own behavior. You can read about three examples of very different personality disorders in Mental Health in the Movies.

This chapter discusses the various types of PDs and the major characteristics of each. Note that the goal of therapeutic approaches is not to restructure the client's basic personality, which is likely to be an impossible task. Instead, interventions are implemented to help those with PDs learn to deal with others in more productive, less stressful ways.

PERSONALITY DISORDERS

There are three major categories of PDs, called *clusters* by the American Psychiatric Association (APA). Each cluster is discussed separately in this section. Even though there are some differences among the three clusters, the following three traits are common to people with all types of PDs:

- Lack of insight—Individuals lack understanding of the impact of their behavior on others.
- External response to stress—When feeling threatened, individuals try to change the environment instead of changing themselves.
- Failure to accept the consequences of their own behavior—They do not view their lifestyles as abnormal and tend to project blame onto others for their own actions.

The essential characteristics of personality disorders are chronicity, pervasiveness, and maladaptation. The individual with a PD often goes through life repeating the same dysfunctional pattern. The PD affects every dimension of life and seriously impairs interpersonal and functional abilities.

Other problematic behaviors that are characteristic of people with PDs include manipulation, narcissism, and impulsiveness. **Manipulation** is control behavior; the manipulative individual uses and exploits others for personal gain. **Narcissism** is self-centered behavior in which the individual feels entitled to special favors due to a mistaken perception of oneself as the "center of the universe." **Impulsiveness** describes the actions of those who act without considering the consequences of their behavior.

MENTAL HEALTH IN THE MOVIES
Girl Interrupted

This film highlights the experiences of three young women with personality disorders, hospitalized on a psychiatric unit. The story is told from the frame of reference of Susanna (Winona Ryder) who was admitted to a psychiatric hospital (where she lived for 18 months) after a suicide attempt. Susanna has a diagnosis of borderline personality disorder. In addition to having attempted suicide, she self-mutilates, and engages in impulsive sexual behavior. She experiences depersonalization several times, and on one occasion bites open the flesh on her hand because she is terrified that she has lost her bones. Although she pushes others away, she is the one who feels abandoned and has low self-esteem.

Lisa (Angelina Jolie) has antisocial personality disorder, and takes pleasure in ordering the other clients around. She preys on the others, breaks down their self-esteem, and uses their disorders against them. Lisa argues and fights with the staff on a daily basis and is frequently taken to the isolation room, kicking and screaming. Lisa has no qualms about hurting herself or others. In fact, she often finds those activities pleasurable, showing no remorse for her actions.

Daisy has obsessive–compulsive personality disorder. Her focus on orderliness and control is seen most clearly in the way in which she handles food. Her social life and daily routine is hindered by her inability to eat in front of others. Eating involves several rituals—peeling chicken off the bone in a certain order, laying the bones out in an orderly fashion, and saving the carcasses. She counts chicken bones and carcasses over and over. Daisy is aware of her obsessional thoughts and her unusual behavior and hides the chicken carcasses so no one will see them.

The personality disorders displayed by the characters in the film are classic and severe enough to warrant hospitalization, not the usual circumstance for people with personality disorders.

Photo courtesy © Columbia/courtesy of Everett Collection.

Essential features of these disorders include significant distress or impairment in at least two of the following areas of functioning:

- Cognition
- Affect
- Interpersonal relationships
- Impulse control

These behavior patterns must be evident by early adulthood and not be a result of other mental disorders or substance abuse (APA, 2000). It is important to distinguish the behaviors that define personality disorders from responses that may emerge as a result of specific situational stressors or transient mental states. Therefore, it is often necessary and important to conduct more than one interview with the client over a period of time. While personality-disordered people display enduring, inflexible, and pervasive maladaptive behaviors in a broad variety of personal, occupational, and social situations, they may not view their lifestyles as abnormal. Typically, they do not seek professional help unless they are extremely anxious.

Although personality disorders are coded on Axis II (see Chapter 11∞ for a description of the axes) of the Diagnostic and Statistical Manual of Mental Disorders (DSM) they may coexist with (be comorbid with) severe psychopathology such as the disorders included in Axis I groupings. In addition, when under stress, the individual with a personality disorder may progressively deteriorate even to the point of psychosis.

Cluster A Personality Disorders: Odd–Eccentric

Cluster A consists of the paranoid, schizoid, and schizotypal personality disorders. They are briefly described in DSM Essential Features. The major features of these disorders are pervasive distrust, social detachment, and subsequent impairment in social and occupational functioning. People with odd–eccentric personality disorders have the most cognitive impairments as well as the most peculiar behaviors and maladaptive defensive styles of all personality-disordered people.

Paranoid Personality Disorder

Clients with **paranoid personality disorder** engage in a pattern of pervasive mistrust of others, interpreting the motives of others as malevolent. They often report that others plot against them or attempt to use or deceive them. They talk about disloyal friends and coworkers and the irreversible harm others' actions have caused. They may be surprised but mistrustful of loyalty shown to them and often refuse to answer questions, saying, "That is no one's business." A frequent theme of clients with a paranoid personality disorder is pathologic suspicion of spousal or partner infidelity. Unrealistic grandiose fantasies often emerge, and clients may discuss activities with others who share their beliefs, such as special interest groups or cults. Client affect may be labile, with hostile, stubborn sarcasm being predominant. Remember that the axiom, "all behavior has meaning," is applicable to individuals with paranoid personality disorder. As the person's fear and anxiety increase, so does their inability to relate well to others.

Suspiciousness and Mistrust Suspiciousness and mistrust reflect an attitude of doubt toward the trustworthiness of objects or people. Suspiciousness is also a way of thinking and includes such manifestations as expectations of trickery or harm, guardedness, secretiveness, pathologic jealousy, and overconcern with hidden motives and special meanings. For example, the suspicious person may perceive a birthday gift as a trick to create an obligation. Legal disputes may arise from the client's response to perceived threats. Note the outcome of having paranoid feelings and behaviors in the following clinical example.

Clinical Example

Jim, a 39-year-old engineer, suspects that his employer is withholding significant data from him pertaining to an important job assignment. Jim began to question others about the reliability and integrity of his boss. He went to the plant one Sunday morning without authorization. A security guard found him going through the filing cabinets of his employer, who confronted him the following day and sent him to the employee assistance program nurse. During the interview, Jim states, "I knew my boss was dishonest from the start. He never could give me a straight answer. As soon as I was almost on him, he sets me up to lose face and maybe my job."

Rigidity People with paranoid personality disorder are inflexible in their perception of the world. They are preoccupied with their expectations of others and relentlessly try to confirm these expectations, often through argumentation. They closely examine information with prejudice. The person with paranoid personality disorder justifies a position by excessive rationalization, rejecting any evidence that refutes the

DSM ESSENTIAL FEATURES

Cluster A Personality Disorders: Odd–Eccentric

Paranoid Personality Disorder: Pervasive distrust and suspiciousness of others: suspecting that others are exploiting, harming, or deceiving him/her; doubting loyalty of others; reluctant to confide in others; reading hidden meanings into remarks; holding grudges; anger reactions.

Schizoid Personality Disorder: Pervasive pattern of detachment from social relationships; restricted range of emotions; engaging in solitary activities; lacks close friends; lacks enjoyment of activities; seems indifferent to praise or criticism; emotionally cold or indifferent with flat affect.

Schizotypal Personality Disorder: Acute discomfort with and reduced capacity for close relationships; cognitive or perceptual distortions. May experience ideas of reference, magical thinking, illusions, and odd patterns of speech and behavior; excessive social anxiety.

distorted thought, and goes to great lengths to prove a point. It is not unusual for a paranoid person to be suspicious of people with opposing ideas. The need to be in control is another characteristic, as is a preoccupation with rank and status. The need to be self-sufficient often results in difficulty working with others. The rigidity in thinking patterns reinforces the individual's need to always be "right."

Hypervigilance An increased state of watchfulness in which the person is always on guard and unable to relax is called **hypervigilance**. There is constant sensitivity to nuances, interpretation of both open and hidden attitudes of others, and scrutiny of others and the environment. As a result, interpersonal relationships are greatly impaired and the person becomes socially isolated.

Distortions of Reality Although paranoid people perceive facts accurately, they may attribute a special significance to events. In this way, they create a private reality. Individuals with paranoid personality disorder have excessive interest in hidden motives, underlying purposes, and special meanings. They do not necessarily disagree with the average observer about the existence of any given fact, only about its significance. Therefore, even severely paranoid people can recognize various essential facts well enough to achieve a limited adjustment to the normal social world. But they often have difficulty distinguishing real from imagined offenses. Their distorted attitudes antagonize others and may lead to real discrimination, as demonstrated in the clinical example that follows.

Clinical Example

Ellen is quick to detect signs of anger, jealousy, and rejection in the actions of her coworkers. She magnifies these negative aspects and overlooks such positive behaviors as humor, support, and empathy. Eventually, Ellen's coworkers begin to snicker when she makes public statements, and they gossip about her.

Projection People who are paranoid attribute their own ego-alien (intolerable) motivations, drives, or feelings to others. Projection is used to attribute to others the harmful intentions that they themselves feel. In this way, the idea that one may be harmed really reflects one's own wish to harm others. Projection and other mental mechanisms (defense mechanisms) are discussed in Chapter 8∞.

Restricted Affect Labile emotional expressiveness and a lack of spontaneity characterize people with paranoid personality disorder. They often appear cold, humorless, and devoid of tender, sensitive feelings. Although they may demonstrate temper outbursts, they pride themselves on remaining objective and reasonable and frequently use intellectualization and rationalization to avoid affective experiences. Some paranoid people may appear friendly, but in fact this friendliness is a "script" that helps them adapt to social situations or achieve their goals.

Alienation Because of the paranoid person's antagonism and suspiciousness, tension develops between the person and significant others. The persistent strain on relationships causes others to define the paranoid person as more than simply "different." Instead, they see the individual as unreliable or untrustworthy, and then begin to interact according to their perceptions. These behaviors reinforce the suspicions and irrational beliefs of the paranoid person. The effects of this process include the following:

- Blocked communication, which increases the process of alienation
- Reinforcement of the paranoid person's beliefs, interpretations, or ideas of reference

Because paranoid people are generally intelligent, persuasive, and creative in justifying their beliefs, they often try to adapt by one of two ways. They may join fringe political groups, esoteric religions, cults, or quasiscientific organizations that reinforce their interpretations of reality. Or they may join organizations that challenge societal norms and trends in an effort to direct and thus control hostile feelings.

You may encounter clients with paranoid personality disorder in any health care setting. Important information for nurses in emergency departments, where clients are under great stress and their usual coping abilities are taxed, is discussed in What Every Nurse Should Know.

Schizoid Personality Disorder

People with **schizoid personality disorder** generally have a detached and aloof social style and display a range of adjustment. Some are fairly well-adjusted individuals who

---

WHAT EVERY NURSE SHOULD KNOW

Client With Paranoid Personality Disorder

Imagine that you are a nurse who works in an emergency department. The coping abilities of clients are taxed when they are in an emergency department. If you observe that a client may have signs of paranoia (e.g., hypersensitivity, guarding, suspiciousness) incorporate the following suggestions in your dealings with the client:

- Avoid personalizing the client's remarks.
- Approach the client with a calm, quiet demeanor in order to increase the client's sense of security.
- Avoid laughing or whispering within the client's line of vision.
- Explain the parameters of confidentiality to the client.
- Maintain reasonable safety precautions at all times when dealing with this client, depending on the extent of the client's paranoia (e.g., if the client is highly paranoid, face the client at all times rather than turning your back on the client; avoid being cornered by ensuring that you have an available exit).
- Call for security immediately if the client's behavior shows signs of escalation.

are loners; others live out their lives in protective environments, such as group homes, mental hospitals, and prisons.

Schizoid personality disorder is found in about 3% of the population (APA, 2000). Individuals who are diagnosed with schizoid personality disorder are rarely seen in clinical settings, but when they are it is usually for treatment of symptoms associated with anxiety, depression, or dysphoric affect. They may experience transient psychotic episodes that last from a few minutes to several hours.

Individuals with schizoid personality disorder show a preference for solitary interests—they claim to enjoy being alone—and occupations that require minimal social interaction. They tend to choose solitary hobbies such as solitaire and computer games, and jobs such as night security guard or bridge tender. They may decline job promotions because social demands (meetings, supervisory responsibilities) accompany the promotion. When questioned about sexual activity, clients with schizoid PD usually deny interest or involvement in intimate relationships. They may appear cool, aloof, or bored, and may seem to be cognitively impaired. When asked if they think their loner-type behavior is unusual, a typical response is, "I never thought about it much . . . it doesn't much matter to me." Schizoid clients acknowledge that they rarely become excited, angry, upset, or joyful. Indifference and humorlessness are hallmarks of the individual with schizoid personality disorder. It is important to be culturally sensitive when working with clients who exhibit odd–eccentric behaviors; see Developing Cultural Competence.

Schizotypal Personality Disorder

Suspicion, including paranoid ideation, is usually noted in the schizotypal client. Maintaining eye contact may be difficult, and communication strategies such as humor to defuse anxiety may be met with a stare and questions about the meaning or purpose of the joking. Be careful about using humor with mentally disordered people. Their interpretation of humor or joking will not always match yours.

Clients with **schizotypal personality disorder** report a great deal of subjective anxiety in social situations, have cognitive or perceptual distortions, and display eccentric behavior. They often report bizarre fantasies, especially of paranormal events. During an interview, they may remark, "I know what you're going to ask me before you say it," believing they are endowed with special powers or have the ability to control others' behavior by simply "willing it to happen." Often, these clients have speech patterns that are so loose, digressive, or vague that an interview is difficult to conduct. The client may acknowledge this behavior by stating, "I was never talkative" (APA, 2000). Clients with schizotypal PD appear absentminded; they daydream, are vague about goals, are indecisive, and lack social skills. Often, they act as if they are in a fog. They fail to respond in the usual manner to social cues and seem like social misfits.

The schizotypal personality-disordered client demonstrates eccentricities in communication and behavior not seen in a person with schizoid personality. Examples include such oddities of thought as magical thinking and ideas of reference;

DEVELOPING CULTURAL COMPETENCE

Assessing Clients With Schizoid and Schizotypal Personalities

Culture determines the meaning of behavior. When assessing both schizoid and schizotypal clients, it is imperative to consider the person's ethnicity, cultural milieu, and spiritual belief system. Within many cultures, speaking in tongues and psychic phenomena are natural experiences and you should not deem them pathologic. People who are making a transition from one environment to another—from a rural to an urban setting, for instance—may seem different because of their constricted affect and solitary activities. You must assess immigrants from a multicultural viewpoint in order to differentiate between lack of understanding and indifference. What may seem odd in Parker, Georgia, may be commonplace in New York City.

CRITICAL THINKING QUESTIONS

1. When would such experiences as speaking in tongues or being guided by a guardian angel be considered cultural and not psychopathological?
2. What does it indicate if a client from an Asian culture such as China does not ask questions when you offer the opportunity?

altered perceptions, such as illusions, **depersonalization** (a feeling of strangeness or unreality about the self), and **derealization** (a feeling of disconnection from the environment); speech alterations, including circumstantiality (giving detailed, factual but nonessential information), digression, metaphoric speech patterns, and overly concrete or abstract responses; and an odd or unkempt manner of dress, which includes ill-fitting, stained, and mismatched clothing.

Individuals with schizotypal personality disorder have a history of being loners and neither desire nor enjoy close relationships. They are indifferent to feedback and insensitive to others. The detachment from social relationships is also noted in the client's lack of interest in having intimate or sexual relationships.

Onset of schizotypal PD is believed to be in childhood or early adolescence. Clients report poor academic achievement and poor peer relationships as well as social anxiety, even as children. Schizotypal personality disorder is strongly associated with adverse childhood experiences (Lentz, Robinson, & Bolton, 2011). Clients with schizotypal personality disorders may experience psychotic episodes of very short duration, lasting from a few minutes to several hours (APA, 2000).

Cluster B Personality Disorders: Dramatic–Emotional

People with borderline, histrionic, narcissistic, and antisocial personality disorders can be characterized as dramatic, emotional, and erratic. Individuals with these disorders are often in conflict with society because of their impulsive behavior. Impulsive people view the world as a discontinuous, fragmented collection of opportunities, frustrations, and affective experiences. They live only in the present moment and, therefore, lack the ability to formulate long-range plans. They

DSM ESSENTIAL FEATURES

Cluster B Personality Disorders: Dramatic–Emotional

Borderline Personality Disorder: Characterized by unstable relationships, affect, and self-image; intense fear of abandonment; identity disturbance; impulsivity; chronic feelings of emptiness; intense anger and/or rage.

Histrionic Personality Disorder: Pattern of attention-seeking and excessive emotionality; a need to be the center of attention; uses physical appearance and provocative behavior to draw attention to self; exaggerated expression; easily suggestive.

Narcissistic Personality Disorder: A pervasive pattern of grandiosity (in fantasy or behavior), need for admiration, and lack of

empathy. Characterized by a grandiose sense of self-importance and a belief that one is "special"; preoccupied with fantasies of success, power, and brilliance; a strong sense of entitlement and a need for admiration. Exploits others, is envious, and lacks empathy.

Antisocial Personality Disorder: Pervasive pattern of disregard for and violation of others' rights. Characterized by deceitfulness, impulsivity, irresponsibility, and aggressiveness. Shows reckless disregard for safety of self and others.

---

act without critical evaluation of consequences. The focus of their intellectual and emotional goals is to achieve immediate satisfaction. This lack of impulse control and inability to delay gratification often result in both verbal and nonverbal outbursts of anger, which may be self-directed or other directed. Indeed, clients with dramatic–emotional personality disorders may experience rapid escalation of anxiety when their own angry impulses are not controlled by others. As interpersonal difficulties increase, they often resort to manipulation and acting out as ways to get their needs met. See DSM Essential Features for cluster B personality disorders.

Borderline Personality Disorder

Individuals with **borderline personality disorder (BPD)** have unstable interpersonal relationships, self-image, and affect, and are impulsive. It is common for such clients to experience psychotic breaks from reality whenever they experience severe stress. Prevalence of this disorder is about 2% (APA, 2000).

Approximately 50% of individuals with BPD also have other coexisting mental disorders, such as major depression, bipolar disorder, eating disorders, and substance abuse (National Alliance on Mental Illness [NAMI], 2011). Research indicates that the risk is high for substance abuse disorders in people affected by BPD (Walter et al., 2009). Many individuals with BPD have experienced traumatic events during childhood. There is a strong relationship between a history of childhood physical and/or sexual abuse and the development of BPD (Kim, Cicchetti, Rogosch, & Manly, 2009). Emotional pain as a result of childhood abuse is prevalent among individuals with BPD (Holm, Begat, & Severinsson, 2009). The more trauma experienced by the child, the more likely the child becomes fearful. This fear may then manifest as symptoms of BPD in adulthood.

Individuals with BPD may also have coexisting physical problems. According to a contemporary study (El-Gabalawy, Katz, & Sareen, 2010), individuals with BPD have a high incidence of arteriosclerosis with resultant hypertension, hepatic disease, gastrointestinal disease, venereal disease, and arthritis. Medical–surgical nurses may meet them as clients in general hospital settings. Helpful guidelines are given in What Every Nurse Should Know.

Impulsivity Impulsivity may be expressed in many ways, including self-damaging acts, lack of responsibility, and disregard for the consequences of one's behavior. The responses of individuals with BPD fluctuate in situations that are subjectively interpreted and often distorted. Impulsivity is reinforced by the borderline personality-disordered individual's inability to learn from past experiences. Impulsiveness is manifested in spending habits, sexual promiscuity, abnormal eating habits, shoplifting, frequent job changes, and substance abuse. Responses such as "I don't know why I did it, I just did" are common when clients are questioned about the reasons for particular actions. "I just told my boss to take this job and shove it" may be the response to a work situation that is perceived as intolerable. "I just got another credit card with a $5,000 limit, so I don't have to worry about going over the limit on my other three cards." "I only drink wine when I'm driving, so I don't worry about DUIs." "I don't worry about

WHAT EVERY NURSE SHOULD KNOW

Client With Borderline Personality Disorder

Imagine that you are a nurse working in a medical-surgical setting, and you meet a client with symptoms of BPD. Take note of the following:

- When a client constantly makes demands, look for the underlying meaning (e.g., does the client really want more water or is it a bid for your attention?).
- Assess the client's anxiety level; expect that the demands will increase as anxiety escalates.
- Teach the client relaxation techniques and encourage their use as soon as you notice an increase in anxiety level.
- Provide attention to the client when appropriate behaviors are exhibited in order to avoid reinforcing the unacceptable behaviors.
- Be sure to communicate often with coworkers about the client in order to reduce the possibility of manipulation.

AIDS; all my partners come from high-rent districts, so they are clean and safe."

Intense Anger Clients with BPD tend to instigate problems as they become involved in therapeutic relationships. The anger may manifest itself in accusations, frequent displays of temper, inability to control anger (acting out), irritability, sarcasm, argumentativeness, devaluing others, and over-reaction to minor irritants. Such behaviors usually sabotage their treatment.

These clients are unable to tolerate their own "bad" image and, therefore, project it onto others, often raging at the perceived attributes of the other. Anger tends to be greatest toward those people who remind them of a nurturing/frustrating parent, as shown in the following clinical example.

Clinical Example

During a community meeting on an inpatient unit, Raul, a 34-year-old client, states, "I can't stand that fat slob of a nurse. She acts like God went on vacation and appointed her to substitute for Him." When confronted by the group leader, Raul responds, "So what if I yell when I get angry? I'm paying a lot of money to be here. If you don't like it, leave."

Identity Diffusion Erikson (1964) coined the term **identity diffusion** to describe the failure to integrate various childhood identifications into a harmonious adult psychosocial identity. Clients with BPD display behaviors that show confusion about values and goals in life. These clients are described as chameleon-like because they are constantly changing their behavior to match the behavior of those around them. An intense fear of rejection causes borderline individuals to say what they think others want to hear and to behave in a manner that they believe will win them popularity or special favors. It is difficult to determine what borderline individuals really think or feel. They cannot genuinely experience feelings and emotions; their core personality is hollow. They do not assume responsibility for their actions but project blame and credit onto others.

Problems of identity diffusion are also apparent in the areas of sexual intimacy and gender identity. Sexual intimacy is disturbed as a result of the person's fears of being either engulfed and destroyed, or else abandoned by another. An approach–avoidance conflict emerges as a consequence of the parent or caretaker having thwarted independence and rewarded dependent behavior. As a result, the borderline client develops two major fears: the fear of abandonment, which leads to clinging behavior, and fear of engulfment, which leads to distancing from others. The client desperately wants intimate relationships but is terrified of losing the self. These fears are reminiscent of the early choice between the parent's love and one's own autonomy, which is the core of the borderline conflict. This conflict is managed by using the primitive dissociation defense, also called **splitting**, which can best be described as the inability to integrate contradictory experiences. Splitting is based on dichotomous thinking, a cognitive distortion in which

the person has an "all-or-none" mentality about others; people are viewed as either all "good" or all "bad."

Gender identity disturbance may be manifested by the selection of rejecting or abusive partners, the preference for homosexual relationships while maintaining a heterosexual lifestyle, and bizarre fantasies.

Another area of identity diffusion is temporal discontinuity, which is manifested by a searching for one's origins or keeping detailed chronologic journals. Borderline individuals seem unable to integrate past, present, and future into a continuum. They may frantically plan for the future while reminiscing about past events. These behaviors often lead to difficulty in choosing long-term goals, making career choices, and reassessing personal values. "I can't make up my mind if I should stay in nursing or try interior design" (after completing 1 year in a 2-year nursing program).

Unstable Interpersonal Relationships Clients relate stories of "one-night stands" in search of the perfect partner. Any real or perceived threat of abandonment results in the client's "switching" to another partner. "He's never there when I need him" may be used in conjunction with "I always see to it that his shirts are ironed and his dinner is ready when he gets home from work." These clients need a payback in return for any giving they do. The failure to resolve the separation–individuation process described by Mahler, Pine, and Bergman (1975) in their classic work is reflected in the person's attitudes toward self and others.

Interpersonal relationships of individuals with BPD may include such behaviors as the following:

■ Manipulation of others
■ Pitting individuals against one another

- Intense attachment
- Explosive separations
- Sudden shifts in attitude toward others perceived as good or bad
- Clinging, demanding
- Controlling, exploiting
- Sadism or masochism in close relationships
- Relationships motivated by a need to avoid being alone rather than a need to be with others
- Lack of empathy
- Diminished capacity to evaluate others realistically
- Transient, superficial relationships

Affective Instability The failure to resolve the issues described previously is also related to the inability of the person with BPD to maintain a consistent, satisfying, affective state. Characteristics of this disorder include intense fluctuations of mood, normally of short duration (a few hours or a few days); intense, discrete episodes of depression with accompanying suicidal ideation and gestures; and hypomanic or elated episodes. "Of course I knew I wouldn't kill myself when I took those pills—do you think I'm stupid or something?" "I only told him [partner] I was HIV positive to see if he really cared for me as much as he said."

Feelings of Emptiness and Aloneness Individuals with borderline personality disorder report hollow, empty feelings, lack of peaceful solitude, a sense of being disconnected, and anhedonia (absence of pleasure in performing ordinarily pleasurable acts). The person may attempt to combat these feelings by compulsive eating, drinking, drug abuse, sexual encounters, and self-mutilation. "I get depressed and I think about taking some pills, but then my boyfriend calls and we'll go out and I won't be depressed anymore," or, "I feel so totally empty inside. I burned my wrist with the cigarette just to see if I could still feel."

Self-Mutilation Impulsiveness, together with identity disturbances, often leads to self-destructive behaviors (also called *self-mutilation*). People with BPD are often depressed, but they may make self-destructive gestures in an attempt to affirm their reality and relieve tension rather than to express a wish to die. People who have experienced early childhood neglect, abuse, or trauma frequently have difficulty understanding how to process feelings verbally and how to solve problems effectively. Many of these individuals will mutilate themselves to deal with anxiety and distress; see the clinical example of Katy's self-mutilating behavior.

Clinical Example

Katy, 29 years old, has had trouble adjusting and being a part of things since "as far back as I can remember." She has no idea how to effectively manage her life problems and her increasing levels of stress. She often cuts her abdomen or her arms. Katy is quick to point out that this is in no way a plan to kill herself. Instead, she finds it helps relieve tension and changes her perspective.

FIGURE 22-1 ■ Cutting is a frequently used self-mutilating behavior. Self-mutilating acts should alert you to the need for suicide risk assessment.
Photo courtesy of Leila Cutler/Alamy.

The exact reason for self-mutilating behavior is unknown, although there is much speculation about it. Several interpretations of the behavior are possible. For example, it may help people cope with a crisis, or deny mental pain, or cope with emotional pain, thus avoiding depression. Self-mutilating behavior may also result from impulsivity whereby people are unable or unwilling to consider the long-term effects of their behavior. Another possible explanation is that the behavior is a coping mechanism that raises low self-esteem by counteracting helplessness. A self-punishing act often relieves unconscious guilt.

Remember that the majority of people who demonstrate self-mutilation do not intend to end their lives; instead, the self-damaging behavior is a way to help decrease emotional pain. Self-damaging behaviors such as those illustrated in FIGURE 22-1 ■ include self-mutilation (cigarette burns, cutting, taking drug overdoses), recurring accidents, and physical fights. Williams and Bydalek (2009) identify the following as risk factors for self-mutilation: female gender, adolescent age, history of being abused, living in a violent environment, poor self-esteem, inadequate impulse control, anger, and disappointment with self.

Distortions of Reality When identity diffusion reaches panic proportions, the borderline individual may experience both depersonalization and derealization.

Histrionic Personality Disorder

People with **histrionic personality disorder (HPD)** show a lifelong tendency for dramatic, egocentric, attention-seeking response patterns. Their seeming lack of sincerity and emotional commitment contributes to disturbances in interpersonal relationships. Individuals with HPD appear to be continually acting a role on stage. Their coping patterns are based on repression, denial, and dissociation. In the following clinical example, Linda exhibits many of the characteristic behaviors of histrionic personality disorder.

Clinical Example

Linda, a 33-year-old woman who is twice divorced, was observed at the outpatient clinic responding flirtatiously to male staff members. She was neatly groomed and seductively dressed in a low-cut peasant blouse, a tight miniskirt, and bright red knee-high boots. When called by the female therapist for her appointment, Linda screamed that the wait was too long and complained loudly about patients' rights to rapid treatment. She quickly captured the attention of others in the waiting room. Then Linda feigned dizziness and "fell" as she arose from her chair. During the ensuing session, Linda complained that several men had made passes at her on the bus. When the therapist failed to share her outrage, Linda accused her of being jealous. Linda terminated the interview at that point and left the office, slamming the door behind her and stating, "My problems are physical, and no one cares whether I live or die. You'll be sorry for treating me this way!"

As with other personality disorders, it is important to consider the client's cultural and ethnic background before assuming that the diagnosis of HPD is correct because norms for interpersonal behavior, dress and appearance, and emotional expression vary widely among cultures, genders (sex role stereotyping), and age groups. Approximately 2% of the general population is diagnosed with this disorder, which affects more females than males (NAMI, 2011).

Dramatic, Exhibitionistic, and Egocentric Responses The behaviors of individuals with HPD are characterized by exaggerated emotional expression. They demonstrate an excessive craving for attention, activity, and excitement. Often, these individuals behave frivolously, acting silly and making nuisances of themselves. When confronted with minor stressors, the individual with HPD overreacts with irrational emotional outbursts and temper tantrums.

Dysfunctional Interpersonal Relationships People with HPD constantly need love, reassurance, and validation of their existence because of their feelings of dependence and helplessness. For this reason, they have problems with significant relationships. They are likely to manipulate others in order to hold on to them while at the same time being highly inconsiderate and lacking in empathy.

Impaired Sexual Expression People with HPD are generally provocative and seductive and use sexual expression to manipulate and control others in relationships. Clients are often unaware of this flamboyance and how others perceive it. They are often competitive with those of the same sex and seductive with members of the opposite sex. A potential problem is promiscuous sexual activity and the risk of developing and spreading sexually transmitted infections. Disregard for the welfare and safety of others may be noted in sexual acting-out, including intimate relationships with others on the unit. When confronted, the client may say, "I've been talking to the social worker about the need for conjugal visits; maybe now you'll understand how important it is for us to get sex as well as therapy."

Dysphoric Mood Clients may express dysphoria as a sense of disquiet or restlessness. Histrionic clients may experience dysphoria when their demands for attention and affection are not met. They may act out in a suicidal fashion to manipulate or coerce others.

Cognitive Alterations Clients with HPD are much more interested in creative or imaginative pursuits than in analytic or academic achievements. They tend to be impressionable and highly suggestible and tend to look to authority figures for magical solutions to problems.

Impaired Health Patterns Regression and the development of somatic and/or dissociative symptoms are frequent among histrionic people. These disabling symptoms may serve the purpose of calling attention to themselves. Generally, the symptoms occur when an audience is present or when an unpleasant situation is anticipated. Substance use, depression, seizure-like activity, blackouts, falling, dizziness, or reactive psychoses may lead to hospitalization.

Narcissistic Personality Disorder

People with **narcissistic personality disorder (NPD)** engage in a pattern of grandiosity, have difficulty regulating self-esteem, and need admiration and attention from others. Their self-evaluation is dependent on admiration and devotion from others. The constant desire to be the center of attention is based on a strong sense of entitlement; narcissistic people feel they deserve to be treated in a special manner. When their need for constant attention is not met, the narcissistic person feels rejected and may retaliate through acting-out behavior. Characteristics most frequently observed include a sense of entitlement, lack of empathy, indifference toward others, and interpersonal manipulation, as described in the following clinical example.

Clinical Example

Michael and his spouse have frequent arguments about his sense of entitlement and his need to be at the center of the family's universe. Michael does not believe that his wife treats him the way he should be treated. He expects her to put his needs above her own, as well as the needs of their children. When Michael feels rejected, he shouts at family members, refuses to talk to them, or leaves the house after banging shut the door. After Michael refused to entertain the notion of family or couples counseling, his wife said she could not tolerate his behavior any longer and threatened to leave him. Michael's response was "You'll regret leaving me. You'll never find anyone else like me."

About 1% of the general population has NPD, and the incidence is increasing steadily. Of those diagnosed, 50% to 75% are male (APA, 2000). There may be a higher than usual risk in children of narcissistic parents who impart to them an unrealistic sense of omnipotence, grandiosity, beauty, and talent (Sadock & Sadock, 2010). Narcissistic traits are quite common (and developmentally appropriate) in adolescents and the majority of teens who exhibit narcissism do not necessarily develop NPD as adults (APA, 2000).

Grandiosity Grandiosity is evidenced by expressions of exaggerated self-importance, self-absorption, and egocentricity. This inflated self-concept may be a compensation for feelings of diminished self-worth. Isolating a child from the feedback of others and the parents' failing to mirror the child's behavior may contribute to the development of grandiosity.

Mirroring, or mirror images, reflects the parents' perception and treatment of the child. When coming in contact with people outside the home, the child may discover a discrepancy between treatment from others and the mirror images developed at home. Excessive boasting may result from the inconsistency in self-concept. Humility is not a characteristic of people with NPD, as shown in the following clinical example.

Clinical Example

Alicia is a 40-year-old teacher who seeks professional counseling after dropping out of a graduate program. When questioned about dropping out of graduate school, Alicia rationalizes her failure by blaming it on a "hostile major professor" and further proclaiming, "I know more than he does." She describes herself as the "leader" in her group of six graduate students and interprets this to mean that they have great respect for her.

Exhibitionism Exhibitionistic behavior is demonstrated by the constant seeking of support and admiration from others. Because of their limited interests, these clients boast about themselves to the point of boring others. Concern over declining physical attractiveness and occupational limitations often lead them to seek cosmetic surgery.

Labile Affective Response Despite the narcissistic individual's extensive use of rationalization for failures, there is an underlying sense of rage, shame, and diminished self-esteem. The perceptive nurse may observe cool indifference, emptiness, humiliation, uncontrolled anger, or desire for revenge. The following clinical example illustrates the lack of empathy typically experienced by people with NPD.

Clinical Example

Alicia tells the therapist that she attempted to call two friends following her withdrawal from school. She dramatically and self-righteously expresses anger and disappointment that they were not available to her. (One was vacationing out of state and the other was hospitalized for major surgery.) When the therapist inquired how her friend was doing following surgery, Alicia responded, "How in the world should I know? That's not my problem. She never even bothered to call me back."

Dysfunctional Interpersonal Relationships Clients with NPD feel entitled to special favors and attention. Further, they refuse to assume mutual responsibilities in relationships and tend to exploit and disregard the rights of others. They lack empathy, especially toward those whom they perceive to be of lower status. The following clinical example describes the characteristics of entitlement and exploitation.

Clinical Example

Alicia requests Saturday morning appointments (no office hours are normally scheduled on this day) because she becomes very tired in the afternoons and always takes a nap. When the therapist refuses to meet this request, Alicia becomes angry and shouts, "You're just like all the rest of them. No one considers my needs! I'll see to it that your supervisor hears about this, and I'll let all my friends know how incompetent you are as a therapist."

Impaired Sexual Expression Perverse sexual fantasies and promiscuity may be associated with NPD. There may be confusion regarding sex-role behavior. Sexual favors may be used as bartering tools with partners.

Antisocial Personality Disorder

Antisocial personality disorder (ASPD), a pattern of disregard for and violation of the rights of others, was one of the earliest personality disorders to be identified. It has been labeled *psychopathy, sociopathy, dyssocial disorder,* and *moral insanity.* Most people with ASPD do not seek medical help. Instead, they often come to the attention of authorities because of criminal activity that leads to judicial commitment to psychiatric facilities or incarceration in correctional facilities. In clinical settings, 3% to 30% of the population may have this disorder. Higher prevalence rates are found in substance abuse treatment centers and forensic settings (APA, 2000).

Manipulation, which is a hallmark of the antisocial client's behavior, can be a normal, nondestructive method of meeting one's needs. However, when used to control others, manipulation interferes with interpersonal relationships. In antisocial clients, the drive to manipulate others is paramount, because these clients feel a need to be "number one" at all times. Manipulation may be evident in the client's attempt to form alliances with the staff. Once alliances are formed, splitting among the staff occurs (playing one staff member against another; not to be confused with the term to describe the dissociative defense discussed on page 486) and the client is in control, as shown in the following clinical example.

Clinical Example

"You know, you are the only nurse on this unit who knows anything about the meds that we get. I always feel so safe when you are at the med station. You know when I really need my tranquilizers. The other nurses look at me suspiciously like I'm some kind of criminal. Thank goodness you're on duty tonight." This same client may tell the nurse on the following shift, "That night nurse does nothing but pass pills all night long; she never spends time with the patients or even tries to talk to them before she drugs them up. I think something should be done about her."

In your contacts with antisocial people, you may find them initially charming. They are often intellectually bright, conversationally glib, and they tell you what you want to hear. Because they are so astute in identifying others' vulnerabilities, nurses are frequently amazed at the "empathy" these clients show for others. These behaviors are manipulative and are used to create a situation that the person with ASPD can control.

During the initial assessment interview, it is common for the person diagnosed with ASPD to refuse responsibility for admission to the mental health or forensic facility. In fact, this individual will probably claim that the victim of his or her actions is at fault; in addition, no remorse will be shown, as in the following clinical example.

Clinical Example

Jason says to his arresting officers, "Well, you know, the only reason I'm here is because those cops made a mistake and thought I was the one who was assaulting that woman. Actually I stopped to help her and she told them I was trying to rape her. You know, if she hadn't parked her car in the mall garage, then she wouldn't have been at risk for an attack in the first place."

Impulsiveness is manifested in the client's making quick decisions without regard for the consequences. Aggression may be exhibited by instigating fights with other clients, often when the client feels a need for excitement or has not received sufficient attention from the staff. The client's explanation might be: "Hey, if you guys would get more sports going for us here, we wouldn't be getting on each other's nerves so much."

Lack of anxiety is notable with antisocial individuals, unless there is extreme external stress, in which case they may act out in ways that put them at high risk for accidents, physical injury, or suicidal acts. History of violence toward others is very common, including sex offenses (i.e., rape, child pornography, child molestation) and murder. These clients often have histories of drug dealing, prostitution, homelessness, erratic job histories, and exploitive sexual relationships. While these individuals can identify what is correct and appropriate behavior, they do not believe the rules apply to them.

People with ASPD need immediate gratification in most situations but can delay rewards to the extent that they need planning time to achieve what they want. They are often admitted to mental health facilities for depressive symptoms, suicidal attempts, substance abuse, somatic disorders, and/or anxiety disorders.

Cluster C Personality Disorders: Anxious–Fearful

Personality-disordered individuals who are primarily anxious or fearful may be diagnosed with avoidant, dependent, or obsessive–compulsive personality disorder. Anxious–fearful people generally experience both social and occupational impairments as a result of their restricted affect, nonassertiveness, problems expressing feelings, unrealistic expectations of others, and impaired decision making and problem solving. The lifestyle of the anxious–fearful person is characterized by intense emotional repression and behaviors that are socially isolating and self-defeating. The behaviors of anxious–fearful personalities tend to overlap, and common diagnostic features are described in DSM Essential Features.

Avoidant Personality Disorder

The essential characteristic of people with **avoidant personality disorder (APD)** is a pattern of social withdrawal along with a sense of inadequacy, fear, and hypersensitivity to potential rejection or shame. These are people who withdraw socially even though they deeply desire affection and acceptance. Their avoidant behavior results in visiting public places (movies, museums, and ballparks) simply to experience the presence of other people because they do not enjoy being alone. When in public places, however, they maintain a safe distance from others. For example, in a movie theater, one can be physically close to people without feeling that one's personal space is being invaded.

Avoidant people devalue their own achievements. They appear overly serious, humorless, and painfully shy. Speech is often slow, and they do not readily express their feelings. Thought content is generally serious. In the following clinical example, Mary Jane exhibits the characteristics of APD.

Clinical Example

Mary Jane is a 27-year-old single female who sought counseling because she felt lonely and lacked friends. She describes herself as having grown up on a midwestern farm where she was "pretty much a homebody." In high school, she made good grades but did not participate in any extracurricular activities. She studied library science in college and admits to receiving secondhand pleasure from reading about others' experiences. Currently employed as a reference librarian in a large computer software company, she has minimal contact with other people.

She says she wants to establish both male and female friendships but feels afraid that people will laugh at her. Mary Jane joined the company bowling team at the suggestion of a coworker but quit after the first evening because she felt she would "hold them back." Mary Jane rationalized her decision by stating, "I think I would be more comfortable pursuing an intellectual hobby."

DSM ESSENTIAL FEATURES

Cluster C Personality Disorders: Anxious–Fearful

Avoidant Personality Disorder: Pervasive pattern of social inhibition, feelings of inadequacy, and hypersensitivity to negative evaluation. Characteristics include avoidance of activities due to fear of criticism or rejection; unwillingness to establish interpersonal relationships; self-perception of inadequacy; reluctance to try new things because of fear of embarrassment.

Dependent Personality Disorder: Pervasive and excessive need to be taken care of, resulting in submissive, clinging behavior; fears of separation/abandonment; needs others to assume responsibility for major decisions; fears disapproval; lacks self-confidence; feels helpless when alone; exaggerated fears of being unable to care for self.

Obsessive–Compulsive Personality Disorder: Preoccupation with orderliness, perfectionism, and control. Characterized by focusing on details to the extent that the major point of the activity is lost; perfectionism interferes with task completion; excessive devotion to work; overly conscientious, scrupulous, and inflexible; hoards money and worthless objects; reluctant to delegate tasks due to need for control. Demonstrates rigidity and stubbornness.

Dependent Personality Disorder

The essential features of **dependent personality disorder (DPD)** include a pervasive, excessive, and unrealistic need to be cared for; fear of separation; lack of self-confidence; an inability to make decisions; and an inability to function independently. In sharp contrast to the avoidant person, dependent people cling to others and passively accept their dictates and leadership. Dependent people view themselves as "helpless" or "stupid" and seek out dominant others to rely on for guidance, control, and support as well as for "permission" to behave. These individuals have difficulty initiating projects and function adequately only when assured of approval and supervision. Infrequently, folie à deux (a shared delusion) may develop. The dependent person incorporates delusional beliefs of the dominant individual in the relationship. Folie à deux is an example of extreme psychopathology shared by two individuals.

In people with dependent personality disorder, the normal symbiotic parent–child relationship has been excessively prolonged, impairing their capacity for thinking, feeling, and responding on their own. They believe they must be taken care of and consequently rely on others to mirror their feelings to them.

Dependent people subordinate their desires and needs to the wishes of others in order to maintain relationships; they often appear friendly, helpful, and indispensable. Indeed, they will volunteer for unpleasant tasks if they think they will be reciprocated with nurturing. When the dominant other is unavailable, or perceived as unavailable, dependent people experience intense anxiety. This may lead to feelings of unhappiness, anger, resentment, or depression. It is also noteworthy that significant others may eventually respond to dependent people with anger and resentment because of their continuous clinging and ingratiating behaviors. The following clinical example illustrates how a dependent client might behave.

Clinical Example

Marie is a 40-year-old single parent of two teenage daughters. She has gained 70 lb since her divorce 2 years ago. Currently, Marie is sporadically attending a group for displaced homemakers, where she has shared a great deal of information about herself. She states that she is essentially a "homebody" and feels most satisfied when baking, cooking, and sewing for her daughters. Marie describes her secondhand pleasure in their activities, including ballet, gymnastics, and modeling. In fact, Marie becomes visibly saddened when she discusses her daughters' eventual departure for college. When her daughters expressed concern about Marie's weight gain and general health, Marie giggled and said, "Better to be fat and jolly than skinny and mean."

Marie has made no attempt to develop new friendships or social outlets since her divorce. She is poorly groomed and haphazardly dressed, in contrast to her impeccably groomed daughters. When confronted by group members about setting priorities and the need to direct some energy toward herself, Marie responded, "My life is devoted to my daughters. Their needs are more important than mine, and that's why I agreed to make 30 costumes for their dance recital next week."

Like people with other personality disorders, the dependent person may have multiple DSM Axis II diagnoses. Because DPD is among the most frequently reported of the

WHAT EVERY NURSE SHOULD KNOW

Client With Dependent Personality Disorder

Imagine that you are a maternal–child health nurse:

- Be alert for signs of depression in the new mother.
- Assess the woman's history for indicators of domestic abuse.
- Women who are excessively dependent may have difficulty in assuming care for a newborn.
- Be attuned to your own feelings of helplessness to ensure that apathy does not interfere with your ability to deliver quality care.
- Avoid the tendency to rescue the dependent client; this will only reinforce the woman's sense of helplessness.
- Encourage the client to do as much for herself and her infant as possible.
- Praise the client's assumption of personal responsibility.

personality disorders (APA, 2000), you may encounter dependent persons in other health care settings. For example, maternal–child nurses should be aware of the key factors outlined in What Every Nurse Should Know.

Obsessive–Compulsive Personality Disorder

People with **obsessive–compulsive personality disorder (OCPD)** demonstrate fear and anxiety concerning loss of control over situations, objects, or people. They demonstrate perfectionism, preoccupation with details, and hoarding behavior. The person with OCPD strives at all times to keep the world predictable and organized. The major features of this disorder are an excessive need for order, extreme dedication to work and productivity, and perfectionism to the exclusion of feelings and pleasure. A person with OCPD may be likened to a drill sergeant in the military who is rigid, serious, detail-oriented, and stingy with emotions.

People with OCPD tend to focus on trivial details. Although they may be highly praised for their organizational skills and work ethic, eventually their rigidity causes them to fear making mistakes. Because they repeatedly check their work, they are not good time managers; thus, projects may not get completed. They are self-critical and adhere strictly and concretely to rules. Consequently, they postpone making decisions. To manage their procrastination, obsessive–compulsive people often initiate work on a project far in advance of the due date.

They tend to resent authority but rarely express this resentment openly. Instead, they may engage in passive–aggressive behavior, such as procrastination and stubbornness.

People who are excessively conscientious and rigid often exhibit a contradictory pattern of slovenliness, which is also compulsive. Thus, a compulsive housewife may scrub her kitchen floor daily but allow bags of garbage to accumulate and become infested. When clients with OCPD describe their lifestyle, you will quickly become aware of their rigidity, concreteness, and need for order and perfection. In the following clinical example, John demonstrates extreme orderliness, Jerlinda shows that obsessive–compulsive tendencies may be confined to certain areas of life, and Peter is really more concerned with checking off his list than in his relatives' enjoyment of their gifts.

Clinical Example

John explained, "I have all my clothes hanging in the closet according to the day of the week, including my shoes, socks and underwear, so I know that if it's a Tuesday after a long weekend with a Monday holiday I need to bypass the clothing on the hanger marked Monday and wear the clothing on the hanger marked Tuesday."

Jerlinda has her linen closet and her silverware drawer scrupulously organized. The towels and washcloths are all folded and stacked in the same direction. The forks are lined up in a row in the silverware drawer. However, Jerlinda's kitchen and bathroom floors are a mess.

Peter set himself an early-fall deadline every year for ordering his family's Christmas gifts. His family found this deadline something of an annoyance. Yet Peter persisted in his attempts to get commitments from everyone about what they wanted. Often he was unable to make his early purchases before Christmas and would rush out to do last-minute shopping anyway.

People with OCPD are also keenly aware of other people's expectations; of the threat of possible criticism; of the weight and direction of authority; of rules, regulations, and conventions; and of a great collection of moral principles. They feel required to fulfill unending duties, responsibilities, and tasks. Obsessive–compulsive people do not view taking work home and working long hours as an imposition, because work organizes their lives and binds their anxiety. Indeed, they will manage to make work out of pleasurable activities.

OCPD appears in males more often than females and in about 1% of the general population (APA, 2000). Because many cultures emphasize and positively reinforce adherence to a strong work ethic, it is important that you consider cultural factors when assessing clients with OCPD.

BIOPSYCHOSOCIAL THEORIES

As the individual experiences life, adaptive mechanisms solidify, ultimately resulting in an automatic response style. When the response style is based on misperceptions or distortions, a personality disorder may develop. Therefore, the psychiatric–mental health nurse using a biopsychosocial model views clients with personality disorders as people whose communication and behavior are greatly influenced by past experiences, a need to maintain self-direction and control, neurobiology, and a unique style of interpreting their world.

Biologic Factors

Contemporary research addresses the role of biologic factors in the genesis of BPD. Hormones are being implicated to the extent that increased levels of testosterone, 17-estradiol, and estrone have been observed in people with impulse control

problems. Dexamethasone suppression test (see Chapter 6∞) findings have also been abnormal in some people with depressive symptoms who are diagnosed with BPD. The serotonin metabolite 5-HIAA has been shown to be low in people who attempt suicide and in those with aggression and impulse control problems (Sadock & Sadock, 2010). The following are some examples of brain research findings that support neurobiology as a major contributing factor to PDs:

- In some personality-disordered individuals, there are alterations in hormone levels and platelet monoamine oxidase (MAO) levels, smooth-pursuit eye movements, levels of endorphin and 5-HIAA (a metabolite of serotonin), and electroencephalographic (EEG) changes (Sadock and Sadock, 2010).
- Neurobiologic studies show that some symptoms and behaviors common in BPD are associated with alterations in the glutamatergic, dopaminergic, and serotonergic systems (Dell'Osso, Berlin, Serati, & Altamura, 2010).
- Neuroimaging studies of BPD clients indicate activity variations in the cingulated cortex, amygdala, and hippocampus, areas of the brain that regulate emotion and impulse control (Dell'Osso et al., 2010).
- A study using positron emission tomography (PET) indicated that an alteration in the opioid receptors is different in individuals with BPD as compared to a control group. The receptor sites are influential in regulating emotional responses (Prossin, Love, Koeppe, Zubieta, & Silk, 2010).

Genetic Theories

Following are some current research studies that support a genetic cause of personality disorders:

- Reviewing studies from 15,000 pairs of monozygotic and dizygotic twins in the United States, Sadock and Sadock (2010) identified significant familial correlations of schizotypal personality disorders among people with family members who are schizophrenic.
- A study of monozygotic twins, dizygotic twins, and siblings indicates a genetic risk of developing BPD (Distel et al., 2009).
- Cluster B disorders (borderline, histrionic, narcissistic, and antisocial) are often correlated with histories of mood disorders, alcoholism, and somatization disorders among family members (Sadock & Sadock, 2010).
- Research indicates strong familial tendencies toward antisocial PD. It is more common among first-degree relatives; having a female biologic relative with the disorder tends to increase the risk. Adoption studies show that both genetic and environmental factors contribute to the risk (APA, 2000).
- Schizoid and schizotypal PDs are significantly more common among first-degree relatives of schizophrenic clients. At this time, however, there is no substantial evidence that these PDs are early indicators of a future schizophrenic process (Sadock & Sadock, 2010).

Psychosocial Theories

The sense of self originates with the earliest parent–child interactions. If parents are not sensitive and attuned to the child's needs, they fail to confirm the child's emerging sense of reality. Consequently, the child distorts reality and develops an unreal "as-if" personality that shifts to meet the demands of cues in the outer world. A study by Gibbon, Ferriter, and Duggan (2009) indicates that children who experience severe adversity and familial criminality experience high rates of personality disorders.

Parental deprivation; inadequate, excessive, or inconsistent discipline; and failure of the child to develop integrated cognitive, affective, and behavioral modes in early life may lead to Cluster B disorders. Clients have generalized feelings of low self-esteem, need to control people and situations, and are unable to delay gratification. In response, dramatic–emotional clients tend to interact by negatively manipulating others. Although manipulation is a standard response in the repertoire of people with these PDs, its occurrence escalates with increased stress.

According to intrapsychic theory, psychological fixations in the genital stage of development may account for many of the behaviors noted in some PDs. For example, it is developmentally appropriate for a toddler to expect immediate gratification of needs. However, many adults with PDs display developmental immaturity through an inability to postpone immediate gratification of needs and wants. Impulsive and self-centered behaviors are examples of this type of developmental fixation.

Individuals with PDs have serious impairments related to establishing and maintaining healthy interpersonal boundaries. Intimacy is characterized by the ability to be close to another while maintaining a sense of separateness. Those with PDs generally have issues related to enmeshment and/or abandonment, which interfere with intimacy. *Enmeshment* refers to a feeling of being engulfed by others or of being overpowered by dominant others. Common signs of enmeshment include speaking for another person, answering for someone else, or responding to an event as another person would. Enmeshment in families is discussed in Chapter 29∞. *Abandonment* refers to feelings of being left alone; many people with PDs are vulnerable to feelings of abandonment because their sometimes bizarre, demanding behaviors push others away, resulting in alienation and isolation. Due to a fear of intimacy, some individuals sabotage relationships by provoking rejection while simultaneously fearing it.

In his classic work on narcissism that remains the standard for understanding this disorder, Kernberg (1975) emphasizes that chronic, intense envy and defenses against envy lead to idealization or devaluation of others. Responses to others may include lack of concern, mistrust, lack of intimacy, accusations of incompetence, and demand for unattainable perfection. Clients with NPD see interpersonal relationships as a means of enhancing their own self-esteem. A narcissistic person often selects a spouse or partner who will be dutiful and subservient in return for assurances of security and faithfulness. More recently, Kernberg (2007) has identified what he calls the "almost untreatable" narcissistic client. These are clients who combine the characteristics of NPD and BPD, and possibly antisocial personality disorder as well, representing the most severe cases of pathologic narcissism. In relationship to BPD, Kernberg (1975) suggests that when, as children, borderline clients perceive the parenting figure as both nurturing and punishing, they learn to reduce anxiety and resolve resulting conflicts by such primitive defensive strategies as splitting, projective identification, primitive idealization, omnipotence, devaluation, and denial.

Humanistic Theories

Individuals need to feel that they are a part of something greater than themselves. In their search for meaning, some individuals with personality disorder often engage in self-damaging acts. For example, after slitting her wrists with a razor, a client may state, "When I hurt, I feel real." While attempting to negate existential emptiness, the client actually threatens his or her own well-being. The fear of abandonment and alienation that is experienced by many people with personality disorders leads to existential dilemmas, such as "Am I real?" and fear of discovering emptiness within if left alone.

When considering the cause of personality disorders, it is wise to think of a culmination of factors. There is no one definitive cause of personality disorders. However, the humanistic holistic perspective considers that a variety of factors contribute to the problem.

NURSING SELF-AWARENESS

Self-awareness is the first step in developing therapeutic approaches to clients with any personality disorder. By examining your responses and feelings toward the client, you will be better able to prevent countertransference from occurring (see Chapter 4∞). Your Self-Awareness will direct you toward introspection. The behaviors demonstrated by personality-disordered clients often evoke strong negative feelings and responses in nurses, which puts clients at risk for stigmatization.

YOUR SELF-AWARENESS
Exploring Your Thoughts and Feelings Toward Clients With Personality Disorders

Pay attention to your feelings when interacting with clients with PDs. The following questions will help you assess your reactions:

- How do you respond when you become angry with a client?
- What do you do when you feel helpless to effect change?
- What do you do when you feel guilty about being unable to help a client?
- Can you detect your early physiological and emotional responses to stress?
- How great is your need to rescue or "save" clients from unhealthy situations?
- How do you know when you are becoming defensive?
- What is your behavioral response when you feel that you have been "used"?

Clients may be labeled or stereotyped, which leads to depersonalization and inadequate treatment.

The arousal of feelings of anger, powerlessness, a sense of having been "conned," disappointment, and even guilt and shame is common among nurses who work with PD clients. Nurses are often unaware of their own beliefs, which may be countertherapeutic. By using introspection and clinical supervision, you can become more aware of the impact of your feelings and behaviors on others. Only then will you be able to respond more appropriately to all clients.

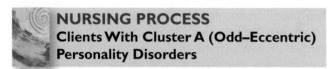

NURSING PROCESS
Clients With Cluster A (Odd–Eccentric) Personality Disorders

This section focuses on information specific to the nursing care of individuals with Cluster A personality disorders: schizoid, schizotypal, and paranoid types.

Assessment

Of the disorders in this group, the one most commonly seen in inpatient psychiatric settings is paranoid personality disorder. You will also see clients with paranoid personality disorders in outpatient settings, emergency departments (refer back to What Every Nurse Should Know on page 483), and prisons. When conducting assessment interviews with clients with paranoid personality disorder, it is very important to remember that behavior is culturally defined. Many individuals, particularly those from minority and/or immigrant groups, are erroneously labeled mentally ill because their behaviors are not congruent with the expected standards of the health care team. Indeed, the clinical evaluation may reinforce suspiciousness, hostility, and acting-out behavior because the client is unfamiliar with and frightened by the assessment process. Remember that paranoid traits may be adaptive in threatening situations.

Nursing Diagnosis: NANDA

Effective nursing diagnosis depends on collecting accurate data in a thorough, organized assessment. There is much overlap among the problematic behaviors in the various types of personality disorders, and in addition, a person can have more than one personality disorder at the same time. Nursing diagnoses are focused on the client's response to a disorder rather than on a specific diagnostic category. Because nursing is client centered rather than disease oriented, the primary nursing diagnoses for clients with Cluster A (odd–eccentric) PDs are as follows:

- Ineffective Coping
- Impaired Social Interaction

Outcome Identification: NOC

Individualize expected outcomes for each client, considering the unique situation and cultural context. The major goal is that clients with Cluster A (odd–eccentric) PDs will interact with others in a socially appropriate manner. Specific outcomes that indicate progress toward achievement of this goal include the following:

- Participates in activity groups
- Copes effectively with stressful situations
- Approaches staff and other clients without encouragement
- Verbalizes thoughts and feelings that interfere with socialization
- Identifies behaviors that maximize social interaction
- Verbalizes trust in other clients, staff, and family

Planning and Implementation: NIC

When interviewing a client who has paranoid personality disorder, maintain an open, nonthreatening style of questioning. The example in Rx Communication gives some suggestions.

Do not argue with or interpret the client's responses. Because these clients may hold grudges and are quick to attack, consider safety provisions for yourself and other staff as well as the clients. For other intervention guidelines, see Your Intervention Strategies: Guidelines for the Client With Paranoid Personality Disorder.

Anger and Aggressive Behavior

Clients with paranoid personality disorder, antisocial personality disorder, and borderline personality disorder are those most likely to demonstrate angry and aggressive behavior. You need to help clients learn to differentiate anger and aggression. Anger is an emotion, and aggression is a behavior. Everyone is entitled to feel the way they feel; however, the

---

R̪ₓ COMMUNICATION

Client With Paranoid Personality Disorder

CLIENT: "What did you mean by that remark? People are always making fun of me."

NURSE RESPONSE 1: "That remark was not meant for you, Jerry. It was directed at everyone in the group." *RATIONALE:* This response provides a simple explanation without being argumentative or overly detailed in explanation. It also reinforces reality for the client.	**NURSE RESPONSE 2:** "You feel others are picking on you." *RATIONALE:* This statement encourages the client to verbalize feelings of mistrust. It is stated in a nonjudgmental manner while maintaining appropriate eye contact, which is a behavior that promotes trust.

YOUR INTERVENTION STRATEGIES Guidelines for the Client With Paranoid
Personality Disorder

Nursing Intervention	Rationale
■ Respect personal space.	■ Promotes a sense of security.
■ Respect the client's preferences as much as is reasonable.	■ Increases self-esteem.
■ Give feedback to the client based on observed nonverbal cues of responsiveness, such as eye movement, posturing, and voice tones.	■ Improves interpersonal effectiveness.
■ Provide the client with a daily schedule of activities and inform the client of changes.	■ Activity schedules will diminish anxiety about social interactions and may help ensure participation.
■ Help the client identify adaptive diversionary activities (leisure, recreation) in one–to–one sessions and groups.	■ Participation in groups may increase the client's support system.
■ Use role-playing to help the client identify feelings, thoughts, and responses brought on by stressful situations.	■ Rehearsing social behaviors in a safe environment provides immediate feedback and time for altering responses.
■ Encourage the client to evaluate how his or her behaviors led to the current crisis.	■ Points out cause-and-effect aspects of interaction.
■ Use an objective, matter-of-fact approach with the client.	■ The client will identify the nurse as a reliable person who gives respect without argument.
■ Use concrete, specific words rather than global abstractions.	■ Keeps the intended message clear by decreasing ambiguity.
■ Respond to suspicious ideas by focusing on feelings: "It must be distressing." "You see him as vindictive."	■ Communicates empathy.
■ Conduct brief one–to–one sessions daily (avoid lengthy sessions).	■ Shortened sessions decrease fear and anxiety.
■ Gradually introduce the client to group situations.	■ Trust building is a slow process.

way in which those feelings are expressed must be modified to avoid causing harm to others. Limit setting (discussed in Chapter 10) and assertiveness training (discussed in Chapters 3 and 35∞) are important interventions for helping clients learn to change aggressive acts to behavior that is appropriate. Another important facet of nursing intervention and psychiatric treatment is helping clients understand and appreciate the rights and needs of others; these concepts can be effectively taught in group settings.

It is important to avoid personalizing the client's aggression. "Taking it personally" will increase your defensiveness, which in turn increases the client's perception of threat and can result in escalation of inappropriate behavior. Nurses who personalize clients' behavior lose their professional credibility. When you look at clients' inappropriate behavior as a clinical manifestation of a disorder instead of an act deliberately intended to harm, you are less likely to personalize the behavior.

When working with aggressive clients, safety is of utmost importance. Many clients with PDs—especially borderline, antisocial, and paranoid types—are at high risk of hurting themselves or others. See Chapter 35∞ for a thorough discussion of theories and strategies that relate to anger and violence.

Evaluation

Remember to use all your observation and interviewing skills when evaluating the progress of clients with Cluster A PDs. Such clients tend to share little of their feelings and will go to great lengths to avoid interacting with staff members. For more

information on evaluating care provided to clients with PDs, see the other evaluation sections on pages 499 and 501–502.

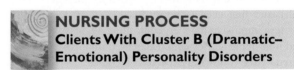

NURSING PROCESS
Clients With Cluster B (Dramatic–Emotional) Personality Disorders

Your responses to clients who have Cluster B personality disorders may be similar to the behaviors displayed by the clients themselves. You may often experience feelings of frustration and helplessness when caring for clients with Cluster B personality disorders (borderline, narcissistic, histrionic, and antisocial). For example, you must be attuned to your own feelings and reactions when working with clients with NPD. Do not criticize their haughty, uncaring attitude, but demonstrate by actions that they are accepted regardless of wealth, position, or status. Following the structure the nursing process provides will help you remain objective, focused, and organized when providing care.

Assessment

When assessing clients with dramatic–emotional PDs, be sure that your words and actions are congruent—that is, be sure that your nonverbal behaviors match what you say. To avoid being drawn in by a client's manipulative behaviors, you must maintain professional distance by using empathy. Specific

---

YOUR ASSESSMENT APPROACH   Clients With Dramatic–Emotional Personality Disorders
and Their Families

Use the following statements with the client:

How often do you notice rapid mood changes?

Tell me about one time you lost your temper.

Describe how you get along with others.

Give me an example of what happens when things do not go as you wish they would.

How do you describe your ability to make decisions?

Describe what you do when you feel bored.

What important lessons did you learn from your last mistake?

Tell me about one time you felt depressed.

Use these statements with the client's significant others:

Do you often feel that the client takes advantage of you?

Explain how the client expresses feelings of concern for others.

What does the client do when he or she becomes angry?

Is the client able to postpone getting what he or she wants?

Describe the client's judgment.

Is the client able to share attention with others, or does he or she need to be the center of attention?

---

questions you can ask clients and their families are outlined in Your Assessment Approach.

Nursing Diagnosis: NANDA

Individuals with Cluster B (dramatic–emotional) personality disorders are likely to experience the following:

- Chronic Low Self-Esteem
- Risk for Self-Directed Violence
- Risk for Other-Directed Violence

Note that these nursing diagnoses may apply to a client with any type of PD. Clients may also have several other diagnoses, based on their unique situations.

Outcome Identification: NOC

Clients with dramatic–emotional personality disorders have several issues that need to be resolved, such as learning to act in a less impulsive manner, controlling aggressive behavior, and improving self-esteem. Decreased impulsivity can be measured by the following expected outcomes:

- Identifies consequences of impulsive behavior
- Verbalizes the need to act less impulsively
- Uses techniques to control impulsive behavior (e.g., deep breathing, counting to ten before acting, taking a "time out" for decision making)
- Demonstrates a decreased incidence of impulsive acts (e.g., criminal acts, substance abuse, sexual promiscuity)

The following expected outcomes help measure the client's potential for violence directed at self and others.

- Identifies feelings of anger and/or frustration
- Verbalizes feelings appropriately
- Copes effectively with feelings
- Remains injury free

Expected outcomes that are relevant to self-esteem include the following:

- Identifies own positive characteristics
- Gives and receives compliments

- Demonstrates assertive behavior
- Demonstrates appropriate eye contact

Planning and Implementation: NIC

Manipulation, impulsivity, and self-destructive behaviors are characteristic of individuals with Cluster B personality disorders. Providing care to individuals with BPD is especially difficult for some nurses, primarily as a result of manipulative attempts by the client. This section provides guidelines for responding to clients who exhibit such behaviors.

Manipulation

Manipulation is pervasive in the life of someone with a personality disorder, and it is extremely difficult for most clients to change behaviors that are so ingrained. Learning to meet one's needs directly is the major challenge for those who demonstrate manipulative behavior. By establishing an interpersonal relationship with the personality-disordered client, you will be better able to role-model appropriate behavior.

Because of their charm, air of superiority, and persuasiveness, people with ASPD sometimes manipulate nurses to assume the roles of nurturers and rescuers. These clients have lifelong patterns of victimizing and exploiting others. Never give out your telephone number, assign special privileges, or make yourself available to these clients outside the therapeutic relationship. Specific guidelines and rationales for responding to clients with ASPD are discussed in Your Intervention Strategies.

Incorporate clear, concise, and consistent limit setting and directions into all intervention strategies. Develop these strategies using a team approach, and contract with the client. When infractions of the rules or manipulative behavior occur, apply consequences immediately.

Splitting of staff is a common manipulative ploy used by clients with PDs. A team approach is the only way to successfully counter this behavior. You must communicate continuously with colleagues, both individually and in team meetings, in order to know what the client is telling each staff member. Responding consistently to the manipulative behavior will help

YOUR INTERVENTION STRATEGIES   Guidelines for the Client With Antisocial Personality Disorder

Nursing Intervention	Rationale
■ Use a concerned, matter-of-fact approach.	■ A nonargumentative response decreases manipulative attempts.
■ Set, communicate, and maintain consistent rules and regulations for all clients.	■ Provides a sense of security.
■ Do not argue, bargain, or rationalize.	■ Decreases power struggles.
■ Confront inappropriate behaviors without anger, punitiveness, or personalization.	■ Addresses the behavior, not the person.
■ Do not seek approval, or coax; use choices and consequences.	■ A professional relationship increases client self-control.
■ Be alert for flattery or verbal attacks.	■ Being prepared decreases the chance of being manipulated.
■ Use contracts to help the client delay immediate gratification and impulsiveness.	■ Increases the client's personal responsibility for behavior.
■ Use peer pressure (groups, buddy systems) to modify manipulative behaviors.	■ Peer feedback is a better reinforcer than staff input.
■ Role-model self-discipline.	■ The client can pattern new behaviors after those of others.

gradually lessen its intensity. Examples of appropriate verbal responses to manipulative behavior are listed in Rx Communication: The Client With Borderline Personality Disorder.

A major intervention in dealing with manipulative behavior is limit setting. It is important to set limits only on the behavior that is most dysfunctional and problematic. If limits are imposed globally, the client is more likely to rebel and the dysfunctional behavior will escalate. Limit setting is done for the following three fundamental reasons:

1. To prevent escalation of negative behavior
2. To establish boundaries
3. To counteract resistance

Boundaries are established by providing consistent expectations and guidelines for self-control. Nursing interventions that provide structure encourage a sense of security in the client; thus, the need to manipulate is decreased. Trying to coerce a client to change is nontherapeutic and counterproductive. The use of confrontation and appropriate self-disclosure are techniques that may help reduce the client's resistance. A set of multiple intervention strategies is suggested in Evidence-Based Practice.

In addition to consistency and limit setting, other strategies for dealing with manipulative behavior are teaching the client relaxation skills (Chapter 33∞ provides specific guidelines) and encouraging the client to ask directly for what is needed instead of demonstrating the need through acting-out behavior. All of these approaches require your commitment and patience, whether you are working on an inpatient psychiatric unit, on a forensic unit, or in an outpatient setting. A variety of intervention strategies and their rationales are suggested in Your Intervention Strategies: Guidelines for the Client With Manipulative Behavior.

Impulsiveness

Clients with PDs often act before thinking about the potential consequences of their actions. As a result, many clients find themselves in dangerous situations that could have been prevented with forethought and planning. Safety maintenance is a primary concern when working with impulsive clients. Helping clients learn to face the consequences of their own actions is difficult for nurses who want to always protect clients. Implementation of consequences must be done consistently by all staff to be effective. Behavioral contracts can be

Rx COMMUNICATION

Client With Borderline Personality Disorder

CLIENT: "You're the sweetest nurse on the unit. I know you can help me get a pass for next Friday."

NURSE RESPONSE 1: "Darlene, whenever you compliment me, you usually want something from me."	**NURSE RESPONSE 2:** "Darlene, when you compliment people because you want something from them, they are not likely to trust anything you say."
RATIONALE: Confronting the client about her manipulative behavior will help her identify maladaptive approaches. If the nurse fails to confront the behavior consistently, the client will assume the behavior is tolerated and acceptable.	*RATIONALE:* This response points out the negative consequences of the manipulative behavior. It encourages the client to consider other ways of interacting.

EVIDENCE-BASED PRACTICE

Intervention Options in Borderline Personality Disorder

Darlene is a 28-year-old woman admitted to an inpatient psychiatric unit from the emergency department, where she was treated for a fractured arm, black eye, and multiple bruises as a reported result of being beaten by her boyfriend. She also had several slashes on her wrists that she stated she inflicted herself in order to "feel real." On this admission, Darlene is screaming hysterically, "Leave me alone. Just let me die because no one loves me." Darlene has been married three times and is currently in an abusive relationship with a man who sells drugs. "I hope you go to prison this time!" Darlene yelled at her male partner; however, she refuses to file criminal charges against him.

This is Darlene's fourth admission to the unit, where staff members are very familiar with her history and diagnosis of borderline personality disorder (BPD). On the last admission, Darlene manipulated the staff through splitting. She told three nurses that they were "special" and said, "You are the only one who ever really cared about me" to each nurse.

Your plan for intervention options is based on current research results. For example, in your review of cognitive–behavioral therapy (CBT) and BPD, you understand that Darlene will likely experience positive, long-lasting effects by participating in dialectical behavior therapy (DBT) groups. After observing Darlene in the group sessions, you determine to spend one–to–one time with her in order to establish a trusting relationship, which you know is a foundation for therapeutic intervention with clients experiencing BPD.

The multidisciplinary treatment team working with Darlene understands that current research shows the efficacy of antipsychotic medications in the treatment of BPD. Therefore, Darlene is prescribed quetiapine as an adjunct to the DBT sessions and other cognitive treatment approaches.

This set of multiple intervention strategies is based on the following research:

Goldman, G. A., & Gregory, R. J. (2010). Relationships between techniques and outcomes for borderline personality disorder. *American Journal of Psychotherapy, 64*(4), 359–371.

Ripoli, L. H., Triebwasser, J., & Siever, L. J. (2011). Evidence-based pharmacotherapy for personality disorders. *International Journal of Neuropsychopharmacology, 15*, 1–32.

Westwood, L., & Baker, J. (2010). Attitudes and perceptions of mental health nurses towards borderline personality disorder clients in acute mental health settings. *Journal of Psychiatric and Mental Health Nursing, 17*(7), 667–672.

CRITICAL THINKING QUESTIONS

1. What are the positives and negatives in having Darlene on a unit where she has been hospitalized before?
2. Is it helpful to know ahead of time that a client has attempted to split the staff?
3. On what basis is quetiapine helpful for clients with BPD?

YOUR INTERVENTION STRATEGIES   Guidelines for the Client With Manipulative Behavior

Nursing Intervention	Rationale
■ Assign one staff member as primary resource person.	■ Consistency reduces opportunities for splitting staff.
■ Make limits realistic, with enforceable consequences.	■ Unpleasant consequences may help decrease negative behavior.
■ Give reasons for limits and consequences.	■ Helps the client make appropriate choices.
■ Model respect, honesty, openness, and assertiveness.	■ Demonstrates expected behavior.
■ Interact with the client when the client is not acting out.	■ Reinforces positive behavior.
■ Confront the client each time manipulation occurs.	■ Consequences must follow behavior closely.
■ Discuss with the client alternative ways of dealing with people or situations.	■ Promotes personal responsibility.
■ Help the client identify assets.	■ Promotes self-esteem.
■ Remove limits from the treatment plan when the client adheres to objectives consistently.	■ Rewards appropriate behavior.
■ Evaluate the effectiveness of limit setting.	■ Clarifies discharge planning goals.
■ Jointly develop contracts for behavioral change.	■ Establishes client responsibility.
■ Offer support to other clients who may be targets of manipulation.	■ Ensures the safety of all clients.
■ Teach stress-reduction techniques (guided imagery, relaxation, thought stopping).	■ Defuses anxiety and reinforces ability for self-control.
■ Involve the client in assertiveness training and problem solving.	■ Teaches assertion as opposed to aggression.

useful for some clients in curbing their impulsive urges. The group setting is often a safe place for impulsive clients to learn to increase their capacity to tolerate frustration.

Self-Destructive Behavior

As a result of impulsiveness and low self-esteem, many clients with PDs inflict harm on themselves. Such behavior is upsetting to many nurses. Never dismiss or negate a suicidal gesture or self-mutilation as "just" attention-seeking behavior. You must thoroughly assess all acts of self-mutilation or verbalizations of intent to harm oneself (assessment of clients at risk for suicide and self-destructive behavior is thoroughly discussed in Chapter 23 ∞).

Individuals who engage in self-mutilating behaviors often experience boundary disturbances and lack insight. Consider the following statements as signals of the need for further assessment of clients with PDs. "I don't see what the big deal is. So I tried to cut my wrists a couple of times—doesn't everybody?" "Yeah, I vomit after I eat; it keeps my weight down and I still get to have all the desserts I want."

Milieu maintenance is one of the most effective nursing interventions in preventing clients' self-destructive behaviors. Physical precautions (e.g., locking doors, removing sharp objects) are some basic measures to ensure client safety. Establishing an environment that is psychologically safe is equally important; see Rx Communication for the client who self-mutilates.

Nurses who demonstrate trustworthiness help clients feel more secure. Clearly explaining expectations and consequences for inappropriate behavior also adds to a sense of stability. Letting clients know that they are in a safe environment and will not be allowed to harm themselves is especially crucial for people with BPD. The use of no-harm contracts is often therapeutic. A no-harm contract is an agreement between you and the client that the client will contact you or another staff member whenever the feeling to hurt him- or herself is experienced. A sample no-harm contract is illustrated in Your Intervention Strategies on page 519 in Chapter 23 ∞.

Dialectical behavior therapy (DBT) is an effective treatment approach for clients with BPD, especially those who are suicidal (Feigenbaum, 2010). DBT combines broadly based behavioral strategies—skill training, exposure, and problem solving—with the more general principles of supportive psychotherapy. The goal is to help the client improve interpersonal relationships, tolerate distress, and regulate emotional responses. See Chapter 30 ∞ for more detailed information on DBT. Also, the Nursing Care Plan at the end of this chapter is developed for a client experiencing borderline personality disorder.

Evaluation

When evaluating any client with a PD, consider the potential existence of major psychiatric conditions such as depression and anxiety-related disturbances. For example, people with obsessive–compulsive personalities often seek treatment for subjective distress, and the course of treatment may be ineffective as a result of the rigidity of the client's defensive operations. If the behavior is confronted directly, the client might develop acute psychiatric conditions because of intense anxiety. For more information about evaluating care provided to clients with PDs, see the evaluation section under Cluster C Personality Disorders.

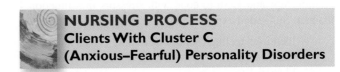

NURSING PROCESS
Clients With Cluster C (Anxious–Fearful) Personality Disorders

The clinging, demanding, excessively helpless, perfectionist, and rigid behaviors typically demonstrated by clients with anxious–fearful personality disorders (avoidant, dependent, and obsessive–compulsive PDs) may create distance between you and the client. However, establishing a therapeutic relationship is your key to helping clients cope more effectively.

Assessment

Because anxious–fearful people tend to be nonassertive and have problems expressing feelings, an accurate assessment will require enough structure and direction to help clients explain themselves and their situations. Rely on the communication techniques discussed in Chapter 10 ∞ to encourage clients to provide the information you need. The sense of inadequacy and fear of rejection or shame that many clients feel may interfere with their responses. Also, remember that speech is often slow, especially for clients with avoidant PD.

Dependent clients, because of their cloying, clinging, and demanding behaviors, have experienced dislike and

---

Rx COMMUNICATION

Client Who Self-Mutilates

CLIENT: "I just had to cut myself. There's no other way I can feel anything."

NURSE RESPONSE 1: "I'm wondering how you felt when you cut yourself."	**NURSE RESPONSE 2:** "Let's talk about what led up to your cutting yourself."
RATIONALE: Gathering more data will help you to understand the client better. You can help the client consider triggers and behaviors if you first encourage the client to identify and describe feelings and emotions around the event.	*RATIONALE:* While this response validates the behavior as real, it also asks the client to begin examining cause and effect.

avoidance in social, as well as health care, settings. This avoidance response tends to reinforce the clients' perceptions that other people are unwilling to help and that they are unable to help themselves. As a result, clients increase their clinging responses because they know no other way to behave. This increased clinging only leads to further avoidance by others. Therefore, self-awareness is your key to being effective in working with clients who demonstrate dependent behavior.

Nursing Diagnosis: NANDA

Several nursing diagnoses apply to those with anxious–fearful personality disorders. However, the two primary diagnoses are as follows:

- Social Isolation
- Defensive Coping

Outcome Identification: NOC

Clients with Cluster C (anxious–fearful) personality disorders primarily need to develop more appropriate interpersonal relationships and learn to cope with stressors in a functional manner. Suggested expected outcomes include the following:

- Identifies feelings about threatening events and situations
- Identifies the consequences of perfectionist tendencies on relationships
- Identifies feelings and beliefs that interfere with asking for help in an appropriate manner
- Makes decisions independently
- Demonstrates ability for self-care

Planning and Implementation: NIC

When you interact with clients experiencing anxious–fearful PDs, you need to consider the impact of your communication on them. Your patience will often be challenged by clients with these disorders. Examples of therapeutic communication techniques are shown in Rx Communication: The Client With Dependent Personality Disorder.

Impaired Social Interaction

Whether it is the paranoid individual who mistrusts others, the borderline person who makes numerous demands, the antisocial person who exploits others, the obsessive–compulsive person who orders others about, or the dependent person with an excessive and unrealistic need to be cared for,

dysfunctional interpersonal relationships are typical of persons with personality disorders. Intervention strategies and their rationales for the client with DPD are in Your Intervention Strategies: Guidelines for the Client With Dependent Personality Disorder.

Nurses often experience a range of responses to obsessive–compulsive clients, including pity, disgust, anger, frustration, anxiety, and intense discomfort. Always consider how clients with OCPD will react to the realization that years of denying themselves satisfaction, working hard, saving, and restricting their quality of life have not produced the expected rewards (e.g., career advancement, status, promotions). This realization often leads to the potential for depression, especially during middle life. Because anxiety may be contagious, it is wise to limit the duration of one–to–one sessions and make contracts with clients to avoid spending an entire session on obsessional material.

Confront the client's illogical perceptions of others as the first step in helping the client increase his or her capacity for intimacy. Establishing a therapeutic relationship with personality-disordered individuals is challenging because it goes against the basic nature of most personality-disordered clients to trust others and express their true feelings. It is helpful to start with a one–to–one interaction in a therapeutic nurse-client relationship (see Chapter 4 ∞), then encourage the client to interact in a group setting (see Chapter 28 ∞). Assertiveness training, which is appropriate for helping clients differentiate aggressive, dependent, and healthy functional behaviors, involves learning how to say "no" and how to get one's needs met without violating others' rights. (Assertiveness is discussed in Chapters 3 and 35 ∞.)

Remember to use a matter-of-fact approach when responding to the client. It is also important to provide feedback to the client about emotional cues sent to others (e.g., suspiciousness, contempt, intimidation). Role-play and group process are tools that are often useful in helping clients understand the impact of their behavior on others.

Chronic Low Self-Esteem

A common thread in all personality disorders is a pervasive sense of inferiority. Nursing interventions aimed at helping clients develop higher levels of self-esteem is appropriate for all those with PDs. It is important to confront clients' negative beliefs about themselves and help clients learn to replace the thoughts with

---

R̲ₓ COMMUNICATION

Client With Dependent Personality Disorder

CLIENT: "You must help me right now! It's too hard for me to do by myself."

NURSE RESPONSE 1: "Nancy, you have made your appointments on your own in the past."	**NURSE RESPONSE 2:** "Nancy, demanding help with tasks you can do for yourself will cause others to leave you alone. It's more effective to ask for help only with tasks that are really difficult for you."
RATIONALE: This response reinforces the client's sense of mastery by pointing out previous success.	*RATIONALE:* This response confronts the client with the clinging, demanding behavior and points out the results of such behavior.

YOUR INTERVENTION STRATEGIES   Guidelines for the Client With Dependent Personality Disorder

Nursing Intervention	Rationale
■ Evaluate the client's ability to perform self-care activities; encourage grooming and personal hygiene.	■ Fosters independent living skills.
■ Avoid doing for the client those things the client is capable of doing without help.	■ Promotes independence.
■ Schedule regular sessions as a way to anticipate client needs *before* the client demands attention through inappropriate responses.	■ Anticipatory guidance minimizes anxiety and acting out.
■ Help the client identify assets and liabilities, including plans for change; emphasize strengths and potential.	■ Self-assessment can enhance a positive self-concept.
■ Encourage the client to take responsibility for own opinions; point out when the client negates own feelings or opinions.	■ Fosters independence.
■ Share with the client your observations of the client's manipulative behavior.	■ Feedback from staff and peers fosters self-awareness.
■ Set realistic limits on what will and will not be done for the client.	■ Minimizes the client's dependence on others.
■ Explore with the client the consequences of behavior (e.g., clinging tends to result in avoidance by others).	■ Increases the client's self-awareness.
■ Discuss personal responsibilities and the fact that the client has choices.	■ Choices optimize independent functioning.
■ Give positive reinforcement for successful achievements.	■ Reinforces the client's ability to succeed.

more realistic ones. Cognitive–behavioral techniques (such as thought stopping) are useful in countering the irrational thoughts; these are discussed in detail in Chapter 30∞.

Another way to help clients develop greater self-esteem is to encourage them to identify their strengths. Once identified, these assets are the tools for building a better view of themselves. Using the classic concept of unconditional positive regard (Rogers, 1957) with all clients helps them feel more valued as individuals. Other techniques that can help clients improve self-esteem include journaling, exercise, and relaxation skills such as those discussed in Chapter 33∞.

Evaluation

Whenever possible, include family members or significant others in some aspects of therapy. Families and significant others can be taught in every setting, both inpatient and outpatient. Inclusion of families helps increase the support necessary for clients to function more independently. Psychoeducation guidelines for teaching clients and their families about personality disorders are listed in Partnering With Clients and Families. Chapter 29∞ discusses a wide range of family interventions.

Clients should be able to identify and verbalize their fears and some specific areas in which change is indicated. The following are among the factors that influence the likelihood of successful change:

- The severity of the client's emotional deprivation
- The rigidity of the client's personality structure
- The client's ego strengths
- The client's motivation to change

PARTNERING WITH CLIENTS AND FAMILIES

Teaching About Personality Disorders

- Provide information about the specific disorder.
- Help the client learn to verbally express needs instead of acting out.
- Provide social skills training (cooking, money management) as needed.
- Teach problem-solving techniques, including goal setting, identifying alternative responses, and evaluating consequences.
- Teach stress-reduction techniques (e.g., guided imagery, relaxation).
- Provide instruction in cognitive–behavioral techniques (e.g., thought stopping).

- Teach the client and family members about the proper use of medications, including: target symptoms, side effects and adverse medication reactions, contraindications, and when to call for help.
- Practice and/or role-play newly acquired skills (e.g., assertiveness).
- Teach the client and family members about signs of relapse or indicators for emergency treatment.
- Emphasize the importance of follow-up care as indicated.

- The nurse's skill and commitment
- Social support systems in the client's family or milieu that favor the desired change

Evaluation focuses on both the client's expected outcomes and the process of nursing care delivery. When assessing personality-disordered clients for progress, it is essential that the outcome criteria focus on resolution of short-term crises rather than global changes in the client's lifestyle. Keep in mind that PDs are lifelong traits and behaviors, so it is unrealistic to expect a client to change easily or in a short period of time. Using specific outcome criteria for measurement is necessary for evaluation to be meaningful. It is also important to include the client and significant others in evaluating the response to treatment.

When evaluating the delivery of nursing care, do not judge your effectiveness only by the client's progress or lack thereof. Instead, your evaluation of nursing interventions should consider how you responded to the client, what milieu you maintained for the client, and whether you consistently set appropriate limits in an attempt to teach the client the skills necessary for living as an independent adult. A determination of whether stability and safety were maintained is just as important as considering the client's response to the treatment plan.

CASE MANAGEMENT

The case manager plays an essential role by collaborating with clients and families/significant others by providing information on when and where to seek help. The case manager also monitors clients for adherence to the aftercare plan, including the client's medication usage. Clients usually need help in identifying community support services and in developing a support system. You can facilitate these tasks by asking the client to identify one family member or friend he or she would trust to help with personal needs.

COMMUNITY-BASED CARE

Individuals with personality disorders lack insight about their behavior; that is, they are generally unaware that their behaviors are problematic to themselves and others. As a result, few people with PDs voluntarily seek inpatient treatment unless they are experiencing a crisis. Many people with PDs are, therefore, treated in the community—in mental health clinics, crisis centers, and through routine visits to therapists' offices. Early intervention and long-term follow-up care are of primary importance for clients with personality disorders. Early identification of severe personality disorders and anticipatory planning help improve client outcomes.

When working with personality-disordered clients on an outpatient basis, it is especially important to help them identify their personal strengths to use as building blocks for therapy. Referral to outpatient classes on dialectical behavior therapy is especially appropriate. Also, you need to help clients develop a realistic time frame in which to achieve expected outcomes.

HOME CARE

Nurses who provide psychiatric–mental health care in the home setting are significant in helping clients with personality disorders improve their social interactions and in helping to shape behavior. Role-play can be an effective tool for helping clients learn to detect social cues given by others. Predictable environments (schedules, consistent caregivers, etc.) decrease anxiety and foster trust. The following interventions are especially helpful for homebound clients experiencing PD:

- Meet with the client and a family member or significant other to discuss realistic expectations for the client.
- Teach the client home management skills necessary for independent living.
- Ask if the client desires testing, placement services, or job skill retraining.
- Refer to community agencies as needed.

NURSING CARE PLAN: CLIENT WITH BORDERLINE PERSONALITY DISORDER

Identifying Information

Wendy is a 27-year-old divorced woman who was admitted to the hospital after threatening to commit suicide. She is a dental hygienist who has been employed for 6 months. Her employer confronted her 1 week ago about her rapid mood swings, irritability, and absenteeism related to chemical dependence.

History

She states that her employer, a female dentist, is jealous that the male patients are attracted to her. Wendy thinks it is unfair that her employer asked her not to see patients socially after hours. She also states that her

employer's jealousy of Wendy's physical appearance prompted her to say that Wendy needs to be treated for an alcohol problem (that Wendy denies having). Wendy states that she only drinks to unwind.

Wendy reports a history of being unable to relate well with previous female employers. She prefers the company of men, even though she states she was abused physically and sexually by males as a child. Wendy does state that she began drinking more often after her second abortion.

Current Mental Status

The mental status assessment shows Wendy to be hyperactive. She is oriented to time,

place, and person. Her judgment is impaired, and her affect is labile. Mood swings alternate between crying and excessive smiling. She denies delusions or hallucinations. Her speech is clear and coherent, though pressured at times. Wendy states she is being treated unjustly and blames others for her hospitalization.

Other Clinical Data

Wendy states that she does not need to be in a psychiatric unit because she really was not going to kill herself; she was merely looking for some attention.

NURSING CARE PLAN: CLIENT WITH BORDERLINE PERSONALITY DISORDER (*Continued*)

Nursing Diagnosis: Ineffective Coping related to inadequate level of confidence in ability to cope

Expected Outcome: Wendy will demonstrate the ability to self-control impulsive behaviors.

Short-Term Goals	Interventions	Rationales
Wendy will verbalize the decreased need to act impulsively.	■ Point out incidences of impulsive behavior to client. ■ Use active listening during all interactions with client. ■ Assign nonjudgmental staff to work with Wendy.	Confrontation makes the client more aware of problematic behaviors. Active listening promotes expression of feelings. A nonjudgmental approach helps the client feel accepted and more willing to express feelings.
Wendy will use relaxation techniques to control impulsive behaviors.	■ Teach relaxation techniques (e.g., deep breathing, visualization). ■ Have Wendy demonstrate newly learned techniques.	Anxiety interferes with the ability to plan ahead. Demonstration and repetition reinforce learning.
Wendy will demonstrate a decreased incidence of impulsive acts.	■ Encourage Wendy to state negative outcomes of impulsive behavior. ■ Allow time for Wendy to modify old patterns of behavior. ■ Set limits on Wendy's behavior to maintain safety.	Considering negative consequences of behavior is an incentive to change. Changing ingrained behaviors is a gradual process. Setting external limits establishes boundaries for behavior that are appropriate and safe.

Nursing Diagnosis: Ineffective Coping related to manipulative attempts to control others

Expected Outcome: Wendy will state needs directly and engage in active problem solving independently.

Short-Term Goals	Interventions	Rationales
Wendy will demonstrate a decreased incidence of manipulative behaviors.	■ Inform Wendy of acceptable behaviors. ■ Consistently enforce limits when Wendy attempts to manipulate. ■ Avoid seeking Wendy's approval. ■ Remain neutral to Wendy's comments, being neither flattered nor offended. ■ Use group techniques to teach self-responsibility. ■ Avoid rescuing or rejecting Wendy. ■ Provide feedback to Wendy about the effects of her behavior on others.	Knowledge of expectations increases likelihood of adherence. Consistency reduces effectiveness of manipulative attempts. People-pleasing behavior provides opportunity for manipulation to occur. Flattery is a form of manipulation; using a matter-of-fact approach removes the effect of manipulative attempts. Peer feedback is often effective in shaping behavior. Rescuing behaviors reinforce Wendy's sense of powerlessness and inadequacy; rejecting behaviors increase Wendy's perception of threat. Both behaviors lead to escalation of manipulation. Awareness of consequences of behavior may serve as catalyst to change.
Wendy will demonstrate independence in daily activities.	■ Encourage Wendy to be independent while being available to help only when necessary.	Providing assistance only when absolutely necessary encourages Wendy's self-reliance.

(Continued)

NURSING CARE PLAN: CLIENT WITH BORDERLINE PERSONALITY DISORDER (*Continued*)

Short-Term Goals	Interventions	Rationales
	■ Give positive reinforcement for achievement of goals.	Encourages development of a sense of mastery and boosts self-esteem.
	■ Help Wendy evaluate personal progress (e.g., through one–to–one, group, journaling).	Seeing progress encourages independence and success.

Nursing Diagnosis: Risk for Self-Directed Violence related to intense rage

Expected Outcome: Wendy will remain free from self-inflicted injury.

Short-Term Goals	Interventions	Rationales
Wendy will verbalize feelings of anger and self-destructive ideation.	■ Establish a trusting relationship with Wendy.	Trust encourages the expression of feelings.
	■ Use a nonjudgmental attitude when Wendy discusses suicidal/self-destructive thoughts.	A nonjudgmental attitude promotes continued dialogue.
	■ Assess history of previous suicidal/self-mutilating thoughts.	Previous self-damaging acts increase the potential for such behavior to be repeated.
Wendy will remain safe from harm.	■ Inform Wendy that she is in a safe place and will be protected from self-harm.	Reassurance decreases anxiety.
	■ Set limits on destructive behavior.	External limits maintain safety until Wendy learns inner control of impulses.
	■ Implement safety precautions (e.g., close observation of behavior, searching Wendy's belongings for contraband, suicide precautions).	Precautions maintain Wendy's safety at all times.

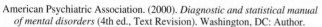

Pearson Nursing Student Resources

Find additional review materials at **nursing.pearsonhighered.com**

Prepare for success with NCLEX®-style practice questions, interactive assignments and activities, web links, animations and videos, and more!

REFERENCES

American Psychiatric Association. (2000). *Diagnostic and statistical manual of mental disorders* (4th ed., Text Revision). Washington, DC: Author.

Dell'Osso, B., Berlin, H. A., Serati, M., & Altamura, A. C. (2010). Neuropsychobiological aspects, comorbidity patterns and dimensional models in borderline personality disorder. *Neuropsychobiology, 61*(4), 169–179.

Distel, M. A., Trull, T. J., Wilemsen, G., Vink, J. M., Derom, C. A., Lynskey, M.,...Boomsma, D. I. (2009). The five-factor model of personality and borderline personality disorder: A genetic analysis of comorbidity. *Biological Psychiatry, 66*(12), 1131–1138.

El-Gabalawy, R., Katz, L. Y., & Sareen, J. (2010). Comorbidity and associated severity of borderline personality disorder and physical health conditions in a nationally representative sample. *Psychosomatic Medicine, 72*(7), 641–647.

Erikson, E. H. (1964). *Childhood and society.* New York, NY: Norton.

Feigenbaum, J. (2010). Self-harm—the solution not the problem: The dialectical behavior therapy model. *Psychoanalytic Psychotherapy, 24*(2), 115–134.

Gibbon, S., Ferriter, M., & Duggan, C. (2009). A comparison of the family and childhood backgrounds of hospitalized offenders with schizophrenia or personality disorder. *Criminal Behaviour and Mental Health, 19*(3), 207–218.

Goldman, G. A., & Gregory, R. J. (2010). Relationships between techniques and outcomes for borderline personality disorder. *American Journal of Psychotherapy, 64*(4), 359–371.

Holm, A. L., Begat, I., & Severinsson, E. (2009). Emotional pain: Surviving mental health problems related to childhood experiences. *Journal of Psychiatric & Mental Health Nursing, 16*(7), 636–645.

Kernberg, O. (1975). *Borderline conditions and pathological narcissism.* New York, NY: Aronson.

Kernberg, O. F. (2007). The almost untreatable narcissistic patient. *Journal of the American Psychoanalytic Association, 55*(2), 503–539.

Kim, J., Cicchetti, K., Rogosch, F. A., & Manly, J. T. (2009). Child maltreatment and trajectories of personality and behavioral functioning: Implications for the development of personality disorder. *Development and Psychopathology, 21*(3), 889–912.

Lentz, V., Robinson, J., & Bolton, J. M. (2011). Childhood adversity, mental disorder comorbidity, and suicidal behavior in schizotypal personality disorder. *Journal of Nervous & Mental Disorders, 198*(11), 795–801.

Mahler, M. S., Pine, F., & Bergman, A. (1975). *The psychological birth of the human infant: Symbiosis and individuation.* New York, NY: Basic Books.

National Alliance on Mental Illness. (2011). *Borderline personality disorder.* Retrieved from http://www.nami.org/Template.cfm?Section=By_Illness&Template=TaggedPage Display

Prossin, A. R., Love, T. M., Koeppe, R. A., Zubieta, J. K., & Silk, K. R. (2010). Dysregulation of regional endogenous opioid function in borderline personality disorder. *American Journal of Psychiatry, 167*(8), 925–933.

Ripoli, L. H., Triebwasser, J., & Siever, L. J. (2011). Evidence-based pharmacotherapy for personality disorders. *International Journal of Neuropsychopharmacology, 15,* 1–32.

Rogers, C. (1957). The necessary and sufficient conditions for therapeutic personality change. *Journal of Consulting Psychology, 21,* 95–103.

Sadock, B. J., & Sadock, V. A. (2010). *Kaplan & Sadock's pocket handbook of clinical psychiatry* (5th ed.). Philadelphia, PA: Lippincott Williams & Wilkins.

Walter, M., Gunderson, J. G., Zanarini, M. C., Sanislow, C. A., Grilo, C. M., McGlashan, T. H.,...Skodol, A. E. (2009). New onsets of substance use disorders in borderline personality over 7 years of follow-ups: Findings from the Collaborative Longitudinal Personality Study. *Addiction, 104*(1), 97–103.

Westwood, L., & Baker, J. (2010). Attitudes and perceptions of mental health nurses towards borderline personality disorder clients in acute mental health settings. *Journal of Psychiatric and Mental Health Nursing, 17*(7), 667–672.

Williams, K. A., & Bydalek, K. (2009). Self-mutilation: The cutting truth. *American Nurse Today, 4*(8), 29–32.

5
UNIT

VULNERABLE POPULATIONS

VONDA and EDZIU are dancing "Cinderella" with other members of their folk song and dance ensemble, Warszawianka, on the occasion of the anniversary of the birth of Chopin celebrated each year in Warsaw, Poland. Vonda loves the glamour associated with this social and recreational activity that she loves, but finds little glamour in being a social and civil rights activist. Before the Chopin celebration began, Vonda helped her colleagues at the Polish division of the International Association Against Psychiatric Assault draft an open letter to the Council of Europe demanding attention be given to the abuse and violation of fundamental human rights of Polish citizens with mental illness.

Many of Vonda's friends and neighbors disagree with her social activism. In their view, mental illness is shameful. They believe that people with mental illnesses are incurable, incapable of leading independent lives, unable to work, and should be isolated in treatment facilities away from town centers. If you have a mental disorder, you may be called *gupi*–crazy, loony, cuckoo, or idiot. For some mentally ill people, this stigmatization means lifelong social exclusion. Growing poverty, unemployment, and crime often lead to alcohol abuse, one of the most important social and mental health problems in Poland. Vonda and her colleagues believe that the stigmatizing attitudes of psychiatric professionals themselves result in the abuse of psychiatric clients, coerced treatment, and extended involuntary hospitalizations.

23

Clients at Risk for Suicide and Self-Destructive Behavior

EILEEN TRIGOBOFF
CAROL REN KNEISL

LEARNING OUTCOMES

After completing this chapter, you will be able to:

1. Identify the social, demographic, and clinical variables that influence suicidal or self-destructive behavior.
2. Compare and contrast the similarities and differences in suicide rates among various demographic groups.
3. Discuss the sociocultural, interpersonal, and biologic theories that enhance our understanding of self-destructive behavior.
4. Formulate a lethality assessment.
5. Distinguish between the crucial components of basic suicide precautions and maximum suicide precautions.
6. Develop nursing intervention strategies to prevent suicide that can and should be implemented in any health care setting.
7. Integrate family members into the plan of care for the suicidal client.
8. Develop nursing intervention strategies that may be helpful to survivors of suicide.

CRITICAL THINKING CHALLENGE

You are responsible for an intake assessment with Jared, a 35-year-old single male client. He is being admitted to inpatient care from an emergency room after driving his car off a highway into a building. His psychiatric diagnosis is major depression with psychotic features, and he has had prior hospitalizations for "suicidal gestures," as noted in his chart. Most guidelines for conducting a mental status intake examination emphasize the importance of a suicide assessment that includes questions such as "Have you ever thought of ending it all?", "Have you ever considered suicide?", or "Do you plan to hurt yourself?"

In your interview you ask if he is considering hurting himself again, and he says, "No." He seems anxious and does express feelings of hopelessness. You also know he's been on the Internet and has been to the Hemlock Society website.

1. What recommendations would you make for Jared's first few days on the psychiatric inpatient unit, and why?
2. What would your purpose be in specifically asking Jared what he learned from the Hemlock Society website?
3. How would Jared's antidepressant medication affect the likelihood that he is dangerous to himself?

Self-destructive behavior has been a part of the human experience since time began. **Self-destructive behaviors** are maladaptive measures a person uses to restore inner equilibrium when overwhelmed or unable to cope with stressful life events. Distressed and unable to see that they have other options, people attempt to harm themselves or commit suicide thinking that they can take away unbearable emotional pain. Did you know that **suicide**, the willful act of ending one's own life, is the 11th leading cause of death among Americans and that over 34,000 people kill themselves a year? That equals one suicide every 15 minutes. Over 90% of people who commit suicide have a psychiatric illness, and over 50% are under active psychiatric or mental health care.

Suicide ranks differently as the cause of death for different age groups. Suicide is the leading cause of death for those 25 to 34 years of age. It is the second leading cause of death for people 15 to 24 years of age, and third for children 10 to 14 years of age and adults 35 to 44 years of age. Suicide is the fourth and seventh leading cause of death (respectively) for adults 45 to 54 and 55 to 64 years of age. There are a number of health problems that cause death in the oldest age group; therefore, suicide might erroneously appear to be of less concern. However, the risk for suicide is quite high for this group (all data are from 2007, the latest data available).

There are gender and method differences to suicide, as well. FIGURE 23-1A ■ shows that people aged 10 to 24 years are most likely to suffocate themselves. Firearms are more likely to be used by the oldest group (65 years and older) and by men (by more than twice the percentage of women). The rate of suicide since 1991 for females remains basically the same, but is slightly lower for males. Ethnicity is represented in FIGURE 23-1B ■ (Centers for Disease Control and Prevention, 2009a).

Stigma and ignorance about mental illness, depression, and suicide may embarrass, shame, and silence individuals who want to speak with others about their pain. Clients may believe that others, including nurses and other health care providers, will label them "crazy" if they speak of suicide. In fact, discussions of suicide do arouse intense and complicated emotions in others.

Suicide is a major public health problem in North America and in many countries around the globe. Suicide affects all age groups, both genders, and all cultures, religions, and socioeconomic classes. Be aware that any client in a health care, occupational, or community setting may, given the right circumstances, contemplate suicide. Box 23-1 shows facts about suicide.

As psychiatric–mental health nurses, we frequently find ourselves face to face with suicidal or self-destructive people. Few clients elicit such intense feelings of anxiety and helplessness. Suicidal individuals will cause you to question your abilities to help others and preserve life. Thus, it is critically important to be prepared for all the emotional reactions—fear, anxiety, anger, and so on—that a suicidal client may evoke in you. Unless you understand them, these reactions may interfere with your ability to establish rapport. This chapter will help you to understand self-destructive people more clearly so that you can be more comfortable in assessing and intervening with suicidal clients.

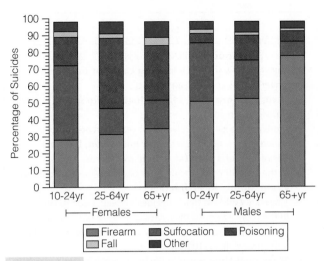

FIGURE 23-1A ■ Death by suicide according to age, gender, and method. Note the differences in the gender, age group, and the type of suicide method used. Note also how many younger males and females die from suffocation (or asphyxiation) and older men kill themselves by gunshot.

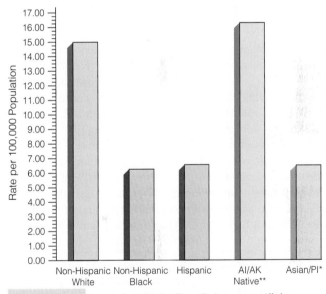

FIGURE 23-1B ■ Rates of suicide for five ethnic groups. All three figures are completed suicides for survey period 2000–2006 (the latest data available).
Source: Centers for Disease Control and Prevention, National Center for Injury Prevention and Control. http://www.cdc.gov/ViolencePrevention/index.html and Centers for Disease Control and Prevention, National Center for Injury Prevention and Control. Web-based Injury Statistics Query and Reporting System (WISQARS). http://www.cdc.gov/injury/wisqars/index.html

SELF-DESTRUCTIVE BEHAVIOR

In addition to suicide, other typical self-destructive behaviors and self-damaging acts include, but are not limited to, nail biting, hair pulling, self-mutilating behaviors such as scratching or cutting one's wrist or another part of the body, smoking cigarettes, driving recklessly, gambling, drinking alcohol, and using drugs. **Chronic self-destructive behavior** is behavior that harms the self, is habitual, and generally poses a

---

Box 23-1 Suicide Facts

- Every **15 minutes**, a life is lost to suicide.
- Suicide is now the **11th leading cause of death** in the United States across all age groups.
- There are **more than 34,000 deaths** from suicide in North America each year.
- More people kill themselves each year than are murdered; for every **two people who are murdered**, there are **three persons who take their own lives**.
- In the past 50 years, the number of deaths from **suicide in young adults has tripled**.
- There are **twice** as many suicides as deaths due to HIV/AIDS.
- In the month prior to their suicide, 75% of older suicide victims **had visited a primary care provider**; many had a depressive illness that was not detected.
- **More men than women** die by suicide; the gender ratio is four males to every one female.
- Over half the deaths from suicide are in **adult men ages 25–65**.
- Many suicidal people **never** seek professional care.

Source: National Institute of Mental Health. (2011). *Suicide facts.* Retrieved from http://www.nimh.nih.gov/health/publications/suicide-in-the-us-statistics-and-prevention/index.shtml. Retrieved August 26, 2011.

---

low level of lethality. In general, these behaviors range from relatively innocuous acts at one end of the continuum, such as overeating and gambling, to more lethal ones at the other, such as driving recklessly in a blinding snowstorm. Such self-destructive behaviors can injure one's health and sometimes hasten one's death.

A completed suicide is the most violent self-destructive behavior. It is important to understand that not all self-destructive individuals (in fact, only about 10% of those who purposefully injure themselves) go on to kill themselves. People who are suicidal may manifest several of the behaviors listed in Box 23-2. Another self-destructive behavior is

---

Box 23-2 Continuum of Suicidal Behavior

- **Suicidal ideation:** Having thoughts of harming or killing oneself.
- **Suicide threat:** A threat that is more serious than a casual statement of suicidal intent and that is accompanied by other behavior changes. These may include mood swings, temper outbursts, a decline in school or work performance, personality changes, sudden or gradual withdrawal from friends, and other significant changes in attitude.
- **Suicide attempt:** A nonfatal, self-inflicted destructive act with explicit or inferred intent to die. The attempt may be thwarted by another person or by circumstances, it may be planned to avoid serious injury, or it may be one in which the outcome depends on the circumstances and is not under the individual's control. For example, someone who takes a heavy overdose of sleeping pills may or may not be discovered in time.
- **Suicide:** A fatal, self-inflicted destructive act with explicit or inferred intent to die.

---

self-mutilation; see Chapters 22 and 24∞ for information related to specific diagnoses and age groups.

Ethics and Suicide

Do people have the right to commit suicide, and can or should nurses intervene when people try to kill themselves? The traditional belief is that mental health care professionals should do everything possible to prevent suicide. You should know that, ethical concerns aside, you may be prosecuted under state laws that make it a crime to aid or abet a suicide under any circumstance, even when a terminally ill person decides to end his or her life. Questions about a client's right to suicide and society's right to control suicide are still being debated. Engaging in the process of ethical reasoning presented in Chapter 12∞ will help you in your search for a personal position.

Meaning and Motivation in Suicide

Suicide is not a random act. Whether committed impulsively or after painstaking consideration, the act has both a message and a purpose. In general, unless it was an accidental overdose or involved substances of abuse, the purpose or reason for suicide was to escape or end an intolerable situation, crisis, or relationship, such as:

- A terminal (especially painful) illness (refer to What Every Nurse Should Know)
- Being a burden to others
- An untenable family situation
- An untenable personal situation
- Punishment or exposure of socially or personally unacceptable behavior

Needing to end intolerable situations is the motivation in the clinical examples of these five individuals.

Clinical Example

Antwon's lung cancer has metastasized to his bones; any exertion causes spontaneous fractures and he is in constant pain. He has asked friends, family, and health care workers to help him escape his illness by ending his life.

Joan, a widow, fell three times last year and is now in a nursing home. She decided on suicide so that she would no longer be a burden to her family. Joan has not eaten in 7 days.

Jeremy, age 7, attempted to run into the path of a car. He had heard his mother say many times, "If it weren't for you, Daddy and I would never have broken up." Jeremy believed that if he were dead, his parents would reunite, thus solving what he believes to be an untenable family situation.

Serena, age 33, had been admitted for the third time to a psychiatric unit because of thoughts of suicide. Jorge, her husband, has broken the last two family therapy appointments and went on vacation when she came into the hospital this time. Serena believes that she is unlovable and will attempt to leave the hospital tonight to finally stop the pain.

Fletcher, 34, was a successful businessman. Last night, he was charged with drunken driving and vehicular homicide. Horrified that his unacceptable behavior would be exposed, he committed suicide after learning that his picture and the story would be in the morning newspaper.

WHAT EVERY NURSE SHOULD KNOW

Suicidal Ideation in Primary Care

Imagine you are a primary care nurse. It is not unusual in primary care settings to see clients with suicidal ideation or at high risk for suicide. It is also not unusual for primary care providers to fail to recognize those at high risk for suicide. Suicidal risk is increased in both physical and psychiatric illness, especially when both are present. Remember that there is also a strong association between depression, risk for suicide, and chronic medical illness. Consider the possibility of suicide risk in all chronically ill clients, including those with solely physical symptoms.

Although there are more effective medications available to primary care practitioners to treat depression, the suicide rate has not declined, and neither has the incidence of unexplained deaths. In instances where mystery surrounds a person's death, a psychological autopsy may be performed. A **psychological autopsy** is an assessment tool that reviews the circumstances and events that preceded an individual's completed suicide. A review of psychological autopsies revealed that more than 90% of suicide victims have a comorbid mental disorder (most of them mood disorders and/or substance use disorders) and, furthermore, that they were undertreated, despite contact with psychiatric or other health care services. Recognizing this association, screening for it, and providing treatment is a primary care imperative and may prevent unnecessary tragedies.

Many people who are self-destructive have lifelong difficulties communicating their needs to others. Some people cannot express their needs or feelings; or, when they do, they do not obtain the results they hoped for. For them, self-mutilation or suicide becomes a clear and direct, if violent, form of communication. The message inherent in suicide tends to be complex and complicated, and is likely to be aimed at a specific person, usually the significant other. Interrupting a suicide plan or suicidal thoughts requires hearing, understanding, and responding appropriately to messages of pain, loneliness, and hopelessness. Rx Communication has an example of communicating with a client who is suicidal.

BIOPSYCHOSOCIAL THEORIES

Suicide and self-destructive behavior are still not well understood by the public or by the scientific community. In fact, many people's understanding of suicide has been influenced by misconceptions. These myths, and the corresponding explanatory facts that negate them, are discussed in Box 23-3.

Suicide is a complex phenomenon, and there is no single explanation for its complicated process; however, sociocultural, interpersonal and intrapsychic, cognitive, and biologic theories seem to contribute the most to our understanding of suicide. In addition to the section that follows, careful study of Chapters 17 and 22 ∞ will help you to understand the behaviors discussed in this chapter.

Sociocultural Theory

Sociocultural theories about suicide propose that the social and cultural contexts in which the individual lives influence the expression of suicidality. The following clinical examples describe two possible social and cultural contexts for suicide:

- Experiencing a precipitous deterioration in one's relationship with society (such as the loss of a job or a close friend)
- Considering self-inflicted death as honorable

Clinical Example

Emma, who is without family or friends, had decided that life was not worth living after retiring from her job with the federal government. She realized that no one would even know or care if she succeeded in killing herself.

In the Gaza Strip, a suicide bomber detonated explosives strapped to his body as he rode his bicycle into an Israeli checkpoint, killing himself and three soldiers and wounding several Israeli civilians. Those who claimed responsibility for the attack indicated their belief that the suicide bomber's death was an honorable one, and that he is rewarded in Heaven.

People in nonwestern countries are less willing to express their emotional distress. Many cultures consider somatic symptom complaints to be more acceptable than psychological ones (Seo et al., 2011). Be sure to take this difference into account. It differs from the typical suicidal symptoms of a North American who experiences an anxious depression.

R℞ COMMUNICATION

Client Who Attempts Suicide

CLIENT: "I just had to do it. There's no way I can take this pain another day."

NURSE RESPONSE #1: "I'm wondering how you felt when you tried to kill yourself."	**NURSE RESPONSE #2:** "Let's talk about what led up to your trying to kill yourself."
RATIONALE: Gathering more data will help you to understand the client better. You can help the client consider triggers and behaviors if you first encourage the client to identify and describe feelings and emotions around the event.	*RATIONALE:* While this response validates the behavior as real, it also asks the client to begin examining what may have caused an overload or an inability to cope.

Box 23-3 Suicide Myths Versus Suicide Facts

Myth: A suicide threat is just a bid for attention and should not be taken seriously.

Fact: All suicidal behavior should be taken seriously; a bid for attention may be a cry for help.

Myth: It is harmful for a person to talk about suicidal thoughts. The person's attention should be diverted when this occurs.

Fact: Of prime importance in helping a suicidal person is talking with that person in order to assess the lethality of the person's suicide plan.

Myth: Only psychotic people commit suicide.

Fact: The majority of completed suicides are committed by people who are not psychotic.

Myth: People who talk about suicide won't do it.

Fact: Most people do talk about their suicide intention before making a suicide attempt.

Myth: A nice home, good job, or an intact family prevents suicide.

Fact: People of all social and economic backgrounds commit suicide.

Myth: A failed suicide attempt should be treated as manipulative behavior.

Fact: Failed attempts are more likely evidence of a person's ambivalence toward suicide.

Myth: People who commit suicide are always depressed.

Fact: People who commit suicide are not always depressed, although depression is common. People can also be psychotic, agitated, organically impaired, or have personality disorders.

Myth: Suicide is more common in the winter months.

Fact: Contrary to popular belief, suicides peak during spring and early summer months in the Northern hemisphere.

Myth: There is no connection between alcohol or drug use and suicide.

Fact: Alcohol, drugs, and suicide are often closely connected. A person who commits suicide may have become depressed, impulsive, and suicidal after using alcohol or other drugs.

Myth: Once suicidal, always suicidal.

Fact: Suicide attempts are often made during particularly stressful times in people's lives. If the suicide attempt is managed properly, people can and do go on with their lives without recurrent thoughts of suicide.

Myth: Suicidal people rarely seek medical help.

Fact: According to studies, 50% to 60% of suicidal people sought help within the 6 months that preceded the suicide.

Age and Gender

Similarities and differences exist in suicide rates among people of different ages. Adolescent suicide is the third leading cause of death in North America. A nationwide survey of youth in grades 9 through 12 in public and private schools in the United States found that 15% of students reported seriously considering suicide and 7% reported trying to take their own life in the 12 months preceding the survey (CDC, 2009b). What we have learned over the past decade is that depressed adolescents need treatment. Appropriately prescribed antidepressants reduce suicide risk. Low rates of suicidality exist in adolescents taking fluoxetine (Prozac). A similar low risk exists for adolescents who take fluoxetine, are in cognitive–behavioral therapy, or in combination-treatment groups.

When gender is considered, the rate of suicide was slightly lower for males during the last survey period (2000–2006) while the rate of suicide for females rose slightly higher. The overall rate of suicide, regardless of gender, continues to trend down.

Alcohol and Substance Use

Alcohol consumption is estimated to cause adolescent males to be up to 17 times more likely to attempt suicide, and adolescent females 3 times more likely to attempt suicide. Alcohol use among adolescents has been consistently associated with increased suicidal behavior. The explanations include the psychologically depressive impact of alcohol, alcohol's disinhibiting effects, adolescent impulsivity heightened by alcohol, as well as the individual's high level of arousal and aggression (including past suicidal behavior) (Dubovsky, 2010). Alcohol use and subsequent suicidal ideation and suicide attempts among preteens suggests that efforts to delay and reduce early alcohol use may reduce suicide attempts. Regardless of age, alcohol is a risk factor for completed suicides (Vijayakumar, Kumar, & Vijayakumar, 2011). Your Assessment Approach in Chapter 15∞ on page 300 on blood alcohol level (BAL) demonstrates alcohol's effect on human physiology and subsequent behavior.

Substances of abuse also increase the risk of suicide. When an individual is intoxicated, rational thought and judgment are impaired and impulsivity is heightened to the point where, if the person has difficulty resolving a dilemma, suicide may seem the best course of action. Mental Health in the News has an example of such a situation.

Ethnicity

In general, there are commonalities in all cultures: Suicides occur when people are stressed, have poor resilience or poor coping skills, use substances, and have symptoms of depression. With that in mind, the CDC's (2009b) latest ethnicity data show that the highest suicide rates were among American Indians/Alaskan Natives with 16.25 suicides per 100,000 and non-Hispanic Whites with 15.02 suicides per 100,000. Refer back to Figure 23-1b on page 509. Further epidemiologic evidence shows Caucasian adolescents twice as likely as African-American adolescents to have used alcohol before committing suicide.

Suicide and suicide attempt rates vary across different ethnicities. African-American and European-American participants were studied by Walker, Alabi, Roberts, and Obasi (2010) for suicide risk based on cultural worldview. The results showed that resilience within ethnic groups, regardless of their worldview, gave individuals more reasons to live. These results give us direction for our psychoeducational interventions.

Interpersonal and Intrapsychic Theory

The notion that suicide is an expression of interpersonal and intrapsychic as well as societal conflict is perhaps the most

MENTAL HEALTH IN THE NEWS

Artie Lange

Artie Lange is a stand-up comic and was the main humor writer for The Howard Stern Show (terrestrial radio, TV shows, and satellite radio program). He has been open in discussing his struggles with years of drug abuse and eating disorder problems. During one show he had a major on-air physical altercation with his assistant. Violence was averted when several people physically intervened. Artie later talked about how his use of heroin destroyed his self-control and led to that unfortunate incident. He later went into rehabilitation for his drug use, completing the program just before the New Year's holiday.

On New Year's Day of 2010 his mother found him in his apartment with self-inflicted stab wounds. He stabbed himself nine times in an apparent suicide attempt. Lange was reported to have sustained six "hesitation wounds" and three deep plunges in the chest and abdomen from a 13-inch blade. Surgeons managed to save Lange despite heavy bleeding. He has not yet returned to his position on the show, but has made personal appearances and discussed his suicide attempt in what he calls his "most personal revelation" to the world. Loneliness, poor coping, and continued struggles remain major features in his life.

Photo courtesy of Jeff Dowder/ZUMA Press/Newscom.

---

significant contribution that psychiatry and psychology have made to our understanding of suicide. The following clinical examples describe some possible interpersonal and intrapsychic contexts for suicide:

- Having no close relationships with others
- Having no personal freedoms and no hope of getting them

Clinical Example

Daniel thought that suicide was the best way to solve his problems after he lost his job at a local factory and his girlfriend of 10 years precipitously broke off their engagement, left the area, and married someone else.

Jamie, who is a battered woman, believes that it doesn't make any sense to go on living. She has no close friends or relatives. Her husband will not allow her to drive, go shopping, or go to work. She is unable to see an alternative and decides that a life regulated to this extent is not worth living.

According to the classic work of Edwin Schneidman (1996), a clinical psychologist and leading authority on suicide, suicide is more accurately described as a dyadic event between two unhappy people, motivated by real or perceived rejection, abandonment, guilt, revenge, or pity. Suicide can be better understood if viewed in the context of the relationship between two people: the suicidal person and the significant other. Broadly defined, the significant other can be a spouse, child, boss, landlord, friend, nurse, or other health care worker.

Suicidal people almost always communicate their intent to significant others before the fact or attempt, although the meaning of the message may not be clear until after the attempt or death. Schneidman found a clear communication of intent in 80% of cases studied. A suicide threat or suicide attempt can arouse feelings of sympathy, anger, hostility, anxiety, or desire for connectedness on the part of a significant other, thus altering the current relationship to meet the need of the suicidal person. Although there is no one cause associated with suicide, there are several interpersonal and intrapsychic elements that are commonly associated with it. The list in Box 23-4 summarizes common characteristics based on Schneidman's work (1996).

Biologic Theory

Several biologic and medical markers have been studied in relation to the biologic foundation of suicidal behavior. The most promising biologic markers to date appear to be decreased central serotonergic function, reduced serum cholesterol levels, decreased platelet 5-HT, low cerebrospinal fluid 5-HIAA, and hypothalamic–pituitary–adrenocortical axis (HPA axis) dysfunction. These biologic markers are discussed next.

Neurotransmitter Receptor Hypothesis

The neurotransmitter receptor hypothesis of depression (see Chapters 7 and 17∞) holds that errors in the receptors for the specific neurotransmitter, serotonin, are critical in the development of depression and suicide. Lower levels of

---

Box 23-4 Characteristics Most Closely Associated With Suicide

1. The common purpose of suicide is to seek a solution to what appears to be an otherwise insoluble problem.
2. The common goal of suicide is cessation of consciousness or oblivion.
3. The common stimulus in suicide is unbearable psychological pain that may arise from any number of sources.
4. The common stressor in suicide is frustrated psychological needs that often result from family turmoil and occupational and interpersonal difficulties.
5. The common emotion in suicide is a pervasive sense of hopelessness coupled with helplessness.
6. The common cognitive state in suicide is ambivalence—desiring to die, but wishing there were another way out of the dilemma.
7. The common perceptual state in suicide is constriction of thought (tunnel vision) that prevents effective problem solving.
8. The common action in suicide is escape from intolerable circumstances.
9. The common interpersonal act in suicide is communication of intention (estimated to be 80% in completed suicides).
10. The common pattern in suicide is consistency of lifelong styles; suicidal people generally employ the same coping styles they have used throughout their lives.

serotonin (called *serotogenic hypofunction*) are associated with suicide and serious suicide attempts. There is considerable evidence that the serotonergic system is partly under genetic control. As yet unknown genetic factors—thought to be independent of the factors responsible for the heritability of major psychiatric conditions associated with suicide—are likely to contribute to the risk for suicidal behavior.

Normally, serotonin is released from one nerve cell, received by the next nerve cell, and then reabsorbed back into the first nerve cell. Many factors influence how much serotonin is passed from the first cell to the second cell, and how much is reabsorbed back into the first cell. Transmission can be influenced by the following:

1. The number of receptors
2. The ability of the receptors to function properly
3. Whether the body produces monoamine oxidase, which catabolizes serotonin (as well as norepinephrine and dopamine)

Whatever the exact mechanism may be when serotonin and serotonin metabolic activity are reduced, more violent lethal suicides and attempted suicides occur in these circumstances. Therefore, enhancing serotonin function may reduce suicide risk.

Genetics

A family history of suicide is a recognized marker for the increased risk of suicide, suggesting that there may be a genetic trait that predisposes some people to suicidal behavior. Various studies provide consistent evidence for a genetic component in suicidal behavior (von Borczyskowski, Lindblad, Vinnerljung, Reintjes, & Hjern, 2011). Genetic studies at the molecular level have concentrated on the genes of the serotonergic system because there is evidence, discussed earlier, that serotonergic neurotransmission is implicated in suicidal behavior.

Cognitive Theory

Suicidologists have speculated about the cognitive style (method of thought processing) of clients who commit or attempt suicide. Although there is no single suicidal logic, some cognitive styles predispose to suicidal behavior. *Dichotomous thinking* (the belief that there is only an either/or choice) is commonly seen in the suicidal person. The person falls into an imminently suicidal state when death seems to be the only escape. The thought processing of suicidal clients is generally constricted; that is, people who are suicidal have great difficulty (if they can do it at all) considering alternatives to their current dilemma. *Constriction in thought* generally results in the belief that there are only two choices: a magical solution or death.

People who are considering suicide are divided within themselves. They have two conflicting desires at the same time (**ambivalence**): to live and to die. Understanding the thinking of someone who is acutely suicidal requires an understanding of the concept of ambivalence. Ambivalence accounts for the fact that a suicidal person often takes lethal or near-lethal action but leaves open the possibility for rescue, allowing for the possibility of intervention. Failing to intervene and provide life choices increases the person's desperation, and death becomes the more focused choice.

The effectiveness of cognitive–behavioral therapy (CBT) in moderating suicide risk in people with significant mental disorders (major depressive disorder, for example) is a subject of current study. One such study (Curry et al., 2011) revealed that CBT provided significant recovery in adolescents with major depressive symptoms. The effectiveness of CBT was sustained at follow up. Further research is indicated to substantiate these findings and determine how and why CBT works.

SUICIDE PREVENTION

Suicide, a serious public health problem, is often preventable. In the 1960s, the federal government established the first special suicide unit at the National Institute of Mental Health in Bethesda, Maryland. Since that time, we have seen the growth of prevention efforts. Suicide prevention programs have developed at both the micro and macro levels in mental health agencies, with the development of suicide crisis centers and hotlines at local levels; in schools, colleges, and universities; at work sites; in correctional institutions; in aging programs; and in family, youth, and community service programs.

Risk Factors and Protective Factors

A combination of individual, interpersonal, community, and societal factors contribute to the risk of suicide as well as to the protective factors for suicide. Risk factors are the characteristics that are associated with suicide. They may or may not be direct causes. Protective factors serve as buffers from suicidal thoughts and behavior. Both are equally important, and both need more extensive and rigorous research.

Identifying people at risk allows us to engage them in effective treatments, support the presence of protective factors, and improve clinical practices. Risk factors and protective factors for suicide are discussed in Box 23-5.

National Suicide Prevention Initiative

The National Strategy for Suicide Prevention, developed in 2001, is the first coordinated effort of resources and culturally appropriate services between all levels of government and the private sector. It is a collaborative, multiproject initiative designed to incorporate best practices and research toward reducing the incidence of suicide nationwide. The goals and objectives of that effort have been summarized (2008) to guide the development of services and programs to reduce suicide. They are as follows:

- Changing procedures and policies in hospital emergency departments, substance abuse treatment centers, and mental health treatment centers designed to assess suicide risk
- Incorporating suicide-risk screening in primary care
- Ensuring that those who provide services to suicide survivors (emergency medical technicians,

---

Box 23-5 Risk Factors and Protective Factors for Suicide

Risk Factors

- Family history of suicide
- Family history of child maltreatment
- Previous suicide attempt(s)
- History of mental disorders, particularly depression
- History of alcohol and substance abuse
- Feelings of hopelessness
- Impulsive or aggressive tendencies
- Cultural and religious beliefs (e.g., suicide is a noble resolution of a personal dilemma)
- Local epidemics of suicide (cluster suicides)
- Isolation (feeling cut off from other people)
- Barriers to accessing mental health treatment
- Loss (relational, social, work, or financial)
- Physical illness
- Easy access to lethal methods
- Unwillingness to seek help because of the stigma attached to mental health and substance abuse disorders or to suicidal thoughts

Protective Factors

- Effective clinical care for mental, physical, and substance abuse disorders
- Easy access to a variety of clinical interventions and support for seeking help
- Family and community support
- Support from ongoing medical and mental health care relationships
- Skills in problem solving, conflict resolution, and the nonviolent management of disputes
- Cultural and religious beliefs that discourage suicide and support the instinct for self-preservation

Source: Adapted from: Centers for Disease Control. (2009b). *Injury prevention and Control: Suicide Prevention.* Retrieved from http://www.cdc.gov/ViolencePrevention/suicide/index.html

---

firefighters, police, funeral directors) have been trained to respond appropriately to their unique needs

- Increasing the numbers of people with mood disorders who receive and maintain treatment
- Ensuring that persons treated for trauma, sexual assault, or physical abuse in emergency departments receive mental health services
- Fostering the education of family members and significant others of those receiving care for the treatment of mental health and substance abuse disorders with risk of suicide
- Eliminating barriers to health care (financial, structural, personal, and cultural)

Reducing barriers to health care is an important advocacy strategy for all nurses. Large numbers of people have inadequate health insurance and do not have the financial capacity to pay for services outside their health plan or insurance program. Others have no health insurance at all. Structural barriers are the lack of primary care providers or other health care

professionals and a lack of health care facilities to meet needs. Cultural and spiritual differences, language, and concerns about confidentiality or discrimination are personal barriers.

Suicide Hotlines and Crisis Centers

For people contemplating suicide or families concerned about loved ones, the *National Suicide Prevention Lifeline 1-800-213-TALK* circumvents the barriers described earlier and provides immediate assistance around the clock. This lifeline consists of a network of more than 120 crisis centers in communities around the country that are committed to suicide prevention. Standards for the assessment of suicide risk to effectively guide crisis hotline workers in assessing callers have been developed. Having empathy, respect, a supportive approach, good contact, and collaborative problem solving are helper behaviors and intervention styles that are significantly related to positive outcomes in telephone suicide intervention.

Individual states also have suicide hotlines and suicide prevention web pages with information about suicide prevention efforts, including statistical data, suicide prevention plans, and suicide prevention coalitions. Links to individual state websites can be found at the website of the Suicide Prevention Resource Center (SPRC) at http://www.sprc.org. As a collaborative effort, SPRC and the American Foundation for Suicide Prevention maintain a best-practices registry for suicide prevention at the SPRC website to disseminate information about the best practices that address the National Strategy for Suicide Prevention.

NURSING SELF-AWARENESS

When working with a suicidal client, it is imperative that you are aware of, and monitor your own reactions to, this potentially life-threatening situation, because your reactions may interfere with your ability to accurately assess the situation and intervene. The suicidal client presents a unique challenge and will call on all your resources. You must be able to ask the right questions and make the right decisions as well as manage your own fears and anxieties. Helping a person who not only may not want your assistance but wants deliberately to harm or kill himself is a very complicated process.

You must be compassionate enough to be able to form an effective link with a suicidal client. The goal is to encourage the client to see you as an ally, yet maintain enough detachment to avoid being overwhelmed by the client's pain. The client will also bring many feelings into the interaction. Whether the feeling is anger, fear, anxiety, irritability, or hostility, remember that all emotions need to be tolerated, worked through, and evaluated.

Our attitudes toward suicidal clients have many sources. In addition to direct experience with suicidal clients, societal, familial, and ethical issues, as well as historical antecedents, influence what we think and how we feel about suicide and self-destructive behavior, euthanasia, abortion rights, the right to commit suicide, and the responsibility to prevent suicide. We can get caught up in the dilemma of how much responsibility to take for the self-destructive person and for

YOUR SELF-AWARENESS
An Attitude Inventory for Working With Suicidal Clients

To increase self-awareness about managing your own anxiety when working with clients who are suicidal, ask yourself the following questions:

- What kinds of things frighten me?
- How do I feel about asking for someone else's help with a client if I'm unsure of myself or uncomfortable?
- Are suicidal clients asking me to take responsibility for their behavior?
- Are suicidal clients able to assume responsibility for their own behavior?

To increase self-awareness of your own feelings about self-destructive people, ask yourself the following questions:

- How do I feel about people who deliberately harm themselves?
- How do I understand self-destructive behavior?
- Do I believe that clients are capable of change?
- Do I believe that people ultimately have the responsibility for their own lives?
- Can a person who is mentally ill choose suicide as a reasonable course?

To increase self-awareness about your own anger, ask yourself the following questions:

- What kinds of things make me angry?
- How do I deal with my own anger? Do I tend to ignore it or hide it?
- How do I react to others when they are angry?
- How do I feel about people who don't change immediately?
- How do I deal with people who appear to do illogical things?
- How do I feel when people don't change their behavior when I've asked them to or when I talk to them about it?

To increase self-awareness about your own feeling of control, ask yourself the following questions:

- In what areas of my life and my work do I feel the need to take control?
- How do I feel when interventions do not go the way I would like them to?
- How do I handle control issues with clients?
- How do I feel about control issues with clients?
- How do I feel about my lack of control over others?

how long. (Ethical issues about suicide are discussed in Chapter 12∞.)

All nurses must be competent not only to assess but also to intervene effectively with a suicidal client. This is not easy. Suicidal and self-destructive people seemingly defeat our best efforts by choosing death over life, or by being self-destructive. Although it is our responsibility to promote and maintain life, we cannot force the client to stay alive. Instead, we encourage clients to examine and understand how it is that they have reached this point and to expand their repertoire of coping methods.

Your attitudes when working with self-destructive, self-injurious, or suicidal clients may include a variety of feelings—frustration and anger among them. Before working with someone who is suicidal or self-destructive, it is critically important to assess personal feelings, experiences, conflicts, and memories that may either impede or facilitate your effectiveness. Clients report a more positive experience in treatment when we have a greater understanding of the client's experiences of self-harm (McHale & Felton, 2010). The inventory in Your Self-Awareness will help you to explore your own attitudes.

NURSING PROCESS
The Suicidal or Self-Destructive Client

Working effectively with a self-destructive client requires understanding the meaning the self-destructive behavior has for the client, performing a lethality assessment, keeping the client safe, and helping enlarge the client's repertoire of adaptive coping behaviors. An example of how this can be done in clinical practice is in Evidence-Based Practice.

Review these other chapters for information on suicide in specific populations: children, Chapter 25; adolescents, Chapter 26; elders, Chapter 27; people who abuse substances, Chapter 15; people with mood disorders, Chapter 17∞.

Assessment

A thorough assessment always includes a self-assessment by the nurse, the identification of clues or cries for help, and an accurate lethality assessment. Because assessment of suicide risk involves a degree of clinical judgment, you should seek sound mentorship if you are a novice practitioner.

Clues or Cries for Help

People intent on suicide almost always give either verbal or nonverbal clues of their plans or ideas. Up to 80% of all individuals who commit suicide may signal their need for help by making a social contact or with someone in the health care system. Unfortunately, the cry for help is not always clear until after the event (Dimirci, Dogan, Erkol, & Gunaydin, 2009). Because people do want help, it is important that you ask questions about depression and suicide. Always be alert to patterns that may at first seem coincidental, as in the following clinical example.

Clinical Example

Yusef, a 21-year-old man, was referred to a therapist by his physician. Although he described chronic "aches and pains" and "not feeling well," a physical exam revealed no physical problems. He did talk about how life was just not worth living, and he had a recent history of driving recklessly. After further discussion, he said that he had recently broken up with his girlfriend and admitted that his reckless driving had a suicidal intent.

EVIDENCE-BASED PRACTICE

Finding Alternatives to Suicide

Carolyn D., a 19-year-old college student majoring in theater arts, has been admitted to the inpatient unit after a heavy night of drinking alcohol that culminated in a suicide attempt. Carolyn's boyfriend has just dropped out of the college they attend—well-known as a "party school"—and returned to his hometown, 1,375 miles away. Within the 3 months prior to this admission, she experienced a major injury to her knee. The injury was severe enough to prevent her from achieving her life plan—being a dancer. Her family reports that she became increasingly despondent, saying she had nothing left to live for. They also worry that Carolyn will revert to the drinking problem she had in high school.

While on the unit, she has been unwilling to attend group therapy, saying that she "can't talk right," that her "head isn't working," and that she "can't talk in front of others." Her diagnosis is major depression, and she has begun taking appropriate antidepressant medications. As her psychiatric–mental health nurse, you formulate a nursing care plan that addresses the following considerations:

1. Carolyn is depressed and is working through multiple losses. In order to be able to find alternatives to suicide, she will need to think and process her feelings in a less rigid fashion.
2. Providing a less-demanding but secure environment will allow time to demonstrate to her that she has the flexibility to develop new coping skills and behaviors in response to her losses.

3. Cognitive–behavioral therapy can help Carolyn learn to identify and respond more appropriately to circumstances that elicit maladaptive responses (alcohol abuse, depression).
4. Helping her to express feelings and perceptions will increase her self-awareness and her ability to plan methods for meeting her needs in the future. Validating Carolyn's perceptions provides reassurance and can decrease her anxiety.
5. Carolyn's hospitalization is likely to be short term. The likelihood of suicide attempts is elevated in the month after starting treatment when Carolyn will be back at school. Referrals in her college and in the community for suicide prevention and alcohol abuse prevention services for both Carolyn and her family will be important.

The interventions for Carolyn are based on the following research:

Curry, J., Silva, S., Rohde, P., Ginsburg, G., Kratochvil, C., Simons, A.,...March, J. (2011). Recovery and recurrence following treatment for adolescent major depression. *Archives of General Psychiatry, 68*(3), 263–269.

Seo, H.-J., Jung, Y.-E., Kim, T.-S., Kim, J.-B., Lee, M.-S., Kim, J.-M.,... Jun, T.-Y. (2011). Distinctive clinical characteristics and suicidal tendencies of patients with anxious depression. *Journal of Nervous and Mental Disease, 199*(1), 42–48.

CRITICAL THINKING QUESTIONS

1. If Carolyn needs to become less rigid in her thinking and more flexible in her coping skills, how can a structured program such as cognitive–behavioral therapy help her?
2. Is a short-term hospitalization such as Carolyn's appropriate for someone at increased risk for suicide? Should Carolyn remain hospitalized until the threat of suicide is over? Why, or why not?

The cry for help may be indirect or subtle. Examples of what a person might say are: "I just can't take it anymore," "There's no reason to go on," "Sometimes I think I'd be better off dead," "I won't be seeing you anymore," "Take care of my dog and cat," "Too bad I won't get to see my little brother grow up," and "Will you be sorry when I'm gone?" Sometimes the behavior of people intent on suicide provides the clue. They may do the following:

- Give away prized possessions
- Make out or change a will
- Take out, or add to, an insurance policy
- Cancel all social engagements
- Be despondent or behave in unusual ways
- Be unable to sleep
- Feel hopeless
- Have trouble concentrating at school or on the job
- Suddenly lose interest in friends, organizations, and activities
- Have a sudden, unexplained recovery from a depression
- Plan their funeral
- Cry for no apparent reason

Be alert to both clear and veiled communications about suicide. Once you have identified clues, the next step is to perform an accurate lethality assessment. You should *always* perform an assessment for suicide whenever you suspect suicidal thought or intent.

Lethality Assessment

A **lethality assessment** is an attempt to predict the likelihood of suicide. An accurate lethality assessment is essential in formulating a plan for helping a suicidal person. Assessment of risk factors is essential in order to determine the client's need for hospitalization or the extent of watchful precautions to take when clients are hospitalized. Carrying out a lethality assessment requires direct communication with the client about the client's intent. Your Assessment Approach presents a lethality assessment scale.

Another component of assessing lethality is a consideration of the lethality of the proposed suicide method. Box 23-6 compares the lethality of various suicide methods. There are some gender differences in suicide methods. Women tend to use less violent methods—drugs and carbon monoxide poisoning—while men tend to use more violent methods—firearms and hanging. The top three methods used in suicides of

YOUR ASSESSMENT APPROACH
Lethality Assessment

Danger to Self	Typical Indicators
No predictable risk of immediate suicide	No suicidal ideation or history of attempts; satisfactory social support network; in close contact with significant others.
Low risk of immediate suicide	Has considered suicide with less lethal method; no history of attempts or recent serious loss; satisfactory support network; no alcohol problems; basically wants to live.
Moderate risk of immediate suicide	Has considered suicide with highly lethal method but has no specific plan or threats; or has plan with less lethal method; history of less lethal attempts; tumultuous family history; reliance on drugs or medications for stress relief; is weighing the odds between life and death.
High risk of imminent suicide	Current highly lethal plan with obtainable means; history of previous attempts; unable to communicate with close friends; drinking problem; feels depressed and wants to die.
Very high risk of imminent suicide	Current highly lethal plan with obtainable means; history of highly lethal attempts; cut off from resources; depressed and uses alcohol to excess; threatened with a serious loss (unemployment, divorce, failure in school).

Box 23-6 Lethality of Suicide Methods

Less Lethal Methods

- Wrist cutting
- House gas
- Nonprescription medications (excluding aspirin and acetaminophen [Tylenol])
- Tranquilizers

Highly Lethal Methods

- Gun
- Jumping
- Hanging
- Drowning
- Carbon monoxide poisoning
- Barbiturates and prescribed sleeping pills
- High doses of aspirin and acetaminophen (Tylenol)
- Car crash
- Exposure to extreme cold
- Antidepressants (tricyclic and monoamine oxidase inhibitor classes)

---

young people are hanging/suffocation, poisoning, and firearms (CDC, 2009b).

It is critical that you evaluate the client's ability and intent to act on an idea or plan. Beyond inquiring into the existence of a plan for suicidal action, ask questions and pay particular attention to whether the client has already taken steps to implement such a plan. For example, has the person already stockpiled medication, written a suicide note, obtained (or have access to) knives or guns, spoken to others about purchasing a gun, written a will, given away valued objects, or recently purchased insurance? Also obtain information about prior suicide attempts as well as the client's history of violence and impulsiveness, alcohol and drug use, and family history of suicide or violence.

Assessment of suicide risk is not easily accomplished. One barrier is the fear inexperienced nurses have of asking inappropriate or possibly harmful questions. It is important that you understand that *it is not possible to "cause" a person's suicide by assessing feelings and thoughts.* Inquiring about suicidal thoughts may alleviate a person's anxiety about considering suicide, not "give them the idea."

These are some suggestions for questions that you might ask:

- "How bad are things for you?"
- "How down do you get?"
- "Are you worried about yourself?"
- "Do you ever think of harming yourself when you're down?"

Then proceed with questioning the client gently, but directly asking questions such as:

- "Have you ever thought of taking your own life?"
- "Have you ever been so sad that you wanted to end it all, maybe by dying?"
- "How long have you been feeling that way?"
- "How are you thinking of hurting/harming yourself?"

Do not use euphemisms—be direct and clear in your communication.

The client who asks you to promise not to tell anyone about a suicide plan poses a serious assessment problem. Never promise to keep clinical information of any kind a secret, and explain to the client that information is shared with the treatment team. You will probably need to discuss the issue of confidentiality further and explore the dynamics of the nurse–client relationship.

A comprehensive assessment, including a lethality assessment, will help you decide which interventions are indicated for the client. For example, a complete assessment of level of lethality can prevent unnecessary hospitalizations. Hospitalizations in and of themselves can create a crisis. However, when the suicide plan is lethal and there are inadequate supports to maintain the client in the community, hospitalization is the optimal option.

Nursing Diagnosis: NANDA

The following core nursing diagnoses apply to most self-destructive clients:

- Risk for Self-Directed Violence
- Risk for Suicide

- Risk for Self-Mutilation
- Powerlessness
- Hopelessness
- Spiritual Distress
- Ineffective Individual Coping
- Low Self-Esteem

Several other nursing diagnoses (Anxiety, Impaired Verbal Communication, Dysfunctional Grieving, Impaired Thought Processes, and Dysfunctional Family Processes, among others) may be appropriate, depending on the situation.

Outcome Identification: NOC

Following are outcome criteria for the self-destructive client:

- Acknowledge self-harm thoughts.
- Admit to use of self-harm behavior if it occurs.
- Be able to identify personal triggers.
- Learn to properly identify and tolerate uncomfortable feelings.
- Choose alternatives that are not harmful.
- Admit to the use of self-harm behavior if it occurs.
- Attempt to identify stressors.
- Cooperate with interventions designed to reduce suicidal thoughts and control behavior.

Planning and Implementation: NIC

The nursing interventions in the following section are based on the belief that mental health care professionals should do everything possible to prevent a suicide. The descriptions of all clinical interventions strive for the ideal outcome; however, recognize that ideal circumstances are not always available and therefore ideal outcomes do not always result.

General Guidelines for Any Setting

The priority task is to work with the client to stop the constricted processing of suicidal thinking, long enough to enable the client and family members to consider alternatives to suicide. The nature of the nursing interventions is in large part determined by the setting in which you encounter the suicidal client. The following list of interventions and suggestions offers general guidelines that are applicable in most settings.

- Take any threat seriously. Evaluate the threat before dismissing it.
- Talk about suicide openly and directly. Remember, asking about it will not put the notion into the client's head.
- Implement suicide precautions/restrictive status (discussed in greater detail later in this chapter).
- Search the client's room, especially if suicidal thoughts or a suicide attempt occur after admission.
- Decide (along with other members of the team) if a no self-harm/no-suicide contract will be used (a sample contract is in Your Intervention Strategies).
- House the client in an area that is accessible for easy observation. Select a room that is near the nurses' station. A two-person room is best.
- Be careful not to encourage staff behaviors that give clients or staff members a false sense of security.
- Organize a plan of care with the client. Discuss all important problems, prioritize them, and list several approaches to each problem. Write down this plan, noting who is responsible for which actions.
- Do not make unrealistic promises such as, "Don't worry, I won't let you kill yourself." Remain honest but hopeful. Making unrealistic promises diminishes your credibility with the client.
- Encourage the client to continue daily activities and self-care as much as possible. Assign tasks for the client that are distracting but not taxing.
- Decide with the client which family members and friends are to be contacted and by whom.

YOUR INTERVENTION STRATEGIES   How to Develop No Self-Harm/No-Suicide Contracts

No self-harm/no-suicide contracts are effective in many situations, and they work well with certain clients. They can be used in hospital or outpatient settings as a means of providing additional support to people who are likely to harm themselves.

- Perform a thorough assessment before developing a no-suicide contract.
- Establish a relationship with the client prior to initiating the contract.
- Specify in the contract the intervals for re-evaluation. In outpatient settings, the interval may be 1 week; the inpatient interval may range from every shift to every 1 to 3 days.
- Have the client write out the contract if at all possible. Be creative if a client is unable or unwilling to write it out (the contract could be audiotaped, or the client and the nurse might each write half).
- Have both nurse and client sign the contract and date it.

- Use the contract as a way of connecting with and staying connected to the client.
- Place more trust in or emphasis on clinical judgment than on a contract.

Clients who are acutely suicidal may agree to the contract even though they have no intention of adhering to it.

Sample No Self-Harm/No-Suicide Contract

I, Cathy Smith, will not harm myself in any way. If I feel as if I am going to lose control, I will tell the staff (inform my nurse, call the crisis unit, call my therapist, etc.).

I will not bring, nor will I ask others to bring, harmful articles or substances onto the unit.

This contract lasts until _____ (date) and is renewable at that time.

Signed (and dated)

_____, Client

_____, Nurse

- Be prepared to deal with family members who may be confused, angry, or uninterested. Strive to remain neutral, and do not make assumptions about the family's behavior.
- Expect that the client will be experiencing shame, and work to help the client toward self-acceptance.
- Remove the client from immediate danger by confiscating pills or other harmful objects in the client's possession, or by moving the client to a physically safe environment.
- Relieve the client's obvious immediate distress. Does the client need a bath, clean clothing, food, sleep?
- Find out what, in the client's view, is the most pressing need. This may be seeing a friend or family member, or arranging for someone to pick up the children after school.
- Assume a nonjudgmental, caring attitude that does not engender self-pity in the client.
- Ask why the client chose to attempt suicide at this particular moment. The client's answer will shed light on the meaning suicide has for the client and may provide information that can lead to other helpful interventions.
- Provide for the client's safety through close observation and careful monitoring (see the section on client safety).
- Review the safety of the environment (see the section on safety in the therapeutic environment).
- Evaluate the client's need for medication.
- Evaluate the plan developed in collaboration with the client, and arrange for appropriate follow up.
- Monitor your personal feelings about the client, and decide how they may be influencing your clinical work.
- Work with other team members to evaluate the issues fully. You do not always have all the pieces of the puzzle.
- Perform a physical examination. One woman had cut herself severely prior to coming to the hospital, but this injury was not discovered until the physical examination was performed.
- Recognize that people can and do hang or strangle themselves with shoelaces, brassiere straps, pantyhose, robe belts, craft materials, and so on. Remain alert: Razor blades may be found in pages of books; matches are relatively easy to hide; pills may be hidden in plastic wrap in a cake box or stuffed animals; light bulbs can be broken and used to cut oneself, as can wire from spiral notebooks. Clients are also able to drown in a bathtub, throw themselves through a plate-glass window, set themselves on fire, or drink bleach from the cleaning person's cart.

General Guidelines for the Emergency Department

Suicidal behavior is prevalent in the psychiatric emergency department. As many as 44% of psychiatric emergency department clients are thought to be at increased risk for suicide (Pompili et al., 2009).

In the emergency department, whether in a psychiatric hospital or a general hospital medical center, the main goal of treatment is to save the person's life. Although the emergency staff may be excellent at technical interventions, they may voice or feel contempt for the client who is a "repeater," especially if the attempt is not a serious one. The client needs a professional, nonpunitive approach and a smooth transition to other caregivers or agencies. One–to–one observation and a psychiatric evaluation by an experienced clinician is the standard of care. Leaving the person alone or with access to harmful objects is obviously a hazard to be avoided in a busy emergency department.

Suicide Precautions/Restrictive Status

Maintain the client's safety in the least restrictive manner possible (right to treatment in the least restrictive setting is discussed in Chapter 12∞). The length of time on restrictive status is of concern to the client as well as the staff. Remember that restrictions meet the client's safety needs, but they do not constitute treatment. On an inpatient unit, times of highest risk for suicide are evenings, nights, and weekends. Two factors account for this. During these periods, clients' time is less structured, and fewer staff members are available.

Suicide Protocols Most psychiatric inpatient units have developed a set of protocols or guidelines for observing and monitoring client behavior, often called **suicide precautions**. Systems of observation may have three to six levels. Restrictions may require a physician's order but can and should be implemented on an emergency basis by nurses or other clinical staff. These protocols are often labeled to reflect the rationale for their use. In addition to suicide precautions, they may be known by such names as *special awareness, observation, constant observation*, and *constant visual observation*. Examine sample protocols in Your Intervention Strategies.

It is of critical importance that all staff members be familiar with the system being used and understand the rationale for its use. Maintaining and observing clients on these protocols is an important nursing responsibility.

Reserve restrictive status for managing the safety of suicidal clients. Restrictions can confound therapeutic management, and their use simply to restrict the free movement of clients diminishes their effectiveness. In general, privileges and other components of unit restriction are better dealt with by other measures such as privilege systems. If there is doubt about the appropriate safety status, the client should remain on a more restrictive status until the team decides what measures are appropriate. If there is doubt or concern about moving a client to a different status, it is best to retain the more restrictive status until the clinical direction of treatment is clarified.

Signs of Clinical Improvement Once you have recognized a client as a suicide risk and you have implemented a safety plan, you must begin the therapeutic work of addressing depression, psychosis, and precipitating factors. The treatment focus shifts as the client begins to show signs of clinical improvement.

YOUR INTERVENTION STRATEGIES   Sample Protocols for Suicide Precautions

Note that these are sample protocols. Check with the policies and procedures of the specific mental health facility.

Basic Suicide Precautions

You may start basic suicide precautions without a physician's order, but you must obtain a psychiatric consultation as soon as possible.

- The client is to remain in the room with the door open unless accompanied by a staff or family member. The client may use the bathroom alone.
- Check the client's whereabouts and safety every 15 minutes. Place a check-off sheet on the client's door to document safety checks.
- Stay with the client while all medications are taken.
- Look through the client's belongings for potentially harmful objects. Make the search in the client's presence, and ask for the client's assistance while doing so.
- Check all articles brought in by visitors.
- Allow the client to have a regular food tray, but be sure to check whether the glass or any utensils are missing when collecting the tray.
- Allow visitors and telephone calls unless the client wishes otherwise.
- Check that visitors do not leave potentially dangerous objects in the client's room.
- Maintain the protocol until it is canceled by a psychiatrist.
- Inform the client of the reasons for, and details of, precautionary measures. You and the psychiatrist both must make this explanation and document it in the chart.

Maximum Suicide Precautions

You can institute maximum suicide precautions without a physician's order under emergency conditions, but you must obtain a psychiatric consultation as soon as possible.

- Provide one–to–one nursing supervision. You must be in the room within arm's reach of the client at *all* times. When the client uses the bathroom, the bathroom door must remain open. A staff member should sit next to the client's bed at night.
- Do not allow the client to leave the unit for tests or procedures.
- Allow visitors and telephone calls unless the client wishes otherwise. Maintain one–to–one supervision during visits.
- Look through the client's belongings in the client's presence, and remove any potentially harmful objects, such as pills, matches, belts, shoelaces, pantyhose, brassieres, razors, tweezers, mirrors or other glass objects (such as light bulbs), wire, and craft materials.
- If suicide precautions are initiated after the client has been on the unit for any length of time, make a complete search of the room.
- Check that visitors do not leave potentially harmful objects in the client's room.
- Serve the client's meals in an isolation meal tray that contains no glass or metal silverware.
- Prior to instituting these measures, explain to the client what you will be doing and why. A physician must also explain this to the client. Document the explanation in the chart.
- Do not discontinue these measures without an order from a psychiatrist.

The following signs usually indicate clinical improvement and signal the need to review or change treatment plans, grant privileges, or plan discharges:

- Verbalizing a range of options other than suicide
- Making long-term plans or discussing future events
- Verbalizing hope
- Responding to antidepressant and/or antipsychotic medications
- Wanting to reconnect or moving toward reconnecting with family or significant others
- Showing more energy
- Sleeping better
- Feeling less hopeless
- Demonstrating a wider range of affective responses to situations that occur on the unit

Removing Suicide Precautions/Restrictive Status Change restrictions gradually, rather than all at once. A realistic plan is to change one or, at the most, two variables at a time while observing, monitoring, and documenting client responses. As the team begins to move the client off special status, it is important for all team members to keep communicating openly about the client (Addo et al., 2010). As the client begins to improve, the risk of suicide increases temporarily (especially if the client has increased energy and ability finally to act on

the suicidal ideation). The following times are critical and call for careful evaluation:

- *When the decision is made to move the client off suicide precaution status.* Clients, especially those who have come to depend on the around-the-clock safety, comfort, and nurturance provided by a staff member, may experience the discontinuing of suicide precaution status as a loss. Gradual removal from suicide precaution status and careful monitoring of its impact on clients is indicated in these cases.
- *When the decision is made to increase access to "sharps" (dangerous objects).* This increased access may make it possible for a client to act on a suicidal impulse. Assess the client carefully before granting this access.
- *During the second or third week of antidepressant medication therapy.* At this time, clients have increased energy but their depression has not been resolved.
- *When the decision is made to grant a pass.* Carefully evaluate decisions to grant pass privileges. Where is the client going, and with whom? What time frame is being considered, and why? Perform a careful assessment both before and after the client goes on a pass. Additional searches may be needed at these times.

■ *Prior to discharge and while formulating the discharge plan.* Remember that while clients are inpatients, they have staff available to them at a moment's notice. This is not the case once the client is discharged. It is crucial to evaluate the "holding environment" in the community. Refer the client to resources in the community, and schedule a follow-up appointment at the time of discharge. Family and significant others should participate in discharge planning. It is generally not a good idea to discharge a client (especially one who lacks immediate family support and must rely on agencies or clinics) on a Friday, over a long weekend, or when the mental health care provider will be on vacation or otherwise unavailable.

Monitoring Safety of the Therapeutic Environment

Periodically evaluate the safety of the therapeutic environment. Does it meet the needs of the current client population, and is the level of restrictions consistent with the milieu philosophy? Here are specific questions to consider:

■ Are areas free of glass or sharps?
■ Are hazardous objects and areas kept locked?
■ Are closet or shower rods of the breakaway type?
■ Are craft items safe?
■ How many clients are there? What is the client population like now? Do they have character disorders? Serious depression?
■ If the therapeutic environment is temporarily deemed to be unsafe—that is, if there are objects (such as liquor, razors, drugs) on the unit that can harm others—is there also a need to conduct a thorough "health-and-welfare search," in order to completely examine all areas of the unit for further contraband or other potential hazards?

It is also very important to educate the client's family and visitors about safety measures and their rationale. Taking this step helps ensure that family members and other visitors do not bring unsafe objects on the unit. Visitors must understand visit limits and unit policies in relation to passes. It is also necessary to explain the need for searches. Families and friends who repeatedly violate safety measures of the unit may require additional attention, and their visiting privileges may have to be restricted.

Documenting Client Behavior and Treatment

Documentation is essential for those working with suicidal clients on an inpatient unit. Documentation helps all staff members understand the rationale for changes and comply with ethical and legal requirements. In general, follow agency rules about documentation. Also be sure to document the following:

■ All team reviews of client status and the names of the team members involved
■ Any decision to remove the client from a more restrictive status to a less restrictive one
■ The rationale for any changes in the treatment approach, especially changes in the level of restriction
■ Statements from clients about self-harm or denial of self-harm
■ Client responses to changes, passes, family, visitors
■ All telephone calls or interactions with family members
■ All searches carried out and the reason for them

Working With Families

Including family members in the plan of care for the client is extremely important. Hospitalizations for suicidal ideation or a suicide attempt may be brief and may be terminated before antidepressant medication has had a chance to work. There are two important strategies that families need to know:

1. How to prevent suicide
2. How to help their loved one avoid acting on suicidal thoughts when those thoughts occur

Guidelines for families in preventing suicide are given in Partnering With Clients and Families. You can also

---

PARTNERING WITH CLIENTS AND FAMILIES

Helping Families Prevent Suicide

If family members strongly believe that someone is close to a suicidal act, or the person has indicated that he or she is close to acting on a suicidal impulse, teaching them these steps can help prevent suicide.

■ **Take the person seriously.** Stay calm, listen, but don't under-react. Express concern.
■ **Listen attentively.** Maintain eye contact. Use body language to show concern, such as moving close to the person or holding his or her hand, if appropriate.
■ **Do not promise secrecy.** You may need to speak to the person's health care professional in order to protect the person from him- or herself. Don't make promises that would endanger your loved one's life.

■ **Ask direct questions.** Find out whether the person has a specific plan for suicide. If you can, determine what method of suicide the person is considering.
■ **Offer reassurance.** Stress that suicide is a permanent solution to a temporary problem. Remind the person that help is available and that things will get better.
■ **Involve other people.** Don't try to handle the crisis alone or jeopardize your own health or safety. Call 911 if necessary. Contact the suicidal person's mental health professional, a crisis intervention team, a suicide hotline, a hospital emergency room, or others who are trained to help.
■ **If possible, do not leave the person alone.** Make sure that arrangements are made for your loved one to be in professional hands.

suggest some helpful websites to family members, such as American Association of Suicidology, American Foundation for Suicide Prevention, and Suicide Prevention Action Network USA. Direct links to these resources can be found on the Online Student Resources for this book. The websites in the section on Suicide Prevention will also be useful to family and friends.

Evaluation

Suicide, like all crisis situations, calls for ongoing evaluation of the plan made by the nurse and client. Because events often occur rapidly, you may need to change initial care plans almost daily. In addition to evaluating individual care plans, staff members who work with suicidal clients need to evaluate their overall approach and philosophy periodically.

CASE MANAGEMENT

Case managers can ensure that planned therapeutic linkages occur once the client has been discharged. Linkages might be established with public health or home health nurses, community mental health nurses, or psychiatric–mental health nurse practitioners. Discharged suicidal clients should also be linked with a mobile crisis unit.

Make sure that discharged clients and their families have all the telephone numbers they need—suicide/crisis hotline, mobile crisis unit, therapists, community resources. Case managers can also find other appropriate resources in the community to meet an individual client's needs. Clients should also have the time and date of their follow-up appointment.

COMMUNITY-BASED CARE

The treatment team needs to have a realistic approach when planning the care of a suicidal client. It is usually not possible to meet all therapeutic goals in an inpatient setting. Even clients who are suicidal are often discharged well before antidepressant medication is at full therapeutic response (see Chapters 7 and 31 ∞ for a discussion of antidepressant medications). These clients will need intensive monitoring in the community and should be encouraged to maintain contact with a mental health professional in a mental health facility, private office, or suicide and crisis center. A good case manager will have armed the client with hotline and mobile crisis unit telephone numbers.

Day hospital and continuing day treatment programs, where available, can be options. These activities structure and focus the day so the client can learn adaptive coping mechanisms, socialize as tolerated, and develop goals in a safe environment. These programs can have open-ended enrollment or be time limited.

HOME CARE

In addition to helping family members learn how to be gatekeepers to prevent suicide (such as in Partnering With Clients and Families: Helping Families Prevent Suicide), the suicidal client and the family should have a suicide crisis plan in place that will help the client avoid acting on suicidal impulses. Parents and friends can be instrumental in preventing suicide. Most symptoms of depression and hopelessness are universally recognized by parents and friends, although friends tend to be better able to recognize symptoms of substance abuse, which increase the risk for suicidal behavior. Partnering With Clients and Families below emphasizes a role for clients in developing a family suicide crisis plan.

SURVIVORS OF SUICIDE

The act of suicide has long-lasting ramifications for the survivors. Nurses who are working with the families or staff who have worked with the deceased must be alert to the potential aftereffects of the death. (Staff reactions are described later in the chapter.)

American Association of Suicidology

Resources for Survivors

PARTNERING WITH CLIENTS AND FAMILIES

Helping an Individual Develop a Family Suicide Crisis Plan

For most people, thinking about committing suicide is temporary. It is important that when suicidal ideas occur to clients that they have a crisis plan in place. This plan will help them avoid acting on suicidal thoughts when those thoughts occur. Teach clients that their plan should contain the following elements:

- **Tell those you trust about your condition.** It is important for the people close to you to be totally familiar with your condition before it becomes a crisis. Discuss your plan with family and friends so that they can respond quickly and effectively if you need their help.
- **Recognize the earliest warning signs of a suicidal episode.** Learn to be sensitive to subtle warnings of illness. This is a time to take care of yourself with the utmost care. Try not to become angry or disgusted with yourself.

- **Avoid drugs and alcohol.** Most deaths by suicide are the result of sudden, uncontrolled impulses. Because drugs and alcohol contribute to such impulses, it is essential to avoid them. Drugs and alcohol also interfere with the effectiveness of medications prescribed for depression.
- **Don't despair if your suicidal thinking recurs.** Suicidal thinking is the signal of a neurochemical imbalance. Call for help.
- **Contact your mental health provider, primary care provider, or clinic.** Have these phone numbers with you along with a backup number such as a psychiatric emergency room or a suicide crisis line.
- **Set your telephone speed dial feature with emergency numbers.** Having these numbers available will get you help sooner if you are feeling desperate.

Farberow (1992), a suicidologist who studied the effects of suicide on survivors, identified these emotional experiences of survivors of suicide that remain relevant to today:

- Strong feelings of loss accompanied by sorrow and mourning
- Anger at being made to feel responsible for the behavior of the suicidal person
- Feelings of separation because their help was refused
- Anxiety, guilt, shame, or embarrassment because the person committed suicide
- Relief that the nagging, insistent demands of the suicidal person have ceased
- Feelings of desertion
- The arousal of impulses toward suicide
- Anger caused by the belief that the suicide represents a rejection of social and moral responsibilities

Survivors rarely seek assistance from mental health care professionals. They may be angry and believe mental health care professionals "should have prevented this." Those who work with survivors, including nurses, must be prepared for this reaction. The American Association of Suicidology maintains a website for professionals and suicide survivors at http://www.suicidology.org

Family and Friends Who Are Survivors

Families and friends may not receive the same degree of support as bereaved people whose loved ones died because of illness or accident. People in the support network (including other family members or friends) may be uncomfortable and embarrassed and may stay away rather than help. If there is shame associated with suicide, that shame may be directed toward the survivors of suicide. Comments may be made about the family not being attentive enough or that they should have prevented the suicide. Options for establishing an alternative network of support exist with Internet support groups (Feigelman, Gorman, Beal, & Jordan, 2008). This process is available 24/7 and has less, if any, stigmatization associated with this source of comfort and support.

Very often, suicide is denied or concealed by family members who wish to avoid feelings of shame or avoid being blamed for the death. This secrecy further impedes grief work, because survivors cannot resolve the loss unless they discuss it openly. Suicide exacerbates dysfunctional family dynamics, such as scapegoating or blaming other family members. If grief is not allowed to proceed, mental health problems ensue for the survivors. Personal growth can arise from healing after a suicide loss (Feigelman, Jordan, & Gorman, 2009).

Besides making the usual preparations after death, which are stressful enough in themselves, families must deal with police investigations, the media, and insurance companies. This can precipitate extreme stress, especially if only limited support is available.

Families and all significant others who survive a suicide need nursing intervention, but it is especially warranted for the following:

- Families who lack support from usual sources
- Dysfunctional families who react by blaming, scapegoating, or covering up the death as an accident
- Children whose parent has committed suicide
- Adolescents exposed to the suicide of a friend

Plan outreach services for these groups. A typical plan might include telephoning the family immediately after the suicide and periodically until the first anniversary of the death, and arranging for staff or a staff representative to attend services, if appropriate. Consider involving the family in a bereavement support group. Families (first-degree relatives, spouses, and significant others of someone who committed suicide) may experience a significant reduction in maladaptive grief reactions and perceptions of blame in cognitive–behavioral counseling programs. Psychoeducational services and family network intervention have also been helpful. Families who need assistance toward the positive resolution of grief can contact Compassionate Friends at http://www.compassionatefriends.com. Peer support services for people affected by a death by suicide of a child of any age may wish to access http://www.friendsforsurvival.org

Child and Adolescent Survivors

Children who experience a loss as the result of a parental suicide require urgent intervention to deal with the trauma. Be

WHY I PLAN TO BECOME A PSYCHIATRIC–MENTAL HEALTH NURSE

Robin's Story: I have decided to become a psychiatric–mental health nurse once I complete a year in medical–surgical settings following my graduation. One of the reasons for this plan is the suicide of a fellow student last year. I was assigned a project by my clinical nursing faculty to be completed with JP, another student I knew only slightly. She seemed pleasant and bright and I thought we made a good team. Our project was to develop an intervention program on a clinical topic and then present it to the class.

JP and I worked twice a week together for 4 weeks. The work went well, but JP kept stressing about the public speaking aspect of the presentation. She was fine with the content of the project, but time and again she said she wished she didn't have to talk in front of a lot of people. We both were nervous about it and came up with ways to support each other and minimize our stress.

The day before our speech JP was unusually happy and smiling during our rehearsal. She said she knew it would all be fine and for me not to worry. We finished on a good note, confident the project would be well received when we presented the next morning. JP went out to the parking lot after our meeting and killed herself. I learned later that this was why she seemed so happy during our last meeting—she had decided to end her life rather than face something too difficult for her. This experience, along with a number of positive associations I now have about counseling and the workings of the mind, are of great interest to me and I would like to explore the rich intricacies of our thoughts and feelings as a psychiatric–mental health nurse.

particularly sensitive with these children, because they often have problems with grieving. A child who loses a parent is also at greater risk for suicide and depression.

Adolescents who are exposed to the suicide of a friend are at high risk for development of major depression. You should carefully screen, observe, and treat for depressive symptoms. A close relationship with the victim, visual exposure to the victim at the scene of death, having a conversation with the victim the day of the suicide, and both a personal and a family history of depression are all predictive of the development of depression subsequent to the suicide.

Cluster Suicide

Cluster suicide—an excessive number of suicides occurring in close temporal or geographic proximity to each other—is a phenomenon of great concern to those who work with adolescents. Clustering is most prevalent in the age group of 14 to 24, where it is two to four times more frequent than in older age groups.

Because of the influence of, and close connections with, their peer group, adolescents are at risk for cluster suicide. At highest risk are hospitalized or institutionalized adolescents. Clustering has been estimated to account for about 5% of teenage suicides in the United States. While that may seem at first glance to be a small number, it is an important one and a particular public health concern.

Staff Survivors of Client Suicide

Staff members are also survivors of a client's suicide. Client suicide during a course of treatment has sometimes been called an "occupational hazard."

The reactions of staff members can be as varied as the roles they perform with clients. For example, the exact memories and reactions will vary with a nurse who finds a client hanging and administers first aid, a therapist who saw a client for his or her last session, and a psychiatrist who was the last person to evaluate the client. All are likely to experience the suicide as a traumatic event.

Support for staff members is critical after client suicide. Typical reactions to the suicide of a client may include sadness, anger, denial, and shame. Some may have the erroneous belief that if you are "a good enough" nurse or therapist, you will be able to effectively prevent all suicides. Ethical concerns may be the focus of guilt if the client requested, and was refused, an assisted suicide (Levene & Parker, 2011). Staff members may lack confidence and be unable to function. This would be a good time for nurses to review their reasons for becoming nurses in the first place. Thoughts of reconsidering what they do or where they work are common. The range of other common reactions among nurses, therapists, and physicians range from refusing to admit suicidal clients to their caseloads or units to recognizing what the particular problems were and how they might manage them better in the future. Clinicians who have lost a client to suicide can access the American Association of Suicidology's website created by its Clinician Survivor Task Force via the Online Student Resources for this book.

Outside therapists or crisis workers can be helpful for counseling and implementing critical incident stress debriefing (CISD). CISD is a seven-stage structured group in which those who have been affected by a traumatic event are given the opportunity to discuss their thoughts and feelings. See Chapter 28∞ for a complete discussion of CISD.

Staff members with little medical training or experience suffer more than those who have previously encountered illness and death. These workers need extra attention.

Pearson Nursing Student Resources
Find additional review materials at
nursing.pearsonhighered.com
Prepare for success with NCLEX®-style practice questions, interactive assignments and activities, web links, animations and videos, and more!

REFERENCES

Addo, M. A., McKie, A., Kettles, A. M., Gibb, J., Gass, J., & Yule, M. (2010). Are nurses empowered to make decisions about levels of patient observation in mental health? *Nursing Times, 106*(9), 26–28.

Centers for Disease Control and Prevention. (2009a). Web-based Injury Statistics Query and Reporting System (WISQARS). Retrieved from http://www.cdc.gov/violenceprevention/suicide/statistics/

Centers for Disease Control and Prevention. (2009b). Suicide facts at a glance. Retrieved from http://www.cdc.gov/violenceprevention

Curry, J., Silva, S., Rohde, P., Ginsburg, G., Kratochvil, C., Simons, A., . . . March, J. (2011). Recovery and recurrence following treatment for adolescent major depression. *Archives of General Psychiatry, 68*(3), 263–269.

Dimirci, S., Dogan, K. H., Erkol, Z., & Gunaydin, G. (2009). Unusual suicide note written on the body: Two case reports. *American Journal of Forensic Medicine & Pathology, 30*(3), 276–279.

Dubovsky, S. (2010, January 4). Suicide—New data on causes and cures. *Journal Watch Psychiatry*, Jan 4. Retrieved from http://psychiatry.jwatch .org/cgi/content/full/2010/104/7

Farberow, N. L. (1992). The Los Angeles Survivors After Suicide program: An evaluation. *Crisis, 13,* 23–24.

Feigelman, W., Gorman, B. S., Beal, K. C., & Jordan, J. R. (2008). Internet support groups for suicide survivors: A new mode for gaining bereavement assistance. *Omega Journal of Death and Dying, 57*(3), 217–243.

Feigelman, W., Jordan, J. R., & Gorman, B. S. (2009). Personal growth after a suicide loss: Cross-sectional findings suggest growth after loss may be associated with better mental health among survivors. *Omega Journal of Death and Dying, 59*(3), 181–202.

Levene, I., & Parker, M. (2011). Prevalence of depression in granted and refused requests for euthanasia and assisted suicide: A systematic review. *Journal of Medical Ethics, 37,* 205–211.

McHale, J., & Felton, A. (2010). Self-harm: What's the problem? A literature review of the factors affecting attitudes towards self-harm. *Journal of Psychiatric and Mental Health Nursing, 17*(8), 732–740.

Pompili, M., Innamorati, M., Del Casale, A., Serafini, G., Forte, A., Lester, D., . . . Girardi, P. (2009). No cathartic effect in suicide attempters admitted to the emergency department. *Journal of Psychiatric Practice, 15*(9), 433–441.

Seo, H.-J., Jung, Y.-E., Kim, T.-S., Kim, J.-B., Lee, M.-S., Kim, J.-M., . . . Jun, T.-Y. (2011). Distinctive clinical characteristics and suicidal tendencies of patients with anxious depression. *Journal of Nervous and Mental Disease, 199*(1), 42–48.

Schneidman, E. S. (1996). *The suicidal mind.* New York: Oxford University Press.

Substance Abuse and Mental Health Services Administration. (2008). National Strategy for Suicide Prevention: Summarized Goals and Objectives. Retrieved from http://store.samhsa.gov/product/National-Strategy-for-Suicide-Prevention-Full-Report-/SMA01-3517 on August 25, 2011.

Vijayakumar, L., Kumar, M. S., & Vijayakumar, V. (2011). Substance use and suicide. *Current Opinion in Psychiatry, 24*(3), 197–202.

von Borczyskowski, A., Lindblad, F., Vinnerljung, B., Reintjes, R., & Hjern, A. (2011). Familial factors and suicide: An adoption study in a Swedish National Cohort. *Psychological Medicine, 41*(4), 749–758.

Walker, R. L., Alabi, D., Roberts, J., & Obasi, E. M. (2010). Ethnic group difference in reasons for living and the moderating role of cultural worldview. *Cultural Diversity and Ethnic Minority Psychology, 16*(3), 372–378.

Intrafamily Violence: Physical and Sexual Abuse

24

EILEEN TRIGOBOFF
KAREN LEE FONTAINE

LEARNING OUTCOMES

After completing this chapter, you will be able to:

1. Describe the biopsychosocial causes of intrafamily physical abuse and intrafamily sexual abuse.
2. Discuss the short-term and long-term effects on victims of intrafamily violence.
3. Distinguish who is at greatest risk for intrafamily physical and sexual abuse.
4. Integrate the main principles for treating victims of violence into a treatment plan.
5. Explain why spiritual recovery is important for persons who have been victims of violence.
6. Incorporate into your nursing role the specific advocacy actions you would take to reduce family violence.
7. Formulate a plan for managing personal feelings and attitudes that may affect professional practice when caring for victims of violence.

CRITICAL THINKING CHALLENGE

Beth is a 40-year-old professional woman in a long-term abusive relationship with Pat. Each time Pat beats Beth, he screams at her that she made him so angry that he had no choice but to hit her. Even though she is a competent professional, Beth has difficulty seeing that she is not responsible for Pat's loss of control.

Much of the current sociocultural climate encourages beliefs and practices about abuse that can subtly, or overtly, support abuse.

1. Is Pat abusive because Beth has made him angry? Why, or why not?
2. If a person yells at or nags another incessantly, does that individual have a right to strike out? Why, or why not?
3. Does violence in families continue to exist because the legal and criminal justice systems tolerate it? Why, or why not?

Violence that occurs as physical or sexual abuse within the family is a national health problem that confronts nurses in every clinical setting. Victims are seen in the community, in pediatric units, in intensive care units, in medical–surgical units, in maternal care settings, in ambulatory care facilities, in geriatric units, and in psychiatric–mental health settings.

As nurses, we assess and provide appropriate intervention for the emotional and physical consequences of violence and abuse. We may be called on to give legal evidence in the prosecution of a perpetrator. Within the community, we can establish, or refer victims to, support groups. We can also become active in increasing public awareness of intrafamily violence through formal and informal teaching activities. Because of our unique position, we can be active in the prevention of intrafamily violence and the treatment of survivors.

It is important to develop a knowledge base and be able to identify factors that contribute to domestic violence in order to assume this preventive role. Part of this role is providing public education and advocating for changes in public policy. This knowledge, along with increased awareness of the extent of the problem, helps us arrive at earlier, more accurate detection of intrafamily violence. When intrafamily violence is detected, nurses must comply with state laws on the reporting of violence and referral for treatment. Nurses with advanced education in family therapy are part of the treatment teams intervening with violent families.

INTRAFAMILY VIOLENCE: PHYSICAL ABUSE

Domestic violence—violence within the family—occurs at all levels of society. The myth is that violence occurs only among the poor and undereducated; the reality is that violence also occurs among the middle and upper classes as well as the professional elite. In the past, these problems among wealthy or prominent people were kept hidden from the general public. With an increase in national concern, however, more publicity is being given to cases of domestic violence at all socioeconomic levels.

In this text, the word *family* refers to any one of these three categories of people who are:

- Related by birth, adoption, or marriage
- In an intimate relationship
- In a domestic relationship; that is, sharing the same household

Although the image of the American family is one of happiness and harmony, this ideal is often in conflict with the underlying reality of domestic violence. The home is the most frequent place for violence of all types. **Physical abuse** is the nonaccidental use of physical force that results in bodily injury, pain, or impairment. **Psychological abuse** takes the form of verbal assaults, threats, humiliation, and/or harassment. Women and children are more likely to be assaulted, raped, and killed by people who claim to love them than they are by strangers. Perpetrators of violence do to intimates in their homes what they would not dare do anyplace else. Our culture does not condone violence in schools, at work, or on the streets, but continues to "allow" it within the privacy of the family despite the relatively recent criminalization of spousal rape (Adinkrah, 2010). Family members often appear to believe they have a license to strike other family members. **Battering**, a pattern of repeated physical assault, can be considered an epidemic in North America. Mental Health in the Movies discusses a disturbing example of intrafamily violence, both psychological and physical.

The incidence of domestic violence can only be estimated. Studies often include only those people who are willing to respond to surveys. Typically under-represented in such studies are those who do not speak English or are illiterate, the very poor, the homeless, and those who are hospitalized or incarcerated at the time of the survey. The actual rates of domestic violence are much higher than reported (Rhodes et al., 2011). A good source of information on domestic violence is the National Institutes of Health (NIH) website (http://www.nlm.nih.gov/medlineplus/domesticviolence.html) and the Office on Violence against Women, in the U.S. Department of Justice, has a website of interest (http://www.usdoj.gov/ovw) that

MENTAL HEALTH IN THE MOVIES
Sleeping With the Enemy

This psychological thriller stars Julia Roberts as the battered and psychologically abused Laura Barney who is married to an abusing, controlling man with very definite obsessions and compulsions. Laura has been attempting to abide by her husband's compulsive rituals and demands since their marriage. However, when Martin physically assaults her as punishment for what he perceives as flirting with another man, Laura develops a complicated plan in which she fakes her own death in a storm at sea near her Cape Cod home. In her desperation, she flees to Cedar Falls, Iowa, adopts a different identity, and attempts to create a new life for herself. The calculating Martin eventually traces Laura to her new home, confronting Laura and her new boyfriend. In the struggle that ensues, Martin is shot and killed. The movie's chilling and haunting music theme (Carl Orff's *Carmina Burana O Fortuna*) is a constant reminder of the sinister nature of their relationship.

Despite not having received the most positive of accolades from movie critics, the movie has been remade four times in India, once in Pakistan, and appears to have inspired similar movies in several other countries around the world. It leads one to believe that the movie touches upon a universally important topic.

Photo courtesy © United Archives GmbH/Alamy.

can also be accessed through the Online Student Resources for this book.

Domestic violence is a violent crime against which the victim has the right to be protected and for which the perpetrator can be arrested and prosecuted. In all 50 states of the United States, nurses are required by law to report suspected incidents of child abuse, and in every state there is a penalty— civil, criminal, or both—for failure to report child abuse. In addition, not reporting child abuse is considered to be nursing malpractice. Laws on reporting the abuse of adults and elders vary by state; be sure to know the laws in your state. The far-reaching impacts of violence on a child's life are explored in Evidence-Based Practice.

Sibling Abuse

A form of domestic violence that is very common but not necessarily acknowledged occurs between siblings. Many people assume it is natural and even appropriate for children to use physical force with one another. Parents may say, "It's a good chance for him to learn how to defend himself," "She had a right to hit him; he was teasing her," and "Kids will be kids." With these attitudes, children learn that physical force is an appropriate method of resolving conflict among themselves. Children who are hit by their parents exhibit more than double the rate of violence against siblings than children whose parents do not hit them. Hitting children increases the probability that they will be violent. Parents should not be complacent about sibling aggression; siblings cause 3% of all child homicides in the United States. Most adults in a position to know about violent confrontations and relationships (parents,

faculty, police, medically trained personnel) have an awareness of sibling and peer violence that is very low (Finkelhor, Ormrod, Turner, & Hamby, 2011). As nurses, we need to focus on identifying child and adolescent victims.

Child Abuse

Each year, more than 3.3 million children are abused or neglected in the United States. One in five U.S. children experience some form of maltreatment, with the statistics being slightly higher for girls than for boys. Children who live in a home with an abusive parent are 1,500 times more likely to be abused than the national average. Younger parents are more likely to engage in physical abuse against children than older parents, and the abuse is often disguised as discipline. For many, hitting begins when they are infants and does not end until they leave home. Younger children are spanked, punched, grabbed, slapped, kicked, bitten, and hit with fists or objects. Adolescents are more likely to be beaten up and have a knife or gun used against them. Men and women are equally likely to abuse young children. Adolescents who abuse others are more likely to be male.

Acts of violence against children range from a light slap, to a severe beating, to homicide. In some families or cultures, hitting or spanking children is condoned and even approved as being necessary and good for the child. Many parents, however, do not realize the underlying messages they are giving the child by hitting:

- If you are small and weak, you deserve to be hit.
- People who love you hit you.

WebLink Application: Parenting in the Context of Domestic Violence

---

EVIDENCE-BASED PRACTICE

Childhood Violence and Its Effects on Dating Relationships

In your role as a community health nurse, you have been conducting health classes for adolescents at a local high school and are aware that many adolescents have interpersonal relationship difficulties, especially when it comes to dating. They are unsure how best to handle strong feelings and impulsivity, and some of the students are involved in physical violence and abuse. During your class discussions, several students spoke about having been exposed to abuse and violence when they were younger. It is not hard to imagine how violence can become "normalized" when it was common during childhood. It becomes apparent to you that there may be a way to predict, and possibly prevent, continuing relationship violence.

Your review of the literature found that adolescents in violent dating relationships had sexual abuse (14%), interparental violence (12%), and parent mental illness (11%) during their childhood. Childhood adversity predisposes people to physical

dating violence, and almost half the adolescents in one study were involved in dating violence. The prevalence of violence in young children's lives is fairly high, as are the negative effects on subsequent relationships. As a nurse, you can talk with adolescents about better ways to communicate, help guide them through challenges without resorting to violence, and promote effective coping and conflict resolution.

You should base action on more than one study, but in this situation the following study was helpful in developing appropriate interventions:

Miller, E., Breslau, J., Chung, W. J., Green, J. G., McLaughlin, K. A., & Kessler, R. C. (2011). Adverse childhood experiences and risk of physical violence in adolescent dating relationships. *Journal of Epidemiology and Community Health.* Advance online publication. doi:10.1136/jech.2009.105429

CRITICAL THINKING QUESTIONS

1. Whom would you identify as important to contact in order to initiate an effort to reduce dating violence?
2. Why would it be useful to identify the major role models in a child's life?
3. How would an increased awareness of childhood violence make a difference?
4. Why would involving adults in reducing childhood violence likely be helpful?
5. What would be the purpose of talking about violence as if it were not normal?

- It is appropriate to hit people you love.
- Violence is appropriate if the end result is good.
- Violence is an appropriate method of resolving conflict.

Generally, violence against children can compromise the child's physical and mental health (Lyden, 2011). Research shows that violence against children affects the type of, quality of, and assumptions made in later relationships (Miller, et al., 2011). For information about child abuse, see http://www.nlm.nih.gov/medlineplus/childabuse.html, which can also be accessed through the Online Student Resources for this text.

Shaken Baby Syndrome

Shaken baby syndrome is one of the most serious, yet frequently overlooked, forms of child abuse. It involves the vigorous shaking of a baby held by the extremities or shoulders that causes whiplash-induced intracranial and intraocular bleeding. It is estimated that one third of victims have significant and permanent brain damage, and one third die. Not recognizing the danger, many parents shake rather than hit the child, mistakenly believing it is less violent.

Child Neglect

Neglect is the most frequently reported type of child maltreatment. It differs from abuse in that it is an act of omission that results in harm. Neglect includes lack of adequate physical care (including not medicating as prescribed), nutrition, and shelter. It also includes unsanitary conditions that often contribute to health and developmental problems. Lack of human contact and nurturance is considered emotional neglect.

Homicide of Child

In the United States, homicide is one of the five leading causes of death before the age of 18. Sixty-one percent of children who are killed by their parents or caretakers are under the age of 4 years of age, and 40% are less than 1 year of age. Most of these deaths are the result of battering in response to colic in the infant and toilet training difficulties in the toddler. A small percentage of children are killed because they are unwanted, as the result of mercy killings, at the hands of a mentally ill parent, or in retaliation when one parent kills the child to inflict hurt on the other parent. Compared to other developed countries, the United States has the highest rate of child homicide at all ages.

The children of parents who have psychiatric disabilities are at relatively high risk for homicide. A 5- to 10-fold increase in risk for being murdered was seen in young and older children of affected mothers or fathers. In judicial documentation, mothers who killed their children were frequently mentally disordered. Postpartum depression has been documented as the primary cause of infanticide. A disproportionately large number of biologic mothers who killed their offspring, especially older children, had a mental illness and received relatively short sentences, if convicted.

Murder of a son or daughter by biologic fathers was disproportionately accompanied by marital discord, suicide, and murder of a wife by her husband. Murders of children by stepparents were disproportionately common and likely to involve ongoing abuse and death by beating. Moreover, if parents also had biologic offspring, their stepchildren were at increased risk of ongoing abuse and neglect prior to death.

Homicide of Parent

Although it is a rare event, each year more than 300 parents are killed by their children in the United States. This number accounts for 1.5% to 2.5% of all homicides. Both victims and perpetrators tend to be European Americans, and 30% of the perpetrators are under age 18. The most frequent situation—90% of the cases—is one in which the teen has been severely abused and/or the mother is a victim of abuse. The adolescent's attempts to get help have failed, and the family situation becomes increasingly intolerable prior to the murder. A critical factor is the easy availability of guns in the home. The other 10% of cases involve either severely mentally ill children who experience hallucinations and delusions or dangerously antisocial children who have extreme conduct problems.

Partner Abuse—Heterosexual

Although no socioeconomic class, ethnic group, religion, or age group is immune to domestic violence, most victims are women. If the abused are mothers of dependent children, their children are also likely to be victims. Female partner abuse in heterosexual relationships is the most widespread form of family violence in the United States. It is thought that one woman in five is physically abused by her partner, and that 3 to 4 million women are severely assaulted every year. Half the women who are abused suffer beatings several times a year. The other half may be beaten as often as once a week. The intensity and frequency of attacks tend to escalate over time. If verbal and emotional assaults were included, the numbers would be much higher. Violence is the single largest cause of injury to women in the United States, with 20% of women's emergency department visits resulting from physical abuse. Three to four battered women are killed every day in the United States.

Overwhelmingly, the first acts of partner violence occur in dating relationships. Physical abuse occurs among as many as 30% to 50% of adolescent and college students who are dating. Sadly, many victims and offenders interpret violence as a sign of love. Common reasons teens and young adults give for the violence is betrayal and jealousy.

It is important to be aware of female abuse of heterosexual males. It is estimated that 100,000 to 150,000 heterosexual male partners are abused by women who initiate the violence. They are generally not recognized as "real" victims, and when they do tell others, they are criticized for not standing up for themselves or for not fighting back. This may account for under-reporting by male victims; admitting the occurrence would be a sign of weakness or a cause for embarrassment.

Partner Abuse—Homosexual

Until very recently, the existence of physical abuse in lesbian and gay relationships has been downplayed or even denied. This denial has been supported by the myths that women are not violent people and that men can defend themselves. In reality, violence does occur in some gay and lesbian families, for the same reasons as in heterosexual families: to demonstrate, achieve, and maintain power and control over one's partner (Wang, 2011). In addition to physical or emotional abuse, the violent partner may use homophobic control—the threat of telling ("outing") family, friends, neighbors, or employers about the victim's sexual orientation.

In the United States, domestic violence is the third largest health problem for gay men, following substance abuse and AIDS. It is estimated that 20% to 25% of coupled gay men are victims. Men rarely talk about being victims for fear of being considered feminine if they admit that their partners are hurting them. Violence in same-sex relationships demonstrates clearly that violence is not a gender issue but rather a power issue.

Homophobia and hatred of homosexuals in the United States contribute to the difficulties of battered lesbians and gays. They are cut off from the usual support systems available to heterosexual victims such as specialized counseling services and shelters. Most state laws regarding domestic violence exclude gays and lesbians by using limiting terms such as *spouse* and *battered wife*. Gays and lesbians of color and those who live in rural areas are even more isolated than their counterparts. Because same-sex partnerships are not recognized as "legitimate," victims have no access to the legal system. Being victimized by one's lover can be less frightening than being victimized by the legal system. Fear of being identified as gay or losing custody of children adds to the silence about the violence. Members of lesbian and gay communities are currently making an attempt to intervene with and support victims.

Elder Abuse

Two million older adults are mistreated each year nationwide (Pearsall, 2005). Elder abuse is any deliberate action or negligence that harms an older adult. Some older adults may be exposed to physical abuse or have their basic physical needs neglected and suffer from dehydration, malnutrition, and oversedation. They may be deprived of necessities such as glasses, hearing aids, and walkers. Emotional neglect can mean leaving a person alone for long periods of time or failing to provide social contact. Some older people are subjected to psychological abuse. Remarks such as "One of these days I am going to poison your food and you won't know when" and "I am the only thing standing between you and a nursing home" are considered psychological abuse.

Families may violate an older person's rights by refusing appropriate medical treatment, forcing isolation or unreasonable confinement, denying privacy, providing an unsafe environment, or demanding involuntary servitude. Some elders are financially exploited through theft or misuse of property or funds. Others are beaten and even sexually abused or raped.

The perpetrator of elder abuse may be a spouse, child, grandchild, niece, nephew, some other relative, or a non-related caretaker. The abuse is most likely to be inflicted by a person with whom the victim lives. A number of factors contribute to the abuse of older adults. Perpetrators may have personal problems such as lack of support in caring for the older family member, alcohol or drug addiction, or a family history of violence. Family factors include unresolved previous conflicts and power struggles. The perpetrator may be retaliating for previous abuse suffered at the hands of the older person. Elders are often resistant to intervention because they fear that losing a caregiver will mean having to be put in an institution.

Emotional Abuse

Although the focus of violence in this chapter is on physical abuse, remember that emotional abuse is often equally damaging. Words can hit as hard as a fist, and the damage to self-esteem can last a lifetime. Emotional abuse involves one person's shaming, embarrassing, ridiculing, or insulting another either in private or in public. It may include destruction of personal property or the killing of pets in an effort to frighten or control the victim. Such statements as "You can't do anything right," "You're ugly and stupid—no one else would want you," and "I wish you had never been born" are devastating to one's self-esteem.

Abuse of Pregnant Women

Pregnancy is a time of increased risk for abuse. There are more incidents of violence during pregnancy than of hypertension, gestational diabetes, or placenta previa, all of which are screened for regularly. Indeed, 13% to 43% of women report abuse during pregnancy (Mitra, Manning, & Lu, 2011). A past history of abuse is one of the strongest predictors of abuse during pregnancy. Nonpregnant women are usually beaten in the face and chest. But pregnant women tend to be beaten in the abdomen, which can lead to miscarriage, placenta abruptio, fetal loss, premature labor, fetal fractures, pelvic fractures, rupture of the uterus, and hemorrhage. Battering during pregnancy is associated with severity of abuse. The man who beats his pregnant partner is an extremely violent and dangerous man. Battering during pregnancy is also a risk factor for eventual homicide of the female partner.

The timing of the first prenatal visit is often related to abuse status. Abused women are twice as likely to delay prenatal care until the third trimester. Many abused women report that the abuser forced them to avoid prenatal care by denying them access to transportation. What Every Nurse Should Know gives you specific questions to ask and cues to incorporate into your assessment of the pregnant woman.

Physical abuse during pregnancy may be related to ambivalent feelings about the pregnancy, competition for attention with the developing fetus, increased vulnerability of the

WHAT EVERY NURSE SHOULD KNOW

Assessing for Emotional and Physical Abuse During Pregnancy

Imagine you are a women's health nurse at an obstetrics office. At the first prenatal visit, you should explain to the client that you will ask her questions related to emotional and physical abuse throughout her pregnancy because pregnancy is a time of increased risk for abuse. Determine if there is a prior history of physical or emotional abuse in the current relationship. Avoid making assumptions based on cultural myths (upper-class women are not abused, lesbian women do not abuse their partners, women could leave abusive situations if they choose to, and so on). In addition to assessing for physical injuries, at each prenatal visit, ask the following questions:

- Do you feel valued as a person by your partner?
- Do you feel safe in your home?
- Are you isolated from others for long periods of time?
- Have you been hurt in any way since your last visit here?

woman, increased economic pressures, and decreased sexual availability. Unfortunately, the abuse of pregnant women is often overlooked by health care professionals even when the victim appears in the emergency department with bruises, cuts, broken bones, and abdominal injuries.

Stalking

The term *stalking* has become not only a part of the American vocabulary but also a new classification of crime, and all 50 states have passed stalking laws. **Stalking** is the act of following, viewing, communicating with, or moving threateningly toward another person. Property damage and assault may accompany stalking. Victims often feel trapped in an environment filled with anxiety, stress, and fear that often results in their having to make drastic changes in how they live their lives.

Domestic stalking occurs when a former partner, spouse, or family member threatens or harasses a person. The stalker often makes it clear that the victim is his "property." The stalker is usually motivated by a desire to continue the relationship, which can evolve into an attitude of "If I can't have her/him, no one can." In some cases the stalker is angry and retaliating against the victim, whom he perceives as rejecting him. Frequently, there is a history of domestic violence, and the stalking often ends in a violent attack on, or killing of, the victim.

Cycle of Violence

Domestic violence is the deliberate and systematic pattern of abuse used to gain control over the victim. The behavior is always intentional. Perpetrators choose to be violent and give themselves permission to be violent. Perpetrators are not out of control, as is commonly assumed. They may be enraged or cool and calculating, but in either case they have made a choice. The victim cannot "make them do it." Generally,

perpetrators of domestic violence are law-abiding citizens who are dangerous only to their loved ones.

To the victim, domestic violence often happens without warning and without a buildup of tension. A pattern of violence usually develops. The first incident may be precipitated by frustration or stress. If the victim immediately refuses to accept the violence and seeks outside help, there are often no further episodes. If the victim submits to the violence, then physical force, without the stimulus of frustration or stress, becomes a way of relating, and the pattern becomes resistant to change. A typical cycle occurs when conflict escalates into a violent episode, after which the perpetrator begs for the victim's forgiveness. The victim stays in the system because of promises to reform. With the next episode of conflict, the cycle of violence begins again and becomes part of the family dynamics.

Violent people are often extremely jealous and possessive. They view other family members in terms of property and ownership. Abusers use violence in an attempt to prove to themselves and others that they are superior and in control. Their use of physical force temporarily obliterates their sense of inadequacy and compensates for a lack of internal resources.

The abuser is the most powerful person in the life of the abused. The abuser's purpose is to enslave the victim, while simultaneously demanding respect, gratitude, and love. Control over the victim is established by repetitive emotional abuse that instills terror and helplessness. Threats of serious harm or threats against other family members keep the victim in a constant state of fear.

In order to have complete domination, the abuser isolates the victim. She often is forced to give up work, friends, and family. He may stalk her, eavesdrop, and intercept letters and phone calls. Control and scrutiny of the victim's body and bodily functions, finances, and transportation further destroy her sense of autonomy. She is shamed and demoralized when told what to eat, when to sleep, what to wear, when to go to the bathroom, and so on. For a victim who has been deprived long enough, the hope of a meal, a bath, or a kind word can be a powerful reward. This ongoing abusive behavior is punctuated by unpredictable outbursts of physical violence. Such domestic captivity of women, along with traumatic bonding to the abuser, often goes unrecognized. Recognize also that some abusers may adopt only one or two of these behaviors.

Victims can be further immobilized by feelings of anxiety and depression. Feelings of self-blame may be expressed in such statements as "If I hadn't talked back to my mother, she wouldn't have hit me," and "If I were a better wife, he wouldn't beat me." Guilt can contribute to depression, which further immobilizes victims and keeps them from leaving or seeking help for the family system.

Fear contributes to women's inability to leave abusive relationships. Often threatened with death at the idea of leaving, they live in fear of physical reprisal. Fearing loneliness, some women may believe that being in a bad relationship is better than being alone, and leaving the relationship would not necessarily ensure the end of the abuse. They may become dependent and believe they are incapable of "making it on my own."

The abuser is often most dangerous when threatened or faced with separation. The following clinical example illustrates the tragic outcome in one situation.

Clinical Example

Sandy, age 20, met Jack at work. In the beginning of their dating relationship, Jack bought her small gifts and said sweet things to her. He told Sandy he'd never loved anyone else as much. Sandy believed him, quickly fell in love, and moved in with Jack. Several months later she called her parents from work and begged them to come and get her. Sandy told them that she didn't like the relationship with Jack but she didn't know how to get out of it. Jack had taken over Sandy's life, even controlling the use of the car her parents had helped her buy. He followed her everywhere and rarely let her out of his sight.

Sandy insisted on returning to the apartment that night to get her car, telling her parents that Jack was not a violent person. However, Jack brutally beat her for having called her parents. Sandy moved back home and began trying to put her life back together. Even so, Jack continued to make harassing phone calls to Sandy. Because she had moved out so quickly, there were still financial matters she and Jack needed to clear up, so Sandy agreed to meet with him one evening. But instead of allowing her to end their 16-month relationship, Jack pulled out a gun and shot Sandy once in the back of the head.

For a partial list of reasons people remain in abusive relationships, see Box 24-1.

Fear also contributes to the inability to leave a partner in an abusive gay or lesbian relationship. Because many couples share close friends within the same community, victims may fear shaming their partners. They may also fear that friends will either deny the problem or take the abuser's side. Homophobia contributes to the victim's reluctance to seek help. Calling the police may result in ridicule or hostile responses from the officers. Victims may not seek help from family members to avoid reinforcing negative stereotypes about homosexuality, which might exacerbate the family's homophobia.

BIOPSYCHOSOCIAL THEORIES

Domestic violence is easy to describe but difficult to explain. There is no single cause of this type of violence. It results from an interaction of neurobiologic, personality, situational, and societal factors that have an impact on families.

Neurobiologic Theory

Neurobiologic theorists propose that genes and neurotransmitters may contribute to causing violent behavior. Although a genetic predisposition may make certain behaviors more likely, it does not make them inevitable. Serotonin (5-HT) plays an important role in mood and aggressive behavior. 5-HT calms us through inhibitory control over aggression. Abnormally low levels of 5-HT result in a lack of control, loss of temper, and explosive rage.

Childhood abuse and neglect lead to permanent alterations in the parts of the central nervous system that are known to be stress responsive. Corticotropin-releasing factor (CRF) is a major regulator of the endocrine, autonomic, immune, and behavioral stress responses. It is thought that stress early in life results in sensitization of the brain to even mild stressors in adulthood, thus contributing to mood and anxiety disorders long after the abuse or neglect has stopped. As a result, changes in the way CRF performs its function make it more difficult for the adult to cope with stress.

Intrapersonal Theory

Intrapersonal theory suggests that the cause of violence lies in the personality of the abuser. It is thought that people who are violent are unable to control their impulsive expressions of anger and hostility. As many as 80% of male abusers grew up in homes in which they were abused or observed their mothers being abused. With these family dynamics, the child sees the father as frightening and intimidating and sees the mother as helpless and nonprotective. This early emotional deprivation contributes to the formation of an adult who has an excessive need for nurturing and support. He comes to adult relationships with unrealistic demands for time and attention. As the relationship develops, he discourages his partner's relationships with other people because of his low self-esteem and fear of abandonment.

Box 24-1 Why Do They Stay? Why Do They Go Back?

Fear: Victims are afraid of physical reprisal if they resist, of being found and beaten again, and of their children being hurt. Those who attempt to leave risk suffering worse violence and even death.

Learned helplessness: Victims believe they have no choices and no control; they have come to believe that violence is an acceptable way of life.

Traumatic bonding: Victims stay loyal in the relationship, hoping and searching for meaning in the indifference and abuse. Traumatic bonding results from alternating good and bad treatment; the victim has no sense of autonomy and puts energy into keeping the relationship intact.

Emotional dependence: Victims are convinced they are weak, inferior, and do not deserve better treatment; they are insecure about their potential autonomy.

Financial dependence: Victims may not have a source of income; if the abuser is arrested, he may lose his job and the family will have no income. Victims have been taught that they must be submissive in exchange for financial support.

Guilt and/or shame: Victims have been convinced that they provoked the abuse. They feel guilt over the failure of the relationship or shame for remaining in the relationship despite the abuse. They may feel pressured by family, religious, or cultural values against divorce or separation.

Isolation: Victims have few, if any, friends; little support from family; and/or no car, phone, or mail.

Children: Victims may believe two parents are better than one. They may be threatened with loss of custody; the abuser may threaten to harm or kidnap the children.

Hope: Victims hope that if they change in the way the abuser wants them to, the abuse will stop. They hope the abuser will keep his promise to stop the assaults.

Social Learning Theory

Social learning theory proposes that violence is a learned behavior and people are conditioned to respond aggressively and violently. Children learn about violence from observing it, from being victims, and/or from behaving violently themselves. If the use of violence is rewarded by a gain in power, the behavior is reinforced. If there is immediate negative reinforcement within the family, a decrease in violent behavior will result. Learning to abuse is the first step in the battering process, but it does not necessarily lead vulnerable individuals to abuse. The social environment affects how the potentially abusive person behaves: The person must have the *opportunity to abuse* without suffering negative consequences. He has the perception that he can "get away with it." Although learning may have occurred and opportunity is present, the potentially abusive person makes a *conscious choice* to abuse. The batterer is solely responsible for the violence.

In addition to family models, the media provide many models of violence to which children are exposed. Some movies and television shows demonstrate that "good" people use force to achieve "good" ends. Many of the stories make no attempt to justify the use of force for "good" ends; they simply present endless, senseless acts of cruelty by one human being upon another—violence without consequences. With these types of family and media examples, children develop values that tolerate, and even accept as normal, everyday violence between people.

Gender Bias Theory

The sexist structure of the family and society is an important factor in domestic violence. It is a common belief that men have the right to keep women subordinate through power and privilege (Duran, Moya, & Megias, 2010). If there is nothing to contradict this ethos within the family system, then reaching the goal of maintaining female subordinance will be accomplished using any means possible. Domestic violence is a way to promote that goal, because it uses the power automatically granted a male in that family system. Victims are sometimes labeled as codependent in the abusive relationship, but such labeling is just another way of blaming the victim for the abuse.

The economic system helps entrap women, who are often forced to choose between poverty and abuse. It is often difficult for women to find advocates and solutions within the male-dominated legal, religious, mental health, and medical systems. Society sanctions male violence by neglecting female victims. The ultimate outcome of the cycle of abuse from which women cannot extricate themselves is that they become a built-in, ready target. Statistics validate this outcome by documenting that women are being murdered on a regular basis, not by strangers, but by husbands and lovers.

NURSING PROCESS
Intrafamily Physical Abuse

Addressing abuse that occurs within the family system requires an approach that is sensitive and effective.

Assessment

Nurses in all clinical settings must routinely assess clients for evidence of intrafamily violence. Considering how extensive this problem is, ask one or two introductory questions of every client. In assessing a child, say, for example, "Moms and dads try to help their children learn how to behave well. What happens to you when you do something wrong?" Or ask, "What is the worst punishment you ever received?" In assessing adults, you may begin with this approach: "One of the sources of stress in our lives is family disagreement. Could you describe how disagreements affect you? What happens when you disagree?" If the responses to these questions are indicative of violence, conduct a more in-depth nursing assessment. Guidelines for assessment are given in Your Assessment Approach nursing history tool.

Nursing Diagnosis: NANDA

The most important outcome of nursing assessment is identifying the existence of domestic violence. You must give priority to critical and serious physical injuries. Consider the severity and potential fatality of the situation, as well as the needs of dependent children and legal issues surrounding the case. Consider the following nursing diagnoses when analyzing your assessment data:

- Disabled Family Coping related to an inability to manage conflict without violence
- Ineffective Coping related to being a victim of violence
- Impaired Parenting related to the physical abuse of children
- Powerlessness related to feelings of being dependent on the abuser
- Situational Low Self-Esteem related to feeling guilty and responsible for being a victim
- Social Isolation related to shame about family violence
- Risk for Other-Directed Violence related to a history of the use of physical force within the family

Outcome Identification: NOC

Achievement of the following outcome criteria is evidence that the intervention plan was successful. The victims have:

- Recognized that they are not to blame for the violence of others
- Ended the denial and minimization of domestic violence
- Demonstrated an awareness of their own strengths, skills, and competence
- Re-established a sense of power over their own lives
- Verbalized their right to express their own needs and to satisfy them
- Established social networks to decrease isolation and secrecy

---

YOUR ASSESSMENT APPROACH   **Nursing History Tool for Assessing Victims of Family Violence**

Behavioral Assessment

- Tell me about how people communicate within your family.
- What types of things cause conflict within your family?
- How is conflict managed or resolved?
- Who in your family loses control of themselves when angry?
- Have you received verbal threats of harm?
- Have you ever been threatened with a knife or gun?
- What happens to you when a family member has violent outbursts? Are you slapped? Hit? Punched? Thrown? Shoved? Kicked? Burned? Beaten up?
- Who in your family has needed emergency medical treatment?
- In what ways have you attempted to stop the violence?
- Have you attempted to leave the situation in the past?
- What happened when you attempted to leave?
- Describe the use of alcohol in your family.
- Describe the use of drugs in your family.

Affective Assessment

- Who do you think is responsible for the use of physical force within your family?
- In what way is this person(s) responsible?
- How much guilt are you experiencing at this time?
- Tell me about your fears. Lack of security? Financial problems? Child care problems? Living apart from your spouse? Further physical injury?
- What factors contribute to your feeling of helplessness to leave or stop the abuse?
- How hopeless do you feel about your situation?
- How would you describe your level of depression?

Cognitive Assessment

- Describe your strengths and abilities as a person.
- If you were describing yourself to a stranger, what would you say?
- What are your beliefs about keeping your family together?
- Tell me about your reasons for remaining in this situation. Promises of reform? Material rewards?
- Do you believe or hope the violence will not recur?
- What are your expectations of how children should behave?
- What rights do parents have with their children?
- What rights do spouses have with each other?
- What are the rules about physical force within your family?

Sociocultural Assessment

- How did your parents relate to each other?
- Who enforced discipline when you were a child?
- What type of discipline was used when you were a child?
- What was/is your relationship like with your mother?
- What was/is your relationship like with your father?
- How did you get along with your siblings?
- In your present family, who is the head of the household?
- How are decisions made in your family?
- How are household jobs assigned in your family?
- Describe recent and current stresses on your family. Unemployment? Financial problems? Illness? New family members? Deaths or separations? Child-rearing problems? Change in job status? Increase in conflict? Change in residence?
- To whom can you turn for support in times of stress?
- Describe your social life.
- What types of contact have you had with the legal system? Phoned police? Obtained an order of protection? Obtained a lawyer? Court cases? Protective services?

Planning and Implementation: NIC

Most victims of domestic violence would like it to end, but they may not know how to seek the help they need. It is extremely important that you be nonjudgmental in your interactions with all family members. Initially, clients may be unwilling to trust you because of family shame and fear of being judged for remaining in the violent relationship. It is vital that you not impose your own values by offering quick and easy solutions to the very complicated problem of domestic violence. Your Self-Awareness and Partnering With Clients and Families will help you to debunk myths about family violence and understand your own feelings and attitudes.

The treatment of families experiencing violence requires a multidisciplinary approach, with a broad range of interventions. Nurses, social workers, physicians, family therapists, vocational trainers, police, protective services personnel, and lawyers must coordinate to intervene effectively in a situation of intrafamily violence.

In the initial contact with family members, ensure their physical safety as much as possible. It is critical to assess the level of danger for the victim; homicide may be a real possibility if previous threats have been made. Also assess the level of danger for the abuser. The severity and duration of the violence are the factors that contribute most directly to victims killing their abusers in self-defense. If the level of danger is high, contact protective services or the police for emergency custody placement or removal to a shelter.

YOUR SELF-AWARENESS
Working With Victims of Domestic Violence

Take some time to think about and consider your reactions to the following questions:

- Is American culture violent compared to other cultures?
- The United States was founded by violence. How has this influenced the values and behavior of present-day Americans?
- What is the difference between spanking a child and beating a child?
- Do you think the stalking laws are decreasing the level of violence in the United States?
- Are you for or against gun control?
- Would it be more difficult for a person to stab a family member than to shoot that person?

PARTNERING WITH CLIENTS AND FAMILIES

Teaching About Domestic Violence

Myths and Facts

Myth: Family violence is rare.

Fact: Every year, 10 million Americans are abused by a family member.

Myth: Family violence is confined to mentally disturbed or sick people.

Fact: Fewer than 10% of all cases involve an abuser who is mentally ill. The vast majority seem totally normal and are often charming, persuasive, and rational.

Myth: Violence is trivial—a joking matter.

Fact: A woman is beaten every 15 seconds in the United States, and 2,000 to 4,000 women are murdered by their husbands or boyfriends every year. Every year, 2.5 million children are abused, and 1,200 die from the abuse. There are 1 million cases of elder abuse annually.

Myth: Family violence is confined to the lower classes.

Fact: Social factors are not relevant. There are doctors, ministers, psychologists, and nurses who beat their family members. Violence occurs at least once in two thirds of all marriages.

Myth: All members of the family participate in the family dynamics; therefore, all must change in order for the violence to stop.

Fact: Only the perpetrator has the ability to stop the violence. A change in the victim's behavior will not cause the abuser to become nonviolent.

Myth: Family violence is usually a one-time event, an isolated incident.

Fact: Violence is a pattern, a reign of force and terror. It becomes more frequent and severe over time.

Myth: Abused women like being hit; otherwise, they would leave.

Fact: Abused women are forced to stay in the relationship for many reasons. The perpetrator dramatically escalates the violence when a woman tries to leave.

Providing Psychoeducation

Provide interventions to improve communication. Families experiencing violence often have poor communication skills. Teach active listening with feedback (see Chapter 10∞), clear and direct communication, and communication that does not attack the personhood of others.

Identify the normality of conflict within all families by discussing how disagreements are inevitable. From there, discuss the use of the democratic process in conflict resolution and decision making. It is best to practice with simple, unemotional family problems at first.

Help family members identify methods to manage anger appropriately. All family members must assume responsibility for their own behavior. They can practice talking about angry feelings as they occur. Make suggestions for appropriate expression, such as relaxation, physical exercise, and striking safe, inanimate objects (a pillow, a couch, or a punching bag). Guide the family in establishing limits and defining consequences if violence recurs. Emphasize that violence within the family will not be tolerated.

Help parents who are physically abusive develop and improve their parenting skills. Begin by recognizing their current positive parenting skills to increase their self-worth and help them engage in the learning process. Share your understanding that the use of violence is often a desperate attempt by parents to cope with their children. Confirming that they care about their children will increase the likelihood of their active participation in the treatment process.

Because domestic violence is often transgenerational, discuss with the parents how they were punished as children. Teach them about the normal growth and development of children. Unrealistic demands for children to comply beyond their developmental ability often result in violence. The first step in the problem-solving process is helping parents identify specific problems they experience with raising children. They can then go on to identify solutions, other than physical force, that are age-appropriate for their children. They need support in implementing, practicing, and evaluating these new skills.

Empowering Survivors One of the primary goals of therapy is the empowerment of victims. The process of violence removes all power and control from the victim, resulting in low self-esteem, anxiety, depression, and somatic problems. The following principles are basic to the empowerment of victims:

- A commitment to the belief that women and men are inherently equal
- An egalitarian approach to the nurse–client relationship: The client is viewed as an equal partner rather than a helpless recipient of nursing interventions.
- An emphasis on the victim's strengths and abilities
- Respect for the victim's ability to understand his or her own experiences
- An emphasis on altering destructive roles and expectations within the family system
- A willingness to state clear value positions about domestic violence

Through this approach, clients can become aware that they have choices in, and control over, their lives. Avoid trying to convince adult victims to leave their abuser. As difficult as it may be, you must be willing to support clients in their pain, rather than telling them what to do about their problems. For the most positive adaptive outcome, adult victims must be their own rescuers and take charge of their own safety and protection plan. If they need help with this process, teach them to ask for that help directly. This is not meant to imply in any way that you would abandon clients; rather, you stand by, support, and affirm the positive choices and decisions they make.

Help adult clients begin identifying ways in which they are dependent on their abusers. High levels of dependence make it difficult for victims to leave abusers without intense support. You can help them identify intrapersonal and interpersonal strengths to decrease their feelings of powerlessness. From there, clients can move on to identifying aspects of life that are under their control. Offer assertiveness training to help them develop new skills for relating to others in the future (see Chapters 3 and 35∞). If they are still in the abusive relationship, however, caution them that assertive behavior may escalate the violence.

Treating the Abuser

Most abusers do not seek treatment unless it is court ordered or there are custody issues involved. It is frustrating to intervene with abusers who deny the reality of, or responsibility for, the violence. Group therapy for abusers is sometimes helpful. The group setting is more effective than individual therapy because interactions with a number of people more successfully address the anger and control problems. The responsibility for aggression is always placed on the aggressor. Issues regarding the patriarchal and power views of relationships are discussed in great depth. Participants are asked to specify their abusive behaviors, identify the intentions behind those behaviors, and examine the effects of the abuse on their victims. Abusers learn that anger can be controlled and that violence is always a *choice*.

Evaluation

Nurses in acute care settings may not have the opportunity for long-term evaluation of the family system. Short-term evaluation focuses on the following:

1. The identification of domestic violence
2. The family's ability to recognize that a problem exists
3. The willingness of the family to accept assistance by following through with referrals
4. The removal of the victim from a volatile situation

Nurses in long-term settings or within the community have an opportunity to evaluate the effectiveness of the multidisciplinary treatment plan over an extended period of time. When violence no longer exists within the family system, the plan has succeeded. Sharing in the process of family growth and adaptation can be a tremendous source of professional satisfaction.

All nurses should evaluate their professional obligations and practice in counteracting those aspects of society that foster domestic violence. Domestic violence is a mental health problem of national and international importance, and we can be leaders in helping prevent it in future generations. Primary prevention includes the nursing interventions of parent education, family life education in schools, referral for appropriate child or elder care, establishment of support groups, and education of fellow nurses about the problem of domestic violence. It also includes community education about the pervasive effects of media violence on individuals and society. An example of a cultural perspective on domestic violence can be found at the website of the Institute on Domestic Violence in the African American Community (http://www.dvinstitute.org/).

Secondary prevention of domestic violence includes working with children who are victims or who have seen their mothers beaten, and making referrals for multidisciplinary intervention. Nurses must be community advocates in supporting hotlines, crisis centers, and shelters for victims of domestic violence. On the political level, nurses must make their voices heard in regard to policies and laws affecting children, women, and older people. Questions to guide the evaluation of nursing practice and the extent of your advocacy activities include the following:

- Have I, as a nurse, assessed each client for possible abuse?
- What actions have I taken to decrease violence in the media?
- Have I considered the issue of gun control?
- Have I confronted the use of physical punishment within families?
- Have I volunteered to teach parenting classes at grade schools and high schools?
- Have I written to legislators to protest funding cuts in programs designed to help children, women, and older people?
- Have I spoken out on the need to increase the number of bilingual/bicultural counselors, lawyers, nurses, and physicians to attend to the needs of ethnic families?

CASE MANAGEMENT

Case managers coordinate care for victims of domestic violence. The goal is to focus on the immediate problems. Intervention is directed toward developing rapport with the victim, clarifying the presenting problems, and enhancing the victim's existing problem-solving ability. Safety of the victim(s) is of primary importance. Once safety is ensured, case management interventions include the following:

- Identification of effective and ineffective coping skills
- Emphasis on victim's strengths and abilities
- Development of problem-solving skills and new coping behaviors
- Identification of available support systems
- Group therapy with other victims and survivors of domestic violence
- Evaluation of the effectiveness of new coping strategies (Burriss, Breland-Noble, Webster, & Soto, 2011; McCloskey & Bulechek, 1996)

Although necessary, case management services present certain issues. Unless attention is paid to the contexts of the problems, these marginalized women's complex needs will be ill-served. A more holistic approach to case management can ease overall struggling (Graham-Bermann, Sularz, & Howell, 2011; Smyth, Goodman, & Glenn, 2006).

COMMUNITY-BASED CARE

Prevention of child abuse is a community function that involves the identification of risk factors and crisis intervention. Risk factors include the following:

- Parents who were abused as children
- Adult relationship dysfunction
- Poor self-esteem
- Social isolation
- Unrealistic expectations of children's abilities
- Having a child with special needs

Interventions are geared toward improving adult–adult relationships as well as adult–child relationships. Helping families connect with other families decreases their sense of isolation. Parenting classes help families develop realistic expectations of their children according to developmental levels. It is very important that families of special-needs children be referred to appropriate support groups.

Prevention of elder abuse involves supporting older individuals and caretakers in identifying and expanding social support networks. Community resources may be able to help with activities of daily living (ADLs), transportation, financial advice, and assistance with personal problems. Assist the caretakers in exploring their feelings about the older people in their care. Help them identify factors that are disturbing to them and that may contribute to neglect or abuse. Determine the caretakers' ability to meet their loved one's needs, and provide appropriate teaching. Provide community resource information, including addresses and phone numbers of agencies that offer senior service assistance.

The federal Gun Control Act of 1968 prohibits anyone who has been convicted of a felony from owning or possessing a firearm or ammunition. The 1996 amendment to the Act prohibits anyone who has been convicted of a misdemeanor involving domestic violence from owning or possessing a firearm or ammunition. There are no exceptions to this law, including police or military personnel. Violation of this Act results in 10 years in prison and a fine of $250,000. Victims of domestic violence should be able to turn to the police and have their perpetrator arrested. This law, however, has been difficult to enforce.

HOME CARE

Nurses involved in home care can help women develop a "safe plan" or an "escape plan" to use when their safety is threatened. They should plan a quick, safe exit from their home and have a safe place to go once they do leave. The plan should be easy and complete, and it must be taught to their children. As part of the plan, you may suggest that they have all important documents (such as birth certificates and orders of protection), some money, a list of important phone numbers, and a couple of days' clothing gathered in one secure location. They should have a second set of car keys so they can leave quickly if the need arises.

INTRAFAMILY VIOLENCE: SEXUAL ABUSE

Childhood sexual abuse is a major health problem in the United States. The majority of cases are probably unreported. **Sexual abuse** is defined as inappropriate sexual behavior, instigated by a perpetrator, for the purpose of the perpetrator's sexual pleasure or economic gain through child prostitution or pornography. Behavior ranges from exhibitionism, peeping, explicit sexual talk, touching, caressing, masturbation, oral sex, vaginal sex, and anal sex to forcing children to engage in sex with one another or with animals.

Health care professionals, as well as families, have used denial to cope with ambiguous evidence of the cultural taboos of incest and sex with children. (Use Your Self-Awareness to help understand your own feelings and attitudes.) In order to respond appropriately to cues that signal sexual abuse, you need to understand the characteristics and dynamics of families involved. A note of caution, however: With the recent increased publicity about the prevalence of child sexual abuse, there is a real danger of jumping to conclusions; any hint or accusation of sexual abuse may be interpreted as absolute proof of guilt. Rumors and false accusations have destroyed individuals and families. You must assess carefully and maintain a balance between the extremes of denial and automatic belief of guilt (Everson & Sandoval, 2011).

Sexually abused children and adult survivors of childhood sexual abuse (hereafter called *adult survivors*) are crying out for help. A few cry out loudly in protest, but most cry inwardly in silence. It is thought that as many as one in three girls and one in seven boys are sexually abused before the age of 18. Many of these are single, isolated incidents. Boys are more frequently molested outside the family system than are girls. Adolescent males who sexually abuse tend to have been sexually abused as children and were exposed to trauma and pornography at young ages (Burton, Duty, & Leibowitz, 2011).

Sexual abuse occurs in all ethnic, religious, economic, and cultural subgroups. Affinity systems—immediate family, relatives, friends, neighbors, clergy, scout leaders—account for 75% to 90% of the abusers. Male perpetrators are involved in 90% of reported cases. Although father–daughter incest

---

YOUR SELF-AWARENESS
Working With Victims of Child Sexual Abuse

Take some time to think about and consider your reactions to the following questions:

- Do you think the rate of child sexual abuse is increasing, or is there just better reporting?
- Do you think sex education can decrease the rate of sexual abuse?
- Which situation do you think is more devastating in child sexual abuse—when force is used or when no force is used?
- Does the fact that most perpetrators were sexually abused as children excuse their behavior? What if the perpetrator is only 11 years old?
- Far fewer women than men are accused of sexually abusing their children. How do you explain this?
- What needs to be done to decrease the incidence of child sexual abuse?

is most reported, it is believed that sibling incest is the most widespread. Some siblings turn to each other for emotional nurturance and acceptance. In other instances, a sibling uses coercion or violence to perpetrate the abuse. More than 41% of sexual assaults occurred in or near the victim's home and 41% of sexual assaults were reported to law enforcement (National Center for Victims of Crime, 2008; Murphy, Potter, Stapleton, Wiesen-Martin, & Pierce-Weeks, 2010).

Types of Offenders

Some offenders prefer girls, others prefer boys, and some abuse both, as long as the victim is a child. Some are interested in adolescents or preteens, some in toddlers, and some in infants. Some offenders do not abuse until they are adults, but more than half start in their teens.

Juvenile Offenders

Many, if not most, cases involving juvenile offenders are unreported. Family members often want to protect and shield the young offender. Sometimes the behavior is rationalized as adolescent male experimentation. Between 50% and 60% of juvenile offenders were sexually abused as children; they gradually develop offending behaviors as they reach adolescence. The other 40% to 50% show fairly high rates of other delinquent behaviors, and most are diagnosed with conduct disorder. Those offenders who were child victims tend to begin abusing at a younger age, to have more victims, and to have male victims when compared with nonabused teen sex offenders. Juvenile offenders may seek victims within or outside the family system. The type of sexual offense often parallels their own experiences of abuse. The most frequent offense is sexual touching, which often escalates to rape and other sex crimes.

Male Offenders

One research study focusing on fathers who abused their daughters established the following five types of incestuous fathers (Greenberg, Firestone, Nunes, Bradford, & Curry, 2005; Schetky, 1999):

1. *Sexually preoccupied abusers* (26% of the fathers) have a conscious and often obsessive sexual interest in their daughters. Many of them regard their daughters as sex objects, in some cases as early as birth. Stepfathers were more sexually aroused by their stepdaughters than biologic fathers, although this was the only difference between the two groups.
2. *Adolescent regressors* (33% of the fathers) become sexually interested in their pubescent daughters. These men sound and act like adolescents around their daughters.
3. *Self-gratifiers* (20% of the fathers) are not sexually attracted to their daughters per se, and during the abuse, they fantasize about someone else. In effect, they are simply using their daughters' bodies.
4. *Emotional dependents* (10% of the fathers) see themselves as failures and feel lonely and depressed. They see their daughters as romantic figures in their lives.
5. *Angry retaliators* (10% of the fathers) abuse out of anger, either at the daughter or at the mother. This type of offender is most likely to have a criminal history of assault and rape.

Female Offenders

Female perpetrators are now less likely to be overlooked and commit between 3% and 13% of sexual abuse cases. The most common types of sexual abuse by women are fondling, oral sex, and group sex.

Female offenders fall into the following four major types:

1. Teacher–lovers are older women who teach children about lovemaking.
2. Experimenter–exploiters are often girls who have had no sex education growing up. Babysitting is often an opportunity to explore younger children. Many of the girls in this group do not even realize what they are doing or that it is inappropriate.
3. Predisposers usually come from a family with a long history of physical and sexual abuse. These families have been dysfunctional over many generations.
4. Women coerced by males abuse children because men have forced them to abuse. Usually, they have been victims as children and are easily manipulated and intimidated.

There is agreement that there is sex abuse in the female perpetrator's history (Tsopelas, Spyridoula, & Athanosios, 2011; McCloskey & Raphael, 2005).

Abusive Behavior Patterns

Typically, adult perpetrators initiate sexual behavior in a manipulative or coercive manner. Often, the adult misrepresents the abuse as a game or "fun" activity. The behavior usually follows a progression of sexual activity, from exposure and fondling to oral, vaginal, and/or anal sex. Secrecy is imposed on the child by persuasion or threat. The abuser may make threatening statements such as those in Box 24-2. Secrecy and silence are used by abusers to escape accountability. When secrecy fails and the child victims or adult survivors begin to talk to others about the abuse, perpetrators usually attack the credibility of the victims and try to make sure no one will listen. Other perpetrators acknowledge the abuse but minimize the impact, while some use the defense mechanism of projection and blame the child for the abuse. Your awareness of the trauma and the effects of these experiences will help you assess more accurately (Sarmiento, 2011).

Child Victims

Children know that adults have absolute power over them, so they obey. When they have been threatened with abandonment or harm, they frequently choose to protect others. When asked, "Why didn't you tell sooner?" the answers are, "I didn't know who to tell," "I was scared," and/or "I did tell and no one believed me."

Children often feel responsible for the adult's behavior and ashamed that they have not been able to stop the abuse.

Box 24-2   Typical Threatening Statements by Sexual Abusers

To Obtain Secrecy and Silence

- "If you tell, you'll be sent away."
- "If you tell, I won't love you anymore."
- "If you tell, I will kill you."
- "If you tell, I'll do the same thing to your baby brother."

To Attack the Victim's Credibility

- "It never happened, she's lying."
- "He's exaggerating some innocent touching."

To Acknowledge the Abuse While Minimizing the Impact

- "Better for her to learn about sex from her father than from some horny teenager."
- "She didn't really mind; in fact, we have a very close relationship."
- "Even if it did happen, it's time to forget the past and move on."

To Use the Defense Mechanism of Projection and Blame the Child

- "She's a very provocative child, and she seduced me."
- "If he hadn't enjoyed it so much, I wouldn't have kept doing it."

This is her description of the abuse: "Whenever I was alone with him in the car, he would fondle me and expose his penis to me. He would tell me I could touch it, it would be all right.

So much of the time I tried to block everything out—it's hard for me to recall exactly what happened. Some of the things I remember clearly. I remember Grandpa's easy chair. When we were alone he would make me sit on his lap in that chair, and he would stick his fingers in me. This happened many times. One time he parked in an isolated area and played with me and made me touch him and kiss his penis. He tried to coax me to have intercourse. He told me it wouldn't hurt. But I cried and he masturbated into his handkerchief instead. He made me promise never to tell anyone.

He always bought me things or gave me money. I remember the day he died. I came home from school and when my mom told me, I cried. But deep down I was glad. I was really safe from him now. And I hated him for hurting me and making me tell lies all the time."

Secrecy and guilt keep these children isolated, causing them to feel alienated from their peers. They may act out sexually by initiating oral or genital sex with other children or adults. The feeling of powerlessness is extremely potent because what the victim says and does makes no difference. If the abuser has an adult partner who does not protect the child, the child may receive the message that this behavior is normal. When the child's repressed rage comes to the surface, it may be directed against the self in self-defeating and self-destructive ways, such as substance abuse, high-risk sexual behavior, and suicide (Champion, 2011; Denton, Newton, & Vandeven, 2011).

Adolescent victims may run away from home to escape an intolerable situation. Because they have learned, at home, that sexual behavior is rewarded by affection, love, and attention, some turn to prostitution. Others are forced into prostitution as a way to support themselves while living on the streets.

Some child victims use denial to cope with the trauma. Acknowledging the abuse would mean acknowledging that the world is dangerous and that those who are supposed to protect and nurture failed instead and caused harm. Other victims minimize the impact, saying things like "It's not so bad; it only happens once a month" or "It's all right because it stopped when I was 11 years old." The following clinical example illustrates the impact on one child victim.

Clinical Example

Sonja describes her current sexual life as one of promiscuity and relates this to being sexually molested from age 4 through age 7 by her grandfather.

Frequently, dissociation is the victim's major defense. The mind is "separated" from the body so the victim is not emotionally present during the sexual attack. Dissociation is evidenced by such statements as "I put myself in the wall, where he couldn't reach all of me" and "When he would come into my room, I would close my eyes and go to my favorite place. Only my body stayed on the bed; the rest of me wasn't there." When sexual abuse is severe and sadistic, the victim may develop dissociative identity disorder (DID). DID is discussed in Chapter 22 ∞.

Adult Survivors

Many adult survivors continue to believe that they were to blame for the abuse and should have been able to resist the adult. This self-blame often contributes to depression, anxiety, panic attacks, and low self-esteem. They feel worthless and different from other people. For some, anger is the only emotion experienced and expressed; all other feelings are repressed. Many adult survivors continue to hate their perpetrators, as well as the nonabusing significant adults who did not protect them.

Sexual Difficulties

Adult survivors may believe they are only sex objects, to be used and abused by others. Some have a very strong aversion to sex and are filled with terror in sexual situations. Some are sexually inhibited and experience discomfort with sexual thoughts, feelings, and behaviors. Some engage in compulsive sexual behavior, perhaps as an unconscious way to validate their shame and guilt, or as a way to feel powerful. Many adult survivors go through a period of celibacy as they try to manage fear, anger, and distrust.

Confusion about sexuality is very common among male survivors. Sexual victimization of a male by a male carries a hidden implication that the victim is less than a man. Heterosexual survivors fear that the abuse has made, or will make, them homosexual. Intense homophobia and/or hypermasculine behavior may be an effort to disprove their fears. Gay survivors worry that their sexual preference may have caused the abuse. Remember that childhood sexual abuse is not related to adult sexual orientation.

Self-Mutilation

Some adult survivors engage in *self-mutilation,* as in cutting, slashing, or burning themselves. It is important to understand the meaning of such behavior. For some, the pain of self-mutilation proves their existence and reassures them that they are alive and real. Self-mutilation may be a plea for nurturance, because they come to the emergency department seeking care. Others nurture themselves by cleaning up the wounds after self-mutilation. For those who dissociate, self-mutilation may be a way to stop the dissociation, to focus on the here-and-now with physical pain. Others self-mutilate as a form of self-punishment and a way to decrease guilt feelings. And finally, some self-mutilate as a way to reduce emotional pain through the feeling of physical pain. It is important to understand the function of the behavior in order to replace it with healthier behaviors that satisfy the same need.

Memory of Sexual Abuse

Research shows that many memories of past events are not reports but reconstructions. It is the difference between remembering facts and remembering events. What is remembered is the overall impression rather than the specific details. The details we add when we reconstruct our experience depend on our personality traits and cognitive styles. We may also create pseudomemories of events that never actually occurred, especially after being told of such "events" by trusted individuals. Reports of remembered child abuse in adults, therefore, should ideally be corroborated by other people. See Caring for the Spirit on page 154 in Chapter 8 ∞.

BIOPSYCHOSOCIAL THEORIES

There is no single cause of childhood sexual abuse. Rather, the abuse results from a combination of personality, family, and cultural factors.

Intrapersonal Theory

There are many types of perpetrators of sexual abuse of children. Some traits are contradictory, and there is no agreement on a composite personality. Certain characteristics apply to many people, not just abusers. The descriptions that follow are guidelines for assessment, not proof that the person actually committed sexual abuse:

1. Perpetrators usually have low self-esteem and feel more secure in interactions with children than with adults.
2. Some were emotionally deprived as children and thus have a great need for constant, unconditional love, which is more easily obtained from children than from adults.
3. Some perpetrators are described as lacking impulse control and the ability to experience feelings of guilt.
4. Some are described as rigid and overcontrolled, while others are dominant and aggressive.

If perpetrators were sexually abused themselves as children, they may have learned to associate all feelings of love with sexual behavior. Most people who were sexually abused as children do not go on to sexually abuse others. Some victimized children, however, develop offending behavior in late childhood, adolescence, or adulthood. Most likely, there are a number of factors involved in why some abuse and others do not. The world of abuse is comprised only of victims (powerless) and perpetrators (powerful). Victims become perpetrators in an unconscious attempt to master the trauma of their own experiences and retrieve power. The move from victim to offender may also result when anger and hostility concerning the past are externalized and projected onto new victims.

Family Systems Theory

Intrafamily sexual abuse most typically occurs in families that have difficulty with structure, cohesion, adaptability, and communication.

Family structure is usually hierarchical according to age, roles, and distribution of power. Typically, the adults, who are older, assume the parental roles and are the most influential. The structure of incestuous families, however, is often quite different as the result of dysfunctional boundary patterns. An adult may move "down" in the structure or a child may move "up" in terms of roles and influence (boundaries). If the father moves downward, he assumes a childlike role and is cared for and nurtured like a child in the family. In this position, the father assumes little parental responsibility. He may then turn to the daughter as a "peer" for sexual and emotional gratification.

As another example, the daughter may move upward and replace the mother in the hierarchy. The mother does not usually move downward but rather moves out of the structure by distancing herself emotionally or physically from the family. As the daughter assumes the parental role and responsibilities, the father may turn to her for fulfillment of his emotional and sexual needs.

Families that are enmeshed—that is, the members are immersed in and absorbed by one another—may be at risk for sexual abuse. In addition, incestuous families tend to be either rigid or chaotic in their adaptability. Rigid family systems have strict rules and stereotyped gender-role expectations, with minimal emotional interaction. Children have no power or authority, even over their own bodies. They are not allowed to question or protest inappropriate sexual behavior. In contrast, chaotic family systems have either no rules or constantly changing rules. Within the chaotic system, there may be no assigned roles or no rules regarding appropriate sexual behavior, which may contribute to the incidence of sexual abuse. Enmeshed and rigid family structures and family dynamics are discussed in Chapter 29 ∞.

Communication patterns within the family system may contribute to the occurrence of sexual abuse. Incest depends on keeping the secret within the family. In family systems that avoid conflict, accusations of sexual abuse are not tolerated. Peace, and therefore silence, must be kept at all costs.

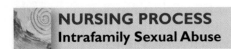

NURSING PROCESS
Intrafamily Sexual Abuse

A nursing care plan for an adult survivor of childhood sexual abuse is at the end of the chapter.

Assessment

It is vitally important that you acknowledge the reality of childhood sexual abuse. Nurses who deny the existence of the problem will miss the cues and fail to complete a detailed assessment. If you are knowledgeable about the incidence and

YOUR ASSESSMENT APPROACH   Nursing History Tool for Assessment of Individuals and Families for Intrafamily Sexual Abuse

Behavioral Assessment
Individual Child

- Have there been any signs of regressive behavior in the child?
- Is the child having sleeping problems?
- Is the child exhibiting clinging behavior to the parents or others?
- Does the child have friendships with other children?
- Has there been any sexual acting-out on the part of the child?
- Has the child ever run away or threatened to run away?
- Has the child ever attempted suicide?

Perpetrator

- Describe how discipline is handled in the family.
- Do you see yourself as the dominant person in the family?
- At what age do you believe parents should give up control of their children?
- How many adult friends do you have?
- Describe your relationships with these friends.
- Describe your relationship with your spouse.
- What kinds of sexual difficulties are you and your spouse experiencing?
- When you were young, who was the closest family member with whom you had any sexual activity?

Family System

- Describe who has responsibility (mother, father, both parents, or children) in the following areas of home management:
  - Caring for the younger children
  - Cooking
  - Cleaning
  - Paying bills
  - Shopping
  - Outside home maintenance
  - Budget planning
  - Decisions about leisure time
  - Supervising children's homework
  - Taking children to activities
  - Putting children to bed
- Who are the best communicators in the family?
- Who talks to whom the most?
- Who is unable to talk to whom very much?
- How are secrets kept from one another within the family?
- How are secrets prevented from leaking outside the family?

Affective Assessment
Individual Child

- How helpless does the child feel about changing any of the family's problems?
- Does the child feel responsible for family problems?
- Does the child get enough love within the family?
- Is the child more loved than the other children in the family?

- Ask about the fears the child may have if any family secrets are told:
  - Fear of not being believed
  - Fear of being blamed for the problems
  - Fear that your parents will not love you
  - Fear that you will be moved to a foster home
  - Fear that your parents will be taken away
  - Fear of physical abuse

Perpetrator

- Who loves you most within the family?
- Who is able to give you unconditional support and affection?
- Do you see yourself as responsible for family problems?
- How does fear of failure affect your life?

Family System

- Describe the emotional relationships among family members.
- Does everybody know each family member's business?
- How is privacy protected within the family?
- Do you have any fears of the family unit disintegrating?
- What will happen if the family is separated?

Cognitive Assessment
Individual Child

- Tell me about your nightmares.
- How would you describe the family's problems?
- What effect do these problems have on you?
- What effect do these problems have on the rest of the family?
- Who do you believe is responsible for these problems?

Perpetrator

- Describe what kind of a person you are.
- What are your personal strengths?
- What are your personal limitations?
- Describe how you handle new situations.
- Do you enjoy changing situations?

Family System

- Who sets the family rules?
- Tell me about the most important family rules.
- How do rules get changed within the family?
- What are the expectations of the males in the family?
- What are the expectations of the females in the family?

Sociocultural Assessment

- What significant events have occurred for your family in the past year?
- What support systems do you have outside the family?
- How often do you visit with friends?
- Who are the problem drinkers in the family?
- How is the issue of drugs managed within the family?

Case Study: Assessing the Needs of a Victim of Sexual Abuse

characteristics of the problem, you will be alert for cues that demand nursing assessment. Guidelines for assessment are given in Your Assessment Approach.

When assessing children, remember that some will exhibit most of the symptoms presented in this chapter, others will exhibit only some, and still others will exhibit none. Also remember that these same behavioral, affective, and cognitive characteristics may be symptoms of other emotional problems. Once it has been discovered that one child in a family is a victim of sexual abuse, suspect the abuse of siblings, both boys and girls, as well. Sometimes entire families are sexually abused before someone "tells."

You must appreciate the power of secrecy and how difficult it is for adult survivors to disclose such information, especially for men, who, in our society, are expected to be anything other than victimized. Routine questions on nursing histories may provide an opportunity for survivors to share their pain and obtain treatment as adults. See Your Assessment Approach on conducting a physical assessment of a sexual abuse victim; the topics included may be easier for the survivor to discuss than details of the actual abuse.

Be responsible for initiating the topic. Shame and confusion may keep the adult survivor from doing so. If you avoid the topic, you will contribute to pathology by supporting the client's denial of reality. Failure to initiate a discussion of sexual abuse sends a message to clients that such abuse does not occur or does not matter. Now that childhood sexual abuse has been identified as a major health problem, nurses in every clinical setting must be alert for cues from both individuals and families.

When working with adult survivors, you must continuously assess the client's comfort level with the physical setting. Closed doors increase anxiety in some clients, while other clients request that doors never remain open. Some are uncomfortable in a room with a couch or a bed rather than chairs. How close you sit can be an issue for some clients. Even normally appropriate physical contact, such as a handshake, may increase anxiety. Always ask permission before touching a client.

YOUR ASSESSMENT APPROACH
Physical Assessment of the Sexual Abuse Victim

Complete a head-to-toe physical assessment with emphasis on the following:

- Weight and nutritional status
- Throat irritation
- Gag reflex
- Episodes of vomiting
- Abdominal pain near diaphragm
- Smears of the mouth, throat, vagina, and rectum for sexually transmitted infections
- Genital irritation or trauma
- Rectal irritation or trauma
- Chronic vaginal infections
- Chronic urinary tract infections
- Pregnancy

Nursing Diagnosis: NANDA

Based on assessment data, nursing diagnoses are formulated for the individual child victim, the family members, and/or the adult survivor. Possible diagnoses for the child victim include the following:

- Ineffective Individual Coping related to being a victim of sexual abuse
- Powerlessness related to being helpless to stop the abuse
- Post-Trauma Syndrome related to being a victim of sexual abuse
- Social Isolation related to keeping the family secret of sexual abuse

For families experiencing sexual abuse, some possible diagnoses are as follows:

- Compromised, Family Coping related to a child being sexually abused
- Disabled Family Coping related to an enmeshed family system that is either rigid or chaotic
- Impaired Parenting related to being a perpetrator of sexual abuse
- Dysfunctional Family Process related to disruption of the family unit when abuse is discovered

For adult survivors of childhood sexual abuse, some possible diagnoses are as follows:

- Post-Trauma Syndrome related to being an adult survivor
- Spiritual Distress related to issues about fairness and justice in life or not being protected by a supreme being
- Chronic Low Self-Esteem related to self-blame for the abuse
- Ineffective Denial related to amnesia for childhood events
- Social Isolation related to difficulty in forming intimate relationships, mistrust of others
- Sexual Dysfunction related to the trauma of abuse

Outcome Identification: NOC

Once you have established outcomes, you, the client, and the family mutually identify goals for change. Goals are specific behavioral measures by which you, clients, and significant others determine progress toward healing. The following are examples of some of the goals appropriate to people who have experienced childhood sexual abuse:

- Remains safe and free from harm
- Utilizes a variety of therapies to express feelings about the sexual abuse
- Verbalizes improved self-esteem
- Manages negative emotions in an appropriate manner
- Verbalizes a feeling of connectedness to significant others
- Verbalizes improvement in sexual functioning
- Utilizes community resources

Planning and Implementation: NIC

The first priority of care with child victims is to ensure the safety of the child. Nurses are mandated by law to report any suspected child sexual abuse. See the Case Management section for details on a plan.

When families are enmeshed and either rigid or chaotic, help family members move to a moderate position between the extremes. Teach the family the problem-solving process. With a rigid family, problem solve ways in which the members can increase their flexibility of roles and rules. With a chaotic family, problem solve ways to organize appropriate roles and formulate consistent rules. Seek out resources to creatively and effectively intervene in cases dealing with domestic violence (Hassija & Gray, 2011).

Working With Children

Facilitate the child's ability to talk and to think about the abuse with decreasing anxiety. Create a safe and predictable environment in which the child feels supported. Make it clear to the child that you understand that talking about the abuse is difficult.

Plan interventions that will encourage affective release in a supportive environment. Child victims must be able to experience a range of emotions. Play therapy helps these children play out traumatic themes, fears, and distorted beliefs. It is a nonthreatening way to process thoughts and feelings associated with the abuse, both symbolically and directly. Art therapy provides an opportunity to express feelings for which there are no words. Therapeutic stories present the traumatic issues of abuse, link victims' feelings and behavior, and describe new coping methods. Journal writing can help children over age 10 cope with intrusive thoughts and feelings. They often choose to bring their journal into the one–to–one sessions with their therapist.

Empowering Survivors

Because the process of sexual abuse is disempowering, it is important to empower survivors. The focus on traumatic stress therapy treats the trauma while acknowledging the process and result of victimization. Developmental therapy focuses on the "gaps" in the personality that occurred during the abusive process such as trust issues, identity issues, and relationship issues. Loss therapy focuses on helping the survivors identify and grieve over the things they have lost during their childhood sexual abuse such as innocence, trust, nurturing, and memories.

In working with adult survivors, remember that they have been robbed of a sense of power and feel detached from others. Recovery includes restoring power and control. Be sure to avoid becoming a "rescuer," as that might send the message that clients are not capable of acting for themselves. Your role as a nurse sets up a collaborative relationship, unlike a powerful authority relationship that occurred with the abuser. The most helpful approach is being an ally, partner, and supporter as clients struggle through the healing process. Point out instances in which they have taken control of their lives, and help them identify situations in which they are able to make self-respecting choices.

Supporting Spiritual Recovery

To recover from sexual abuse, survivors must place responsibility for the abuse where it belongs—100% with the offender. If they fail to do this, they will continue to be paralyzed by self-blame and guilt. For this reason, it is essential that you support the client's need for spiritual healing. Strategies for doing so are in Caring for the Spirit.

Increasing Self-Esteem

Design interventions to increase self-esteem. Adult survivors have a continuous internal monologue of negative statements such as "You're weak, stupid, incompetent, unlovable, and unattractive." Negative statements become self-administered abuse and keep the survivor weak and powerless. Help clients become aware of the frequency and intensity of these negative thoughts. Teach them to consciously replace negative thoughts with positive ones. While this is often difficult at first, it becomes easier with practice.

CARING FOR THE SPIRIT

Supporting Spiritual Recovery from Sexual Abuse

Betrayal by abusing adults is a spiritual issue. Therefore, be sure to acknowledge a client's need for spiritual healing. Victims and survivors are consumed with spiritual questions such as "Why did it happen to me?", "What's wrong with me?", and "Am I an evil person?" When people are sexually abused, they must struggle with questions of a God who either overlooked their pain and did not respond or did not even see their pain at all. Questions arise, such as "What's wrong with God?" and "Why didn't God stop it?" It is not unusual for survivors to be angry with God and hold God responsible for the abuse. This anger may in turn trigger fear and guilt for hating someone so powerful.

Spirituality includes a sense of connectedness to others. Survivors must begin the long journey of developing trusting relationships. The adult self needs to reach out and care for the hurt inner child by breaking down the walls that have isolated that child. Fully experiencing the rage and grief enables the survivor to move on to self-forgiveness and more complete healing. Survivors need to experience human contact and the warmth of the nurse–client relationship. When requested, refer clients to religious counselors who understand the emotional issues surrounding sexual abuse and who are sensitive to the need of survivors to work slowly through their spiritual struggles.

Reducing Anxiety

Because adult survivors are often anxious, interventions to reduce anxiety are also necessary. Clients who learn progressive relaxation and controlled breathing are often able to avoid full-blown panic attacks. Teach the process, and talk clients through the stages of relaxation until they are able to reduce anxiety by themselves. When they are relaxed, instruct them to imagine a scene in which they feel safe and comfortable. Anytime they need to, they can return to this safe scene where they are in total control. Daily practice increases the effectiveness of these techniques (see Chapter 33∞).

Facilitating Healing

Art therapy helps adults in the healing process. Making group murals to express both individual progress and a sense of unity among clients can be very effective. Music therapy, combined with movement or dance, may be a way for clients to experience very early memories. Journal writing is used more than any other expressive therapy and can be expanded to include poetry, songs, and plays.

Group therapy allows survivors to share their feelings and experiences with others who believe their stories. The group setting fosters mutual understanding and decreases the sense of isolation. Many adult survivors find self-help groups to be very supportive in the process of healing (see Chapter 29∞).

Evaluation

Nurses in acute care settings may not have the opportunity for long-term evaluation. Short-term evaluation focuses mainly on identifying child victims and adult survivors and referring them to appropriate community resources.

Nurses in long-term or community settings can evaluate the effectiveness of the treatment plan over an extended period. Questions to guide the evaluation of the child victim and family include the following:

- Has the child remained safe from further harm?
- Has the child returned to functioning at an appropriate developmental level?
- Is the child able to express feelings either verbally or through play or art therapy?
- Is the child verbalizing decreasing feelings of guilt and/or responsibility?
- Is the child developing peer friendships?
- Has the family structure become more flexible?
- Is communication more open within the family?

As a nurse, you have the opportunity to influence the care of adult survivors of childhood sexual abuse. Explain to others that the survivors' behavior is a post-trauma response that makes sense as an adaptation to trauma and to a possibly dysfunctional family. Intervene if staff members recreate the dynamics of the abusive relationship by assuming a position of power and control.

Questions to guide the evaluation of adult survivors include the following:

- Has the client remained safe from further harm in adult relationships?

- Is the client able to talk about the childhood trauma? If not, is art therapy, music therapy, movement therapy, or journal writing effective in facilitating expression?
- Is the client able to identify situations in which he or she has been able, or hopes to be able, to make self-respecting choices?
- Is the client verbalizing increased spiritual comfort regarding the trauma?
- Is the client verbalizing less self-blame?
- Is the client verbalizing improved self-image?
- Is there evidence that the client is able to develop trusting and respectful relationships with adults?

Although, as a culture, we say that we protect our children, we do not in reality live out this value. We do not invest many of our energies—time, caring, and money—in the prevention of childhood sexual abuse. Our present approaches to treatment and to the social control of sexual abuse are not yet effective enough so we are assured of the long-term safety of children. Be encouraged to become active in the battle to stop childhood sexual abuse.

CASE MANAGEMENT

Case management in these cases typically involves protective services for the child/children, spouse/cohabitants, and elders. Protective services for children will implement one of the following four plans if the abuse is occurring within the family system:

1. The most frequent option is removing the abuser from the family. The nonabusing parent must protect the child from any contact with the abuser.
2. When the nonabusing parent is unable to protect the child, both the child and the abuser are removed from the home. This option maximizes the child's safety and decreases the child's feelings of responsibility.
3. In a few cases in which families have not used physical violence, there is no substance abuse, and there is someone who can ensure the child's safety, the family may be allowed to remain intact while participating in intensive therapy.
4. In a few instances, the child may be removed from the family when that is the safest option. Unfortunately, this decision may place additional guilt on the child.

COMMUNITY-BASED CARE AND HOME CARE

A community issue that touches the lives of women, in particular, is how women are treated by men in the workplace. If the environment is one that tacitly supports keeping women subordinate, then those women are being discriminated against. Sexual harassment of women in the workplace and in schools has always existed as a hidden crime. Only recently has it been recognized for what it is—discrimination against and violation of the victim. It is on one end of the continuum of sexual violence, the other end being childhood sexual abuse and rape. Girls and boys and women and men must be taught that they do not have to tolerate harassing behaviors. These behaviors include the following:

- Engaging in sexual teasing, jokes, remarks, or demeaning comments
- Making sexually stereotypical comments
- Showing offensive pictures
- Asking invasive questions regarding personal life
- Pressuring persistently for dates
- Communicating through letters, telephone calls, or e-mails of a sexual nature
- Making sexual gestures
- Deliberately touching, cornering, or pinching
- Watching invasively (such as leering, staring, following all actions)

- Pressuring for sexual favors
- Attempting or committing rape

Sexual harassment can lead to severe stress in the victims. Many experience depression, isolation, feelings of powerlessness, helplessness, fear, restlessness, inability to concentrate, somatic complaints, sexual problems, and loss of self-esteem. At its most severe, harassment resembles the other sexual traumas of child sexual abuse and may result in post-traumatic stress disorder. The U.S. Equal Employment Opportunity Commission (EEOC) is the government agency that interprets and enforces employment laws. In 1980, the EEOC issued a position statement clearly stating that sexual harassment is a form of sexual discrimination and, therefore, an unlawful employment act. The intent of the law is to ensure a work environment that is free from sex-based discrimination and harassment.

NURSING CARE PLAN: AN ADULT SURVIVOR OF CHILDHOOD SEXUAL ABUSE

Identifying Information
Jill is a 35-year-old woman who is a full-time homemaker. Her husband, John, is president of an advertising firm. Jill and John have been married for 15 years and have three children, ages 14, 12, and 7.

Jill was sexually abused by her grandfather from a very young age until she was about 11 or 12. Sometimes the grandfather would involve Jill's brother, who is 3 years older, by forcing Jill and her brother to have sex for the grandfather's enjoyment. She states that she told her mother about the abuse when she was 9 or 10 but that her mother just ignored it. Her mother now denies that Jill told her about the abuse when it was occurring. Jill has tried to ignore her abuse history until several months ago when she saw a television program about incest. She has periods when she is filled with rage at her parents and grandfather.

History
No prior psychiatric history.

Jill was born and raised in Ohio and is the third child of five in an intact family. Jill describes her mother as "strict . . . she would threaten by saying 'wait until your dad comes home.'" When asked about her father, Jill states, "He wasn't around . . . he was working . . . he was always distant." She describes the family communication as "dysfunctional; only certain people talked to certain other people. For

example, none of us kids could talk directly to our father. We always had to go through our mother."

Jill describes herself as a "homebody." In the past, she attended social functions with her husband as required by his professional position. These functions were not a great source of pleasure for her, however. Lately she has had no desire to participate in any activities outside the home. She states that she has never had close friends. Her only friend is her husband, and she feels somewhat intimidated by him. She has a very close relationship with her children.

Jill has no current or past medical problems. She states she is in good health except for feeling "terrible at times."

Current Mental Status
Jill is oriented to person, place, and time. Her affect appears dysphoric, irritable, and constricted in range. At times she is filled with rage, saying, "I am mad . . . mad at the world in general and at having to deal with all of this." She states that during her entire life she has spent much of her energy in "not thinking," "not imagining," and "not remembering" the abuse. She has attempted to keep a sense of distance from her inner emotional life. After viewing the television program on incest, she now experiences "painful, bitter, brooding thoughts about the abuse." Jill is an anxious

and angry woman with extremely low self-esteem and intense feelings of inadequacy. She views herself as unable to function in an autonomous, self-directed, and self-reliant fashion and sees the world as untrustworthy, betraying, and often cruel. Unable to rely on her own resources or depend on the support of others, Jill feels a sense of bitter futility and resignation. She identifies herself as a victim who is inevitably betrayed and disappointed. Many of her dynamics are consistent with those of adult survivors of sexual abuse. She feels intense rage at her parents for being unsupportive, unprotective, and unable to provide her with a sense of safety and security in herself and in the world around her. This contributes to Jill's fear of autonomy and the conflict between her need to depend on others and her intense mistrust of the sincerity and commitment that others can offer. There is no evidence of psychotic illness or of a manifest thought disturbance.

Other Clinical Data
Jill states that she needs more emotional support from her husband. Her husband states that he has been unable to give it to her lately because he is often irritated at the mess and dirt in the house. She thinks he is being perfectionistic. He has offered to hire someone to help, but Jill sees that as another failure on her part.

(Continued)

NURSING CARE PLAN: AN ADULT SURVIVOR OF CHILDHOOD SEXUAL ABUSE (*Continued*)

Nursing Diagnosis: Post-Trauma Syndrome related to being an adult survivor of incest

Expected Outcome: Jill will resolve associated anger and anxiety.

Short-Term Goals	Interventions	Rationales
Jill discharges the energy of her anger appropriately.	▪ Discuss feelings of guilt. Repeat often that children are never responsible for the incest but rather that her grandfather is totally responsible. ▪ Discuss her feelings of anger toward the grandfather and her parents for not protecting her as a child. ▪ Connect feelings of low self-esteem to feelings of guilt and anger. ▪ Assign journal keeping for recording feelings, thoughts, and memories. ▪ Help Jill identify and grieve over things lost in childhood, such as innocence and trust.	Jill needs to place the responsibility for this abuse where it belongs. Survivors of abuse frequently take blame for the incest. Jill's current interactions with others are based on what she learned from these experiences as a child.
Jill uses relaxation exercises.	▪ Teach anxiety-reducing techniques such as muscle relaxation, deep breathing, and physical exercise.	Handling stress and taking care of herself were not taught to her as a child by the adults who raised her.

Nursing Diagnosis: Social Isolation related to withdrawal and decreased desire to interact with others

Expected Outcome: Jill will increase interactions with people outside her family.

Short-Term Goals	Interventions	Rationales
Jill will be able to initiate relationships outside the family.	▪ Help Jill identify the benefits of social interactions. ▪ Help Jill identify a variety of available supportive people. ▪ Give Jill positive feedback when she expresses an interest in or engages in interactions with others. ▪ Provide assertiveness training.	Jill may not know that she could feel better when she is in regular contact with other people. Jill will respond to positive feedback and be likely to continue to discover others by answering where, how, and when questions on social interactions. Jill's ability to say "No" comfortably through assertiveness training will increase her comfort in relationships with others.
Jill will receive support and help from a self-help group.	▪ Provide information on self-help groups for adult survivors where Jill can share with others and establish trusting relationships.	Self-help groups provide the opportunity to realize that one is not alone.

REFERENCES

Adinkrah, M. (2010). Criminalizing rape within marriage: Perspectives of Ghanaian university students. *International Journal of Offender Therapy and Comparative Criminology*. Advance online publication. doi: 10.1177/0306624X10371800

Burriss, F. A., Breland-Noble, A. M., Webster, J. L., & Soto, J. A. (2011). Juvenile mental health courts for adjudicated youth: Role implications for child and adolescent psychiatric mental health nurses. *Journal of Child & Adolescent Psychiatric Nursing, 24*(2), 114–121.

Burton, D. L., Duty, K. J., & Leibowitz, G. S. (2011). Differences between sexually victimized and nonsexually victimized male adolescent sexual abusers: Developmental antecedents and behavioral comparisons. *Journal of Child Sexual Abuse, 20*(1), 77–93.

Champion, J. D. (2011). Context of sexual risk behaviour among abused ethnic minority adolescent women. *International Nursing Review, 58*(1), 61–67.

Denton, J., Newton, A. W., & Vandeven, A. M. (2011). Update on child maltreatment: Toward refining the evidence base. *Current Opinion in Pediatrics, 23,* 240–248.

Duran, M., Moya, M., & Megias, J. L. (2010). It's his right, it's her duty: Benevolent sexism and the justification of traditional sexual roles. *Journal of Sex Research, 14,* 1–9.

Everson, M. D., & Sandoval, J. M. (2011). Forensic child sexual abuse evaluations: Assessing subjectivity and bias in professional judgments. *Child Abuse and Neglect, 35*(4), 287–298.

Finkelhor, D., Ormrod, R., Turner, H., & Hamby, S. (2011). School, police, and medical authority involvement with children who have experienced victimization. *Archives of Pediatrics and Adolescent Medicine, 165*(1), 9–15.

Graham-Bermann, S., Sularz, A. R., & Howell, K. H. (2011). Additional adverse events among women exposed to intimate partner violence: Frequency and impact. *Psychology of Violence, 1*(2), 136–149.

Greenberg, D. M., Firestone, P., Nunes, K. L., Bradford, J. M., & Curry, S. (2005). Biological fathers and stepfathers who molest their daughters: Psychological, phallometric, and criminal features. *Sexual Abuse: A Journal of Research and Treatment, 17*(1), 39–46.

Hassija, C., & Gray, M. J. (2011). The effectiveness and feasibility of videoconferencing technology to provide evidence-based treatment to rural domestic violence and sexual assault populations. *Telemedicine Journal & E-Health, 17*(4), 309–315.

Lyden, C. (2011). Uncovering child abuse. *Nursing, 41,* 1–5.

McCloskey, J., & Bulechek, G. M. (1996). *Nursing interventions classification (NIC)* (2nd ed.). St. Louis, MO: Mosby.

McCloskey, K. A., & Raphael, D. N. (2005). Adult perpetrator gender asymmetries in child sexual assault victim selection. *Journal of Child Sexual Abuse, 14*(4), 1–24.

Miller, E., Breslau, J., Chung, W. J., Green, J. G., McLaughlin, K. A., & Kessler, R. C. (2011). Adverse childhood experiences and risk of physical violence in adolescent dating relationships. *Journal of Epidemiology and Community Health*. Advance online publication. doi:10.1136/jech.2009.105429

Mitra, M., Manning, S. E., & Lu, E. (2011). Physical abuse around the time of pregnancy among women with disabilities. *Maternal and Child Health Journal*. Advance online publication. doi:10.1007/s10995-011-0784-y

Murphy, S. B., Potter, S. J., Stapleton, J. G., Wiesen-Martin, D., & Pierce-Weeks, J. (2010). Findings from Sexual Assault Nurse Examiners (SANE): A case study of New Hampshire's pediatric SANE database. *Journal of Forensic Nursing, 6*(4), 163–169.

National Center for Victims of Crime. (2008). Domestic violence statistics. Retrieved from http://www.ncvc.org

Pearsall, C. (2005). Forensic biomarkers of elder abuse. *Journal of Forensic Nursing, 19*(4), 182–186.

Rhodes, K. V., Kotari, C. L., Dichter, M., Cerulli, C., Wiley, J., & Marcus, S. (2011). Intimate partner violence identification and response: Time for a change in strategy. *Journal of General Internal Medicine*. Advance online publication. doi: 10.1007/s11606-011-1662

Sarmiento, I. (2011). Rape stereotypes and labeling: Awareness of victimization and trauma. *Psychological Reports, 108*(1), 141–148.

Schetky, K. H. (1999). Sexual victimization of children. In J. A. Shaw (Ed.), *Sexual aggression* (pp. 107–128). Washington, DC: American Psychiatric Press.

Smyth, K. F., Goodman, L., & Glenn, C. (2006). The full-frame approach: A new response to marginalized women left behind by specialized services. *American Journal of Orthopsychiatry, 76*(4), 489–502.

Tsopelas, C., Spyridoula, T., & Athanosios, D. (2011). Review on female sexual offenders: Findings about profile and personality. *International Journal of Law and Psychiatry, 34*(2), 122–126.

Wang, Y. W. (2011). Voices from the margin: A case study of a rural lesbian's experience with woman-to-woman sexual violence. *Journal of Lesbian Studies, 15*(2), 166–175.

Children

EILEEN TRIGOBOFF

25

LEARNING OUTCOMES

After completing this chapter, you will be able to:

1. Compare and contrast the similarities and differences between generalist and specialist roles in child psychiatric nursing.
2. Synthesize the key ideas in the biopsychosocial theories that help you understand the development of childhood psychiatric disorders.
3. Differentiate between the multicausal and interactive models of child mental illness.
4. Incorporate an understanding of the potential risk factors for childhood mental illness into working with children in community settings.
5. Modify a care plan according to the signs and symptoms associated with common children's psychiatric disorders.
6. Conduct an assessment of a child with a mental health problem.
7. Incorporate various therapeutic approaches that child psychiatric–mental health nurses might use in working with children.
8. Incorporate various therapeutic approaches that child psychiatric–mental health nurses might use in working with the parents of child clients.
9. Compare and contrast the various psychopharmacologic agents for children at each major developmental level.
10. Analyze your own attitudes and behavior toward child psychiatric clients and their parents.

CRITICAL THINKING CHALLENGE

You are checking your clients' records. A nurse who is finishing her shift says to you as she is leaving, "So you will be working with Kevin tonight, the little red-haired guy with autism. I warn you, his mother is a real pain. She is constantly asking questions and telling the staff what to do. I don't think they should even let her visit. If you ask me, she is the reason for all the kid's problems."

1. How might the nurse's attitude influence the care that Kevin and his family receive?
2. What are the possible effects of autistic disorder on family relationships?

There are more children in need of psychiatric care than ever before. About one in ten children in the United States suffers from mental illness (National Institute of Mental Health [NIMH], 2011) but fewer than one in five of these children receive treatment. Available resources for prevention and treatment of mental illness are minimal and the number of mental health professionals prepared to work with children has dwindled. To promote mental health in children and treat problems more effectively, nurses in every area can do the following:

- Improve assessment and recognition of children's mental health needs.
- Eliminate racial/ethnic and socioeconomic disparities in access to care.
- Educate primary care providers and families to better recognize and manage children's mental health issues.

A number of mental health problems can appear in childhood and these problems may continue into adulthood, or lead to other psychiatric disorders later in life. Mental Health in the Movies discusses a classic movie, *David and Lisa,* in which childhood disorders are managed into adolescence. The disorders we explore in this chapter are commonly found in childhood.

CHILD PSYCHIATRIC–MENTAL HEALTH NURSING AS A SPECIALTY

Nurses have a variety of important roles in child psychiatry. Our unique perspective of both mental and physical health allows us to assess psychological and physical symptoms in children, explain laboratory tests to children and their families, administer medications that require strict and systematic monitoring, and work with children having a dual medical and psychiatric diagnosis (such as diabetes and conduct disorder). Child psychiatric–mental health nurses educate children about their illness and in the process, promote wellness, self-esteem, and more effective interpersonal relationships. When we help children identify and label their feelings, deal with stress, and manage anxiety we are preparing them to cope effectively for the rest of their lives.

As a specialty, child psychiatric–mental health nursing had its inception in the early 1950s, when graduate programs opened and training funds became available through the National Institute of Mental Health (NIMH). As the community mental health movement developed, programs specifically for children expanded. Child psychiatric–mental health nurses are involved in treatment, consultation, education, and medication supervision and are the mainstay of hospital treatment programs where they are responsible for daily treatment plans, ongoing one–to–one or group counseling, and management of the child's medication regimen. You will see advanced practice nurses as the primary caregivers for children with mental health problems, providing direct psychotherapy, working with the family, and managing the child's medications. This comprehensive role is especially common in rural or inner city areas.

A growing role for child psychiatric–mental health nurses involves promotion of infant mental health in high-risk families in which infants who have medical complications or the parents have a history of mental illness or substance abuse. They also function as liaisons to pediatric inpatient and outpatient settings, providing psychiatric consultation to the pediatric staff. In most cases, the nurse functions as part of an interdisciplinary team, along with child psychiatrists, social workers, psychologists, occupational therapists, recreational therapists, special educators, pediatricians, and child care workers. (For more information, visit the website of the Association of Child and Adolescent Psychiatric Nurses via the Online Student Resources for this book.) Other specialists are used for consultations as indicated, particularly child neurologists, speech and language specialists, child protective services, clergy, and physical therapists.

DEVELOPMENTAL DISORDERS

All **developmental disorders** involve either a failure to develop as expected or a regression after normal development. These impairments can occur in single areas or involve a spectrum of deficits.

MENTAL HEALTH IN THE MOVIES
David and Lisa

David and Lisa is a black-and-white, independent film made in 1962, and is based on a novel written by Theodore Isaac Rubin, a psychiatrist. It was adapted as a stage play in 1967, finally released to DVD in 1999, and remade as a television movie in 1998 with Sidney Poitier playing the role of the psychiatrist.

In the original, David (Keir Dullea) has an extreme phobia (fear of being touched) and obsessive–compulsive disorder. Lisa (Janet Margolin) is diagnosed as schizophrenic. The two adolescents make contact with each other in a residential facility for disturbed youth. As their relationship deepens from antagonism to trust, they are able to help one another come to terms with their mental disorders. Eye-catching dream sequences, flashbacks to their childhood, and a melancholy mood clearly convey the isolation that both young people experience.

The film caused quite a stir when it was released in 1962 and was nominated for several awards. Despite the fact that some mental health professionals have criticized the film for its suggestion that David's obsessive–compulsive behavior was caused by his mother's domination, it is an insightful character study. When compared to other films about mental illness made prior to it, this film offered an intelligent and sensitive study of mental illness. It looked at several possible explanations—parental culpability, childhood trauma, and individual sensitivity to the environment. It is a film that encourages people to take charge of their own mental health.

Photo courtesy of Everett Collection, Inc.

Intellectual Developmental Disorders

The major feature of **intellectual developmental disorders** (also known as *mental retardation*) is significantly subaverage intellectual functioning (an IQ below 70 in children, or, in infants, clinical judgment based on cognitive tests). The degree of severity of intellectual impairment is described as mild (IQ 50/55–70), moderate (IQ 35/40–50/55), severe (IQ 20/25–35/40), or profound (IQ below 20/25). The child must also show deficits or impairments in adaptive functioning in at least two areas of life—for example, communication, social/interpersonal skills, or safety. The onset of this disorder occurs before the age of 18.

Intellectual disability is found in approximately 1% of the population (American Psychiatric Association [APA], 2000). The major risk factor for retardation is the early alteration of embryonic development as a result of exposure to toxins in utero (maternal drug use, for example) or chromosomal changes (such as Down syndrome). Other predisposing factors include inherited errors of metabolism (such as fragile X syndrome), pregnancy and perinatal problems such as prematurity or trauma, medical conditions acquired in infancy or childhood, and early environmental influences such as deprivation of nurturance or other stimulation.

Specific Developmental Disorders

Three categories of developmental disorders involve specific cognitive impairments that are presumed to result from dysfunctions in the cortex of the brain: learning disorders, motor skills disorder, and communication disorders. These dysfunctions have been associated with genetic vulnerabilities, organic damage, and delayed maturation. Children from disadvantaged socioeconomic circumstances tend to receive these diagnoses more frequently, particularly boys.

Learning Disorders

A learning disorder (LD) may be diagnosed when a child's achievement on standardized tests in reading, mathematics, or written expression is substantially below what is expected for his or her age, schooling, or intelligence level. LDs affect 2% to 10% of the population and about 5% of all public school students (APA, 2000). Reading is the major learning problem. The problems are so major as to significantly interfere with the child's activities of daily living or academic progress.

Motor Skills Disorder

A motor skills disorder, where there is marked impairment in the development of motor coordination, occurs in approximately 6% of all children (APA, 2000). You may first notice this problem in a child's delay in achieving motor milestones such as walking or crawling, in "clumsiness," and in poor handwriting or sports performance. To be considered a psychiatric disorder, the impairment must significantly interfere with the child's academic achievement or activities of daily living and not be the result of a physical health problem such as cerebral palsy.

Communication Disorders

Communication disorders can be one of four different problems: impairments in language expression, in the understanding of language, in phonology (how sounds are pronounced), or stuttering:

1. Problems in language expression may include a markedly limited vocabulary, errors in tense, or difficulty recalling words or producing sentences of developmentally appropriate length or complexity.
2. Problems in understanding language include difficulty understanding words, sentences, or specific types of words.
3. The symptom of a phonologic disorder is the failure to use developmentally expected speech sounds appropriate for a child's age and dialect. For example, the child may substitute one sound for another ("t" for "k") or omit sounds in words.
4. Stuttering is a disturbance in the normal timing and fluency of speech; for instance, frequent repetitions, prolonged sounds, or pauses in the middle of a word.

Word substitution is often used by a child to avoid problematic words (see FIGURE 25-1 ■). These impairments must be severe enough to interfere with academic achievement or social communication.

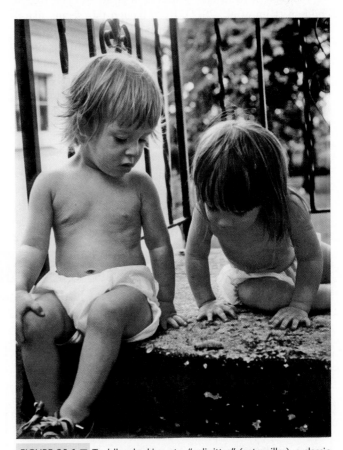

FIGURE 25-1 ■ Toddlers looking at a "calipitter" (caterpillar), a classic language flip.
Photo courtesy of Eileen Trigoboff.

While stuttering occurs in about 1% of prepubertal children, the prevalence of the other communication disorders is somewhat greater: about 3% to 5% of all children. Remember to evaluate any communication problems within the child's cultural and language context, especially if the child is bilingual. The only known predisposing factor for the development of a communication disorder is a family history of the disorder. For stuttering, especially, family and twin studies provide strong evidence of a genetic factor in its etiology.

AUTISM SPECTRUM DISORDERS

The **autism spectrum disorders (ASD)**, called *pervasive developmental disorders (PDD)* in the DSM-IV-TR (2000), include autistic disorder, Rett's disorder, childhood disintegrative disorder, and Asperger's disorder. Each of these psychiatric conditions usually arises in the first years of life and is characterized by severe developmental impairment in several areas.

Autistic, disintegrative, and Asperger's disorders are much more common in boys, with rates of autism four to five times higher than for girls. Rett's disorder has been found to occur only in girls. The reasons for these gender differences are not yet understood for autistic, disintegrative, and Asperger's disorders. A probable explanation for the occurrence of Rett's disorder in girls is explained later in this section.

All of these disorders are rare, with autistic disorder having the highest incidence. It occurs in up to 180 per 10,000 children (Kim et al., 2011). Even though this seems like a large range, it is a very small percentage of children affected. Pervasive developmental disorders have an enormous effect on children and their families. They also represent a substantial segment of the families to whom child psychiatric–mental health nurses provide care, because the problems these families encounter are severe and require significant professional support (see Rx Communication).

Autistic Disorder

Sometimes called **autistic disorder**, autism is a lifelong condition that involves difficulties in the quality of the child's social interactions and communication. In social interactions, the child may have problems making eye contact and have

a repetitive repertoire of interests or behaviors (as in folding a piece of tissue repeatedly or flapping both hands up and down). DSM Essential Features describes the specifics of this disorder.

About 75% of children with autism also have a diagnosis of intellectual disability, usually in the moderate range. Autism appears prior to age 3. Parents may tell you that their baby does not want to cuddle, shows indifference to touch and affection, does not make eye contact, or is not facially responsive. Children may also have many associated behavioral problems such as hyperactivity, aggressiveness, self-injurious behaviors such as head banging, temper tantrums, and unusual sensitivity to sensory stimuli (such as an oversensitivity to touch or a high threshold for pain). You may notice abnormal mood or affect as well; for example, a child may over-react or not react at all to the environment.

Autism is a serious developmental disability. Based on statistics from the U.S. Department of Education, the Centers for Disease Control and Prevention, and other government agencies, we can expect the following:

- Autism is the fastest growing developmental disability with 10% to 17% annual growth.
- One in every 110 children will have some form of autism (approximately 1 in 70 boys).
- Between 1 and 1.5 million Americans have some form of autism.
- The prevalence of autism may reach 4 million Americans in the next decade (Autism Society of America, 2011).

These and other facts about autism are available at the website of the Autism Society of America, which can be accessed through a link on the Online Student Resources for this text.

Several current clinical trials for ASD are listed in the National Institute of Mental Health (NIMH) clinical trials registry (NIMH, 2011). They include studies of the effectiveness of medications such as atomoxetine (Strattera), olanzapine (Zyprexa), aripiprazole (Abilify), D-cycloserine (Seromycin, a drug more commonly used for the treatment of tuberculosis), methylphenidate (Ritalin), fluoxetine (Prozac), and risperidone (Risperdal). Autism clinical trials of school- and

---

℞ COMMUNICATION

Communicating With the Parent of a Child With Autism

PARENT: "I've had it. I just can't take this anymore. Kaetlin screams and flaps her arms every time I touch her. I can't even give her a bath without a huge scene. It's exhausting."

NURSE RESPONSE 1: "I hear how frustrated and exhausted you are. Let's talk about your needs for a bit and figure out ways to get you some support and relief."

RATIONALE: This response shows the parent that the nurse empathizes with the parent's situation. It also provides an opportunity (a) for the parent to discuss her feelings in more detail, and (b) for the nurse to make concrete suggestions for decreasing the burden the parent is experiencing.

NURSE RESPONSE 2: "Yes, it can be very exhausting. Other families I work with have these same experiences. Let's talk about some approaches that you might use to help Kaetlin handle her bath without getting so upset."

RATIONALE: First, this response provides comfort to the parent that the problem is not unique to her family but is shared by others. The nurse then offers her the opportunity to learn some specific strategies to better manage the child's behavior.

DSM ESSENTIAL FEATURES

Childhood Disorders

Each of these diagnostic categories is used only when symptoms are not due to any other developmental or childhood medical or psychiatric problem.

Autistic Disorder: Social impairment through problematic nonverbal behavior, poor friend making, absence of sharing enjoyment with others, or a lack of social or emotional reciprocity (asking others about their lives or interests). Communication is delayed or there is no spoken language, there is an inability to sustain a conversation. There are notable inflexible nonfunctional routines or rituals.

Attention Deficit Hyperactivity Disorder: Multiple symptoms of inattention or hyperactivity, for 6 months or more. Symptoms start before age 7 and are present in two or more settings. Significantly impairs social, educational, or occupational functioning.

Reactive Attachment Disorder of Infancy or Early Childhood: Markedly disturbed and developmentally inappropriate social relatedness starting before age 5. Manifested either by failure to initiate or respond appropriately to most social interactions, and/or by indiscriminate sociability. Arising in a context of neglectful, abusive, or unreliable care thought to be contributory. There are two types discussed on page 557.

Feeding Disorders: Either a failure to eat adequate amounts of food with subsequent lack of weight gain, or significant weight loss within at least 1 month. Begins before age 6 and is not related to a problem with the esophagus or stomach.

Separation Anxiety Disorder: Excessive anxiety concerning separation from home or from people to whom the individual is attached. This happens for at least 4 weeks, onset before age 18. Symptoms when separation is anticipated or occurs include potential refusal to go to school or elsewhere, persistent refusal to sleep without being near a major attachment figure, and complaints of physical symptoms.

Stereotypic Movement Disorder: Repetitive nonfunctional motor behavior (i.e., hand waving, self-biting, body rocking, or head banging) that interferes with normal activity or risks self-inflicted bodily injury. These behaviors are seemingly driven and protective measures are usually needed so that medical treatment will not be necessary. Lasts 4 weeks or longer.

Tourette's Disorder: Multiple motor tics and at least one verbal tic, not necessarily concurrent, happening many times on most days for a year or more. During that time any tic-free period lasted less than 3 months, and tic onset was before age 18. Not due to substance abuse.

---

home-based early intervention for toddlers, relationship training for children and their peers, factors that distinguish autism from delayed development and normal development, and the interaction of diet and behavior are also in the NIMH pipeline (NIMH, 2011). You can counsel parents to obtain information on current clinical trials through the NIMH website via a link on the Online Student Resources for this book.

Recent attention has been given to autism with the made-for-TV movie about Temple Grandin, a very accomplished woman born with autism. It called attention to the media

reports of a number of people who have some symptoms on the autism spectrum as well as the possibilities when someone is autistic. See Mental Health in the News for Dr. Grandin's story and her website for more information about autism at http://www.templegrandin.com/

Rett's Disorder

Rett's disorder is the accumulation of multiple developmental deficits by a child following normal development during the first 5 months of life. Within the first or second year of life,

---

MENTAL HEALTH IN THE NEWS

Temple Grandin

Temple Grandin was first diagnosed in 1949, at age 2, with brain damage. She was then diagnosed with autism when she was 3 years old. Her parents placed her in a structured nursery school with what Temple considers to have been good teachers. Her mother spoke to a doctor at the time who suggested speech therapy, and she hired a nanny who spent hours playing turn-based games with Temple. Within a year she began speaking and making progress.

Middle and high school were very difficult times for Temple socially. Temple was the "nerdy kid" and she was teased a great deal. At times, while walking down the street, people would taunt her by calling her "tape recorder," because she would repeat things over and over again. Temple describes these experiences, "I could laugh about it now, but back then it really hurt."

Because of the support Temple received from her family and her teachers' educational focus on her skills (visual thinking and design), she earned her bachelor's degree in psychology, and her master's and doctoral degrees in animal science. Her forte is constructing sweeping, curved pens to reduce the stress animals feel while penned, and during their entry into a slaughter house.

Dr. Grandin is listed in the 2010 Time magazine list of the 100 most influential people in the world. Her category is "Heroes." She regularly presents at conferences and other public speaking venues. Dr. Grandin describes those of us without autism as "neurotypical" and, even though she feels like an alien around us, she knows how to soothe herself and behave appropriately with others.

Photo courtesy of Nancy Kaszerman/ZUMA Press/Newscom.

the baby begins to show deceleration in head growth, loss of previously acquired hand skills and eventual stereotypic hand movements (repetitive movements that serve no purpose), loss of social engagement, poorly coordinated gait or trunk movements, and severely impaired language development with psychomotor retardation. Rett's disorder primarily affects females. The disorder is lifelong, with persistent and progressive loss of skills. Only modest developmental gains have been noted in a few children later in their childhood or adolescence.

Childhood Disintegrative Disorder

Childhood disintegrative disorder (CDD) is quite similar to Rett's disorder except that its period of normal development is much longer, with symptoms not appearing until ages 2 through 10. In addition, there is no head growth deceleration or loss of hand skills. Instead, the losses involve skills in expressive or receptive language, social skills, play, and bowel or bladder control. Some of the functional abnormalities that develop are similar to those in autistic disorder, such as impairments in social interaction, communication, and repetitive, restricted, stereotypic behavior. However, in autistic disorder, the abnormalities are usually noticed within the first year of life and do not reflect the pattern of developmental regression found in CDD.

Asperger's Disorder

Asperger's disorder has some, but not all, of the features of autism. Children with this disorder show the same problems with social interaction and restricted, repetitive behavior as in autism. However, there is no delay in language, in cognitive development, in age-appropriate self-help and adaptive skills, or in curiosity about the environment. The onset of the disorder is also later than in autism, most commonly in the preschool period. In contrast to CDD, there is no loss of previously acquired skills in Asperger's disorder.

ATTENTION DEFICIT AND DISRUPTIVE BEHAVIOR DISORDERS

This category of child psychiatric problems includes attention deficit hyperactivity disorder and two disruptive behavior disorders: conduct disorder and oppositional defiant disorder. Disruptive behavior disorders are a group of mental disorders in which behavior problems cause significant impairment in social, academic, or occupational functioning. The symptoms common to all of these disorders involve behavior that is externally manifested or directed, often called *externalizing disorders*.

Attention Deficit Hyperactivity Disorder

The most distinctive features of **attention deficit hyperactivity disorder (ADHD)** are the child's inattention to the surrounding environment, and hyperactivity and/or impulsiveness. Symptoms must be inconsistent with the child's developmental level, and cause clinically significant impairment in functioning. To determine whether inattention exists, look for behaviors such as not listening when spoken to and disliking

tasks that require sustained mental effort. You will be able to observe hyperactivity in signs of impulsivity. Most children with this disorder have a combination of symptoms indicating both inattention and hyperactivity–impulsiveness, but some children have predominantly one or the other. Girls are more likely to have symptoms only of inattention. See DSM Essential Features on page 553 for details.

ADHD is most commonly diagnosed in early school years, when demands for sustained attention increase. (See What Every Nurse Should Know.) By late childhood and adolescence, excesses in gross motor activity become less apparent, and symptoms may reflect primarily fidgetiness or even inner feelings of restlessness without any observable signs. A clinical example that includes ADHD is in the next section on conduct disorder.

Controversy has grown about the number of children being diagnosed with ADHD. National statistics indicate that approximately 3% to 7% of all children have ADHD, but many more children are diagnosed than this figure represents (Storebø et al., 2011; Smith, et al., 2011). Concerns have developed regarding possible overdiagnosis and overtreatment of ADHD. Some mental health professionals question whether the growing trend toward assessment and management of the disorder by pediatricians and family physicians is problematic because they may not be skilled in the differential diagnosis or treatment of psychiatric disorders. Another concern relates to the pressures by school personnel to control children's behavior, pressures that may influence parents and/or primary care practitioners to prescribe medication for ADHD when psychosocial management of the behavioral problems would be better. Yet another possibility is the difficulty in differentiating between ADHD and childhood bipolar disorder. There are some diagnostic differences, although the reticence about, and cautions against, diagnosing bipolarity in youngsters may be the issue.

In response to these public and professional concerns, a number of studies have assessed the effectiveness

WHAT EVERY NURSE SHOULD KNOW

ADHD Assistance

Imagine you are a school nurse. Children with ADHD may be eligible for assistance under the Individuals with Disabilities Education Act (IDEA) of 2004 or section 504 of the Rehabilitation Act. To help children receive accommodations, families often need the following:

- Education about the school district's protocol for identifying, assessing, and intervening with children with ADHD
- Help finding a provider who is knowledgeable about ADHD
- A nursing liaison between their child's teacher and the child's psychiatric or primary care provider, especially when children are on medication and need monitoring to determine the optimal dose and schedule

of stimulants. Outcomes of these studies suggest that psychostimulants are highly effective at reducing symptoms, improve the child's quality of life, and typically have mild and short-lived side effects. Some adjunctive therapies have also been helpful for children with a suboptimal response to psychostimulants alone (Spencer, Greenbaum, Ginsberg, & Murphy, 2009).

Conduct Disorder

Conduct disorder (CD) is also one of the most frequently diagnosed problems for children. Boys have an incidence three to five times greater than girls. There is a high prevalence of CD in inner-city areas because of high crime, chaotic family lives, and limited access to some mental health services (Ståhlberg, Anckarsäter, & Nilsson, 2010). The central feature of CD is repetitive and persistent behavior in which the basic rights of others or major age-appropriate societal norms or rules are violated. Look for behaviors that show aggression toward people and animals, destruction of property, deceitfulness or theft, or serious violation of parental or school rules. These symptoms may appear as early as 5 to 6 years of age, but occur more typically in later childhood or early adolescence. The diagnosis of CD is made only when the behavior is symptomatic of a problem within the child and not a reaction to a social context of war, poverty, high crime, or fear for one's well-being.

There are two subtypes of conduct disorder: childhood onset and adolescent onset. Childhood onset must show at least one symptom prior to 10 years of age. In the majority of cases, the disorder remits by adulthood, but individuals with childhood onset are more likely to develop adult antisocial personality disorder (APD; see Chapter 22 ∞) than are those with onset in adolescence.

Children with conduct disorder may have little empathy toward others, and in ambiguous situations they often misinterpret the intentions of others as hostile and threatening, responding with aggressive behavior that they view as reasonable and justified (see Rx Communication). Self-esteem is commonly low, but covered up by a façade of toughness.

Boys with the disorder are more likely to fight, steal, vandalize, or have school problems, whereas girls are more likely to run away, be truant, use drugs, or become involved in prostitution. It used to be that girls did not show confrontational behavior, although in recent years confrontation has become more common. While almost all cases of CD in childhood involve boys, there is a more even gender balance in adolescent onset. The following clinical example illustrates the constellation of symptoms often found in boys.

Clinical Example

Rob, a 9-year-old boy, was recently diagnosed with CD in addition to an earlier diagnosis of ADHD. Rob has been in numerous fights at school for the past 2 months. His grades have dropped substantially, and he was caught vandalizing school property. At home, he refuses to talk to his parents and hit his mother when she was yelling at him for stealing money from her purse.

Rob's long history of behavioral problems began with temper tantrums at 6 months of age. At the age of 3, he cut up the family sofa. His parents took him out of preschool because the teachers couldn't handle his behavior, especially the shoving of other children and running around. During his early school years he had difficulty concentrating and focusing on an activity for a sustained period of time and interrupted ongoing class activities. He has almost no friends in school.

Rob views his problems as the result of others' hostility and threats toward him. He expresses much anger toward the "school bullies" and all authority figures in his life.

Oppositional Defiant Disorder

All the features of **oppositional defiant disorder (ODD)** are usually present in conduct disorder, so it is not diagnosed if it meets the criteria for CD. ODD is a recurrent and hostile pattern of behavior toward authority figures. However, it does not involve the physical aggression, destructive behavior, deceitfulness, theft, or serious violation of rules shown in CD.

ODD has a prevalence rate of 2% to 16% (APA, 2000). It is more common in children from families in which the child experiences many different caregivers; in which harsh, inconsistent, or neglectful child-rearing practices are used; in which mothers are depressed; or in which serious marital discord exists. The disorder is associated with problematic temperament in the preschool years and a high degree of motor activity. ODD usually becomes apparent before age 8, with symptoms

Care Plan: Oppositional Defiant Disorder

R̲x COMMUNICATION

Communicating With a Child With Conduct Disorder

CHILD: "I'm going to beat the crap out of that kid!"

NURSE RESPONSE 1: "You sound very angry at him. What is it that has made you feel so angry?"

RATIONALE: This response reflects back to the child the feelings underlying the aggressive behavior and helps to facilitate the child's awareness of his anger. The follow-up question encourages the child to develop some insight regarding his anger and is general enough to allow issues to surface that may actually be unrelated to the other child.

NURSE RESPONSE 2: "You know, Rob, that you will not be allowed to hurt anyone on the unit. If you're angry about something, I'll help you find ways to deal with your anger."

RATIONALE: This response clearly establishes limits on the child's behavior, reinforcing what is appropriate versus inappropriate behavior. The nurse also makes it clear that there are constructive ways to handle anger and that she will be there to help the child learn how to manage his feelings more effectively.

first appearing in the home and then later within other settings. The child may show low self-esteem, minimal frustration tolerance, swearing, mood lability, and precocious use of tobacco, alcohol, or illegal drugs.

FEEDING AND EATING DISORDERS

Three feeding and eating disorders—pica, rumination disorder, and feeding disorder of infancy or early childhood—are persistent feeding and eating disturbances that include problems with what is being eaten, how much is being eaten, and the activities and behaviors around eating. Anorexia nervosa and bulimia nervosa may also occur during later childhood. These disorders are not unique to childhood, nor do they necessarily first appear in childhood. See Chapter 21∞ for details of those eating disorders.

Pica

In **pica** the child persistently eats nonnutritive substances (such as paint, plaster, string, hair, cloth, animal droppings, insects, or leaves). To be considered a disorder, the behavior must be inappropriate for the developmental level of the child and not part of a culturally sanctioned practice. This disorder is most frequently seen in preschool children and in individuals who have intellectual disability. Lack of adequate supervision, neglect, and poverty increase the possibility of the problem. Usually, the disorder lasts only for a few months, but it can continue into adolescence or adulthood.

Rumination Disorder

Rumination disorder is the repeated regurgitation and re-chewing of food. It appears after a period of normal eating behavior in an infant or child. The child brings up partially digested food into the mouth, with no evidence of nausea or retching, and then chews and re-swallows it. Sometimes the food is spit out. These symptoms are not associated with any medical condition or with any other eating disorder. Rumination disorder is most common in male infants between 3 and 12 months of age. You will observe a characteristic straining and arching of the back in these babies, and they make sucking movements with the tongue, appearing to enjoy the process very much. However, between regurgitations, babies are often irritable and hungry, and they eat a lot when fed. Because they regurgitate immediately after eating, either weight loss or failure to gain expected weight is common.

Certain factors place an infant at risk for the disorder, including lack of stimulation, neglect, and problems in the parent–child relationship. In turn, the unsuccessful nature of the feeding experience and the aversive nature of the regurgitation may result in a parent's difficulty in providing responsive or loving care.

Feeding Disorder of Infancy or Early Childhood

In a **feeding disorder**, there is a persistent failure to eat adequately, accompanied by either a failure to gain weight or significant weight loss. This state is described sometimes as "failure to thrive." Resulting malnutrition can threaten the child's life. As with other disorders in this category, there is no medical condition causing the behavior.

Children with this problem are particularly irritable and difficult to console during feeding. At other times, they may appear apathetic or withdrawn. Infants who have pre-existing developmental impairments or problems with regulation of the nervous system (for example, sleep–wake irregularities) may be less responsive to the parent, creating difficulties in the feeding process. DSM Essential Features lists feeding disorder elements for diagnosis on page 553.

In addition, parent behavior can make the feeding problem worse. For example, a parent may force the food into a baby's mouth too roughly or at too rapid a pace. There is a high incidence of parental psychopathology as well as child abuse or neglect associated with the condition. Although the disorder is most common in infancy (about 1% to 5% of all pediatric hospital admissions are for failure to thrive), it may have its onset as late as age 2 to 3 years (APA, 2000). Most children eventually achieve improved growth patterns. The following clinical example illustrates how both child and parental factors can contribute to a feeding disorder.

Clinical Example

Chang, an 8-month-old Asian-American boy, was referred to the child psychiatric clinic by pediatrics for an assessment. Chang's mother was dependent on alcohol and had several bouts of drinking during her pregnancy with Chang. As a result, he had low birth weight and many neurobehavioral problems at birth. Chang continued to have tremors and an increased startle response throughout his first 6 months of life. He was also highly irritable and difficult for his mother to console, especially during feeding. His health care was being conducted by a nurse practitioner, Dawn, since the time he was 3 months of age.

Dawn reported that he had not eaten well from the time he was born, was quite undernourished, and failed to gain weight. Chang's failure to thrive became such a concern that Dawn hospitalized him for treatment of a number of resulting medical problems. During his hospitalizations, an extensive diagnostic workup produced no clear reasons for his failure to eat and develop normally. The pediatric nurses, however, had noted his mother's frustration with Chang's lack of interest in eating. Her frustration was often accompanied by impatience and she would simply stop trying to get Chang to eat. They also charted some concern about her current alcohol use. They could smell alcohol on her breath when she came to the unit and sometimes she was verbally abusive to the staff.

The child psychiatric–mental health nurse noted that, most of the time, Chang's mother related to him with very little emotion. His mother commented to the nurse, "Chang has always been a difficult and stubborn baby, never happy with anything. I've given up trying to please him. He has a personality just like his father." The nurse also noticed that Chang's facial expression was solemn and he rarely made eye contact with anyone. He seemed listless and lethargic much of the time. When attempts were made to feed him, Chang would become very distressed, crying, and trying to bang his head against the wall or floor. His mother commented that, because of such behavior, she rarely tried to pick him up anymore and would prop the bottle during his feeding.

When parents are interacting with a child who has these responses, it is not uncommon for the parents to become less involved.

REACTIVE ATTACHMENT DISORDER OF INFANCY OR EARLY CHILDHOOD

Reactive attachment disorder (RAD) of infancy or early childhood is a markedly disturbed and developmentally inappropriate way of relating that is presumed to be the result of extremely inadequate or negligent caregiving. Inadequate or negligent care may involve any of the following:

■ Persistent disregard of the child's basic emotional needs for comfort, stimulation, or affection

■ Persistent disregard of the child's basic physical needs

■ Repeated changes of caregivers that prevent the formation of stable attachments

However, not all children who experience extremely inadequate care develop the disorder. See DSM Essential Features for information about reactive attachment disorder on page 553.

The two types of this disorder are distinctly opposite in their symptoms. The *inhibited type* involves a failure to initiate and respond to most social interactions in a developmentally appropriate way. Children show excessively inhibited, hypervigilant, or ambivalent responses. Examples are a look of frozen watchfulness, resistance to comfort, and a mixture of approach and avoidance. In contrast, the *disinhibited type* involves an indiscriminate sociability or lack of selectivity in the choice of attachment figures. The child may be excessively familiar with strangers—hugging and cuddling an adult stranger in a store, for example—or may seek comfort and affection from a variety of adults who are not well known to the child.

The severity and duration of the disorder depend on the degree of psychosocial deprivation and the nature of any intervention. If a supportive environment is provided, improvement does occur. Children with this disorder commonly have a feeding and eating disorder as well. Evidence-Based Practice demonstrates how parental detachment and interruptions in the parent–child relationship affect the child's ability to form attachments to others.

SEPARATION ANXIETY DISORDER

Separation anxiety disorder involves a developmentally inappropriate and excessive anxiety over separation from home or from attachment figures. Symptoms may include fear and worry about possible harm befalling attachment figures or about being separated from them. Children with this disorder frequently come from close-knit families and are often described as demanding, intrusive, or in need of constant attention. They may also be unusually compliant, conscientious, or eager to please. You may also see a depressed mood that increases over time.

The disorder occurs in about 4% of children and may appear after a stressful life event such as the death of a pet, a family illness, or immigration (APA, 2000). There are periods of exacerbation and remission over the course of the disorder that persist for many years, including into adulthood. DSM Essential Features on page 553 describes separation anxiety disorder.

ELIMINATION DISORDERS

The elimination disorders (problematic behaviors associated with urination and defecation) are encopresis and enuresis. **Encopresis** is the repeated passing of feces by the child into inappropriate places such as clothing or a corner of the room. **Enuresis** is the repeated voiding of urine into the bed or clothes, either during the day or at night. In order to be

---

EVIDENCE-BASED PRACTICE

The Effect of Disengagement Between Parents and Children

Elena Vasquez is being seen at your family mental health clinic for PTSD and depression. She is a recent refugee who experienced many traumatic events, most notably seeing her parents shot and killed. She was also the victim of domestic violence, being frequently beaten by her partner. You notice that Ms. Vasquez regularly brings her 2-year-old son Mario with her to her treatment sessions. He sits in the hallway while his mother meets with her therapist. You are concerned that Mario shows very little facial expression, seems uninterested in his toys, and is distant toward his mother. You are concerned about Mario's affect. You also recently read a research report that identified disengagement between mother and child as a sign of potential attachment problems. Concerned about Mario, you propose that Mario have a clinical assessment.

When an adult has been severely traumatized in some form or another, this changes the urge to be close and nurturing. Sometimes

that change is toward detachment. When exposed to detachment early in life, children may perceive it as the norm, making it difficult for the child to attach appropriately to others.

With the mother's agreement, you perform a mental status examination with Mario and interview the mother about his behavior. The assessment indicates that Mario has symptoms of major depression as well as indications of reactive attachment disorder. Based on the assessment, you then develop a care plan that includes both play therapy and child–parent psychotherapy. Your interventions are based upon the following classic and recent publications:

Shlafer, R. J., & Poehlmann, J. (2010). Attachment and caregiving relationships in families affected by parental incarceration. *Attachment and Human Development, 12*(4), 395–415.

CRITICAL THINKING QUESTIONS

1. When is assessment of children of traumatized adults appropriate in clinical practice?
2. How would you expect a 2-year-old child to react to play therapy?
3. When would you expect Mario's symptoms of depression and attachment disorder to improve? To resolve?

classified as a mental disorder, these problems must not be due to any medical condition or to the physiological effects of a laxative, diuretic, or other substance. For both encopresis and enuresis, there is a primary and secondary type:

- With the *primary type,* the child has never been toilet trained.
- In the *secondary type,* the disturbance develops after a period of using the toilet appropriately.

Of course, the problem is not diagnosed as a mental disorder unless the child has reached a chronologic age at which elimination problems should not be apparent (at least age 4 for encopresis and age 5 for enuresis). Predisposing factors for both disorders include inconsistent or lax toilet training, or psychosocial stressors such as entry to school or a sibling birth. In contrast to encopresis, about 75% of all children with enuresis have a parent or sibling who had the disorder (APA, 2000).

Both disorders are more common in boys, with prevalence rates for enuresis being higher (5% to 10% of 5-year-old children) than for encopresis (1% of all 5-year-old children) (APA, 2000). Neither disorder is typically chronic. Most children become continent by adolescence. The degree of immediate and long-term impairment depends to a great extent on the amount of resulting peer rejection, punishment and rejection by the caregiver, and a child's overall self-esteem.

Encopresis

This is usually involuntary behavior, but it may be intentional in some situations. There are two subtypes of the disorder. The first involves constipation and continuous leakage of feces during the day and during sleep. Incontinence stops once the constipation is treated. The constipation may develop for psychological reasons, often related to a general pattern of anxious or oppositional behavior that leads the child to avoid defecation. Health problems causing dehydration, or the side effects of medication, may also initially create the constipation, but once it has developed, a child may retain stool because of painful defecation or anal fissure. The second subtype does not involve constipation or incontinence. Feces are normal and soiling is intermittent, with feces usually found in an obvious place. Children with this subtype often have a dual diagnosis of ODD or CD. With either subtype, smearing the feces may result from attempts to clean or hide the feces, or it may be a deliberate effort to make a mess.

Enuresis

There are two types of enuresis:

- The *nocturnal type* is most common and typically occurs during the first part of the night.
- The *diurnal type* (during waking hours) happens most typically in the early afternoon of school days. This type may be related to social anxiety and a resulting reluctance to use the toilet, or it may be because the child becomes preoccupied with play or other activities.

Some children show a combination of both day and night enuresis.

OTHER IMPORTANT DISORDERS OF INFANCY OR CHILDHOOD

Two other disorders are typically diagnosed in childhood and rarely continue past childhood. Features or components of these disorders may have relevance for adult behaviors.

Selective Mutism

Selective mutism is the persistent failure to speak in specific social situations, even though the child can speak in other situations. Of course, the failure to speak must not be the result of a lack of normal language skills or knowledge of a certain language. The child can be excessively shy, fearful of embarrassment, withdrawn, clinging, and negative; or you may observe temper tantrums or oppositional behavior, especially at home. Mutism is rare, but slightly more common in girls. Usually, the disturbance lasts for only a few months, but it can continue for several years.

Stereotypic Movement Disorder

Stereotypic movement disorder is a pattern of motor behavior that is repetitive and nonfunctional and one that the child appears driven to do. Examples of such movements are rocking, twirling objects, head banging, self-biting, picking at skin or body orifices, or hitting parts of one's own body. The specific behaviors may change over time from one type to another. The disorder can result in self-injurious behavior (see Chapter 22∞) that causes tissue damage or is life threatening. The behavior is frequently associated with intellectual disability; however, it may also occur in children with severe sensory deficits—blindness or deafness, for example—or in institutional environments without sufficient stimulation.

Sometimes children try to restrain themselves from the behavior—for example, by putting their hands in their pockets—but if the restraint is interfered with, the behaviors resume. Onset of the disorder may follow a stressful event. See DSM Essential Features describing stereotypic movement disorder on page 553.

TIC DISORDERS

The following three disorders are classified as tics:

1. Tourette's disorder
2. Chronic motor or vocal tics disorder
3. Transient tic disorder

Tic disorders are characterized by rapid, recurring, stereotypic movements or vocalizations that occur suddenly and involuntarily. Tic disorders are worse during stress but occur less frequently when the child is focused intently on an activity such as reading. Most tic disorders appear to be transmitted through a genetic or constitutional factor, creating a vulnerability to the disorder. However, about 10% of children with the disorder have a "nongenetic" form; these children frequently have a dual diagnosis with another mental disorder or a medical condition such as epilepsy (APA, 2000). Regardless of type, boys are more likely to develop tic disorders than girls.

The symptoms of children who have tic disorders (or other disorders such as obsessive–compulsive disorder) may worsen following streptococcal infections (e.g., strep throat). The mental health problems resulting from such an exacerbation of symptoms are referred to as PANDAS (pediatric autoimmune neuropsychiatric disorders associated with streptococci). (See Chapter 18∞ for a more detailed discussion.)

Tourette's Disorder

Tourette's disorder involves multiple motor tics and one or more vocal tics, which can occur simultaneously or at different periods during the illness. The diagnosis requires that there is never a tic-free period longer than 3 months. Vocal tics are words or sounds such as yelps, barks, snorts, or coughs. *Coprolalia* is a specific type of vocal tic in which obscenities are uttered. *Motor tics* include such behaviors as eye blinking, protruding the tongue, sniffing, retracing steps, or twirling when walking.

The disorder may begin as early as age 2, but more often it begins during childhood or early adolescence. Tourette's disorder normally lasts for a lifetime with periods of remission, but in most cases the symptoms decrease during adolescence and adulthood. DSM Essential Features on page 553 describes the disorder.

Chronic Versus Transient Tic Disorders

Chronic motor or vocal tic disorder differs from Tourette's disorder in that it involves *either* motor tics or vocal tics, but not both, as is required for a diagnosis of Tourette's disorder. Transient tic disorder differs from chronic motor or vocal tic disorder and Tourette's disorder in its duration. While the others require that the problems have occurred for at least a year, transient tic disorder does not last longer than 12 months.

ADULT DISORDERS THAT MAY BEGIN IN CHILDHOOD

A few disorders that are diagnosed more frequently in adulthood may begin in childhood. These include anxiety disorders, mood disorders, and schizophrenia.

Anxiety Disorders

In addition to separation anxiety, which was described earlier, children can have many other anxiety disorders (anxiety disorders are thoroughly discussed in Chapter 18∞). Panic disorder and agoraphobia are rare in children. Specific phobias, however, may be seen in children even before age 5 and are common childhood anxiety disorders. Children develop fears, especially of animals and blood-related events. Severe social phobia is also found in children and may lead to school avoidance.

The onset of obsessive–compulsive disorder (OCD) is common for children aged 9 to 11. Because children may not have developed "insight" yet, the requirement for OCD that they recognize the excessive nature of their behavior is waived for children. Generalized anxiety disorder (GAD) and post-traumatic stress disorder (PTSD) are also found in

WHY I PLAN TO BECOME A PSYCHIATRIC–MENTAL HEALTH NURSE

Averi's Story: Something clicked for me when I was on an outpatient clinical rotation last month. I made a home visit with the community mental health nurse from a local psychiatric center to a client who has schizophrenia. This client has been doing fairly well for a year and Jill, the nurse, told me that we would be assessing how the client is doing, as well as how her 4-year-old daughter was doing. When we got to their home I was impressed by the neat kitchen and playroom and how well the client and her daughter were interacting.

On the ride back to the clinic, Jill asked me what I noticed about our visit. I told her I thought the client was doing very well and that, given the neatness of the environment and the nice interactions, I thought all was good. Jill agreed—to a point. When we looked a little more deeply into what I saw, I was struck by how intricate a nursing assessment must be. Jill noted that the playroom was neat because the 4-year-old child was not playing with any of the toys; she wasn't even touching them. And the two of them were interacting nicely as long as the 4-year-old child was being almost adult-like. The child was being the adult in the relationship and that is too big a burden for such a small child. Jill subsequently planned parenting classes for her client and play dates for her client's daughter so the child would have social contacts more appropriate for her age. This is the type of forward thinking and holistic care I am interested in doing with my clients.

children. Children with GAD are often shy and may act more mature and serious than expected for their age. They often are perfectionistic and highly compliant to demands of authority figures.

PTSD in children is often associated with child abuse. In contrast to the adult experience of "flashbacks" of the traumatic event, children typically re-experience traumatic events as nightmares or through repetitive reenactment during play. Remember that children can have strong memories of events even though they cannot describe them verbally. These memories can be brought forth in play or dreams by children who are as young as 2 or 3 years of age.

Early treatment of all types of anxiety disorders in children is very important because they can lead to many social problems, including rejection or neglect by peers, academic failure, and inadequate development into an autonomous, secure adult. In general, the symptoms of anxiety disorders are similar in children and adults.

Mood Disorders

Mood disorders are discussed fully in Chapter 17∞, however, a few issues related to mood disorders in children are important to note here. Diagnoses of mood disorders are usually not made during infancy, because developmentally children often do not have the ability to reflect on their feelings even if the feelings are strongly affecting them. Remember also that children may not be able to accurately report symptoms even if they are experiencing them. Bipolar disorder was considered very rare in childhood but this disorder is now being better recognized and diagnosed. Hyperactivity can easily be confused with symptoms of mania in children. Children with bipolar disorder often have a chronic mixed state of depression and mania or rapid cycling. In addition to hyperactivity, observe for aggressive, long-lasting temper outbursts, excessive risk taking, and highly energized affect as signs of mania in children.

Depressive disorders are quite common in children, with depressive symptoms occurring even in the first year of life. Although there is a greater incidence of depressive disorders among women in adulthood, the prepubertal incidence is about 2% for both boys and girls (APA, 2000). The two types of depressive disorders are major depression and dysthymia. Major depression involves a definite change in behavior from the child's normal functioning. The child begins to show a depressed or sad mood or a lack of pleasure (anhedonia) in almost all activities at least 50% of the time.

There are some important differences in how children and adults may manifest these symptoms. Children may describe things as bad, gloomy, blue, or empty when they are depressed. You may see a bland, frozen look on their faces or only fleeting smiles, as if they are smiling because it is socially expected rather than because they feel like smiling. On the other hand, you may see no evidence of sadness in children but rather a persistent irritability around even small matters. Pervasive boredom is a common sign of anhedonia in children. Another sign is social withdrawal, especially when a child avoids or rejects opportunities to play.

Other symptoms of depression in children include unexplained somatic complaints, poor school performance, sleep and appetite changes, and/or psychomotor agitation and increased risk taking. The most common type of depression in children is called *reactive depression,* which occurs in response to a particular situation, such as the trauma of hospitalization or an extended separation from a parent.

Dysthymia is a chronic disorder with periods of depressed affect interspersed with normal mood. Symptoms of later adult dysthymia often begin in childhood, even if not diagnosed until later. Because of this early and chronic quality, the person is often described as a "depressive personality." Although the symptoms of dysthymia are the same for children and adults, children are likely to show greater evidence of irritability, not simply depressed affect, and may react negatively or shyly to praise. They may respond to positive relationships with testing, anger, or avoidance. Other symptoms of dysthymia are similar to major depression, except that the child may show more evidence of low energy and low self-esteem. A key predisposing factor for childhood dysthymia is the presence of an inadequate, rejecting, or chaotic home environment.

Schizophrenia

Occurring as early as age 5 or 6, childhood-onset schizophrenia is rare. The features of schizophrenia (delusions, hallucinations, disorganized speech and behavior, and negative symptoms) are the same in children as adults. Be aware, however, that failure to reach expected levels of speech and behavior may be seen in children rather than a deterioration into disorganization. (Schizophrenia is discussed fully in Chapter 16∞.) The following clinical example illustrates one girl's symptoms that led to the diagnosis of schizophrenia.

Clinical Example

Shauna, an 11-year-old child, described hearing the voice of her mother calling her name and yelling at her, although her mother was not present. At times, she heard her own voice telling her to do things such as chores for her mother. She experienced her mother's voice as coming from outside her head and her own voice as coming from inside her head. She reported seeing a woman who looked like her mother and who she thought was her mother. She also believed that her mother was watching her.

Shauna described going to the bathroom in the morning and "daydreaming" that objects were weapons (e.g., cotton swabs were sticks to stab people, and washcloths were used to smother people). All these experiences seemed real to Shauna as they happened. Shauna also believed that the world was coming to an end. She described hearing on the news that a hole was breaking apart pieces of the earth, and she thought this was going to happen. She also expressed concern that a heat wave might result in there not being enough air to breathe.

It is difficult to make the diagnosis in children, however, because delusions and hallucinations are less detailed and more accepted developmentally as normal fantasy or imaginary playmates. Visual hallucinations are more common in children than in adults but are almost always accompanied by auditory hallucinations. Disorganized speech (such as in communication disorders) or disorganized behavior (as in ADHD or autistic disorder) may result in other diagnoses when they are actually symptoms of schizophrenia.

BIOPSYCHOSOCIAL THEORIES

Major theories guide existing views of childhood psychopathology and the therapeutic approaches. These are psychodynamic theory, attachment theory, cognitive–behavioral theory, and biologic theory. The central features of these theories will be presented.

Psychodynamic Theory

Psychodynamic theory originated with Sigmund Freud in his conceptualization of psychoanalysis but has evolved substantially since its original formulation. Much of Freud's speculation regarding psychosexual stages of development has been rejected, but components of his personality theory serve a purpose for assessing and treating children. *Psychic determinism* proposes that the child's initial perceptions of the world are defined substantially during the first 5 to 6 years of life and will influence the child's later views and behavior. While this stance seems almost a given in today's world, the concept was unheard of when Freud first proposed it.

Because the ego and superego prevent the id from getting all needs met, Freud proposed that children attempt to cope with the anxiety associated with need deprivation through the unconscious mental processes known as defense mechanisms (see Chapter 8∞). Defense mechanisms commonly employed by children are regression, repression, reaction formation, and projection. The child comes to deal with the world through these distorted views in an attempt to defend against painful unconscious issues. However, the unconscious content continues to influence the behavior and conscious thoughts of the child, often in ways that severely impair his or her ability to function in life. The focus of treatment is attempting to bring repressed conflicts and issues into awareness so that they can be addressed and resolved.

Attachment Theory

In attachment theory, relationships are the organizing principle for the child's well-being in attachment theory. *Attachment* is the child's socioemotional bond to another person (the attachment figure) who is perceived as strong or powerful and who can be turned to for protection and support in situations of perceived danger or adversity. Attachment behaviors (proximity or contact-promoting behaviors such as calling, approaching, or clinging) help the child acquire a sense of security. Four major patterns of attachment have been identified (see TABLE 25-1 ■).

Cognitive–Behavioral Theory

The origins of cognitive–behavioral theory stem from psychologist B. F. Skinner's behavioral learning school of thought. However, current views integrate cognitive theory and social learning theory. The basis of this theory is the importance of the environment (family, school, and neighborhood) in the child's psychological development. Modeling is important; children learn by watching others. They also learn about the consequences of behavior.

Cognitive theorists emphasize that psychopathology results from particular mental sets or cognitions that involve distortions of reality. Biased or inaccurate ways of thinking or processing information include the following:

- Interpreting things as worse than they are
- Overgeneralizing
- Selective perception
- Disqualifying the positive
- Jumping to conclusions
- Personalizing events that are not actually related to the child

Treatment is focused on a relearning process to correct inaccurate thinking.

Biologic Theory

The exact relationship between various biologic factors and mental illness is not fully understood.

Neurobiologic Factors

There is considerable evidence for the role of neurobiologic factors in the development of disorders such as autistic disorder and childhood-onset schizophrenia. Children with these disorders have more physical anomalies, neurologic soft signs,

TABLE 25-1 ■ Patterns of Attachment		
Attachment Pattern	**Characteristics of the Child**	**Characteristics of the Caregiver**
Secure	■ Readily seeks out caregivers in times of stress and is reassured by the caregiver's presence.	■ Is available and responsive to the child's attachment needs. ■ Encourages the child to seek security through proximity and contact.
Insecure–avoidant	■ Appears indifferent to stress and uncertainty, although physiological responses suggest otherwise. ■ Actively avoids the attachment figure during stressful times and focuses on other things, such as play.	■ Is insensitive to the child's needs. ■ Actively rebuffs the child's attempts to be comforted during distress.
Insecure–resistant	■ Resists interaction and contact with caregivers when it is available. ■ Shows proximity-seeking behavior when contact is unavailable. ■ Shifts between seeking comfort excessively and being difficult to settle or soothe when contact is acquired.	■ Tends to be unpredictable in accessibility to child. ■ Is less able to adapt than typical children, is hesitant, and is occupied with caregiving routines.
Disorganized	■ Shows unexplainable or disoriented behavior toward the attachment figure during distress (e.g., frightened expressions and freezing while greeting the parent with raised arms, smiling while forcefully striking the parent's face, or extended rocking or ear pulling).	■ May behave in frightening or threatening ways toward the child. ■ May reverse roles, acting timid or deferential toward the child.

and brain abnormalities on electroencephalograms (EEGs) and in computed tomography (CT) and magnetic resonance imaging (MRI) scans. Similarly, lead poisoning, central nervous system (CNS) trauma, and infections in childhood have all been implicated as possible causative factors. There had been concern among parents, consumer advocacy groups, and health care professionals that vaccines given to infants may be linked to an increase in autism. Because of these concerns some parents had been reluctant to have their children protected from childhood diseases through vaccination. The data do not support the hypothesis that vaccines cause autism.

Nervous System Responsiveness

Studies indicate that problems with nervous system responsiveness may be related to certain psychiatric disorders. For example, children with schizophrenia have unusually high autonomic system reactivity when in baseline or resting states, and children with attention deficit disorder with hyperactivity (ADHD) appear to have a lowered excitability in the reticular activating system of the brain, requiring more stimulation in order to feel optimally aroused.

Neuroendocrine Reactivity

A related biologic vulnerability is the child's neuroendocrine reactivity. The hypothalamic–pituitary–adrenal axis regulates the nervous system's release of stress hormones such as cortisol. The feedback mechanism controlling these hormones appears dysfunctional in certain psychiatric disorders. For instance, children with post-traumatic stress disorder (PTSD) tend to show excessive levels of stress hormones, with neurotoxic effects on brain development and function.

Genetic Predisposition

Twin and adoption studies continue to provide evidence in support of genetic etiology for many disorders, including pervasive developmental disorders, schizophrenia, and depression. Rett's disorder has been found to be an X-linked dominant inheritance disorder associated with mutations in the MECP2 gene (van Bon et al., 2010). In addition, there is evidence that other milder mutations in the MECP2 gene may predispose to autism and intellectual disorder.

Research into autism spectrum disorders (ASD) has been a rich field. NIMH Autism Genome Project Consortium and the Autism Genetics Group continue to explore this complex topic (2011). Glutamate has been implicated as involved in ASD, as has chromosomal defects/damage, and biologic processes. Some cases of genetically-caused autism are due to a random accident while the egg or sperm is being formed, and not to heritability.

Perinatal Complications

Perinatal complications, including perinatal asphyxia, congenital anomalies, deficient treatment of the pregnant mother for major mental illness, and intrauterine exposure to drugs of abuse and alcohol, have also been associated with psychiatric disorders (Schieve et al., 2010). Refer to What Every Nurse Should Know regarding potential effects of premature birth.

WHAT EVERY NURSE SHOULD KNOW

Prematurity and Mental Health Problems

Imagine you are a neonatal nurse. Infants born prematurely are at greater risk of developing mental health problems. Neonatal nurses who help parents learn parenting skills in caring for their infant can improve the child's mental health outcomes. Important parenting skills include attending to the infant's behavioral cues, understanding the potential meaning of various infant behaviors, and reducing the infant's distress through soothing, consoling, and other stress reduction techniques.

Brain Structure and Function

Finally, there is a growing body of research that suggests that early psychological trauma from severe neglect or abuse may create deficits or abnormalities in brain structure and function. It was previously thought that a child's biologic makeup could influence his or her psychosocial outcomes, but not the reverse. Evidence indicates that psychological trauma in the first few years of life can create changes in the size of the brain, the number of neuronal pathways affecting certain brain functions (such as emotion), and the amount and function of neurotransmitters in the brain (Cole & Lanham, 2011).

Multicausal Model

There is growing acceptance of a multicausal, multidimensional nature of mental illness. Box 25-1 lists potential risk factors that have been identified for childhood mental illness. Although specific risk factors surface in the literature, FIGURE 25-2 ■ illustrates how life experiences influence mental health outcomes.

Many children show tremendous hardiness and resilience in the face of horrible life experiences, while other more vulnerable children may be severely affected by even a minimally stressful or adverse experience. In a multicausal model, there is

---

Box 25-1   Risk Factors for Developing Mental Health Problems in Childhood

- Inherited metabolic deficiencies or nervous system abnormalities
- Injury, toxic exposure, or physical complications in utero or during the perinatal period
- Medical conditions of infancy or childhood (such as epilepsy, low birth weight)
- Early deprivation of nurturance or stimulation (parental absence or loss, neglect or rejection, large family size, foster placement)
- Traumatic experience (such as abuse or life-threatening event)
- Family history of a psychiatric disorder
- A chaotic home environment (family violence or severe marital discord)
- Disadvantaged socioeconomic status (poverty, violence, hopelessness)

Genetic Predisposition
• Metabolic Deficiencies
• Nervous System Abnormalities

Interaction Between Genotype and Experience → **Child Mental Illness**

Life Experience
• Injury/Illness
• Toxic Exposure
• Deprivation/Neglect
• Abuse/Rejection
• Other Major Stressors (e.g., death of a parent)

FIGURE 25-2 ■ Interactive model of child mental illness.

no certain etiology, no predictable set of risk factors, and no specific therapeutic approach with a standard outcome. Consider the unique fit that is possible between a particular child and a particular set of life experiences to understand the child's mental health problems and develop an appropriate intervention.

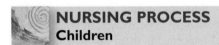

NURSING PROCESS
Children

The assessment, diagnosis, planning, implementation, and evaluation activities undertaken by the child psychiatric–mental health nurse are always in collaboration with the child, the family, and professional colleagues who are part of the child's care. The degree to which these individuals are active partners in the nursing process will influence the resulting quality and efficacy of your nursing care.

Assessment

The basics of an effective assessment include gathering cultural and developmental information, eliciting a history from the parents, and undertaking a clinical assessment of the child.

Cultural and Developmental Context

Your ability to perform a valid assessment depends on your knowledge of developmental norms and your cultural sensitivity to appropriately frame a child's behavior. Assess within the context of a child's cultural background and developmental stage. (See Developing Cultural Competence for guidelines.) As the clinical example illustrates, you may also need to help family members reconcile different cultural beliefs within the family.

Clinical Example

The maternal grandmother of a suicidal child who was scheduled for admission to an inpatient unit tried to block the admission. She insisted that the child was possessed by a demon and wanted the child to stay with her so she could pray over her and give her healing herbs.

The child psychiatrist and the child psychiatric nurse spent time with the parents discussing the pressure they experienced from the child's grandmother. They mentioned to the parents that psychiatric services were unfamiliar to the grandmother's generation and cultural beliefs. They also reviewed the basis for the recommendation of hospitalization. The parents were encouraged to make their own decision based on their experience with their child and their concerns for her safety. Ways to involve the grandmother and her traditional medicines were suggested, and the professionals offered to be available to discuss the grandmother's questions and concerns.

Regarding developmental norms, you must determine whether a behavior (such as temper tantrums or separation anxiety) is understandable or appropriate based on the

DEVELOPING CULTURAL COMPETENCE

Perception of Temper Tantrums

Nursing assessments of children occur within the context of a child's cultural background and the child's developmental stage. What can be defined as "normal or functional" versus "abnormal or dysfunctional" is relative to the meaning certain behaviors have within a culture and the child's developmental capabilities. For instance, temper tantrums can be viewed very differently within different cultures, as in the following examples:

■ In one culture, tantrums may be viewed as the result of a nervous temperament or a fragile personality.
■ Families of another culture may think that tantrums are the disobedient acts of a stubborn child.

These different perceptions bring about different responses by the parent, which may, in turn, affect the child's behavior over time.

Ask families what they believe about the cause of their child's problems. This is a good way to assess their culture-specific beliefs. You can also find out what their parents and grandparents have said about the problems as well as traditional resource people within their communities (such as spiritual advisors or healers). Another good discussion point is where any traditional remedies or cultural practices have been used to deal with the child's problems. Show respect for a family's unique views of mental illness, and build a mutually acceptable approach to discussing the child and his or her behavior.

CRITICAL THINKING QUESTIONS

1. How can multigenerational perspectives be useful in assessing a child's behavior?
2. How might your view and feelings about temper tantrums affect your approach to the child, parents, grandparents, and greatgrandparents?

child's age. Stage of development affects the symptoms you will see, a child's expected responses to life stress, and the child's ability to understand and communicate with you about certain problems. Allow adequate time for full responses to open-ended questions, active listening, and careful observation of patterns of behavior. Assessment should be an ongoing process rather than a one-time session. You typically cannot generalize your observations to other times and settings.

The History-Taking Interview

Include the child as well as the parents in discussing the history of the problem. Although parents are a better source of facts such as onset, developmental milestones, or context surrounding the symptoms, including the child is helpful because it has the following effects:

- It decreases the child's feelings of being left out, talked about, or powerless in the situation.
- It helps you learn the child's perspective. Children are the best informants regarding their feelings and thoughts. You will also find it very useful to hear an older child's response to the parents on certain issues or how the child's view may differ.
- It allows you to observe the nonverbal communication among family members. Their interactions give important clues regarding the family's functioning in areas such as closeness, conflict, decision making, and flexibility.

Because parents may not be comfortable discussing certain information in front of their child, be sure to give them some time with you alone in addition to this total family approach. Specific areas to cover in the history-taking interview are outlined in Your Assessment Approach. You may also wish to refer to Chapter 29 ∞ for suggestions on assessing family process.

Clinical Assessment of a Child

The clinical assessment of a child involves a mental status examination by the nurse and referral of the child for a complete physical and neuropsychologic evaluation. These latter evaluations are important in order to rule out any medical conditions and identify any neurologic or cognitive problems that may be associated with the child's psychiatric symptoms.

A mental status examination consists of both a semi-structured interview and an unstructured play session with the child. Areas for assessment during the mental status examination are shown in Your Assessment Approach: Guidelines for Assessing Children. If the child is nearing adolescence or is ambivalent about unstructured play, try games instead as a medium through which you can observe the child's way of relating and approaching various situations.

For both aspects of the examination, a relaxed, conversational approach is the most effective, where the child has the opportunity to tell you his story about problems he may be having and his relationships with family, peers, and teachers. Research shows that children are a better source than their parents regarding the nature and extent of their symptoms. Frame questions in ways that are developmentally appropriate for the child. Even 3- to 6-year-old children can give excellent feedback about their symptoms if questions are developmentally appropriate. Asking simple, informal questions such as what kind of animal they would like to be, what they would want if they could have three wishes, or what was the saddest thing that ever happened to them can provide a great deal of information regarding speech, modes of thinking and perception, and feeling states. Having children draw and discuss pictures of themselves and their family can be very useful for understanding their view of the world. The drawing in FIGURE 25-3 ■ by a 6-year-old girl named Emma is an excellent example.

Observing a child at play with puppets, clay, or a sand tray can also provide invaluable information about motor behavior, thought content, affect, and impulse control. In addition, there are many children's books using stories about abuse, depression, divorce, or hospitalization as themes. These stories portray children and animals with problems that relate to a variety of mental health challenges faced by children. They can serve as a stimulus for questions such as "How

---

YOUR ASSESSMENT APPROACH   Areas to Cover in the History-Taking Interview

1. **The child's current problems.** Discuss the history of the problem(s), including major concerns or complaints, how long it has been since the problem(s) first began, the specific symptoms, and the parents' previous and current efforts to address the problem(s).

2. **Family history and process.** Talk with the family about their own history and family process. This aspect of the assessment can include a genogram or family time line (see the description in Chapter 29 ∞), discussion of child-rearing beliefs and behaviors, supports and stressors for the family, the history of any separations between parents and child, and any psychiatric or other illness in the family.

3. **The child's medical history.** Find out about any childhood illnesses, allergies, medications, and physical health problems.

4. **The child's developmental history.** Starting with pregnancy or birth complications, progress through the child's development to identify any lags or events in achieving developmental milestones.

5. **The child's characteristics and psychosocial environment.** Find out both the parents' and the child's view of the child's temperament, interests, and skills. During this aspect of the interview, also identify the nature of the child's sociocultural environment (home, neighborhood, school) and how it may support or inhibit the achievement of developmental tasks. Be sure to find out about the number and type of friends the child has.

YOUR ASSESSMENT APPROACH   Guidelines for Assessing Children

Areas to Assess During the Mental Status Exam

General Appearance and Demeanor
- Grooming, alertness, eye contact, and overall attitude toward clinician

Motor Behavior and Coordination
- Activity level, gross motor and fine motor control, nature of movements, posture

Mood and Affect
- Overall mood state, manner of expressing feelings, range and intensity of emotions, evidence of dysphoric state (anger, anxiety, sadness)

Speech and Language
- Clarity and articulation, rhythm and organization, appropriateness of word choice

Thought Process
- Ability to understand and express meaning in an age-appropriate way, evidence of any loss of connectedness

between ideas (loose associations), repeated behaviors or mannerisms (perseveration), or tangentiality of child's response to your questions

Thought Content
- Themes in play and talk, fears, evidence of beliefs that have no basis in reality

Perceptual Disturbances
- Threshold and tolerance for sensory input, evidence of hallucinations or illusions

Cognitive Function
- Orientation to person, time, and place; ability to follow through on requests; attention and concentration; distractability

Impulse Control
- Ability to manage behavior appropriately in response to needs and desires

---

do you think that puppy might feel?" or "What would you do if you were that little girl?" These stories offer children opportunities to project their own thoughts and feelings onto the characters in the stories and share them with you.

FIGURE 25-3 ■ Family drawing by Emma, a 6-year-old girl. Emma's drawing has a number of distinctive features. She has placed herself at a distance from the rest of the family, suggesting feelings of isolation, rejection, or perhaps fear. The heavy lines around her father's body may indicate that he is seen as aggressive or angry. This interpretation is supported by the father's mouth, which appears to be open as if shouting or showing his teeth. Her brother looks happy, and her mother's downturned mouth looks a bit sad. Emma's drawing of herself is quite small, in contrast to others in the family (especially her brother, who is actually younger and smaller than Emma). Her smallness could indicate some insecurity, low self-esteem, or perhaps a desire to withdraw from the world and not be noticed. The center of Emma's body is shaded, suggesting some anxiety about that part of her body. She is also missing her mouth and hands. This could imply a sense of inadequacy or powerlessness to act or speak.

Assessing Possible Maltreatment

You should always be alert for possible signs of maltreatment during your psychiatric assessment. Maltreatment can be identified in emergency departments as well (see What Every Nurse Should Know). Important signs of maltreatment in a child are detailed in Your Assessment Approach: Signs of Maltreatment of a Child.

Maltreatment can involve child neglect or outright abuse. In neglect, parents fail to recognize when a problem exists or to meet their child's normal emotional and physical needs.

WHAT EVERY NURSE SHOULD KNOW

Assessing Physical Abuse in Children

Imagine you are an emergency department nurse. Physical abuse of children can be addressed through careful observation in the emergency department (ED). Take special notice if any of the following occurs:

- A child seems hypervigilant or hyperreactive to your touch.
- A parent seems evasive, unconcerned, or resistant to your questions or any follow-up procedures.

Collect further information if the following risk indicators are present:

- The child has been admitted to the ED for previous injuries.
- There are inconsistencies between your clinical exam and the parent's or child's description of what occurred.
- There was a delay in bringing the child for medical attention.

Abuse can take many forms. It may be physical, involving severe disciplinary practices (e.g., beatings) or unexplained injury to the child (e.g., burns or bruises). Before age 12, boys are at greater risk of physical abuse but girls are more at risk as teenagers. Abuse can also be emotional, such as a child being verbally demeaned or rejected. And, of course, sexual abuse is possible. Sexual abuse can include exposure to exhibitionism, molestation or fondling, intercourse, or rape. Girls are more likely than boys to be victims of sexual abuse by a 10-to-1 ratio. Chapter 24 ∞ has more information on physical and sexual child abuse.

Assessing Suicide Risk

Suicide by children, while always a difficult and devastating situation, has become more of a problem because we are not entirely sure what causes the rate to rise or fall. There is a continuing discussion over the role of antidepressants in youth suicide (see Chapter 23 ∞). There is a decline in suicide attempts and completed suicides among adults and adolescents who are prescribed antidepressant medications.

Some people cannot believe that children can be depressed or would want to end their lives. Suicide attempts by children belie the myth of the "happy child" in our culture. The following clinical example illustrates denial and lack of information on the part of the parents of a suicidal child.

Clinical Example

A 7-year-old boy set up a rope over a door to hang himself. His attempt was stopped by his parents. The door, a second entrance to the room, was nailed shut and painted, but the subject of suicide was not discussed. His parents failed to recognize the same symptoms in the child 2 years later. At this time, however, severe behavioral problems in school, and pressure by school personnel, forced the parents to seek a psychiatric evaluation.

Although suicide in children under 12 occurs infrequently, suicidal ideation or suicide threats by a child always deserve attention and merit careful study. Even the most obvious gesture can prove fatal, especially in a child whose assessment of physical danger is immature and unrealistic. Children commit suicide by simple but lethal methods such as poisoning, shooting themselves with firearms, hanging, or darting into the path of moving cars.

It is unclear what drives a child to suicide. However, there are characteristic presuicidal symptoms and life circumstances of the suicidal child. The symptoms are known as depressive equivalents; that is, the symptoms may indicate a masked depression (see What Every Nurse Should Know). Life circumstances that put the child at higher risk for suicide are experiences of significant loss, family discord, abuse, neglect, or the presence of other psychiatric problems, such as depression and related disorders.

Perform a careful assessment of suicide risk whenever a child expresses ideas about suicide or makes an attempt. The assessment interview should consider the degree of risk while exploring the family situation and the external events that preceded the thoughts or the attempt. Explore the meaning behind the attempt. Young children are less able to verbalize, and need more structure and planned activities before you can complete an appropriate assessment. You may, for example, use books that help children talk about suicide. Also see Chapter 23 ∞ for a discussion of youth suicide and child survivors of the death by suicide of a parent.

Nursing Diagnosis: NANDA

Nursing diagnoses are the critical foundation underlying all planning, implementation, and evaluation activities with a child. Once you identify a child's problems, determine which of the NANDA diagnoses best match the problems. Then, prioritize the diagnoses based on their urgency or their need for attention before you can address other problems. There are some diagnoses specific to children in the NANDA classification system, such as the following:

- Disorganized Infant Behavior
- Risk for Delayed Development
- Risk for Impaired Parent/Child Attachment

Many other general diagnoses are relevant to children, such as Impaired Verbal Communication, Anxiety, Disturbed Sensory Perception, Ineffective Coping, Impaired Social Interactions, Risk for Violence, Post-Trauma Syndrome, and Chronic or Situational Low Self-Esteem. Many family and parent-related diagnoses are also quite relevant.

WHAT EVERY NURSE SHOULD KNOW

Childhood Depression

Imagine you are a pediatric nurse. Parents are often unaware of their child's sadness or depression and do not recognize suicide risk. A confidential discussion with the child is essential in assessing suicidal thoughts or actions. Signs of depression can be masked, so take note if a parent or child reports the following symptoms:

- Boredom or lethargy
- Irritability or restlessness
- Difficulty concentrating
- Purposeful misbehavior
- Somatic preoccupation
- Isolation from others or excessive dependence on others

Outcome Identification: NOC

After determining your nursing diagnoses, identify outcomes that are important for the child and/or family to achieve specific to each diagnosis. These outcomes are behaviors or skills that are necessary to bring about positive mental health changes. For instance, you may have identified a diagnosis of disturbed sensory perception in a young child with autism who is highly sensitive to being touched. You could then work with the child's parents to identify specific outcomes they would like to achieve, such as the child being able to receive an affectionate stroke from the parent or have her hair cut without becoming agitated and emotionally distressed.

Planning and Implementation: NIC

Treatment approaches most commonly used by child psychiatric–mental health professionals are shown in Your Intervention Strategies, along with a rationale for when each is likely to be useful.

Therapeutic Approaches

Therapeutic interventions usually involve both the primary caregiver (typically the mother) and the child, focusing on three components: the child's behavior, the parent's attitudes and feelings about the child, and the interaction between parent and child. Depending on the particular problems being addressed, greater focus may be placed on one of these components.

Therapeutic Play Therapeutic play can be used as part of assessment and as an intervention for a variety of mental health problems. Role-play, as a way for a child to communicate feelings difficult to articulate, can occur through the child taking on a character himself or projecting that character onto a puppet or doll.

Cognitive–Behavioral Therapy Cognitive–behavioral therapy approaches focus on the child's conscious, rather than unconscious, issues with emphasis on more effective coping in the present rather than on mastery over unresolved feelings associated with the child's past experiences. Cognitive–behavioral approaches have been particularly successful in treating children with problems associated with depression, conduct disorder, ADHD, and anxiety (Bidwell, McClernon, & Kollins, 2011). Re-education and relearning are processes leading to more adaptive and functional behaviors for the child. Behavioral therapy is based, to a great extent, on pairing a negative stimulus (such as a feared situation or animal) with a positive stimulus (such as candy or relaxation exercises). The clinical example illustrates how a program of rewards and sanctions helped one boy learn to control his anger at his peers.

Clinical Example

Jervis was a strong, very large 8-year-old boy with intellectual disability. He was on a child psychiatric unit for evaluation after he severely injured another child during a fight. When the other children on the unit made fun of him or made faces at him, Jervis would strike out at them, often punching and knocking them to the floor.

The unit staff met to develop a behavioral program for Jervis. They also met with Jervis to discuss a behavioral contract with him. Part of this discussion was to identify the things Jervis liked most and least on the unit because these would be used as part of his rewards or sanctions for fulfilling his part of the contract. For instance, he loved his television time, making cookies with the staff, and playing ball outside in the courtyard. But he disliked helping with cleanup after meals and sitting in the corner for a time-out from games or other activities.

The purpose of the contract was to help Jervis learn to better control his anger when other children teased him. If he ignored the children or came to one of the staff to express his frustration or seek their help in resolving the problem, he got a red star. If he struck out at the children, he got a blue dot. These were kept on a bulletin board in his room. For each red star, he could negotiate with staff for an extra something on his list of "likes." For each blue dot, he would either lose a chance to participate in one of his favorite activities or he would have to do something on his list of "dislikes."

Family Therapy Family therapy is used when interactions among family members need attention in order to address specific problems exhibited by the child. The goal is to increase the likelihood that improvements in the child's mental health will occur and will be supported in the home. The following clinical example illustrates how parents may need to be involved in order for treatment to progress.

Family therapy is described fully in Chapter 29 ∞.

Clinical Example

The staff on an inpatient unit found they needed to help the parents of Nathan, a 12-year-old boy with conduct disorder, plan his weekend day passes. Nathan reported that he barely saw his parents while home on pass. Both parents worked most of the time, and when they were home, they argued a lot. So Nathan hung out at the local mall with his friends and got into trouble. This situation was interfering with Nathan's recovery and his transition back into the home.

The family therapist and primary nurse brought the family together to talk about the issues related to Nathan's use of time on his weekend passes. The overt goal of the first meeting was to help the family better structure Nathan's time and their availability to him. But it became clear that there was a great deal of conflict between the parents as well as much hostility directed at Nathan during the family discussions. Because the family conflict had implications for the success of Nathan's treatment, the entire family was scheduled for a number of therapy sessions.

YOUR INTERVENTION STRATEGIES
Guidelines for Various Treatment Approaches Used With Children

Approach	Focus for Intervention
Child–parent psychotherapy	Parent's caregiving style or relationship problems between the parent and child
Play therapy	The child's emotions and previous experience
Cognitive–behavioral therapy	The child's attitudes, beliefs, and behaviors
Family therapy	The dynamics of family interaction
Medication	A neurobiologic deficit or abnormality

Psychopharmacology

There are important considerations in using medications with children. First, never assume that the actions and side effects of any medication will be the same for children as for adults. The size of a child's liver relative to the child's overall body size is different proportionately than in adults. This means that dosing for children could be lower than for adults of the same size.

Only recently have studies been undertaken to carefully examine the impact of medications on children at various developmental stages (Masi & Liboni, 2011). Not only do children at various stages have different medication needs in terms of rates of absorption, excretion, sites of action, and toxicity, but these may change for the same child as he or she develops. Monitor children in your care carefully, with ongoing titration if they are kept on a medication over extended periods of time.

The classes of psychiatric medications most commonly used with children include stimulants, antidepressants, low-dose antipsychotics, mood stabilizers, and antianxiety agents. TABLE 25-2 ■ outlines these major classes of medications, their uses, and common side effects. You can refer families to the American Academy of Child and Adolescent Psychiatry website (http://www.aacap.org) for information on children and psychiatric medications.

Nurses play an important role in monitoring the child on medication and educating the child and parents about the medication. The following are vital actions:

- Monitor side effects daily in inpatient settings and weekly in outpatient settings.
- If the child is being treated in an outpatient setting, work closely with parents and teachers to observe and record the child's behavior.
- Assess the child's concerns about side effects and stigmatization by peers related to the medication.
- Take time to assess the parents' beliefs and fears about the medication. Parents are often concerned about side effects and the potential for dependency. Give them an opportunity to discuss their worries and questions as you educate them about the medication.
- Prepare the child and the parents for the possibility that symptoms will worsen when a medication is removed or decreased. Plan other interventions to help the child and family at this time.

TABLE 25-2 ■ Classes of Medications Used With Children		
Medication Class	**Disorders Treated**	**Side Effects**
Stimulants	ADHD PDD Intellectual disability (ID)	Anorexia and weight loss Abdominal pain Headache Sadness or mood lability, irritability Insomnia
Antidepressants	Major depression OCD Enuresis Separation anxiety ADHD Tourette's disorder PTSD Panic disorder Phobias	Fatigue, drowsiness, insomnia Nausea, upset stomach, diarrhea Cognitive dulling Tachycardia and hypotension Weight gain Restlessness, agitation Headaches, dizziness Dry mouth
Antipsychotics	Schizophrenia Tourette's disorder Severe aggression in PDD and CD	Sedation, lethargy Cognitive dulling Tremor, rigidity, drooling Nausea, diarrhea or constipation, abdominal discomfort Weight gain
Mood stabilizers	Bipolar disorder Intellectual disability PDD	Tremor Weight gain Polyuria Nausea, abdominal discomfort, diarrhea Hypothyroidism Fatigue, lethargy, cognitive dulling
Antianxiety agents	Anxiety disorders Sleep disorders	Fatigue, drowsiness Addiction Disinhibition

■ Discuss any risk that the medication may increase suicidal tendencies in the child, and review signs of masked depression with the parents (see the section "Assessing Suicide Risk" on page 566).

Antipsychotics Antipsychotic medications are effective in treating childhood psychoses such as schizophrenia and in managing the behavior problems associated with intellectual deficits. Antipsychotics may also be used to treat bipolar disorder, severe aggression, and Tourette's disorder. The general principle of reduced dosage is again applicable. The upper limit of the usual daily dosage for children under 12 might be 200 mg/day of chlorpromazine (Thorazine) or 20 mg/day of trifluoperazine (Stelazine). Keep amounts of individual IM injections of chlorpromazine at 0.25 mg per pound of body weight every 6 to 8 hours, or not over 40 mg/day for up to 50 lb and not over 75 mg/day for children weighing 50 to 100 lb.

The developmental impact of a medication on a child must be weighed alongside its potential benefits for a specific mental health problem. Some research has shown that the developing neurotransmitter systems of young children can be very sensitive to medications and it is unclear how this sensitivity may affect their brain development (National Institute for Health and Clinical Excellence, 2011). Medications are often used to address a behavioral problem that may be disturbing to the child's family or teachers, yet their use may interfere with the child's developmental capacity. For instance, antipsychotic medications such as chlorpromazine cause cognitive dulling and may interfere with learning. They also cause tardive dyskinesia, a movement disorder that can occur after chronic use. Such risks have significant implications for children who are developing and who may experience cumulative effects of medications over many years. You must balance all the benefits and risks against one another in a full and open discussion with the child's family.

The newer atypical antipsychotics have fewer of these side effects than the typical antipsychotics such as haloperidol (Haldol) or thioridazine (Mellaril) and also appear to be more effective in reducing psychotic symptoms in children. Risperidone (Risperdal) and aripiprazole (Abilify) have the most support for use with children (Masi & Liboni, 2011).

You should be aware of the sometimes inappropriate use of antipsychotics to reduce agitated behavior or sedate children with intellectual disorder (ID) or pervasive developmental disorders (PDD). Although medications like haloperidol may be appropriate for some children who could injure themselves or others, do not use medications as a substitute for careful supervision or behavioral interventions that could modify and control problem behaviors.

Stimulants The stimulants most frequently used with children are methylphenidate (Ritalin, Concerta), dextroamphetamine sulfate (Dexedrine), and mixed amphetamine salts (Adderall), primarily for the treatment of ADHD. Some stimulants have been approved only for children over 6 years of age, while others may be used for ages 3 and up. Methylphenidate appears to have fewer side effects, although dextroamphetamine sulfate has a longer duration of action and is less expensive. A nonstimulant medication, atomoxetine (Strattera), is effective for some children and adults with ADHD. It is very important to monitor for vital sign changes or signs of depression. An increase in symptoms (rebound effect) may occur as each dose wears off every 3 to 4 hours, so maintaining a consistent schedule for taking the medication is important for the parent or for you as the nurse who manages a child's medication.

There has been a fair amount of controversy regarding the long-term effects of stimulants on the growth of children. Some studies have found deficits in weight and height for children treated with these medications while other research suggests that growth catches up once the stimulant is discontinued. Little is known about the effects of stimulants on children treated continually from childhood through adolescence. As a result, we cannot be sure about the persistence of growth deficits and whether they are the result of stimulant use versus maturational delays related to ADHD itself.

Antidepressants Antidepressants are used primarily to treat major depressive disorder and many anxiety disorders in children. They may also be used for enuresis, bulimia, and ADHD. Until recently, tricyclic antidepressants (TCAs) have been the most widely used with children, especially imipramine (Tofranil). But they can create cardiac rate and rhythm changes (a greater risk for children than adults) and can be highly toxic if overdosed accidentally by a child. So adults must closely supervise their administration and keep the medication in a safe place.

Because they have fewer side effects and low risk, selective serotonin reuptake inhibitors (SSRIs) have become the first-line medications of choice for treating depression, anxiety, and obsessive–compulsive behavior in children. The SSRIs used with children include fluoxetine (Prozac), paroxetine (Paxil), citalopram (Celexa), sertraline (Zoloft), and fluvoxamine (Luvox). Because of the disinhibition that can occur when using antidepressants, some children may become more impulsive and uninhibited about harming themselves. Therefore, you will need to assess regularly the child's suicidal ideation and risk-taking behavior and teach the parents to monitor these as well.

Monoamine oxidase inhibitors (MAOIs) are rarely used for children because they require careful dietary control to prevent untoward interactions. The foods restricted are commonly ingested by children (i.e., processed foods with MSG, pizza, common submarine sandwiches, etc.). Such control is very difficult for anyone to maintain and is especially burdensome for family members or guardians when children are being treated.

Mood Stabilizers Lithium carbonate (Lithobid) is the mood stabilizer used with children. Its primary use, however, is for severe aggression and agitation across a variety of disorders (e.g., intellectual disability or PDD) rather than for managing mania. In general, children have a poorer response to lithium than do adults. In addition, children under 7 are more prone to toxic side effects of lithium than are older youth or adults, so you must cautiously consider its use. Seizures and coma may occur; it can be lethal in overdose. Potential hypothyroidism from the use of lithium has especially negative consequences for a child because of the impact of thyroid disease on so many facets of development. Selected anticonvulsants such as carbamazepine (Tegretol) and valproic acid (Depakote) are also effective mood stabilizers for children.

Antianxiety Medications Benzodiazepines such as clonazepam (Klonopin) and lorazapam (Ativan) are only infrequently used with children. Most clinicians believe that symptoms of anxiety or sleep disturbances should be treated first with psychosocial interventions or perhaps SSRIs unless these methods have proved unsuccessful and the symptoms are causing severe impairment or distress for the child. Remember that benzodiazepines can become addictive if used over a period of time, so they are normally discontinued after a few weeks.

Responding to Suicide Risk

If your assessment of a child indicates the child is at risk of attempting self-harm, you must take immediate action. Determine the seriousness of the attempt by talking to the child confidentially and asking questions such as:

- Do you have a plan to hurt yourself? If so, tell me about it.
- What would you do if you were thinking about hurting yourself? Would you let someone know before you did anything?
- Do you want to be dead?

Well-thought-out plans that avoid discovery and plans to use lethal methods indicate a greater risk for suicide completion.

If you are concerned by the child's responses, be sure that the child is seen by a psychiatrist or an advanced-practice psychiatric nurse for a comprehensive evaluation. The treatment team must consider the need for hospitalization. If there is agreement by the psychiatric team that the child does not require hospitalization, you can do the following:

- Obtain a promise from the child, in the form of a contract, not to cause self-harm for a specified period of time (see the discussion of no self-harm/no-suicide contracts on page 519 in Chapter 23 ∞).
- Obtain the support of the family in creating a safe environment for their child by making sure that all potentially lethal objects and medications are secured and out of sight.

If the child and family are unable or unwilling to agree to the contract or to create a safe home environment, it may be necessary to hospitalize the child.

Evaluation

The purpose of evaluation is to determine whether interventions are effective and how you should modify your care if necessary. Focus your evaluation on the nursing outcomes you have identified in your work with a particular child. But it is important to choose concrete and observable aspects of the child's behavior. Tangible changes or improvements are more readily assessed than vague statements that cannot be measured or observed in some way. For example, assessing an increase in the child's self-esteem is very difficult, but evaluating specific behaviors indicating esteem (such as positive statements about self or improved grooming) will make your evaluation easier and more useful.

Acquiring input from as many sources as possible is also essential to effective evaluation of the child. Have you obtained information from the child, parents, other nursing staff, or school personnel? Depending on the situation, it may or may not be possible to conduct a comprehensive evaluation, but it should be your goal whenever possible.

Remember that you must ensure that the outcome criteria for evaluation are congruent with appropriate developmental and sociocultural expectations. Frustration tolerance, for example, is much lower in the 4-year-old child than the 14-year-old child. For this reason, an accurate evaluation must consider the norms for age appropriateness. Similarly, expectations should take into consideration the child's sociocultural norms. For instance, a child who exhibits aggressiveness or informality with adults may have had such behaviors encouraged at home but is viewed by the larger society as disrespectful toward authority. Children need to fit in with their own communities and social context as well as society as a whole, so you must weigh these factors as various outcomes are identified for interventions.

NURSING SELF-AWARENESS

In addition to the outcome criteria you establish to assess the effectiveness of your interventions, another critical feature of evaluation is the ongoing review and evaluation of your own process as a child psychiatric nurse. This clinical example illustrates one instance where you must address staff feelings in order to work effectively with a child and her family.

Clinical Example

Eleven-year-old Luisa had a history of living with extended family and several hospitalizations. Luisa's mother was ambivalent toward her, often openly rejecting her (by visiting rarely, missing family sessions, and so on). Luisa's predicament stimulated a lot of feeling among the staff about bad mothers and good mothers, and staff members were protective of the child and angry at the mother. They were encouraged to examine the mother's own deprivation by an abusive mother and her difficulties in raising this very troubled child.

Are you aware of your attitudes and behaviors in working with specific children? How are these affecting your interventions with each child? For some key areas to consider in evaluating your potential impact, see Your Self-Awareness.

Working with children, particularly children with emotional problems, may activate feelings about your own unresolved issues with your family of origin or current family. You may then react as if the child is feeling or acting in ways that you might have felt or acted, and project your own issues onto the child, rather than responding to the child's actual therapeutic needs. Nurses may also respond to children or parents with certain stereotyped attitudes or beliefs, rather than being open to each child and parent as individuals. Self-awareness and ongoing self-monitoring and self-evaluation are essential skills for child psychiatric nurses. Without this capacity, you have little assurance that you can provide truly therapeutic nursing care.

CASE MANAGEMENT

Community-based care and home care are dependent on effective case management. Case management by a child psychiatric–mental health nurse includes multiple responsibilities. In a full-service model, the nurse may work with a multidisciplinary team to provide most, if not all, of the major clinical and support services needed by a child. In another type of case management, the nurse serves as a broker for the child and family, identifying and arranging services that are then provided by other agencies or professionals. Advanced-practice child psychiatric nurses can provide psychiatric assessment, medication prescribing and monitoring, symptom management, direct psychotherapy, supportive counseling, teaching, and coordination of overall care.

Case management is especially useful for children with serious mental illness or those who do not respond well to standard treatment programs. As part of community-based care, a major feature of case management is collaboration with other agencies to improve care across the continuum of services. Effective collaboration requires nursing skills in communication, relationship building, and conflict resolution. See Partnering With Clients and Families for examples of useful information to share with families at various stages in the child's treatment.

COMMUNITY-BASED CARE

The focus of this chapter is on the care of children in both inpatient and outpatient settings. Because mental health work with children entails close relationships with parents and school systems, the nurse's role in the community typically involves visits to the home and school as well as contacts with the juvenile justice system, family shelters, foster care placements, and social services. Child psychiatric nurses work in clinics, daycare programs, residential treatment programs, and school-based mental health programs. These sites may provide general mental health services or specialized care such as treatment for children who have been sexually abused, children in correctional facilities, or children with life-threatening illnesses.

HOME CARE

Resources for inpatient care have been reduced in recent years. As a result, children with serious mental health problems are often living at home. Home care presents numerous challenges that family members must face. You must engage parents as active members of their child's treatment. Develop a strong relationship with the family and work closely with the parents to help them learn strategies for managing their child's symptoms while promoting his or her mental health. Develop a care plan with parents for the daily management of the child's illness. Adherence to the plan will be enhanced if you do the following:

- Discuss the purpose and goals of each aspect of the child's treatment with the family. Be sure they understand what you have said by asking questions to assess their understanding.
- Educate the family about the child's symptoms and ways to manage them. Give the information in simply written handouts that will reinforce what you tell them.

- Give the family written reminders of days and times for therapy sessions, medications, and other treatments the child may have.
- Give the family information about whom to call if the child's mental health deteriorates or emergency management is needed.
- Schedule regular visits with the family to reinforce, support, and monitor their care of the child.

Involving parents as active members of their child's treatment team has a profound impact on the degree to which the treatment is effective.

Pearson Nursing Student Resources

Find additional review materials at
nursing.pearsonhighered.com
Prepare for success with NCLEX®-style practice questions, interactive assignments and activities, web links, animations and videos, and more!

REFERENCES

American Psychiatric Association. (2000). *Diagnostic and statistical manual of mental disorders* (4th ed., Text Revision) (DSM-IV-TR). Washington, DC: Author.

Autism Genetics Group, Department of Psychiatry, Trinity College Dublin. (2011). Gene-ontology enrichment analysis in two independent family-based samples highlights biologically plausible processes for autism spectrum disorders. *European Journal of Human Genetics.* Advance online publication. doi:10.1038/ejhg.2011.75

Autism Society of America. (2011). Defining autism. Retrieved from http://www.autism-society.org

Bidwell, L. C., McClernon, F. J., & Kollins, S. H. (2011). Cognitive enhancers for the treatment of ADHD. *Pharmacology, Biochemistry, and Behavior, 99*(2), 262–274. doi:10.1016/j.pbb.2011.05.002

Cole, S. Z., & Lanham, J. S. (2011). Failure to thrive: An update. *American Family Physician, 83*(7), 829–834.

Kim, Y. S., Leventhal, B. L., Koh, Y. J., Fombonne, E., Laska, E., Lim, E. C., . . . Grinker, R. R. (2011). Prevalence of autism spectrum disorders in a total population sample. *American Journal of Psychiatry.* Advance online publication. doi:10.1176/appi.ajp.2011.10101532

Masi, G., & Liboni, F. (2011). Management of schizophrenia in children and adolescents: Focus on pharmacotherapy. *Drugs, 71*(2), 179–208.

National Institute of Health and Clinical Excellence. (2011). Clinical guidelines. Retrieved from http://www.nice.org.uk/

National Institute of Mental Health. (2011). *Clinical trials: Autism spectrum disorders (pervasive developmental disorders).* Retrieved from http://www.nimh.nih.gov/health/trials/autism-spectrum-disorders-pervasive-developmental-disorders.shtml

Schieve, L. A., Baio, J., Rice, C. E., Durkin, M., Kirby, R. S., Drews-Botsch, C., . . . Cunniff, C. M. (2010). Risk for cognitive deficit in a population-based sample of U. S. children with autism spectrum disorders: Variation by perinatal health factors. *Disability and Health Journal, 3*(3), 202–212.

Shlafer, R. J., & Poehlmann, J. (2010). Attachment and caregiving relationships in families affected by parental incarceration. *Attachment and Human Development, 12*(4), 395–415.

Smith, A. K., Stasi, S. M., Rhee, S. H., Corley, R. P., Young, S. E., & Hewitt, J. K. (2011). The role of attention-deficit/hyperactivity disorder in the association between verbal ability and conduct disorder. Frontiers in Psychiatry 3: 2–3.

Spencer, T. J., Greenbaum, M., Ginsberg, L. D., & Murphy, W. R. (2009). Safety and effectiveness of coadministration of guanfacine extended release and psychostimulants in children and adolescents with attention-deficit/hyperactivity disorder. *Journal of Child and Adolescent Psychopharmacology, 19*(5), 501–510.

Ståhlberg, O., Anckarsäter, H., & Nilsson, T. (2010). Mental health problems in youths committed to juvenile institutions: Prevalences and treatment needs. *European Child and Adolescent Psychiatry, 164*(10), 930–934.

Storebø, O. J., Pedersen, J., Skoog, M., Thomsen, P. H., Winkel, P., Gluud, C., & Simonsen, E. (2011). Randomized social-skills training and parental training plus standard treatment versus standard treatment of children with attention deficit hyperactivity disorder – the SOSTRA trial protocol. *Trials, 21*, 12–18.

van Bon, B. W., Koolen, D. A., Brueton, L., McMullan, D., Lichtenbelt, K. D., Adès, L. C., . . . deVries, B. B. (2010). The 2q23.1 microdeletion syndrome: Clinical and behavioral phenotype. *European Journal of Human Genetics, 18*(2), 163–170.

Adolescents

CAROL BRADLEY-CORPUEL

26

LEARNING OUTCOMES

After completing this chapter, you will be able to:

1. Compare and contrast the biopsychosocial theories important to understanding adolescents.
2. Incorporate relevant biologic and developmental data in the assessment of adolescents.
3. Illustrate how a humanistic–interactionist perspective contributes to a comprehensive assessment of adolescent problems.
4. Design intervention strategies for adolescent clients who act out.
5. Formulate intervention strategies for adolescent clients who are angry or hostile, test the staff, scapegoat others, engage in problematic sexual behaviors, or abuse substances.
6. Construct a client contract for use with an adolescent in treatment.
7. Analyze personal feelings and attitudes or unresolved issues about adolescence that may affect your professional practice with adolescent clients.

CRITICAL THINKING CHALLENGE

Your 15-year-old client, Angela Cook, informs you that her mother has sent her to your community clinic for contraception and information on "safe sex." Your own personal beliefs advocate sexual abstinence before marriage for religious as well as preventive health reasons. Moreover, you feel compelled to be a "better parent" to this young girl than her mother has been and feel inclined to dissuade her from sexual intercourse at this early age.

1. Why do you suppose Angela's mother sent her to the community clinic rather than educating Angela at home?
2. How might your own personal convictions interfere with or influence the preventive health care and education you provide?
3. Can you be a "better parent" to Angela? Should you? Why or why not?

What is adolescence? Some sources define it simply as the time of physical and psychosocial development between the ages of 12 and 20. Others describe it as a period of "normal psychosis." Still others see it as an attempt by a tyrannical subculture to overtake adult America. It is not necessary to accept the latter two definitions verbatim to understand their implications. Most people recognize the immense stress that occurs during adolescence and the importance to an adolescent's future of managing that stress.

Trying to understand adolescents is a challenge for anyone. Recollect your own experiences and reactions during this tumultuous time—it may help you better appreciate the dilemmas that adolescent clients face. Nurses who choose to work with adolescents find considerable rewards from the challenge. Whether the nurse functions as a generalist, a clinical nurse specialist, or a nurse practitioner, today's health care settings integrate professional capabilities, skills, and roles to intervene with adolescents. The goal is to achieve optimal social, emotional, cognitive, and physical development. Adolescents are emotionally and economically dependent on several systems (family, school, community, and institution) and we nurses work closely with them all to identify relevant deviations in the developmental process.

The *Healthy People 2020* initiative presents a special opportunity to promote the health, safety, and well-being of adolescents and young adults. The link to the site is available through http://www.healthypeople.gov/2020/topicsobjectives 2020/pdfs/AdolescentHealth.pdf and through the Online Student Resources for the text. Nurses in school and community settings are vital to establishing more effective health programs and other policy and programmatic interventions to reduce risk, highlight protective factors, and improve health outcomes among adolescents.

MENTAL DISORDERS AND ADOLESCENTS

There is a broad range of mental disorders for people from 13 to 18 years of age. Approximately one in every five youth in North America meets criteria for a mental disorder with severe impairment across their lifetime. Mental disorders common in adults likely first emerged in childhood and adolescence. This highlights the need for increased focus on prevention and early intervention during adolescence. See Mental Health in the News for a description of a troubled teen.

Anxiety disorders, the most common condition (31.9%), is followed by behavior disorders (19.1%), mood disorders (14.3%), and substance use disorders (11.4%). The median age of onset for a mental health issue was earliest for anxiety disorder (6 years of age), followed by 11 years of age for behavior disorder, 13 years of age for mood disorder, and 15 years of age for substance use disorders (Merikangas et al., 2010). Given these statistics, it is highly likely that you will be working with mental disorders within your youthful client population in a variety of settings. See the following chapters for a discussion of these diagnoses: Chapter 15, Substance-Related Disorders; Chapter 17, Mood Disorders; Chapter 18, Anxiety Disorders; and Chapter 22∞, Personality Disorders.

BIOPSYCHOSOCIAL THEORIES

A sound theoretic knowledge base helps you differentiate between the "normal" and the "abnormal," or the usual and unusual, behaviors of adolescents. When you do a comprehensive assessment you focus on the psychological development of the individual and the evolution of the adolescent as a biopsychosocial being. You can accomplish the first task with an understanding of developmental theory, and the second with an appreciation of biologic and humanistic–interactionist theories.

Biologic Theory

Psychiatric–mental health nursing requires you to integrate a biologic focus into your practice, to accommodate both changing client needs and an expanding biologic knowledge base.

MENTAL HEALTH IN THE NEWS

Lee Boyd Malvo

Lee Boyd Malvo, a 17-year-old sniper, terrorized the Washington, D. C. area in 2002, shooting 13 people and leaving 10 of them dead. Together, Malvo and John Allen Muhammad, 48 years old, shot people from a specially contrived car so they would not be detected. Muhammad, who masterminded the serial murders and whom Malvo's defense lawyers claimed had brainwashed the young man, was executed by lethal injection in November 2009.

When Malvo was arrested for his role in the deadly attacks, many questions were asked about how a 17-year-old boy could kill without compunction. Two theories proposed were a pseudo-father/son arrangement, and the adolescent's thrill of being in a powerful position—holding life and death in his hands. As an immigrant from Jamaica, Malvo may have been specifically identified as susceptible by Muhammed. Muhammed's plan (unfulfilled) was to travel with the intent to access and recruit impressionable young boys like Malvo, who have no parents, lacked guidance, and would likely be found at YMCAs and orphanages. Muhammad believed he could be their father figure as he was with Lee Boyd Malvo. He would begin their training once he recruited a large number of young boys and made his way to Canada. Malvo described how Muhammad allegedly intended to train the youths with weapons. After their training was complete, Muhammad planned to send them to carry out mass shootings in many different cities.

Malvo lived with Muhammed in Tacoma, Washington for a year prior to the Washington, D. C. crimes. He used the alias John Lee Malvo on more than one occasion. Many questions about these crimes are unanswered. He is serving a life sentence without parole for his role in the murders.

Photo courtesy of Luke Frazza/AFP/Getty Images/Newscom.

An appreciation of hormonal changes, growth spurts, stress, immune function, chronic illness, depression, and other mental disorders can help you evaluate adolescents from a more effective and comprehensive perspective.

Neurobiology and Biochemistry

In recent years, clinician researchers have carried out studies using neuroimaging, magnetic resonance imaging (MRI), and spectroscopy in children and adolescents in order to better delineate the anatomic, functional, and biochemical imbalances of mood disorders and other behaviors in children and adolescents. As a result, we have data that depressed adolescents without a comorbid psychiatric disorder exhibit an abnormally hyperactive amygdala compared to healthy controls (Arnold, Hanna, & Rosenberg, 2010). Equally important, neuroscientists have identified structural brain changes in correlation with emotional neglect and other early life stress experiences (Frodl, 2010). Researchers recognize that this developmental phase, with its risky behaviors, makes this population even more vulnerable to neurobiologic problems, such as substance dependence and abuse (Rutherford, Mayes, & Potenza, 2010).

Advancements in molecular biology and biochemistry allow investigations of gene expressions in specific neuronal systems of the brain. Apply these advances to a common and important health issue for adolescents, metabolic functioning, and you see the interconnecting systems. Neurobiologic systems and specific neuropeptides and hormones are as important as behavioral and familial habits in abnormal body weight regulation. We now know that neurochemical and humoral substances are related to the traits of overeating, weight gain, and eating disorders. These discoveries are important in themselves for clinical treatment. In addition, knowledge regarding the biochemical and physiological etiology for these physical conditions could help positively influence society's tendency to discriminate against people who have these conditions. Realizing that biochemical and neuronal systems are contributing to these medical conditions could alleviate some of the bias and prejudice that, for example, the obese adolescent receives from his peers who believe "All he has to do is push himself away from the table" or that the adolescent with an eating disorder endures from her peers who may say, "Doesn't she know that's disgusting?"

Chronic Illness

Of equal importance is the effect of chronic illness on the adolescent's mental health. Asthma, head injury, diabetes, epilepsy, and many of the less common chronic physical diseases can result in depression. Equally at risk for depression are adolescents with various learning disabilities or specific neuropsychiatric illnesses, such as attention deficit/hyperactivity disorders (ADD/ADHD), disruptive behavior disorders, tic disorders, eating disorders, anxiety disorders (including obsessive–compulsive disorder [OCD] and post-traumatic stress disorder [PTSD]), and schizophrenia (American Psychiatric Association, 2000).

The proportion of obese and overweight children and adolescents in North America more than tripled in the last

WHAT EVERY NURSE SHOULD KNOW

Allaying the Stress of Parents and Family Members of Adolescents

Imagine you are a pediatric nurse. In the pediatric acute care or critical care arenas where adolescents are treated, emotions and fears can run high. Parents and family members frequently feel guilt, anger, and helplessness as they watch their adolescent undergoing invasive procedures. You can help allay their fears as well as obtain much-needed assessment data by talking with them about their stress. Consider comments such as, "This must be very stressful for you. The diagnosis of diabetes was such a shock. This is beyond the usual day–to–day stressors. How do you usually cope?" Such questions can yield adaptive measures and they can draw on or reveal maladaptive measures, such as physical abuse.

three decades. Specifically, among adolescents between the ages of 12 and 19 years, obesity increased from 5% to 18% in the same time period (Ogden, Carroll, Curtin, Lamb, & Flegal, 2010). In addition to the more publicized comorbid medical conditions (such as diabetes, cardiac abnormalities, hypertension, and metabolic syndrome) associated with excessive weight, there is the psychological impact of depression and peer discrimination that burden the obese teen. Health care professionals who treat adolescents, including pediatric practitioners, need to be aware of the stressors inherent in having a chronic illness. See the What Every Nurse Should Know features, which provide some of this information for a variety of settings.

WHAT EVERY NURSE SHOULD KNOW

Helping Adolescents Cope With the Stress of a Cancer Diagnosis

Imagine you are an oncology or hospice nurse. It is estimated that in 2010 in the United States 10,700 children under the age of 15 will be diagnosed with cancer. Prior to the 1970s, the 5-year survival rate was less than 50%. However, due to major treatment advances in the last four decades, 80% of these children are now expected to survive 5 years or more (American Cancer Society, 2010). Considerations for the physical, cognitive, emotional, social, and spiritual strategies are key to helping your young clients and families cope during this stressful time. Moreover, you should familiarize yourself with evidence-based standards for end-of-life care for young clients in order to prepare both the client and the family for the process of dying. Tending to the physical symptoms of distress (such as dyspnea, fatigue, and nutritional concerns) will provide you with the opportunity to deal with the psychological and spiritual distress as well.

Psychopharmacology

There is increasing impetus to study the clinically significant effects that various psychotropic medications may have on the brain when administered during the developing phase that spans the time period from birth through adolescence. The study of psychotherapeutic medications and treatment of children and adolescents remains a priority area of the *Healthy People 2020* initiative. The U.S. Public Health Service is committed to achieving the health promotion and disease prevention objectives of this comprehensive, nationwide agenda (U. S. Department of Health and Human Services [USDHHS], 2010).

Controversy continues regarding use of psychotropic medications during this vulnerable period of development, especially the value and safety of psychotropic drugs in the primary care treatment of children and adolescents. While clients with various mental disorders benefit from medication, there are serious concerns among mental health professionals that an undue amount of prescriptions are written for adolescents in the primary care setting without a comprehensive psychological evaluation of symptoms and without sufficient studies of the efficacy and adverse effects of the drugs (Morrato et al., 2010). Of equal concern is the practice of prescribing drugs without offering the benefit of evidence-based, effective, and safe treatments, including psychotherapy. Ongoing studies suggest that cognitive–behavioral therapy (CBT) and even bibliotherapy could offer alternative treatments for depression in adolescents and adults, especially when considering the implications of receiving unmonitored medications from primary care providers (Naylor et al., 2010). Nurses in various settings can be helpful to adolescents and their parents by making them aware of the risks as well as the benefits of pharmacologic agents and helping them to make informed decisions about their usage.

Developmental Theory

An understanding of developmental theory helps you identify deviations in adolescent growth and development processes and intervene appropriately. The theories of Freud and Erikson provide considerable insight into the adolescent's struggle to attain adulthood. These developmental theories are discussed in Chapter 5∞.

The development of an adolescent's sense of identity entails a preoccupation with self-image. It also entails a connection between future role and past experiences. In the search for a new sense of sameness and continuity, many adolescents must repeat the crisis resolutions of earlier years to integrate these past elements and establish the lasting ideals of a final identity. According to Erikson, these crisis periods or stages are reviews of the adolescent's sense of trust, autonomy, initiative, and industry, in that order.

Equally important for an adolescent's development is cognition. Piaget's research revealed three stages of cognitive development. The third stage, called *formal operations,* develops between ages 12 and 14 and results in the adolescent's ability to conceptualize on an adult level. The

---

YOUR ASSESSMENT APPROACH
Exploring the Meaning of an Adolescent's Identified Problem or Behavior

Asking yourself the following questions will help you determine the meaning of an adolescent's behavior:

- What meaning does this behavior or problem hold for the adolescent?
- What message is he or she conveying through this behavior?
- What impact does this problem have on the client in this developmental stage? Is this a usual or unusual problem or behavior for the adolescent's peer group?
- How have resulting changes, if any, affected the adolescent and his or her relationships with others?
- What goals does the client have for the immediate and distant future?
- What personal strengths does the adolescent have to help deal with this problem?
- What considerations have you and the client given to other developmental, familial, biologic, or sociocultural factors involved?

---

adolescent has the capacity to think abstractly, to be self-reflective, and to adopt a multidimensional perspective on problems.

Humanistic–Interactionist Theory

As a psychiatric–mental health nurse, you not only need knowledge about psychobiology and developmental theories, you must also integrate humanistic–interactionist principles into your assessments and interventions to develop a trusting, caring interpersonal relationship with adolescent clients. The adolescent developmental period is a time when identity, values, and goals are in a state of flux. The immediate situation and the developmental stage are taken into account along with the social, ethnic, and cultural factors; family influences; and psychodynamic conflicts. To accomplish this, explore the meaning of the identified problem or behavior. See Your Assessment Approach for a list of questions to explore the adolescent's problem.

It is insufficient to base nursing interventions solely on adolescent behaviors without a more comprehensive evaluation of the other factors. Only by considering all aspects of the adolescent client as a biopsychosocial being can you truly understand the meanings of such behaviors to the client and intervene effectively. Also, you may find Caring for the Spirit to be useful as you gain an increased understanding of your teen clients and what is most important to them.

THE ROLE OF THE NURSE

Psychiatric–mental health nurses assume numerous roles within a variety of treatment modalities. The goal is to identify abnormal or problem-causing behavior during this difficult period of development and help maintain the health

CARING FOR THE SPIRIT

Grappling With Life's Meaning and Purpose During Adolescence

Many adults with years of life experience may feel "settled" with their spiritual beliefs and ritualistic practices, their attitudes about health and healing, and their perspective on optimal living and a peaceful death. For many, turning to their spiritual, religious, or philosophical resources is both a proactive and reactive strategy, particularly when faced with an acute stressor, a chronic illness, or a life-threatening diagnosis. For adolescents, life may have offered little such experience or at least few "hard facts" in dealing with life's challenges. Whereas you may turn to meditation, ritual, yoga, or prayer for support during times of stress or illness, the adolescent is still grappling with life's meaning and purpose.

If asked, it may be appropriate to offer your beliefs or practices to the wondering teen, but otherwise, the best thing you can do in your health provider role is to serve as a positive role model. Rather than imposing your own beliefs or practices on the developing teenager, the most helpful stance you can take is to be objective and receptive to the teen's explorations and experimentation. You can help the curious teen to ponder the interconnectedness of the body with the mind and spirit with some well-considered questions.

Increase their appreciation for physical reactions when emotionally upset. Ask the emotionally distraught teen, "Where in your body are you feeling stressed right now?" and then after a response that could range from a curt reply to a veritable inventory of bodily sensations, guide the client to remember times past when the teen felt this before, asking what worked at that time to improve the upset feelings.

You might encourage deep breathing or progressive muscle relaxation as an immediate means to relaxing the body and to lessening the focus on the emotions. This will improve the teen's sense of confidence in having greater self-control over an upsetting event or situation, at least in the moment before trying to be more rational in designing a plan for intervention.

Increase their cognitive understanding of events or realization of emotional stressors that can contribute to physical complaints. Rule out any medical source of pain or discomfort before inviting the teen to consider, "What was happening just before you realized that your stomach was upset?" To recall an upsetting text message may open a flood of emotional responses from the teen, lessening the need for somatic symptoms and yielding the opportunity for some rational problem solving.

Increase their awareness of positive experiences, daily practices, regular rituals, or helpful spiritual resources that have given them support in their daily lives or with unusually threatening events. Discover who the adolescent is before a crisis hits. Explore with them what has given solace and support in the past and respect their answers. The adolescent may have found camaraderie at a local youth group or found comfort in talking to a member of the clergy. On the other hand, the teen may tell you that reading a good book, listening to favorite music, or immersing oneself in a television situation comedy is as helpful as "talking it out" with you or another authority figure. You can learn more by allowing the teen to educate you than by believing that you must have all of the answers to teach them at a time of need.

---

and well-being of adolescent clients. In the past decade, studies have determined that as many as one in five youth between the ages of 9 to 17 have a mental illness (Kurtz, 2011). Many times these mental health problems are identified in primary care and community health settings. Early intervention for adolescents with depression and other mental health issues promotes better outcomes (Asarnow & Albright, 2010).

Whether dealing with typical adolescent stress or with the challenge of a mental disorder, parents and families can experience the gamut of emotions, from feeling mildly frustrated to feeling overwhelmed with the unpredictability of their adolescent's behaviors. Collaborative treatment helps families understand why adolescents behave so differently from adults. Dealing with impulsivity, problem solving, and decision making can be more productive and less stressful with some guidance. Partnering With Clients and Families is a helpful tool in this regard. In fact, this excerpt, taken from *Facts for Families*, is one of numerous topics offered by the American Academy of Child and Adolescent Psychiatry (AACAP, 2010). The AACAP provides this vital information as a public service and allows you to duplicate and distribute copies free of charge as long as you give proper credit to the AACAP and do not have monetary gain from their use. The AACAP has

produced the *Facts for Families* in English and in Spanish. You can save to your hard drive, unzip the file, and open each *Facts for Families* individually as a PDF document. Also, independently created files (but without benefit of AACAP review) are available on the web in other languages such as Malaysian, Arabic, Hebrew, Polish, Icelandic, and Urdu.

In Outpatient Settings

In the changing world of health care, the outpatient arena for services to adolescents yields numerous diverse roles for the psychiatric–mental health nurse.

Community Health Nurse

In the school, clinic, or community health agency, the community health nurse has excellent opportunities to observe adolescents engaging in normal activities. The nurse who knows how to deal with typical adolescent problems will also be adept at identifying obstacles to effective resolution of emotional problems and suggesting treatment. There are frequent occasions to counsel adolescents about solutions to the problems that confront them daily, such as teen pregnancy and substance abuse, and to advise school or clinic staff members on their encounters with adolescents.

PARTNERING WITH CLIENTS AND FAMILIES

Teaching About the Teen Brain

This excerpt from *Facts for Families* from the AACAP can give you some quick pointers in teaching parents and families about the adolescent's behaviors. However, you may want to access the full sheet of information in order to provide your audience with more facts, such as the developmental conflict between the impulsive (and early developing) amygdala and the more rational (and later developing) frontal cortex. Based on the stage of their brain development, adolescents are more likely to:

- Act on impulse
- Misread or misinterpret social cues and emotions
- Have accidents of all kinds

- Become involved in fights
- Engage in dangerous or risky behavior

Adolescents are less likely to:

- Think before they act
- Pause to consider the potential consequences of their actions
- Modify their dangerous or inappropriate behaviors

This information is not intended to lessen the adolescent's responsibility for actions, but may provide parents and family members with a greater understanding of developmental challenges and increase tolerance in dealing with their adolescent's behaviors.

With the increasing number of ethnic minority teens predicted to comprise one third of all persons younger than 20 years of age early in the 21st century, we realize the importance of designing culturally sensitive interventions related to reproductive health needs, unplanned pregnancies, and risk factors that contribute to adverse outcomes (Champion & Collins, 2010). Partnering with schools and other community agencies will be crucial in providing effective education and treatment to this increasing population.

Within the School School is the most influential experience in an adolescent's life outside the home. Adolescents spend more waking time in school activities than in any other activity, and most of their successes, problems, and conflicts are demonstrated in the school setting. Even adolescents who are supposedly truant from school are often on the school grounds, perhaps meeting their friends at lunchtime, playing cards in the library, or "hanging out" on the school steps. Such an "absent" student may suddenly appear at the school nurse's door because of "boredom" or a physical complaint.

Unfortunately, the school nurse's role in the early recognition and treatment of predelinquent individuals has been minimized or has gone unrecognized. There are several reasons for this. One reason is that school administrators and teachers tend to view the school nurse as a person who deals only with physical sickness and medical emergencies. They may not be aware that because of the intimate quality of a nurse–client relationship or the comprehensive and holistic nature of nursing assessments, the nurse may be helpful in exploring an area of conflict in an adolescent's life or intervening with a disruptive student. Such early intervention could prevent more serious problems in later years. Box 26-1 outlines problems in the school setting that should warrant early intervention.

Another reason for the school nurse currently being an unexplored asset is that administrators may limit the nurse's activities to the school itself. They may see no need for the nurse to make home visits to meet with a sick student's family or view problems firsthand. Many school districts lack the time and money to provide for counseling families or individuals in a formal setting. As the role of the independent nursing practitioner expands, and as legislation for third-party reimbursement for independent practice becomes a reality in more states, nurses will be better able to assume more autonomy and responsibility in meeting student needs more comprehensively and effectively.

Within Community-Based Care The nurse who is employed in a community agency can seize every opportunity to provide an active school health program and educate school administrators and faculty members about the importance of preventive care. For example, the nurse in a viable school health program can provide preventive counseling not only to troubled adolescents in school but also to their preschool siblings during routine home visits when possible. Nurses can establish productive relationships with teachers, help other faculty members, encourage parent–teacher conferences, take an active part in developing the curriculum, and help adolescents on probation or parole return to school.

Within Social Programs The many problems encountered by today's youth—substance abuse, teenage pregnancy, family and school violence, street crime, and school failure—are increasingly being recognized in professional, community, and social arenas. As mentioned earlier in this

---

Box 26-1 Adolescent Behaviors in the School Setting That Call for Early Intervention

- Antisocial behaviors such as stealing, setting fires, bullying others
- Avoidance behavior
- Chronic illness
- Depression
- Disruptive classroom behavior
- Substance abuse
- Excessive daydreaming
- Hypochondriasis
- Learning difficulties
- Poor school performance or a dramatic shift in school performance
- Temper tantrums

Box 26-2 Youth Violence: Facts at a Glance 2010

The following is a summary of the information collected by the CDC on youth violence-related behaviors.

In 2007, among young people ages 10 to 24:

- 5,764 people were murdered—an average of 16 each day.
- Homicide was the second leading cause of death.
- 86% (4,973) of homicide victims were male and 14% (791) were female.
- 84% were killed with a firearm.

In a 2009 nationally-representative sample of youth in grades 9 through 12:

- 3.8% reported being in a physical fight one or more times in the previous 12 months that resulted in injuries requiring treatment by a doctor or nurse.
- 17.5% reported carrying a weapon (gun, knife or club) on one or more days in the 30 days preceding the survey.
- Males were more likely than females to carry a weapon (27.1% versus 7.1%) on one or more days in the preceding 30 days.

Regarding health disparities among various ethnic groups in the 10 to 24 age range:

- Homicide is the leading cause of death for African Americans, the second leading cause of death for Hispanics, and the third leading cause of death for Asian/Pacific Islanders, American Indians, and Alaska Natives.

- Homicide rates among non-Hispanic, African-American males (60.7 per 100,000) exceed those of Hispanic males (20.6 per 100,000) and non-Hispanic males, and White males in the same age group (3.5 per 100,000).

In the 12 months preceding the survey:

- 15.1% of male students and 6.7% of female students reported being in a physical fight on school property.
- 7.7% reported being threatened or injured with a weapon on school property one or more times.
- 19.9% reported being bullied on school property with the prevalence higher among females (21.2%) than males (18.7%).

In the 30 days preceding the survey:

- 5.6% reported carrying a weapon (gun, knife, or club) on school property on one or more days.
- 5% did not go to school on one or more days because they felt unsafe at school or on their way to or from school.

In the time span studied from 1999 to 2006:

- Most school-associated homicides included gunshot wounds (65%), stabbing or cutting (27%), and beating (12%).

Source: Centers for Disease Control and Prevention. *Youth risk behavioral surveillance—United States, 2009.* Copyright 2010.

---

section, the American Academy of Child and Adolescent Psychiatry (AACAP) has developed various tools to disseminate information, including the AACAP fact information sheets on various topics and the AACAP *Facts for Families.* Another excellent source for information and quick reference is the Centers for Disease Control and Prevention (CDC). See Box 26-2 for a summary of Youth Violence Facts at a Glance (CDC, 2010a).

The Youth Risk Behavior Surveillance System (YRBSS) monitors priority health risk behaviors among youth and young adults. This includes a national school-based survey conducted by the CDC and state, district, tribal, and territorial surveys. The YRBSS monitors the following six categories of priority health risk behaviors in youth (in addition to obesity and asthma):

- Behaviors that contribute to unintentional injuries and violence
- Tobacco use
- Alcohol and other drug use
- Sexual behaviors that contribute to unintended pregnancy and sexually transmitted diseases (STDs), including human immunodeficiency virus (HIV) infection
- Unhealthy dietary behaviors
- Physical inactivity

The 2009 YRBSS survey was conducted among students in grades 9 through 12 during October 2008 through February 2010. Box 26-2 presents a summary of the survey results pertaining to school violence including incidence of bullying. For a more comprehensive discussion on bullying, see the section on Reducing Scapegoating.

Nurse Counselor/Therapist

Whether in the clinic, home, school, or community health setting, the psychiatric–mental health nurse has many opportunities to organize individual, group, or family counseling sessions. Nurses can function within a variety of treatment roles, according to their experience and capabilities.

Individual Therapist The nurse's qualifications and role in the clinic, school, or community setting may allow for counseling adolescents on an individual basis. Sometimes the nurse can establish a trusting alliance and facilitate communication with the client. (Chapter 4∞ discusses establishing a therapeutic relationship and Chapter 10∞ provides facilitative communication strategies.) Sometimes, however, the adolescent is too threatened to talk openly with the nurse in this intimate setting. Some adolescents view the nurse as an authority figure and resist all efforts to communicate. You may make more headway with this mode of treatment when you use it in conjunction with group therapy. Unless educated at the graduate level and certified to provide this service, you should counsel the adolescent only for the purposes of identifying the problem area and referring the client to a qualified professional for individual psychotherapy.

Group Therapist It is usually more effective to work with adolescents in a group. Because the values, acceptance, and recognition of peers are so important during adolescence, the group can provide support for dealing with problems and effecting change. In addition, involving the adolescent's peers helps dilute the conflict with adults that may exist in one–to–one work. In the school setting, health education groups can provide an acceptable forum for peer interaction and discussion of difficult topics such as teen pregnancy as in What Every Nurse Should Know. In other settings, nurses seek out advanced-practice nurses to supervise their practice as a group therapist or they complete graduate preparation as an advanced-practice nurse. Knowledge of group dynamics is crucial to being an effective group leader. Chapter 28∞ discusses the group leader role for generalist nurses and the group therapist role for advanced-practice nurses.

Family Therapist Being a parent of a "normal" adolescent is difficult, at best. As the child grows into adulthood, with all its perplexing questions and problems, parents normally worry about the child's safety and well-being. They may feel rejected because they are no longer needed in the same way. Because many parents of relatively normal adolescents share this plight, they can usually find receptive listeners who will give them comfort and support.

The problems of the parents of emotionally disturbed adolescents are more complicated. Many of these parents have a strong sense of failure because their children did not turn out "right." Their feelings of guilt, frustration, and helplessness are likely to increase if their child is institutionalized. They may have felt confused and resentful when offered advice when presented in a noncollaborative manner. Unlike the parents of other adolescents, these parents may have no one in whom to confide, either because they lack the support and understanding of others or because their own self-reproach prevents them from seeking out confidantes.

Meetings with family members may be indicated if the adolescent's role in the family seems to compound the problems presented in the school or agency setting. An important part of the problem-solving process is organizing initial interviews with parents and family members. Use the information gathered during these meetings to determine whether the problems stem from difficulties posed by the larger system (the family), and, if so, whether family therapy is indicated (refer to Chapter 29∞).

Show compassion and understanding for the parents' dilemma without blaming them or their offspring. Parents will be more receptive to family therapy and to exploring their part in the adolescent's problems if they sense that you will support them, too. Stress and psychological symptoms evidenced by parents can serve as markers for emotional or behavioral problems in adolescents.

Any tendency to feel self-righteous or superior to the disturbed adolescent's parents is an obstacle to effective treatment. These feelings are readily communicated to parents and can only validate their fear of blame and increase their reluctance to participate in therapy with their child. By the same token, resist any temptation to overidentify with the parents—this inadvertently perpetuates the family system's problems. The adolescent and the family need a neutral party who can play an objective, knowledgeable, and supportive role in helping them change. The adolescent's chances for resolving the underlying conflicts and maintaining a healthy life are virtually nonexistent if the family system remains unchanged.

Parents, school, and agency staff must understand the objectives and goals of treatment to appreciate the progress the client has made and avoid reinforcing the client's previously maladaptive behavior. The following clinical example illustrates the problems that arise when parents and school authorities, particularly those who must deal directly with behavior problems in the classroom, lack psychological sophistication.

WHAT EVERY NURSE SHOULD KNOW

Teen Pregnancy

Imagine you are a school nurse. The prospect of more than a million pregnancies in females under the age of 20, with fewer choices for alternatives to continuing the pregnancy, is of utmost concern. Recent challenges in the court system to the adolescent's right to access abortion and contraception are eroding the *Roe v. Wade* decision. Regulation enforcement under HIPAA (Health Insurance Portability and Accountability Act) is further complicating adolescent care for those younger than 18 who are unemancipated minors. Individual state laws have an impact on disclosure of health information, as well. Nurses need to familiarize themselves with legal issues pertaining to their specialty areas in order to fully address the health and psychological needs of adolescents.

Clinical Example

Jeremy, a 13-year-old boy, was referred to the school nurse because he was introverted and isolated. He made no contact with either his peers or his teachers and rarely spoke unless addressed directly. After he had spent 3 months in group and individual counseling sessions with the nurse, Jeremy started going to the grade counselor's office of his own accord to talk about his depression and the problems he had been having in his family. Both the grade counselor and the boy's family believed this to be an indication that his difficulties had worsened, and they began to complain to the nurse about his illness! Not only were Jeremy's parents and counselor ignorant of the goals of treatment and the behaviors expected to come with change, but apparently they were also uncomfortable with the changes in Jeremy's behavior and with the implications of these changes for their relationships with him.

The client's siblings may experience many different feelings. Sometimes they share in the parents' guilt and shame. Sometimes, however, they are pleased and relieved when the "troublemaker" is out of the family and hospitalized. You should extend the same understanding to the siblings as to the parents, helping them see how each member of the family contributes to the problem. If the troubled adolescent is hospitalized, another member of the family, usually a sibling, may assume the role of the "bad" or "sick" person in the family because the identified "bad" person is no longer at home. Be aware of this tendency. If you are not skilled in assessing the need for family therapy or in providing this service, refer the family to a competent family therapist.

You may identify a need for all of these therapies in dealing with a client's problems. In some cases, an informal discussion with you is all that is warranted. In other cases, you may identify problems that require considerable attention. For problems that do not threaten the safety of the adolescent or the family, sometimes a period of unsuccessful treatment is necessary to determine that outpatient therapy is ineffective and that hospitalization is indicated. Before making such a recommendation, you need to establish a trusting relationship with the client and the client's parents. An excellent resource referred to several times in this chapter, AACAP's *Facts for Families,* has been developed by the AACAP and will help you provide concise and current information on issues that affect adolescents and their families. You can access this on the web via http://www.aacap.org or through the Online Student Resources for this text.

In the Inpatient Setting

Admission into a hospital or other residential treatment facility may be indicated under the following circumstances:

- If the adolescent is unable to control impulsivity
- If the degree of destructive or antisocial behavior escalates beyond normal limits
- If the adolescent cannot form meaningful, stable relationships within the everyday environment (as in the case of family dysfunction)

The existence of any of these conditions warrants counseling or professional treatment. A combination of two or more is likely to make treatment on an outpatient basis virtually ineffective, indicating the need for hospital or residential treatment.

Hospitalization of the disturbed adolescent has these possible advantages:

- It provides additional structure within which to handle the physically and psychologically destructive elements of the adolescent's behavior.
- It removes the individual from the stresses of a disturbed family environment.
- It offers opportunities for supporting existing ego strengths and promoting whatever ability the client has for forming relationships.

Your Intervention Strategies will help you encourage parents to be more effective.

Adolescents are sometimes institutionalized because their ideas are strange or threatening to their families, or because the responsible authorities seek to punish the adolescent's unacceptable behavior. The results can be disastrous. Therefore, it is important to make accurate assessments and to implement early treatment when indicated. You can play a crucial role in making assessments, undertaking appropriate interventions, and educating parents, teachers, and school officials to recognize these needs.

Staff Nurse in a General Hospital Setting

Adolescents with emotional problems may have symptoms of physical illness and as a result may be admitted to a general hospital setting for evaluation and treatment. Clients with anorexia nervosa, in particular, may be referred for inpatient treatment on general adolescent medical units. As a medical unit staff nurse, you can take the opportunity to reach out to adolescents who have emotional problems.

Consultant in a General Hospital Setting

Staff nurses from a psychiatric inpatient unit of a general hospital may be consulted by other nursing staff about emotionally disturbed adolescents who have been admitted to their general medical or surgical units. Some general hospital settings have advanced practice registered nurses (APRNs) who are clinical nurse specialists or nurse practitioners in psychiatric liaison positions as consultants.

Staff Nurse or Advanced Practice Nurse in a Psychiatric Setting

In inpatient psychiatric settings, the staff nurse or APRN may assume any of the previously mentioned roles. Nurses in inpatient settings also have numerous opportunities to observe and assess the family dynamics among the adolescent's family members and possibly to intervene. Nurses involved in family therapy sessions can perceive maladaptive ways of relating and take direct steps to work toward change. However, you need not work within the structured format of a therapy hour to have an impact on the family system.

Because inpatient nursing entails around-the-clock care, the nurse has the responsibility to maintain the therapeutic environment. The role of the inpatient staff nurse includes the following:

- Maintaining physical and psychological safety of the unit
- Setting verbal and physical limits on client behavior
- Establishing meaningful one–to–one relationships with clients
- Identifying client strengths and promoting more adaptive coping skills
- Role-modeling socially acceptable behaviors
- Participating in group therapies and other structured activities

Milieu Therapist

Many authors have described the importance of the therapeutic environment, indicating the strong influence of the treatment environment on the treatment outcome. (For a complete discussion, see Chapter 13∞.) Because of

---

YOUR INTERVENTION STRATEGIES   Encouraging More Effective Parenting Behaviors

Parent Behavior

- Initiates loud verbal arguments during visits with adolescent

Nursing Interventions

- Stop the immediate behavior, pointing out the disruptiveness to the unit.
- Refer adolescent and family to a family therapist to resolve differences and learn more adaptive ways of relating in supportive atmosphere of family therapy.
- Suggest that family therapist contract with family for one or more of the following:
  - Staff will monitor visits.
  - Family will bring up potentially volatile topics only within the structure of family meetings and not on the unit during visits.
  - Staff will intervene if arguments ensue on the unit.
  - Staff may limit visiting time on the unit.

Parent Behavior

- History of physical violence against adolescent

Nursing Interventions

- Upon admission, contract with adolescent and family for no acts of violence against people or property.
- Monitor parent visits with adolescent on the unit.
- Limit or deny passes with parents until progress is demonstrated.
- Depending on the parent's level of self-control, refuse visiting privileges with adolescent until progress is seen in family therapy.

Parent Behavior

- Unable to set limits with adolescent during unit visits (is adversely influenced by manipulative attempts, tolerates verbal abuse, etc.)

Nursing Interventions

- Intervene if demands or behavior could lead to physical harm, unit rule breaking, or other negative results.
- Point out problem and refer adolescent and parents to family therapy.
- Role-model appropriate and effective limit setting with adolescent, if necessary.
- Offer to discuss situation with parents and adolescent if desirable in the immediate situation.
- Offer emotional support to parent who needs to talk.

Parent Behavior

- Limited interaction with adolescent during unit visits

Nursing Interventions

- Initiate discussion among adolescent and family members related to visit and treatment goals.
- Communicate observations to family therapist.
- Initiate discussion with parents to allow exploration of difficulty, if desired.
- Suggest that family members and adolescent discuss the problem in family therapy.
- Plan outings or special-occasion celebrations to include family, if appropriate.

---

adolescents' needs for peer acceptance, their overwhelming uncertainties and fears, and their ever-changing behaviors and attitudes about identity, their chances for success in inpatient treatment are increased by a peer group setting. Much has been written about the value of the therapeutic environment in dealing with adolescent problems, including the problems of substance abuse and similar destructive activities. Without the social interaction and living–learning situations provided by the peer group, psychotherapy may be ineffective. Of course the nature of the psychotherapy, the treatment modalities and intervention strategies, will be largely determined by the theoretical base of your treatment setting and the training of the staff. Specifically, most adolescent units use behavioral management principles to be the basis for work with clients. Units that specialize in treating specific disorders or problems use relevant treatment modalities that studies have shown to be effective. As one example, the use of CBT has been used to treat adolescents with depression, anxiety, PTSD, and eating disorders. Another example is dialectical behavior therapy (DBT) that has been used successfully in individual and group therapy with adolescents with chronic suicidal thoughts or self-harm behaviors. See Chapter 30∞ for a more complete discussion of cognitive–behavioral interventions.

The therapeutic environment provides valuable experiences for adolescents for the following reasons:

- Adolescents more readily hear and accept limits from peers than from adults.
- Adolescents more readily respond to feedback, both negative and positive, from peers than from adults.
- Shared goals and objectives facilitate group processes and the development of cohesion among adolescent group members.
- Group interaction allows for the expression of appropriate feelings and identification with peers with similar feelings.
- Group interaction provides opportunities for learning how to develop relationships with others.
- Group structure allows for the testing of new, more adaptive behaviors.
- Adolescents receive feedback from the peer group and have the opportunity to give feedback in a supportive environment.
- The group format provides an opportunity to work out specific issues of conflict with adult group leaders while receiving the support and understanding of peers.

NURSING PROCESS
Adolescents

Adolescents present behaviors and problems unique to their developmental stage. Without knowledge and understanding about potentially difficult areas, you may respond with confusion, anger, and even hostility, which will cause feelings of frustration and failure for both yourself and your adolescent clients. The following pages contain numerous examples of either typical behaviors expected of the "normal" adolescent or problem behaviors that may provide the impetus for referral to a treatment setting, or both. In many situations, you may simply need to focus on the difficult issues encountered in working with adolescents. That information is given in the Assessment section. Situations that represent an identified problem necessitating treatment are discussed under Planning and Implementation.

Assessment

It is important for you to keep in mind that over the course of normal development, children and adolescents experience symptoms of anxiety, dysphoria, oppositionality, or conduct disorder. On the other hand, there are factors that can contribute to missed or inaccurate diagnoses in the assessment of an adolescent:

- Symptom overlap, which can blur diagnostic boundaries
- Effects of normal development on symptom presentation
- High rates of comorbidity in youth with mental illness
- Perception of informants (i.e., parents/guardians, teachers, or other family members)

Moreover, two other factors that can minimize the effectiveness and comprehensive nature of an adequate assessment in the adolescent are:

- The impact of managed care, with its emphasis on brevity of client contact in inpatient and outpatient settings
- The emphasis in some clinical training on the rigid adherence to DSM criteria without the exploration of developmental stages, risk and protective factors, current stressors, temperament, cultural issues, and/or family dynamics

Accurate and comprehensive assessments can be obtained only by viewing the adolescent as a biopsychosocial being. Only by integrating knowledge from biology, psychology, and humanistic–interactionist theory can you understand what a particular behavior means to an adolescent. If you can remember your own adolescent experiences—the conflicts and uncertainty as well as the elation and the triumphs—you will better appreciate the adolescent's turmoil. It is equally important that you discover who the individual adolescent is.

Meanings of behavior, values, and actions can vary from client to client and may not reflect meanings or values that you hold. For example, the client who has trouble with competitive feelings may be reluctant to accept an invitation to play a game of Trivial Pursuit. And because adolescents are developmentally between childhood and adulthood, they frequently have the feelings and choices of adulthood without an adult's abilities in verbal discourse and impulse control. As a result, adolescents may "act out" feelings and decisions nonverbally, in a childlike way. This is particularly true of the emotionally disturbed adolescent. In settings where tension and anxiety are typically high, such as the emergency department of a hospital, the high emotionality of an adolescent can be potentiated. See What Every Nurse Should Know about helping adolescents when they are upset.

Acting Out

The concept of acting out is complex. The term has been used to describe a variety of behaviors, ranging from antisocial, destructive acts to unconscious impulses expressed in action rather than in symbolic words or symptoms. Acting out may, and often does, include destructive actions and seemingly undefinable behaviors. The term describes a re-creation of the client's life experiences, relationships with significant others, and resulting unresolved conflicts.

These are all components of what is commonly called the client's *life script*, which unfolds as the client relates, reacts, and behaves in accustomed ways. Through observation of and interaction with the client, you can uncover the meanings that various behaviors and actions hold for the individual. For example, the child who has assumed the "black sheep" role in the family seeks to re-create that familiar role with others outside the home, particularly in the inpatient setting. This

WHAT EVERY NURSE SHOULD KNOW

Helping Upset Adolescents

Imagine you are an emergency department nurse. If the hospital is often a frightening place for adults, you can imagine what the emergency department (ED) is like for an adolescent. Adolescents come to the ED as clients, as family members of a client, or as friends of a client. In fact, if there is an injury or accident at the local school, an onslaught of teens may show up to support their injured or sick schoolmate. Whether as clients or supporters of a client, adolescents can be histrionic and exaggerate the nature of a problem. You may find it helpful to deal with the upset adolescent by suggesting deep-breathing or de-escalation techniques. Having the teens focus on their breathing can provide a focus for their anxiety, allow them to concentrate, and increase their oxygen level. When they are able to "hear" what you have to say, ask questions with simple answers while also encouraging positive expectations. An example might be, "Have you felt this way before?" If the answer is yes, ask, "What did you do to help yourself at that time?"

clinical example illustrates one girl's relationship with her parents as replayed with the staff on an inpatient unit.

Clinical Example

Liza is 14 years old. She has been on the unit for 6 days. She is an attractive, engaging young person who has been friendly with both staff and clients. Liza has been on the periphery of several rule-breaking incidents but has not been directly involved. She has begun to establish close ties with Jim, a nurse, and engages in frequent lengthy discussions with him about her innermost feelings and fears. One evening she candidly talks to him about the callous way in which she was treated by one of the other nurses, a woman, in regard to a gynecologic problem. Liza says with undisguised fear and embarrassment that she is afraid the situation will repeat itself. She expresses great respect for Jim's knowledge and style and asks him to attend to any subsequent problems himself so that she does not have to interact with Jane, the other nurse.

The implications for treatment are many. The most important factors for Jim to consider are what meaning Liza's behavior has for her and what would be the most therapeutically effective way to deal with the situation. The client's presenting problems and the expectation that the client will act out previous conflicts and life scripts have provided Jim adequate information on which to base an appropriate intervention. The client's attempt to manipulate (seduce) the nurse, and the need for nurses to examine their own behavior and motivations, are discussed in detail later in this chapter.

Clinical Example

In the previous clinical example, Jim recognizes how Liza is unconsciously acting out her life script by re-creating her relationships with her parents with Jim and Jane, a female nurse on the unit. Jim remembers that Liza's home situation is chaotic. Liza's mother and father frequently fight over who is the better parent. Jim surmises that Liza also plays a part in these fights. Jim recognizes the "pull" from Liza to feel that only he can adequately handle the situation. The present situation seems to indicate that he is about to be pitted against Jane, just as Liza perhaps plays one parent against the other. Jim responds by reiterating his concern for her dilemma and suggesting that Liza speak with Jane about the situation that is causing her concern.

In this example, it is clear that the client is attempting to re-create her home situation, using two of the nurses to re-enact the roles of her parents. Had Jim been seduced into playing the father's role in the script, he would have re-created the family's conflict on the unit. The ideal solution is for staff to interrupt this pathologic process by substituting a healthier way of resolving the problem. Thus, Jim does not react with compliance or with anger to Liza's attempts. Instead, he recognizes the significance of her behavior and deals with the situation in a concerned yet healthy way, suggesting a resolution to the immediate problem that demonstrates respect for both Liza's and Jane's abilities to resolve the conflict.

Such situations are commonplace with adolescents. They require nursing staff to evaluate the client's psychodynamics and psychopathology as well as their own inner feelings and behavior. For these reasons, it is imperative to identify transference and countertransference issues and to discuss them with your clinical supervisor. Transference and countertransference are discussed in Chapter 10∞, but these situations are not limited to the inpatient setting. This fact alone obliges you to be alert in observing and assessing verbal and nonverbal communication and to understand your own feelings and behavior in order to make accurate assessments and appropriate interventions. In this way, you will be most effective when working with adolescents. An illustration of how research can help shape interventions to maximize resilience in an adolescent who is acting out a self-destructive life script is in Evidence-Based Practice.

Communication

Communication with adolescents is an art in itself. To become proficient in this area, you must accept and understand the following:

- Adolescents tend to act out feelings and conflicts rather than verbalize them.
- Adolescents have an unconventional language of their own.
- Adolescents, especially disturbed ones, may use profanity frequently.
- Many clues can be obtained simply by observing an adolescent's behavior, dress, or environment.

If you learn the verbal and nonverbal communication skills discussed in Chapter 10∞, you can use them comfortably and naturally in communicating with adolescents.

Nonverbal Cues Adolescents give many nonverbal cues to their specific emotional struggles, underlying confusion, or transitory moods. A glance around their rooms or a brief study of their dress can tell you more than what several direct questions would elicit. Sometimes adolescents give obvious cues. A client who wears a coat around the unit may be planning to run away. Other less obvious behaviors, which are often outside the client's conscious awareness or control, can also yield vital information. A sudden escalation of horseplay among the boys around bedtime is an example. You would probably be correct in identifying this behavior as an expression of anxiety related to sexual identity and fears of homosexual feelings. Interactionist theory holds that the adolescent boy's newfound sexual feelings and changing body image provide unfamiliar ways of relating to members of his own gender. As a result, he regresses to preadolescent behavior, which served him well in handling close feelings then, but now proves inappropriate. In this instance, firm limit setting is in order. Avoid interpreting the behavior or paying undue attention to the specifics. (Testing and limit setting are discussed later in the chapter.)

Slang and Obscenities Adolescents create a language all their own. This takes some understanding and acceptance. In seeking their identity, adolescents establish a form of communication unique to the group. To gain acceptance into the

EVIDENCE-BASED PRACTICE

Maximizing Resilience

Danny is a slightly underweight 15-year-old boy who was admitted to the crisis unit in your community after treatment in the ED for an "accidental" overdose of his insulin. After admitting to his parents that he had intentionally drawn up too much insulin in a suicide attempt "to get what's coming anyway" he was admitted to the unit for observation and treatment.

Your initial nursing assessment revealed that Danny's depression and guilt seem to have evolved over time as he endured the loss of several relatives close to him, who died following complications from diabetes. He fears for himself and also feels guilty for "surviving" the illness that has taken his loved ones. Talking to him and his family about his diabetes condition reveals a similarly fatalistic attitude among his family members.

Your plan for intervention options is based on current research results. For example, in your review of studies of building resilience in adolescents, you know that optimism is a trait that contributes to resilience and has been identified as the most influential adolescent cognitive factor to moderate the effects of life stressors. Danny's parents commented that they had always regarded him as the "most positive" of their three children. Prior to puberty (his female cousin with diabetes died at age 12) he had been active in all sports and was "upbeat in every way." You recall that the design and delivery of an intervention to maximize resilience in adolescents require gender-specific strategies that are attractive, engaging, and easily accessible. You ask his parents to bring in pictures of him when he was active in sports. You encourage him to talk about his exploits and remind him about his physical abilities and competitive nature. You encourage him to be conscientious about managing his diabetes while inviting him to envision his goals for the future after high school. You

incorporate these values and resiliency-building interventions in the nursing care plan and in all staff treatment meetings.

Furthermore, your readings and experiences have yielded information regarding the financial and staffing limits of community and school resources. As a result, you understand that local resources may tend to be problem focused and disease oriented because they do not have the funds or time to provide preventive or creative activities. You expect to put a plan in motion that will use pre-existing resources as well as connect Danny with new supports, perhaps even identifying a program or resource to enhance Danny's school and social environments. With the help of Danny's school nurse, you set up a "surprise" visit from a local sports celebrity, an adult who has managed his diabetes since childhood. Danny is thrilled to meet him but, more importantly, is surprised to learn of his lifelong diabetes self-management and to see firsthand the positive results of his efforts. Over the next few weeks of his treatment, Danny demonstrates renewed optimism and displays a newfound autonomy and self-assurance in his diabetes self-management skills. Moreover, he agrees to explore serving as a counselor to younger kids in a local diabetes camp who might feel the way he "used to." This set of multiple intervention strategies is based on the following research:

Macgowan, M. J., & Engle, B. (2010). Evidence for optimism: Behavior therapies and motivational interviewing in adolescent substance abuse treatment. *Child and Adolescent Psychiatric Clinics of North America, 19*(3), 527–545.

Yancey, A. K., Grant, D., Kurosky, S., Kravitz-Wirtz, N., & Mistry, R. (2010, August 26). Role modeling, risk, and resilience in California adolescents. *Journal of Adolescent Health Online.* Retrieved from http://www.jahonline.org/article/S1054-139X(10)00227-2/-fulltext

CRITICAL THINKING QUESTIONS

1. How would knowing how the adolescent has coped with earlier problems in life help you to design strategies for intervention?
2. Would an increased awareness of ways to be resilient make a difference in an adolescent client's life? How?
3. Why would involving others in Danny's goal of increased resilience be helpful?
4. Of what value are reminders of earlier active times in Danny's life? Would they be discouraging rather than encouraging?

---

adolescent world, the adult must accept this need to use ambiguous (to the adult) yet specific (to adolescents) terms to express themselves. In many cases, you must communicate with adolescents by using their slang.

This slang often includes obscene and profane words. This is particularly true of disturbed adolescents, who have an especially difficult time expressing anger and fear appropriately. The words they use often reveal the nature of the emotional conflict. For example, a young male adolescent grappling with his sexual identity and aggressive feelings may resort to sexually graphic words when he feels anxious or afraid. You may sometimes find it productive to use similar words to give explanations or to clarify communication. Understandably, some nurses have difficulty tolerating profane or sexually graphic language. However, you must evaluate your

clients' underlying reasons for using such language, to help them understand their feelings. Only then can you encourage clients to use more appropriate means of expression. If clients sense that the reason you want them to speak more appropriately is only to make you, the nurse, feel more comfortable, the end result will not be satisfactory. Rx Communication: Client Using Profanity or Obscenities further demonstrates two examples of this.

The adolescent psychiatric client often has symptoms of disturbed communication, which can affect all realms of daily living, particularly in relationships with peers, family members, and nonparental authority figures. Giving information is one way you can help decrease communication deficits and facilitate relationships with others. Other nursing behaviors are outlined in the Planning and Implementation section.

R̲ₓ COMMUNICATION

Client Using Profanity or Obscenities

CLIENT: "Hey, bee-atch! [Slang word for "bitch."] When is dinner served around this hell-hole? [Other clients are snickering in the background.]"

NURSE RESPONSE 1: [with an exaggerated look of surprise] "Rocky, you're new to the unit. I will give you information about the unit and about mealtimes but you need to understand something first. Profanity is not an acceptable way to get to know anyone here. I expect you to treat me with respect, as I will you. Now I'll show you your room and you can put your things away." [She then proceeds with him to a less public space where she talks with him without the other clients for an audience.]

RATIONALE: A newly admitted client may be attempting to over-compensate for his anxiety and fears as "the new kid" with bravado and intimidation. Giving information may allay his anxiety while verbally setting limits on his provocative behavior avoiding escalation and the need for physical controls.

NURSE RESPONSE 2: [with an obvious look of surprise] "Rocky, you need to learn about the unit. That includes information about acceptable behaviors as well as mealtimes. Let that be the last time you address me or anyone else here that way. If you have trouble controlling your behavior we can assist you in taking a time out until you're able to control yourself and are ready to be with the rest of the group. Steve and I will show you to your room, and you can ask us any other questions there." [She and a male staff member escort him to his room, soliciting information as they evaluate his reactions and degree of control.]

RATIONALE: The client was newly admitted to the unit. Immediate limit setting and spelling out consequences may deter further provocative behavior to assert domination over staff and intimidate other clients.

Confidentiality An emerging body of research underscores the importance of discussing confidentiality with the adolescent. There will be health concerns, thoughts, and feelings that the adolescent client will want to keep private. Assurances of confidentiality will increase the likelihood that the adolescent will disclose sensitive personal information to you. Confidentiality, however, cannot be unconditional in that some information, such as sexual abuse, must be disclosed by law, and other information, such as a suicide plan, must be discussed with the parents and the rest of the treatment team. In discussing confidentiality with the adolescent, one way of clarifying this dilemma might be to simply state, "What you and I discuss is confidential. However, you need to know that *if it means harm to you or to someone else* [emphasize these words], it will be important for me to talk it over with your parents/other members of the team [whoever is most appropriate to the situation]. In that case, I will first discuss it with you to determine the best way to present our concerns to others."

Anger and Hostility

Expressions of anger and hostility are common on an adolescent unit. Anger expressed verbally usually takes the form of profanity. How effectively you deal with expressions of anger and hostility depends on how effectively you handle your own angry or hostile feelings. You will compromise your effectiveness as a nurse if you are uncomfortable with expressions of anger or hostility, or view anger and hostility as negative or to be avoided at all costs.

Nurse's Self-Assessment A subject that is rarely considered is anger felt and expressed by the nurse toward the client. The general focus on the client's need for understanding and good care seem to make it unacceptable to display negative feelings toward the client. In the nursing care of adolescents, however, a constant all-giving and all-accepting attitude by the nurse, particularly during times of testing, would be not only nontherapeutic but also illogical and dishonest, and adolescents need honest feedback. The adolescent sometimes escalates the provocative behavior to test your response or to evoke an angry reaction. For you to pretend that you are not angry in such a situation is as undesirable for treatment as it would be to pretend that you are fond of the client when you are not.

Being honest about your feelings is a prime prerequisite in establishing and maintaining meaningful and productive relationships with adolescent clients. This does not mean that you should vent all your thoughts or impulses. Be aware of your reactions, and use good judgment in handling them. This is also an opportunity to model adult modes of anger expression. The questions in Your Self-Awareness: A Self-Awareness Inventory for Working With Adolescents will help you assess your own ways of dealing with anger.

Anxiety and Resistance

Normal adolescents frequently feel anxious as they experience change and inner turmoil in adapting to a new identity. The anxiety evidenced by disturbed adolescents in treatment can indicate many other things. The changes required are much more threatening to disturbed adolescents than to normal adolescents. If treatment is to be successful, clients must look at the meaning of their behavior and must change many of their earlier interactional patterns. This can be frightening. For example, it is more comfortable to play the role of the "bad seed" or "bad kid," with its known pitfalls and expectations, than to attempt a change that entails many uncertainties and unknowns.

Clients feel threatened and anxious when the nurse does not act according to their expectations, because they must then find other ways of handling the situation. They must also deal with the anxiety. Frequently this anxiety is channeled into a game of "cops and robbers," as the client once again assumes

YOUR SELF-AWARENESS
A Self-Awareness Inventory for Working With Adolescents

To increase self-awareness about your own way of dealing with anger, ask yourself these questions:

- What kinds of things make me angry?
- How do I deal with my anger? Do I tend to ignore or hide it, or do I show that I am angry?
- Do I sometimes use profanity or act out my feelings in a physical way? How do I feel about others who do this?
- What do I think about how I handle anger? Am I proud of the way I handle anger?
- How do I react to others when they are angry?

To increase self-awareness about your tendency to be seduced or manipulated, ask yourself these questions:

- Is this client's friendliness compromising the professional role boundaries between us and "personalizing" our relationship?
- Do I feel compelled to respond in a personal rather than therapeutic way, possibly revealing information about my own life and lifestyle?
- Do I feel uncomfortable with the client's flattering comments or probing questions?
- Do I tend to forget that this person is a client?
- Is the client encouraging me to keep secrets from other staff or to "side" with the client against other staff?

To increase self-awareness about your own sexual attitudes and feelings, ask yourself these questions:

- How would I describe my adolescence as it related to my developing sexuality?
- What do I remember about the development and changes in my body?
- How did I feel about these changes?
- How would I describe my adolescent relationships with members of my own sex?
- How would I describe my adolescent relationships with members of the opposite sex?
- What events stand out in my mind when I recall my sexual experiences during adolescence?
- How have these past relationships, events, and feelings influenced me today?

a familiar role and maintains the negative or unhealthy image. The anxiety caused by unfamiliar roles is dissipated by further testing and acting out. Do not take this as an indication that therapy is not working. It may simply indicate that the client needs to move ahead more slowly with insightful discoveries and needs your support to do so.

Keep in mind that to these adolescents, "opening up" in a trusting way does not hold the same positive promise that it might for you. Adolescents who have been rejected or have experienced loss following close relationships in the past will be wary of your expressions of interest or concern and will be cautious about repeating such experiences. They may respond to you with testing behaviors, anger and mistrust, or outright rejection. Adolescents who expect rejection gain some control

over the relationship if they reject others before being rejected themselves.

Nurse's Self-Assessment Sometimes nurses find it difficult to allow adolescents to grapple with their anxieties and fears. At other times, you may not recognize the client's behavior as a symptom of anxiety or depression. The following clinical example demonstrates the value of a comprehensive assessment, of exploring all possible reasons for a client's resistance to your efforts, before implementing action.

Clinical Example

Kathy was the quietest and most aloof client on the unit. She had isolated herself from the other clients during the week that followed admission and avoided conversing with staff members outside meetings. One evening she seemed unusually receptive to the new nurse, Ellie, who was able to interest her in a sewing project. Ellie, who was a new graduate, felt pleased that Kathy had responded warmly to her during their time together. The next day, Kathy did not speak to Ellie and seemed to avoid her at all costs. Later, Ellie noticed that the dress Kathy had been sewing had been torn into shreds and stuffed into the wastepaper basket. Ellie interpreted this quite personally. She felt deeply hurt and rejected.

In her discussion with her supervisor, Ellie showed her disappointment and anger. Her supervisor observed that, although the good time and feelings that Ellie and Kathy had shared the evening before were genuine, Kathy had not experienced many such times before with her parents or other adults. She suggested that Kathy was probably angry with Ellie for pointing out what she, Kathy, had missed. The supervisor suggested that Ellie be patient with Kathy. Perhaps later Ellie could re-establish the bond, and they would be able to talk about what had happened.

Fortunately, Ellie did not act on her angry feelings. Had she done so, she might have impulsively assessed Kathy's behavior as "hopeless," interpreting Kathy's anxiety and resistance as an inability to trust, or she may have begun to relate to the client in a vindictive way, withdrawing from Kathy in turn. Instead, she sought advice. Ellie's supervisor recognized that Ellie wanted to do well and needed positive feedback. She also realized that Ellie did not understand the nature of giving to emotionally disturbed adolescents. Had Ellie not sought advice, she might have acted on her angry feelings, further alienating Kathy and causing herself more anger and frustration. Without an understanding of Kathy's actions, Ellie would have continued to expect kindness in return for kindness and would have been keenly disappointed.

Seduction and Manipulation of the Nurse

In working with adolescents, there is always the risk of **seduction** of the nurse—that is, manipulation of the nurse by the client into relating in a nontherapeutic way. (Thus, the word *seduction* is not necessarily linked to *sexual* in psychiatric settings.) These factors contribute to the problem:

- The intimate nature of the nurse's involvement with the adolescent client
- The narcissism inherent in this age group
- The nurse's all-accepting attitude in working with the adolescent client

Narcissism in this age group is caused by the child's withdrawal from the parents and their value system. This withdrawal leads to a general self-centeredness, overevaluation of the self, heightened self-perception, decreased ability for reality testing, and extreme self-absorption. The result is that the people to whom adolescents turn become all-important and perfect in their eyes. Nurses may be strongly tempted to respond accordingly.

Nurse's Self-Awareness The dangers inherent in this situation are not simply the two possible extremes: total submission to temptation, resulting in a sexual relationship with the client; or strong denial of temptation by maintaining a rigid, unapproachable stance that makes it impossible to establish a meaningful, trusting relationship. Neither of these extremes is unknown. The questions in Your Self-Awareness: A Self-Awareness Inventory for Working With Adolescents on page 587 will help you assess how you deal with seduction and how you deal with your own sexual attitudes and feelings.

It is tempting to respond to the adolescent's idealized view, to be the "savior" who succeeds with this difficult person where everyone else has failed, to feel superior to the imperfect parents, the harassed school teacher, the skeptical juvenile judge, or other members of the staff on the unit. However, you should not give in to such temptations. Complications will most certainly develop that at best will temporarily compromise your effectiveness and at worst will render the treatment program completely ineffective. Liza's example of acting out demonstrates this. Jim, the evening nurse, could have been seduced by Liza to collude with her against the day nurse, Jane, had he not been keenly aware of that possibility.

Nurses who work intensively with adolescents often face situations in which their own unresolved feelings are aroused. You must choose whether to act on these impulses or to explore their origin. Of course, one is not always conscious of these unresolved feelings. It would be unrealistic to expect you to be totally aware of the meaning of your behavior at any given moment. Nonetheless, the skilled clinician is usually acquainted with the issues or conflicts that have caused problems in the past. In doubtful cases, the knowledgeable nurse will seek consultation from a clinician. The clinician can help you assess the situation and understand what part you may have played in initiating it. Nurses who wish to explore their personal conflicts further may then seek counseling or therapy.

Nursing staff would benefit from establishing one or more of the following to provide a consistent format for assessing and evaluating ongoing situations with adolescent clients:

- Each nurse's own ongoing supervision with a preceptor or nurse supervisor
- A regularly scheduled meeting (perhaps monthly) for all nursing staff to discuss difficult situations and conflicting feelings
- Staff meetings (perhaps weekly) in which all disciplines identify interpersonal obstacles and plan interventions toward more optimal treatment

Sexual Behavior of the Adolescent

The biologic changes that occur in late childhood and early adolescence are rapid and pervasive. Do not underestimate the importance of the adolescent's experimentation and attitude in sexual matters. Likewise, evaluate your own attitudes and feelings about sexual issues as they relate to past experiences and current activities. Conflicts in such matters or resentments left over from the past will certainly affect your decisions or interactions with clients regarding sexual matters. Again, while it is not necessary for you to resolve all these issues, it is highly desirable to be aware of areas of conflict that might make it difficult to view a situation objectively or to set rational limits. What Every Nurse Should Know offers suggestions on creating a youth-friendly environment for talking about sexuality with this age group.

Until adolescents master their anxieties and fears about their sexual identity and gain control over sexual urges, they will exhibit a variety of behaviors and attitudes that may confuse or trouble you. In the past decade, rates of sexual activity, pregnancy, and live births among adolescents had stabilized and perhaps even begun to decline as there appears to have been a decrease in intercourse as a sexual activity among youth and a reported increase in the use of more effective contraceptive methods. Although these trends were encouraging, in this decade it seems that the pregnancy rate is again increasing. Moreover, it is estimated that each year there are approximately 19 million new STD infections, and almost half of them among youth aged 15-24 (CDC, 2010a).

Heterosexual Behavior Heterosexual activity is normal and desirable during adolescence. However, nurses working with either normal or disturbed adolescents will sometimes see them engage in sexual activities that do not seem healthy or growth producing. For example, the adolescent girl who seeks

WHAT EVERY NURSE SHOULD KNOW

Discussing Sexuality With Adolescents

Imagine you are a community health nurse. Discussing sexual matters with adolescents may be easier and more practical if you use a structured, user-friendly tool to "break the ice" and acquire the information you need. One helpful research-based publication, "Best Practices for Youth Friendly Clinical Services," can provide you with the guidelines and key components of a youth-friendly clinic or other community setting that provides health care to adolescents. The paper provides detail related to the need for all staff training regarding confidentiality with the adolescent and gives extra attention to the needs of special subgroups, such as HIV-positive youth, gay, lesbian, bisexual, and transgender youth, pregnant or parenting teens, and various ethnic minority groups. This is only one of many publications provided by Advocates for Youth that can be ordered through their website at http://www.advocatesforyouth .org/ (Alford, 2009).

℞ COMMUNICATION

Client With Sexual Acting-Out Behavior

CLIENT: [A male and female client are discovered making out in a closet on the unit.] "Hey, a little privacy, if you don't mind!"

NURSE RESPONSE 1: "Laurie, Bill, not cool, guys. What's going on? You knew I was coming in here to get more towels. Laurie, does this have to do with your pass home tomorrow? Let's talk about this in the office. C'mon." [She escorts the two clients to the office to talk.] *RATIONALE:* Both adolescents are "veterans" on the unit and know full well the rules and expectations. The nurse believes that the behavior is a display of Laurie's anxiety about her pass home tomorrow and may be an attempt to sabotage the privilege. Rather than addressing the rules as the focus for their discussion, she talks with them about the underlying meaning of their behavior.	**NURSE RESPONSE 2:** "Knock it off. Stop what you are doing now, and we are going to talk about appropriate behavior on the unit." *RATIONALE:* This intervention is particularly appropriate if the offenders have repeated this inappropriate behavior.

punishment rather than true pleasure in her sexual exploits will display them in an overt, exhibitionistic way in a place where a particularly moralistic person will discover her and give her the reprimands she desires. She may be testing a parent's values in an attempt to resolve her own inner conflicts.

Adolescents in an inpatient treatment setting where sexual intercourse is forbidden may engage in sexual intercourse where you or another staff member will be sure to discover them. The experience may reinforce their image of sexual behavior as "bad" behavior. Or it may simply provide a means of acting out their defiance of the rules, thereby earning the familiar "bad kid" label. The incident involving clients Laurie and Bill in Rx Communication is an excellent example of this situation.

Homosexual Behavior Homosexuality is the persistent sexual and emotional attraction to someone of the same gender. It is part of the range of sexual expression and has existed throughout history and across cultures. Preadolescents usually choose a member of the same gender with whom to experience intimate or loving feelings. This does not necessarily mean that a sexual relationship will ensue, although it often does. Homosexual activity may continue into the adolescent years. Many gay, lesbian, and bisexual individuals first become aware of their sexual thoughts and feelings and may have their first experiences during adolescence. Recent changes in society's attitude toward sexuality, including homosexual issues, have helped gay, lesbian, and bisexual youth feel more comfortable with their sexual orientation. On the other hand, much more needs to be accomplished. Numerous incidents of electronic bullying resulting in the suicide of young people engaged in homosexual activities have been well publicized. Research suggests that 9% to 35% of youth report being victims of this type of violence (CDC, 2010b). AACAP has designed a fact sheet to assist parents and professionals alike in meeting the developmental needs of the homosexual or bisexual adolescent (AACAP, 2010). Although the causes of homosexuality or bisexuality are not fully understood, the AACAP position makes it clear that sexual orientation is not a mental disorder. Nor is it a matter of choice. Individuals are no more

able to "choose" whether or not to be homosexual than to be heterosexual.

Like their heterosexual counterparts, gay, lesbian, and bisexual teens have many concerns, including: feeling different from their peers; fearing ridicule, rejection, or harassment by others; worrying about a negative response from their families or loved ones; and worrying about sexually transmitted diseases, including HIV infection. Moreover, they have an additional fear of discrimination due to their sexual orientation when seeking employment, applying to college, or joining clubs or sports activities. They can become socially isolated, withdraw from friends and activities, have trouble concentrating, develop low self-esteem, become depressed, and feel suicidal. Counseling may be helpful for teens who are uncomfortable with their homosexuality or who are unable to express it. Regardless of setting or sexual orientation, adolescents do have a choice about how and where to express their sexual feelings, just as they do their other emotions.

Generally speaking, however, adolescents view homosexual feelings as a threat to the development of their identity. As a result, they may ward off such feelings by engaging in frantic sexual activity with a member of the opposite sex. This is particularly true for boys. It is normal for an adolescent boy to be afraid of feelings of passivity and to label these feelings as homosexual. Some boys may have been brought up to identify with physical displays of strength or aggressive displays of power. If that is the case, an incident where he feels threatened or powerless would produce feelings of sexual impotence, a feeling of dependence or weakness, and a greater fear of homosexuality. The adolescent boy in treatment may act out these feelings, or he may attempt to reaffirm his masculinity with inappropriate displays of aggression or destructive behavior. Likewise, the adolescent girl who feels a need to ward off intense feelings for female peers may engage in frantic sexual activity with numerous male partners for similar reasons. Clients who use homosexuality to express hostility toward their parents will undoubtedly act out with the staff as well.

Nurses who work with adolescents may encounter any of these situations and they must attempt to understand the meaning that homosexual behavior has for the client. The clients may need to explore their feelings and anxieties openly. Open discussion with an understanding yet knowledgeable professional may help resolve many of the concerns and conflicts inherent in adolescent sexual behavior. Remain objective and nonjudgmental with these clients, allowing them to deal with the feelings of anger or depression that may result from addressing the conflict.

Although homosexual behavior during adolescence does not predict adult sexual preference, some adolescents make a lasting identification as homosexuals during these years. These adolescents will not experience conflicts about homosexual relationships or need to flaunt them or act out with the staff in an angry or hostile way. In these cases, however, you may have to deal with your own negative feelings about homosexuality, if any exist. It is important for you to consider what clients' relationships mean to them and to respect them.

Pregnancy Adolescent pregnancy may reflect social and family expectations and unconscious motivations. Some teenage girls are quite pleased to be pregnant and suffer no emotional consequences from motherhood. In general, however, a conscious, deliberate decision to become pregnant at this age is manipulative. The goal may be to escape a difficult family situation, to express hostility toward parents, or to act out a life script in which the daughter is seen as "bad." The adolescent girl who did not receive adequate nurturing as a child could be acting out dependency needs by giving her baby the love and caring she herself did not receive. In so doing, she feels loved and cared for in turn.

Be sensitive to motivational factors in dealing with emotionally deprived adolescents. Use existing educational tools and interpersonal relationships to help adolescent girls understand their needs and motivations to become pregnant. It is also important to educate adolescents of both genders about sex and birth control. Many high schools are now recognizing this need and providing information in birth control clinics or through health education classes. Too often parents and professionals alike deny the adolescent's sexual activity until an unwanted pregnancy occurs.

Dietary Problems and Eating Disorders

The eating habits and food preferences of disturbed adolescents can reveal a great deal about the nature of their inner turmoil. A comparison between the client's diet and that of a normal, healthy adolescent may show little difference in variety but probably a great difference in quantity.

Adolescents who have been deprived of early nurturing tend to eat more than others and probably place a higher value on mealtimes and on receiving their "share" of the food. You may notice that adolescents consume more milk than usual during periods of stress or anxiety. In general, girls want to follow food fads or unreasonable dietary regimens to become slim and attractive. This usually gives you an opportunity to engage in health teaching about nutrition and exercise, and to express a cooperative interest in their developing feminine identity. (Eating disorders are discussed in Chapter 21∞.)

Depression and Suicide

Both depression and suicide are thought to be under-reported among adolescents. DSM Essential Features highlights the criteria necessary for adolescents to be diagnosed with depression. For youth between the ages of 10 and 24, suicide is the third leading cause of death. It results in approximately 4,400 lives lost each year. The top three methods used in suicides of young people include firearm (46%), suffocation (37%), and poisoning (8%). Yet youth deaths from suicide are only part of the problem. It has been reported that more young people survive suicide attempts than actually die. A nationwide survey of youth in grades 9 through 12 in public and private schools in the United States found that 15% of students reported seriously considering suicide, 11% reported creating a plan, and 7% reporting trying to take their own lives in the 12 months preceding the survey. Each year, approximately 149,000 youth between the ages of 10 and 24 receive medical care for self-inflicted injuries at emergency departments across the United States (CDC, 2010a) The presence of self-injurious behavior should always trigger a suicide assessment. (See Chapter 23∞ for a complete discussion of suicide.)

Substance Use and Abuse

According to the 2009 Monitoring the Future survey of approximately 50,000 students in 8th, 10th, and 12th grades,

DSM ESSENTIAL FEATURES

Adolescent Depression

Depression: Core symptoms are the same for children and adolescents as adults, although the prominence of symptoms may change with age. Somatic complaints, irritability, and social withdrawal are particularly common in children and younger adolescents whereas psychomotor retardation, hypersomnia, and delusions are less common in prepuberty than in adolescence and adulthood. In adolescents, depression is frequently associated with disruptive behavior, attention deficit disorders, anxiety disorders, substance-related disorders, and eating disorders. Rather than a depressed mood during depression, adolescents display an irritable mood. In addition to depressed and/or irritable mood, you will see: lack of interest or pleasure in activities during most of the day, weight change of more than 5% in a month, psychomotor changes, loss of energy, concentration difficulties, feeling worthless, inappropriate guilt, durable thoughts of suicide. With adolescents it is important to consider problematic sleep patterns (insomnia or hypersomnia nearly every day) as a sleep change.

there was a gradual decline in the use of most illicit drugs except marijuana. The exception to this was the 30-day use of smokeless tobacco that rose in 2009. More importantly is the slight increase in marijuana usage. Lifetime, annual, and 30-day usage of marijuana that had leveled in 2008 began to rise in 2009. This increase for the three grades for 30-day usage from 12% to 14% is significant over the 2-year period of 2007 to 2009. As had been speculated by some experts, this increase was preceded and accompanied by a decrease in the subjects' belief regarding the degree of risk posed by marijuana usage. Although alcohol, like most illicit drugs, continues to show a decline, its usage continues to be widespread among teens. Nearly three quarters (72%) of students have consumed alcohol (more than a few sips) by the end of their high school years and more than one third (37%) report this experience by the end of 8th grade. Equally significant is the report that more than half (57%) of 12th graders and one sixth (17%) of 8th graders have been drunk at least once in their young lifetimes (Johnston, O'Malley, Bachman, & Schulenberg, 2010).

Adolescents give many reasons for using drugs: to experiment, to get high, to "get inside my head," to have fun, to understand more about life. Adolescents may also use drugs to cope with feelings of worthlessness or loneliness or to avoid uncomfortable feelings, as in the following clinical example.

Clinical Example

Cindy is a 15-year-old high school sophomore who has been abusing drugs since age 12. According to Cindy, her 3-year history of substance abuse has involved regular marijuana use one to two times a week, occasional use of Valium (which she sneaks from her mother's 5-mg tablet prescription bottle), Seconal ("street reds") on two occasions, and LSD on two occasions.

Cindy describes herself as a "loner" who has few friends and keeps to herself at home and at school. She leaves the house each morning for school before the others are awake "to avoid the hassles with my mother and sisters." She describes one female classmate to whom she feels close but states that their time together is usually brief and usually involves smoking marijuana in the morning just before school. Cindy has recently been suspended from school as a result of the school principal's discovery of Cindy and her friend smoking marijuana outside the cafeteria.

Cindy is lonely and depressed, and has extreme feelings of worthlessness. She characterizes herself as "bored," "bad," and "hopeless." Cindy says that when she uses drugs, her situation doesn't seem as bad.

Although the general public may disagree about whether drugs are harmful, the fact remains that using drugs—or at least experimenting with them—is acceptable to many adolescents.

Assessing Drug Abuse How can you determine when drug *use* becomes drug *abuse*? Generally, the adolescent who abuses drugs or alcohol exhibits at least one of these following characteristics:

- The adolescent's performance at school or work increasingly deteriorates.
- The adolescent is frequently caught high or in the act of getting high by parents or other authority figures.

- The adolescent increasingly resorts to alcohol or drugs in times of stress or boredom.
- The adolescent has seriously deficient interpersonal relationships and can relate only when under the influence of drugs or alcohol.
- The adolescent may lose interest in interpersonal relationships altogether, preferring to be high alone rather than to be with others.

Nurses are most effective when they can determine what the particular drug or high does for the client. A boy with a poor self-image and low-esteem may say that it makes him "feel like a man." A particularly shy or introverted girl may say that it makes her "outgoing and friendly." You may discover that being high helps rid disturbed adolescents of angry or depressed feelings. Indeed, in the treatment setting, the client frequently resorts to smoking marijuana or "popping" uppers or downers to escape uncomfortable feelings. Your Assessment Approach highlights some of the behavioral changes that may be observed in adolescents using drugs.

Nursing Diagnosis: NANDA

The use of nursing diagnoses with adolescent clients can lend meaning and substance to the clients' behavior that might be overlooked with a DSM diagnosis alone. For example, look back at Cindy, the 15-year-old girl with a 3-year history of substance abuse. Limiting your assessment to a DSM diagnosis alone might yield a substance use disorder, a cannabis (marijuana) use disorder, or a substance-induced mood disorder. While this tells you something about her drug history, it does not reveal any specifics such as current

YOUR ASSESSMENT APPROACH
Behavioral Changes Associated With Teenage Drug Abuse

- Unexplained periods or reactions of moodiness, depression, anxiety, irritability, oversensitivity, or hostility
- Strongly inappropriate over-reaction to mild criticism or simple requests
- Lessening in warmth toward family; avoids interaction and communication with parents, withdraws from family activities
- Preoccupation with self, less concern for the feelings of others
- Loss of interest in previously important hobbies, sports, activities
- Loss of motivation and enthusiasm (amotivational syndrome)
- Lethargy, lack of energy and vitality
- Loss of ability to self-discipline and assume responsibility
- Need for instant gratification
- Change in values, ideals, beliefs
- Changes in friends, unwillingness to introduce friends
- Secretive phone calls; callers refuse to identify themselves or hang up when someone other than the adolescent answers
- Unexplained absences from home
- Disappearance of money or items of value from home; handling of money becomes secretive
- Desire for increased sensory stimuli

stressors; temperament; or cultural, social, or family dynamics that might contribute to or even underlie her drug abuse.

Specifically, your assessments (and interventions) become more comprehensive and universally informative with an exploration of any or all of the following: Ineffective Coping, Compromised Family Coping, Chronic Low Self-Esteem, and/or Hopelessness. By using the various subsystems provided by nursing diagnoses, you can establish a more comprehensive picture of the client's difficulty and immediately become more goal oriented in assessing and planning care.

In many treatment settings, mental health care professionals are reluctant to give adolescents a DSM diagnosis during these formative years to avoid labeling them (possibly erroneously). Such labeling may result in inadequate treatment, self-fulfilling prophecy, or both, in subsequent mental health care contacts (see also Your Self-Awareness on standardized terminology interfering with individualized client care on page 222 in Chapter 12∞). For a more thorough discussion of DSM diagnoses with psychiatric clients, see Chapter 11∞.

For nurses, the dilemmas described here make the language of nursing diagnosis even more beneficial and user friendly. We can use nursing diagnoses as tools to adequately describe the client's behavior without rigidly adhering to a medically diagnostic label. We can then communicate the adolescent's experience to family, lay personnel, and non–mental health professionals without having to resort to specialized terminology.

Outcome Identification: NOC

Your choice of NOC expected outcomes and NIC interventions will depend primarily on your individualized assessment and the adolescent's stated goals. As a result, your goals and your interventions for the client have depth and are more likely to be effective.

With 15-year-old Cindy, for example, an expected outcome that she will no longer use drugs after discharge might be unrealistic. Expected outcomes that would yield more success, yet demonstrate client improvement, might be one or all of the following:

- Approaches a nurse to discuss temptation to use drugs
- Attends and participates in family meetings
- Verbalizes negative feelings
- Correlates negative feelings with temptation to use drugs
- Demonstrates alternative ways of dealing with stressful situations, such as talking to others, becoming involved in peer group activities, or using "quiet time" in anticipation of family meetings

Successful treatment with adolescents may translate into their use of new skills the vast majority of the time, but not 100% of the time. Adolescents will take some time to "try out" new behaviors and coping mechanisms. It is important to acknowledge that clients may need to take two steps forward and one step backward as progress is made. Moreover, as stressful situations arise, adolescents will be inclined to resort to previous and maladaptive patterns of behavior. In Cindy's situation, she may resist attending a difficult family meeting or may even bolt from the room when confronted with her behaviors or feelings. Either behavior alone does not mean that she is not showing progress or improvement.

Likewise, correlating interventions to support these expected outcomes might include one or all of the following:

- Establish a no-drug contract with the client.
- Adopt a neutral, matter-of-fact attitude when discussing drug usage.
- Encourage the client to seek out a nurse when feeling tempted to use drugs.
- Draw a parallel for the client between drug usage and sad or angry feelings.
- Encourage the client to talk about feelings in individual therapy, group meetings, and family meetings.

Planning and Implementation: NIC

Nurses in numerous roles and diverse settings are in prime positions to recognize and intervene early with pathologic symptoms and behaviors.

Prevention Plans

By preventing certain circumstances in the early stages of life, such as smoking or drug use as coping mechanisms, health improvements are more probable at later stages. The progression from primary prevention (education/self-care) to secondary prevention (early problem recognition and treatment) to tertiary prevention (more complicated and serious forms of illness and risky behaviors) includes services that become increasingly more technologic, expensive, and exclusive.

Establishing a Contract With the Adolescent

Contracts can be particularly useful with adolescents. Adolescents can feel powerless in a treatment setting, especially when referred to treatment by parents or the legal system. Moreover, with this increased sense of involvement in their treatment and control over their own behavior, adolescents become your collaborators in, rather than objects of, your treatment plan.

With most adolescents a written contract is best, for these reasons:

- The goals and expectations are less easily forgotten.
- The process seems more formal and "serious."
- The adolescent has more responsibility as a signee, indicating increased awareness of responsibility and choice of behavior.
- There is less room for misinterpretation and manipulation.

Contracts seem especially helpful in situations of substance abuse, eating disorders, suicidal behavior, and impulsive or manipulative behaviors. Whether verbal or written, the contract can be simply stated to promote clarity, consistency, and cooperation. Here is an example:

- I will not take drugs or bring drugs onto the unit.
- I will not call or accept calls from my drug friends while in the treatment program.

- I will go directly to my outpatient therapy appointment and return immediately to the unit.
- I will not harm myself or others. If I feel like hurting myself, others, or property, I will tell the staff.

If written, the contract is signed by the client, dated, and cosigned by you. The contract is renegotiated at regular intervals (hourly, daily, or weekly), depending on the goals, the severity of the symptoms, and the degree of adherence with the agreement. The form of the contract is less important than the way you and the client jointly set the goals and expectations, carry out the contract, set limits and renegotiate changes, and evaluate the final outcome. Chapter 23∞ discusses and illustrates no-suicide contracts.

Moderating Anger and Hostility

Depending on the degree to which the client is experiencing and expressing anger and hostility, you may choose any of a variety of interventions. These range from observing and assessing the client's behavior to physically restraining someone who is attempting destructive action (see Chapter 35∞).

Choosing an Appropriate Intervention In some situations, a disturbed adolescent's ability to express anger directly to another person can be a sign of success in treatment. The choice of interventions also depends on your own experiences with these feelings, your knowledge and understanding of this client's life experiences with anger, and the external limits imposed by the mental health agency.

Attempt to discover what meaning anger and hostility have for the client by asking the following questions:

- How has this client handled anger in the past?
- Does the client have a history of aggression toward objects or people?
- If so, what were the consequences of this behavior?
- What does this adolescent describe feeling after such a reaction?
- What kinds of things make this client angry? Which of these would be most likely to occur on the unit or in this setting?

This clinical example illustrates a situation in which you might choose to observe and assess rather than intervene in response to a client's anger and hostility.

Clinical Example

Steve had expressed great interest in building a model airplane. He saved up his money and took a long time to choose "just the right one" at the hobby shop. After spending most of the afternoon constructing and painting it, he was interrupted by a phone call from his mother. She told him that she would not be able to attend the family meeting that week, giving a number of reasons. This was the third consecutive week that she had missed a family meeting. Each time, she gave questionable reasons for being unable to attend.

Steve was disappointed and angry. He slammed down the receiver, yelling obscenities in response to the nurse's questions, and ran into his room. There he destroyed the plane by throwing it repeatedly against the floor.

In this example, Steve was not hurting himself or another. Although he did destroy property, the plane belonged to him, and he was free to do with it as he chose. The nurse resisted any impulse to stop Steve from damaging his plane. Because it was of significant value to him, he later regretted having taken out his anger on it. However, the situation provided Steve with an opportunity to explore his actions, and he later asked the nurse why he would destroy something that he valued so much after his mother had disappointed and angered him. The parallel between this situation and hurting himself with drugs right after he had argued with his mother was only too apparent.

Anger Directed Toward the Nurse Incidents in which the nurse bears the brunt of a client's anger or hostility do not offer obvious solutions. Disturbed adolescents may not think twice about addressing a female nurse as "bitch" and coupling such a greeting with a request for a favor. Adolescents direct insults and hostile remarks at nurses for many reasons, most of which have little to do with the nurses as people but a lot to do with nurses as adults or authority figures.

In choosing interventions, consider the meaning behind the client's behavior, your own relationship with this client, your immediate feelings, and the desired result. For example, if the client calls you "bitch" the first time you meet, you may interpret this as a form of testing and may choose to respond immediately with a bewildered look at this unwarranted display of hostility. Later, you may approach the client,

WHY I BECAME A PSYCHIATRIC–MENTAL HEALTH NURSE

Carol Bradley-Corpuel, RN, MS

Like so many new graduates, I wanted "to make a difference" in people's lives and believed that the only way to do that was in the medical–surgical acute care arena. Starting out in the ICU soon after graduation, I was thrust into the thick of things in an ICU multispecialty trauma unit where clients and their families grappled with bleak prognoses and the need to cope with a loved one's new disability. Despite the diverse technical and clinical challenges, collegial relationships, and great on-the-job education, I still felt dissatisfied. Something was missing. I wanted my nursing care to have a greater interpersonal impact than what my meds, IVs, or physical procedures were doing.

I feel truly blessed as a psychiatric–mental health nurse to be able to get to know my clients intimately and to help them to more fully know themselves. I have been afforded opportunities for satisfaction and diverse roles in varied employment settings. Having expertise as a psychiatric–mental health nurse can open doors for you that didn't exist before—in hospitals, private offices, the corporate world, schools, and the community. I encourage you to talk to psychiatric nurses. Conduct an information interview with them to explore their daily challenges and rewards and discover how you can be the best you can be in your professional life.

expressing a naïve curiosity as to the origin of the hostile feelings: "Hey, I don't understand what happened between us a few minutes ago. We just met, and you're calling me a bitch. What's that all about?" This simple question conveys two messages. First, it indicates to the client that you are not accustomed to this kind of salutation. Second, it indicates that you are more interested in the motivation for the remark than in curtailing its use.

If the client resorts to name calling only when angry or under stress, you may decide to ignore the words and deal only with the feelings involved. For example, if a client has angrily left an ongoing family meeting and then calls you a bitch, you can probably assume that the anger is displaced. It is probably a result of overwhelming feelings experienced during the meeting. You may elect simply to say, "I know you're not angry at me right now. It seems like the meeting was pretty heavy, though. Do you want to talk about why you don't want to be in there now?" In neither situation is the name calling intended as a personal affront. However, the way you handle it determines both the outcome of the immediate situation and your chances of furthering your relationship with the client.

Client Reactions The adolescent's reaction to your intervention largely determines its effectiveness. For example, with Steve, the boy who destroyed his plane, the nurse's goal was to help Steve understand the impulsive reaction that destroyed something he loved and to encourage a more appropriate and direct expression of anger at his mother. He was able to do this as well as draw a parallel between anger at his mother and his drug abuse, which hurt himself. If the nurse's goal had been simply to stop the destruction of his property, Steve could have felt even greater anger and frustration, and he might have turned his aggression toward himself, the nurse, or the environment. Certainly if Steve had escalated his destructive behavior, turning his aggression toward himself or others, then direct limit setting, up to and including physical restraints, would have been indicated.

In first-time encounters with any client new to the setting, do not be surprised or dismayed about less-than-optimal success with interventions. It may take some time and trial and error to assess the client's behaviors and choose the most effective interventions.

Moderate Testing and Setting Limits

As young adolescents attempt to adjust to the upheaval in their emotional lives and begin to emancipate themselves from parental figures, a good deal of testing is to be expected. This is normal. However, the meaning that testing holds for the disturbed adolescent is a more complicated matter.

Adolescents who lack early nurturing have difficulty with interpersonal relationships. In many cases, parents were emotionally unable to provide adequate parenting. In other cases, they chose not to impose their values on their children. In either case, the children never developed the internalized values that reduce conflict and avert crisis during adolescence. This causes identity diffusion (the failure to maintain a cohesive self-concept), which in turn results in emptiness, a lack of basic trust, and difficulties with intimacy on any level.

In the treatment setting, these clients test by making limitless and absolute demands. Although these clients often react to imposed limits with cries of injustice, they often really seem to be asking for limits as an indication of caring, as Julie did in the clinical example that follows.

Clinical Example

Julie had been on the unit only 2 days. During that time she had seen several of the older clients run away from the unit, commonly known as "going AWOL," and had witnessed the staff members' attempts to encourage those remaining on the ward to deal with whatever feelings they were experiencing. Toward the end of her second evening, Julie abruptly jumped up from a conversation with a nurse and ran toward the open door. The surprised nurse immediately followed, running down the stairs after her. A smiling Julie was waiting at the bottom step when the nurse arrived, breathless and confused, asking why Julie ran away. Julie quickly answered, "I just wanted to see if you cared enough to come after me."

In this situation, no further action was necessary.

Sometimes the client may use annoying or destructive behavior to test you. At these times, setting firm limits without further interpretation or exploration may be indicated. In other instances, the client may be reacting to some real threat or to an uncomfortable situation.

Clinical Example

Joanne was quietly playing pool by herself when she noticed her therapist talking to a new female client. Joanne's volatile nature gave rise to jealousy and rage, and she began to hit the billiard balls off the table, making a lot of noise and startling everyone around her.

The nurse who had been observing her witnessed the change in her behavior and understood it as a reaction to sharing her therapist's attention with the new client. Without questioning Joanne's apparent anger, she stepped up to the table and challenged her to a game, which Joanne immediately accepted. Because Joanne prided herself on her pool-playing ability, she quickly channeled her energy and competitive feelings into the game and won. She then sought out her therapist and happily announced her victory.

Had the nurse not understood what had triggered Joanne's outburst, she might have become angry with her for making noise and set limits on her privilege to play pool. This would certainly have produced a helpless and even angrier Joanne, whose destructive behavior probably would have escalated. Because of the nurse's perceptive action, Joanne was able to save face by winning at pool and was not forced into a situation that would have made her feel more helpless.

Think about what other interventions might have been equally effective with Joanne. In your relationships with adolescent clients, you might find yourself inclined to respond with myriad, seemingly unrelated, interventions. With a combination of increased clinical experience, a personalized assessment of the adolescent and the immediate situation, and knowledge of current practice studies, you will be most effective in your interventions.

Reducing Scapegoating

Scapegoating—a process by which an individual or group of individuals is identified as different from others and becomes the object of the group's fears, frustrations, or anger—is common in many groups, but particularly in adolescent groups. It occurs in three stages:

1. Frustration generates aggression.
2. The aggression is then displaced onto other people.
3. A process of blaming, projecting, and stereotyping follows. This displaced aggression is rationalized and finally justified, because the identified scapegoat is "different" in some real way.

The members of a group tend to attack the scapegoat because they are afraid to attack the person, group, or institution on whom their feelings are actually focused. Adolescents readily identify peers who are "different" and project on them their own fears and insecurities about their changing images. The client identified as the scapegoat is the object of much teasing and many hostile remarks.

In general, refrain from attempting merely to rescue the scapegoat, because this may augment the other clients' anger and frustration and encourage an escalation of the hostility. Set limits on the behavior and then ask the group to focus on what is going on, to acknowledge the anxiety or other uncomfortable feeling that preceded the scapegoating incident. If possible, anticipate the occurrence of scapegoating in times of stress and try to circumvent the process before it gets out of control.

Also be aware that identified scapegoats share some responsibility for their predicament by presenting themselves to the other clients in a different or provocative stance. In some instances, the scapegoat is accustomed to this role or has an inner need to be punished, and the scapegoat meets the group's urgent need to punish as well. You can be valuable to these clients by helping them explore whatever function this role serves for them.

Reducing Bullying

A discussion of scapegoating would be incomplete without some information on bullying. Teasing and bullying are a major concern among youth. As a child or teenager, you may have been the object or the instigator of such behavior. Prior to the electronic age, such behaviors took the form of verbal taunts or physical challenges and typically were limited to the school or social group setting, events known only to you or perhaps your family or closest circle of friends. Such behaviors were generally perceived by parents and authorities as unfortunate but typical expressions of youthful insecurities and part of growing up. However, in more recent times, with Internet access, the prevalence of cell phones, the advent of online social networks, and the capability of communicating with literally hundreds of others in your peer group with the touch of your computer mouse, the term *bullying* has taken on more dramatic meaning that has sometimes resulted in tragic outcomes.

One National Institutes of Health (NIH) study of 6th through 10th grade students revealed that 20.8% of U.S. adolescents were bullied physically at least once in the last 2 months, 54% were bullied verbally, 51% were bullied socially (excluded or ostracized), and 14% were bullied electronically. Being bullied interferes with scholastic achievement, development of social skills, and general feelings of well-being.

A more contemporary form of bullying, **cyber bullying**, refers to any form of electronic harassment. Cyber bullying is discussed in Developing Cultural Competence.

Because society has become more sophisticated about technology and there are a great number of social media outlets, the opportunity to express emotions electronically is more accessible. Consider the environment of a communicating adolescent. The following experiences are quite common:

- Insecurity
- Inexperience managing strong emotions
- Communication difficulties
- Anger
- Fear of the unknown or unfamiliar
- Anxiety
- Impulsivity
- Hostility and resentment

DEVELOPING CULTURAL COMPETENCE

Cyber Bullying

Cyber bullying may include harassing emails, provocative cell phone messages or images, and aggressive behaviors communicated through online social networks. Notably, victims of cyber bullying reported higher rates of depression than cyber bullies or non–cyber victims. Unlike traditional bullying that usually involves a face–to–face confrontation, cyber victims may not see or identify their harasser and, as a result, may be more likely to feel isolated, dehumanized, or helpless at the time of the attack (Wang et al., 2010). Moreover, according to a national survey commissioned by Care.com, Inc., bullying and cyber bullying have eclipsed kidnapping as the greatest fear parents have regarding their child's safety. Nearly one in three (30%) parents of youth 12 to 17 years of age fear bullying and cyber bullying over kidnapping, domestic terrorism, car accidents, suicide, or any other incident (PRNewswire, 2010). See Partnering With Clients and Families for information that you can use in helping your clients and their parents with incidents of cyber bullying.

CRITICAL THINKING QUESTIONS

1. Why do you need to keep up to date with electronic media issues with adolescents?
2. In what ways would cyber bullying affect the mental health of an adolescent?
3. Are you familiar with recent news items regarding cyber bullying? Why, or why not?

PARTNERING WITH CLIENTS AND FAMILIES

Preventing and Dealing With Cyber Bullying

Encourage parents and their teens to design rules for disclosure as well as rules of privacy and confidentiality with all electronic communications. Teens will be more likely to initiate conversation and engage with their parents if they can take part in the "rules of the game." Visit the websites that your teenager frequents. You may join a social networking site to see firsthand the activities of your teen and the social connections they have made. Know that such technology is not a passing fad. Moreover, many such websites and online activities can be very helpful to the student in obtaining information and in making beneficial connections with peers with similar interests.

Suggest that parents talk regularly with their teen about their online activities. You can offer "what to say" suggestions to the parent that show sensitivity but also convey concern: "I'm aware of stories of cyber bullying. I want to trust you and hope that you will tell me if you are the victim of cyber bullying, stalking, or any other illegal or troublesome online behavior. I will not take away (that technology) if you confide in me a problem that you are having."

Explain to the parent to allow the teen to respond and to take part in a dialog with the parent before rushing to give limits or warnings: "My concern for your safety may over-ride my concern for your privacy and I may need to look at your online communications if I think you are in danger."

With incidents of cyber bullying, you can help teen victims and their parents with the following suggestions:

1. Encourage them to not respond directly to the cyber bully.
2. Do not erase the messages or images. They may be needed by authorities. Save them in a way that avoids subjecting the teen to them again and again.
3. Try to identify the sender. Even if cyber bullies are anonymous, there may be a way to identify them through their internet service provider, website, or cell phone company.

4. If the behavior/threat is criminal, contact your local police and ask them to do the tracking. While laws of states and jurisdictions may vary, in general the following constitute criminal activity:
   a. Obscene or harassing phone calls or text messages
   b. Threats of violence
   c. Harassment, stalking, or hate crimes
   d. Child pornography
   e. Sexual exploitation
   f. Extortion
   g. Taking a photo of someone in a place where the teen expects to have privacy
5. Contact the school. If the cyber bullying is coming through the school's Internet system, the administrators have an obligation to intervene.
6. Even if the behavior is happening off campus, the school authorities may be able to identify and resolve the cyber bullying or at least be watchful for an escalation of the aggressive behavior, as with physical or verbal bullying within the school.
7. Talk with the teen and the family to see if professional counseling is needed to help deal with the stress and upset of cyber bullying. As with traditional forms of bullying, electronic aggression has been associated with emotional distress in general and conduct problems at school. Moreover, depression is a foremost concern for the cyber victim.
8. As a preventive measure or postevent intervention, consider working with parents and school officials to present a class on electronic aggression, develop a zero-tolerance policy for cyber bullying, and encourage a collaborative relationship among all parties.

Once a powerful feeling is felt by an adolescent who does not have competent skills, the path of least resistance is to resolve the situation with the comfortable and easily maneuvered cyberspace option.

Managing Sexual Behaviors

With self-awareness and an understanding of your feelings and attitudes about sexual issues, you can more readily plan interventions to deal with the sexual behaviors of the adolescent client.

Masturbation Masturbation is a normal sexual activity for people of all ages, from the beginning of sexual awareness to senescence. If you have a relatively healthy attitude toward masturbation, you are not likely to run into problems unless the client masturbates in inappropriate places or uses masturbation to express hostility.

You may be confronted with an adolescent boy who fondles his genitals when he is anxious or feels threatened. Understanding his behavior as an indication of anxiety, you may elect to ignore the gesture and explore the nature of his anxiety with him. At other times, the boy may make a masturbatory gesture to convey contempt or hostility. In this case, it would be ludicrous to feign indifference in response.

Your reaction depends on all the previously mentioned factors, such as the nurse–client relationship and the behavior that preceded the gesture. Generally, however, it is wise to comment on the client's gesture—for example, by mentioning it as an attempt to "make me uncomfortable"—and then to allow the client the opportunity to express his feelings verbally. It is unlikely that this intervention will produce a tumultuous outpouring of feeling resulting in immediate resolution. However, it does allow you to acknowledge both the client's and your own feelings, perhaps paving the way for a more appropriate exchange in the future.

Heterosexual Behavior The adolescent often uses sexual behavior as a means of acting out other conflicts and as a testing ground for the nursing staff's feelings and attitudes. The clinical example of Barbara and Laurie illustrates both issues.

Clinical Example

This was the third time Barbara, a nurse, had gone into Laurie's room to check on two clients, Laurie and Bill, who were an identified couple on the unit. Although there was a rule against clients having sexual intercourse with each other, Laurie and Bill had been discovered in the act each evening Barbara was on duty. Barbara found these discoveries disconcerting. She wondered if she was the only staff member who checked on clients, because no one else had reported any sexual activity. She decided to bring up the subject at the next treatment planning meeting to find a more effective way to deal with the situation.

Imagine Barbara's surprise when her peers agreed that Barbara was actually partly responsible for Laurie and Bill's acting out. It seemed that her frequent checking on clients conveyed her expectation that they were "up to something." Barbara acknowledged that she expected that sort of behavior and was quite afraid of discovering Laurie and Bill in the act of intercourse.

The team helped Barbara see that her own expectations were being met. Laurie and Bill were doing exactly what she expected them to do—maybe even wanted them to do. Laurie and Bill were following their scripts of being "bad" and expressing their hostility toward Barbara. When Barbara heard how other staff members spent time with the couple to encourage them in indirect ways to join the larger group activities, she realized how obvious her anxiety and unconscious messages actually were. She then began to question her own attitudes about sexual matters and to explore why she feared discovering the couple engaged in sexual intercourse.

In this example, the client couple used sexual behaviors to act out their own underlying feelings. Had Barbara's assessment been limited to each immediate situation, she would have focused only on the couple's unacceptable behavior and would not have been open to the implications their behavior had for her. By seeking out information and feedback from her peers, she made a discovery about herself and realized it was more effective to anticipate and possibly circumvent such client behaviors than to intervene after the fact. Had Barbara not asked for feedback, the problem would have continued with an increase in the sexual behaviors and in Barbara's frustration. The situation would then have required intervention by an astute supervisor or an empathic colleague.

Homosexual Behavior In situations in which homosexual behavior is an expected developmental step or a lifestyle without expressions of anger or hostility toward parents or staff, little or no intervention may be indicated. As mentioned in the Assessment section, it is as important for the nurse to understand and provide emotional support for the homosexual or bisexual teen as for the heterosexual teen dealing with sexual identity and other developmental issues. Moreover, allow adolescents to decide when, and to whom, to disclose their sexual orientation.

Counseling directed specifically at insisting that the counselor's sexual orientation be the norm, when it is not, may be traumatic and cause lasting harm for an unwilling adolescent. Professionals and laypersons alike can obtain understanding and support from organizations such as Parents, Families, and Friends of Lesbians and Gays (PFLAG, http://www.pflag.org).

The term *metrosexual* is frequently used in young adult references. The term, a combination of the words "metro" meaning *urban* and "sexual," has nothing to do with the man's sexuality as much as his lifestyle choice. The term *metrosexual* refers to the urban lifestyle of a man who typically spends a great deal of time and money on his appearance and lifestyle. While his fastidious grooming, beauty treatments (which can include nail care and facials), and fashionable clothes might stereotypically be identified with a homosexual lifestyle, he is heterosexual. The term was introduced in 1994 by Mark Simpson, a British journalist, who explores male and female roles and lifestyles in his writings and in the popular media (Hagood, 2010).

On the other hand, when homosexual behavior is used to act out feelings of impotence, or aggressive behavior is used to counteract feelings of intimacy, limits must be imposed. Try to anticipate this behavior and provide other ways for the adolescent client to work with the anxiety. As one example, with a male needing to demonstrate his masculinity, perhaps you could organize a game of football or tennis, if he is fairly proficient at these skills, or engage him in some other activity in which he excels. With a female who fears intimate feelings, anticipate and circumvent a similar display of acting out, perhaps with a group activity where intimate or competitive feelings can be channeled in a more socially appropriate way. The point is to re-establish the adolescent's feeling of competence and control. Without these interventions, feelings of impotence will escalate to the point where the client will act them out in a negative way. The client who uses homosexuality to express defiance toward authority figures will flaunt homosexual activities and consistently incur the anger, embarrassment, or both, of staff and clients alike.

Reducing Substance Abuse

You will benefit from self-awareness and an understanding of the feelings that working with substance abusers can evoke. For example, the nurse who feels angry and punitive with the client who abuses drugs, or who overidentifies with the client and finds adventure in the client's drug stories, cannot establish a therapeutic relationship with the client. Feelings of disdain or envy can compromise nursing care and, indeed, may make the client's treatment ineffective. Only by viewing substance abuse as a symptom of a broader illness can you be effective in dealing with adolescents. Cultural and generational factors are important in understanding your client's choice of drug as well. You may wonder why the current teen population had not learned lessons from your generation or previous generations. The wide historical divergence seen in the ongoing Monitoring for the Future studies indicate that there is a phenomenon known as **generational forgetting**. This occurs as a result of older drugs being rediscovered by a newer generation of young people. Such drugs make a comeback from previous years when they fell from popularity because the adverse consequences are unknown or forgotten by the next generation. Such drug examples that were popular in the 1960s and that saw a resurgence in the 1990s were LSD, methamphetamine, heroin, cocaine, and crack (Johnston et al.,

2010). Nurses who have contact with adolescents, especially in school or community settings, should familiarize themselves with the general effects of various drugs and the first aid treatment for each (see Chapter 15∞).

Interventions are determined to be effective or ineffective by the use of subjective and objective behavioral criteria, as described in the outcome identification section on page 592. These criteria should reflect your individualized plan of care and the goals you and the client agreed on. Only then can you expect to see the merits of your professional interventions and reap the rewards that can come from working with this special population.

Evaluation

Evaluating nursing interventions with adolescent clients can be tricky for numerous reasons:

- The adolescent client may need to test the limit one more time following a nursing intervention to avoid appearing "too compliant" or to "save face" with the group.
- Although it is important to set limits, it is equally important to be flexible. To set a limit and immediately "draw the line" with the next infraction is to invite the client to step over that line to test its seriousness.
- This is a slow process. Do not make quick judgments if immediate results are not obtained.
- The behaviors that brought the adolescent to psychiatric treatment will continue long after treatment and nursing interventions have begun. Despite a well-designed nursing care plan and client contract, the adolescent will resort to previous maladaptive ways, immature and impulsive acts, or destructive behaviors in the face of change, particularly if this change represents improvement or growth (such as an increase in privileges or an impending discharge). The nurse who thinks this means that the nursing interventions are not effective may feel hopeless about progress and convey that hopelessness to the client and the rest of the treatment team.
- Using a behavioral contract without understanding the underlying reasons or factors contributing to the adolescent's problems will result in a superficial approach with an equally superficial evaluation.

If the adolescent had the desire or the impulse control simply to "act right" after being given the rules and consequences, then the client would be doing so, and psychiatric treatment would not have been necessary. The adolescent needs the structure and consistency of a nursing care plan and a client contract without the rigidity that can be imposed by a "now or never" behavioral plan with absolute consequences.

You can make a more adequate evaluation if you are aware of the social context and the meaning of the behavior to the adolescent. For example, you may be wrong in determining that an indicator of increased self-esteem for a female client would be to stop dyeing her hair purple. Dyeing one's hair an unusual color may have been an indication of low self-esteem during *your* adolescent years, but for the client in question, that may or may not be the case. For that adolescent client and her peer group, purple hair may be a well-defined status symbol.

CASE MANAGEMENT, COMMUNITY-BASED CARE, AND HOME CARE

Psychiatric–mental health nurses who work with adolescents need to be able to function as case managers and to work in community-based and home care settings. The skills required in these roles include the following:

- Assessing conflicted adolescents and problematic families wherever you encounter them
- Educating faculty, school administrators, and parents about the importance of preventive attention and the resources available to help teens and their families
- Preventing youth violence and drug abuse if possible
- Advocating for home-based therapy models
- Refining skills as an individual, group, and family therapist with adolescents and their families
- Teaching about sensitive health topics such as drug use, STDs, unwanted pregnancy, and the consequences of violence
- Advocating for social policies and programs that help keep families out of poverty, a major risk factor for adolescents

Psychiatric–mental health nurses are most likely to encounter troubled adolescents in community-based settings such as schools, emergency rooms, jails and detention centers, detoxification programs, STD clinics, and other outpatient settings that provide programs for angry, abused, neglected, or otherwise troubled teenagers. Psychiatric–mental health nurses may also encounter adolescents who are experiencing a temporary crisis and are in need of support and counseling while in abortion clinics, group homes, homes for young mothers, and drunk-driver programs. The earlier section in this chapter on psychiatric–mental health nursing roles in outpatient settings addresses in detail the skills you will need to address these client problems.

Of particular interest to psychiatric–mental health nurses who are committed to advocating for troubled and troublesome teens are opportunities to effect change at the state and national level. AACAP has been particularly effective in advocating for youth through postings on its website, also accessible via the Online Student Resources. We know that despite treatment advances and improved early identification, most youth with mental illnesses do not receive treatment. Some of the barriers to treatment include a severe shortage of child/adolescent psychiatrists and psychiatric–mental health nurses, lack of adequate coverage of mental health services within health care systems, lack of research funding, and lack of community mental health services. See the AACAP website for their extensive legislative agenda to help eliminate these barriers: http://www.aacap.org/

On a global scale, youth of all nations should be recognized for the hope they bring to the health and vitality of their countries. The World Health Organization states that child and adolescent mental health is a necessary priority for the healthy development of societies. In particular, child and adolescent mental health is central to the future development of low-income countries throughout the world (WHO, 2010). Developing Cultural Competence details serious challenges faced by youth of other nations, challenges that impact not only low-income countries but North America and other developed countries as well. The accompanying critical thinking questions might challenge you and your clinical peers to be dissatisfied with the status quo in your clinical setting, your neighborhood, or your state.

Discussion among your colleagues might prompt you to make changes to improve the quality of care provided to teens of minority groups or immigrant populations within your local areas in particular. You might want to access numerous WHO publications that are available free online from the WHO library database in numerous languages. One example, The Adolescent Job Aid, is a handy desk reference tool for nurses and other health workers who provide services to teens to help them deal more effectively and with greater sensitivity with their adolescent clients. It contains step-by-step guidance on how to address frequently asked questions and how to deal with more common health concerns such as STDs, pregnancy-related conditions, and mental health concerns. The tool is used in numerous countries and can be downloaded at http://www .who.int/child_adolescent_health/documents/9789241599962

With the promise for change that these innovations bring, community health nurses are in a prime position to play a key role in the movement toward proactive partnerships among schools, families, and the community in enhancing the health and ensuring the future of our nation's youth. Moreover, with an increased appreciation and knowledge of the challenges facing adolescents on a global scale, we can hope to improve the quality of life in our multicultural communities, the mental health of youth throughout the world, and the future of human societies.

DEVELOPING CULTURAL COMPETENCE

Cultural and Societal Obstacles to Displaced and Disenfranchised Youth

In low-income countries, such as sub-Saharan Africa, the health and societal challenges of AIDS orphans, AIDS infected youth, displaced populations of child combatants, reintegrated child soldiers, and youth marginalized because of lack of economic opportunity are all jeopardizing the future of these nations. Furthermore, the voluntary and forced migration from Africa and other parts of the world affected by internal conflict brings to the shores of North America and elsewhere youth who are unable to integrate into these new societies because of mental health and health-related problems (WHO, 2010). Seeking health care from you in your clinical setting may be a daunting challenge for any adolescent for the usual developmental reasons, but for these displaced and disenfranchised youth, cultural and societal reasons pose added obstacles as well. Moreover, the stigma associated with certain medical problems, such as HIV infection and mental health disorders, particularly in ethnic minority groups and/or immigrant populations, cannot be overestimated.

CRITICAL THINKING QUESTIONS

1. How youth friendly is your clinic, office, or other practice setting? Do you have literature available to prompt a discussion with adolescents about awkward or embarrassing topics?
2. What are your attitudes and biases related to teens with a different cultural background from yours?
3. How might the unknown practices or unfamiliar customs of a different race, religion, or ethnic group affect the assessment and care given to a minority member teen at your clinical setting?
4. What actions can you take on your local, regional, or state level that might impact a multicultural teen population?

Pearson Nursing Student Resources
Find additional review materials at
nursing.pearsonhighered.com
Prepare for success with NCLEX®-style practice questions, interactive assignments and activities, web links, animations and videos, and more!

REFERENCES

Alford, S. (2009). *Best practices for youth-friendly clinical services.* Advocates for Youth. Retrieved from http://www.advocatesforyouth.org/index .php?option=com_content&task=blogcategory&id=106&Itemid=336

American Academy of Child and Adolescent Psychiatry. (2010) *Facts for families.* Retrieved from http://www.aacap.org/galleries/FactsForFamilies/

American Cancer Society. (2010). *Cancer facts and figures 2010.* American Cancer Society. Retrieved from http://www.cancer.org/acs/groups/content/ @epidemiologysurveilance/documents/document/acspc-026238.pdf

American Psychiatric Association. (2000). *Diagnostic and statistical manual of mental disorders* (4th ed., Text Revision) (DSM-IV-TR). Washington, DC: Author.

Arnold, P. D., Hanna, G. L., & Rosenberg, D. R. (2010). Imaging the amygdala: Changing the face of gene discovery in child psychiatry. *Journal of the American Academy of Child & Adolescent Psychiatry,* 49(1), 7–0.

Asarnow, J. R., & Albright, A. (2010, October 13). Care management increases the use of primary and medical care services by people with severe mental illness in community mental health settings. *Evidence-Based Nursing, 2010*(4), 128–129.

Centers for Disease Control and Prevention. (2010a). Youth risk behavioral surveillance—United States, 2009. *MMWR, 59* (No. SS-5), 1–142. Retrieved from http://www.cdc.gov/ViolencePrevention/pdf/yv-datasheet-a.pdf

Centers for Disease Control and Prevention. (2010b). *Youth violence: Electronic media and youth violence—A CDC issue brief for educators and caregivers.* Retrieved from http://www.cdc.gov/violenceprevention/youthviolence/electronicaggression/index.html

Champion, J. D., & Collins, J. L. (2010). The path to intervention: Community partnerships and development of a cognitive behavioral intervention for ethnic minority adolescent females. *Issues in Mental Health Nursing, 31*(11), 739–747. Retrieved from http://informahealthcare.com/doi/abs/10.3109/01612840.2010.512697

Frodl, T. (2010). Childhood stress, serotonin transporter gene and brain structures in major depression. *Neuropsychopharmacology, 35*(6), 1383–1390.

Hagood, C. (2010, April 13). Wo-metrosexuality and the city: My chat with Mark Simpson. *Huffington Post.* Retrieved from http://www.huffingtonpost.com/caroline-hagood/metrosexuality-and-the-ci_b_535333.html

Johnston, L. D., O'Malley, P. M., Bachman, J. G., & Schulenberg, J. E. (2010). *Monitoring the future, a continuing study of American youth. National results on adolescent drug use: Overview of key findings, 2009* (NIH Publication No. 10-7583). Bethesda, MD: National Institute on Drug Abuse.

Kurtz, B. (2011). Adolescent mental health disorders. In M. A. Goldstein (Ed.), *The Massachusetts General Hospital for children adolescent medicine handbook* (pp. 167–188). Massachusetts: Springer Science. Retrieved from http://www.springerlink.com/content/thn3622634205311/

Macgowan, M. J., & Engle, B. (2010). Evidence for optimism: Behavior therapies and motivational interviewing in adolescent substance abuse treatment. *Child and Adolescent Psychiatric Clinics of North America, 19*(3), 527–545.

Merikangas, K. R., He, J., Burstein, M., Swanson, S. A., Avenevoli, S., Cui, L., . . . Swendsen, J. (2010). Lifetime prevalence of mental disorders in U.S. adolescents: Results from the National Comorbidity Survey Replication–Adolescent Supplement (NCS-A). *Journal of the American Academy of Child and Adolescent Psychiatry, 49*(10), 980–989.

Morrato, E. H., Nicol, G. E., Maahs, D., Druss, B. G., Hartung, D. M., Valuck, R. J., . . . Newcomer, J. (2010). Metabolic screening in children receiving antipsychotic drug treatment. *Archives of Pediatric and Adolescent Medicine, 164*(4), 344–351.

Naylor, E. V., Antonuccio, D. O., Litt, M., Johnson, G. E., Spogen, D. R., Williams, R., . . . Higgins, D. L. (2010). Bibliotherapy as a treatment for depression in primary care. *Journal of Clinical Psychology in Medical Settings, 17*(3), 258–271. Retrieved from http://www.springerlink.com/content/93qr8335907n37k5/

Ogden, C. L., Carroll, M. D., Curtin, L. R., Lamb, M. M., & Flegal, K. M. (2010). Prevalence of high body mass index in U.S. children and adolescents, 2007–2008. *Journal of the American Medical Association, 303*(3), 242–249.

PRNewswire. (2010, October 20). *New study finds bullying and cyber bullying are parents' #1 fear more than kidnapping, domestic terrorism and suicide.* PR Newswire for Journalists. Retrieved from http://www.prnewswire.com/news-releases/new-study-finds-bullying-and-cyberbullying-are-parents-1-fear-more-than-kidnapping-domestic-terrorism-and-suicide-105335413.html

Rutherford, H. J. V., Mayes, L. C., & Potenza, M. N. (2010). Neurobiology of adolescent substance use disorders: Implications for prevention and treatment. *Child and Adolescent Psychiatric Clinics of North America, 19*(3), 479–492. Retrieved from http://www.ncbi.nlm.nih.gov/pubmed/20682216

U.S. Department of Health and Human Services. (2010) *Healthy people 2020.* Rockville, MD: Office of Disease Prevention and Health Promotion. Retrieved from http://www.healthypeople.gov/hp2020/Objectives/TopicArea.aspx?id=11&TopicArea=Adolescent+Health

Wang, J., Nansel, T. R., & Iannotti, R. J. (2010, September 22) Cyber and traditional bullying: Differential association with depression. *Journal of Adolescent Health Online.* Retrieved from http://www.jahonline.org/article/S1054-139X(10)00343-5/pdf

World Health Organization. (2010, August). Media Centre/Fact Sheets. *Young people: Health risks and solutions.* Fact Sheet #345. Retrieved from http://www.who.int/mediacentre/factsheets/fs345/en/index.html

Yancey, A. K., Grant, D., Kurosky, S., Kravitz-Wirtz, N., & Mistry, R. (2010, August 26). Role modeling, risk, and resilience in California adolescents. *Journal of Adolescent Health Online.* Retrieved from http://www.jahonline.org/article/S1054-139X(10)00227-2/fulltext

Elders

EILEEN TRIGOBOFF

27

LEARNING OUTCOMES

After completing this chapter, you will be able to:

1. Identify the age-related demographic projections that have implications for planning future mental health services for elders.
2. Discuss the major theories of aging and the ideas associated with each one.
3. Differentiate the normal physical and psychosocial changes that accompany aging from mental disorders affecting elders.
4. Synthesize the key components of a biopsychosocial assessment into the plan of care for an older client.
5. Develop treatment plans including reminiscence therapy, life review, reality orientation, and socialization enhancement for elders.
6. Incorporate available community support programs such as adult day care, restorative programs, and assisted living for elders and their families into your plan of care.
7. Analyze personal biases, feelings, and attitudes that may be experienced in professional practice when caring for elders who suffer from mental disorders.

CRITICAL THINKING CHALLENGE

A recently retired 65-year-old man is brought to your clinic by his wife, who states he "just sits around all day watching TV and won't do anything." She tells you that he had a very active career and loved it. He also played golf or spent time in his garden on the weekends. She reveals that he has changed considerably in that he now seems unable to concentrate and has become bitter and difficult. Upon interviewing the client, you find that he had been a successful owner of a small hardware store with his younger brother, who recently died of a heart attack while working at the store. Your client retired from the business soon thereafter at his family's insistence. He goes on to tell you that his memory is impaired, he has difficulty sleeping, and he has lost his robust appetite. You would like to gather further data, including assessing his grieving skills (for his younger brother, for his career, for confidence in his own longevity), and assessing for depression and dementia.

1. What areas of his functioning and interactions with others are important to assess?
2. How would you determine whether physical problems contribute to his symptoms?

The population of elders is growing in every nation. Improvements in health care, preventive medicine, and overall longevity have increased the numbers of people living to older and older ages. Also, the population explosion that took place in many countries in the mid-20th century is visible in the sheer numbers of people entering the stage we call being an elder. Estimates for the world population are that by the year 2050 people over 85 years of age will continue to increase dramatically, especially in North America, China, and India.

With this booming section of the population, the term "elderly" or even "geriatric"—meaning those over the age of 65—is insufficient to discuss a group of people whose ages may span four decades. The descriptive terms used to specifically group elders into relevant age categories include *young-old* (65 to 74), *middle-old* (75 to 84), and *old-old* (85 and older).

The norm is that elders live independently with healthy lifestyles and satisfying experiences for all of their lives. As a consequence of improved pharmacologic and other treatments, individuals affected by dementia and mood disorders (once associated with decreased longevity) will experience a relatively normal life span. An unprecedented growth in the number of elders with chronic mental illness will have a significant impact on the need for quality geropsychiatric care. **Geropsychiatry** is the treatment of psychiatric problems in elders. At the same time, family caregivers, who themselves are aging, will also strain geropsychiatric care resources. You can access nursing care information for elders who do not have psychiatric issues in fundamentals and geriatrics nursing resources.

It is important to examine the age distribution of the over-65 population carefully. Grouping elders into an aggregate of all persons over the age of 65 tends to blur important distinctions. The old-old group tends to have the greatest incidences of depression, delirium, dementia, and other chronic disabling conditions (Mackenzie, Reynolds, Chou, Pagura, & Sareen, 2011; Unverzagt et al., 2011). The frail elders who consume many health care resources and maintenance services constitute only 5% of the over-65 population. A large proportion of healthy elders, particularly single older women (who outnumber single older men by 2.5 to 1), will benefit most from supportive psychosocial services often provided by psychiatric–mental health nurses.

Anticipating the varied mental health needs of a growing population of aging "baby boomers" is important for program planning and funding allocation. The data clearly underscore a need for an increased number of health professionals who recognize that elders have multiple needs. Nursing's role in psychogerontology and in geriatrics is expanding as the needs and real numbers of elders increase (Berlau, Corrada, Peltz, & Kawas, 2011; Brooks, 2011). **Psychogerontology** is a subspecialty within gerontology that studies the psychosocial needs of elders.

The aim of this chapter is to provide a comprehensive discussion of health promotion and advocacy for elders

with mental health needs. Contemporary issues including end-of-life care, restorative programs, and community-based support are also addressed. We do not discuss the nursing care of elders with cognitive disorders in this chapter. Refer to Chapter 14 for nursing care strategies for cognitively impaired elders. Only a small percentage of elders have physical or mental health issues. This chapter will focus on that small percentage of elders who have psychiatric–mental health problems.

ROADBLOCKS TO MENTAL HEALTH SERVICES FOR ELDERS

Elders are the most underserved population in need of supportive and tertiary mental health care. This discussion highlights four roadblocks to mental health care services—ageism, myths, stigma, and health care financing—and examines the demographic realities that compel us to break through these disabling roadblocks through self-awareness, health promotion, and client advocacy (see FIGURE 27-1 ■).

Ageism

A primary roadblock to adequate mental health services for elders is ageism—prejudice against people because they are old. In many contemporary Western cultures, aging is often viewed with disdain, dislike, and trepidation. Elders are criticized for being unattractive, incompetent, socially irrelevant, and unhealthy. Nunney, Raynor, Knapp, and Closs (2011) found a paternalistic attitude among health care providers who assumed elders would not be able to understand and function as well as younger people. That type of ageism marginalizes and dehumanizes elders, and has the potential to undermine selfhood and self-worth. Ageism stems from the belief that elders present a financial and emotional drain on the family and society. Ageism results from our fears of facing our own aging process and mortality. Ageist attitudes can be internalized by elders, causing decreased self-worth and self-esteem, whatever the source.

When caring for elder clients, be aware of their feelings and your own. Your personal biases can influence your clinical assessment and your decisions about interventions. You can provide invaluable support, insight, and feedback to colleagues who are working with elders. Consider using Your Self-Awareness as a discussion point. We know that elders are as responsive to mental health services as are members of any other age group (Lysack, Lichtenberg, & Schneider, 2011). By modeling positive attitudes toward aging and by advocating quality of life and health care for elders in all settings and at all levels of function, you can help dispel ageist influences. See FIGURE 27-2 ■ for a photograph of an elder and the supportive, candid, and loving comments her family made about her.

Myths

Mental health care professionals and elders themselves often equate growing old with growing sad, lonely, disengaged, inactive, socially isolated, and dependent. Such myths all too often inhibit people from seeking treatment for feelings

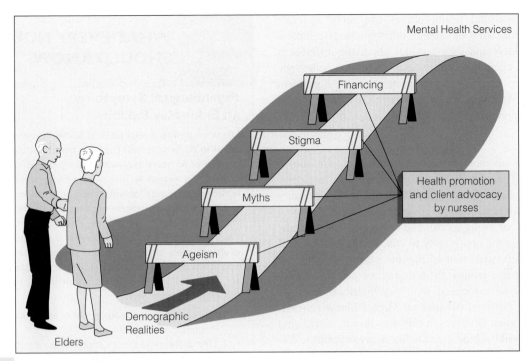

FIGURE 27-1 ■ Roadblocks to mental health services for elders.

and behaviors that they believe are a normal part of aging. Misled by these myths, health professionals can be less inclined to refer elders for mental health services. We know that advancing age does not condemn an individual to senility, social isolation, loneliness, or dependence. Most elders live independently and contentedly—well into late life—unless they can no longer drive and live alone, live in rural areas without transportation, or live in urban areas with limited access to health care resources.

YOUR SELF-AWARENESS
Attitudes Toward Aging

A bias against elders because of their age can result in discrimination against them even by mental health professionals. Ask yourself the following questions and discuss your responses with other students, faculty, or colleagues.

1. Am I uncomfortable around people who are old, infirm, or confused?
2. Do I have positive role models for aging with grace?
3. Do I dread growing old myself?
4. Should elders be encouraged to do as much as possible for themselves or be cared for by others?
5. How do I feel about old people who are sexually active and insist on trying to look and act young?
6. What are my specific ideas about how elders should look and act?
7. Do most elders become rigid and set in their ways once they age?
8. Am I well informed about the differences between mental disorder in elders and the normal aging process?
9. Do I equate advanced age with unattractiveness, incompetence, and senility?
10. Am I well informed about community resources and support systems available for elders and their family caregivers?
11. How do I feel when caring for an elderly person who is demanding and dependent?

Reflecting on questions such as these can promote your awareness of attitudes that might interfere with quality care for elders.

FIGURE 27-2 ■ In the eyes of her family and friends, this was a woman worthy of respect and admiration. She was "strong willed" and "the epitome of aging with style and grace." "She had a sense of humor, kept moving, spent 96 years living a full life rather than 50 years preparing to die, and enjoyed it to the last." "She was her own person, no matter what."
Photo courtesy © Dr. Eileen Trigoboff

Psychiatric–mental health nurses can serve as elder advocates by educating the public, other health care professionals, and elders and their families about the differences etween normal aging and changes associated with pathologic conditions. Recognizing that aging itself is not a problem increases the likelihood that problems that do arise will be assessed and appropriately treated (Mezey & Mitty, 2011).

Stigma

Despite recent advances in mental health care, the stigma associated with mental illness remains very real to elderly people. Elders may not seek mental health services as readily as they should and may hide their psychic pain for fear of being labeled "crazy" or losing control and being institutionalized.

Nurses have the opportunity to educate the public about mental disorders and state-of-the-art treatments that are available to all age groups. In so doing, we can help to decrease the stigma associated with psychiatric illness and treatment. The National Alliance on Mental Illness (NAMI) has made important advances in this direction by circulating information about the biologic basis for many psychiatric disorders. You can refer elders who feel reluctant about acknowledging a psychiatric problem to the NAMI website at http://www.nami.org, which can be accessed through a resource link on the Online Student Resources for this text.

As people learn more about research that confirms brain mechanisms associated with psychiatric disorders, traditional stigma associated with seeking mental health services is likely to decrease. At the present time, however, the primary care provider for many mentally ill elders is their family physician or adult nurse practitioner.

Elders are seen by their general health care providers, surgeons, specialists for chronic illnesses such as arthritis or diabetes, and in clinics where they receive medications and have laboratory tests evaluated on a regular basis. Because of the likelihood that they will need specialized care, nurses specializing in a variety of settings need specific information about elders. What Every Nurse Should Know has information that is useful for nurses, especially those in rehabilitation services.

Health Care Financing

Financial barriers, physical disability, and transportation problems are some factors that limit access to services, especially elders diagnosed with mental disorders. The financial barriers are particularly serious. Medicare, the major form of health care financing for elders, covers only a portion of the costs for its beneficiaries. Long-term care coverage and coverage for chronic conditions are sorely lacking.

Medicare initiated its Part D program to address the costs of pharmaceutical management of health care problems. Expensive prescription medication plans and large copayments for services reimbursed through Medicare add to an older person's psychosocial stressors. Although Medicare Part D provides options for elders in an effort to minimize costs and maximize treatment adherence, the program is

WHAT EVERY NURSE SHOULD KNOW

Psychological Symptoms an Elder May Exhibit

Imagine you are a rehabilitation nurse. A rehabilitation nurse needs to be familiar with the likely symptoms that people over the age of 65 years may exhibit when placed in rehabilitation centers. The reason for the placement—poststroke care, joint replacement, respite for family members, recovery from a fall—can direct you to anticipate what is likely to occur emotionally with the individual. Each of these events carries meaning for an elder that would not apply to someone younger. Stress, being in an unfamiliar environment, and struggling to adapt to body and emotional changes take a larger toll on older adults. There are three reasons rehabilitation nurses should be familiar with the following symptoms:

1. These symptoms could be part of an emotional response requiring treatment.
2. The presence of these symptoms can distort or mask symptoms of physical illnesses.
3. Severe psychiatric distress can impair healing from medical and surgical procedures and injuries.

When a rehabilitation client has symptoms that appear to be behavioral or psychiatric, be prepared and able to document, classify, and report these symptoms correctly so that the client receives necessary treatment. Knowing the proper interventions, pharmacologic and nonpharmacologic, can speed stabilization and improve the quality of life your clients experience.

difficult to understand. Working through the many options can be daunting, and high costs are still very likely.

Community and home-based care for elders is limited at best, and Medicare does not cover many mental health services. Few practitioners across the nation specialize in ongoing psychotherapy for the elderly. As baby boomers reach old age and require long-term care services, these gaps and lack of coverage will reach crisis levels unless service needs are addressed and resolved. For mentally ill elders, the crisis is even more acute as long-term care facilities selectively admit identified geropsychiatric clients. It is important for us to become active voices in lobbying for policy changes to improve financing for elder care that covers the broad range of acute and chronic illnesses. The American Association of Retired Persons (AARP) is an excellent source of information related to these topics. The AARP website, http://www.aarp.org, can be found through a resource link on the Online Student Resources for this text.

BIOPSYCHOSOCIAL THEORIES OF AGING

Distinguishing between changes associated with aging and mental disorder in later life is a challenge. Many variables affect mental health as a person ages. Not all theories identified here have been fully confirmed through systematic research, and some, such as the disengagement theory, remain controversial.

Biologic Theories

Biologic theories of aging include genetic, wear-and-tear, immunology, nutritional, and environmental theories.

Genetic Theory

Throughout the Human Genome Project (initiated in 1990) of the Department of Energy and the National Institutes of Health, which aimed to map and sequence the human genome in its entirety, definitions of health, illness, and healthy aging have been transformed by knowledge of genetics (Barzilai & Gabrieli, 2010). According to genetic theories, aging is a process that operates over time to alter cellular structures. Harmful genes activate in late life to stop cell growth and division. This theory supports the idea that the life span is predetermined and people's aging experience is programmed by their genetic makeup. To learn more about this, you can access the website of the National Coalition for Health Professional Education in Genetics (http://www.nchpeg.org), initiated by the American Nurses Association, the American Medical Association, and the National Human Genome Research Institute, can be accessed through this text's Online Student Resources.

Wear-and-Tear Theory

The wear-and-tear theory proposes that the accumulation of waste products from metabolism damages DNA synthesis, leading eventually to organ malfunction. In short, cells wear out. Even though the theory allows for individual rates of cell decline that can be accelerated from abuse and slowed by care, the emphasis is one of loss and decline in later life.

Immunology Theory

The immunology theory explains age-related decline in the immune system. As a person ages, his or her ability to defend against foreign organisms declines, with a corresponding increase in susceptibility to diseases, including cancer and serious infections. Theorists suggest that the changes that take place with aging allow the body to misidentify old, irregular cells as foreign bodies and then attack these cells (Barzilai & Gabrieli, 2010). Multiple neurochemical and viral theories are being developed as cellular research advances. For example, free radical theory posits that free radicals cause the damage to cell membranes as one ages.

Nutritional Theory

Nutritional theory focuses on the idea that diet affects how one ages. The quality of one's diet (amounts of vitamin D, fresh fruits, and vegetables especially) is as important as the quantity because vitamin and nutrient deficiencies or excesses have an influence on disease processes. How an older body metabolizes nutrients is also a theoretical issue. For example, there may be more than enough vitamin D in a meal, but if an elder cannot fully metabolize it, calculations of the actual amount of vitamin D that are bioavailable to that individual would need to be revised.

Environmental Theory

A number of environmental factors are known to threaten health and may be associated with aging. The ingestion of lead, arsenic, pesticides, and other substances can seriously harm the body, as does smoking, exposure to secondhand smoke, and air pollution. Environmental factors such as crowded living conditions and high levels of noise are known to be stressful and do drain a person's coping capacity (Volkers & Scherder, 2011). An elder's primary activities can also be an indication of health status or a threat to health; for example, sedentary TV watching contributes to metabolic syndrome in elders. All these factors can affect one's vulnerability or vigor while aging.

Psychosocial Theories

Psychosocial theories of aging include the activity and disengagement theories, which contrast sharply with each other.

Activity Theory

The activity theory proposes that the way to age successfully is to stay active and involved. Exercise and social interaction are believed to contribute to mental health and satisfaction in late life. Participation in regular exercise programs (both aerobic and strength training) contributes to healthy aging and could play a role in preventing or reducing functional decline in elders (Lobo, Carvalho, & Santos, 2011). Consequently, elders are encouraged to remain as active as possible for as long as possible. A number of consumer products, including computer and card-based activities, have been developed to encourage motor activity and mental activity contributing to successful aging. Evidence-Based Practice discusses types and timing of activities. Elders in assisted living facilities benefit from the newer video games—especially bowling, tennis, and interactive World War II games. They are often inspired by video documentaries of elders surfing in Hawaii, ballroom dancing, and traveling in elder hostel groups.

Disengagement Theory

Disengagement theory is quite the opposite of activity theory. First proposed in the 1960s, the disengagement theory described what was considered an inevitable process in which elders willingly withdrew from social contact and responsibilities, relieved to turn matters over to the younger generation. This theory has become controversial because many older adults continue to be engaged and responsible well into later life unless limited by immobility, which can lead to involuntary social isolation. Recent research discusses the negative impact of apathy on elder health and wellness (Adams, Roberts, & Cole, 2011) and emphasizes the need for continued mental activity in order to sustain health throughout the life span. See the section on restorative care later in this chapter.

EVIDENCE-BASED PRACTICE

Staying Active and Involved While in an Elder Care Program

Doris is 92 years old, lives in her own home, and attends a geriatric care program during the day. Her family is very close to her and wants to make sure that Doris remains active enough to keep her mind and her body in the best possible form.

The program in which Doris is involved includes traditional activities as well as access to technologic tools. Members of the center are encouraged to use all the technology to make their lives better through communication, education, and physical activity. The geriatric day program staff are sensitive and realize that while some elders are technologically sophisticated, others find technology frustrating and avoid it. Nursing staff are trained to be technologically competent and to educate others to become more technologically proficient. The following study noted that, importantly, techno-savvy elders can maintain and achieve health and well-being (associated with bodily comfort, social networks, self-efficacy, and intellectual life) in and beyond their homes. You should base action on more than one study, but for this training program, the following research evidence was helpful.

Loe, M. (2010). Doing it my way: Old women, technology and wellbeing. *Sociology of Health & Illness, 32*(2), 319–334.

CRITICAL THINKING QUESTIONS

1. You have most probably used technology since you were a child. Elders have not. What are the implications of these generational differences?
2. What other evidence would you need to review before designing an intervention for Doris?

PSYCHIATRIC DISORDERS IN ELDERS

Ageist attitudes in our culture account for some of the misconceptions about the prevalence of mental disorders among elders. Older people are believed to be more prone to mental illness than are young people. For several reasons, however, it is difficult to obtain exact incidence and prevalence rates for mental disorders in later life. Elders are often difficult to reach with community-wide surveys, some are reluctant to respond to personal questions that deal with emotional problems, and most either do not seek treatment for emotional problems or consult primary care providers rather than psychiatric professionals.

When physical deterioration becomes a significant feature of an elder's life, the risk of co-morbid psychiatric illness rises. Social isolation and financial burdens are additional common difficulties elders experience. The sequelae of these social and physical pressures can evolve into symptoms of a psychiatric nature, to the extent that psychiatric diagnoses are not unusual. Results of lifetime prevalence indicate that psychiatric disorders and mental health problems such as eating disorders, depressive symptoms, and psychosocial stress are public health concerns for this population.

Symptoms of mental illness in the older population often differ from those in other age groups. While the Diagnostic and Statistical Manual (DSM; American Psychiatric Association [APA], 2000) has enhanced our ability to make valid and reliable diagnoses of mental disorders, there are few age-specific categories. Thus, despite the DSM's detailed descriptions of each category, clinicians and researchers continue to have difficulty applying the written descriptions of symptoms to older adults.

Dementia

Dementia is one of the more common psychiatric–mental health problems experienced by elders. It is an umbrella term covering the vast variety of cognitive impairments that interfere with memory and function. The most common is dementia of the Alzheimer's type (DAT); however, vascular dementia and dementia with Lewy bodies (DLB) are also quite common. Functional difficulties range from minor (such as not being able to do simple math) to extreme (such as the loss of ability to conduct basic hygiene). See Chapter 14∞ for details about cognitive disorders.

Mood Disorders

Mood disorders are primarily characterized by disturbed affect or emotional experience. When they occur in elders they may present as:

- Sustained elation and hyperactivity, such as in a manic episode
- Changes from elation to depression, such as in bipolar disorder
- Pervasive depressed mood not accompanied by mania, such as in major depression

Depression is the most preventable and most treatable mental disorder in later life.

Depression in Elders

Depression among elders is widespread in general practice and even higher in hospitals and nursing homes. Depression robs the person of later-life satisfaction, inhibits ego integrity, and may substantially decrease life expectancy. Elders have the highest rate of suicide of any age group and a range of physical disturbances intensified by depression (Lapierre et al., 2011).

Although the signs and symptoms of depression are relatively consistent throughout the life span, certain characteristics of depression are particular to elders. It is crucial for clinicians to remember that depression in older adults that responds well to treatment may appear with cognitive changes similar to those that accompany other organically based, irreversible disorders. Loss of executive function (often a diagnostic clue to dementia) includes disturbances in planning, sequencing, organizing, and abstracting. Such cognitive impairment can also be a sign of depression.

In addition to cognitive changes, another sign of depression in older adults is an excessive preoccupation with physical symptoms known as *somatization*. Expressing discomfort through the body may be more familiar and comfortable than recognizing and describing psychic pain. Such is the case in the following example.

Clinical Example

Mr. Gambino, a 79-year-old widower, came to his physician's office complaining of "not feeling well." After a physical examination, the doctor told Mr. Gambino that he had a weight loss of 10 pounds, mild chronic obstructive pulmonary disease (COPD), and slight hypertension, but was otherwise in good health for his age. Mr. Gambino responded angrily, "I know I'm dying but it doesn't matter because I have nothing to live for now that my wife is dead. She's been gone for 6 months and everyone says I should be feeling better, but I feel worse! I can't eat, can't sleep, and I don't have enough energy to even wash my car!" Mr. Gambino says he is tired all day but cannot sleep at night. "I'm up at 3:00 a.m. and can't go back to sleep." He says he tries to eat but does not cook well and "the food just doesn't taste right."

Clearly, Mr. Gambino has a number of physical complaints that may shift the focus away from distressing emotions to more acceptable medical conditions that are less stigmatizing. Other possible somatic signs of depression to watch for include:

- Chronic constipation
- Muscular pain
- Chest tightness
- Headaches
- Difficulty breathing
- Chronic gastrointestinal upset

It is important to be persistent and perceptive in looking for signs of depression. Depressed, apathetic elders may believe they are supposed to feel blue and "down in the dumps" as they age. We need to educate them and their families about depression as a pathologic condition often caused by biochemical imbalances that can be corrected. Interventions for depression in older adults should be instituted as aggressively and comprehensively as they are with any other age group.

Depressive symptoms may also result from social and economic circumstances such as social isolation and neglect. They may be the result of an acute or chronic medical condition such as a stroke, Parkinson's disease, or even a hip fracture. Consequently, it is imperative to include a comprehensive geriatric assessment of elders before beginning a treatment regimen. An older person's response to traumatic events may be tied to functional disability and requires multiple areas of intervention.

Suicide Among Elders

Data from nearly all industrialized countries report that suicide rates rise progressively with age. People aged 65 and older comprise about 13% of the U.S. population; however, they account for over 18% of all suicides (Suicide.org, 2011).

Compared with the general population, suicide attempts are more lethal and approached with a greater degree of premeditation and planning when made by elders. Older adults who are at greater suicide risk include:

- Men
- Widowed or divorced people
- Caucasians
- Those of lower socioeconomic status
- Those with chronic pain and terminal illness
- Alcoholics
- Those with mental disorders
- Those with neurologic deficits due to stroke and brain injury
- Those who fear becoming a burden

Suicidal elders have been known to seek help in the emergency department, often for a vague nonspecific physical problem, prior to their self-destructive act. Accurate assessment of suicide potential requires active listening and direct questioning and attending to anxious depression as a particular risk factor (Seo et al., 2011). Assess a suicidal elder when any of the following are present:

- Verbal cues ("I'm going to end it all;" "Life is not worth living;" "I won't be around much longer;" "I won't be here for the next holiday.")
- Behavioral cues (completing a will, making funeral plans, acting out, withdrawing, somatic complaints)
- Situational cues (a recent move, loss of a loved one, the diagnosis of a terminal illness)

For detailed information on suicide and the assessment of suicide potential, including a lethality assessment, see Chapter 23∞.

Schizophrenia

The number and proportion of elders with schizophrenia will increase considerably with the movement of baby boomers into this population group over the next 30 years. This generation of people with chronic mental illness has not spent years in institutions as the mentally ill elders of past generations did. There is limited research on late-life schizophrenia and less on its treatment. This population of clients poses a particularly critical issue—85% of older individuals with schizophrenia live in the community and are approaching the age when long-term care may become necessary. At the same time, nursing homes are severely restricting admission of psychiatric clients.

An individual with *late-life schizophrenia* may be a psychotic person who has grown old or may be a person who did not experience psychotic symptoms until late in life. People with late-onset schizophrenia are often women with less severe negative symptoms, better premorbid functioning in early adulthood, and less impairment in the areas of learning, abstraction, and cognitive flexibility. They also require smaller doses of neuroleptic medication to manage their psychotic symptoms.

Adjustment Disorders

Elders often experience dramatic life changes because of losses due to death, relocation, dependence, loss of autonomy,

Case Study: Late-Life Schizophrenia

retirement, illness, and financial stress. One or a combination of life changes and losses may contribute to the development of an *adjustment disorder*. The essential feature of adjustment disorders is a maladaptive reaction to an identifiable psychosocial stressor or stressors that occurs within 3 months after the onset of the stressor and has persisted for no longer than 6 months (APA, 2000). Mental Health in the Movies discusses a movie about life changes within and between generations. People experiencing adjustment disorders may have a variety of psychiatric symptoms, including the following:

- Anxious mood
- Depressed mood
- Mixed emotional features
- Physical complaints
- Withdrawal

Talk therapies can be enormously successful in the treatment of persons with adjustment disorders.

Anxiety Disorders

Anxiety is common across age groups and increases in frequency with advancing age (Seo et al., 2011). Adjustments to physical, emotional, and socioeconomic changes add to the variety of causes for anxiety. Anxiety reactions in the aging individual may manifest themselves as somatic complaints, rigid thinking and behavior, insomnia, fatigue, hostility, restlessness, confusion, and increased dependence. Physiological indicators of anxiety include increased blood pressure, pulse, respirations, psychomotor restlessness, and frequent voiding. Many of these manifestations are present in the following clinical example.

Clinical Example

Mrs. Pyun, age 82, was rushed to the emergency department by her bridge group with what they think might be a heart attack. She is short of breath and sweating, her pulse is rapid, her hands are shaking, and she cannot sit still during the assessment. She is tearful and cannot tell the triage nurse what is wrong. Mrs. Pyun says, "I don't know why I feel this way. I just know something bad is going to happen. I have to leave and get home. Why are you asking me all these questions? No, I don't have chest pain. I tried to tell them I was just nervous. I get this way sometimes."

Unfortunately, anxiety disorders and panic attacks are often overlooked in elders because, as with depression, these clients have a predominance of physical complaints that mask the underlying disorder. In addition, anxiety in older people often co-occurs with depression. The anxiety is treated but the depression persists, leading to a cycle of anxiety–depression and physical illness.

Delusional Disorders

Delusions in elders are considered a cognitive mechanism for maintaining a sense of power and control. The delusions may be comforting ("I know I'm being guarded by an angel from God") or threatening ("The UPS driver has reported me to Homeland Security because he thinks I am a terrorist"), but whatever the content, they customarily form a structure for understanding a situation that otherwise seems unmanageable. Delusions may also result from internalized ageist attitudes, sensory losses (particularly hearing impairment), and social isolation, as in the following clinical example.

Clinical Example

Ms. Colgán is an 88-year-old woman living alone in a rural suburb of Calgary, Canada. Her cottage is on a country road with few neighbors nearby, and the long winters have kept her indoors and isolated. A sister who has financial power of attorney pays her bills, and she primarily eats canned soups that she heats herself. Ms. Colgán rarely wears her hearing aids and spends most of her time watching TV with the sound turned up to the highest volume. Recently, she called her sister demanding to know "what all these people are doing in my house." She believed people were there to take her money and poison her food. After a careful assessment by the community mental health nurse, it became clear that Ms. Colgán was mistaking the actors on TV for people in her home.

The delusions of elders are often associated with delirium, depression, dementia, or anxiety disorders.

Persecutory delusions involve the belief that one is under investigation, being harassed, or at the mercy of some powerful force. Persecutory delusions may be a response to an older person's diminishing sense of self-mastery. Delusions involving suspiciousness and persecutory ideation are among the most unsettling for elders' caregivers and families. As older

MENTAL HEALTH IN THE MOVIES
The Joy Luck Club

Every week, four older women, all Chinese immigrants, meet to tell stories, play mahjong, and eat. The film reveals their hidden pasts—their brutal lives in feudal China. It is an exploration of the cultural conflict between the women and their daughters, how the mothers' experiences in pre-Revolutionary China continue to influence the lives of their American daughters, and the daughters' belief that they are very different from their mothers.

When one of the older women, Suyuan, dies, the three surviving members invite her daughter, June, to take her place.

Catharsis and emotional fulfillment during the mahjong games come through the telling of the varied difficulties in the mother–daughter relationships. In America, the mothers find it difficult to understand the directions their daughters are taking. The Joy Luck Club reveals the importance of understanding culture and the differences between the generations. It illustrates how family roles and structures can be successfully negotiated when everyone gives a little.

Photo courtesy © Everett Collection.

adults gradually give up important areas of function, such as financial management, driving, cooking, and shopping, they may begin to develop delusions that people are robbing them or poisoning their food. They respond to these delusions by "dismissing" or rejecting their caregivers in an effort to regain control over these areas of life.

With somatic delusions, the predominant theme is an imagined physical disorder or abnormality of appearance. Somatic delusions in older people are frequently characterized by extremely morbid content ("My blood is leaking into my skin and will poison anyone who touches me").

As a psychiatric–mental health nurse, you will find it crucial to establish trust and consistency with delusional elders. It is important to assess the situation to validate that any persecutory and somatic content is not based in reality. Clients need social interaction with caring people and consistent reality orientation. Relieving social isolation and correcting sensory losses may go far to solve the problem. Delusional processes associated with delirium often abate when the cause of the delirium is treated. Medication in small doses, geared toward relieving underlying anxiety or depressive disorder, may be helpful, although adherence is often a problem because of the client's suspiciousness.

Substance-Related Disorders

A growing body of information suggests that substance use disorders, particularly alcoholism and prescription medication abuse, are more serious problems among elders than had been thought in the past (Arndt, Clayton, & Schultz, 2011). Later-life losses and poor coping skills can lead to increased use of alcohol as a self-medication. Alcohol is both a psychological and physical depressant, thereby raising the risk for both depression and substance dependence. The multiplicity of prescription medications elders are frequently given can create problems with side effects, cognitive impairments, drug–drug interactions, and metabolism. Prescribing practices can also inadvertently mask a substance abuse issue. The clinical example discusses an elder's benzodiazepine misuse.

Clinical Example

Agnes Szczechowski, a 78-year-old woman, was brought by her family to an assisted living facility. Over the previous couple of years she has had increasing difficulty taking care of herself at home. The family reported the following problems prior to making the decision to place Mrs. Szczechowski: leaving a stove burner turned on long after she had stopped cooking, putting household objects away in unusual places (frying pan in the dryer, for example), and leaving the house dressed inappropriately for the weather. The family also noticed that medication bottles were in a state of disarray, and she could not give them a coherent account of which medications she was taking or on what schedule.

Several days after Mrs. Szczechowski moved to Green Meadow Assisted Living Facility, staff members noticed that she was developing increasing symptoms of anxiety. These included physiological symptoms such as hyperventilation and diaphoresis, behavioral symptoms such as pacing and an inability to relax, and cognitive symptoms such as catastrophic thinking. However, she was not able to specify any cause for the anxiety. It appeared to be an adjustment disorder related to moving to the facility.

A psychiatric–mental health nurse interviewed Mrs. Szczechowski and found, in the course of researching the problem, that the client's primary care physician had been prescribing diazepam (Valium) for her for at least 5 years prior to admission. In gathering collateral information from family members, the nurse discovered that the client had taken larger doses of diazepam than prescribed over several periods. Recently, Mrs. Szczechowski appeared to be consistently taking more diazepam on a daily basis than prescribed, six to eight pills a day rather than the prescribed three. Since admission to the assisted living facility, the diazepam has been administered by the staff exactly as prescribed. Therefore the client's effective dose of diazepam has suddenly been reduced by 50% to 75%.

The upsurge in Mrs. Szczechowski's anxiety appeared to be a consequence of her previously undetected diazepam abuse, because she had difficulty tolerating the reduction in the dose. To address this problem, the psychiatric–mental health nurse worked with the other health care providers to reformulate the diazepam regimen so that the client could be safely and slowly titrated off the diazepam and be prescribed a safer agent for the treatment of her anxiety.

The extent of alcoholism and drug- and alcohol-related problems among older adults, while a definite problem, is not clearly known. In previous generations it was believed that the elderly constituted the age group with the lowest rate of alcohol and illegal drug use because of influences in early life such as Prohibition and a historic disapproval of drinking by women. With the societal changes in subsequent generations, these beliefs are changing as baby boomers age.

It is important to note that elders are more vulnerable than younger people to the effects of alcohol and other substances and that they consume more over-the-counter (OTC) preparations and prescribed medications than other population groups. Alcohol abuse and drug dependence among elders are serious problems. Alcohol abuse can predispose older people to accidents, nutritional deficiencies, and diseases that may lead to loss of autonomy. When older drinkers seek medical help for alcohol-related problems such as malnutrition, injuries from falls, and sleep problems, they rarely report alcoholism as their primary complaint. Unfortunately, the presenting problems may be treated and other symptoms mistakenly attributed to the aging process.

Clinical manifestations of alcohol abuse in elders include:

- Tolerance (requiring more of the substance for the same effect)
- Alcohol-related physical health problems such as gastritis, liver problems, and pancreatitis
- Physiological dependence on alcohol (the experience of withdrawal symptoms)
- Unexpected reaction to prescription medications
- Poor response to antipsychotic medications
- Multiple social complications (problems with family relationships and social isolation)
- Frequent behavioral problems such as aggression, memory gaps, driving while impaired by alcohol, and traffic accidents
- Self-care neglect such as incontinence, malnutrition, dehydration, and poor hygiene and home maintenance

Alcoholics Anonymous

Be Medwise

Palliative Care

Many late-onset alcoholics are believed to have turned to drinking in response to stressful life events such as bereavement, illness, divorce, retirement, marital stress, or depression. Assessment for drug and alcohol abuse in elders, especially socially isolated elders who have suffered recent losses, should be respectful; approach elders in a nonjudgmental way when addressing this topic. All clients must be educated about the risks of mixing medications with alcohol. Preventing drinking as a reaction to stress may be accomplished by providing social support and mental health services for elders at risk for social isolation and depression. Referral to resources such as Alcoholics Anonymous (http://www.alcoholics-anonymous.org) is a recommended intervention, especially when combined with other psychiatric supports (see Chapter 15∞ for information about treating people with the dual diagnosis of mentally ill chemical abuser).

Disorders of Arousal and Sleep

Elders frequently experience sleep disruptions that may or may not meet the diagnostic criteria for a formal sleep disorder. For example, a lighter sleep phase pattern occurs with less deep sleep, as well as a common circadian rhythm sleep disorder called *advanced sleep-phase cycle* (*advanced* in terms of direction rather than severity, e.g., sleep and wake times are far earlier than desired). The result in elders is an inability to stay awake past 7:00 p.m. and then awakening—unable to return to sleep—at 3:00 a.m. (Gooneratne et al., 2011). This pattern can be mistakenly diagnosed as depression. Because older adults do have a disproportionately high incidence of depression, determining the presence of depression is also important.

The quantity and quality of sleep change with the aging process. For example, the amount of REM sleep decreases with aging. Elders experience more frequent awakenings during the night, spend increased total time awake at night, and take longer to fall asleep. Changes in sleep architecture and resulting sleep patterns are believed to be related to changes in internal body rhythm, emotional stress, physical illness, and the effects of medications or drugs. Over one-third of people over 60 years of age complain of sleep disturbances (Gooneratne et al., 2011). Elders nap more during the day and use a disproportionately high amount of OTC and prescription sleeping aids. Yet the chronic use of sedatives and hypnotics by elders has not been shown to improve their quality of sleep and can lead to many undesirable and dangerous side effects. Elders excrete these medications more slowly than the young and thus are prone to developing toxic effects, including delirium, daytime drowsiness, and loss of equilibrium. Respiration can be significantly disturbed with the use of sleeping medication.

Clinicians and clients alike must be cognizant of the risks associated with medications, especially when combined with alcohol or even herbal and other supplements. Frequently, sleep disturbances are treated with medications that treat the underlying cause of the sleep problem. Examples include mirtazapine (Remeron), an antidepressant that helps with the sleep and appetite problems of depression, and alprazolam (Xanax) if the sleep difficulty is associated with anxiety. The National Council on Patient Information and Education and the Federal Drug Agency launched a campaign called "Be MedWise" to educate consumers on OTC medication use. For information go to http://www.bemedwise.org or use the Online Student Resources for this textbook.

Clients and health care providers should be more willing to try nonpharmacologic therapies if indicated. Nonpharmacologic guidelines that are recommended for improving sleep for elders include the following:

- Consistent daily physical activity
- A cool, well-ventilated room
- A light bedtime snack
- Stress reduction to promote relaxation
- Regular arousal time
- Avoiding long naps during the day
- Clean bed linens
- Avoiding caffeine, tobacco, and alcohol

PALLIATIVE AND END-OF-LIFE ISSUES WITH MENTALLY ILL ELDERS

Death and dying have been characterized in two entirely different directions: as a crisis that is a natural part of life and as a part of life constituting another transition. Death has been referred to as the ultimate loss; a uniquely personal experience that each of us faces alone. While more imminent for older adults, the need for improved care near the end of life is not unique to elders. Each death evokes different needs and behaviors and provides an opportunity for you to address physical, psychological, social, and spiritual needs of clients and their families (Lavoie, Blondeau, & Picard-Morin, 2011). The increased use of technology at the end of life, diminished inpatient care resources, and an aging population have all created a demand for palliative care.

Precepts of Palliative Care

The World Health Organization (WHO) defines **palliative care** as the active total care of clients whose disease is not responsive to curative treatment. Not all palliative care occurs at the end of life, and much of it aims to help clients and their families reach personal goals, reconcile conflicts, and derive meaning at the end of life (Kimble et al., 2011; McSherry, 2011). Addressing such end-of-life issues is especially complicated when an elder client is exhibiting alteration in mental status due to delirium or dementia or associated with a preexisting psychiatric illness.

Palliative care requires attention to helping clients achieve comfort, the amelioration of pain and distress, and the best possible death. While fears of pain, abandonment, and loss of control are among the most common symptoms for which nurses must provide relief, other end-of-life symptoms of particular concern to psychiatric–mental health nurses include the following:

- Delirium
- Agitation
- Anxiety
- Depression
- Loneliness
- Hopelessness
- Grief
- Social isolation
- Suffering
- Spiritual distress

CARING FOR THE SPIRIT

Supporting and Nurturing Spirituality of Elders in End-of-Life Care

The word *spirituality* is rooted in the Greek language as a word for breath, breathing, and inspiration. Spirituality has evolved to mean something more than religiosity in nursing literature due to the influence of holism and humanism (as described in Chapter 5 ∞). Spirituality is recognized as a source of inner peace, hope, trust, faith, meaning, and strength and can be said to incorporate our sense of identity and understanding of our place and status in the world.

Attending to a client's spiritual quality of life and spiritual well-being has emerged as an important role for nurses. Spiritual needs, problems, concerns, distress, and pain all have been considered as nursing diagnoses, particularly among those receiving end-of-life care. In addition to conducting and documenting a spiritual assessment and facilitating religious practices if the client wishes, a number of strategies are available to you as you attempt to provide care that supports and nurtures the spirituality of your clients. Consider learning more about each of them and adding them to your repertoire.

Feelings of wonder, awe, and transcendence; a renewed sense of vigor; increased mindfulness; the sense of being present in the moment; an awareness of humility; and a better perspective all have been recognized as benefits of experiencing nature. Bringing elements of the natural environment to clients who are confined in nursing homes, hospice care, or hospitals can help them draw strength and courage from things as simple as the image of a rainbow or the fragrance of pine needles.

The American Association of Colleges of Nursing (AACN) developed guidelines concerning end-of-life care. These guidelines are considered the definitive statement on the knowledge and skills needed by nurses who are committed to improving palliative care. The statement, entitled *Peaceful Death: Recommended Competencies and Curricular Guidelines for End-of-Life Nursing Care,* can be found at http://www.aacn.nche.edu/Publications/deathfin.htm or through the Online Student Resources for this text. An additional web-based resource can be found at the City of Hope Pain & Palliative Care Resource Center at http://www.cityofhope.org/prc/

An understanding of family dynamics as well as social, cultural, and religious beliefs may result in the need for the additional supportive services of social workers, hospital chaplains, or other members of the interdisciplinary team. The entire team should be aware of the client's wishes and respond in an appropriate manner to his or her requests.

Spirituality and End-of-Life Care

One of the precepts of palliative care is honoring the preferences, values, and culture of the client and family, especially with respect to suffering, whether physical, psychosocial, or spiritual. Spiritual assessment and care are significant components of end-of-life care. Spiritual integrity gives meaning, purpose, and fulfillment to life and death. The spiritual dimension has been described as a striving for self-transcendence or a search for a higher power and meaning that is greater than the self. Spirituality may or may not include formal religious participation. According to The Joint Commission (2011) standards, the dying client requires a comprehensive spiritual assessment and care that maximizes the client's comfort and dignity and addresses spiritual needs. Staff members must be educated about the needs of: (1) clients receiving care at the end of their lives, (2) clients who are being treated for emotional or behavioral disorders, and (3) people in recovery from alcohol or drug dependence. Spiritual care according to hospice philosophy is nonjudgmental and all-inclusive and focuses on healing, forgiveness, and acceptance. Spiritual interventions can include any of the practices identified in Caring for the Spirit.

Suffering is defined as a highly personal state of severe distress that transcends the physical, psychological, social, and spiritual dimensions and threatens the intactness of the person. Efforts to reduce suffering involve collaborative care at this fragile time in the client's life. Responding to the spiritual needs of clients and families coping with end-of-life issues may ameliorate the depth of suffering. McSherry (2011) highlights the theme of "living while dying" in her phenomenologic study of an effective process for guiding and supporting people at end of life. Lewis (2010) discovered that successful aging was defined by Alaskan natives as not reaching an age, but acquiring wisdom, being personally responsible, and making the conscious decision to live a clean and healthy life. The interplay of culture, spirituality, and the meaning of life and death is vital to providing competent end-of-life care.

Historically, the role of the psychiatric–mental health nurse did not require expertise in palliative and end-of-life care. However, as the current population of psychiatric clients age and geropsychiatric care settings expand, addressing end-of-life care issues will become a major challenge and critical to the management of a client's psychiatric illness. Effective communication with clients and their loved ones is essential. Communication strategies require that you accomplish the following:

- Be clear about the client's goals and expectations of care and treatment.
- Avoid euphemisms for words like *death* and *dying*.
- Be specific when using words such as *hope* and *better*.
- Listen to and honor the preferences, values, and cultural beliefs of clients and their loved ones.

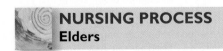

NURSING PROCESS
Elders

The following sections provide specific strategies for applying the nursing process when providing care to elders.

Assessment

Assessment of the elder includes the assessment interview, a biologic assessment, consideration of cognitive status, an assessment of psychological/emotional status, an assessment of strengths and coping strategies, an assessment of sexuality, an attempt to determine social and financial status, and a focused effort to be alert for any indicators of elder abuse.

The Assessment Interview

The variety of theories on aging and the complex interrelationship of physical, emotional, and environmental factors affecting the mental health of elders require an individualized, comprehensive, and multidimensional approach. If feasible, a multidisciplinary team approach is most effective in providing validation of assessment impressions, accurate diagnoses, and appropriate intervention strategies.

The interview is the initial step in the assessment process and important in differentiating between psychiatric disorders and the normal aging process. Chapter 11∞ offers a comprehensive overview of assessment procedures that should be adapted for elders. Specific guidelines for interviewing elders appear in Your Assessment Approach.

Interviewing requires skill and heightened sensitivity and may take more time with older adults than with members of other age groups. Sensory loss, confusion, agitation, wandering, communication disorders, cultural influences, shame, and the fear of stigmatization may inhibit the expression of feelings in elders. They may be unaware of their behavior or expect negative changes as a normal part of aging. It is imperative to solicit interpretations from family and other staff members to help fill in aspects of the clinical picture and validate information provided by the client in the individual interview. See Rx Communication for an illustration of communicating with a confused elder.

A holistic assessment of elders should include objective and subjective data regarding the client's status on a number of levels: biologic, cognitive, psychological, strengths and coping strategies, sexual, social, and financial. In addition to the usual repertoire of screening tools, a variety of self-report screening tools have been designed for use specifically with older clients. These require minimal special training to administer and can help you obtain subjective assessment information. These tools may also be used as objective measures of the outcomes of interventions.

YOUR ASSESSMENT APPROACH
Guidelines for Interviewing Elders

1. Try to make the assessment interview as pleasant as possible by conveying a sense of respect and caring.
2. Be close to the client; use touch when appropriate.
3. Be clear in stating the purpose of the interview and the length of time it will take.
4. Attend to verbal, nonverbal, and environmental cues as well as to the cognitive and behavior status of the client.
5. Repeat the purpose and the time frame of the interview if the client forgets.

Biologic Assessment

Before a definitive psychiatric diagnosis can be made, all medically based illnesses with psychiatric symptoms (depression, confusion, restlessness, and anxiety) must be ruled out. In addition, a complete medical and neurologic examination is necessary to differentiate irreversible conditions from treatable conditions such as pseudodementia (discussed in Chapter 14∞). There are conditions, both chronic and systemic, that can predispose an older individual to confusion. For elders, a urinary tract infection (UTI) is a common and debilitating problem that has accompanying pain and cognitive symptoms. Examine a client exhibiting confusion for anemia, infections, organ failure, or cardiovascular disease. Many emergency department admissions for psychiatric problems in older adults prove to have an underlying biologic etiology such as an infection or dehydration.

Objective assessment information includes laboratory results, a complete history, and physical examination including weight, vital signs, and a description of the physical appearance of the client. Standard diagnostic laboratory analyses appear in FIGURE 27-3 ■. Your medical–surgical nursing or general nursing texts offer specific biologic assessment guides for elders.

Other procedures important for ruling out infections, space-occupying lesions, drug and medication toxicities, and cancers include chest radiography, drug toxicology screening, computed tomography (CT) scanning, positron-emission tomography (PET) scanning, electrocardiogram (ECG), electroencephalogram (EEG), and lumbar puncture. A dementia

---

℞ COMMUNICATION

Communicating With a Confused Elder

CLIENT: "I don't know why I'm here. My brother takes care of my finances. He doesn't think I take proper care of myself, but I am as I am and I want him to leave me ALONE!"

NURSE RESPONSE 1: "Give me an example of something that your brother told you was your 'not taking proper care of yourself.'"	**NURSE RESPONSE 2:** "Why are you here at the clinic?"
RATIONALE: This response focuses on collecting more information about the genuine safety risks faced by this 84-year-old woman who lives alone in a small New York City apartment. She has been referred to your clinic to have her safety skills assessed.	*RATIONALE:* This response requests concrete information from the client rather than any interpretations. It also has the potential to provide a picture of memory impairments the client might have.

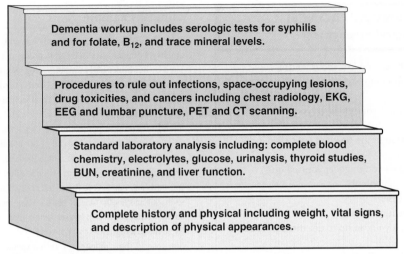

Dementia workup includes serologic tests for syphilis and for folate, B₁₂, and trace mineral levels.

Procedures to rule out infections, space-occupying lesions, drug toxicities, and cancers including chest radiology, EKG, EEG and lumbar puncture, PET and CT scanning.

Standard laboratory analysis including: complete blood chemistry, electrolytes, glucose, urinalysis, thyroid studies, BUN, creatinine, and liver function.

Complete history and physical including weight, vital signs, and description of physical appearances.

FIGURE 27-3 ▦ Levels of biologic assessment for elders.

workup should include serologic tests for syphilis; folate, B₁₂, and trace mineral levels; and a thyroid panel.

Subjective assessment information includes clients' perceptions of their physical health and a description of their chronic illnesses, symptoms, self-care activities, and concerns and fears about their current situation.

Cognitive Status

A thorough mental status examination is essential. Objective information includes the presence and extent of cognitive impairment. Include the family and other caregivers to determine the course of any mental changes. Ask: "Did the changes happen gradually (dementia of the Alzheimer's type, drug/medication toxicity, metabolic imbalances), suddenly (depression, cerebrovascular accident, drug/medication toxicity), or in a graduated, stepwise fashion (multi-infarct dementia)?" Family and other caregivers may have noticed changes at certain times of the day that could indicate specific problems (Gaugler, Roth, Haley, & Mittelman, 2011). Ask: "Have there been changes in mood, or has there been agitation in the late afternoon or early evening (sundowning)?" "Has the client been observed to have or complained of having trouble making decisions or concentrating (depression)?"

The Short Portable Mental Status Questionnaire (SPMSQ) is a simple, reliable, and valid 10-item cognitive performance evaluation tool. It was designed to assess and monitor cognitive changes in an elderly client. Keep in mind, however, three important points when using standardized assessment tools with elders:

1. Older people are sensitive to fatigue, boredom, medications, and environmental influences that can affect results on a mental status measurement tool.
2. Tools like the SPMSQ cannot distinguish delirium from dementia.
3. Assessment instruments designed for use with other age groups may not be accurate or complete for use with elders.

Subjective information regarding cognitive status includes clients' own perceptions of their mental status. Questions to ask include:

- How has your thinking been lately?
- Is your memory as good as it used to be?
- Have you been able to keep track of your medications? The days of the week? Mealtimes?

Psychological/Emotional Status

Objective data about the client's psychological and emotional status require synthesis of impressions from both the content and process of the assessment interview and mental status examination. Avoid the overuse of psychiatric terminology but rather strive for descriptions accompanied by examples of the client's behavior and direct quotations. Be sure to include significant negative findings such as the absence of delusional thoughts, the absence of suicidal ideation, and the absence of hallucinations. Your assessment should include not only pathology and problems but also health, adaptive strengths, and personal assets.

Strengths and Coping Strategies

Aging is a process punctuated by positive and negative stress-producing events. Elders are people who have learned to cope with stress. Data about an elder's coping strategies and strengths are as important as information about psychiatric symptoms. You can shift the conversation in this direction by making a statement such as, "You certainly have lived a long, full life. Would you share with me some of your survival secrets?" Your Assessment Approach provides sample questions to help you gather data about an elder's strengths and coping strategies, such as spiritual practices, playing a musical instrument, or reaching out to help others. With this information you can develop a cogent plan of care that supports weak areas and activates those areas in which the client excels.

Spirituality can be a psychological support and a coping mechanism. Often, people who are facing novel stressors

---

YOUR ASSESSMENT APPROACH
Assessing Psychological Strengths

- What are some of the things you like about yourself?
- What are some of the upsetting, stressful, difficult times you can remember?
- What did you do to comfort yourself when your spouse/ partner died?
- How did you make it through the death of your child (or friend)?
- What kinds of things do you do to cheer yourself up?
- What makes you happy or content?
- How do you nurture yourself?
- What do you do to have fun? To relax?
- What things do you think you can do to get through rough times?
- How have the passing years affected your sexuality?
- What are you most concerned about right now?
- What kind of help do you feel you need?

Clinical Example

Irene is a 75-year-old widow who recently broke her hip while cross-country skiing. At first she felt depressed, embarrassed, and socially isolated by her injury and immobilization. She longed for her usual schedule of hiking, swimming, traveling, and attending plays and concerts. Because Irene had a wide circle of friends, had regularly hosted holiday parties at her home, and was generous with her time and energy with her adult children and grandchildren, her social support network rallied to help her as soon as they learned of her condition.

Friends and family brought in the health food Irene loved and stayed with her to keep her company while she ate. Others sent clever, encouraging cards and notes. One friend telephoned her each day until she was able to be out and about. One of her sons sent her some of his favorite books, and her other son set up Internet and e-mail connections for her computer. Irene made a rapid and full recovery both physically and psychologically. She rose to the challenge of an unexpected injury and recovery period with cheerfulness and resilience. Instead of being derailed by her accident, she emerged even stronger.

---

or significant threats to their security turn to religion or spirituality for the first time in their lives, or after an absence for a significant period of time. Assess clients to determine whether a recent focus on spirituality is a new addition to their support structure. If so, explore the concepts, meanings, and emotions that spiritual expression offers the client.

Sexuality

Sexuality is an important area often overlooked when assessing elders. Remember that sexual activity can and does continue into later life and that sexuality is a broad, multidimensional component of personal identity. Films such as *Harold and Maude* and *Something's Gotta Give* portray richly, and with humor, sexual expression among elders. Sexual expression includes body image, affection, love, flirtation, social roles, and interaction. Older people who do abstain from sexual expression often do so because they lack the opportunity or perceive negative social pressure about sexuality in people their age.

Approach the topic of sexuality in a tactful, caring, and nonjudgmental manner. An elder who does not wish to discuss sexual issues most likely will make that clear by stating it directly, not answering the question, or changing the subject. An elder who was socialized in a different, more conservative era may not be comfortable discussing sex. Older adults who matured in the 1960s, however, may have entirely different attitudes toward their continuing sexuality.

Social and Financial Status

Also assess the quality and quantity of social support (past and present) available to an elder. Social support has been confirmed as important for optimal functioning. If a client is able to maintain a meaningful social network, it suggests the client has strong interpersonal skills that can be mobilized to help negotiate stresses and losses in later life. Formation of a new social network when others have dissolved is easier for an elder with social skills and the personal resources of assertiveness, friendliness, and warmth. Consider the following clinical example.

Elders who get by on a low, fixed income may be plagued by financial problems that affect their mental and physical health. Some communities offer services to help older people manage their finances. The removal of financial strain can dramatically improve the health of an aging person. Learning about available financial aid and assistance programs will help you be an effective case manager for older clients. Sample questions for obtaining information about a client's social and financial status are listed in Your Assessment Approach below.

Elder Abuse

The mistreatment of elders is a serious, underreported, underdetected phenomenon. Elder mistreatment may take many forms, including physical abuse, neglect, exploitation, abandonment, and psychological abuse (see Your Assessment Approach on the next page). Older adults with fewer psychosocial resources or a number of psychosocial deficits seem to have an increased vulnerability to mistreatment. Mistreatment is particularly detrimental to psychological well-being (Luo & Waite, 2011).

YOUR ASSESSMENT APPROACH
Guidelines for Assessing Social and Financial Status

- How many phone calls and e-mails do you get in a week?
- How frequently do you have visitors?
- How frequently do you visit others?
- Are you happily married/partnered?
- How would you describe your relationship with your family members?
- Do you have someone you can trust and confide in?
- Do you find yourself feeling lonely?
- Do you have transportation to get to doctor/nurse appointments or to the hospital if needed?
- How is your financial situation? Do you worry about spending or running out of money?

YOUR ASSESSMENT APPROACH   **Forms of Mistreatment of Elders**

Determine whether the following have occurred:

Physical Abuse	Neglect	Exploitation	Abandonment	Psychological Abuse
▪ Direct beatings ▪ Inflicting pain ▪ Coercion (abrasions, sprains, dislocation)	▪ Withholding food ▪ Withholding fluids ▪ Withholding medication/ treatment ▪ Withholding medical attention	▪ Taking Social Security or pension checks ▪ Taking possessions against elder's will ▪ Removing excess funds from elders' account when purchasing items for them	▪ Dropping off elder at hospital or other health care facility ▪ Leaving incapacitated elder alone at home ▪ Failing to provide for basic services	▪ Degrading comments ▪ Threatening comments ▪ Using scare tactics when the elder cannot provide for his or her own needs

---

Elders who are at greatest risk for abuse and neglect are those who are dependent on others for care (Centers for Disease Control [CDC], 2010). The degree of dependence may overwhelm the caregiver, who may then harm the elder. Stressors related to caregiving can overwhelm any caregiver, but the caregiver of a frail elder is often an adult child with additional family and work responsibilities or a spouse who is also aging. (See Chapter 29∞ for more information on family stress and the burdens of caregiving.)

A growing number of states provide legal alternatives for the removal of an elder to a protective situation. Long-term care centers or respite care placement, discussed later in this chapter, may be necessary. However, most elders react negatively to such placement and want to return to the potentially harmful home situation. In-home assistance is becoming available in most areas, and such home health services can decrease the strain on caregivers. Home visits made by a case manager or community health nurse can provide an opportunity to assess the possibility of elder abuse in any of its forms, or to prevent it by planning for services to meet the needs of elders and their family caregivers.

Nursing Diagnosis: NANDA

Once a comprehensive, multidimensional assessment is accomplished, nursing diagnoses are identified. The NANDA nursing diagnoses likely to be associated with DSM-IV-TR disorders in elders are covered in this section.

Major Depression

NANDA diagnoses associated with the DSM disorder of major depression include the following.

Chronic or Situational Low Self-Esteem Low self-esteem is a hallmark feature of depression. Not only do elders internalize social ageist biases, but they are also often plagued with irrational guilt in the form of intrusive, obsessional, and self-deprecating thoughts.

Risk for Self-Directed Violence Feelings of hopelessness, low self-esteem, obsessive–compulsive symptoms, apathy, and powerlessness often contribute to suicidal ideation and suicide attempts in depressed elders.

Activity Intolerance Psychomotor agitation and/or retardation are both symptoms of depression. Psychomotor agitation affects social interaction, self-care abilities, and the sleep–wake cycle. Psychomotor retardation is a common vegetative sign of depression in elders. People with psychomotor retardation experience compromised self-care abilities and lack of physical exercise, and are at risk for developing complications of decreased mobility.

Feeding Self-Care Deficit, and Imbalanced Nutrition: More or Less Than Body Requirements Many depressed elders lose weight dramatically. A weight gain secondary to overeating and decreased activity occurs less frequently.

Ineffective Health Maintenance Depressed elders are at risk for developing physical health complications secondary to poor self-care and poor health maintenance habits.

Sleep Deprivation or Insomnia Often, older clients with depression experience sleep pattern disturbances, particularly early morning awakening. Occasionally, depressed elders report excessive sleeping.

Disturbed Thought Processes Elders may have cognitive changes such as short-term memory loss that accompany depression. Concentration may be impaired, and lack of motivation hinders the ability to learn new information and avoid social isolation. Chapter 14∞ provides detailed information on memory impairment.

Adjustment Disorder

NANDA diagnoses most likely to be found in elders with adjustment disorder are described next.

Dysfunctional Grieving Elders may become immobilized by stress associated with loss. Often, depression ensues, with an identified stressor as the only factor differentiating an adjustment disorder from major depression.

Self-Care Deficit Individuals may lose interest in self-care activities. Grooming, hygiene, and other activities of daily living are neglected. In some cases, elders are at risk for developing serious physical illnesses as a result of failing to adhere to medication regimens and refusing to eat or engage in other health care practices.

Ineffective Role Performance The experience of losses often leads to changes in social interaction and role performance. Social withdrawal and loneliness as well as changes in mental status can occur due to lack of social stimulation.

Hopelessness The experience of loss, coupled with a pervasive dysphoria, can place an older person at risk for developing dependence and loss of function as self-concept and motivation wane.

Anxiety Disorders

Elders with anxiety disorders may have the following NANDA diagnoses.

Ineffective Coping Anxiety symptoms often impair a person's ability to concentrate and think clearly. Consequently, judgment is affected and the client decreases activities in order to avoid stressful situations.

Activity Intolerance Anxiety is often associated with psychomotor agitation and restlessness.

Delusional Disorders

NANDA diagnoses most likely to be found in elders with delusional disorder are covered next.

Disturbed Thought Processes Older people with delusional disorders often become paranoid and suspect others of trying to rob them, cheat them, or harm them in some way. They may also have delusions about their body or bodily functions. Delusions may be accompanied by feelings of fear, paranoia, anger, and anxiety. Behavioral manifestations of these feelings include suspiciousness, aggression, lashing out, social isolation, and unusual eating behaviors.

Impaired Social Interaction Delusions that are centered on family members and caregivers strain interpersonal relationships and may make them impossible to maintain.

Outcome Identification: NOC

Outcomes associated with NANDA diagnoses common among elders are described in the following section.

Improvement in Disturbed Thought Processes

Subjective indications of improvement in thought processes include client reports of thinking more clearly, improved concentration, and ability to remember recent and remote events. Individuals with delusions and other signs of psychosis will note that they feel more like themselves and will be able to make more accurate, reality-based interpretations. Other NOC outcomes specific to this nursing diagnosis include the following:

- Cognitive orientation: Ability to identify person, place, time, and purpose
- Concentration: Ability to focus on a specific stimulus
- Decision making: Ability to choose between two or more alternatives
- Information processing: Ability to acquire, organize, and use information
- Memory: Ability to cognitively retrieve and report previously stored information
- Consciousness: Ability to arouse, orient, and attend to the environment

Renewed Hope and Self-Acceptance

Expressions of hope and self-acceptance, renewed involvement, and motivation in activities and planning for the future indicate improvement and replace dependence, apathy, and negative self-talk. Other NOC outcomes relevant to this diagnosis in elders include the following:

- Expressions of faith, will to live, reasons to live, meaning in life, optimism, and belief in self and others
- Ability to identify personal strengths
- Ability to recognize behaviors that reduce feelings of hopelessness
- Interest in social and personal relationships
- Interest in, and satisfaction with, life goals

Resumption of Self-Care and Health Maintenance

Elder clients will resume their prior level of self-care and health maintenance. Other NOC outcomes relevant to this nursing diagnosis with elders include the following:

- Ability to perform most basic physical tasks and personal care activities
- Ability to dress self
- Ability to maintain neat appearance
- Ability to maintain own hygiene

Appropriately Paced Activity, Rest, and Psychomotor Activity

Vegetative signs will be replaced with more appropriately paced activities, movement, gait, speech, appetite, and sleep–wake cycle. Anxiety and fear will be replaced with subjective feelings of calm, restfulness, and well-being.

Pleasure in Eating and Normal Weight

Clients will report that their appetites are returning and there is increased pleasure associated with eating. Weight will return to the normal range.

Decreased Preoccupation With Death and Dying

Clients will report that suicidal ideation has markedly decreased if not resolved. Morbid preoccupation with death and dying will also decrease.

Planning and Implementation: NIC

The following psychiatric–mental health interventions are frequently effective when working with elders.

Reminiscence Therapy and Life Review

Reminiscence therapy and life review are useful interventions for elders who are experiencing self-esteem disturbance, grief, hopelessness, powerlessness, altered role performance, and social isolation. **Reminiscence therapy** uses the recall of past events, feelings, and thoughts to facilitate pleasure, quality of life, or adaptation to present circumstances. Although it can be used throughout the life span, it is of special significance when working with elders.

Reminiscing can and should be encouraged for elders individually and in groups. Creative use of food, music, pets,

CARING FOR THE SPIRIT

Listening to Storytelling, Life Review, and Reminiscence

Encouraging a client to make an audiotape, dictate letters, create a photo album or scrapbook, or create other artistic expressions to depict the wholeness of his or her life can help the client establish a sense of satisfaction from a life well lived. Reminiscence and life review are identified as useful nursing interventions later in this chapter. Experts who teach about listening to clients' stories suggest guidelines for nurses using this approach. A major guideline is the idea of developing a list of questions that encourage awareness of positive aspects of a life story and reflection and enthusiasm on the part of the client telling the story. Questions might include: "How would you like the rest of your story to be?" "How has what has happened to you shaped who you are today?" "What do you think are the major themes in your life story?"

Assisting With Journal or Diary Writing

Keeping a journal offers a client a way to express inner thoughts. A journal can consist of narratives on topics such as "What do I stand for?", "What personal quality do I feel best about?", or "What makes me feel joy?" However, a journal can also take the form of sketches, song lyrics, descriptions of dreams, poetry, or prayers that can be original or collected from various sources.

Making and Appreciating Art as Spiritual Expression

Creating art and sharing it with others allow clients to leave a legacy, build a sense of community, and make sense of experiences. You can encourage clients to participate actively by drawing, painting, or sculpting or passively by collecting healing images such as mandalas, icons, or wilderness landscapes or photographs. Listening to music can help decrease anxiety, depression, agitation, and aggressive behavior as well as improve relaxation and peace of mind.

The strategies for supporting and nurturing spirituality described here represent only a sample of the possibilities. They all require self-disclosure on the part of clients who may feel vulnerable. Extreme sensitivity is required of the nurse who uses them in practice. Some clients prefer to discuss these topics with a member of the clergy or a spiritual advisor. You must respect their wishes.

---

and special events can facilitate the process and make it fun. Materials such as photo albums, journals, cameras, and video recorders provide ways for older people to establish a record of their lives, creating a legacy for those who follow. Storytelling, life review, and reminiscence are discussed in Caring for the Spirit.

Life review is a structured process involving the recall of past events in one's life in an effort to find meaning in those events. The process systematically reviews remote memories and addresses the expression of related feelings and the recognition of conflicts. A life review is a chance to re-examine one's life, solve old problems, make amends, establish perspective, and restore harmony. As life review becomes an integral part of clinical care, it provides emotional and spiritual support. Approaching the second half of life with a positive perspective—a journey filled with new possibilities and enriched by wisdom and learning from life experience—provides an opportunity to reflect on personal intentions, values, interpersonal relationships, and a personal legacy (McSherry, 2011). Initiating and therapeutically directing the life review process requires your use of effective therapeutic listening skills (refer to Chapter 10∞) in order to enhance the psychological growth that can emerge as a result of this process.

Reality Orientation

Reality orientation emphasizes awareness of time, place, person, and purpose. The approach provides consistency and a constant reminder to clients of where they are, why they are there, and what is expected. The periodic use of reality orientation tests the elder's level of confusion and disorientation. The rationale for reality orientation is the need to use the part of the person's mind that remains intact.

Socialization Enhancement

Socialization enhancement with elders usually takes place in **resocialization groups** conducted in senior centers, adult day care, rehabilitation, and long-term care facilities. The goal of resocialization groups is to facilitate the elder's ability to interact with others and to renew interest in his or her surroundings. One form of resocialization group focuses on **remotivation therapy**, in which the emphasis is on stimulating interest in the environment and relationships with others. Group discussion focuses on topics chosen by members of the group and may include world affairs, current local activities, and happy experiences. In the discussions, group members are encouraged to pool knowledge and develop stimulating discussions related to the topic at hand.

Animal-Assisted Therapy

Animal-assisted therapy or pet therapy involves the purposeful use of animals to provide affection, attention, diversion, and relaxation to clients. The animals may be certified therapy animals, may be obtained from a variety of sources such as community-based SPCA/Humane Society volunteer programs or the local zoo, or may live on the grounds of the facility. Animals that have physical contact with elders are trained to respond in a calm, nonthreatening manner. Small animals can be held in an older person's lap, larger animals are trained to stand next to a chair and allow the client to stroke or pet them without having to hold them, and aviaries of birds provide sound, movement, and interaction. FIGURE 27-4 ■ shows one such therapy animal.

Exercise and Movement Therapy

Exercise and movement therapy can help induce relaxation, maintain flexibility, restore balance, and enhance joy in older clients. Such interventions may include stretching and reaching

FIGURE 27-4 ■ Therapy animals like Bruno provide unconditional acceptance, and emotional, tactile, and interactional opportunities for even significantly regressed or isolated elders.
Photo courtesy of Anne Garcia

activities, complex exercises such as Tai Chi for those able to mirror the leader, or simple and concrete movements such as handholding for those who are physically or cognitively incapacitated. What Every Nurse Should Know has information on specific challenges posed by elders in the radiology department.

Support Groups

Social support and group interventions are useful when working with clients who experience dysfunctional or interrupted family processes, knowledge deficits, ineffective coping, dysfunctional grieving, social isolation, and spiritual distress. The group situation or social environment provides emotional support as well as information for its members. Groups are the treatment of choice for many older clients,

WHAT EVERY NURSE SHOULD KNOW

Needs of Elders Differ from Those of Other Age Groups

Imagine you are an interventional radiology nurse. Treating an elder in radiology differs from treating younger clients. In a number of ways elders are more restricted in their movements and their ability to accommodate change. For example, many elders have a lower tolerance for cool temperatures than others, and radiology departments tend to be very cool. Do whatever keeps older clients comfortable to ensure their continued interest in treatment. Other issues include positioning difficulties due to injuries, surgery, arthritis, or scoliosis. Make positioning more comfortable with a little extra effort and creativity. Attending to the elder's particular needs will enhance treatment and allow for more effective nursing assessment.

especially those in long-term care facilities, because several people can benefit and transportation is not a problem.

Medication Administration

Used judiciously, medications can be an effective adjunct to other interventions when working with clients with mental disorders in later life. A key axiom to remember about medication dosing with elders is: "Start low, go slow." The high incidence of adverse medication reactions in older clients underscores the need for careful monitoring and conservative dosages. TABLE 27-1 ■ summarizes recommended dosages for categories of psychotropic medications used with elders. In general, information about dose adjustments and special considerations with elders are catalogued in medication references such as drug guides and medication manuals. (See also Chapters 7 and 31∞ of this text for in-depth information.)

It is important that you recognize that elders are more prone to side effects from psychiatric medications and observe for their occurrence. Among these side effects are the following:

- Extrapyramidal symptoms (dystonias, akathisia, tremor, pseudoparkinsonism)
- Constipation
- Anticholinergic effects (urinary retention, cognitive impairments, blurred vision, dry mouth, hallucinations, sexual dysfunction)
- Cardiovascular effects (postural hypotension, arrhythmias)
- Drug interactions resulting in delirium, confusion, or disorientation
- Sedation
- Paradoxical effects, especially common with diphenhydramine (Benadryl) and meperidine (Demerol)

Medications within each psychotropic class vary widely in intensity of side effects and ideally should be monitored by a specially prepared psychogerontologist who is knowledgeable about the appropriate doses and possible side effects of these medications.

Evaluation

Identified outcomes and their measurement in both subjective and objective terms guide the evaluation step in the nursing process. When working with older mentally ill clients, expectations must be realistic. The aging process has normal, nonpathowlogic impacts on behavioral speed, rate of learning new information, and adaptation to degeneration of sensory input. Once these normal characteristics of aging are taken into account, evaluation of an older client's response to nursing interventions can proceed. As with clients in other age groups, psychiatric symptoms are evaluated for reduction in intensity, intrusiveness, and interference with functioning.

Remember that ultimately clients' own values, culture, and preferences, particularly in the late stages of life, should be honored as the gold standard. See Developing Cultural Competence for information on using what elders have learned. Whenever possible, involve families and significant others along with the client in the evaluation process.

TABLE 27-1 ■ Dosage Ranges of Psychotropic Medications Used with Elders

Category	Dosage Range
Antipsychotics: Atypical	
olanzapine (Zyprexa)	5–10 mg/day
risperidone (Risperdal)	0.25–6 mg/day
Antipsychotics: Conventional	
chlorpromazine (Thorazine)	10–800 mg/day
fluphenazine (Prolixin)	PO: 0.25–20 mg/day, IM: 2.5–10 mg/day, Decanoate: 12.5–25 mg/1–4 wk
haloperidol (Haldol)	PO: 0.25–15 mg/day, IM: 2–5 mg q4h PRN, Decanoate: 50–100 mg/4 wk
trifluoperazine (Stelazine)	PO: 0.5–40 mg/day, IM: 1–2 mg q4–6h, Max 10 mg/day
Anxiolytic Agents	
buspirone (BuSpar)	10–60 mg/day
Anxiolytic Agents (Benzodiazepines)	
clonazepam (Klonopin)	1.5–20 mg/day
lorazepam (Ativan)	0.5–2.0 mg/day
oxazepam (Serax)	10–30 mg/day
Mood Stabilizers	
carbamazepine (Tegretol)	400–1,200 mg/day
lithium	300 mg tid
valproate (Depakote)	125 mg bid to max 60 mg/kg/day
Monoamine Oxidase Inhibitors (MAOIs)	
isocarboxazid (Marplan)	10–30 mg/day
phenelzine (Nardil)	15–90 mg/day
tranylcypromine (Parnate)	30–60 mg/day
Sedative–Hypnotic Benzodiazepines	
flurazepam (Dalmane)	15–30 mg/bedtime
temazepam (Restoril)	7.5–15 mg/bedtime
Atypical Antidepressants	
bupropion (Wellbutrin)	50–300 mg/day
nefazodone (Serzone)	50–600 mg/day
trazodone (Desyrel)	25–150 mg/day
Selective Serotonin Reuptake Inhibitors (SSRIs)	
citalopram (Celexa)	20 mg/day
fluoxetine (Prozac)	10–80 mg/day
paroxetine (Paxil)	10–80 mg/day
sertraline (Zoloft)	25–200 mg/day
Tricyclic Antidepressants	
amitriptyline (Elavil)	10–150 mg/day
desipramine (Norpramin)	75–150 mg/day
imipramine (Tofranil)	PO: 75–300 mg/day
nortriptyline (Pamelor)	10–150 mg/day

Source: Trigoboff, E., Wilson, B. A., Shannon, M. T., & Stang, C. L. (2005). *Psychiatric drug guide*. Upper Saddle River, NJ: Prentice Hall. Adapted by permission of Pearson Education, Inc., Upper Saddle River, NJ.

CASE MANAGEMENT, COMMUNITY-BASED CARE, AND HOME CARE

Care of mentally ill elders takes place in a variety of settings, including at home, in day care programs, in geropsychiatric or dementia units of hospitals, in outpatient clinics, in assisted living programs, and in long-term care facilities.

Goals for care provided in the community emphasize the following:

- Maintaining elders in their own homes or apartments for as long as feasible and safe
- Supporting clients and families as clients move from one setting to another

Care Plan: Adjustment to Nursing Home

DEVELOPING CULTURAL COMPETENCE

Generational Commonalities of Elders

Cultural competence in psychiatric–mental health nursing with elders requires sensitivity to not only the ethnic, racial, and cultural heritage of an elder, but also to their generational commonalities. Elders have a history and a perspective in addition to their cultural identity. Even if an elder is of a majority culture, there is nothing routine or mainstream about the decades of experience the individual client has accumulated.

Think about your culture and how you express it through religion, cooking, celebrations, and traditions. What is defined as successful aging in your generation within your culture? Do you think that your parents and grandparents defined successful aging in the same way? Aging well might include: abstaining from drugs and alcohol, having a successful financial portfolio, demonstrating personal responsibility, or having wisdom based upon one's life experiences.

Elders with mental health issues may have gone for years without the benefit of psychopharmacology (not developed until the late 1950s). Or, they may have undergone unmodified electroconvulsive therapy (ECT) when muscle relaxants and anesthesia were not used. They may have lived in underserved areas where therapists were not available or the stigma was so palpable that no one went for treatment. Attitudes in our society toward mental health issues have undergone change, yet much more needs to change. Elders who have had mental health issues through the years have experienced stigma and lack of services. This will inevitably have an influence on their attitudes toward mental health care. Cultural competence takes their perspective into account and increases our ability to establish therapeutic relationships.

CRITICAL THINKING QUESTIONS

1. Why would it be helpful to consider the history of treatment choices for elders?
2. What would you consider as the biggest difference between an elder with psychiatric–mental health issues and a 20-year-old person with psychiatric–mental health issues?

- Maintaining optimal functional independence
- Delaying institutionalization by staging increased levels of care (rehabilitation facility, assisted living, supervised settings, etc.)
- Enhancing self-esteem and personal integrity
- Educating clients and family caregivers about treatment strategies
- Ensuring coordinated supportive daily activities that enhance the client's ability to cope and compensate for deficits

Restorative Care

Restorative care is a planned, systematic program that focuses on restoration and maintenance of optimal function and assisting adults to compensate for impairments. It also emphasizes prevention of deterioration whenever possible.

In order for it to be successful, everyone working in the environment must adopt the philosophy of restorative care.

This approach is particularly relevant in long-term care facilities. Staff from the living units, the social work staff, dietary staff, and activities staff are all involved in promoting and restoring function and ability.

Community-Based Programs

While the philosophy of restorative care is clearly applicable to the care of elders who live in nursing homes or other long-term care facilities, it also guides many other community-based programs. Senior centers, adult day care, respite centers, and community support services such as Meals on Wheels and Whistle Stop Wheels, which respectively bring prepared food and transportation to elders being cared for at home, are all designed to promote the elder's optimal independent functioning and reduce the stress and burden on family caregivers.

Community-based programs offer alternatives to institutionalization. In the case of senior centers, the emphasis is on (1) health and wellness promotion, and (2) social, educational, and recreational activities. Adult day care programs are another alternative to institutionalization. Adult day care programs represent a community resource for elders who need nursing, medical, and rehabilitative services beyond socialization and education. Many adult day care facilities and assisted living centers offer a **respite** option wherein elders can remain overnight in order to relieve family caregivers if they are feeling burdened. Both of these community programs allow elders to continue living at home.

Assisted living communities are a relatively new option for elders who require support and can no longer remain in their own homes. Such communities take several forms but usually offer a range of assistance levels from independent apartment units through nursing home–like complete care. Unfortunately, this option is rarely available to elders who have sparse financial resources.

The next level of care for frail or mentally disordered elders is admission to a nursing home or other long-term care facility. Even when long-term care is an option, the decision to institutionalize a loved one is usually made only when family caregivers have reached the brink of their own tolerance levels, putting their own health at risk; when the elder no longer recognizes them; or when it becomes physically impossible to manage the elder due to violence or incapacity. As a nurse, especially when serving as case manager, you should be well informed about your community's resources for mentally ill elders and their family caregivers.

Resistance to Care

Descriptions such as *uncooperative, stubborn, noncompliant,* and *aggressive* have all been used to characterize elders who are resistant to care. These behaviors are commonly noted as the biggest problems when caring for a mentally disordered elder in a community or home setting. The research by Hodgson, Gitlin, Winter, and Czekanski (2011) examined elders with DAT or a related disorder who resided in the community. The behavior most often demonstrated (66%) by these psychogeriatric clients was resisting or refusing care. Nursing professionals define *resistance to care* as client behaviors that prevent, oppose, or interfere with the caregiver's efforts to provide help. Resistance to care by mentally disordered elders can take the form of pushing, hitting, screaming, and cursing. Suggested potentially useful nursing interventions include the following:

- Consult with the primary caregiver (family member or nursing staff member) who is in most frequent contact with the client about strategies that worked in the past.
- Talk and reason with the client.
- Allow the client to eat or dress independently.
- Distract the client by initiating social activity.

- Wait and return at a later time to resume the activity.
- Allow the client to refuse care, such as getting dressed, that involves few health consequences.

Try to discover the reason for resistance to care. Is it pain? Fatigue? Fear of caregivers who are strangers to the client? Confusion because of an unfamiliar environment? Not knowing what is wanted or expected by caregivers? Dealing with mentally ill elders can be challenging, particularly in the home or community. More nursing research is needed to determine strategies that are effective, especially with elders who are resistant to care.

Pearson Nursing Student Resources

Find additional review materials at **nursing.pearsonhighered.com**

Prepare for success with NCLEX®-style practice questions, interactive assignments and activities, web links, animations and videos, and more!

REFERENCES

Adams, K. B., Roberts, A. R., & Cole, M. B. (2011). Changes in activity and interest in the third and fourth age: Associations with health, functioning, and depressive symptoms. *Occupational Therapy International, 18*(1), 4–17.

American Psychiatric Association. (2000). *Diagnostic and statistical manual of mental disorders* (4th ed., Text Revision). Washington, DC: Author.

Arndt, S., Clayton, R., & Schultz, S. K. (2011). Trends in substance abuse treatment 1998–2008: Increasing older adult first-time admissions for illicit drugs. *American Journal of Geriatric Psychiatry, 0,* 1–8.

Barzilai, N., & Gabrieli, I. (2010). Genetic studies reveal the role of the endocrine and metabolic systems in aging. *Journal of Clinical Endocrinology & Metabolism, 95*(10), 4493–4500.

Berlau, D. J., Corrada, M. M., Peltz, C. B., & Kawas, C. H. (2011). Disability in the oldest-old: Incidence and risk factors in The 90+ Study. *American Journal of Geriatric Psychiatry, 0,* 1–10.

Brooks, C. L. (2011). Considering elderly competence when consenting to treatment. *Holistic Nursing Practice, 25*(3), 136–139.

Centers for Disease Control and Prevention, National Center for Injury Prevention and Control, Division of Violence Prevention and Control. (2010). *Understanding Elder Maltreatment—Fact Sheet.* Retrieved from http://www.cdc.gov/violenceprevention/

Gaugler, J. E., Roth, D. L., Haley, W. E., & Mittelman, M. S. (2011). Modeling trajectories and transitions: Results from the New York University caregiver intervention. *Nursing research, 60*(3S), S28–S37.

Gooneratne, N. S., Tavaria, A, Patel, N., Madhusudan, L., Nadaraja, D., Onen, F., & Richards, K. C. (2011). Perceived effectiveness of diverse sleep treatments in older adults. *Journal of the American Geriatrics Society, 59*(2), 297–303.

Hodgson, N. A., Gitlin, L. N., Winter, L., & Czekanski, K. (2011). Undiagnosed illness and neuropsychiatric behaviors in community residing older adults with dementia. *Alzheimer Disease and Associated Disorders, 25*(2), 109–115.

Kimble, L. P., Dunbar, S. B., Weintraub, W. S., McGuire, D. B., Manzo, S. F., & Strickland, O. L. (2011). Symptom clusters and health-related quality of life in people with chronic stable angina. *Journal of Advanced Nursing, 67*(5), 1000–1011.

Lapierre, S., Erlangsen, A., Waern, M., De Leo, D., Oyama, H., Scocco, P., . . . Quinnett, P. (2011). A systematic review of elderly suicide prevention programs. *Crisis, 32*(2), 88–98.

Lavoie, M., Blondeau, D., & Picard-Morin, J. (2011). The autonomy experience of patients in palliative care. *Journal of Hospice & Palliative Nursing, 13*(1), 47–53.

Lewis, J. P. (2010). Successful aging through the eyes of Alaskan natives: Exploring generational differences among Alaska natives. *Journal of Cross-Cultural Gerontology, 25*(4), 385–396.

Lobo, A., Carvalho, J., & Santos, P. (2011). Comparison of functional fitness in elderlies with reference values by Rikli and Jones and after one year of health intervention programs. *The Journal of Sports Medicine & Physical Fitness, 51*(1), 111–120.

Loe, M. (2010). Doing it my way: Old women, technology and well-being. *Sociology of Health & Illness, 32*(2), 319–334.

Luo, Y., & Waite, L. J. (2011). Mistreatment and psychological well-being among older adults: Exploring the role of psychosocial resources and deficits. *The Journals of Gerontology, 66*(2), 217–229.

Lysack, C., Lichtenberg, P., & Schneider, B. (2011). Effect of a DVD intervention on therapists' mental health practices with older adults. *American Journal of Occupational Therapists, 65,* 297–305.

Mackenzie, C. S., Reynolds, K., Chou, K.-L., Pagura, J., & Sareen, J. (2011). Prevalence and correlates of generalized anxiety disorder in a national sample of older adults. *American Journal of Geriatric Psychiatry, 19,* 305–315.

McSherry, C. B. (2011). The inner life at the end of life. *Journal of Hospice & Palliative Nursing, 13*(2), 112–120.

Mezey, M. D., & Mitty, E. (2011). A Bill of Rights for hospitalized older adults. *The Journal of Nursing Administration, 41*(3), 115–121.

Nunney, J., Raynor, D. K., Knapp, P., & Closs, S. J. (2011). How do the attitudes and beliefs of older people and healthcare professionals impact on the use of multi-compartment compliance aids?: A qualitative study using grounded theory. *Drugs & Aging, 28*(5), 403–414.

Seo, H. J., Jung, Y. E., Kim, T. S., Kim, J. B., Lee, M. S., Kim, J. M., . . . Jun, T. Y. (2011). Distinctive clinical characteristics and suicidal tendencies of patients with anxious depression. *Journal of Mental and Nervous Disease, 199*(1), 42–48.

Suicide.org, Suicide Prevention, Awareness, and Support. (2011). *Elderly suicide.* Retrieved from http://www.suicide.org/elderly-suicide.html

Trigoboff, E., Wilson, B. A., Shannon, M. T., & Stang, C. L. (2005). *Psychiatric drug guide.* Upper Saddle River, NJ: Prentice Hall.

Unverzagt, F. W., Ogunniyi, A., Taler, V., Gao, S., Lane, K. A., Baiyewu, O., . . . Hall, K. S. (2011). Incidence and risk factors for cognitive impairment no dementia and mild cognitive impairment in African Americans. *Alzheimer Disease and Associated Disorders, 25,* 4–10.

Volkers, K. M., & Scherder, E. D. (2011). Impoverished environment, cognition, aging, and dementia. *Reviews in the Neurosciences, 22*(3), 259–266.

6
UNIT

INTERVENTION STRATEGIES

PARVIN and SHARMA are happy to be able to shop for rugs at a market stall in Jalalabad, Afghanistan, and draw their blue burkas even closer about them. They feel much luckier than their friend, Foruzan. Foruzans' husband beat her severely and threw her out of the house because she would not stop crying and threatened to kill herself. She is believed to be possessed by a *jinn*, an evil spirit that causes the symptoms of her depression. Foruzan is now chained to a tree at the Mia Ali Saeb Shrine (a religious site that takes in the mentally ill for 40 days so that God can cure them).

Afghanistan is the only country in the world where the suicide rate is higher for women than it is for men. It is likely that this relates to the culturally sanctioned social deprivation of women through a system of strict gender segregation, frequent domestic and sexual violence, and the effects of living in a combat zone—witnessing violence to others, being injured, experiencing the death or disappearance of close relatives and friends, seeing mutilated or dead bodies, and forced displacement.

Mental illness is misunderstood and stigmatized in Afghanistan. In this socially conservative country people self-medicate with alcohol and opium, which is plentiful in the poppy-growing areas in the south and east. Psychotropic medications are in short supply and there are few psychiatrists, few facilities for mental health care, and virtually no psychiatric nurses.

28

Therapeutic Groups

CAROL REN KNEISL

LEARNING OUTCOMES

After completing this chapter, you will be able to:

1. Apply the general principles of the Johari Window to create opportunities for change and learning in small groups.
2. Encourage the assumption of appropriate task roles and maintenance roles among members of small groups.
3. Improve the dynamics of small groups by incorporating an understanding of the interpersonal needs of inclusion, affection, and control.
4. Explain the purposes that therapeutic groups fulfill.
5. Design a therapeutic group based on the needs and personality characteristics of potential members.
6. Apply the process of here-and-now activation to a therapeutic group.
7. Develop process commentary appropriate to the level and purposes of the group.
8. Maintain a therapeutic group based on the needs of a specific population in inpatient or community settings.

CRITICAL THINKING CHALLENGE

The staff members of a long-term inpatient unit in a state psychiatric hospital were mandated to provide two daily group sessions for all clients. The clients had varying psychiatric diagnoses—mainly bipolar disorder, schizophrenia, major depression, schizoaffective disorder, and obsessive–compulsive disorder. The only area that could accommodate all of the clients (28–30 at any one time) was a large day room in which the chairs were set in a square. The nurses' station desk with telephones, and a locked door through which others entered and exited the unit, were also located in the day room.

1. Which elements of the environment might interfere with the smooth functioning of a group? Why?
2. How would the client characteristics facilitate or hinder the group process?
3. What kinds of group activities would be appropriate given the population of clients and the environmental circumstances?

Why are groups important? Most people are born into a group—the family—and our survival from the moment of birth depends on relationships formed with other human beings. Our sense of self, of being, and of personal identity derives from the ways in which other members of the groups to which we belong perceive and respond to us. We interact with others at all stages of our lives in various groups—family groups, peer groups, work groups, play groups, worship groups. Many of the goals we set for ourselves cannot be achieved without membership in groups. Through cooperation and coordination we can achieve objectives and reach goals that we could not through individual effort alone. In this way, groups help us improve the quality of our lives.

Much of our professional life is spent in groups—groups of clients and groups of colleagues with whom we plan and implement the delivery of health care services. Nurses have long been involved in working with clients in small groups brought together for health teaching, psychoeducation, or supportive purposes in inpatient facilities and in community-based agencies as well. All nurses, regardless of level of education, can lead therapeutic groups or psychoeducation groups as long as they understand and apply group dynamics in their interventions. In fact, group interventions will become increasingly more important in this economy as a result of the need to provide treatments that are also cost effective. However, the role of the psychiatric–mental health nurse as group psychotherapist is reserved for advanced-practice registered nurses prepared at the master's level and above (see Chapter 2∞, which discusses psychiatric–mental health nursing roles in relationship to education, preparation, and certification). Psychiatric–mental health nurses at the generalist level are qualified, with appropriate preparation, to lead the therapeutic support groups described later in this chapter.

To use groups rationally and effectively, you must understand the forces that underlie small group interactional processes. Using group interventions, you can provide psychoeducation for your clients and their families. Therapeutic groups offer clients the opportunity to seek validation, give and receive interpersonal feedback, and test new and different ways of being that may improve the quality of life. Mental health can be preserved, maintained, and restored through interaction with others in productive groups.

SMALL GROUP DYNAMICS

Several forces modify and shape groups, influencing their effectiveness. These forces are discussed in the sections that follow.

Trust

Trust develops in relationships when people disclose more and more of their thoughts, perceptions, attitudes, and reactions to one another and find that their disclosures have been made in a safe environment among persons who respect their self-disclosures. The group member who makes a suggestion; discloses an attitude, feeling, experience, or perception; gives feedback; or confronts another member engages in trusting behavior and assumes the risks inherent in trusting. Trusting and being trusted are intimately linked to risk taking. The level of trust among the members of a group determines the extent of risk-taking behavior in the group. When trust exists, individual members will risk sharing more. Because trust takes some time to build, do not expect that trust will necessarily exist in short-term inpatient groups in which membership changes frequently in a brief period of time.

Self-Disclosure and Self-Awareness

There are many ways to think about self-awareness. Some theorists have used the image of multiple masks that people wear under a variety of circumstances. Others have written about the "true self" versus "the false self" or the "good me," the "bad me," and the "real me." Common to all these concepts is the idea that self-awareness is a complex, multidimensional phenomenon, often contradictory and partly undiscovered. The Johari Awareness Model, often called simply the **Johari Window**, is a theoretical tool used to represent self-awareness and self-disclosure in relation to other people. The notion of self-disclosure has been discussed in general in Chapter 4∞. This section discusses a theory of self-disclosure that can be applied to the understanding of individuals as well as therapeutic groups.

The Johari Awareness Model maintains that interpersonal interaction, in a group setting for example, is facilitated when people have sufficient knowledge about one another's attitudes, beliefs, actions, and opinions to determine how safe it is to self-disclose. The Johari Window is a graphic representation of this self-awareness model. It is described here and illustrated in Figure 28-1 ■ :

■ *Johari Window Quadrant 1:* Open Activity (known to self and known to others). Quadrant 1of the window represents aspects of the self that are known to you and are readily available and known to others as well. This is the part of the self that engages in daily

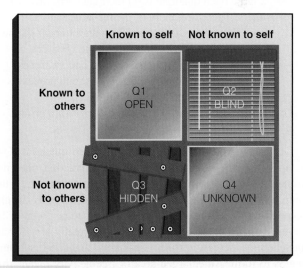

FIGURE 28-1 ■ Johari Window of self-disclosure.
Source: Adapted from Beebe, S. A., Beebe, S. J., & Redmond, M. V. (2011). *Interpersonal communication: Relating to others* (6th ed.). Boston, MA: Allyn & Bacon, p. 54.

social conversation. The more you reveal about yourself, the larger this quadrant will be.

- *Johari Window Quadrant 2:* Blind (not known to self but known to others). Quadrant 2 contains characteristics that are known to others but not to yourself. In this quadrant is information about how you affect others intentionally or unintentionally. It is an aspect of self about which you may get honest, genuine, uncensored feedback from others that may surprise you. In this case, the blind window gets smaller.
- *Johari Window Quadrant 3*: Hidden (known to self but not known to others). Quadrant 3 represents the private life space—knowledge you have about yourself that is not known to others. These are the secrets, the personal and private feelings, thoughts, and fantasies that you have but that you do not want others to know.
- *Johari Window Quadrant 4:* Unknown (not known to self or others). Quadrant 4 contains knowledge about yourself that you do not know *yet* and is also unknown to others. Eventually, some of this knowledge becomes known to you or to both you and others. This quadrant also represents unconscious processes that may be brought into awareness through psychotherapy.

Relations Within the Group

Major elements in this awareness model are its assumptions that humans respond to groups and that change or learning can follow opportunities for new interaction. The primary principle of change in relation to the Johari Window is: A change in one quadrant will affect all other quadrants. Certain other general principles of change that derive from the Johari Window are particularly suited to the understanding of small group behavior. These principles are:

- A large open quadrant (Q1) facilitates working with others. Therefore, more of the resources and abilities of group members can be brought to bear on the group task when members have large Q1 areas.
- The open quadrant can be enlarged and awareness can be increased by learning about group processes as they are being experienced.
- The group's value system influences how a group confronts the unknown quadrant.

In a new and immature group, the open quadrant (Q1) is small because free and spontaneous interaction does not immediately occur in new groups. As the group matures, the open quadrant expands and the private quadrant (Q3) shrinks accordingly. This means that members become freer to be themselves and to perceive others as they really are. An atmosphere of increasing trust, risk-taking, and self-disclosure begins to form. An enlarged area of free activity means that the group uses more energy to work on the group task than to maintain or defend the hidden or avoided area of Q3. The blind quadrant (Q2) also diminishes as members learn more

FIGURE 28-2 ■ Johari Window self-awareness configuration of the immature versus mature group.

about themselves. Dealing with blind spots requires sensitivity, empathy, and timing (Gans, 2011). The unknown quadrant (Q4) changes more slowly and to a lesser degree, because it represents an area in which unknown behaviors and motives reside. FIGURE 28-2 ■ compares the degrees of openness in immature and mature groups.

A group can also be understood and diagrammed according to the Johari Windows of the individual members.

Clinical Example

Sam was a person with limited freedom. Although he was polite, he appeared to be superficial and constricted. He devoted large amounts of energy to walling off the behavior and motivations of the blind, private, and unknown quadrants (Q2, Q3, and Q4) by intellectualizing.

Laura was a group member whose great inner resources allowed her to develop a very large area of free activity.

In contrast, Debbie was what could be termed a "plunger." Debbie's spontaneity and inappropriate openness lacked discretion and created distance in her relationships with other group members.

Van and Maria, the other two members of this group, tended not to take many risks in their interactions with others, although their moderate openness indicated flexibility.

The Johari Window configurations of the group members in the clinical example are illustrated in FIGURE 28-3 ■:

- Sam's window shows a greatly reduced and constricted open quadrant. His behavior and feelings are likely to be limited in range, variety, and scope. His interactions tend to be conventional, and he is likely to be threatened by group behaviors that go beyond the bounds of convention.
- Laura's window represents a person whose interactions are characterized by great openness to the world. Much of her potential has been developed and realized.
- Debbie's window is that of the inappropriately transparent person who deals with others by disclosing too much.
- Maria's and Van's windows show moderately large open areas although Q2, Q3, and Q4 are equally large.

The group members' windows raise an interesting question: What behaviors might be predicted in a group with

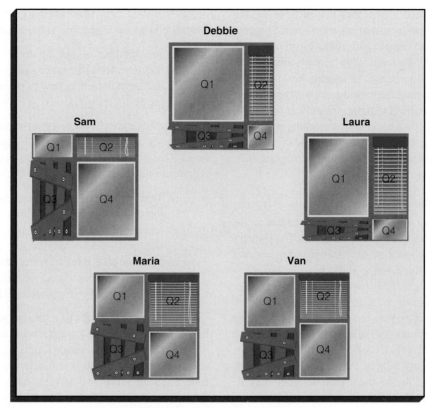

FIGURE 28-3 ▦ Johari Window self-awareness configurations of the members of one group.

members such as these? Obviously, this group needs to resolve several problems. An underddiscloser like Sam reveals too little, thus reserving control for himself. He tends to quell spontaneous reactions in order to double check. He may be one of the last to acknowledge the development of trust.

Debbie's failure to control her overdisclosure means that her relationships with others in the group will be either too smothering (because of being too close) or too demanding because she imposes herself on others without considering their intimacy needs. She discloses to everyone because she has not learned to discriminate among relationships. Her behavior forces others to take responsibility for defining the nature of the relationship. Group members are likely to feel threatened by her early, spontaneous disclosures, which they may experience as overwhelming. Problems of trust, intimacy, and risk taking may arise in her interactions with the other members.

Laura, because of her high degree of self-awareness, will be less preoccupied with defensiveness and differences than other members. She will be able to accept the differences in others and serve as a role model for them.

Van and Maria, whose awareness configurations demonstrate that they have progressed to moderate openness, should continue to move in this direction with minimal discomfort to themselves or the other group members.

Cohesion

Cohesion can be defined as a spirit of common purpose. In groups that cohere (hang together), the members have a desire for mutual association. Cohesion is the primary factor keeping a group in existence and working effectively (Norcross & Wampold, 2011).

A group is cohesive when its members are attracted to it. People are attracted to a therapeutic group for a wide variety of reasons. The group may meet their needs for affiliation, interpersonal security, self-knowledge, or therapy. It may have members who not only are available for human interaction but also have important shared attitudes, values, interests, and beliefs. An attractive group has explicit, mutual, and attainable group goals with clear paths to goal attainment.

What indicates that the spirit of cohesion exists in a given group?

- Attendance is high.
- The members arrive on time.
- The members stay with the group.
- The members engage in an interdependence that is cooperative rather than competitive.
- The activities the group undertakes are satisfying and successful.
- There is a high degree of member participation.
- Communication networks are open, central, and flexible in a warm and friendly atmosphere.
- "We" is frequently heard in discussions.
- The members like and trust one another.
- The members enjoy interacting with one another.
- Participation is high.

Cohesive groups are not born—they are developed. Cohesion does not become evident until the group has come together long enough to have shared experiences that provide the basis for attraction. An outpatient group has an existence lengthy enough to provide time for cohesion to develop. Inpatient groups on acute care units are usually too brief to become cohesive.

How can a group's tendency to cohere be enhanced? Some methods are increasing the trusting and trustworthy behavior of members, the affection expressed among members, the expressions of inclusion and acceptance among members, and the influence that members have on one another. Another method for building cohesion is structuring cooperative relationships among the group members.

Group Roles and Leadership

Leadership is a process of influence. Group roles center on the influence relationships that exist within the group. The primary influence relationship is leadership. An effective group leader is the catalyst for, and facilitator of, the group process. An effective group leader helps focus and shape the group discussion, motivates group members to participate, encourages a group to remain on track, and empowers the group to make creative decisions. In general, a good leader is successful in helping the group accomplish its goals (Harris & Sherblom, 2011).

Group dynamics theory tells us that leadership functions within a group can be fulfilled by the person designated as the leader, and by members who engage in leadership behavior. This approach to understanding leadership behavior is called the *distributed functions approach* and stems from the classic research of Benne and Sheats (1948). The distributed functions approach to group leadership is based on two major beliefs:

1. Any member of a group may become a leader by taking actions that serve group purposes.
2. Different members may perform various roles in a group.

Each member may play more than one role during a meeting of the group and a wide range of roles in successive participations. Any member may play any or all of the roles. The various functional roles may be grouped in two categories:

1. **Task roles** are related to the task of the group. The job of people assuming these roles is to facilitate and coordinate group efforts in the selection, definition, and solution of a group problem.
2. **Maintenance roles** are oriented toward building group-centered attitudes among the members and maintaining and perpetuating group-centered behavior.

Sometimes members of a group satisfy individual needs that are irrelevant to the group task and may also be negatively oriented to group maintenance functions. These are called **self-serving roles**. If a group is to function effectively, it must perform a self-diagnosis to determine what the needs of the group are and how they can be met, so that the self-serving roles no longer present obstacles to effective functioning. Task, maintenance, and self-serving roles are described in TABLE 28-1 ■.

TABLE 28-1 ■ Group Roles and Functions

Role	Function
Task Roles	
Coordinator	Identifies the relationships among the group suggestions and ideas
Elaborator	Fleshes out ideas and suggestions (arranging seating; distributing handouts)
Information giver	Offers facts, ideas, and own experiences
Information seeker	Asks for information that would clarify issues
Opinion giver	States beliefs about group function and group values
Opinion seeker	Asks for beliefs that would clarify group values
Maintenance Roles	
Compromiser	Minimizes conflict by seeking alternatives
Encourager	Moves the group in a positive direction by encouraging and praising the contributions of others
Follower	Goes along with the group
Group observer	Keeps the group records; interprets data
Harmonizer	Keeps the peace; smoothes over conflict
Standard setter	Reminds group of the standards to be achieved
Self-Serving Roles	
Aggressor	Attacks group members, ideas, or values
Blocker	Disagrees, opposes, and resists
Dominator	Manipulates others, seeks control through excessive talking; interrupts others
Playboy	Fails to become involved in group process
Recognition seeker	Boasts, brags about accomplishments, calls attention to self
Self-confessor	Expresses personal and self-oriented, rather than group-oriented, insights and feelings

Source: Adapted from Harris, T. E., & Sherblom, J. C. (2011). Small group and team communication, 5th ed. Boston: Allyn & Bacon, pp. 46–47.

Distributing leadership functions among group members is important because it teaches people the diagnostic skills and behaviors needed to accomplish the group's goals and maintain good interpersonal relationships. Of course, in psychotherapy groups, some functions or activities may be largely, or even solely, the province of the therapist. In psychotherapy groups, the quality of the therapeutic alliance with the group therapist was a consistent predictor of short-term group therapy outcome (Joyce, Piper, & Ogrodniczuk, 2007).

Power and Influence

It is impossible to discuss group dynamics without discussing power because it is impossible to interact without influencing, and being influenced by, others. This process constantly occurs within groups, forcing members to adjust to one another and modify their behavior and, sometimes, their attitudes and beliefs. Power is defined as the ability to do or act, to have possession of command or control over others, or to achieve the desired result. The terms *power* and *influence* are used interchangeably in this chapter.

Power and influence are not negative forces. Do not confuse the judicious use of power in building effective groups with the use of power to control, manage, and manipulate others. Become aware of how you can employ power and influence in serving your clients and your profession.

A group in which certain members have much power and others have little power is likely to be a group in trouble. The unequal distribution of power affects both the task and the maintenance functions of a group. Members who believe they have little influence within the group are unlikely to feel committed to group goals and to the implementation of group decisions. Their dissatisfaction with the group decreases its attractiveness and reduces its cohesion.

Group Developmental Phases

As you will see in this chapter, group development is not always orderly. Not all groups proceed through the stages in the order discussed here, although the following stages describe common experiences.

Forming

In this beginning stage, the members are beginning to know one another, the purpose of the group, and their place or role in the group. Because the group has not yet established its norms (rules), unease, tension, and awkwardness are normal (Harris & Sherblom, 2011). Gradually, people begin to relax and devote themselves to the task. Members are reluctant to self-disclose until issues of confidentiality are understood. Only then can members begin to build interpersonal trust. Getting to know other members of the group helps, but does not remove all anxiety. Concerns about other group members and their intentions, one's own role in the group, and the process, purpose, and goals of the group remain. These concerns lead to the second group stage—storming.

Storming

In this phase, conflict inevitably erupts, usually over such issues as power, authority, and competition within the group. In this stage, the politeness that characterized the first phase (forming) is replaced by more forthright opinions that are not based on keeping things "nice." In other words, the communication among members is more open and authentic. Successfully resolving this stage of conflict allows the group to move toward cohesion as members become more interdependent upon one another. However, groups that avoid or suppress conflicts may create a continuing tension that stifles the development of cohesion, decision-making, and problem-solving abilities. The secret to moving on and becoming an effective group is based on the ability of the group to air their conflicts and work through them.

Norming

Once differences are expressed and conflicts have subsided, the group begins to become more cohesive. The relationships among members are more open and trusting and cooperation among the members has increased. The storming phase has given members the opportunity to test one another's reactions. However, just because conflicts have subsided does not mean that they are totally resolved. It is normal for groups to move back and forth between stages. Norming is an important stage in the group's development. During this stage, the group settles on specific rules—how discussions take place, how decisions will be made, which issues of the storming phase need to be revisited, how the labor in the group is to be divided, and how goals, roles, and expectations are negotiated.

Performing

Performing is the real work phase of the group (Harris & Sherblom, 2011). Members increase their focus on the task at hand. There is an open exchange of information and the giving and receiving of feedback. Social tensions decrease as the group moves toward solving the task of the group. The group identifies possible solutions and looks at what impact the possible solutions can have. They engage in the problem-solving process using the nine-step problem-solving process in Your Intervention Strategies on page 63 of Chapter 4∞. Group members share the facts and data they possess and make sure that all members understand the facts and data. They treat all ideas as welcome and piggyback off one another's ideas. They look at the positive and negative aspects of each solution before devising a plan of action.

Terminating

The final phase in the group process is terminating. Ideally, groups experience termination because they have completed their task and stop meeting together. Termination aspects may be experienced in earlier phases of the group if members leave the group for any reason. Termination is not without its stresses, especially if the group is a long-standing one and its purpose is more interpersonal (psychotherapy, support, self-awareness) than one oriented toward solving a specific problem (determining the unit rules on a psychiatric inpatient unit). Termination is an opportunity for members to say good-bye. Some groups mark the end of the group with a special event to experience a sense of closure.

Clinical Example

A group of eight senior nursing students were ending their 10-week clinical experience on a long-term inpatient unit at a state psychiatric hospital. They planned a special event for their last day—a combination psycho-education experience with a special treat for the clients. The nursing students developed a program for the clients that focused on the benefits to brain function and cognition of certain vitamins and minerals found in fruits. After a poster presentation and a show-and-tell of pineapples, papayas, mango, oranges, cantaloupe, strawberries, and kiwi, the clients were given a bowl of these fruits unlikely to be found on the menus of most long-term inpatient psychiatric facilities.

The activity allowed students and clients to finish on a positive note. The students provided an educational experience, surprised the clients with an unusual treat, and ensured an opportunity for clients and students to say their goodbyes to one another.

GROUP DEVELOPMENT THEORY

The interpersonal needs approach discussed in this section can be used to understand the development, dynamics, and functioning of small groups, from mutual-help or self-help groups to psychoeducation groups to psychotherapy groups. The interpersonal needs approach helps us to understand how groups develop and the factors that determine how effective they are.

The basic assumption of the interpersonal needs approach known as FIRO (fundamental interpersonal relationship orientation), a classic group dynamics theory, is that people need people. In addition, people need to establish some equilibrium between themselves and the others in their environment. This equilibrium is determined by the interaction of three basic interpersonal needs, and it appears to be synonymous with interpersonal compatibility (Schutz, 1958b).

Three Basic Interpersonal Needs

An interpersonal need is one that can be satisfied only through relationships with people. Schutz reasoned that every individual has three interpersonal needs: inclusion, control, and affection.

Inclusion

The interpersonal need for *inclusion* is the need to establish and maintain relationships with others that offer interactions and associations satisfying to you. To put it another way, the **inclusion need** consists of the ability to take an interest in others to a satisfactory degree, and the ability to allow other people to take an interest in you to a satisfying degree to yourself. This need determines whether a person is outgoing or prefers privacy. Compare the inclusion needs illustrated in FIGURE 28-4 ■.

Control

The interpersonal need for *control* is the need to establish and maintain a satisfactory relationship between yourself

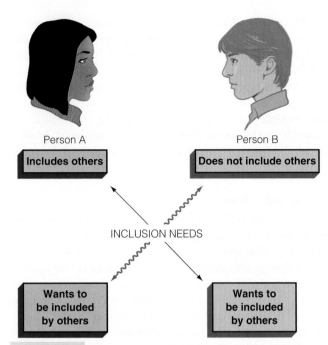

FIGURE 28-4 ■ Inclusion needs. While both people want to be included by others, only one (Person A) includes others. Therefore, Person B's needs for inclusion are met. However, Person A will feel frustrated because her need to be included is not being met.

and other people with regard to power and influence. Stated another way, the **control need** consists of the ability to take charge to a satisfactory degree, and the ability to establish and maintain a feeling of respect for the competence and responsibleness of others to a satisfying degree to yourself. Compare the control needs illustrated in FIGURE 28-5 ■.

Affection

The interpersonal need for *affection* is the need to establish and maintain a satisfactory relationship between yourself and other people with regard to love and affection. Put another way, the **affection need** consists of being able to love other people or to be close and intimate to a satisfactory degree, and having others love you or be close and intimate with you to a satisfactory degree. Compare the affection needs illustrated in FIGURE 28-6 ■.

Interpersonal Group Phases

According to this approach, any group, given enough time, moves through three interpersonal phases—inclusion, control, and affection, in that order—that correspond to the three basic interpersonal needs.

Inclusion Phase

The first, or inclusion, phase is concerned with the problem of *in or out*. People attempt to find their place in the group and are concerned with learning whether they will be acknowledged as individuals or left behind and ignored. Because these concerns give rise to anxiety, this phase is dominated by behavior centered around the self. Overtalking, withdrawal, exhibitionism, and sharing other group experiences and biographies are some examples.

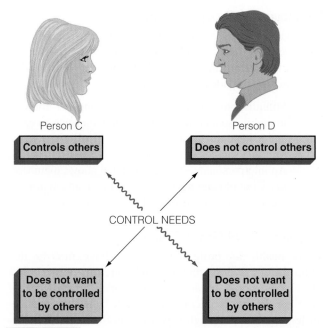

FIGURE 28-5 ■ Control needs. This situation has the potential for great conflict. Person D, who is happiest in a lackadaisical atmosphere, will resent, and perhaps sabotage, Person C's efforts to control. Person C is likely to intensify her control efforts in response.

Frequently, what Schutz (1958a) calls **goblet issues** predominate. These are issues of minor importance to the group that help the members get to know one another better and to test each other out. Goblet issues are a vehicle for sizing people up. Goblet issues may revolve around the weather, sports,

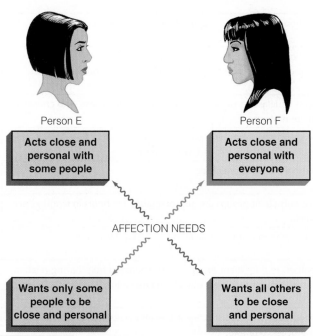

FIGURE 28-6 ■ Affection needs. Both people in this situation are getting some of their affection needs met if Person F is one of the people with whom Person E wishes to be close and personal. If not, Person E could back away emotionally if she views Person F as intrusive. Backing away would likely cause frustration for Person F.

rules of procedure, and so on. If goblet issues continue to a significant extent beyond this initial phase of the group, they will impede group progress.

Control Phase

The second, or control, phase is concerned with the problem of *top or bottom,* which becomes central after problems of inclusion have been resolved. Concern about decision-making procedures predominates. The problems that emerge in this phase center around the following two concerns:

1. How responsibility is shared
2. How power and influence are distributed

There are struggles for leadership and about the structure, rules of procedure, and methods of decision making. Members are attempting to establish comfortable positions for themselves in terms of responsibility and influence.

Affection Phase

The third, or affection, phase is concerned with the problem of *near or far,* and it follows satisfactory resolution of the preceding two phases. Individual members are now faced with the problem of becoming emotionally involved with one another. Concerns about not being liked by, being too close to, or not being close enough to others, become relevant. The behavior in this phase is generally characterized by high emotion—positive feelings, jealousy, hostility, and pairing are some examples. Schutz (1958a) describes this phase as one in which, like porcupines, people attempt to get close enough to receive warmth, yet avoid the pain that sharp quills can inflict.

Interweaving of Phases

None of these phases is distinct, because all three problem areas—in or out, near or far, top or bottom—are present at all times, even though only one predominates. Schutz (1958a) uses a tire-changing analogy, what he calls *tightening the bolts,* to describe the sequence of the phases. Changing a tire is best done by tightening the bolts just enough to hold the wheel in place. Then each bolt is tightened further until it is secured. The leader helps the group work on all three interpersonal need areas in similar fashion, returning to and working over each area to a more satisfactory level than was reached the last time. The interpersonal needs approach of Schutz is based on the belief that the way to attack problems within groups is by investigating what is going on among the individuals in the group and attempting to improve their interpersonal relations. You will discover a parallel between this group development theory and Yalom's group therapy theory, discussed in the next section.

GROUP THERAPY THEORY

There is great diversity and flux in the field of group therapy. Many types of groups are found in mental health care settings or in communities at large. However, certain common principles seem to apply to all therapeutic groups, although specific methods and techniques may vary according to the purpose of the group or the skills and theoretic orientation of the therapist or group leader.

Irvin Yalom (2005) uses the term *interactional group therapy* to describe a process of group therapy in which member interaction plays a crucial role. In **group therapy**, six to eight members come together to learn about themselves and their relationships with others as a means of improving their mental health (see Advantages of Group Therapy in the next section for a complete discussion of the purposes and the common principles that apply to interactional group therapy).

The psychiatric–mental health nurse, even if not an advanced-practice nurse qualified as a group psychotherapist, can incorporate many of these principles of group therapy into the leadership role in therapeutic groups as well as in informal groups in the milieu. The principles will have a sense of familiarity—Yalom, like Hildegard Peplau (see Chapter 2∞) was greatly influenced by the interpersonal theory of Harry Stack Sullivan (see Chapter 5∞). You will need to modify the principles for use in short-term groups, such as those in effect on most inpatient units. Modifications for short-term inpatient groups are discussed throughout this section. Essential differences between inpatient and outpatient groups are identified in TABLE 28-2 ■ .

Advantages of Group Therapy

The advantages of group therapy stem from one major factor: the presence of many people, rather than a solitary therapist, who participate in the therapeutic experience. Specifically, group therapy provides the following:

- Stimuli from multiple sources, revealing distortions in interpersonal relationships so that they can be examined and resolved
- Multiple sources of feedback
- An interpersonal testing ground that allows members to try out old and new ways of being in an environment specifically structured for that purpose

Qualifications of Group Therapists

Mental health care professionals may believe, in error, that group therapy is less complex and therefore "easier" than one-to-one work—because, for example, the presence of more people makes interactions between therapist and client less intense. Although it is true that the interactions between any one member and the therapist may be less intense because interactions are dispersed among others, it does not follow that anyone can be an effective group therapist. Rather, group processes are very complex because the interactions occur among many different personalities. To be

TABLE 28-2 ■ Differences Between Inpatient and Outpatient Groups

Inpatient Groups	Outpatient Groups
The composition of the group changes depending on who has been admitted and who has been discharged.	The composition of the group is stable, usually over its life.
Members may be selected because they happen to be clients on a particular unit or assigned to a particular therapist.	Selection criteria play a major role in designing the group.
Although clients may be assigned to one or another of available groups depending on appropriateness, selection interviews are not usually conducted.	Selection interviews are standard practice to prepare clients for the group experience and to establish and clarify the group contract.
Attendance is compulsory and clients are often wary of, or ambivalent about, attending the group.	Clients usually choose whether to join a group. Those who choose to join are motivated.
Membership length is determined by the length of hospitalization. When the client is discharged, membership in the group ends.	The group continues for a predetermined length of time identified in the group contract—often 1 year or more.
The goal is relief of symptoms, possibly some degree of self-awareness, support, and/or psychoeducation.	The goal is insight-oriented.
Sessions are usually 30–45 minutes long, daily or several times a week, and are based on the clients' tolerance level.	Most outpatient groups are approximately 1½ hours in length, once a week.
Because of the continually changing membership, inpatient groups on acute care units rarely become cohesive.	Group cohesion can be expected to develop over time.
Group members have 24-hour exposure to one another; therefore, what goes on in the milieu outside of the group influences what goes on inside the group.	Members in outpatient groups are discouraged from having relationships with other members outside the meetings.
The inpatient therapist provides a greater degree of structure and takes on a more active role because of the clients' needs.	The outpatient therapist is less active and waits for the structure and the process to unfold.
Because the therapist has limited ability to select who will be in the group, the group tends to be heterogenous in terms of vulnerability or ego strength as well as personality characteristics.	Outpatient therapists usually design their groups to balance the behavior and characteristics the members bring to the group. The members are more likely to be homogenous in terms of their ego strength.

effective, the group therapist should have the following special preparation:

- Education in small group dynamics
- Education in group therapy theory
- Clinical practice with groups
- Expert supervision of the clinical practice (with ongoing supervision and/or consultation, depending on level of expertise)

Experienced therapists report that it is also valuable to have been a member of a therapy or sensitivity training group before becoming a group leader.

The Curative Factors

Yalom (2005) contends that 11 interdependent *curative factors* or mechanisms of change in group therapy help people.

These factors constitute a rational basis for the therapist's choices of tactics and strategies and are identified and defined in TABLE 28-3 ■. Yalom recommends group therapy as a means for achieving genuine encounters with other members and the group therapist (Yalom, 2009).

Types of Group Leadership

Groups can be led by a therapist working alone or by cotherapists working together in a variety of ways.

Single Therapist Approach

Groups led by a single therapist are common. They have an economic advantage in that only one therapist need be involved. A disadvantage is that the therapist cannot compare analyses of the group process with a cotherapist or get instant

TABLE 28-3 ■ Curative Factors of Group Therapy

Factor	Definition
Instilling hope	■ Establishing a sense of optimism for change and the success of the group therapy experience ■ Calling attention to the improvement that group members have made
Universality	■ Confirming that group members experience similar pain and struggles ■ Disconfirming that the client is alone or unique in misery or hurt to provide a powerful sense of relief
Imparting information	■ Sharing didactic information or advice about recovery, strategies, resources, and coping behaviors ■ Providing psychoeducation
Altruism	■ Finding that the members can be of importance to others and have something of value to give ■ Gaining from the act of giving
Corrective recapitulation of the primary family group	■ Reviewing and correctively reliving early familial conflicts and growth-inhibiting relationships in a more supportive environment ■ Challenging and exploring fixed roles ■ Working through unfinished business
Development of socializing techniques	■ Acquiring basic social skills, e.g., preparing for discharge, approaching a prospective employer, asking someone out on a date ■ Acquiring sophisticated social skills, e.g., resolving conflicts, being attuned to process, being facilitative toward others
Imitative behavior	■ Trying out bits and pieces of the behavior of the therapist and the members and experimenting with those that fit well ■ Benefiting by observing the therapy of another member
Interpersonal learning	■ Learning that one authors one's own interpersonal world, and therefore, one has the power to change it ■ Comparing one's interpersonal evaluations with those of others and altering distortions (consensual validation) ■ Learning how to adapt and to take on perspectives other than one's own
Group cohesiveness	■ Being attracted to the group and the other members with a sense of "we"-ness rather than "I"-ness ■ Being included, accepted, and involved meaningfully with the other members
Catharsis	■ Being able to express feeling as a way of acquiring skills for the future ■ Feeling a sense of liberation by being able to get relief in a supportive group
Existential factors	■ Being able to "be" with others, to be a part of a group ■ Taking ultimate responsibility ■ Self-realization

Source: Yalom, I. D. (2005). *The theory and practice of group psychotherapy* (5th ed.). New York, NY: Basic Books.

feedback or validation from a peer. Therapists working alone, however, do not have to direct their energies toward creating and maintaining a relationship with a colleague.

Cotherapy Approach

Groups led by two therapists, who share responsibility for leadership of the group to varying degrees, are gaining in popularity. The two models seen most often are the junior–senior and the egalitarian styles of cotherapy.

Junior–Senior Cotherapy In the junior–senior approach, the therapists have unequal responsibilities toward the group. The senior member of the team is usually the more experienced or educated. Besides having major responsibility for the success of the group, the senior therapist is responsible for training the junior member of the team.

This approach is commonly used in agency settings, because it provides in-service training of new personnel and nonprofessionals under the guidance and watchful eye of an experienced group leader. However, the members of the group may be unclear about the subordinate/superordinate roles and unsure of how to deal with, and respond to, leaders of unequal abilities and responsibilities.

Egalitarian Cotherapy In the egalitarian approach to cotherapy, two therapists of relatively equal ability and status share equally in responsibility for the group. Two nurses considering an egalitarian cotherapy relationship with each other need to engage in preliminary work to determine whether such a relationship is feasible for them. Exploration should include the following:

- Discussing each therapist's theoretic approaches, intervention styles, past experiences with groups, sociocultural background, and personality characteristics
- Considering and resolving such issues as how and when feedback is to be given, how disagreements between them are to be handled in the session, and the general conditions under which they will work together
- Agreeing that decisions on client selection, length and number of sessions, time, and place are made together, and that decisions of an emergency nature made by one therapist in the absence of the other are based on mutually agreed-upon procedures for just such situations

Obviously, egalitarian cotherapists must establish and maintain clear channels of communication. Not only must they expend a great deal of time and energy in preparation for the group experience, they must also plan for presession and postsession meetings, joint analysis of data, and joint supervision or consultation.

Creating the Group

The effectiveness of a group depends greatly on the conditions under which it is created. Much as architects design buildings, therapists design groups with certain functions and characteristics in mind. An interesting example of a group of severely ill clients who manage to achieve their goals is in Mental Health in the Movies.

Selecting Members

Selecting the members is one of the most important functions of group leaders or group therapists, because the quality of the interpersonal relationships among the members constitutes the core of successful group treatment. This is one of the major differences between group and individual therapy.

Clients may be admitted to an inpatient group on the basis of being hospitalized on a particular unit that mandates group therapy for all clients, being assigned to a particular therapist, or because group therapy has been determined to be the most appropriate form of treatment. Group therapists or leaders of therapeutic groups in inpatient units may have little leeway about including specific individuals in the group. Therefore, inpatient

---

MENTAL HEALTH IN THE MOVIES
The Dream Team

Convinced that his four clients at a New Jersey Mental hospital—Billy, Henry, Jack, and Albert—need fresh air and time away from the hospital, Dr. Jeff Weitzman (Dennis Boutsikaris) convinces the administration to allow him to take the group of four to see a baseball game at Yankee Stadium. Billy (Michael Keaton), an easy-to-anger, unpredictable pathologic liar with delusions of grandeur, becomes the "leader" of this group of four. Henry (Christopher Lloyd) is delusional—he believes he is a doctor at the hospital. Jack (Peter Boyle), also delusional, believes that he is Jesus Christ. Albert (Stephen Furst) is a simple and childlike man who needs direction to perform even everyday tasks. (Note that it is unlikely in real life that one staff member alone would independently take four clients with severe psychotic symptoms for such an outing.)

Their plans to attend the baseball game go awry when Dr. Weitzman is knocked unconscious by two crooked cops fleeing the scene of a crime. Stranded, and on their own in New York City without money or a phone, the group is forced to pull together and work in concert in order to cope with their circumstances.

The stereotyping of the clients and their often outlandish, but humorous, behavior are stigmatizing elements of the film. However, the film's saving grace is its portrayal of the ability of four clients to overcome their delusions and disorders in order to work together as a group to save Dr. Weitzman. This positive message overshadows the over-the-top stereotypic portrayals of people with mental disorders.

Photo courtesy of KPA/Heritage Image/Glow Images.

groups tend to have a more heterogeneous composition; that is, the members may vary significantly in terms of their personality characteristics, their vulnerabilities, or their ego strengths. They also tend to be more ambivalent about group therapy. You are encouraged to attempt to apply the following principles, regardless of the nature or location of the group.

It is more difficult to identify the characteristics of people who make good candidates for group therapy than it is to identify people who do not make good candidates. We know that a person's motivation for therapy in general, and group therapy in particular, is of primary importance. Personality variables such as extraversion, openness, and conscientiousness have been found to be directly related to a favorable treatment outcome. Inclusion in a therapy group should also be at least partially determined by the effect a prospective member will have on the others, in terms of the prospective member's ability to bring the curative factors into play (Yalom, 1998). The higher the percentage of members in a therapy group with a history of relatively mature relationships, the better the outcome for the group as a whole.

Selection for a group is also determined by the balance, in terms of behavior or characteristics, a prospective member will bring to the group. Will the person's subdued presentation prevent a member with similar behavior from being marginal and alone in the group? Does the person's age, occupation, cultural background, or sex match another's so that the member will not feel singled out as different or deviant? The factor that appears to be most important, according to Yalom (1998), however, is that members are homogeneous (similar) in terms of their vulnerabilities or ego strengths. Highly vulnerable members retard the progress of the less vulnerable, and vice versa. Yalom's research indicates that, if at all possible, group therapists should avoid including in the group individuals who use denial to a significant extent, differ significantly from others in the group in relation to psychopathology, or have a pervasive dread of self-disclosure (Yalom, 2005).

Selection Interviews

Selection interviews are standard procedure for long-term outpatient groups. They are useful as well for short-term inpatient groups and groups in day hospitals to help determine the most appropriate type of group for each individual client.

The pregroup interview session has two major purposes: selecting the members and establishing the initial contract. Cotherapists should always interview potential members jointly, and both should make all decisions regarding membership. The interview session gives members and therapists the opportunity to be exposed to one another. The therapists should accomplish the following tasks in the selection interview:

- Determine the motivation of the potential member.
- Encourage the client to ask questions about the group.
- Correct erroneous prejudgments or misinformation the client has about group therapy.
- Inquire about any major pending life changes that may prevent the client's full and continued participation in the group.

- Inquire about what hurts—what the client sees as a need to work on.
- Establish and clarify the initial group contract.

During this period, therapists and members have a chance to decide whether they can work together in the specific group under consideration. Many outpatient clients can choose whether they will participate. When clients have the choice of being a member of the group, they tend to be motivated to learn and to change.

Group Contract

The group contract identifies the shared rights and responsibilities of therapists and members. It is a negotiated set of rules or arrangements for the structure and functioning of the group. It may be written or verbal, and it should cover the following elements.

Goals and Purposes The purpose of the group must be clear to all involved. In interactive group psychotherapy, the purpose is to bring about enduring behavioral and character change. The interactive group psychotherapy experience takes place largely in the present, in the here-and-now.

Goals may be long term or short term and are both group oriented and individualized. Some goals may be identified as early as the selection interview, and others may be added as they emerge during the life of the group. You may alter goals as appropriate.

Time, Length, and Frequency of Meetings The time, length, and frequency of meetings should be determined by the therapists after consideration of the clients' needs. Most outpatient clients find one 80- to 90-minute session per week useful. Shorter periods may not allow adequate time for discussion. Longer periods generally tax the endurance and alertness of both members and therapists. Inpatient groups generally meet several times per week, or even daily for about 30 to 45 minutes, although sessions may be longer or shorter depending on the anxiety and tolerance levels of the particular clients.

Place of Meetings The physical environment is important and influences the interaction among members. It is best to choose a pleasant room with comfortable chairs, preferably placed in a circle. The room should be private and free from external distractions.

Starting and Ending Dates If the group has a predetermined life span and the inclusive dates are known, inform the members of the dates. Groups without fixed termination dates usually plan termination individually as each member is ready to move away from the group. Starting and ending dates are determined in inpatient groups by the length of the client's hospitalization.

Addition of New Members Open groups accept members after the first session; closed groups begin with a certain number of members and do not add new members. Open groups maintain their size by replacing members who leave the group. They may continue indefinitely or have a predetermined life span. Open groups are more common in short-term inpatient units where there is rapid turnover. Once the client leaves the inpatient setting, membership in the group ends. This means that because most hospitalizations in acute care settings are of 1 to 3 weeks' duration, there is little time for cohesion to develop. Cohesion develops in outpatient groups and in long-term inpatient units because of their length—1 or more years in duration, and 52 or more meetings.

Closed groups are more common in settings where the stability of membership is likely. Such settings include private practice settings, residential facilities of various types, and prisons. A major problem with the closed group is that it runs the risk of extinction as members leave the group for various reasons.

Attendance It is important that members make a commitment to attend every session. Absences hinder the establishment of cohesion and have a demoralizing effect, especially when perceived as evidence that a member lacks interest or that the group is not attractive and valuable to its members. Stability of membership and high attendance are critical factors in the successful outcome of group therapy (Yalom, 2005).

Confidentiality Establish some rules regarding confidentiality, and explore clients' concerns about who will have access to information about them. Many therapists like to use tape recorders so that their work can be evaluated by supervisors. They must first obtain client agreement before using a tape recorder.

The therapists' employing agency may determine rules about confidentiality and access. In some instances, therapists may be required to make regular notes concerning each member's participation. Therapists may also wish to establish with group members guidelines on confidentiality that allow the therapists to share content with professionals who provide clinical supervision to the therapist, or when clients are dangerous to themselves or others. A good rule of thumb is: *Promise only what you can safely deliver.* You should also hold members accountable for maintaining the confidentiality of the group.

Member Interaction Outside of the Group Members in outpatient groups are discouraged from having relationships with other members outside the meetings. Relationships outside of the group are likely to interfere with the group dynamics because of the formation of social coalitions or dyads. Limiting relationships is impossible in inpatient groups because the members may have 24-hour exposure to one another on the hospital unit or in a residential setting and may also interact with the group therapist while the therapist is functioning in other roles. In fact, interaction with one another is encouraged in inpatient settings.

Participation of Members and Therapists Therapists and clients should reach an understanding about the responsibilities of participants. Clients should be fully informed participants in the therapeutic process. Participants should share their expectations about the behavior and functions of clients and therapists and should clearly understand the modes of participation. Interaction patterns should form pathways among all members and the therapist, as illustrated in FIGURE 28-7 (left) ■.

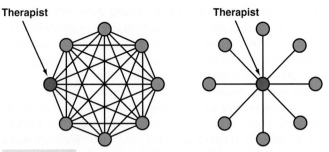

FIGURE 28-7 ■ Comparison of positive and negative interaction patterns in group therapy. The desirable interaction pattern is on the left. The diagram on the right, in which communication is primarily to or through the therapist, is undesirable.

It is important for the inpatient group therapist to provide significantly more structure for the group and to take on a more active role than would be necessary in an outpatient group. Hospitalized inpatients are likely to be in crisis and to be more dysfunctional than outpatients. Passivity on the therapist's part would be destructive to the group and could increase a client's distress. Yalom (1998) suggests a protocol for structuring an inpatient group that is listed in Your Intervention Strategies.

Fees Fees for outpatients should be determined in advance and arrangements for payment made. Most mental health care agencies have a sliding fee scale that is determined by the client's income and ability to pay. Clients should know whether fees will be charged for missed sessions. Fees for inpatients are included in the cost of hospitalization.

Stages in Therapy Group Development

There is comfort in being able to predict, to some extent, the behavior of members at specific points in the group's life. Therapists organize predictions around stages or phases in the therapeutic experience, hoping to be prepared for expressions of behavior. You must bear in mind, however, that human experiences are dynamic and fluid and do not always progress as neatly as predicted.

The Schutz framework, presented earlier, gives clear indications of how group life develops in terms of meeting inclusion, affection, and control needs and the stages of group development discussed on pages 629–631 describe the

---

YOUR INTERVENTION STRATEGIES
Structuring an Inpatient Group

1. 3–5 minutes of orientation, warm-up, or preparation
2. 20–30 minutes for an agenda go-around in which each member may share personal concerns or problems
3. 20–30 minutes in which the therapist attempts to fit the members' agendas together by finding commonalities or threads to work on
4. 3–5 minutes to review the work of the group and to identify the issues or concerns that remain unresolved

Source: Copyright © 1988 Irvin D. Yalom. Reprinted by permission of Basic Books, a member of the Perseus Books Group.

common experiences of group members. This section focuses on the characteristics of member behavior and therapist interventions in the orientation phase (where inclusion needs are more salient), the working phase (where control needs are more salient), and the termination phase (where affection needs are more salient) of interactional group therapy. As members' problems in living are revealed, group life becomes richer and more complex. Therefore, there is no "cookbook" method that a therapist can follow to respond to every situation. Your Intervention Strategies is simply a guide for identifying some common member behaviors and therapist interventions at various points in the life of the group.

Here-and-Now Emphasis

The core of interactional group therapy is the here-and-now. According to Yalom (2005), the here-and-now work of the interactional group therapist occurs on the following two levels:

1. Focusing attention on each member's feelings toward other group members, the therapists, and the group

2. Illuminating the process (the relationship implications of interpersonal transactions)

Thus, group members need to become aware of the here-and-now events—what happened—and then reflect back on them—why it happened. Yalom (2005) calls this the **self-reflective loop** (see FIGURE 28-8 ■).

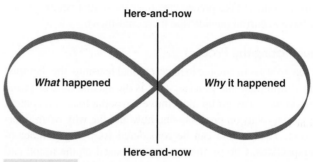

FIGURE 28-8 ■ The self-reflective loop.

YOUR INTERVENTION STRATEGIES   Characteristic Member Behaviors and Nursing Interventions in Phases of Group Therapy

Member Behavior	Nursing Interventions
Beginning Phase	
Anxiety is high.	Move to reduce anxiety; avoid making demands until group anxiety has abated.
Members are unsure of what to do or say; need to be included.	Be active and provide some structure and direction; suggest members introduce themselves; work to sustain therapeutic rather than social role; include all members and encourage sharing but limit monopolizing.
Members are unclear about contract.	Clarify contract; give information to dispel confusion or misunderstandings.
Members test therapists and other members in terms of trustworthiness, value stances, etc., often through goblet issues.	Capitalize on opportunity to "pass" tests by proving trustworthiness and by being open to and accepting the values of others.
Beginning attempts at self-disclosure and problem identification are made.	Focus on related themes; begin exploration; begin to focus on here-and-now experiences in session.
Members have sense of "I"-ness, little sense of "we"-ness.	Encourage involvement with others through curative factor of *universality*.
Middle Phase	
Sense of "I"-ness is replaced by "we"-ness.	Encourage cohesion; provide opportunity for expression of warm feelings.
Self-disclosure increases.	Encourage exploration and move to problem solving.
Members are more aware of interpersonal interactions in the here-and-now.	Encourage members to participate in observing and commenting on the here-and-now; make process comments.
Additions and losses of members evoke strong reactions.	Prepare members for additions and losses where possible; provide opportunity to talk about addition and loss experience.
Ability to maintain focus on one topic increases.	Encourage exploration of topic area in depth.
Termination Phase	
Feelings about separation may run the gamut (anger, sadness, indifference, joy, etc.).	Provide adequate time in as many sessions as necessary to work through affective responses; be sure members know the termination date in advance; help members leave with positive feelings by identifying positive changes that have occurred in individual members and in the group.
Members may feel lost and rudderless.	Explore support systems available to individual members; bridge the gap where possible (to another agency, another therapist, etc.); keep in focus the task of resolving the loss.

Steering the Group into the Here-and-Now

The first task of the therapist is to steer the group into the here-and-now. Yalom calls this process **here-and-now activation**. As the group progresses and becomes comfortable with awareness of the here-and-now, much of the work is taken on by the members. Initially, however, a primary task of the therapist is to actively steer the group discourse toward here-and-now work. In other words, events in the session (the here-and-now) take precedence over those that occur outside or have occurred outside (the there-and-then).

Illuminating the Process

If the group is to engage in interpersonal learning, the therapist must illuminate the process. This is the second task of prime importance. The group must move beyond a focus on content toward a focus on process—the how and the why of an interaction. The process can be considered from any number of perspectives. Choose the perspective based on the mood and needs of the group at that particular time. The members must recognize, examine, and understand the process and be willing to self-disclose (review the discussion of self-disclosure earlier in this chapter). The task of illuminating the process belongs mainly to the therapist, as in the following clinical example.

Clinical Example

Every time Jim makes a comment in group, Al either sneers or smirks. As soon as Jim finishes speaking, Al contradicts whatever Jim has said. The group members focus on the content of the disagreements between Jim and Al. Margaret, the clinical nurse specialist who is the group therapist, steers the group in the direction of analyzing the dynamics of the relationship between these members and the possible purposes their disagreements can serve for the group (e.g., controlling the direction of the group's efforts, meeting Al's control needs, or keeping the group anxiety down by keeping the focus away from other, more anxious members).

Process commentary is anxiety producing for new or inexperienced therapists and group members because there are so many injunctions against it in social situations. For example, commenting on someone's nervousness at a party is generally taboo. It not only makes the nervous person uncomfortable, but also puts the process commentator in a high-risk social situation. The comment may well be taken as criticism or viewed as inappropriate to the social context, and the commentator is vulnerable to retaliation from others. Be aware that process commentary may be difficult for you if you do not understand the differences between social and professional relationships (refer back to Chapter 4 and the discussion on pages 47–49). It is essential to educate group members about these differences and to prepare them to hear, respond to, and eventually initiate process commentary themselves (Ulman, 2011). You will be unable to do so if you have not incorporated this understanding into your professional psychiatric–mental health nursing practice.

The process of focusing on the here-and-now is akin to the process that is called *clearing the air* (making covert interpersonal difficulties overt) in Schutz's framework. Clearing the air is a major step in the interpersonal needs approach. Although this step is initially uncomfortable, the final result is rewarding. The following are common interpersonal difficulties that occur in therapy groups and should be made overt:

- Withdrawal or silence by members
- Inactivity or overactivity by members
- Unintegrated behavior by members
- Destructive behavior by members
- Power struggles between members
- Battles for attention among members
- Dissatisfaction with the leader
- Dissatisfaction with the amount of recognition a member receives for contributions
- Dissatisfaction with the amount of affection and warmth demonstrated in the group

In concert with Yalom's principles, Schutz's interpersonal needs approach is based on the belief that the way to attack problems within groups is by investigating what is going on among the individuals in the group, and attempting to improve their interpersonal relations.

Focusing on the here-and-now experience differentiates interactive group psychotherapy from many other group therapies or therapeutic groups such as those discussed in the next section.

THERAPEUTIC GROUPS

Nurses at all levels have long been involved in working with clients and their families in small groups brought together for health teaching, psychoeducation, or supportive purposes. This section discusses several different types of therapeutic groups that do not require the nurse to be an advanced-practice registered nurse.

Developing and planning a therapeutic group should be a systematic process. FIGURE 28-9 ■ illustrates a step-by-step investigative process that you could use to determine the clinical need for a group and to develop and implement the group.

Mutual-Help Groups

The major operating principle in mutual-help groups (also known as *self-help groups*) is that the help given to members comes from the members themselves. A mental health professional is viewed as unnecessary. In fact, many of these groups developed because of the failure of programs planned and implemented by professionals.

The role of the nurse in mutual-help groups is that of a resource person. You need to be informed about such groups so that you can refer potential members to groups appropriate to their needs, or to provide consultation when invited to do so. Appropriate referral is important. When dually diagnosed clients (substance abuse and psychiatric disorder) were referred to a twelve-step mutual-help group they did better than those not in a mutual-help group (Timko, Sutkowi, Cronkite, Makin-Byrd, & Moos, 2011). In most mutual-help groups, leaders are former members. Alcoholics Anonymous is a well-known example of this principle.

Nursing Process   **Developmental Steps**

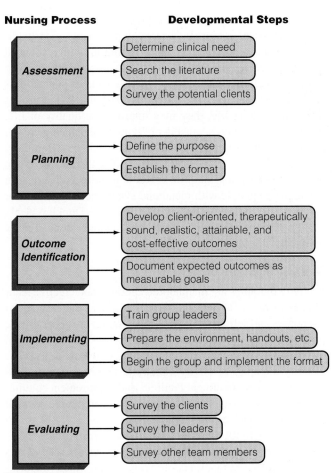

FIGURE 28-9 ■ Planning a client or family time-limited therapeutic group.

There is a wide variety of mutual-help groups, for example:

- Recovery Incorporated, concerned with recovery and rehabilitation for people with serious and persistent mental disorders
- Schizophrenics Anonymous, concerned with people coping with schizophrenia
- Alcoholics Anonymous and Narcotics Anonymous, concerned with people who abuse substances
- Al-Anon and Alateen, concerned with the families of people who abuse alcohol
- Rational Recovery, concerned with people who abuse substances and may be uncomfortable with the philosophy of 12-step programs such as Alcoholics Anonymous
- Overeaters Anonymous, concerned with people who overeat
- Gamblers Anonymous, concerned with people who gamble compulsively
- Gam-Anon, concerned with the families and friends of people who gamble compulsively
- Child Abuse Listening and Mediation (CALM), concerned with people who abuse children

Self-help groups can be located through http://www.mentalhealthamerica.net, formerly the National Mental Health Association. In Canada, a directory of mutual-help and self-help groups is available through the Canadian Mental Health Association, http://www.cmha.ca. All of these resources can be accessed through the Online Student Resources for this book.

Groups for divorced, widowed, or single people, for parents of runaways and troubled adolescents, for parents who abuse their children, and for the recently bereaved are common in most major cities throughout the world. Client clubs for people who have had a colostomy, ileostomy, laryngectomy, mastectomy, or amputation are also popular.

Psychoeducation Groups

Psychoeducation groups led by nurses have the sharing of mental health care information as a primary goal. They also have the secondary benefit of facilitating the discussion of feelings such as isolation, helplessness, sadness, stigmatization, and/or anger and possible strategies for dealing with these feelings. Psychoeducation groups may be specifically designed for family members. Even a brief psychoeducation group can be helpful in reducing the psychosocial burdens that relatives of clients with depression face (Katsuki et al., 2011) or that caregivers of clients with dementia face (Haberstroh, Neumeyer, Krause, Franzman, & Pantel, 2011). Some examples of nurse-led psychoeducation groups follow.

Medication Teaching Groups

Nonadherence to psychopharmacologic prescription medication is the leading cause of relapse or recurrence of psychotic illness. Many studies have shown that the causes of medication nonadherence are related to a lack of insight and understanding by clients or their families of their illness and of their medication treatment. In addition, medication side effects such as dry mouth, blurred vision, impotence, sedation, weight gain, and akathisia can be difficult to tolerate.

Medication teaching groups provide an opportunity for psychiatric–mental health nurses to educate clients about medications, their side effects, the nature and course of their mental disorder, the possibility of relapse (see Chapter 32∞) without continued medication treatment, and the positive effect medications have on their lives. Research has shown that improved attitudes, adherence to treatment, and insight often result from medication teaching groups (Tay, 2007).

Social Skills Training Groups

Groups can effectively provide social skills training for clients as well as for their family members. Small groups provide structure and support, while clients are coached in simple yet essential social interactions. It is best to form groups of clients who function at similar levels. Provide structure by clearly setting the time for group meetings, beginning and ending each session with a statement of goals, and recapping what the group has accomplished. The combination of social skills training with cognitive–behavioral therapy (CBT) or dialectical behavior therapy (discussed in Chapter 30∞) appears to be powerful.

Social skills training continues to be found useful for varying populations. Through cognitive–behavioral training in a social skills depression prevention program, adolescents increased their perception of social support by friends (Stice, Rohde, Gau, & Wade, 2010). Perception of social support by others is inversely related to depressive symptoms—the greater the social support the fewer the depressive symptoms. The positive effects were maintained through 1- and 2-year follow-up (Stice, Rohde, Gau, & Ochner, 2011.) After a 24-session social skills training group, psychiatric outpatients showed an improvement in social cognition (Horan et al., 2011). Decrease in positive, depressive, and anxiety symptoms in first-episode psychosis participants, as well as improved quality of life, and improvement in negative symptoms was found by another group of researchers who also combined CBT with social skills training (Gaynor, Dooley, Lawlor, Lawoyin, & O'Callaghan, 2011). Older people with severe and persistent schizophrenia can also learn and maintain new skills and report improved functioning after cognitive–behavioral social skills training (Granholm et al., 2007). Social skills training groups that focus on communication skills can reduce relationship risk factors for couples by teaching conflict resolution and communication skills.

Groups of Medically Ill Clients and Their Families

Groups composed of medically ill clients are increasingly common, as psychiatric–mental health nurses move into general health care settings offering liaison and consultation services to clients and staff. Group work is useful for chronically ill or disabled clients, preoperative and postoperative clients,

WHY I BECAME A PSYCHIATRIC-MENTAL HEALTH NURSE

Cleo Newton Watkins, RN-C, MS

When I was a senior in high school, my cousin was admitted to a psychiatric hospital. He found talking to me helpful and I began to think that I could help others who were experiencing psychiatric difficulties. After graduating from nursing school, my first clinical experience in psychiatric–mental health nursing was a gratifying one in a private psychiatric hospital. The desire to be a proficient psychiatric-mental health nurse motivated me to enroll in a master's degree program that would prepare me to function as a clinical nurse specialist in psychiatric–mental health nursing. Following graduate school I worked as a teacher and an administrator and then in full time clinical practice as a clinical nurse specialist with ANCC certification in adult psychiatric nursing.

My life and work as a psychiatric–mental health nurse has been filled with autonomy. I am immensely pleased to be able to support clients in their efforts to make appropriate changes and meet their identified goals. I know that I made the right choice to become a board certified clinical nurse specialist in adult psychiatry.

clients with regulative medical problems (such as diabetes, cardiac disease, or kidney disease), dying clients, elderly clients, and clients who have medical conditions with associated psychological factors (see Chapter 8∞), among others. Such groups generally focus on the stress associated with illness and have as their goal the reduction of stress. While groups may not prolong life, they may improve the quality of life, including protection against depression, by enhancing coping skills in, for example, breast cancer survivors (Hamilton, Miedena, Macintyre, & Easley, 2011). The therapeutic group has also been found helpful in teaching primary prevention strategies to people with metabolic syndrome at high risk for cardiovascular disease and type-2 diabetes (Dunkley et al., 2011). Groups may be composed of clients alone, family members alone, or a combination.

Activity Therapy Groups

Activity therapies are manual, recreational, and creative techniques to facilitate personal experiences and increase social responses and self-esteem. Activity therapies are generally the province of health and recreation specialists. Large psychiatric hospitals, especially those with long term care units, have activity therapists. Activity therapy is also important in psychiatric day care treatment facilities and in retirement communities, assisted living facilities, and other long term residential care settings such as nursing homes.

Many activity therapies, such as the creative arts therapies, are organized and conducted in groups. Creative arts therapies provide many people with a comfortable opportunity for social exchange. Although there are specifically educated creative arts therapists, their numbers are small. Nurses may lead such groups or use the principles to reach beyond the ordinary realm of verbal communication with clients.

Poetry Therapy Groups

The goal of poetry therapy groups is to help members get in touch with feelings and emotions through the use of poetry. Poems that are read aloud provide the stimulus for understanding and catharsis. They are selected as the therapeutic medium because they are powerful but not explicit avenues of communication. It is not necessary to be able to write poetry to be a member or leader of a poetry therapy group, although some members or leaders may be stimulated to write poems of their own.

Art Therapy Groups

In art therapy groups, the art produced by each member gives the art therapist or group leader a personal insight into the artist's personality and an opportunity for clients to communicate on a nonverbal level. The art is produced during the session and is used as the basis for discussion and for exploring members' feelings.

Music Therapy Groups

Music therapy consists of singing, rhythm, body movement, and listening. It is designed to increase group members' concentration, memory retention, conceptual development, rhythmic behavior, movement behavior, verbal and nonverbal retention, and auditory discrimination. It is also used to stimulate members' expression and discussion of affect. Some of the most positive results have been found in studies of the effects of music therapy on pain. In a randomized controlled trial of women with breast cancer, music therapy was found to reduce pain in both the short and the long term (Li et al., 2011).

Dance Therapy Groups

Dance therapy combines movement and verbal modes. In dance, members find it easier to express nonverbally the feelings and emotions that have been difficult to realize and communicate by other means. The person's inner sense is often reflected in body movements, and dance therapists work to help members integrate their experiences verbally as well as nonverbally.

Bibliotherapy Groups

In bibliotherapy groups, literature is the means for achieving a therapeutic goal. The purpose of a bibliotherapy group is to assimilate the psychological, sociologic, and aesthetic insights books give into human character, personality, and behavior. Literature provides a stimulus for group members to compare events and characters with their own interpersonal and intrapsychic experiences.

Storytelling Groups

Storytelling groups—a process by which group members create a story together—can stimulate interaction and imagination. For example, the group leader or the group members can choose one person to be the main character in a story. The group leader can give direction to the story by having an opening question in mind that is likely to determine the direction of the story. Questions a group leader could ask include the following:

1. Where would you go if you were given a trip?
2. What would you do if you won the lottery?
3. What would you title your autobiography?
4. What would your epitaph say?
5. If your fairy godmother could grant your wish, what would it be?
6. What is your favorite room in the house you grew up in?

Storytelling can be very effective in helping clients talk about feelings they would otherwise have suppressed and to connect with one another. It can assist elders in reminiscence work. In addition, storytelling can be fun, generate laughter, and reduce stress, no matter the client's age.

Community Client Groups

Psychiatric–mental health nurses in community settings are involved in a variety of community groups. These settings include schools, youth centers, work places (Dietrich, Dechert, Ceynowa, Hegerl, & Stengler, 2011), neighborhood centers, churches, prisons, summer camps, single-room occupancy boarding houses, transitional facilities such as halfway houses, apartments for the elderly, and residential facilities for delinquent youths and runaways. Clients may also be people who have direct contact with these groups, such as teachers, youth counselors, prison guards, police officers, camp counselors, or caregivers of persons with a psychiatric disorder (Haberstroh et al., 2011).

Groups With Nurse Colleagues

Nurses who work together may form discussion and counseling groups to help reduce their job-related stress and to help them deal with problems of interpersonal relationships in more satisfying ways. Nurses in various intensive care and other high-pressure settings identify with increasing frequency the need for group work services that the psychiatric–mental health nurse can provide. The psychiatric–mental health nurse may also identify the need and offer this opportunity to colleagues.

Pearson Nursing Student Resources
Find additional review materials at
nursing.pearsonhighered.com
Prepare for success with NCLEX®-style practice questions, interactive assignments and activities, web links, animations and videos, and more!

REFERENCES

Beebe, S. A., Beebe, S. J., & Redmond, M. V. (2011). *Interpersonal communication: Relating to others*. Boston, MA: Allyn & Bacon.

Benne, K. D., & Sheats, P. (1948). Functional roles of group members. *Journal of Social Issues, 4*, 41–49.

Dietrich, S., Dechert, S., Ceynowa, M., Hegerl, U., & Stengler, K. (2011). Depression in the workplace: A systematic review of evidence-based prevention

strategies. *International Archives of Occupational and Environmental Health*. Advance online publication. doi: 10.1007/s00420-011-0634-7

Dunkley, A. J., Davies, M. J., Stone, M. A., Taub, N. A., Troughton, J., Yates, T., & Krunte, K. (2011). The reversal intervention for metabolic syndrome (TRIMS) study: Rationale, design, and baseline data. *Trials, 12*(1), 107.

Gans, J. S. (2011). Unwitting self-disclosures in psychodynamic psychotherapy: Deciphering their meaning and accessing the pain within. *International Journal of Group Psychotherapy, 61*(2), 218–237.

Gaynor, K., Dooley, B., Lawlor, E., Lawoyin, R., & O'Callaghan, E. (2011). Group cognitive behavioral therapy as a treatment for negative symptoms in first-episode psychosis. *Early Interventional Psychiatry, 5*(2), 168–173.

Granholm, E., McQuaid, J. R., McClure, F. S., Link, P. C., Perivolliotis, D., Gottlieb, J. D., . . . Jeste, D. V. (2007). Randomized controlled trial of cognitive behavioral social skills training for older people with schizophrenia: 12-month follow-up. *Journal of Clinical Psychiatry, 68*(5), 730–737.

Haberstroh, J., Neumeyer, K., Krause, K., Franzmann, J., & Pantel, J. (2011). TANDEM: Community training for informal caregivers of people with dementia. *Aging and Mental Health, 15*(3), 405–413.

Hamilton, R., Miedena, B., Macintyre, L., & Easley, J. (2011). Using a self-talk intervention to enhance coping skills in breast cancer survivors: Lessons from a community-based delivery model. *Current Oncology, 18*(2), 246–253.

Harris, T. E., & Sherblom, J. C. (2011). *Small group and team communication* (5th ed.). Boston, MA: Allyn & Bacon.

Horan, W. P., Kern, R. S., Tripp, C., Hellemann, G., Wynn, J. K., Bell, M., . . . Green, M. F. (2011). Efficacy and specificity of social cognitive skills training for outpatients with psychiatric disorders. *Journal of Psychiatric Research, 45*(8), 1113–1122.

Joyce, A. S., Piper, W. E., & Ogrodniczuk, J. S. (2007). Therapeutic alliance and cohesion variables as predictors of outcome in short-term group psychotherapy. *International Journal of Group Psychotherapy, 57*(3), 260–296.

Katsuki, F., Takeuchi, H., Konishi, M., Sasaki, M., Murase, Y., Naito, A., . . . Furukawa, T. A. (2011). Pre-post changes in psychosocial functioning among relatives of patients with depressive disorders after brief multifamily psychoeducation: A pilot study. *BMC Psychiatry.* Advance online publication. doi: 10.1186/1471-244X-11-56

Li, X. M., Yan, H., Zhour, K. S., Dang, S. N., Wang, D. L., & Zhang, Y. P. (2011). Effects of music therapy on pain among female breast cancer patients after radical mastectomy: Results from a randomized controlled trial. *Breast Cancer Research and Treatment, 128*(2), 411–419.

Norcross, J. C., & Wampold, B. E. (2011). Evidence-based therapy relationships: Research conclusions and clinical practices. *Psychotherapy, 48*(1), 98–102.

Schutz, W. C. (1958a). Interpersonal underworld. *Harvard Business Review, 36*, 123–135.

Schutz, W. C. (1958b). *The interpersonal underworld: FIRO.* Palo Alto, CA: Science and Behavior Books.

Stice, E., Rohde, P., Gau, J., & Ochner, C. (2011). Relationship of depression to perceived social support: Results from a randomized adolescent depression prevention trial. *Behavioral Research and Therapy, 49*(5), 361–366. doi: 10.1016/j.brat.2011.02.009

Stice, E., Rohde, P., Gau, J. M., & Wade, E. (2010). Efficacy trial of a brief cognitive-behavioral depression prevention program for high-risk adolescents: Effects at 1- and 2-year follow-up. *Journal of Consulting and Clinical Psychology, 78*(6), 856–867.

Tay, S. E. (2007). Compliance therapy: An intervention to improve inpatients' attitudes toward treatment. *Journal of Psychosocial Nursing and Mental Health Services, 45*(6), 29–37.

Timko, C., Sutkowi, A., Cronkite, R. C., Makin-Byrd, K., & Moos, R. H. (2011). Intensive referral to 12-step dual-focused mutual-help groups. *Drug and Alcohol Dependency.* Advance online publication. doi:10.1016/j.drugalcdep.2011.03.019

Ulman, K. H. (2011). The present moment and implicit communication in group psychotherapy. *International Journal of Group Psychotherapy, 61*(2), 275–284.

Yalom, I. D. (1998). *The Yalom reader.* New York, NY: Basic Books.

Yalom, I. D. (2005). *The theory and practice of group psychotherapy* (5th ed.). New York, NY: Basic Books.

Yalom, I. D. (2009). *The gift of therapy: An open letter to a new generation of therapists and their patients.* New York, NY: HarperCollins.

Family-Focused Interventions

29

CAROL REN KNEISL

LEARNING OUTCOMES

After completing this chapter, you will be able to:

1. Describe families and their dynamics in terms of relationships, associations, and connections.
2. Differentiate among schism, skew, enmeshment, and disengagement as problems of intimacy and control in families.
3. Carry out a family assessment.
4. Incorporate the data obtained in a family assessment into the care plan for the client.
5. Partner with clients and their families in recognizing when family interventions, referral to NAMI, or family therapy are appropriate.
6. Design family psychoeducation activities to improve client recovery and family well-being.
7. Provide information about family therapy and support to clients and their families while they are engaged in family therapy.

CRITICAL THINKING CHALLENGE

You are present at a multidisciplinary case conference presentation. Mark James, your 22-year-old client, is being discharged from his first hospital admission for schizophrenia to the home he shares with his father and two sisters. Mark has been alienated from his mother since his parents' divorce when he was 17 years old. Mark's mother has failed to show up for the discharge conference. The mental health team has recommended family therapy to the James family. You perceive what you think is annoyance on Mr. James's face, and one of Mark's sisters appears embarrassed. Although you would not be the James family therapist because you are not a clinical specialist, you recognize how important Mark's family can be to his progress.

1. What might be some of the family's unspoken concerns and needs?
2. What actions can you take to address the family's unspoken needs and concerns?
3. Mark is 22 years old, an adult. Why would family therapy be appropriate, rather than individual therapy?

We encounter families in many areas of our practice—in the emergency department, the intensive care unit, the school, the cancer hospital, the community health setting, and the mental health care setting, among others. It is for this reason that the knowledge you gain by reading this chapter will apply no matter what your practice setting will be. To help you in this endeavor, we have also integrated discussions of family dynamics, needs, and functioning in all chapters in this text. This chapter specifically discusses family dynamics, family assessment, family interventions such as psychoeducation and self-help, and family therapy. They are recognized as important components of treatment for psychiatric disorders.

The family is the context in which most people, including nurses, develop their first relationships with other people. Our view of the larger social world outside our own unique family is molded by the events that happen within our families and influence our development. Preventive approaches to family mental health, assessment of families in trouble, and intervention on their behalf must be based on an understanding of how families grow and interact and how family coping patterns develop. The Harry Potter movies are visible demonstrations of how the events that happen within families mold the personalities and actions of the main characters. The threads of family interaction and coping run through the Harry Potter series (see Mental Health in the Movies).

NURSING SELF-AWARENESS

Assessing and intervening with the families of your clients is an essential role. Unfortunately, some mental health care professionals still have a bias against family involvement. This bias is a remnant of now-discredited theories that poor parenting and dysfunctional family interaction patterns give rise to mental illness. A related bias is the belief by some that if families "cause" schizophrenia, then the family's contact with the client should be limited for the client's sake. Besides violating family rights, this bias prevents social interaction with family members that might serve as a normalizing force by confronting clients with reality. That is, circumstances within a family may not be ideal, but they are real and require coping skills. Here is a question you can use to check if you have a bias against the family's rights: *Am I responding to this family any differently than I would to the family of a client with a medical condition?*

In addition, your experiences in your own family influence how you perceive and react to your client's family. Truthfully answering the self-assessment questions in Your Self-Awareness will help you to determine how your own family experiences might influence your behavior with your clients' families.

MENTAL HEALTH IN THE MOVIES
The Harry Potter Movie Series

Themes of family dynamics, family responsibilities and roles, and family coping consistently run through the Harry Potter movie series, especially in relation to four specific characters.

Harry Potter, an orphaned half-blood wizard (his father, James, was born into a wizarding family, but his mother, Lily, was not) was taken in, and brought up by, his Muggle (non-wizard) relatives, the spiteful Aunt Petunia, Uncle Vernon, and Cousin Dudley Dursley. The Dursleys discouraged anything to do with imagination or magic, punishing Harry whenever anything "unusual" occurred, and providing him with ill-fitting hand-me-downs. He was bullied by Dudley and slept in a cupboard under the stairs while Dudley had two bedrooms all to himself. Harry's life was guided by a life script determined by his family circumstances—Lily died while protecting him and he was the only person to live when exposed to Voldemort's death curse. Harry's greatest strength was his ability to feel love despite a miserable childhood of neglect and abuse.

Hermione Granger, the daughter of Muggles, dealt with the prejudice and stigma of being a "filthy Mudblood," a disparaging name used by some people in wizarding society who look down upon those born to Muggle families like her own. Her parents are intelligent and hardworking dentists who, unlike the Dursleys, are proud of their daughter. Strong-willed and relying heavily on logic

as well as magic, Hermione nevertheless feels the need to prove herself. She recognizes prejudice and stigma and becomes an advocate for the better treatment of another stigmatized group—house-elves. She is also the protector of her family and her friends.

Ron Weasley, the sixth son and seventh child of a wizarding family, had a mostly happy childhood in a close and supportive family. Because the Weasleys were poor, Ron's secondhand outdated robes, school books, and wands made him an object of disdain among certain privileged elements of the wizarding society. Ron has been characterized as emotionally immature, insensitive, and embarrassed by his family's less fortunate circumstances. Feeling shunted aside in relation to the popular and admired Harry reawakened Ron's envy and feeling of being "second best" to his older accomplished siblings. Despite these characterizations, Ron is fiercely protective of his siblings and friends and stoutly defends his parents.

Albus Percival Wulfric Brian Dumbledore, the Hogwarts schoolmaster, had a sad family life. His mother's death and his father's incarceration left him with the responsibility of taking care of a damaged sister and a wayward brother. Bitter and angry, Dumbledore nevertheless found a way to become one of the greatest and kindliest wizards of all time. A touching scene with Dumbledore and Harry involves the magical Mirror of Erised, so called because it shows the deepest and most desperate desire of one's heart. Both see themselves in the mirror as happily reunited with their families.

Photo courtesy of Mary Evans/WARNER BROS/JK ROWLING/Ronald Grant/Everett Collection (10382154).

It is helpful when working with families to first come to an understanding of the experiences you bring with you from your own family. Complete the following statements to facilitate your self-understanding and recognition of the biases you bring to your work with families.

1. When someone in my family talks too much, I usually …
2. When one of my family members is silent, I usually …
3. When someone in my family cries, I usually …
4. When my family members are excessively polite and unwilling to confront each other, I usually …
5. When there is conflict in my family, I usually …
6. When one individual in my family is verbally attacked, I usually …
7. If there is physical violence in my family, I usually …
8. My typical intervention "rhythm" is (fast/slow) …
9. My style is characteristically more (nurturing/ confronting) …
10. The things that make me most uncomfortable in my family are …

FAMILY DYNAMICS

While there are common factors and mechanisms of change that undergird most forms of successful treatment, there are several unique dynamics that take place in families and influence both family and individual functioning. A selection of relevant theories that help to explain family dynamics and family treatment are discussed next. The section on family therapy will help you to understand and explain family therapy to clients and support clients and their families during the therapeutic experience. It does not prepare you as a family therapist. As you will learn later in the chapter, the nurse family therapist role is an advanced-practice role.

Family Structures

The traditional nuclear family is a two-parent, two-generation family consisting of a married couple and their children by birth or adoption. In today's society, fewer than one in five children have grown up in the traditional nuclear family structure. Contemporary families may look like any one of the following:

- A mother, a father, and 2 children (traditional nuclear family)
- A couple with five children—two of hers, two of his, and one of theirs (blended family)
- A 32-year-old single electrical engineer and his three foster children
- A divorced woman and her two teenagers
- A widowed man, his child, and his parents
- A grandmother raising her three grandchildren
- Two lesbian mothers and their child

- Three single women friends sharing an apartment none could afford alone
- Two gay men living together in a committed relationship

North American family forms continue to change, making the task of defining the family a difficult one (Anderson & Sabatelli, 2011). For that reason, sensitive psychiatric–mental health nurses reject a narrow definition of family and adapt their clinical practice to the wide variety of family constellations that exists in contemporary society.

Family Life Cycle

The notion of universal family stages has attracted criticism over several decades. Critics of family development theory point to it as a limiting way of thinking about ethnically and racially diverse populations, gender, and families without children (Anderson & Sabatelli, 2011). They propose that the notion of families moving through rigid, predetermined stages is a less productive method of understanding the dynamics that take place in families. Many family therapists believe that it is not necessary to understand a family's past in order to help them (Nichols, 2010). It is also important to recognize that the universality of family life cycle stages and tasks have not been empirically validated through research. Despite these criticisms, the notion of a family life cycle helps us to understand the family's organization in the present. Understanding families requires consideration of the challenges they face in each stage, how well they resolve the challenges, and how well they transition to the next stage.

Theories to explain family development were first formulated after World War II. Probably the most important was that originally proposed by Duvall in 1957 and expanded upon by Duvall and Miller in 1985 (Duvall & Miller, 1985). Duvall's formulations focused on the patterns and changes in family development as families move through stages. Duvalls' framework was enriched by Carter and McGoldrick (2005) whose multigenerational point of view, discussed in TABLE 29-1 ■, expanded the framework to include divorce, remarriage, and culturally diverse patterns. The family life cycle is the period of time in which the structure and interactions of role relationships are noticeably distinct from other periods. The stages are inferred from events spurred on by a change in family membership.

Family Characteristics and Dynamics

Whether they are functional or dysfunctional, families have certain characteristics and dynamics. In a family, each person's behavior is contingent on, and affects the behavior of, the others. This creates some interesting and complex turns in family relationships such as those you learned about in Mental Health in the Movies.

Family Roles

Members of a family must determine how to accomplish family tasks. They do so by establishing roles; patterns of behavior sanctioned by the culture. Jackson (1968) believes

TABLE 29-1 ■ Family Developmental Tasks	
Stage of the Family Life Cycle	**Family Developmental Tasks**
Leaving home as single young adults	■ Accepting emotional responsibility for self ■ Differentiating self from family of origin ■ Developing intimate peer relationships ■ Establishing self in respect to work and financial independence
Becoming a new couple through marriage	■ Forming a marital system ■ Committing to the new system ■ Realigning relationships with extended family and friends to include spouse
Making space for children	■ Adjusting the marital system to include children ■ Joining in childrearing, financial, and household tasks ■ Realigning relationships with extended family to include parenting and grandparenting roles
Increasing flexibility of family boundaries	■ Increasing flexibility of parent-child relationships to support adolescent's independence ■ Increasing flexibility of family boundaries to support grandparents' frailties and caring for older generation ■ Refocusing on midlife marital and career issues
Accepting exits from and entries into the family system	■ Launching children and moving on ■ Renegotiating marital system as a dyad ■ Realigning relationships to include in-laws and grandchildren ■ Dealing with disabilities and deaths of parents (grandparents)
Accepting shifting generational roles in later life	■ Facing physiological decline while maintaining own and/or couple functioning and interests ■ Exploring new familial and social options ■ Supporting a more central role for the middle generation ■ Making room for the wisdom and experience of elders ■ Dealing with losses—of spouse, siblings, and other peers—and preparing for death

Source: Nichols, M. P. (2010). Family therapy: Concepts and methods (9th ed.). Reprinted by permission of Pearson Education, Inc. Upper Saddle River, NJ.

that families set roles by operating as a rule-governed system, an ordered format designed so that members may be aware of their positions in relation to one another. Families decide which roles will exist within the system, socialize members into the roles, and then expend energy maintaining members within their roles.

When members are unable or unwilling to perform assigned roles, the family experiences stress. For the health of the **family system**—which includes not only family members but also their relationships, their communication with one another, and their interactions with the environment—roles often must be negotiated in other than stereotyped ways. When the roles are not negotiated satisfactorily, family disequilibrium results. Refer also to Mental Health in the Movies in Chapter 27 ∞ on page 608 that highlights four families in which assigned roles are renegotiated.

Family Boundaries

Families have *boundaries* as well. Boundaries define who participates in the family, the amount or intensity of emotional investment in the family, the amount and kind of experiences available outside the family, and particular ways to evaluate experiences in terms of the family. Clear, stable, and healthy boundaries allow for personal and meaningful relationships with others. A person with healthy boundaries has a solid sense of self. There are feelings of belongingness to the family as well as to others outside the family.

Boundaries may be clear or conflicting, rigid or diffuse. **Rigid boundaries**—those in which rules and roles are maintained under all conditions—keep members from having meaningful relationships with and understanding one another. People with rigid boundaries can become isolated or withdrawn. The isolation extends to the outside community as a whole and the family is cut off from others.

A **diffuse boundary** is the opposite of a rigid boundary—a person with diffuse boundaries has no clear, definable boundaries with others. In families, diffuse boundaries are characterized by family over-involvement in the lives of its members, leading to loss of independence by one or all family members. Parents and children become increasingly dependent on one another at the expense of relationships outside the family. Diffuse boundaries increase the family's dependence on one another. Families that struggle with boundaries tend to raise children who struggle with boundaries.

Power Structure

Most families have a hierarchical power structure in which the adults wield the power. The power structure is often developed in this way because it creates a safe environment in which young children can grow and develop, and because it is easy to operate. However, stress develops when disagreements exist about who holds the power.

Clinical Example

Tom, the 17-year-old son in the M family, always used the family car without permission. Although some serious arguments ensued between Tom and his father, no restrictions were placed on Tom's behavior, and the car keys continued to hang on a key rack in the front hall. Tom's paternal grandfather, who lived with the M family, took Tom's side in his arguments with his father. Grandfather M took the stance that "boys will be boys."

One evening when the family car was in a repair shop for some minor work, Tom "borrowed" his grandfather's new car. He was involved in a collision about an hour later. Although no one was injured, Grandfather M's car was extensively damaged and had to be towed away. Later that night, the adults of the M family managed to come together to agree on a stance they could mutually support concerning Tom's use of the family cars.

Once the adults in the M family were able to acknowledge their internal power struggle and come to an agreement on what rules were to be set and by whom, the family system was subject to less stress.

When children mature and become capable of assuming greater responsibility for their own functioning, power is often diffused among the members of a family system in a more democratic fashion. Certain families, however, do not allow power to be redistributed, thus hindering the individual development of the members with less power. In some dysfunctional families, there is chronic discord about power.

Relationship Strains or Conflicts

Relationship strains or conflicts can occur in the family or among various parts of the family, or outside of it. This commonly occurs when a previously and unanimously held family view is challenged by one or more members. A strain can exist between the individual members of a family—for instance, between two siblings with differing views on an issue. Conflict or strain can also occur between a member of the family and the rest of the family, or between a minority of family members and the other members.

Clinical Example

Charlene lives in the Florida panhandle near the Alabama border. Her brother lives in Indiana, one sister lives in northern Michigan, and an estranged sister lives in Nevada. Their 94-year-old mother who lives in South Florida and needs increasing amounts of care refuses to consider moving to a nursing home or an assisted living facility. The burden of driving 9 and ½ hours to her mother's home every few weeks to check on her has fallen to Charlene because she lives the closest. Her sisters have begun to pressure Charlene to move to South Florida so that she can take care of their mother. However, Charlene is reluctant to do so. Her friends, church, and job are in the community in which she lives. Currently, the two sisters are pitted against Charlene and her brother.

Strain can also exist between a family and the community when the family view differs from that of the community at large.

Relationship and Communication Intricacies in Families

Some of the relationship complexities described next exist in all families, but dysfunctional families handle them differently than do functional families. Functional families allow for individuation and growth-producing experiences.

Self-Fulfilling Prophecy and Life Scripts

A **self-fulfilling prophecy** is an idea or expectation that is acted out, largely unconsciously, thus "proving" itself. In families, self-fulfilling prophecies are often seen in the guise of family life scripts. A **life script** is a plan decided not by the fates, but by experiences early in life. People with life scripts are following forced, premature, early childhood decisions. Most people live a scripted life, at least to some extent.

There is an endless variety among life scripts. The Miss America script is decided for the 5-year-old girl whose parents enroll her in the Little Miss New York State (or Alabama or Colorado) competition. There are "My Son the Doctor, Delinquent, Alcoholic, Drug Addict" scripts. A person with a script, either "good" or "bad," is terribly disadvantaged in terms of autonomy or life potential. According to self-fulfilling prophecy, unless people recognize what the script is and take steps to change it, they are prevented from living to their potential.

Family Myths and Themes

Family myths and themes help families maintain balance by permitting them to resist change. *Family myths* are well-integrated beliefs, shared by all family members, about each other and their positions in family life. The beliefs are unchallenged, even though family members may have to resort to distortions to maintain the myth. The family myth is related to the family's inner image—how the family appears to its members.

Clinical Example

A myth in the Lundqvist family was that the father had the ability to make wise decisions. Individual members in this family participated to maintain the myth of the father as a wise man by gearing interactions with him in such a way that he appeared to make high-level family decisions single-handedly.

The *family theme* is the family's perception of its development and history. Family themes are important because they shape the fates of individual members and determine the pressures with which each person must contend.

Clinical Example

The Weber family had a theme constructed around second-generation grandparents of Austrian descent, who were able to provide their oldest son with a law school education through their hard work. This family conceived of people on welfare as "lazy," thus reaffirming its view of the value of working hard and becoming educated.

Energy in the family is directed toward upholding particular images of the family—as the most hard working, religious, popular, talented, financially successful, nonconformist, or whatever—in order to maintain the front the family strives to present to others.

Family Coalitions

Of all the forms of communicative exchange, dyadic communication is the most common. In fact, many families begin with a couple, a dyad. The presence of a third person always has an effect on an existing dyad. When the couple gives birth to or adopts a child, or a third person enters the family, the relationship becomes triadic. A triad is not a stable social situation, because it actually consists of a dyad plus one. Shifting alliances characterize triads or triangles in families. For example, adult partners may unite to discipline the child, mother and child may unite to argue for a family vacation, or father and child may join forces to go fishing together. Triangles are dysfunctional when issues are solved by shifting the intimacy among members rather than by working the actual issue through, or when interaction among family members is determined by fixed triangles. Fixed and rigid triangles are an effort to reduce stress and restore balance in a dysfunctional family. In actuality, fixed and rigid triangles perpetuate problems in families. Such coalitions always result in someone feeling "left out" (Bowen, 1988). A problematic family triangle is illustrated in FIGURE 29-1 ▪.

Coalitions arise basically to affect the distribution of power. By joining forces, two people can increase their influence over a third. Parents frequently pair up in order to discipline their child in a consistent manner. However, the child may also attempt to pair up with one parent to avoid discipline. In families with a number of children, typical coalitions involve children closest in age or children of the same sex.

Deviations in the Adult Partners' Coalition

In some families, problems develop from the couple's inability to form a satisfying coalition in terms of intimacy and control. Several common deviations within the family are examined in the sections that follow.

Schism Families in which the children are forced to join one or the other camp of two warring spouses or adult caretakers are called **schismatic families**. The constant fighting in these families is most likely a defense against intimacy or closeness.

Clinical Example

Patty and Krista joined their father in "teasing" their mother whenever she was unclear about the latest news event, historical or geographic fact, movie, or music. Their teasing gradually became increasingly derogatory and public. Patty, Krista, and their father made it clear that they viewed her as incompetent and not very bright.

In schismatic families, the adult partners devalue and undercut each other. This makes it difficult for the children to want to be like either of them.

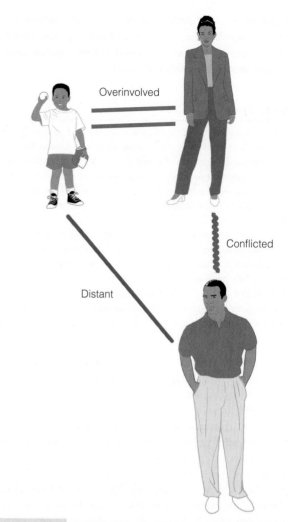

FIGURE 29-1 ▪ A family triangle. In this family, the relationship between husband and wife is conflicted. Mother and son are overinvolved. Father and son have a distant relationship.

Skew Families in which one mate is severely dysfunctional are called **skewed families**. The other mate, who is usually aware of the dysfunction of the partner, assumes a passive, peace-making, submissive stance to preserve the relationship.

Clinical Example

Mick and Cindy loved to join their friends at elegant restaurants known for fine food. Cindy who was anorexic, usually ordered as her one and only entree "a small house salad, lemon only, please, no dressing." At home, Cindy often ate only raw carrots. Dinner for her family was likely to be a scoop of mashed potatoes in a bowl of clear chicken broth. Mick did not acknowledge Cindy's unusual food preferences, her interest in recipes and restaurants, or her anorexia.

The passive partner is caught between effectively responding to the dysfunctional partner's view of "reality" of the outside world and giving up this view within the home, accepting the dysfunctional mate's view. On the surface, a skewed couple may appear to be complementary. However, their relationship is actually lopsided and unsuited to many basic family tasks.

Enmeshment A fast tempo of interpersonal exchange is characteristic of **enmeshed families**. Interactions within the family are of high intensity and are directed more toward issues of power than toward issues of affection.

Clinical Example

Gia is a college student and a single mom with a 1-year-old daughter who lives with her parents, first-generation Americans, in an enmeshed family. Gia has failed to maintain the life script expected of her—Little Miss Innocent—a chaste and innocent young woman who lives at home with her parents while she does her best to be the first in the family to graduate from college, thus improving her own and her family's circumstances. Gia's mother is especially embarrassed by the presence of Gia's young daughter, actually forcing Gia to hide her daughter away when relatives and friends come to visit. Gia and her father have no idea how to deal with her powerful and controlling mother. She feels stymied—unable to move out because of financial reasons and reluctant to do so because of her own dependency needs—and torn, because she recognizes that the family situation is not the best for her daughter.

In enmeshed families, one adult is often overcontrolling and becomes anxious over the possibility of losing control over the children. Enmeshed families have diffuse boundaries. As you saw in this clinical example, none of these categories are discrete. A family characterized as enmeshed may also be dealing with dysfunctional coalitions among the members as well as life scripts that prevent them from living to their potential.

Disengagement Abandonment—at the other extreme from enmeshment—is characteristic of **disengaged families**. Family members seem oblivious to the effects of their actions on one another. They are unresponsive and unconnected to each other. Structure, order, or authority in the family may be weak or nonexistent. The responsibility of controlling and guiding increases the anxiety of the parent, who may feel overwhelmed and depressed. In these families, a child often assumes the parental role.

Clinical Example

Tony and Mary have eight children. Tony is seldom home and works two full-time jobs in order to support his family financially. The little spare time he does have is spent with his friends at the local bowling alley. Mary is tired, sleeps a lot, and is probably clinically depressed. Rita, the oldest, takes care of her seven younger siblings. She can't wait until she is old enough to get married and leave home.

Pseudomutuality and Pseudohostility

A family with *pseudomutuality* functions as if it were a close, happy family. This pattern of relating has the following characteristics:

- Persistent sameness in the structuring of roles
- Insistence on the desirability and appropriateness of the role structures within the family, despite evidence to the contrary

- Intense concern over deviations from the role structure or emerging autonomy
- Marked absence of spontaneity, enthusiasm, and humor in participating together

In these families, the members do not form intimate bonds with one another as individuals. Instead, an inordinate amount of energy is expended in maintaining ritualized and stereotyped ways of behaving and relating. Such a family requires its members to give up their sense of personal identity.

Pseudohostility exists in families characterized by chronic conflict, alienation, tension, and inappropriate remoteness.

Clinical Example

Jim and Ingrid had three children, only one of whom, a daughter, keeps regular contact with them. Their children play out with them the relationships Jim and Ingrid had in their own families of origin. Jim has a brother, Fred, and Ingrid has several brothers and sisters in Finland. Jim is unconcerned about the fact that he has no idea where his brother is, or even whether his brother is still alive. Ingrid left her large family's home in Finland for the United States when she was 16 years old—they do not correspond nor do they visit. This remoteness and lack of connectedness is mirrored in Jim and Ingrid's own family. When they are not ignoring one another, they and their children are in chronic conflict. The spouses of their two sons encourage their husbands to maintain contact with Jim and Ingrid despite knowing that Ingrid undermines them at every opportunity. Occasions when they are together are marred by tension.

As in pseudomutuality, family members deny the problems in an attempt to negate the hostility. Family members view their differences as only minor ones. Both pseudomutual and pseudohostile family environments are stifling milieus.

FAMILY ASSESSMENT

The family who has cared for the client with a mental disorder most likely has an in-depth understanding of the client's illness, history, and ability to function in the community. Include the family's insights in the assessment phase, and, if appropriate, use them in the planning of care, particularly care after discharge. Family members want to be involved at an early stage and to have their opinions heard and their experience with the ill family member respected (Nordby, Kjonsberg, & Hummelvoll, 2010).

Family assessment involves gathering data in several different areas and can be done both formally and informally. Do not overlook natural opportunities to assess families and their needs. During visits, join the family for a few minutes to learn about their understanding of the treatment program, their concerns, and their questions. More formal assessments using interview guides or strategies such as a family genealogy or time line (discussed later in this chapter) are also available. Whichever methods you use, remember that a trusting relationship with key members of the client's family is essential for establishing a flow of information and planning care. Remember, however, to secure clients' permission before releasing information to their families, and encourage clients to involve their families in their treatment. Clients' rights in relation to sharing of information is discussed in Chapter 12 ∞ .

Demographic Information

Obtain data pertaining to gender, age, occupation, religion, and ethnicity. In addition to gathering discrete bits of information (the father is a 39-year-old Latino, physician's assistant, and a member of St. Ann's Roman Catholic parish), it is important to gather more detailed information that will give insight into family functioning:

- How actively does the family pursue religious/ spiritual activities?
- What is the link of religion/spirituality to the family's value system, norms, and practices?
- What is the family's racial, cultural, and ethnic identification in relation to sense of identity and belonging?
- Who in the family is employed? What are their attitudes about employment?

Medical and Mental Health History

Here, you should also gather substantive information. You want to know about past medical and mental health treatment including experiences with psychotropic medications, past and present illnesses, and pertinent health facts in the family of origin, in the extended family, and in the family history.

Gather information about the developmental stage of the family.

- What were (are) the problems in transition from one developmental level to another?
- How has the family solved problems at earlier stages?
- What shifts in role responsibility have occurred over time?

Gaps in the collection of medical and mental health history were important in the unfortunate escalation of the situation summarized in Mental Health in the News.

Family Interactional Data

This is probably the most complex data to obtain. For example, you want to gather information about family rules.

- What family rules foster stability in the family?
- What rules foster maladaptation?
- How are rules modified?
- What happens when all members do not agree about the family rules?

You also need to determine the roles of family members.

- What are the formal roles for each member?
- What are the informal roles (scapegoat [scapegoating is explained in Chapter 26∞], controller, decision maker, and so on)?
- Do the roles seem to have a good fit in the family?

Most important, gather information on how family members communicate.

- What are the channels of communication—who speaks to whom?
- Are the messages clear?
- What is the extent of unclear or ambiguous messages, mixed messages, or missed messages?
- Do members "hear" one another?

Assess levels of cohesion by noting who accompanies the client and who visits if the client is hospitalized. Visits from family are a rich source of information.

- Is it the whole family or just one member?
- Does the client come in alone?
- Who visits, how often, and for how long?
- How do family visitors behave with the client?
- Do the members spend time interacting and sharing activities, do they sit quietly together, or do they maintain physical and emotional distance from one another?

Document these patterns of family interactions, and monitor the effect of family visits on the client.

MENTAL HEALTH IN THE NEWS

The Andrea Yates Case

One of the best-known instances of a mother killing her children is the case of Andrea Yates, a nurse, who killed her five young children (from 6 months to 7 years), by drowning them in a bathtub. She believed that Satan was inside her causing her to be a bad mother, that Satan spoke to her through the cartoons the children watched on television, and that by killing her children she would be saving them from hell. The Yateses were under the influence of a preacher and his wife who emphasized repentence because women have Eve's witch nature. A major controversy in this case was over the question of whether Andrea was ill or evil.

Andrea's delusions and hallucinations began soon after the birth of their first child. She was pregnant every year after that with some miscarriages interspersed among the live births. During these intervening years, she attempted suicide and had been treated by a number of psychiatrists, all of whom prescribed different antidepressants, none of which she took consistently and most of which she flushed down the toilet. She had thoughts about hurting the children for 2 years before she actually did do so.

Eventually, Andrea ended up in the care of a psychiatrist who seemed to have an incomplete knowledge of the history of her treatment for postpartum depression with psychotic features. Andrea's actual diagnosis was the focus of a debate during the court case. Some experts indicated that she also had schizophrenia. During her trial, a family history of depression and bipolar disorder was brought to light. This case highlights the consequences of an incomplete family history, untreated or undertreated mental disorder, and lack of therapeutic family intervention.

Photo courtesy © Reuters/CORBIS.

Family Burden

More than 4 million American families live with severely mentally ill members. Most families of mentally disordered individuals report that caring for the ill member is a very important, largely underappreciated, stigmatized, and frequently expensive, all-consuming, and lifelong task. **Family burden** is a term that refers to the difficulties and responsibilities of family members who assume a caretaking function for relatives with psychiatric disability. Be aware that the burden of care may involve shame, embarrassment, and feelings of guilt and self-blame (Awad & Voruganti, 2008), especially when the burden becomes great. This is the time when families may need the greatest level of support and understanding from professional staff.

You may ask the question: Do all families and all members in a family experience the family burden in the same way? Studies that have examined the role of gender found that relatives of male clients with schizophrenia frequently experience more social dysfunction than those of female clients (Awad & Voruganti, 2008). In addition, the more severe the symptoms the client has, the greater the family burden, although there is no agreement on which cluster of symptoms increases the family burden the most.

Family burdens reported most often are financial strain, violence in the household, reductions in the physical and mental health of family caregivers, disruption of family routines, worry about the future, the impact of stigma, the mental health system itself as a stressor, and feeling over-whelmed or unable to cope. Families also report having the following needs:

- Information about the disorder itself
- Information about how to manage day-to-day problems due to the client's symptoms
- Information and access to resources about medications and their side effects
- Strategies for helping the seriously mentally ill family member accept treatment
- Support in their role as caregiver

Gathering information about the family burden will help you to determine what kind of support would be most helpful to this family. A family support group? Referral to the National Alliance on Mental Illness (NAMI; discussed later in this chapter)? Respite care to give the family a break from their caregiving role? Family therapy?

Remember also that many clients are parents. Unfortunately, children's voices are rarely heard (Maybery & Reupert, 2009) despite the fact that a parent's mental disorder can have a significant psychosocial influence on the development of the children (Korhonen, Vehvilainen-Julkenen, Pietila, & Kattainen, 2009). The family burden is shared by children who should also be included in the support given to the family.

What Families Want from Mental Health Professionals

What better way to find out what families need from us than to ask them directly? When family members and clients with schizophrenia were asked what elements were most important to them when in remission, clients indicated that good subjective well-being was the most important (Karow, Naber, Lambert, & Moritz, 2011). Family members believed that symptom reduction, combined with good subjective well-being, was most important. In another study, Nordby and associates (2010) asked family members in focus group interviews what they wanted from mental health professionals. Family members revealed that they wanted the following:

- An explicit invitation from mental health staff to participate
- The opportunity to get involved at an early stage
- Staff members to treat their ill family member as a person and not a disease
- To be treated as resource people; to have their opinions and experiences respected and taken into consideration
- Expressions of hopefulness from staff members and nurturance of hope, no matter the prognosis
- Psychoeducation to help them learn what to say and how to behave toward their family member
- Individual counseling and support

These family members' requests will guide you in developing a therapeutic alliance (McGhee & Atkinson, 2010) with the client's family and help you to diminish the social isolation and alienation from professional caregivers (Ewertzon, Lutzen, Svensson, & Andershed, 2010) that family members often feel.

Family System Data

Determine how the family interacts with the outside world.

- How permeable or rigid are its boundaries?
- What is the extent to which the family fits into the larger culture of which it is a part?
- To what degree could the family be considered deviant from the larger culture?

Within the family, determine the family alliances.

- Who supports whom?
- Which members are in conflict with one another, or with the family as a whole?
- Are there extended family supports?
- What other social supports are available to the family?

Needs, Goals, Values, and Aspirations

Determine whether essential needs are met.

- Are physical needs met?
- At what level does the family meet the social and emotional needs of its members?
- What are the individual needs of family members, and how do they fit with the family needs?
- Is the family willing or able to meet the individual needs of its members?

Determine the extent to which individual family members' goals, values, and aspirations are articulated and understood by the other members.

- Are the goals, values, and aspirations shared by all?
- Do some members compromise?

■ Do other members simply give up and give in?

■ Does the family as a whole allow individual members to pursue individual goals and values?

Family Genogram

From the study of families in detail, it becomes apparent that patterns are spread over generations. The timeline, or **genogram**, is highly effective as a visual representation of family patterns from one generation to the next. By drawing it on a long, narrow piece of paper and taping it to the wall during a family conference or family sessions, the treatment team or therapist can use it repeatedly as therapy progresses. Colored lines can differentiate individual family members. Colored flags, pins, or stickers can identify and call attention to significant events in the family history. Note births, deaths, marriages, and leave-takings. You can use any of several family tree or genealogic tracing formats for the family timeline. One example is illustrated in Figure 29-2 ■ . You can develop other genograms to explore specific issues.

Cultural Family Genogram

A cultural family genogram is a useful tool for working with culturally diverse families. You can use a cultural family genogram to become more aware of the cultural differences between yourself and the family and between the family and other families, assess a family's strengths, and point to areas where intervention may be useful. A cultural family genogram might include the elements discussed in Developing Cultural Competence.

Spiritual Family Genogram

A spiritual genogram—a multigenerational map of family members' religious and spiritual affiliations, events, and conflicts—enables clients to make sense of their families' religious/spiritual heritage. It also helps them to explore the ways in which their experiences with spirituality affect couple or family issues. A spiritual family genogram could also be a tool in a spiritual issues discussion group for clients that helps them explore their spiritual beliefs, past experiences,

DEVELOPING CULTURAL COMPETENCE

The Cultural Family Genogram

Identifying the following elements will help in developing a useful cultural family genogram:

■ What language is spoken at home and in the community?

■ What significance does race, skin color, and hair play within the group?

■ What role does religion and spirituality play within the everyday lives of the family members?

■ What prejudices or stereotypes does this family have about themselves and other members of their cultural group?

■ What prejudices or stereotypes does this family have about other cultural groups?

■ What are the health beliefs in this family's culture?

■ How does this culture view mental health professionals?

■ What values does this family have about family, education, and work?

■ What are the pride/shame issues of this cultural group? How are they manifested in this family?

CRITICAL THINKING QUESTIONS

1. What benefit is there in knowing the role that religion and spirituality play in this family?

2. How could you use knowledge about how this family views mental health professionals?

3. How might pride/shame issues of this family's cultural group affect the care plan?

and spiritual lives in relationship to their mental illness (Popovsky, 2007).

Forensic Family Genogram

A forensic family genogram is a useful tool for forensic nurses for both assessment and intervention purposes. A two- or three-generational map can help offenders see the patterns in their lives as a way to begin to understand their personal circumstances. As part of the legal chart, it provides the courts

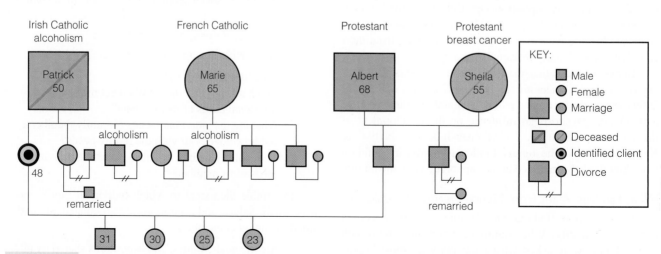

FIGURE 29-2 ■ One example of a family genogram.

with information about the events and factors in the individual lives of offenders in the form of a graphic database.

FAMILY INTERVENTIONS

Three main goals for involving family members in a client's treatment plan are as follows:

1. Enlisting the family as an ally in promoting and bringing about therapeutic progress and reducing relapse
2. Improving the family environment
3. Supporting family caregivers

The main forms of family intervention in current use are: family psychoeducation, referral to NAMI, and family therapy. Also important are availability of crisis management, legally mandated community treatment to help avoid hospitalization, and well-informed advocacy.

Services directed toward supporting the family caregivers of persons with serious and persistent mental illnesses may have the potential to improve outcomes for both the caregivers and the clients (Pahlavanzadeh, Heideri, Maghsudi, Glazavi, & Semendari, 2010). Although there seems to be a consensus about the need for coordinated family-based services, they are not always implemented. Family interventions are not always appropriately integrated in care plans

and are frequently underfunded (Awad & Voruganti, 2008). This is an area for active advocacy by the psychiatric–mental health nurse.

Family Psychoeducation

Family members can benefit from psychoeducation groups designed specifically to help them cope with their loved one's illness. In studies of family caregivers of people with dementia, psychoeducation provided immediate help to reduce the family burden (Pahlavanzadeh et al., 2010) as well as support and information (Wilhelmson et al., 2011). Family psychoeducation programs have emerged as a strongly supported evidence-based practice in the treatment of schizophrenia (Karow et al., 2011) and, when combined with antipsychotics for people who are schizophrenic, is found to be cost effective (Phanthunane, Vos, Whiteford, & Bertram, 2011). Family psychoeducation has also been found to reduce psychotic relapse and rehospitalization (Karow et al., 2011) and to improve client recovery and family well-being. Suggestions for elements to include in a family psychoeducation program are given in Partnering With Clients and Families.

Family psychoeducation groups educate family members about the specific mental disorder, including its signs and symptoms, the medications the client takes, the signs

---

PARTNERING WITH CLIENTS AND FAMILIES

Psychoeducation for Families

To assist families, you need to evaluate the family's current responses to living with and caring for a family member with a mental disorder. The following suggestions apply to the time period shortly after a mental disorder has been diagnosed.

Suggestions	Rationale	Suggestions	Rationale
Discuss the basic nature of the disorder: a disease of the brain, like any other biologic disease.	Families misunderstand mental illness to be a personal failing and are comforted by the fact that it has a biologic basis.	Refer families to structured educational or psychoeducational programs in which they can learn about the disease and its treatment, as well as receive support.	Mental disorders are extremely complex, and their treatment is multifaceted. Families can benefit from structured classes. Programs that offer support to families in addition to education have proven effective in improving the illness course for the ill member.
Help families identify their responses to the early ambiguous signs of the illness and notice how their responses have changed now that the diagnosis has been made.	Families often misinterpret early signs of the disorder as acting out or developmentally appropriate behavior. On learning that these signs are part of the illness, they feel guilty for not seeking help sooner.	Inform families about how to reach the local branch of the National Alliance on Mental Illness (NAMI). Hand out fliers that provide telephone numbers and people to contact.	NAMI is a nationwide family support organization that provides peer support, education, and advocacy for the seriously mentally ill and their families.
Reinforce families for supporting the ill member in seeking treatment.	Stigma about mental illness persists, and families need support for taking action and engaging with treatment systems.	Provide families with access to appropriate, accurate, and up-to-date information in books and manuals, or refer them to their local library. Two examples are listed below.*	It is often useful for family members to have a quick reference book available for help in managing client symptoms and their own distress.

*Mueser, K. T., & Gingerich, S. (2006). *Guide to schizophrenia: Helping your loved one get the most out of life.* New York, NY: Guilford Press.
Torrey, E. F. (2006). *Surviving schizophrenia: A manual for families, patients, and providers* (5th ed.). New York, NY: Harper Collins.

and stages of relapse, the treatment plan, and the fluctuating course of mental illness. They also learn about life events that cause stress for the client, how to prevent relapse, and how to manage behavior that is disturbing to others. Family psychoeducation may also address all family members' emotion regulation and interpersonal skills deficits.

Family psychoeducation groups also serve a supportive function in an accepting environment. Family members are informed about local and national groups and organizations that provide educational and counseling services and respite care. A family psychoeducation program is a good bridge to referral to NAMI or to family therapy.

Unfortunately, the use of family psychoeducation in routine clinical practice is limited. Family members are most likely to receive information about diagnosis and medications and least likely to receive information about the treatment plan. However, nurses can be influential in persuading their agencies to develop family psychoeducation programs, as discussed in Evidence-Based Practice.

Dialectical behavior therapy combined with family skills training is being used more often because of its confirmed effectiveness. It is particularly effective in teaching family members (or couples in marital therapy) how to regulate their emotions and helping them to achieve an understanding of how strong feelings affect, and are affected by, their relationships with one another (Kirby & Baucom, 2007). Behavior therapy is discussed in Chapter 30 and social skills groups are discussed in Chapter 28∞.

Referral to NAMI

NAMI is a grassroots, mutual-help, advocacy, and support organization of families, consumers (a term used by NAMI to describe people diagnosed with and receiving treatment for severe mental illness), and friends of people with severe mental disorders. NAMI provides several services to families and consumers, including general information on mental disorders, psychiatric medications, and mental health policy positions; referral to state and local affiliates and support groups throughout the country; and support from trained volunteers—consumers and family members—who know what it is like to have a mental disorder or to have a family member with a mental disorder. One program of special interest to families is the NAMI Family-to-Family Education Program. The special features of this course, prepared by families for families, have both a personal and a social focus and can be found on the NAMI website provided at the end of this section.

NAMI also provides educational services to mental health care providers. The NAMI Provider Education Program for staff at public agencies who work directly with people with severe and persistent mental illness is a 10-week course to educate providers about how to include families in the care of the client. The program is based on principles of competence (stressing empowerment and collaboration) and adaptation, rather than psychopathology, and shifts the emphasis from the causes to the effects of mental disorders.

You can refer consumers and families in need (as well as other health care providers) to the NAMI HelpLine at 1-800-950-NAMI (6264). You can also suggest the NAMI website at http://www.nami.org, which can be accessed through a direct link on the Online Student Resources for this book.

Family Therapy

In general, family therapists believe that the emotional symptoms or problems of an individual are an expression of emotional symptoms or problems in a family. Therefore, family therapists view the family system as a unit of treatment. Their concerns are basically with the relationships between the family members, not with the intrapsychic functioning of individual family members, and therapy is directed at changing the organization of the family (Nichols, 2010). The discussion of family therapy in this chapter is designed to provide you

---

EVIDENCE-BASED PRACTICE

Decreasing Family Burden Through Psychoeducation

The program development committee at the mental health outreach clinic where you work has challenged you to provide a convincing rationale for your recent proposal. You believe that family psychoeducation helps to reduce family burden. However, in order to commit resources such as staff and funding, the committee has asked you to review the research to determine on what basis the agency can support your proposal.

Your review of the research found significant support for your proposal. Family psychoeducation groups for families with a schizophrenic member show a significant improvement in clients' social relationships, interest in obtaining a job, and management of social conflicts. Family burden significantly improved, as did relatives' social contacts and perception of professional support. Family distress decreased as the confidence and skills of the members increased. Similar results are found with studies of bipolar disorder, depression, suicide, borderline personality disorder, and dementia of the Alzheimer's type.

You should base action on more than one study, but the following research was helpful in developing this proposal:

Karow, A., Naber, D., Lambert M., & Moritz, S. (2011). Remission as perceived by people with schizophrenia, family members and psychiatrists. *European Psychiatry*. Advance online publication.

CRITICAL THINKING QUESTIONS

1. What are the purposes of reviewing the evidence before designing an intervention?
2. What specific areas of research should you review other than studies of family psychoeducation?
3. What might a structured family psychoeducation program look like?

with the information you need to know in order to formulate a referral for family therapy and to educate and support clients and their family members.

Forms of Family Therapy

There are two basic forms of family therapy—insight-oriented family therapy and behavioral-oriented family therapy—into which all schools of family therapy fit on some level. Some examples of insight-oriented family therapy approaches are as follows:

- *Psychodynamic:* Problems are believed to arise because of developmental delays, or current interactions or stresses.
- *Family of origin therapy:* The goal is to foster differentiation among the members and decrease emotional reactivity and triangulation (Bowen, 1988).

Some examples of behavioral-oriented family therapy and the theorists who developed them are:

- *Structural:* The focus is on systems, subsystems, boundaries, and schismatic, skewed, enmeshed, or disengaged families (Minuchin & Fishman, 1981; Navarre, 1998).
- *Strategic:* Problems arise because of inequality of power, flawed communication, and repetitive and maladaptive family interaction patterns (Haley, 1996; Satir, 1983).
- *Cognitive–behavioral:* The focus is on changing thinking and behavior, problem solving, and the development of skills (see Chapter 30∞ for a complete discussion of cognitive–behavioral strategies).

These lists are general, not exhaustive. Discussion of these theories and their specific interventions is beyond the scope of this book.

Qualifications of Family Therapists

Being a family therapist requires a firm and clear understanding of all of the dynamics and forces that influence families. Family therapists should be specially educated in the practice of family therapy and strongly committed to a belief in the importance of the family. Nurse family therapists should be clinical specialists or advanced practitioners prepared in graduate programs that provide both theory and supervised clinical practice in this specialized area. Refer families to qualified nurse family therapists or other qualified family therapists. Families can also receive help in finding a therapist on the website of the American Association for Marriage and Family Therapy, which can be accessed through the Online Student Resources for this book. Consider whether the family discussed in Mental Health in the News on page 650 would have benefitted from family therapy or couples therapy.

The Unit of Treatment

Most family therapists recommend that all people in the family constellation participate in the assessment phase of family therapy. Not all agree on which people comprise the family constellation or the treatment unit. Some include all members of the nuclear family; others include members of the extended family; and still others, large numbers of people in the family's social network. Different coalitions may be seen together at different times to accomplish specific goals. For example, mates are often seen together for the first few sessions.

Children 4 years of age and younger are often not included in ongoing family therapy sessions. They may misinterpret, or be frightened by, the dialogue. In addition, small children tend to be disruptive. Some therapists, however, make it a point to bring all the children into some family therapy sessions to see how the family as a whole operates.

Contract or Goal Negotiation

The negotiation phase of family therapy is begun by identifying what each member would like changed in the family. When each family member and the therapist have identified important goals, they begin negotiating a set of attainable goals that everyone is willing to work on. Compromise is needed to achieve a working goal. At this time, the family therapist, along with the family, may also identify the means—tasks, strategies, and so on—that will be used to reach the negotiated goals.

Intervention

Therapy for a family system involves understanding and use of the here-and-now, and of the basic processes that occur in the system. Guidelines for common interventions employed by family therapists are listed in Your Intervention Strategies.

YOUR INTERVENTION STRATEGIES
The Role of the Family Therapist

- Creating a safe setting in which family members can risk looking at themselves and their actions
- Teaching family members how to share their observations with one another
- Asking for and giving information in a matter-of-fact, nonjudgmental, congruent way
- Responding as a role model whose meaning or intent can be queried without fear
- Setting rules for interaction to ensure that all family members participate; interruptions, acting-out, or making it impossible to converse are not tolerated; no one speaks for anyone else
- Clarifying the content and relationship aspects of messages
- Pointing out significant discrepancies, incongruities, or double-level messages
- Helping everyone speak out clearly so that each can be heard
- Viewing the family as a system and not taking sides
- Validating that anger, pain, and the "forbidden" are safe to examine
- Re-educating family members to be accountable
- Delineating family roles and functions and teaching explicitly about role responses and role choices

American Association for Marriage and Family Therapy

Terminating Family Therapy

Family therapists use various criteria to determine when termination is appropriate. Family therapy is often terminated when family members can do the following:

- See how they appear to others
- Give feedback to others, telling them how they appear
- Share their hopes, fears, and expectations with one another
- Openly discuss problems with one another

- Openly disagree with one another when appropriate
- Give clear messages
- Check meanings with one another
- Ask for clarification
- Support one another
- Achieve the family's goals

Termination in family therapy occurs in a flexible way, helping families achieve realistic goals, thus ending therapy with a feeling of accomplishment.

Pearson Nursing Student Resources

Find additional review materials at
nursing.pearsonhighered.com

Prepare for success with NCLEX®-style practice questions, interactive assignments and activities, web links, animations and videos, and more!

REFERENCES

Anderson, S. A., & Sabatelli, R. M. (2011). *Family interaction: A multigenerational developmental perspective* (5th ed.). Boston, MA: Allyn & Bacon.

Awad, A. G., & Voruganti, L. I. (2008). The burden of schizophrenia on caregivers: A review. *Pharmacoeconomics, 26*(2), 149–162.

Bowen, M. (1988). *Family therapy in clinical practice* (2nd ed.). Northvale, NJ: Jason Aronson.

Carter, B., & McGoldrick, M. (2005). The expanded family life cycle (3rd ed.). Boston: Allyn & Bacon.

Duvall, E. M., & Miller, B. C. (1985). *Marriage and family development.* New York, NY: Harper & Row.

Ewertzon, M., Lutzen, K., Svensson, E., & Andershed, B. (2010). Family members' involvement in psychiatric care: Experiences of the healthcare professionals' approach and feeling of alienation. *Journal of Psychiatric and Mental Health Nursing, 17*(5), 422–432.

Haley, J. (1996). *Learning and teaching therapy.* New York, NY: Guilford Press.

Jackson, D. D. (1968). *Communication, family, and marriage.* Palo Alto, CA: Science and Behavior Books.

Karow, A., Naber, D., Lambert, M., & Moritz, S. (2011). Remission as perceived by people with schizophrenia, family members and psychiatrists. *European Psychiatry.* Advance online publication.

Kirby, J. S., & Baucom, D. H. (2007). Treating emotion dysregulation in a couples context: A pilot study of a couples skills group intervention. *Journal of Marital and Family Therapy, 33*(3), 375–391.

Korhonen, T., Vehvilainen-Julkunen, K., Pietila, A. M., & Kattainen, E. (2009). Preventive child-focused family work: Development of instrument in adult psychiatry. *Journal of Psychiatric and Mental Health Nursing, 16*(9), 804–812.

Maybery, D., & Reupert, A. (2009). Parental mental illness: A review of barriers and issues for working with families and children. *Journal of Psychiatric and Mental Health Nursing, 16*(9), 784–791.

McGhee, G., & Atkinson, J. (2010). The carer/key worker relationship cycle: A theory of the reciprocal process. *Journal of Psychiatric and Mental Health Nursing, 17*(4), 312–318.

Minuchin, S., & Fishman, H. (1981). *Family therapy techniques.* Cambridge, MA: Harvard University Press.

Navarre, S. (1998). Salvador Minuchin's structural family therapy and its application to multicultural family systems. *Issues in Mental Health Nursing, 19,* 557–565.

Nichols, M. P. (2010). Family therapy: *Concepts and methods* (9th ed.). Boston, MA: Allyn & Bacon.

Nordby, K., Kjonsberg, K., & Hummelvoll, J. R. (2010). Relatives of persons with recently discovered serious mental illness: In need of support to become resource persons in treatment and recovery. *Journal of Psychiatric and Mental Health Nursing, 17*(4), 304–311.

Pahlavanzadeh, S., Heideri, F. G., Maghsudi, J., Glazavi, A., & Semendari, S. (2010). The effects of family education programs on the caregiver burden of families of elderly with dementia disorders. *Iranian Journal of Nurse Midwifery and Research, 15*(3), 102–108.

Phanthunane, P., Vos, T., Whiteford, H., & Bertram, M. (2011). Cost-effectiveness of pharmacological and psychosocial interventions for schizophrenia. *Cost Effectiveness and Resource Allocation, 9*(1), 6.

Popovsky, M. (2007). A spiritual issues discussion group for psychiatric inpatients. *Pastoral Care and Counseling, 61*(1–2), 119–128.

Satir, V. (1983). *Conjoint family therapy.* Palo Alto, CA: Science and Behavior Books.

Wilhelmson, K., Duner, A., Eklund, K., Gosman-Hedstrom, G., Blomberg, S., Hasson, H., . . . Dahlin-Ivanoff, S. (2011). Continuum of care for frail elderly people: Design of a randomized controlled study of a multiprofessional and multidimensional intervention targeting frail elderly people. *BMC Geriatrics, 11*(1), 24.

Cognitive and Behavioral Interventions

30

EILEEN TRIGOBOFF

LEARNING OUTCOMES

After completing this chapter, you will be able to:

1. Explain the central features of cognitive–behavioral interventions.
2. Discuss how humans express themselves in cognitive and behavioral ways.
3. Relate conditioning and association to the process of human learning.
4. Design nursing care plans for people with varied diagnoses using cognitive–behavioral therapies.
5. Analyze the effectiveness of a behavioral contract to promote a change in health-related behaviors.
6. Modify a nursing care plan to promote and enhance positive outcomes for cognitive–behavioral therapies.
7. Describe how your personal characteristics might influence your effectiveness in using cognitive–behavioral therapies.

CRITICAL THINKING CHALLENGE

Steven Norah is a full-time college student. He has been depressed for some time and has not made significant progress in long-term psychotherapy specifically focused on his childhood and developmental issues. You discussed his treatment responses with other members of the treatment team during his recent hospitalization for an exacerbation of his depression. Steven has expressed frustration at his inability to "get better and leave the depression behind." His depression and his routine ways of thinking and behaving continue in an unchanged, habitual manner.

The team believes a cognitive–behavioral approach would give Steven a better chance at recovery from depression. Changing his thoughts and behaviors could change his feelings and diminish depressive thinking. Once changes occur, Steven would have the opportunity to feel competent and successful, a distinct difference from his current view of himself.

1. How do you explain the notion that a change in thoughts and behaviors results in a change in feelings?
2. What should Steven know about this therapeutic method?
3. What differences would you expect to see in Steven's behavior if the cognitive–behavioral approach is effective?

Marcy, a person who is most comfortable with structure and routine in her daily life, has finally decided to seek help to overcome her fear of flying. Her friends have invited Marcy to travel with them to Paris, a place she has always wanted to visit. Marcy always has several reasons why she cannot travel with them. Most of the time, she says that she needs to stay home to care for her sister, who has a severe case of arthritis.

How might therapists with a variety of orientations approach Marcy's problem? A biologically oriented therapist would first focus on diagnosing Marcy's problem as a specific phobia—fear of flying—once the presence of other anxiety disorders, specifically panic disorder with agoraphobia, have been ruled out. The biologically oriented therapist would investigate Marcy's family history for the presence of phobias among first-degree biologic relatives and prescribe an anti-anxiety medication to alter her brain chemistry.

In contrast, a psychodynamic therapist would focus on Marcy's defensive style of avoidance. This therapist would identify Marcy's pattern of needing to have structure and control as a way of keeping anxiety in check. Treatment would be a talk therapy in which the therapist provides only minimal direction in the exploration of Marcy's past, her feelings, and her frustrations. The therapeutic goal would be for Marcy to gain insight into her intrapsychic conflicts, interpersonal difficulties, and defenses.

A cognitive–behavioral therapist would be aware of the issues in Marcy's life, but would approach therapy quite differently. A believer in the axiom that "actions speak louder than words," the cognitive–behavioral therapist looks for treatments that work based on research evidence. The therapist would focus on changing behavior in the present rather than focusing on gaining insight into the past. This change-oriented approach would pair relaxation training (discussed in Chapter 33∞) and systematic desensitization (discussed later in this chapter) in Marcy's case.

In this chapter, you will learn that cognitive (thought) and behavioral (action) interventions have their base in human learning theory and are comprised of diverse treatments based on empirical evidence. While not the only effective treatment—medications and talk therapy can also be effective—cognitive and behavioral strategies lend themselves to integration within a plan of care for clients who may be receiving diverse, but effective, treatments for mental disorders. Frequently, cognitive–behavioral therapy (CBT) is recommended for anger management. Mental Health in the Movies describes the media's depiction of an "appropriate" anger management program.

More recently, the term *cognitive–behavioral therapy* has largely replaced the terms *behavior therapy* and *cognitive therapy* as a way of describing these therapeutic techniques. *Cognitive–behavioral therapy* (CBT) focuses on changing thinking and behavior, and improves problem solving and the development of skills. Cognitive and behavioral interventions make use of the principles of cognitive functioning and behavior listed in Box 30-1. Interventions are tailored to individual client needs and may be applied as single therapeutic entities or in combination. You can access the empirical evidence for cognitive–behavioral therapy

---

Box 30-1   Principles of Cognitive Functioning and Behavior

Principles of Cognitive Functioning

1. What people think affects how they feel.
2. What people think is often based on thinking habits.
3. If we change our thinking, we can effect a change in our feelings.

Principles of Behavior

People do things:	When they are rewarded in a way that is meaningful for them When something they don't like is removed
People don't do things:	When they get punished When something they like is taken away from them

---

MENTAL HEALTH IN THE MOVIES
Anger Management

Sometimes media, such as movies, are not accurate primers for conducting cognitive–behavioral interventions. In the movie *Anger Management* the therapeutic process is bizarre and slapstick. However, it makes the point that we think and we behave in ways that can be changed for the better.

After a small misunderstanding aboard an airplane escalates out of control, timid businessman Dave Buznik (Adam Sandler) is ordered by the court to undergo anger management therapy at the hands of specialist Dr. Buddy Rydell (Jack Nicholson). Dave reluctantly accepts anger management counseling, but after another mishap Dr. Rydell steps up his aggressive and unorthodox treatments by moving in with Dave. As Dr. Rydell wreaks havoc with every aspect of Dave's life, Dave must decide whether to crawl back into his shell or finally stand up for himself. By the end of the movie, Dave's unrealistic and irrational thinking gives way to healthier behaviors. He has learned to cope with a disrespectful boss and an aggravating acquaintance by respectful assertiveness.

Photo courtesy © Photos 12/Alamy.

through the National Science Foundation's website specifically dedicated to behavioral and cognitive sciences, which can be accessed through the Online Student Resources for this text.

COGNITIVE THERAPY

We know that our thoughts (cognitions) affect our feelings. Cognitive therapy is based on making cognitive changes, which, in turn, alters feelings. Consider the routine and habitual thinking of most depressed persons: "I'm no good at anything. I'm a failure in life." With enough repetition, the depressed person comes to accept this particular self-evaluation as accurate. The goal in cognitive therapy is to alter these thoughts to: "There are things that I can do well, and there are things that I need to work on." This type of thinking is more realistic and avoids adhering to an unhealthy perspective. Over time, a change in thinking allows the client to replace disturbing and negative thoughts with neutral and positive thoughts; a cognitive change can influence an emotional change for the better. This process is the basis for cognitive therapy (Skinner, 1974, 1989).

Basic Concepts

Three basic concepts are basic to an understanding of cognitive therapy—attributions, modeling, and self-efficacy.

Attributions

As humans, we constantly ascribe causes to the events in our lives. By labeling or assigning meaning to a circumstance or a set of circumstances, we make *attributions* ("I only got a grade of C. I'm no good at anything. Sarah and Francisco got As. They can do anything.") Think of attributions as perceived causes that may or may not be objectively accurate. Depressed people often attribute failure to themselves and success to others. Then they attribute associated features or characteristics to that circumstance or set of circumstances (such as being a poor student or not knowing the material). Next, they expect a certain outcome from that circumstance and they behave consistently with the expectation that they will not succeed. Finally, they have feelings that match, or are congruent with, the experience. The basic idea is that thoughts and behaviors lead to feelings.

Modeling

Modeling involves imitating another (or others) in the expectation that one will receive rewards such as the rewards other people seem to be receiving. See FIGURE 30-1 ■ for an example of how people learn through modeling the behaviors of others. You have likely experienced modeling throughout your education, especially once you selected nursing as your career. You have doubtless observed nurses who are competent and effective, and you strive for that level of skill in order to receive the same rewards.

FIGURE 30-1 ■ Modeling. Imitative learning is a form of complex learning.
Photo courtesy of Elizabeth Crews Photography.

National Science Foundation

Self-Efficacy

Human learning also occurs through self-efficacy. Self-efficacy involves believing that one's own actions are effective. People learn and adapt when they find themselves in circumstances demanding new or different skills. Under those circumstances, people who tend to believe that they can cope successfully with life and problems in living through acquiring skills, practicing them, and observing successful outcomes will gain confidence and a sense of self-efficacy.

Over time, consistently making attributions, modeling behavior, and experiencing self-efficacy set a pattern of thinking in place. The pattern explains events while shaping expectations about interactions and other behaviors. The patterns can be shaped in adaptive or maladaptive ways, depending on the circumstances and the multiple variables that come into play. Unrealistic thought patterns are maladaptive in that they make demands on the individual that cannot be met or cannot be resolved. For example, a 70-year-old woman who was adopted as a child may have believed for decades she has no worth because her birth mother gave her away. In her case, it is unrealistic to assume that the reason her mother gave her up for adoption was a malevolent one, and, because her birth mother is not likely to be found or identified in order to explain the circumstances of the adoption, this negative perception taints her life.

Cognitive Therapy Techniques

The purpose of cognitive therapy is first to identify thoughts that are unrealistic, negative, or otherwise problematic. Once these thoughts are identified, they are examined for their impact on the individual. Nurses are instrumental in helping a client see how a particular set of thoughts can create a problem. When this connection is made, substituting neutral or positive thoughts for problematic thinking takes place over time. Correcting automatic problematic thinking is a retraining experience. The individual must unlearn the maladaptive cognitive style, then learn adaptive cognitions. The following clinical example describes why cognitive changes are important to mental health.

Clinical Example

George is a 45-year-old male being treated for schizophrenia. His symptoms are coming under reasonable control with medications and therapy; however, he has been having difficulty lately with his mother. Whenever she cannot visit him at his apartment, he becomes depressed and agitated. The outpatient clinic nurse spoke with him about his current problems, and together they identified an irrational thought George had about his mother. He believed that if she didn't visit him every 7 days, regardless of whether she had to work overtime, that meant she did not love him. George thought he would never be able to be "a man" without his mother's love.

Once George identified his irrational conclusions about the meaning of her visits, he was able to talk to her about her feelings for him. George had to concentrate and work to replace his automatic and irrational thoughts with more realistic ones; his mother's love does not need to be renewed—it is always there. George recognized that the visiting schedule and their interpersonal relationship were not connected. He prepared a number of neutral and positive statements that he could repeat to himself whenever the old irrational thoughts appeared. Eventually, George was able to tolerate changes in the frequency of his mother's visits.

Positive Imagery

Positive imagery consists of thinking in a positive way about how an event or experience will unfold rather than anticipating disastrous results. This tends to promote the likelihood of a positive outcome.

Positive imagery can also be applied to past events. It is a reframing of actions taken. For example, a woman is attacked at her parked car and blames herself for being weak, unprepared, and frightened. Positive imagery reframes the woman's actions as perfectly understandable under the circumstances and walks her through the events with this different perspective. It gives her permission to react to frightening events with fear.

When directed toward an upcoming event, positive imagery can be a cognitive rehearsal. That is, thinking positively in advance about how a set of behaviors or an event occurs helps the individual perform more competently in a variety of situations and with a wider array of skills.

Mastery Imagery

Mastery imagery shapes the individual's thoughts about being in control or having mastery over a particular situation. The point of this technique is to practice imagined successful behavior change. An example of mastery imagery is imagining interacting competently and in an adult manner with someone who abused you in childhood. In the clinical example that follows, Christine is achieving mastery over her work situation.

Clinical Example

Christine imagines and rehearses interacting with her usually demanding, critical, and agitated supervisor. In the past, she would typically respond haphazardly and with agitation, which resulted in making errors and feeling ineffective. Christine's mastery imagery establishes a new routine that consists of interacting with her supervisor in a consistently calm and organized manner.

Negative Imagery

Another useful cognitive therapy tool to help change maladaptive behaviors is **negative imagery**, or envisioning negative events and outcomes for maladaptive behavior. Envisioning the negative outcome of maladaptive behavior can serve as a powerful educator. The scenario is played out in the client's thinking and can assist the client in predicting what is likely to happen unless changes are made.

The client is taught to identify the imagery invoked (the thoughts) when beginning a maladaptive behavior, such as substance use. It may be something like: "My favorite drug will be fun" or "I am so much more relaxed and able to interact better when I use this stuff." This is positive imagery. In this case, positive imagery promotes use of the substance even though that behavior will interfere with and damage important relationships with others. The real impact of the behavior is understood only when denial is dispensed with and consequences are recognized. Then substituting with negative imagery can begin.

For example, if a client uses cocaine, the positive imagery may be that the drug will make him feel good. Negatively envisioning cocaine use would consist of the client learning to say and think, "If I use cocaine, I will lose control of my thoughts and feelings. It will cost a lot of money, which I don't have, and will put a bigger emotional and physical gap between me and my wife." Replacing positive imagery with negative imagery may reduce the automatic positive associations over time and reduce the urge to use the drug.

Attribution Restructuring

The heart of cognitive therapy lies in recognizing how we think and behave and in identifying problematic learning. People develop patterns of thinking over time, often automatically, without active or conscious effort. Automatic thoughts can develop into specific (and frequently solidly crystallized) sets of automatic thinking. For example, a person who takes the same mental steps over and over comes to the same problematic conclusion. It is important to realize that maladaptive automatic thoughts and attributions require detection prior to intervention.

If a client has had a number of depressive episodes, the resulting *cognitive map* (thinking in a particular path) must be factored into treatment. Each depressive episode generates negative cognitive maps that are likely to be reactivated the next time the client experiences even a mild dysphoric state, so that current experiences are interpreted more negatively. Each successive negative experience breeds another.

Attribution restructuring or retraining involves abandoning intuitive strategies in order to change the meanings associated with people, places, and things. Once maladaptive cognitions are detected, evidence-based cognitive interventions are employed to alter and restructure thinking.

BEHAVIOR THERAPY

Behavior has an impact on feelings and thoughts, as the clinical example demonstrates.

Clinical Example

An older woman with a hearing deficit is living with her daughter and son-in-law. She wears a hearing aid but, to save on battery power, she removes it and turns it off immediately after dinner every night. When they try to talk to her, she cannot hear. She complains to others that her daughter and son-in-law are not interested in talking or interacting with her in the evening. Her behavior isolates her, but she does not see the connection between her attempts at thriftiness and her feelings of loneliness.

The ways in which particular types of behavioral therapy can affect a variety of conditions are discussed next.

Classical Conditioning

Generally, behavior therapy reduces the occurrence of problematic behaviors. Behavioral therapy is very effective when used with a current problem that is relevant to the client's life (Zeidan et al., 2011). It focuses on behavioral learning processes, including *classical conditioning*. The principles of classical conditioning are as follows:

- People learn to associate a particular feeling state with a particular circumstance that then becomes a conditioned stimulus for the feeling.
- Over time, the association between the circumstance and the feeling is strengthened through repetition and rehearsal.

The therapist's goal in behavior therapy is to decrease or eliminate the association of a particular circumstance (the conditioned stimulus) with a particular feeling. See FIGURE 30-2 ■ for an example of a behavior that responds well to conditioning and intermittent reinforcement.

Operant Conditioning

Operant conditioning is another behavioral learning process and is based on the following concepts:

- People are positively reinforced for certain behaviors.
- People learn to seek further positive reinforcement (an environmental event that rewards, and thus increases the probability of, a behavioral response) by increasing that behavior.
- Positive reinforcement results from either obtaining something desirable or avoiding something unpleasant.

FIGURE 30-2 ■ Intermittent reinforcement. Operant conditioning involves an association between a stimulus and a response.
Photo courtesy of Greg Ward/DK Images.

The therapist's goal in operant conditioning is to help the individual increase positive reinforcement through more adaptive and effective behavior. The effort to change health-related behavior can be facilitated with a behavioral contract. An effective behavioral contract must be tailored for the individual, and a comprehensive behavioral assessment is necessary to design such a contract and form practical, measurable, and feasible objectives and goals. Behavioral contracting is covered in the nursing process section of this chapter.

Rational Emotive Behavioral Therapy

Rational emotive therapy (RET) was originated by Albert Ellis in 1975 and emphasizes cognitive causes of emotional problems along with the importance of taking personal responsibility for maintaining health-damaging thought habits and irrational beliefs (Ellis, 2011). An irrational belief is a belief that lacks reason and sound judgment. Box 30-2 is a list of some common irrational thoughts that, when incorporated into an individual's belief system, are known to create unhealthy thoughts and feelings. The clinician who is skilled in RET helps identify irrational thought structures with the client and then helps develop a plan to substitute more rational personal life philosophies and attitudes based on accurately perceived realities. Healthy emotional consequences occur when rational thinking drives adequate functional behaviors.

Rational emotive behavior therapy (REBT), as it is now known, identifies and corrects irrational beliefs. Rational and irrational beliefs, defined by REBT, form the basis of inferences (conclusions based on reasoning) derived to explain life experiences. Those inferences can be more or less functional depending on the beliefs behind them. People who hold rational beliefs form inferences that are significantly more functional than those formed by people who hold irrational beliefs. The Albert Ellis Institute and the Association for REBT (1975, 2011) can be accessed through the Online Student Resources for this text.

The following clinical example illustrates how firmly held irrational beliefs can inhibit functioning.

Box 30-2 Irrational Thoughts

Rational therapy holds that certain core irrational ideas, which have been clinically observed, are at the root of most mental health disturbances. They are as follows:

- The idea that it is a dire necessity for adults to be loved by significant others for almost everything they do—*instead of their concentrating on their own self-respect, on winning approval for practical purposes, and on loving rather than on being loved.*
- The idea that certain acts are awful or wicked, and that people who perform such acts should be severely damned—*instead of the idea that certain acts are self-defeating or antisocial, and that people who perform such acts are behaving stupidly, ignorantly, or neurotically, and would be better helped to change. People's poor behaviors do not make them rotten individuals.*
- The idea that it is horrible when things are not the way we like them to be—*instead of the idea that it is too bad, that we would better try to change or control bad conditions so that they become more satisfactory, and, if that is not possible, we had better temporarily accept and gracefully lump their existence.*
- The idea that human misery is invariably externally caused and is forced on us by outside people and events—*instead of the idea that neurosis is largely caused by the view that we take of unfortunate conditions.*
- The idea that if something is or may be dangerous or fearsome we should be terribly upset and endlessly obsess about it—*instead of the idea that one would better frankly face it and render it nondangerous and, when that is not possible, accept the inevitable.*
- The idea that it is easier to avoid than to face life difficulties and self-responsibilities—*instead of the idea that the so-called easy way is usually much harder in the long run.*
- The idea that we absolutely need something other or stronger or greater than ourselves on which to rely—*instead of the idea that it is better to take the risks of thinking and acting less dependently.*
- The idea that we should be thoroughly competent, intelligent, and achieving in all possible respects—*instead of the idea that we would better do, rather than always need to do, well and accept ourselves as a quite imperfect creature, who has general human limitations and specific fallibilities.*
- The idea that because something once strongly affected our life, it should indefinitely affect it—*instead of the idea that we can learn from our past experiences but not be overly attached to or prejudiced by them.*
- The idea that we must have certain and perfect control over things—*instead of the idea that the world is full of probability and chance and that we can still enjoy life despite this.*
- The idea that human happiness can be achieved by inertia and inaction—*instead of the idea that we tend to be happiest when we are vitally absorbed in creative pursuits, or when we are devoting ourselves to people or projects outside ourselves.*
- The idea that we have virtually no control over our emotions and that we cannot help feeling disturbed about things—*instead of the idea that we have real control over our destructive emotions if we choose to work at changing the musturbatory hypotheses (the destructive idea that all of our needs and expectations must be met) which we often employ to create them.*

Adapted from: Ellis, A. (2011). The essence of rational emotive behavior therapy: A comprehensive approach to treatment. Retrieved from http://www.rebt.ws/albert_ellis_the_essence_of_rebt.htm

Clinical Example

Marvin, a 38-year-old forklift operator, was injured on the job 4 years ago. His back injuries were treated and all tests indicate a complete recovery; however, his ability to function at work is impaired and he continues to complain of back pain. Marvin has been referred to a specialist in psychotherapy for chronic pain.

In an REBT session, he describes an early experience of observing his father's lengthy struggle with cancer, during which his father was largely sedentary and his mother reacted hysterically whenever his father tried to be more active. In therapy it emerged that Marvin had acquired an irrational core belief that problems or fears are best handled with rest, withdrawal, and being sedentary. Marvin's past pain symptoms were uncomfortable enough to trigger this response, consistent with his core belief. As he became more sedentary and less functional, his back became increasingly weak and prone to pain. The greater the pain, the less active he became, until he was caught in a vicious cycle of increasing pain and withdrawal.

REBT helped Marvin learn to identify his irrational belief. This was accomplished through a Socratic question-and-answer format whereby Marvin recognized that withdrawal and inactivity led to more rather than fewer problems. The sources for Marvin's irrational belief were clarified as well. The belief was reframed in a more rational direction—that many problems respond best to constructive and productive activity. Specifically, Marvin's chronic pain was likely to improve with exercise, physical therapy, and daily productive activity. Assignments were given between sessions to help Marvin develop his repertoire in these areas. As he successfully proceeded to do so, his pain symptoms diminished and his self-esteem increased.

The Socratic question-and-answer format is an important aspect of REBT. This method, illustrated in Box 30-3, allows the client to explore how a particular line of reasoning was allowed to develop and how it continues to function. It focuses on a logical perspective, which is an appealing and manageable therapeutic style to which many adults can relate. As with all therapeutic styles, however, there must be a fit between the client and the therapeutic intervention. Not all therapies will be useful, or even therapeutic, with all clients in all situations.

Behavior Modification

Behavior modification frequently focuses on a target behavior that is problematic for the individual (e.g., overeating) or for the community (e.g., loud verbal outbursts). The behavior is observed and tracked in objective and measurable terms, then addressed with a behavior modification plan. Both nonpharmacologic and pharmacologic interventions may be employed to assist in the modification of behavioral disturbances. We will discuss nonpharmacologic behavioral modification interventions here. Pharmacologic interventions are discussed in Chapters 7 and 31 ∞.

A behavior modification program begins with the identification of a specific behavior that requires change. It is important to monitor the target behavior and develop a detailed database about it. The problem behavior is carefully observed for the following:

- Antecedents (what came before)
- Precipitants (what appeared to cause or provoke the behavior)

Box 30-3 The Socratic Question-and-Answer Format

Marvin:	"I spent the day in bed yesterday because my back hurt."
Therapist:	"What did you hope that would accomplish?"
Marvin:	"That my back would feel better."
Therapist:	"Did it?"
Marvin:	"No."
Therapist:	"Can you ever remember a time when inactivity made your back feel better?"
Marvin:	"No, it just gets worse."
Therapist:	"So where and how did you come to believe that inactivity would make your back feel better?"
Marvin:	"In my family we always rested when we were hurt."
Therapist:	"Did that help your family?"
Marvin:	"Come to think of it, not that I ever saw."
Therapist:	"Maybe too much resting doesn't help?"
Marvin:	"I never thought of it that way."
Therapist:	"If too much resting doesn't help, what else might?"
Marvin:	"Once when my back hurt I went to a chiropractor and did some exercises. I remember that helped."
Therapist:	"What does that tell you about resting too much?"
Marvin:	"Maybe it's not such a good idea."

- How the behavior is expressed
- Timing
- Frequency
- Duration
- Personal strengths to be capitalized on in designing the plan

To enable a client to modify behavior that is undesirable or unhealthy, giving support and involving the client in the plan of action are required. One strategy organizes the client's problem behavior into a hierarchy. In this **hierarchy**, the least distressing changes are at the lowest level and the most distressing are at the highest. For example, scores are assigned to levels of distress, ranging from zero, or none, to 100, the highest level of difficulty the client can imagine. Someone who overeats may feel only slight distress, or a score of 15, when thinking about not eating at a movie or a sporting event. A much higher distress level, with a score of 85, might occur when the same client considers being in an unfamiliar or uncomfortable social environment and not being able to eat.

Response Prevention

Guiding an individual through imagining a situation at the lowest level of distress initially and developing and rehearsing adaptive responses to the distress establishes a new pattern that supplants the older, maladaptive response. This is called **response prevention**, meaning the automatic maladaptive responses are

modified and replaced with adaptive behaviors. Gradually, the client advances through his or her hierarchy of distress, learning to develop skills in responding competently at every step.

Systematic Desensitization

Systematic desensitization, another behavioral modification treatment regimen, also uses a hierarchy to arrange treatment. Behaviors are identified and ordered according to level of distress for the client. The client imagines being in certain situations at various levels of distress and learns to cope before moving on to the next level of distress. See Your Intervention Strategies for a desensitization hierarchy for a phobic fear of heights.

Assignments for graded exposures and response prevention are usually completed as homework, accompanied by self-monitoring (through diaries and/or graphs) and clinical assessment of progress through the behavioral programming. The behavior modification plan requires a realistic appraisal of the difficulties facing the person who wants to make a change and includes a plan for handling those difficulties. Clients with significant symptoms can make changes in this manner (Horan, et al., 2011). A sample plan for someone who wants to quit smoking, for example, must include the following three steps:

1. Understanding the mechanisms that trigger the urge to smoke
2. Substituting other activities for the habit of smoking
3. Recognizing supports that will promote success in unlearning the rituals of smoking behavior

For a client trying to quit smoking, the environment should be smoke free and all smoking materials and accoutrements disposed of in order to minimize relapses. Psychopharmacologic supports are available for the smoking cessation process.

YOUR INTERVENTION STRATEGIES
Desensitization Hierarchy for Phobic Fear of Heights

1. Develop 10 to 12 scenes of increasing levels of fear. *Example:* Tell the client to imagine the scene with the lowest level of fear:
   "You are going up a kitchen stepladder. Step to the third rung, and look around."
   "Now you are going up to the top rung. You are at the top. Look around at the cupboards. Look at the floor."
   "Now you are on the second floor of an office building. Walk toward the window and look out."
2. Continue in this manner, increasing the level of fear attached to the scene each time the client is able to visualize without undue anxiety:
   "Now you go to the top of the Sears Tower. Go over to the guardrail and look straight down."
3. The final steps of the desensitization process include encouraging the client to try some of these behaviors in real life, after the client has successfully coped with the imagined scenes.

YOUR INTERVENTION STRATEGIES
Smoking Cessation Behavior Modification Guidance

Use the guidelines below to help a smoker quit:

- Set up a timeline of the typical smoking schedule.
- Develop a tracking mechanism for where the individual smokes (couch, corner bar, car).
- Use checklists for situations and interactions with others in which smoking is involved.
- Suggest a set of behaviors to substitute for smoking.
- Provide self-help literature.
- Encourage those in the environment to also quit smoking.
- Provide motivational material related to the client's current health status.
- Identify stressors.
- Enhance skills for coping with stressors.
- Emphasize positive benefits of smoking cessation.
- Provide individual support.
- Reinforce short-term success.
- Provide support through group therapy.

Your Intervention Strategies lists behavior modification tips for smoking cessation.

COGNITIVE–BEHAVIORAL THERAPY

The goal in cognitive–behavioral treatment is to develop healthier labeling and an expectancy strategy that leads to more desirable feelings and a greater feeling of self-efficacy. Beck (1976; Beck & Freeman, 1990) indicates that behavioral problems arise in childhood when people learn core beliefs and make associations between what they believe and what they expect to happen. Beck's theories are accessible at the website for the Beck Institute for Cognitive Therapy and Research and through a link on the Online Student Resources for this text.

Building on what we learn in childhood, our labels and expectations influence the strategies we select to compensate and cope. Webster copes with the following situation according to the particular pattern that he developed over time.

Clinical Example

Webster is a traveling salesman who must drive long distances to meet with his clients. One day, during a meeting with a client, he experienced a panic attack. His symptoms included shortness of breath, rapid heartbeat, and thoughts of wanting to escape the situation. Afterward he was very tired. He decided to leave work early and drive home. When he got home he felt more relaxed and relieved. He hoped the panic attack was an isolated event that would not happen again.

However, Webster had more panic attacks. He longed to be at home when they occurred because he experienced relief and greater comfort there. He soon began to cut back on face-to-face client meetings and conducted meetings online or by telephone instead. The more he stayed at home, the more anxious he became when he was required to leave. Eventually he became almost completely unable to leave home, whether for business, social, or any other purpose (such as an emergency with a friend). The mere thought of stepping outside the house precipitated a panic attack. Webster had developed diagnosable panic disorder with agoraphobia at a severe level.

Cognitive and behavioral treatment consists of identifying and recognizing maladaptive thinking styles and working toward the acquisition of new skills for managing stressors. Features of treatment include teaching, interpreting, reframing, and learning and practicing new behaviors, and are extremely beneficial for people with mild to moderate depression and anxiety, and post-traumatic stress disorder (Høifødet, Strøm, Kolstrup, Eisemann, & Waterloo, 2011; Cohen, Mannarino, & Iyengar, 2011). Once thoughts and behaviors are realistically and rationally framed and implemented, emotional reactions will be consistent with them. See Evidence-Based Practice for a description of how these treatment strategies are incorporated into a group setting for the treatment of panic disorder.

The cognitive–behavioral approach is important in the contemporary treatment of substance dependence. There is sufficient research evidence supporting both drug-free outpatient treatment programs and treatment methods involving medications such as naltrexone (ReVia) and buprenorphine (Subutex). These programs, combined with psychosocial treatment or behavioral techniques, provide additional promise for outpatient-based drug abuse treatment. CBT can be used to teach new coping skills to people with substance problems as long as the interventions are tailored to the individual's cognitive functioning (Kiluk, Nich, & Carroll, 2011).

People who have psychotic symptoms also benefit from CBT (Thomas, Rossell, Farhall, Shawyer, & Castle, 2011). The presence of auditory hallucinations or a lack of insight into illness does not interfere with CBT nor does it interfere with the reduction of negative symptoms of schizophrenia (see Chapter 16∞). Early intervention with CBT when someone first begins having psychotic symptoms has also been supported in the literature (Gaynor, Dooley, Lawlor, Lawoyin, & O'Callaghan, 2011).

Thought Stopping

Thought stopping is an example of a cognitive–behavioral psychotherapeutic technique that can help a client change thinking processes. Changing the thinking process is important, because feelings can be strongly influenced by the pattern and process of thoughts. Clients sometimes have difficulty with repetitive, maladaptive thinking. For example, one client worries incessantly about things she cannot control; another client repeatedly has inaccurate, negative thoughts about himself. For these clients, the cognitive–behavioral therapist may implement the procedure known as *thought stopping*. The client learns to stop negative or maladaptive thinking by visualizing or imagining a specific image, sensation, or circumstance. Examples of thought stopping include the following:

- Visualizing a traffic stop sign
- Imagining hearing the word "stop" said loudly
- Imagining the tactile sensation of leaning against a closed door
- Visualizing pushing the problematic thoughts out of one's room or off one's lawn

Thought stopping is done whenever the identified negative or maladaptive thought occurs. Over time, the client

EVIDENCE-BASED PRACTICE

Treating Panic Attacks

Otis, a 45-year-old man, experienced panic attacks for 6 years. He tried to control the attacks on his own, but after 2 years finally went for treatment. Otis took medications with only moderate success for 4 years and was ready to try something different to address his problem. He agreed to participate in your cognitive–behavioral therapy group in an outpatient clinic.

It was noted by Otis's pharmacotherapist and reported to you that Otis had a number of automatic responses to his panic attacks. He would think and feel a particular way whenever he became anxious, was exposed to a stressor, or had a panic attack. His defense mechanisms were frequently immature, although he did not describe them as such.

Over 4 months, Otis and several other individuals attended 12 group sessions based on a cognitive–behavioral curriculum. Muscle relaxation, diaphragmatic breathing skills, cognitive restructuring, and homework assignments formed the cognitive–behavioral

aspects of the therapy. There was also a component to the group where the therapist guided participants through exposure to the problematic trigger. At the end of the treatment period, Otis was able to respond to stressors in a more mature, satisfactory manner. His panic attacks and other symptoms were also reduced. Even 1 year after the group concluded, Otis was still benefiting from the cognitive–behavioral therapy he received.

Base your actions on more than one study, but these interventions were developed using cognitive–behavioral principles in conjunction with the following research:

Gloster, A. T., Wittchen, H. U., Einsle, F., Lang, T., Helbig-Lang, E., Fydrich, T., . . . Arolt, V. (2011). Psychological treatment for panic disorder with agoraphobia: A randomized controlled trial to examine the role of therapist-guided exposure in situ in CBT. *Journal of Consulting and Clinical Psychology, 79*(3), 406–420.

CRITICAL THINKING QUESTIONS

1. What elements would you take into consideration when planning to introduce behavioral change?
2. How can Otis and his family benefit from psychoeducation?
3. What exercises and rehearsals would be considered priorities for Otis?

learns to stop such thoughts in an almost reflexive manner. This technique is typically used as part of a larger set of techniques that might also include developing alternative thoughts and mastering behavioral skills to alter outcomes in various problematic circumstances.

Techniques used in CBT such as thought stopping are defined and explained on the website of the National Association of Cognitive Behavioral Therapists, accessible through the Online Student Resources for this text.

Dialectical–Behavioral Therapy

Linehan and associates (1999) specifically developed dialectical–behavioral therapy (DBT) for the outpatient treatment of chronically suicidal people with borderline personality disorder. DBT is a specialized subset of the cognitive–behavioral treatment modalities. The client with borderline personality disorder tends to be crisis prone, with intense relational episodes (Smoski et al., 2011). In other words, interactions with others have the potential to disrupt the client powerfully.

DBT is a biosocial behavioral model of treatment that assumes there is a disorder in how the client regulates emotions and tolerates stress (Grogan & Murphy, 2011). The numerous dysfunctional patterns of behavior common in the diagnosis of borderline personality disorder (see Chapter 22∞), such as self-destructive behavior, the inability to govern impulses, or severe dissociative phenomena, are regarded within the DBT framework as the client's attempts to problem solve. DBT has also been used successfully in treating the multi-problem adolescent who is at highest risk for suicidal behavior and self-injury.

DBT is a psychosocial treatment program that focuses on teaching clients the following four skills:

1. Mindfulness (attention to one's experience)
2. Interpersonal effectiveness
3. Emotional regulation
4. Distress tolerance

This concept of therapy focuses on the continuing balance between the necessity of accepting maladaptive behavior patterns (a cognitive feature) in both an intrapsychic and interactional context while still working to change them (the behavioral feature). DBT is a clearly structured therapy and integrates a wide choice of therapeutic strategies. It is a promising psychosocial intervention for improving interpersonal functioning among severely dysfunctional individuals with borderline personality disorder. For more information, visit the website of the Association for Behavioral and Cognitive Therapies, accessible through the Online Student Resources for this book.

Cultural Aspects of Cognitive and Behavioral Interventions

Cultural considerations involve more than an individual's race or ethnicity. Culture is an envelope that includes, among other characteristics, religion, spirituality, gender, sexual orientation and expression, social status, and age. To be a competent provider of cognitive–behavioral interventions, you must, at a minimum, understand these variables, be self-aware, and be comfortable working with those from a culture that differs from your own. Your Self-Awareness will help sensitize you to the forces of a dominant culture. This section

YOUR SELF-AWARENESS
Influence of the Dominant Culture on Cognitive–Behavioral Interventions

What you think (cognition) and how you act (behavior) are influenced by your culture. Being a member of the dominant cultural group shapes who you are. On the other hand, not being a member of the dominant cultural group also has the power to shape your identity. Determine whether there is a difference between you, your client, and the dominant culture on the major cultural characteristics in the following list. Be alert to the effect these differences will have on your cognitive–behavioral interventions.

- Religion
- Spirituality
- Gender
- Ability/disability
- Sexual orientation and expression
- Social status
- Age
- Race
- Ethnicity

DEVELOPING CULTURAL COMPETENCE

Culture and Cognitive–Behavioral Interventions

Consider what it may be like to have a client discuss the following situation with you. Rachel is upset about being spoken to in a harsh and loud manner by her male supervisor at work. She feels demoralized after every interaction with him. Rachel is willing to make several changes in her thinking and behavior in order to feel and function better and agrees to work with you within a cognitive–behavioral framework. She may require cognitive restructuring, mastery imagery, and assertiveness and communication assignments.

You examine each feature of Rachel's situation and Rachel's characteristics to determine if there are any cultural contributions to the overall problem and identify the following factors. Rachel is young, and therefore may not have a lot of experience with supervisors. She has an untreated 20% hearing loss that may prompt people to speak louder to her than normal to ensure she hears all of what is being said. Because Rachel is Egyptian-American, assess Rachel's comfort level when speaking with males, her expectations when she interacts with males, and whether her heritage could contribute to the difficulties she is having with her supervisor. When you take cultural considerations into account, you may change the overall structure of her plan (or not), but you would certainly shape your interventions around these issues.

CRITICAL THINKING QUESTIONS

1. What cognitive–behavioral changes would you recommend for Rachel?
2. What recommendations would you make for homework or rehearsals that Rachel could practice?

will briefly describe how to implement this consciousness within a cognitive–behavioral intervention framework. Chapter 9 ∞ explores cultural considerations in detail.

The emphasis is on the individual in cognitive–behavioral interventions (what the individual thinks, feels, interprets, assigns meanings to, etc.); therefore, it can be the ideal venue to address multiculturalism in treatment.

There is a further benefit to blending an understanding of cognitive and behavioral interventions and multiculturalism. Developing Cultural Competence indicates some of these.

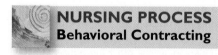

NURSING PROCESS
Behavioral Contracting

The effort to change health-related behavior may be facilitated with competent behavioral contracting. A behavioral contract is a behavior modification plan arranged as a specific agreement between the individual and the team of caregivers who identify the behavior and design the plan. To be effective, tailor the behavioral contract for the individual client. A comprehensive behavioral assessment is necessary to form such a contract, as is the identification of practical, measurable, and feasible objectives and goals. For example, smoking cessation is important to improve the everyday life and future health of clients, especially those in long term care psychiatric facilities for whom smoking can ease anxiety and improve (temporarily) executive functioning. The components of a behavioral contract for quitting smoking in the form of the nursing process follow.

Assessment

A comprehensive assessment interview is the first step in developing a contract with the goal of behavioral change. The purpose of the interview is to assemble a complete picture of the behavior and what maintains it or keeps it going, so that strategies for changing the behavior have the best chance of success. The interview process identifies problem behavior and divides it into four components, to be explored in turn:

- The *behavioral* component asks what the client is doing.
- The *cognitive* component examines what the client is thinking.
- The *affective* component identifies what the client is feeling.
- The *physiologic* component examines the physical realities of the situation.

What precipitates or precedes this client's problem behavior? Try to identify when it occurs. Does it occur only when the client is anxious, with certain people, or in certain places? What are the consequences of the problem behavior for the client? Assess whether the behavior relaxes or angers the client, or if it endangers the client's life.

Environmental factors (family, economic, and social) may have an effect on the problem behavior and therefore on the success of a behavioral contract. If the client's relatives or friends smoke or if social occasions always take place in smoking areas, the behavioral contract should take this into account.

Assessing the intrapsychic factors influencing the problem behavior can be accomplished during the assessment interview. Determine whether the client:

- Has assertiveness skills
- Experiences stress when asserting needs with other people (such as when stating to friends, "I have trouble staying away from cigarettes when others smoke around me")
- Has fragile, dependent, or abusive relationships

Take all of these factors into account to develop a viable behavioral contract.

A comprehensive interview also covers any difficulties with depression, irritability, anxiety, psychotic symptomatology (hearing, seeing, or believing in things that are not real), substance or alcohol use/abuse, or addictive/compulsive behavior). Problematic behaviors could also be uncovered during the interview. Such behaviors would include smoking as a type of addictive behavior or refusing to adhere to bed rest instructions as a compulsive and self-destructive behavior.

Current psychosocial variables are essential features to be investigated in a thorough interview and assessment. These variables include present employment, marital and family status, social and romantic functioning, and avocational pursuits. Hobbies are not always constructive. They can be quite destructive, especially if the hobby revolves around a problematic set of behaviors (e.g., drinking beer and smoking while bowling).

If possible, observe the client demonstrating the problem behavior to confirm or disconfirm the client's self-reports. Collateral information on the problem behavior from family, work records, friends, colleagues, and other treatment providers can offer a different perspective. Ultimately, the assessment interview seeks to identify the client's perception of how behavior change might alter his or her life.

Nursing Diagnosis: NANDA

Examples of nursing diagnoses that may derive from a cognitive–behavioral assessment in preparation for the development of a behavioral contract include the following:

- Deficient Knowledge
- Dysfunctional Family Processes
- Interrupted Family Processes
- Impaired Social Interaction
- Hopelessness
- Ineffective Coping
- Ineffective Health Maintenance

Outcome Identification: NOC

Knowledge about one's disease process, medication, treatment regimen, or health behaviors would indicate a positive outcome for Deficient Knowledge. Displaying hope would indicate a positive change in Hopelessness. Improved family functioning and coping is evidence of a successful outcome in relation to Dysfunctional Family Processes and Interrupted Family Processes. For a client with the nursing diagnosis of Ineffective Coping, identifying harmful behaviors and what triggers them, then avoiding high-risk situations, constitutes a successful outcome.

In general, outcomes for behavioral change are easily identified. Behaviors are objective criteria by which progress can be tracked. They can be compared to previous behaviors for similarities or differences. If problematic behaviors occur less frequently, they may be considered to have a positive outcome. The following clinical example illustrates positive outcomes with a client experiencing anxiety.

Clinical Example

Kim, a 29-year-old man with a diagnosis of obsessive–compulsive disorder, worried obsessively that electrical appliances would cause fires. Kim's nurse taught him relaxation exercises and thought-stopping techniques to use when he found himself becoming anxious. The expected outcomes in Kim's situation are: uses coping strategies to reduce anxiety and reports decreased physical manifestations of anxiety. With practice, Kim found that within 1 week he was less anxious when in the kitchen or near other electrical appliances. Although his thoughts about appliance fires and his anxiety had not completely abated, they were definitely more manageable.

Planning and Implementation: NIC

The planning phase of the nursing process with behavioral contracting requires taking into consideration the client's interactions with you during the assessment interview. Consider these components of the mental status exam: appearance; facial expression; motor behavior; cooperativeness; quality of speech, including spontaneity, pace, volume, response time, coherence, and relevance; and goal directedness. Observations of the client's affect (appropriate or inappropriate), mood, lethality, delusions, hallucinations, and orientation to person, place, time,

WHY I PLAN TO BECOME A PSYCHIATRIC–MENTAL HEALTH NURSE

Treya's Story: My best friend started therapy last year because she was depressed. I was so proud of Bobbie for doing something none of us ever thought of doing—going to therapy—and she got a lot out of it. Her therapist, a psychiatric–mental health nurse, taught her that what you think and what you do affects how you feel. During my clinical rotations at psychiatric–mental health sites, I heard about cognitive–behavioral counseling and psychotherapy, but wasn't able to see how well it worked until Bobbie's experience. One example helped me plan my specialty area in nursing: Bobbie learned that she had some unrealistic expectations of herself and when she couldn't possibly achieve those goals she became sad, ashamed, and depressed. In counseling, Bobbie talked about these goals and gradually came to realize she could think and do things differently. The change in her is remarkable and she is a healthier woman now. That's why I want to be a psychiatric–mental health nurse.

Care Plan: Depression Intervention

and purpose also contribute information essential to developing a plan of care. The client's immediate, short-term, and long-term memory abilities, along with evidence of executive functioning (such as the ability to carry out multistep activities independently), give direction to how the client thinks.

How people think and react and remember is their cognitive style or overall pattern of thought. A cognitive style is the way someone thinks best. For example, some people respond better to audiovisual than to printed material, or they perform tasks more effectively with persistent encouragement versus occasional monitoring. These differences in cognitive style shape several components in your behavioral contract. Planning and implementation with behavioral contracting includes taking the family into account. Partnering With Clients and Families provides some pointers on helping the family improve their communication with CBT. The website of the National Association of Cognitive Behavioral Therapists has information about cognitive behavioral therapy and its uses in treatment and is accessible through the Online Student Resources for this text.

Forming Practical and Measurable Objectives and Goals

Formulating practical and measurable objectives and goals is the next step in developing a behavioral contract. Objectives are small steps leading to goal attainment; goals represent the overall desired outcomes. Prioritizing the behavioral objectives involves the following four main features:

1. The goal should contribute directly to the desired result. In other words, how will tracking every cigarette the client smokes, and under what circumstances, help the client stop smoking? (It will sensitize the client and you to factors that contribute to smoking behavior and exactly how much and when the client smokes.)
2. The goal can be objectively monitored. (You know the objective is reached when the client completes the tracking mechanism.)
3. The goal is easily understood by the client and all supportive significant others. (The client knows how to fill out the tracking mechanism and knows why he or she is tracking the behavior.)
4. The goal can be accomplished in the available time. (The client can fill out the form daily for 1 week.)

Behavioral goals should be objectively verifiable as contributing to positive treatment outcome. The change is necessary and relevant, not outlandish (it is relevant to track how often one smokes through daily journaling; it is outlandish to set a goal of never having another craving to smoke). The client, all significant others, and the treatment team agree to and understand the goal. Also, the goal is not likely to negatively affect other important aspects of the client's health or psychosocial, interpersonal, or intrapersonal functioning. Remember with whom you are formulating this contract—for example, you will not be asking a lifelong introvert to engage in sensitive self-disclosure in an intense psychotherapy group.

An obtainable goal could be for the client to develop better social skills. The combination of social skills training with cognitive–behavior therapy (CBT) or dialectical–behavior therapy (DBT) appears to be powerful. Social skills training is discussed in Chapter 28∞.

Negotiating a Behavioral Contract

The basic rules for negotiating a behavioral contract include engaging the client and family as colleagues, avoiding complex terminology or coercive formats, and making sure the client and the family completely understand, agree to, and, to the extent possible, feel comfortable with the contract.

Potential problems can have a minimal impact if they are detected early in the process. If you anticipate and address them, the client does not have to experience failure simply because the contract was poorly designed. Possible problems include a lack of understanding, lack of commitment, lack of adequate follow-up monitoring, and lack of a defined format or contingency plan for unforeseen problems. A contract is poorly designed when it is in conflict with important and unchangeable aspects of the client's psychosocial functioning. Your Intervention Strategies summarizes the behavioral contracting process.

Continuing assessment, regular evaluations, and troubleshooting meetings will determine whether adjustments to the contract are necessary. Designing a contract to which the client can adhere will maximize the chance of success. Contracts can be adjusted in many ways, including formal supports, prioritization of various objectives, and appropriate revisions of goals. Creativity is an essential component in negotiating an effective behavioral contract.

PARTNERING WITH CLIENTS AND FAMILIES

Promoting the Effectiveness of CBT With Families of Clients With Schizophrenia

This list can give you some quick pointers about the best ways families can promote the effectiveness of cognitive–behavioral therapy (CBT) with clients who have schizophrenia.

- Explain how what we think (cognition) and what we do (behavior) form the basis of CBT.
- Explain the difference between a thought and a feeling.

During family contacts with someone who has schizophrenia:

- Talk about thoughts and behaviors with the client.
- Describe practical issues.

- Use words that do not create emotional responses (neutral words such as "unusual" instead of "odd," "unexpected" instead of "frightening").
- Reinforce functional behavior.
- Recognize that some behavior may be the result of misread or misinterpreted social cues.

Talking about thoughts and behaviors, instead of feelings, is not intended to lessen problematic behaviors, but may provide clients and family members with a structure for conversations when the client is symptomatic.

YOUR INTERVENTION STRATEGIES   Developing a Behavioral Contract

Step	Purpose	Action	Strategy
1	Comprehensive behavioral assessment	Interviewing	Collecting data on which the contract will be based
2	Formulating practical and measurable objectives and goals	Prioritizing	Evaluating abilities
3	Negotiating a behavioral contract	Setting basic rules Identifying potential problems	Making adjustments Evaluating the relevance and usefulness of the behavioral contract
4	Optimizing the client's ability to adhere to a behavioral contract	Determining barriers <ul><li>Intellectual</li><li>Emotional</li><li>Motivational</li><li>Physiological</li></ul>	Including constructive catalysts <ul><li>Psychotherapy</li><li>Relaxation training</li><li>Biofeedback</li><li>Family involvement</li></ul>

Data on how well the client adheres to the contract can be collected through client self-monitoring, client self-reports at regular meetings, discussions in counseling sessions, and natural or scheduled observations of the client. Further information can be collected from relatives, friends, colleagues, and other treatment providers.

Optimizing the client's ability to adhere to a behavioral contract requires careful determination and assessment of any potential barriers. Check for overall intellectual functioning as well as cognitive style. Emotional perspectives can influence performance and outcome. Does the client manifest depression, irritability, or anxiety that would interfere with contract adherence? It is important to design supports that will address these problems and promote success (Stice, Rohde, Gau, & Ochner, 2011). Motivation can also play a large part in outcome. Was the client poorly motivated to begin with? What was done to address this problem? If design features to address motivation were implemented, check to see how they are working. Is the client demonstrating a decline in motivation? If so, why (psychiatric, social, economic, or medical causation)? Address all underlying causative factors.

Physiology can affect outcome. Is the client experiencing side effects, or is the main effect of a medication (such as mood stabilization for symptoms of mania) bothering the client? If the client perceives this behavioral change as threatening to an established lifestyle and interaction pattern or if the client becomes uncomfortable with the independence or responsibilities expected of him or her following the behavioral change, this could also sabotage adherence.

Provide constructive catalysts—those tools that will enhance the process without interference. Some psychotherapeutic interventions are useful with most clients undergoing stress. These include general stress management, preparing for the likely emotional consequences and adjustment difficulties that changes in health behaviors can cause, providing the opportunity to ventilate and disclose feelings, and support services. More specialized treatment and techniques include relaxation training and biofeedback. Family involvement is a powerful and useful catalyst for promoting and maintaining behavioral change. Significant others, particularly those with whom the client resides or will reside, are likely to provide important input about the level of contract adherence. It is therefore important to involve them as much as appropriate in formulating and implementing the behavioral contract. If the details of the contract do not work for the involved family, they will not work for the client.

FIGURE 30-3 ■ is a sample behavioral contract format and gives an overview of how the process of combining medications and behavioral change can be documented. Sections may be expanded or eliminated depending on the targeted behavior and client needs. Imagine a health behavior of your own that you could change and walk yourself through this contract. If you can develop a plan to change your behavior, you may very well be successful in helping others to change theirs.

Providing Physiologic Support With Medications

Often, clients feel anxious when faced with making behavioral changes. This anxiety is best handled through supportive and instructive interactions. However, some individuals require physiologic support to prevent their anxiety from reaching panic levels. Anxiolytics, or antianxiety medications, could be administered in sufficient quantities to reduce the problematic affect yet leave the client with enough motivation to learn behavioral techniques for anxiety management where appropriate. Recall from Chapter 8 ∞ that some anxiety is necessary for learning to take place. Therefore, levels of anxiolytics that completely eliminate anxiety are countertherapeutic.

Evaluation

Evaluating client abilities and strengths, particularly with regard to learning and making changes, will help in the design of the contract. Discover what other situations requiring behavioral change the client has mastered and what specific personal or social strengths the client employed in implementing the change. Evaluate the client's weaknesses with regard to learning and making changes as well. What has the client attempted to change without success? Try to ascertain the specific factors that interfered with the success of that goal.

Formulated objectives and goals should draw on the client's strengths and prior patterns of successful change. What the client is asked to do should mirror as closely as possible

Sample Behavioral Contract

Client Name _____ Date _____

Problem Behavior: _____

Problem Behavior Components

Behavioral	Affective
Cognitive	Physiological

Interview Findings

Depression	Anxiety	Substance or Alcohol Use/Abuse
Irritability	Psychotic Symptomatology	Addictive/Compulsive Behavior

Psychosocial Variables

Present Employment	Social/Romantic Functioning	Typical Daily Routines
Marital/Family Status	Avocational Pursuits	Eating/Sleeping/Exercise Habits
The Client's Expectations of How This Behavior Change Might Alter Any of the Above		

Collateral Information _____

_____

Cognitive Style _____

_____

Which of the following apply for this contract?

☐ Psychotherapy for any current psychological problems
☐ Relaxation training/biofeedback
☐ General stress management
☐ Preparation for likely emotional consequences and adjustment difficulties
☐ The opportunity to ventilate and disclose feelings
☐ Support

Contract Objectives and Goals

This goal is agreed upon and understood by the client, all significant others, and the treatment team.

Signature _____
Signature _____
Signature _____
Signature _____

FIGURE 30-3 ■ Sample behavioral contract.

what the client has previously done successfully. The best predictor of future behavior is past behavior.

Carefully crafted contracts to lead to successful outcomes. Frame the components of a behavioral contract in the success (e.g., will maintain abstinence) rather than failure (e.g., will not relapse into use) mode.

CASE MANAGEMENT

It is important to focus on maintaining the routines and schedules of cognitive–behavioral interventions once a plan of care has been established. Homework assignments and practicing more competent responses will ensure that the client retains the skills developed in therapy. The case manager can be helpful in sustaining that structure. The variety of interventions, such as group or individual therapy, behavior modification, and self-study, can all be promoted and supported through case management.

COMMUNITY-BASED CARE AND HOME CARE

Each of the problems addressed with cognitive–behavioral interventions benefits from maintaining those interventions in the client's natural setting. Counseling, psychotherapy, and other treatments discussed in this chapter are frequently conducted in the community. The behavioral contract can be designed to address inpatient issues and community living and to enhance the transition from inpatient treatment to an outpatient setting. Additional supports can be built into the contract to ensure the client's success after the transition. These interventions in the community maximize both the quality of life and management of symptoms.

Family psychoeducation can be an integral feature of community-based care and home care. Teaching about symptoms and how to address them with the planned interventions is supportive and reassuring. Involving significant others increases the likelihood that the plan of care is implemented and that frustrations and misunderstandings are minimized.

REFERENCES

Beck, A. T. (1976). *Cognitive therapy and the emotional disorders.* New York, NY: International Universities Press.

Beck, A. T., & Freeman, A. (1990). *Cognitive therapy of personality disorders.* New York, NY: Guilford Press.

Cohen, J. A., Mannarino, A. P., & Iyengar, S. (2011). Community treatment of posttraumatic stress disorder for children exposed to intimate partner violence: A randomized controlled trial. *Archives of Pediatrics & Adolescent Medicine, 165*(1), 16–21.

Ellis, A. (2011). The essence of rational emotive behavior therapy: A comprehensive approach to treatment. Retrieved from http://www.rebt.ws/albert_ellis_the_essence_of_rebt.htm

Ellis, A., & Harper, R. (1975). *A new guide to rational living.* Chatworth, CA: Wilshire Book Co.

Gaynor, K., Dooley, B., Lawlor, E., Lawoyin, R., & O'Callaghan, E. (2011). Group cognitive behavioral therapy as a treatment for negative symptoms in first-episode psychosis. *Early Interventional Psychiatry, 5*(2), 168–173.

Gloster, A. T., Wittchen, H. U., Einsle, F., Lang, T., Helbig-Lang, E., Fydrich, T., . . . Arolt, V. (2011). Psychological treatment for panic disorder with agoraphobia: A randomized controlled trial to examine the role of therapist-guided exposure in situ in CBT. *Journal of Consulting and Clinical Psychology, 79*(3), 406–420. doi: 10.1037/a0023584

Grogan, S., & Murphy, K. P. (2011). Anticipatory stress response in PTSD: Extreme stress in children. *Journal of Child & Adolescent Psychiatric Nursing, 24*(1), 58–71.

Høifødet, R. S., Strøm, C., Kolstrup, N., Eisemann, M., & Waterloo, K. (2011). Effectiveness of cognitive behavioural therapy in primary health care: A review. *Family Practice.* Advance online publication. doi: 10.1093/fampra/cmr017

Horan, W. P., Kern, R. S., Tripp, C., Hellemann, G., Wynn, J. K., Bell, M.,... Green, M. F. (2011). Efficacy and specificity of social cognitive skills training for outpatients with psychiatric disorders. *Journal of Psychiatric Research, 45*(8), 1113–1122.

Kiluk, B. D., Nich, C., & Carroll, K. M. (2011). Relationship of cognitive function and the acquisition of coping skills in computer assisted treatment for substance use disorders. *Drug & Alcohol Dependence, 114*(2–3), 169–176.

Linehan, M. M., Schmidt III, H., Dimeff, L. A., Craft, J. C., Kanter, J., & Comtois, K. A. (1999). Dialectical behavior therapy for patients with borderline personality disorder and drug-dependence. *American Journal on Addictions, 8,* 279–292.

Skinner, B. F. (1974). *About behaviorism.* New York, NY: Knopf.

Skinner, B. F. (1989). The origins of cognitive thought. *American Psychologist, 44,* 12–18.

Smoski, M. J., Salsman, N., Wang, L., Smith, V., Lynch, T. R., Dager, S. R., . . . Linehan, M. M. (2011). Functional imaging of emotional reactivity in opiate-dependent borderline personality disorder. *Personality Disorders: Theory, Research, & Treatment, 2*(3), 230–241. doi: 10.1037/a0022228

Stice, E., Rohde, P., Gau, J., & Ochner, C. (2011). Relationship of depression to perceived social support: Results from a randomized adolescent depression prevention trial. *Behavioral Research and Therapy, 49*(5), 361–366. doi: 10.1016/j.brat.2011.02.009

Thomas, N., Rossell, S., Farhall, J., Shawyer, F., & Castle, D. (2011). Cognitive behavioural therapy for auditory hallucinations: Effectiveness and predictors of outcome in a specialist clinic. *Behavioural and Cognitive Psychotherapy, 39*(2), 129–138.

Zeidan, M. A., Lebron-Milad, K., Thompson-Hollands, J., Im, J. J., Dougherty, D. D., Holt, D. J.,...Milad, M. R. (2011). Test-retest reliability during fear acquisition and fear extinction in humans. *CNS Neuroscience & Therapeutics.* Advance online publication. doi: 10.1111/j.1755-5949.2011.00238.x

31

Psychopharmacologic Nursing Interventions

EILEEN TRIGOBOFF

LEARNING OUTCOMES

After completing this chapter, you will be able to:

1. Assess the effectiveness of medications in psychiatric–mental health settings.
2. Integrate an understanding of the positive and negative effects of psychiatric medications into the administration of pharmacologic treatment.
3. Incorporate the different perspectives and beliefs clients have about pharmacology into treatment regimens.
4. Educate clients and their families about acute extrapyramidal side effects.
5. Implement a plan of care for a client who will be taking these medications for an indefinite period of time.
6. Formulate nursing interventions to address the major side effects associated with psychotropic medications.

CRITICAL THINKING CHALLENGE

Frank is a 42-year-old married man who has had repeated episodes of depression. His symptoms have responded well to SSRI antidepressants in the past. He has been taking fluoxetine (Prozac) as prescribed and has experienced a substantial improvement in his symptoms. Frank and his wife are here to talk with you about a sexual problem they are having. After attempting to deal with it on their own, unsuccessfully, they finally decided to speak with you about it. Frank has had a substantial delay in ejaculation and sometimes he is not able to have an orgasm. Both he and his wife are concerned that the problem indicates he is not enjoying sexual activity as he should (one of the symptoms of depression he had in the past). The couple also is concerned that if he is not depressed, then Frank may be losing interest in his wife as he recovers from depression. Frank denies losing interest, but they have been through so much with his illness that they feel unsure of many previously held convictions.

1. How would you explain the experiences Frank is having?
2. What key elements should be included in a program designed to address Frank's side effects?

Unlike medications for medical illnesses, psychiatric medications are stigmatizing. Telling a man with diabetes that he must take insulin for the foreseeable future, or possibly suffer unmanageable and life-threatening symptoms, is not equal (yet) in our society to telling a man with bipolar disorder that he must take psychiatric medications for the same purpose. Treating mental illness with psychiatric medications is still relatively new.

It is also more difficult for people to understand the similarities between physical problems and psychological problems. For example, both physical and psychological problems may require medications to help healing, prevent serious problems, and save lives. Because clients can benefit greatly from the neuroprotective effects of psychopharmacologic agents and from the reduced disruption and increased stability that they bring to clients' lives, remember to add advocacy to reduce stigma to your repertoire of nursing interventions related to psychiatric medications.

The safe and effective management of medications by nurses, clients, and family members is the focus of this chapter. We discuss nursing interventions to promote client and family coping with medication side effects or adverse effects, with drug interactions, and with the psychosocial impact of medications. We also focus on specific psychoeducational activities that demonstrate how you can cooperatively interact with clients and their families in meeting the goal of medication management. An important example of cooperation is in Evidence-Based Practice.

Medication management is a therapeutic challenge that requires you to marshal complex nursing knowledge and resources within a holistic framework. Your goal is to design psychopharmacologic nursing interventions that promote recovery and wellness (Sulosaari, Suhonen, & Leino-Kilpi, 2011). Well-designed psychopharmacologic nursing interventions require your understanding of the science of pharmacology, which is discussed in Chapter 7∞. The science of psychopharmacology—medication categories, how they work, safe dosage ranges, and so on—will not be repeated here; therefore, be sure to review Chapter 7∞ before continuing.

EVIDENCE-BASED PRACTICE

Medication Psychoeducation Groups

You are conducting an outpatient psychoeducation group of seven people in treatment for depression. The goal is to educate clients about symptoms of depression, available treatments, and prevention or reduction of relapse.

In this group, everyone has a different viewpoint about medications. Several of the group members ask you about the latest information on these treatments. You report that research indicates that a combination of talk therapies and antidepressants works well in treating the symptoms of major depression. Other group members wonder about criticisms they have heard about some studies. The popular media occasionally report that antidepressants are no better than placebo treatment, that results indicating otherwise are illusory, or that antidepressants are dangerous.

You tell them that the literature shows that antidepressant treatment is safe and effective and that a variety of psychopharmacologic strategies help individualize treatment in particularly exacting ways. Medication categories and doses can be adjusted and adjunctive therapies such as mood stabilizers, electroconvulsive therapy (ECT), or stimulants can be employed. Importantly, you share with group members that numerous studies show that inadequate treatment of depression puts people at unnecessary risk.

When group members mention how some medications were of no use to them (their symptoms did not resolve), the discussion turned to how some people have an agitated depression versus a vegetative depression and that different symptoms require different treatment. Also, individuals respond differently to medications. It came to light that many group members had family members who responded well to a particular medication, and when they took the same or a similar medication, they had reasonable relief from their symptoms. A clinician may prescribe the same or similar medication that worked for a blood relative to take advantage of the biologic commonalities.

Psychoeducation groups provide a very important function beyond giving facts about mental illness and treatment. Examining and discussing what the layman hears and reads allows for correction of misconceptions and support for the scientific basis of care. When public statements strongly assert that a treatment definitely will or will not be successful, this can be misleading and thereby become a public health concern. If a public figure or a media outlet declares that treating depression is wrong for nonscientific reasons (religion, personal opinion, fear, superstition, politics, or economics), clients may assume the public figure is correct and refuse treatment. Keeping current with research so that you can counter misleading information and actively engaging in critical thinking skills benefit your clients. Findings from antidepressant research, such as the following references, are usually valid.

Connolly, K. R., & Thase, M. E. (2011). If at first you don't succeed: A review of the evidence for antidepressant augmentation, combination and switching strategies. *Drugs, 71*(1), 43–64.

Gibbons, R. D., & Mann, J. J. (2011). Strategies for quantifying the relationship between medications and suicidal behavior: What has been learned? *Drug Safety, 34*(5), 375–395.

CRITICAL THINKING QUESTIONS

1. Why is it important for clients to know how to evaluate research?
2. What do the clients in your group need to know and what do you need to teach them to best interpret research results published in the popular media?
3. Should you refer group members directly to the research articles with which you are familiar? Why, or why not?

THE NURSING ROLE IN PSYCHOPHARMACOLOGY

Because psychopharmacology is an integral and important part of a client's life for years, and perhaps a lifetime, psychiatric–mental health nurses must know as much about the many ways that psychiatric medications affect a client as they do about the characteristics of a client's mental disorder. Psychopharmacologic medications affect the client's behavior, body, and thought processes.

In general, psychopharmacologic treatment is not the only answer. It is combined with various psychological and social therapies to achieve the goal of promoting hope and recovery from a mental illness. Many clients can manage some symptoms by activating certain thought processes (cognitive therapy), changing beliefs or incorporating different beliefs (which contribute to the effectiveness of cognitive therapy), and changing or activating specific behaviors (behavioral therapy). Chapter 30∞ discusses cognitive–behavioral therapy. Certainly, when psychiatric symptoms are severe or hospitalization is required, medication management is a must.

Theorists and clinicians hold a variety of attitudes, beliefs, and philosophies about psychiatric medications. Medications many times are used as a complement to the psychotherapeutic process to decrease overwhelming arousal (feelings of being overwhelmed by matters raised in psychotherapy), to improve judgment that has been impaired by psychosis, to improve information processing, to reduce anergia (lack of energy), and to improve thinking and motivation. Clients and their family members also hold specific attitudes and beliefs about psychiatric medications. These are discussed in Chapter 7∞.

When added to a medication regimen, talk therapies (psychotherapy) are used to treat demoralization and lethality in the interim period before medication has a chance to take effect. Talk therapies can improve medication adherence, decrease irrational thinking, address problems in relationships, modify the triggers that cause a recurrence of symptoms, and treat residual symptoms. With any psychiatric problem, relapse is an issue. Psychotherapy reduces the risk of relapse by preparing the client for vulnerabilities, identifying prodromal symptoms, teaching coping mechanisms, and managing residual symptoms or rebound symptoms after pharmacotherapy is discontinued. See Chapter 32∞ for discussions of strategies to reduce relapse risk.

A variety of terms are used to refer to psychiatric medications. The terms **neuroleptic** and **psychotropic** both describe medications that address psychiatric symptoms. The terms can be, and often are, used interchangeably to describe any medication for a psychiatric diagnosis. For example, antidepressants, anxiolytics, and mood stabilizers could all be called neuroleptics or psychotropics. Clients and family members often report having taken "a psychotropic for years." This statement tells you that psychiatric symptoms were being addressed. It does not tell you the category or categories of medication prescribed.

The ongoing assessment of a psychiatric client includes determining how well the medications are helping the client to cope with psychiatric symptoms. An additional observation

WHY I BECAME A PSYCHIATRIC–MENTAL HEALTH NURSE

Eileen Trigoboff, RN, DNS
Textbook Author

What attracted me to psychiatric–mental health nursing was recognizing the powerful link between the emotional and physiological aspects of my clients. I began my nursing career as a pediatric ICU nurse, talking to parents and siblings about injuries, illnesses, surgery, and recovery. The most demanding interactions were with parents who had abused their children so severely they ended up in the ICU. My colleagues pointed out to me that when I spoke to these parents—not avoiding them, not judging them, and not scolding—I was performing the therapeutic role of a psychiatric–mental health nurse.

The idea of psychiatric–mental health nursing interested me so much that I enrolled in a clinical nurse specialist graduate program in psychiatric–mental health nursing; met some wonderful faculty who shared, taught, and mentored (one of them is my coauthor on this book); became a clinical nurse specialist in psychiatry and mental health; then got my doctorate in psychiatric–mental health nursing and have never looked back. Working in this field has been wonderfully fulfilling and enriching.

to be made is whether the psychiatric medication is causing a side effect or an adverse effect. Managing side effects behaviorally and pharmacologically is crucial to our clients' health and to their quality of life. Effective medication management is a vital process that depends upon your understanding of the content in this chapter as well as the content in Chapter 7∞. What Every Nurse Should Know will help you to evaluate how well you carry out your responsibilities in relationship to pyschopharmacology.

The nursing functions described in the next three sections—assessing clients, administering medications, and educating clients and families—are general and can be applied to the care of any client receiving a psychiatric medication. Specific nursing functions are described in the drug category sections later in this chapter.

Assessing Clients

Our responsibilities as nurses to clients receiving psychotropic medications are very different from our responsibilities to clients in nonpsychiatric settings. A nurse working with clients having cardiac difficulties, for example, may have clear physiological indicators for the administration of drugs such as isosorbide dinitrate (Iso-Bid) or nitroglycerin (Nitroglyn), but psychiatric nurses rarely have comparable consistent complexes of symptoms on which to base clinical judgments.

In psychiatric work, nurses must often observe client behaviors closely to be aware of the sometimes subtle nature of the presenting symptom. Pacing, mild diaphoresis, slight increases in blood pressure or pulse, heightened muscle tone, and hypervigilance may indicate escalating anxiety, but they may also point to other problems such as caffeine toxicity,

WHAT EVERY NURSE SHOULD KNOW

Guidelines for Psychopharmacology

Imagine that you are responsible for administering a psychopharmacologic agent. Nurses of every specialty perform the following functions related to psychopharmacology:

1. Describe and discuss the variety of psychopharmacologic agents and their actions
2. Apply the science of psychopharmacologic agents used to treat symptoms of mental disorders and disabilities
3. Identify the side effects and drug interactions that may occur with psychopharmacologic agents
4. Assist clients in managing side effects through nonpharmacologic interventions
5. Design psychopharmocologic nursing interventions that promote recovery and wellness
6. Synthesize knowledge of psychopharmacologic agents in developing psychoeducation for clients and their families.
7. Advocate to reduce stigma related to psychiatric medications so that clients can benefit from their neuroprotective effects.
8. Incorporate into your professional practice an understanding of the holistic effects of psychopharmacologic agents on the client's life and lifestyle.

excessive use of tobacco, or side effects of psychopharmacologic agents. Accurate nursing assessment of client behavior is crucial in order to give medications effectively and appropriately. Psychiatric nurses must also be attuned to the circumstances of adjunct pharmacotherapy (taking different medications at the same time). This clinical example demonstrates how symptoms can become unmanageable for a client when adjunctive therapy is discontinued.

Clinical Example

Evan, a 33-year-old man with a diagnosis of bipolar disorder, decided to stop taking his risperidone (Risperdal) and lamotrigine (Lamictal) as mood stabilizers because he did not like the way they made him feel—emotionally stunted and less creative. Evan has difficulty when his manic symptoms are reduced as a result of the main effect of the medication. As he put it, "I miss feeling on top of the world."

Within 2 weeks of stopping the medication, he was unable to sleep and berated his neighbors in the middle of the night for their choice of house siding. Although he liked his job at the local playhouse and knew he would likely earn more money in the near future, he refused to go to work because "they just don't understand my potential as an actor, dancer, and director." He was fired because of poor attendance and belligerence toward other workers. His spiraling symptoms and the loss of a structured schedule exacerbated his deterioration and Evan relapsed, requiring hospitalization.

Assessment is not a static process. It takes shape over time and depends upon activating a wide range of nursing knowledge. A sleepy, isolated client with schizophrenia may be experiencing paranoid ideation, may have negative symptoms of the illness, may be experiencing sedating side effects of the antipsychotic medication, or may be depressed as well as schizophrenic. The behaviors may be similar, but they come from a wide array of vastly different sources. Your assessment of this client and your clinical judgment will direct the nursing care. Whether you decide to administer a PRN (given when needed) antipsychotic, hold the next dose of antipsychotic, develop a treatment plan that includes motivational aspects, or discuss the possibility of depression with the other treatment team members depends on your ongoing assessment of this client.

Administering Medications

Administering psychiatric medications demands more than the six rights: the right medication, the right client, the right dose, the right route, the right time, and the right technology. These aspects of medication administration are confounded by the psychiatric illness. Knowing the side effects of the medication in addition to the interactive effects with other psychiatric and medical–surgical medications is crucial in psychiatric–mental health nursing.

Administering the right medication in a psychiatric setting depends on your assessment skills. The right medication may be one of a number of choices. A medication may be ordered by mouth (PO) for routine administration, but the client may refuse it. Assessment skills come into play here as well; you must determine whether the client needs a liquid, a pill, a quick-dissolving formulation, or a PRN injection.

Making sure you are administering medications to the right client, a client identification issue, is different than it is in medical–surgical settings. In psychiatric settings, clients usually do not wear wristbands. Clients may be confused or have psychiatric symptoms that encourage them to spontaneously assume the identity of another client for any number of reasons, including an effort to please the staff.

Assessing, Documenting, and Evaluating the Effects of Medications

Assessing your client's need for additional or PRN medication involves nursing judgment. The symptom your client is having difficulty with may be anxiety, psychosis, or even a side effect from other medications. Your decision is based on your observations of the client and your discussion with the client of the current difficulty. Selecting the appropriate PRN medication for the problem depends on your assessment.

Documenting the effect of medications is an important nursing responsibility. Follow-up documentation on a medication that was given as a PRN medication helps to evaluate its effectiveness and will simplify treatment decisions for the client. Did the PRN medication work? How did you determine the value of the PRN medication's effect? What behavioral indicators are you using in your evaluation of a medication's effectiveness? Your documentation describes the regularly

Client Education on Medications

YOUR INTERVENTION STRATEGIES   Medication Teaching Checklist

Be sure to teach clients and families about the following regardless of the category of medication the client is taking. Do not hesitate to repeat instructions. Repetition is a useful tool in psychoeducation.

- Keeping all medications and information about them together in one dry, cool, place (not the bathroom or the kitchen)
- When to report side effects

- How to report side effects
- Strategies and tools for managing side effects
- Strategies and tools for managing residual symptoms
- The effect of mental illness and psychiatric medications on life goals
- Reinforce learning by providing an opportunity at some point for the client to teach others about medications

---

administered medication as well as stat (immediate administration) and PRN doses.

Educating Clients and Families

Nursing responsibilities include educating clients and family members about medications. Your Intervention Strategies includes guidelines for medication teaching strategies and reminders of general information to include for all clients and their families, regardless of the category of psychiatric medication.

Information on client education is also available from a variety of sites. For example, PsychNet-UK and the University of Iowa Virtual Hospital websites offer accessible and relevant information on various psychopharmacologic topics and can be accessed through the Online Student Resources for this text.

Addressing Individual Differences

As a psychiatric–mental health nurse, address individual differences in the course of the teaching–learning process. Partnering With Clients and Families suggests learning strategies and methods.

An issue of great concern to many nurses is the planning of teaching–learning experiences for severely and persistently

mentally ill clients. Although this population has learning needs, teaching is often difficult, depending on the severity and chronicity of the illness. See Box 31-1 for common learning problems or interferences associated with specific psychiatric diagnoses.

Another concern for nurses working with psychiatric clients is the need to assess the client's learning capacity at different points in the chronology of the disorder. For example, when clients are first admitted to an inpatient unit, they may be too disorganized and symptomatic to focus on specific learning tasks. Depressed clients may have severe psychomotor retardation because of hormonal shifts and dysfunctional neurotransmission and may be unable to learn. Given appropriate treatment and care, however, a client's psychobiologic disequilibrium may be corrected, making learning possible.

Perceiving that a client is ready to learn—that is, that the client's cognitive abilities are intact—does not necessarily mean that learning will occur. Many nurses conduct medication groups on an acute psychiatric unit to not only address the importance of assessing cognitive abilities but also to explore affective and social issues that may contribute to effective learning experiences. Once you have considered the client's readiness, knowledge, background, environment, beliefs, preferences, and lifestyle, involving the client and significant

---

PARTNERING WITH CLIENTS AND FAMILIES

Strategies and Methods for Teaching About Medications

Before you begin teaching clients and their family members about medications, identify which learning methods have already proven successful for them:

- **Repetition:** Rehearsing or practicing the skill repeatedly can place it in several areas in the memory, thereby increasing the chances of retrieval.
- **Primacy:** Some learners more easily retrieve the *first* item learned or the first skill performed.
- **Recency:** Some learners more easily retrieve the *last* item learned or the last skill performed.
- **Association:** Learning by hinging one memory to another.
- **Coding:** Shaping a thought in one's memory in a particular way to facilitate retrieval for skill performance.
- **Background information and explanation:** Describing a skill by giving specific details can assist many to learn the skill

and perform it reliably. Incorporating the client's value system into this method is most effective.

- **Reminder boxes:** Physical prompts are helpful for clients who need concrete environmental hints.
- **Lists, notebooks:** Making lists and keeping track of tasks and events in a notebook can be a powerful tool for clients with executive functioning deficits.
- **Videos:** Visual learners can make use of a multimedia presentation of materials.
- **Positive transfer:** If the client learned to do task *A* well, and it is similar enough to task *B*, then task *B* can be accomplished through transferring that learned behavior.
- **Positive reinforcement:** The client either obtains something desirable or avoids something unpleasant as a result of a behavior.

Box 31-1 Common Learning Challenges With Specific Psychiatric Diagnoses

Schizophrenia and Schizoaffective Disorder

- Cognitive difficulties secondary to thought disorder
- Motivational problems secondary to negative symptoms
- Unpleasant side effects from medication
- Persistence of positive symptoms (delusions) mitigating against adherence

Mood Disorders

- Persistent dysphoria leads to amotivation
- Self-destructiveness–lethality
- Manic irresponsibility as a result of impulsivity, thoughtlessness, and cognitive symptoms
- Loss of manic or hypomanic egosyntonic excitement (energy around ideas in harmony with an ideal self-image)
- Unpleasant side effects from medications
- Substance use/abuse

Anxiety Disorders

- Addiction to antianxiety medication
- Quick action of many antianxiety agents leads to positive reinforcement of increasing dosages
- Lack of consistent provider knowledge of and expertise in application of effective nonmedication treatment strategies for anxiety problems

Personality Disorders

- Addictive or abusive use of medications
- Sensation seeking
- Manipulation

---

others in the design and implementation of the medication treatment plan will help ensure the client's active collaboration in his or her care. In many ways, psychiatric clients are no different from other learners. When presented with material that has clear benefits for them, they are more likely to be interested in the learning process.

Recidivism, the tendency to relapse into a previous mode of behavior requiring readmission to a treatment program, can be linked to a psychiatric client's psychoeducation. Helping a client change health-related behavior requires a thoughtful, comprehensive approach. Relevant interventions designed to match the client's learning style can reduce recidivism and promote healthier behavior. Contracting with a client for behavioral change can also help to avoid relapse. See "Developing a Behavioral Contract" in Chapter 30∞ on page 669.

Evaluating the Teaching–Learning Process

An evaluation of teaching efforts and the client's knowledge of the information taught is essential to completing the teaching–learning process. You will not be able to evaluate a client's understanding of information unless, at minimum, the client verbally reiterates information or performs a return demonstration of the skill. A change in behavior over time is a powerful indication that learning has taken place.

If you desire a more extensive evaluation, you may consider using a "pretest/posttest" format. You can develop a written test that the client completes to cover the content before you begin teaching (a pretest). This provides a written measure of the client's learning needs and level of knowledge. After you implement the teaching plan, the client completes the same examination (a posttest). Comparison of the pretest and posttest results yields a documented measure of how much learning has occurred as a result of your teaching intervention.

Ethical Concerns

Several ethical issues are: Should children and adolescents take psychiatric medications? Do conflicts of interest influence the prescribing of psychiatric medications? Should clients be informed of the risks of taking psychiatric medications and the alternatives to medication? These issues, as well as questions of impaired decision making, are discussed here. Issues such as limiting individual freedom through chemical controls and an individual's right to refuse treatment are discussed in the ethics and legal sections of Chapter 12∞.

Children and Adolescents

The question of whether children and adolescents are helped or harmed by psychiatric medications continues to arouse concerns, which are often accompanied by intense feelings. Some of the ethical issues are: Should young persons be treated with psychopharmacologic agents because they prevent symptoms from overwhelming and traumatizing the child or adolescent? Or, should children and adolescents not be given psychopharmacologic agents because of their unknown long-term effects? Current clinical practice supports treating symptoms with the minimal effective amount of medication.

Elders

Medication planning for elders is different than it is for other age groups. Specifically, elders—because of aged organs, injuries, and comorbidities—metabolize medications differently than younger clients. Medications pose several challenges to the physiological functioning of older clients because medications:

- Are metabolized at a somewhat slower rate
- Take longer to reach therapeutic levels
- May interact with the many other medications elders tend to take
- May cause side effects or adverse effects at lower doses than for other age groups
- Take longer to clear the system

When older clients begin a regimen of psychotropic medications, the strategy followed is often based on the principle, "Start low; go slow." Frequent assessment of the effect of the medication on the targeted symptoms is important. Your vital role is to observe elders to assess and monitor their physiological functioning along with the effectiveness of the medication.

Pharmaceutical Advertising

The potential impact of advertising in the popular media by the pharmaceutical industry has engendered debate. (This issue is central to the discussion in Evidence-Based Practice on page 673.) We are exposed to innumerable print, radio, and television commercials for over-the-counter and prescription agents to address any number of physical and psychological ailments. Two major ethical concerns are as follows:

1. Individuals who are unable to think critically because of psychiatric symptoms could make decisions based on the advertisement.
2. Prescribers, influenced by the media or by those who have a financial interest in the outcome (such as a pharmaceutical representative, for example), may prescribe a medication without considering all the options or accessing the available research evidence.

Both concerns can be minimized with proper action.

When clients approach you with questions about a medication they heard about on the Internet or saw on television, you can give them fair and balanced information. In order to do so, your knowledge about available pharmaceuticals must be thorough and complete. Keep up-to-date and absorb relevant information from reliable sources. Employ your critical thinking skills to determine if you have adequate information to satisfactorily address the issue.

Conflicts of Interest

Professionals are required to monitor their relationships for conflict of interest (COI). COI is defined as a situation in which there is an opportunity for bias not in the client's best interests. These are usually situations in which your personal interests, such as a hobby or an investment, can be advanced by what you decide to do professionally. It would be considered a COI if a prescriber who owns stock in a pharmaceutical company recommends that company's medication to the exclusion of similar medications manufactured by other pharmaceutical companies. COI is especially worrisome in psychiatry, where clients with interactional

and interpersonal difficulties and impaired decision-making abilities may be swayed by subtle influences such as trademarks and branded items. Does COI affect the objectivity of your interactions? See Your Self-Awareness for information on tracking COI.

Right to Refuse Medications

Another ethical issue involves our duty to inform the client of the risks of, and alternatives to, the proposed treatment, and to accept the client's decision to authorize or refuse that treatment. We do not assume that clients with psychiatric disorders lack capacity; mentally disordered clients can make unimpaired decisions. Even a diagnosis of dementia does not inevitably mean that clients do not retain some abilities to decide for themselves. Impairment in decision-making capacity does not equal legal incompetence to make a decision. When the deficit makes it unlikely or impossible to understand the specific information needed to make a decision, then the deficit is relevant. We should also be concerned about whether the refusal to accept treatment places a member of the community at risk. Community safety is a responsibility nurses share with other health care professionals and may involve coerced treatment for the client (Galon & Wineman, 2010). Be sure to work closely with the client's designated decision maker if the client has a psychiatric advance directive (see Chapter 12∞).

THE CLIENT'S CULTURAL PERSPECTIVE

A vital component of competent care is accounting for the client's cultural perspective. People can have strong feelings about psychopharmacology that arise from their cultural background. Refusing to take medication may indicate more than paranoia or misunderstanding; it may be intrinsically representative of a cultural standard—for example, the perception that any mental strain or mental illness indicates a weakness of spirit or personality. In another culture, its members may believe that illness is caused by a supreme being, and therefore prayer is the only acceptable route to healing.

Learning as much as you can about the culture's ideas about mental health and illness, its perspective on medications, and its belief systems related to mental health care and treatment will help to minimize miscommunication. Summaries of cultural health beliefs and practices for six major cultural groups (Hispanic, African-American, Native American and Alaska Native, Asian-American, Pacific Islander, and Anglo-American/European-American populations) are in Partnering With Clients and Families in Chapter 9∞ on pages 172–173. This table also provides helpful suggestions to consider when working toward cultural competence.

Cultural Self-Awareness of Nurses

An awareness of the issues relating to your own, as well as the client's, culture helps minimize cultural interferences with communication and is necessary for providing quality mental health care. See Developing Cultural Competence to determine how your cultural inclinations influence your attitudes toward medications.

YOUR SELF-AWARENESS
Conflict of Interest (COI)

Does COI affect your objectivity? Review the following and think about what impact each has, if any, on your clinical judgment.

- Your professional and facility policies on ethics
- Your financial interests (monetary or percentage interests in products or sponsors), board memberships, or relationships that may make conflicting demands
- How your financial interest in a product could influence your professional judgment
- Professional, government, and agency or facility policies on the financial amount or percentage of interest you can have in a product, business, or stock
- Whether your loyalties could be divided

Once you have carefully considered these points, expunge the opportunities for bias.

DEVELOPING CULTURAL COMPETENCE

Cultural Competence in Psychopharmacology

Check your cultural competence in psychopharmacology by thinking about your perspective on the following statements.

1. I learn as much as I can about how members of other cultures view mental health symptoms, their perspective on medications, and their belief system on health care.
2. I avoid using medical euphemisms and Anglocentric health concepts when I teach clients and families about psychiatric medications.
3. I am clear and descriptive when I give information on psychiatric medications.
4. I recognize the validity of cultures and values other than Western and their influences on client and family attitudes toward, and beliefs about, psychopharmacology.
5. I promote client rights and advocate for clients of all cultures in issues of psychopharmacology.
6. I maintain awareness of the issues and controversies that involve culture and psychiatric medications.

CRITICAL THINKING QUESTIONS

1. How likely is it that you are using mainstream cultural terms that are not as meaningful for all clients?
2. How would you go about selecting common Anglocentric terms you use and converting them to global terms?

Ethnicity and Metabolism of Psychiatric Medications

Cultural influences can have enormous consequences for the recovery of clients. In addition to assessing for cultural influences on behavior, you must also assess for the biologic effects of medications on ethnically distinct groups. Different races and ethnicities do metabolize psychiatric and other medications in a variety of ways. Dose levels, side effects even at low dose levels, toxicity effects, and physical impacts will be different with diverse groups. Recognizing how ethnicity determines a client's response to medications promotes the provision of culturally competent care. Be sure to discuss the nature of the client's responses to psychopharmacology with the client, and remember that focused and specific documentation of unusual responses to medications communicates the culture-related reality to the interdisciplinary team. The biologic effects of medications on ethnically distinct groups are explored in detail in Chapter 7∞ on page 115.

NURSING RESPONSIBILITIES WITH ANTIPSYCHOTICS

Detailed information on the category of psychiatric medications known as antipsychotics is in Chapter 7∞. This section discusses the important clinical considerations for psychiatric–mental health nurses.

Medications are frequently referred to in terms of their generation (their discovery, or birth) as a way of characterizing the major features of the medication. Once a newer, more sophisticated and powerful medication is developed, the previous grouping is called the *first-generation antipsychotics* and the newer group as the **second-generation antipsychotics (SGAs)**. Although the first- and second-generation classifications can apply to other classes of medications, the terms are most often used when discussing antipsychotics. Generational designations can also be determined not just by timing but also by the neurologic pathways they use and their effects on neurotransmitters.

Side effect issues can and do occur with psychiatric medications. Side effects are sometimes called *adverse effects*. They are interchangeable terms, although *side effects* may be a more recognizable phrase for your clients.

Continuous contact with clients in the inpatient psychiatric setting gives nurses an advantage over other mental health professionals who may see a client only every other day or, at best, once a day. Both the dangerous and the more uncomfortable side effects frequently have a rapid onset and require immediate attention (Masi & Liboni, 2011; Koreki et al., 2011). TABLE 31-1 ■ lists the side effects of various antipsychotic medications in common use.

Autonomic Nervous System Side Effects

All antipsychotics possess anticholinergic and antiadrenergic side effects; that is, they interfere with the normal transmission of nerve impulses by acetylcholine and epinephrine, in both central and peripheral nerves. **Anticholinergic side effects** and adverse effects are the most common and are generally drying to the various tissues and systems. They are usually more pronounced in older adults. See Your Assessment Approach for a list of the various anticholinergic side effects that result from interference with acetylcholine transmission.

Constipation

Constipation, a burdensome problem for many people, is also a side effect of many psychiatric medications. Medications and supplements that can cause constipation include opioids, anticholinergics, antihistamines, tricyclic antidepressants, antispasmodics, calcium channel blockers, iron supplements, aluminum antacids, and antiemetic, chemotherapeutic, and antiparkinsonian medications (Bliss, Savik, Jung, Whitebird, & Lowry, 2011). Strategies for coping with this common and frustrating side effect can be found in your fundamental nursing texts.

YOUR ASSESSMENT APPROACH
Anticholinergic Side Effects

- Nervousness, drowsiness, headache
- Tachycardia
- Blurred vision
- Dry mouth, constipation, nausea, vomiting
- Under rarer circumstances, paralytic ileus
- Urinary hesitancy/retention
- Cognitive functioning impairment and hallucinations (especially with older adults)

TABLE 31-1 ■ Side Effects of Antipsychotic Medications

Effect	Chlorpromazine (Thorazine)	Haloperidol (Haldol)	Loxapine (Loxitane)	Risperidone (Risperdal)	Clozapine (Clozaril)	Thioridazine (Mellaril)
Akathisia	Occasional	Frequent	Occasional	Occasional	Occasional	Occasional
Allergic skin reactions	Occasional	Rare	Rare	Rare	Occasional	Not reported
Anticholinergic effects	Frequent	Not reported	Rare	Occasional	Occasional	Frequent
Blood dyscrasia	Occasional	Occasional	Not reported	Not reported	Occasional	Rare
Cholestatic jaundice	Occasional	Rare	Not reported	Not reported	Not reported	Rare
Dystonias	Occasional	Frequent	Rare	Rare	Occasional	Occasional
Impotence	Occasional	Not reported	Not reported	Rare	Rare	Occasional
Parkinsonism	Occasional	Frequent	Frequent	Rare	Rare	Frequent
Photosensitivity	Occasional	Rare	Not reported	Not reported	Not reported	Occasional
Postural hypotension	Frequent	Occasional	Rare	Occasional	Frequent	Frequent
Retinitis pigmentosa	Not reported	Not reported	Not reported	Not reported	Not reported	Occasional
Sedation	Frequent	Not reported	Occasional	Rare	Frequent	Frequent
Effect	Thiothixene (Navane)	Trifluoperazine (Stelazine)	Fluphenazine (Prolixin)	Olanzapine (Zyprexa)	Quetiapine (Seroquel)	Ziprasidone (Geodon)
Akathisia	Occasional	Frequent	Frequent	Frequent	Rare	Occasional
Allergic skin reactions	Rare	Rare	Rare	Rare	Rare	Frequent
Anticholinergic effects	Occasional	Frequent	Frequent	Frequent	Not reported	Common
Blood dyscrasia	Rare	Rare	Rare	Rare	Rare	Rare
Cholestatic jaundice	Rare	Rare	Rare	Not reported	Not reported	Not reported
Dystonias	Occasional	Frequent	Frequent	Not reported	Rare	Occasional
Impotence	Not reported	Occasional	Occasional	Not reported	Not reported	Occasional
Parkinsonism	Occasional	Frequent	Frequent	Not reported	Not reported	Occasional
Photosensitivity	Rare	Occasional	Occasional	Not reported	Not reported	Frequent
Postural hypotension	Occasional	Rare	Rare	Frequent	Occasional	Frequent
Retinitis pigmentosa	Not reported	Not reported	Not reported	Not reported	Not reported	Not reported
Sedation	Frequent	Not reported	Occasional	Frequent	Occasional	Common

Orthostatic Hypotension

Orthostatic hypotension, also known as *postural hypotension,* is a common antiadrenergic effect. The primary danger here is injury from a fall. Clients receiving parenteral medications, such as chlorpromazine intramuscularly, must have their blood pressure monitored both lying down and standing, before and a half hour after each dose. Advise clients to rise from a supine position gradually and to sit down if they feel faint. Support stockings and a large intake of fluids may be indicated. Orthostatic hypotension is much less significant with oral administration of the drug. However, nurses working with clients receiving oral antipsychotic medications should take both baseline and routine vital sign readings at regular intervals. This practice establishes the client's tolerance for medications without the untoward side effects of orthostatic hypotension and subsequent falls. This is an important evaluation of cardiac functioning with certain neuroleptic medications. Review the technique for measuring orthostatic blood pressure in your fundamental nursing textbook.

Extrapyramidal Side Effects

Another common and sometimes frightening group of adverse reactions results from the effects of antipsychotics on the extrapyramidal tracts of the central nervous system, which are involved in the production and control of involuntary movements. This group of reactions is known as **extrapyramidal side effects (EPSEs)**. The abbreviation for extrapyramidal side effects is sometimes erroneously written as EPS instead of EPSE. Keep in mind there is a fundamental difference between extrapyramidal syndromes (EPS) such as naturally occurring Parkinsonism, and the side effects of psychopharmacology (EPSE) such as drug-induced Parkinsonism. Your Assessment Approach details each EPSE.

The first-generation, conventional, or typical antipsychotics such as haloperidol (Haldol), trifluoperazine (Stelazine), and chlorpromazine (Thorazine) tend to be harsher on the body and cause significant EPSEs. Although many clients are taking second-generation antipsychotics, some respond well to first-generation antipsychotics and must continue taking

YOUR ASSESSMENT APPROACH   Extrapyramidal Side Effects (EPSEs)

Acute Dystonic Reaction, or Dystonia

- Usually occurs within 48 hours after beginning treatment but may occur at any time.
- Described by the client as "Sometimes my back tightens up," or "I get tongue-tied when I try to talk."
- Characterized by abnormal tonic contractions of muscle groups.
- Characterized by odd posturing and strange facial expressions such as torticollis (twisting of the neck or pulling the neck down into the shoulders), opisthotonos (spasms of the neck and back, forcing the back to arch and the neck to bend backward), and oculogyric crisis (a fixed gaze that cannot return to lateral once raised vertically).
- Is more common in young males.
- Treated prophylactically by anticholinergics. Some clients may experience a "high" from this treatment.

Parkinsonian Syndrome, or Drug-Induced Parkinsonism

- Usually occurs after 3 or more weeks of treatment.
- Characterized by rigidity (cogwheeling), tremor, or regular rhythmic oscillations of the extremities, particularly the distal parts, and in the hands (a pill-rolling movement of the fingers).
- Clients are more susceptible to aspiration or to injury by falling.
- Treatment consists of decreasing the medication dosage or administering anticholinergics.

Akathisia

- Usually occurs after 3 or more weeks of treatment.
- Described by the client as "My nerves are jumping," or "I feel like jumping out of my skin."

- A subjective need or desire to move, not a type of pattern or movement.
- Mild akathisia: vague feelings of apprehension and irritability.
- Severe akathisia: an inability to sit (or the feeling one cannot sit) for more than a few seconds, resulting in running, rocking, or agitated dancing.
- Not always responsive to anticholinergics; lowering the medication dosage may be necessary.
- There is an associated dysphoria not treated by anticholinergics or benzodiazepines.

Tardive Dyskinesia (TD)

- Late onset during the course of treatment with antipsychotics, with frequently irreversible abnormal movements or a neurologic syndrome.
- Characterized by coordinated, arrhythmic, involuntary movements (lip smacking, tongue protrusion, rocking, foot tapping).
- Complications include inability to wear dentures, impaired respirations, weight loss, and impaired gait and posture.
- Treatment is primary prevention through careful initial assessment of the client's needs, as well as continual evaluation of the course of treatment.

Dopamine–Acetylcholine Imbalance in the Extrapyramidal System

- Uncommon side effect.
- Diificult to recognize.
- Characterized by hallucinations, dry mouth, blurred vision, decreased absorption of antipsychotics, decreased gastric motility, tachycardia, and urinary retention.

---

them. Managing the EPSEs as a long-term treatment option involves careful nursing intervention and client and family education. Four major types of EPSEs are discussed in the following section and in Your Assessment Approach; each EPSE has distinguishing clinical characteristics and times of onset after the initiation of drug therapy. A fifth category, dopamine–acetylcholine imbalance in the extrapyramidal system, is an uncommon type of EPSE and is also discussed in Your Assessment Approach.

There are several different types of EPSEs that take unique and distinctive forms. They are discussed next. First, be aware of the frequency with which these syndromes complicate treatment. Report any suspicious sign or symptom to the prescriber. Finally, reassure the client of the reversibility of the syndrome in almost all cases.

Acute Dystonic Reactions

The earliest and most dramatic EPSEs are the *acute dystonic reactions*, which are forms of dystonia. These occur in the first days of medication treatment, sometimes after a single dose of medication. They involve bizarre and severe muscle contractions. These reactions can be physically painful and are almost always frightening to the individual. They are readily reversible. The term *dystonia* describes the experience of the side effect. The prefix *dys-* typically means bad, and *-tonia* means muscle tone; essentially, these are muscle spasms.

Dystonic movements can occur abruptly and co-occur with other extrapyramidal side effects (Fontenelle, Oostermeijer, Harrison, Pantelis, & Yücel, 2011). Treatment to resolve the EPSEs is effective in many instances, although the impact on the client is taken into account. Continued experiences that are painful and unpredictable tend to shatter trust in psychophamacology, and discontinuing the medication may be necessary. This clinical example describes one way to address dystonic reactions.

Clinical Example

Nino has been treated with antipsychotic medications for fixed delusional beliefs that include believing that he must rid the planet of people attempting to "steal" its vibrations and use them as weapons. Years ago, Nino had a dystonic reaction during which he could move his eyes from side to side but, when he raised them to look at the ceiling, could not lower them again. The spasms in his eye muscles frightened and angered him. Because Nino requires medication to think more clearly, it is important to prevent dystonic events that might cause pain and damage his trust in both the medication and the prescribers. A prophylactic regimen of the anticholinergic medication trihexyphenidyl (Artane) has proven most effective for Nino.

Parkinsonian Syndrome

Parkinsonian syndrome, or drug-induced Parkinsonism (so named because of its striking resemblance to true

Parkinson's disease) commonly occurs after a week or two of the medication therapy. It is the result of dopamine blockade caused by psychiatric medications. Treatment with oral medication is usually sufficient, because urgency is seldom a consideration in the management of this syndrome. Your accurate observation of the course of therapy can promote prompt recognition and proper interpretation of EPSEs. If care is not taken, the health care provider may misinterpret the increasing withdrawal, emotional blunting, apathy, and lack of spontaneity (observations of Parkinsonian syndrome) as an increase in the severity of schizophrenic symptoms.

Akathisia

A third reversible extrapyramidal side effect is known as **akathisia**. The word *akathisia* is derived from the Greek word *kathisia,* meaning "ability to sit" (the prefix *a-* indicates "not" or "without"; hence "inability to sit still"). Akathisia is a motor restlessness perceived subjectively by the client and experienced as an urge to pace, a need to shift weight from one foot to the other, or an inability to sit or stand still. Akathisia can occur weeks to months into the course of therapy.

Akathisia can also be confused with psychotic agitation, and this error in interpretation may lead to a mistaken increase in the dosage of antipsychotic medication, which will aggravate the condition. Clients with akathisia require a reduction in the dosage of offending agents and/or treatment with an antiparkinsonian drug. You can save the client many uncomfortable and worrisome days.

Tardive Dyskinesia

The last EPSE to emerge in the course of treatment, **tardive dyskinesia (TD)**, is also the most severe because it can be irreversible. TD frequently appears after years of antipsychotic drug treatment, although it can occur earlier. It usually appears after a maintenance dose is discontinued or reduced, and it can be masked—but not treated—by reinstituting the medication or increasing the dosage, or by switching to another drug. The term *tardive dyskinesia* is formed from the word *tardive,* meaning "late onset" or "slow" (from the root for tardy and retardation); the prefix *dys-,* and the word *kinesia,* meaning movement. It is essentially a late-arriving bad movement. TD is a neurologic syndrome involving the innervation of muscle groups. Typical tardive dyskinesia movements include thrusting the tongue out of the mouth and facial grimacing.

Current estimates put the incidence of TD at 5% per year for young adults and as high as 25% after 1 year in older adults. The limited evidence available clearly indicates that atypical antipsychotics cause less tardive dyskinesia, approximately 1%. Atypical antipsychotics are being studied for antidyskinetic properties in individuals with pre-existing TD. The underlying mechanisms remain unclear, and without such information it is impossible to say under what clinical conditions, if any, these advantages might be diminished or even eliminated (Bhidayasiri & Boonyawairoj, 2011). Early detection through regular examinations (at least every 6 months) is recommended.

There is no known cure for the adverse event of TD. The recommended intervention is to stop all medication to see if the

syndrome resolves spontaneously. This course of action must be weighed against the client's need for medication and the likelihood of relapse into psychosis. Using vitamin E, antioxidants, botulinum toxin, and surgery, among other options, would need to be thoroughly discussed with the client and considered in light of the latest research (Bhidayasiri & Boonyawairoj, 2011).

With the emergence of the newer antipsychotic medications such as clozapine (Clozaril), aripiprazole (Abilify), and paliperidone (Invega), which have been found to reduce TD, the available choices are expanding. See Chapter 7∞ for detailed discussions of these medications. The seventh and newest antipsychotic, paliperidone, is currently being evaluated in this regard.

Prophylactic Treatment of EPSEs

In view of the relatively high incidence of EPSEs, the question of whether clients should be treated prophylactically with antiparkinsonian agents is open to debate. Some argue that the use of antiparkinsonian agents eventually leads to relatively higher antipsychotic doses, because the prescriber assesses the client as able to manage more comfortably the higher antipsychotic dose thereby increasing the probability of serious side effects. Another argument is that antiparkinsonian agents also pose risks and thus should be used only to counteract EPSEs, not to guard against their possible emergence. Moreover, a great many clients never develop the syndromes. If the likelihood of an extrapyramidal reaction is high (if, for example, the client has a history of them) and the possible consequences are significant (the client may discontinue medication or drop out of treatment altogether), antipsychotic and antiparkinsonian agents are frequently initiated simultaneously. TABLE 31-2 ■ lists the commonly used antiparkinsonian medications for addressing EPSEs.

Assessment of EPSEs

Nursing assessment of EPSEs is important to the quality care of clients receiving psychotropic medications. One difficulty is consistency of assessment among caregivers. For example, nurses usually assess for the presence of **cogwheeling** (muscle movement that demonstrates a clicking into place instead of a smooth, gliding muscle movement) or muscle rigidity in clients receiving psychotropic drugs. However, those assessments are not necessarily reliable or consistent; what one nurse may consider moderate to severe side effects may be assessed as mild to moderate by another nurse. Repeating the assessment after

TABLE 31-2 ■ Antiparkinsonian Medications

Generic Name	Trade Name	Maximum Daily Dosage	Available in Injectable Form?
Amantadine	Symmetrel	300 mg	No
Benztropine	Cogentin	8 mg	Yes
Biperiden	Akineton	8 mg	Yes
Diphenhydramine	Benadryl	100 mg	Yes
Procyclidine	Kemadrin	15 mg	No
Trihexyphenidyl	Artane	15 mg	No

the medication is given helps you assess the amelioration of the side effect. These assessment data chart the course of a client's side effects and the effectiveness of medications to decrease them and are vital to quality nursing care.

Two assessment tools that lend greater objectivity to the assessment of EPSEs are the Simpson Neurological Rating Scale for the assessment of extrapyramidal side effects and the Abnormal Involuntary Movement Scale (AIMS) for the assessment of iatrogenic movements resulting from particular psychotropic drugs. These assessment tools can be found on the Online Student Resources for this book. They are helpful in quantifying EPSEs prior to administering a medication to counteract the side effects.

An example of the AIMS tool is in Your Assessment Approach. Directions on the assessment tool and the accompanying examination procedure guide you through a careful and

---

YOUR ASSESSMENT APPROACH
The Abnormal Involuntary Movement Scale (AIMS)

Examination Procedure

Either before or after completing the Examination Procedure, observe the client unobtrusively, at rest (e.g., in waiting room). Use a chair that is hard and firm without arms.

1. Ask the client to remove shoes and socks.
2. Ask the client whether there is anything in his/her mouth (e.g., gum, candy, etc.) and if there is, to remove it.
3. Ask the client about the current condition of his/her teeth. Ask client if he/she wears dentures. Do teeth or dentures bother the client *now*?
4. Ask the client whether he/she notices any movements in mouth, face, hands, or feet. If yes, ask to describe and to what extent they *currently* bother client or interfere with his/her activities.
5. Have the client sit in the chair with hands on the knees, legs slightly apart, and feet flat on the floor. (Look at entire body for movements while in this position.)
6. Ask the client to sit with hands hanging unsupported. If male, between legs, if female and wearing a dress, hanging over knees. (Observe hands and other body areas.)
7. Ask the client to open his/her mouth. (Observe tongue at rest within the mouth.) Do this twice.
8. Ask the client to protrude his/her tongue. (Observe abnormalities of tongue movement.) Do this twice.
9. Ask the client to tap his/her thumb, with each finger, as rapidly as possible for 10–15 seconds; separately with the right hand, then with the left hand. (Observe facial and leg movements.)
10. Flex and extend the client's left and right arms (one at a time). (Note any rigidity.)
11. Ask the client to stand up. (Observe in profile. Observe all body areas again, hips included.)
12. Ask the client to extend both arms outstretched in front with palms down. (Observe trunk, legs, and mouth.)
13. Have the client walk a few paces, turn, and walk back to the chair. (Observe hands and gait.) Do this twice.

---

complete TD screen. It is helpful to use a gooseneck lamp to see minute movements, particularly in the oral/facial areas. Clinical practice dictates that an AIMS be completed every 6 months during treatment. Using a video camera allows clinicians to record the client examination and compare results over time.

Sedation and Reduction of the Seizure Threshhold

Central nervous system (CNS) side effects of antipsychotic medications are sedation and reduction of the seizure threshold. Because antipsychotics vary in their sedative effects, these side effects are troublesome, but can be managed by changing to a less sedating agent. Seizures are not a contraindication for using these medications; however, their use in the presence of seizures requires close observation.

Allergic Effects

The principal allergic manifestation of the antipsychotics is cholestatic jaundice. This occurs much less frequently than in the early days of psychopharmacology, and it is usually a benign and self-limiting condition. Chlorpromazine (Thorazine), tricyclic antidepressants, and phenothiazines can all cause cholestatic jaundice, which is not universally thought to always be an allergic reaction. It is suggested that chlorpromazine exerts a direct toxic effect on the bile secretory mechanisms of the liver.

Some clients may have a record of what is thought to be an "allergic" reaction to a psychotropic medication but without documented evidence of cholestatic jaundice or other allergic reactions. When these circumstances are more carefully analyzed, it may turn out that the client either experienced neuroleptic malignant syndrome (NMS; discussed later in this chapter) or a dystonic reaction. The dangers associated with NMS may have prompted an explanation to the client along the lines of the dangers associated with an allergic reaction. This communication may have been misinterpreted and not detected or corrected.

Sometimes clients report dystonia as an allergic reaction to a psychiatric medication. A painful side effect such as dystonia is a negative experience to be avoided and clients may report it as an allergy in an attempt to ensure that the offending medication is not prescribed for them. Carefully scrutinize reports of allergies regularly to determine true allergies not only to protect the client from contact, but also to make sure no effective medications are removed from the array of treatments for that client.

Cardiac Effects

Antipsychotics can have an impact on the length of time it takes the heart to go through its electrical and muscular cycle. This cycle is abbreviated as the QT complex, referring to the length of the interval between the first wave identified in an ECG—there are Q, R, S, and T waves—and the last wave. A standardization of the length of this cycle is referred to as the QTc (a corrected QT interval). An interval longer than 450 to 500 msec can indicate a cardiac problem. An elongated QT interval can lead to arrhythmias and a drug-induced cardiac condition called torsades de pointes. Elongated QT intervals can also be traced to a family history of QT prolongation, non-psychiatric medications that prolong the QT, and lifestyle factors such as exercise, activity level, and nutrition (Vigneault et al., 2011; Dabiesingh, Psevdos, & Sharp, 2011). High doses of antipsychotics can contribute to the prevalence of QT interval abnormalities. However, the incidence of cardiac side effects is low and the increased risk of QTc abnormalities can be managed (Hough et al., 2011).

The highest risk for significant QT prolongation is with thioridazine (Mellaril). This medication was given a black box warning by the FDA to call attention to the risk. Pimozide (Orap), droperidol (Inapsine), and haloperidol (Haldol) also increase cardiac risk. The atypical antipsychotic aripiprazole (Abilify) was first marketed with FDA direction to monitor QTc. Ultimately, as with all other antipsychotics, use aripiprazole with caution in clients with known cardiovascular disease (history of myocardial infarction or ischemic heart disease, heart failure, or conduction abnormalities), cerebrovascular disease, and conditions that increase the likelihood of hypotension or hypertension. In clinical trials of aripiprazole, the incidence of QT prolongation was comparable to placebo (Pae, Forbes, & Patkar, 2011).

Blood, Skin, and Eye Effects

Among the other side effects in this category, one called *agranulocytosis* is the most serious. It is both potentially fatal and, fortunately, extremely rare (Barnes & Paton, 2011). The term means the body is not producing enough of the particular white blood cells (WBCs) called *granulocytes* (grainy cells), which are needed to fight infections. Usually the person acquires an infection and deteriorates rapidly or begins to bleed spontaneously, requiring emergency medical attention. Many medications cause agranulocytosis, including benzodiazepines and antibiotics. (See the discussion on page 121 in Chapter 7∞.)

Skin eruptions, photosensitivity leading to severe sunburn, blue-gray metallic discolorations over the face and hands, and pigmentation changes in the eyes are all potential side effects. Clients are generally advised to avoid prolonged exposure to sunlight or to use a sunscreen agent when outdoors. These conditions usually remit. An important feature of skin eruptions for people who have a serious and persistent mental illness is what it means to them. Delusions may be exacerbated as a result of eczema, rashes, or other eruptions. They can be frightening to someone who has paranoia, or perceived as justice and punishment by someone who has unrealistic guilt for some minor misdeed.

One serious and permanent eye change is retinitis pigmentosa. This condition may occur in clients receiving dosages of thioridazine exceeding 800 mg/day. The condition may lead to blindness. Therefore, doses exceeding 800 mg per day are contraindicated.

Endocrine Effects

Lactation in females and gynecomastia and impotence in males lead a list of endocrine changes that can occur with antipsychotic drug treatments. Hyperprolactinemia is a common side effect that will affect many aspects of the client's sex life. Difficulties with libido, arousal, excitation, orgasm, male ejaculatory volume, and overall performance can occur to a disturbing degree with hyperprolactinemia. You can imagine how these side effects would affect the regular or long-term use of the medication. Hyperprolactinemia is also responsible for oligomenorrhea or amenorrhea in women, galactorrhea in women and rarely in men, and, in cases of prolonged hyperprolactinemia, osteoporosis (Veselinović et al., 2011). Be alert to these endocrine changes; you are most likely to be the professional the client will tell about such problems.

Another endocrine problem is diabetes in people who have schizophrenia. The baseline occurrence of diabetes is elevated with schizophrenia (twice the rate of the general population), and seems to be further escalated by endocrine changes from psychotropics. Although weight gain raises the risk of diabetes, some studies show diabetes occurring in clients who have not gained significant weight. The particular medication used may be a contributing factor. Be alert to any changes in body functions reported by clients taking these medications.

Weight Gain

Weight gain is a significant side effect that affects self-esteem and poses health risks for the client. Certain antipsychotics, tricyclic antidepressants, lithium, anticonvulsants, and other classes of medications can cause an increase in weight. As mentioned earlier, an increase in weight can put an individual at risk for health problems such as diabetes, hypertension, and coronary artery disease. The impact of weight gain can be more disturbing to clients than EPSEs. Over time, this side effect can be a devastating blow to long-term treatment and quality of life. Paying careful attention to the potential for weight gain from the inception of treatment can help minimize this particular side effect.

Neuroleptic Malignant Syndrome

Although we discuss **neuroleptic malignant syndrome** (muscle rigidity, hyperpyrexia, altered consciousness, and diaphoresis) in this section on antipsychotic medications, be aware that it is a severe and potentially life-threatening side effect of all psychotropic medications. This extreme condition is believed to be the result of either dopamine blockade in the striatum of the brain or dopaminergic antagonism in the CNS (Thompson & Johnson, 2011). NMS occurs in 0.2% to 0.5% of clients taking psychiatric medications. Approximately twice as many men are affected as women, and younger clients appear to be more susceptible than older ones (Seitz & Gill, 2009). NMS typically occurs within the first 2 weeks of treatment with a new medication or a return to a previously used medication, or when a dosage has been increased. NMS has also been reported months after a new medication regimen has begun. Nurses are in the best position to assess for this condition. Because NMS often occurs in clients whose presentations are already complex, the nursing assessment can be difficult.

Treatment for NMS includes discontinuing all psychotropic medication immediately and supporting the client medically through the crisis. If cooling and rehydration are not achieved quickly, the client may die. Follow-up care is, of course, important. The pathology of NMS is complex and not completely understood at this time beyond the knowledge that its major symptoms are caused by the blockade of the dopamine receptors.

Client and Family Education

Client and family education about antipsychotics centers upon the individual client's medications, responses to it (or them), side effects exhibited, the client's and family members' abilities to learn about medications, and their interest in learning. Partnering With Clients and Families discusses common questions that clients and families ask and suggests responses that you can make.

NURSING RESPONSIBILITIES WITH ANTIDEPRESSANTS

Detailed information on the category of psychiatric medications known as antidepressants is in Chapter 7∞. This section discusses the important clinical considerations for psychiatric–mental health nurses. Atypical antidepressants such as mirtazapine (Remeron) and bupropion (Wellbutrin) are referred to in Chapter 7∞.

Antidepressant medications are not effective in all cases of depressed mood. Evidence from research and clinical practice indicates that only a portion of depressive disorders respond to this category of drugs. For example, tricyclic antidepressants (TCAs) and monoamine oxidase inhibitors (MAOIs) are generally contraindicated in depression related to grief reaction or pathologic grief. Other types of depression may be more amenable to psychopharmacologic intervention. Therefore, accurate diagnosis is necessary to ensure maximum effectiveness.

Clients for whom antidepressants are indicated usually have characteristic symptoms: a severely depressed mood, loss of interest, an inability to respond to normally pleasurable events or situations, a depression that is worse in the morning and lessens slightly as the day goes on, early morning awakening (and an inability to fall asleep again), marked psychomotor retardation or agitation, appetite and weight changes, and excessive or inappropriate guilt. These symptoms are known as *melancholia*. In fact, the symptoms of melancholia are the features that most reliably predict a person's response to drug therapy. A significant, and commonly overlooked, clinical consideration is that antidepressants have a delayed-reaction onset. A client will not show lessening of depressed

---

PARTNERING WITH CLIENTS AND FAMILIES

Teaching About Antipsychotics

This teaching plan points out the major areas to address when educating clients and their families about antipsychotic medications. Individualize each teaching plan for the following issues: the client's specific medication(s), responses to it (or them), side effects, and the client's and family members' abilities and interests in learning. Your documentation of client and family education can be a narrative note or a checklist of the topics discussed.

"What does this medication do?"	"Antipsychotic medications help treat the emotional and thinking problems of schizophrenia or psychosis. It helps organize thinking, keeps you in touch with reality, and reduces the symptoms of your illness. It is not a cure. When you stop taking this medication, the benefits wear off over time and you will have these problems again, possibly at a more disturbing level."
"How should I take this medication?"	"Take it as prescribed on a regular basis. If you feel that you cannot or do not want to continue, notify your therapist or prescriber before you take action."
"What if I miss a dose?"	"Take the dose as soon as you remember if it's only been a few hours. But if it is almost time for your next dose, do not take double or extra doses."
"What other medication does not mix with this antipsychotic?"	Tailor this response to the specific medication prescribed. Mention the major drug interactions with prescribed medications, over-the-counter substances, alternative and complementary supplements, and, of course, alcohol and recreational drug use. There may even be interactions with caffeine, nicotine, and food items that you should discuss in detail.
"What side effects can I expect?"	A discussion of the client's previous side effects with the substance drives this conversation. Although there is no need to overwhelm the client with excess information, the client should know what actions to take when side effects occur. Describe ordinary and extraordinary side effects as well as the actions that the client should take in response to the side effects. Some standard side effects are important to cover, and include: dystonia, akathisia, agitation, confusion, sensitivity to sunlight, and changes in sexual expression.
"Where can I keep my medication?"	"In a safe place at room temperature. Do not keep it in the bathroom where there is a shower or bathtub, in the kitchen where there is a dishwasher, or above or right next to the kitchen sink. Do not keep medications in a motor vehicle, because temperatures can reach extreme levels within such an enclosed area. Moisture, light, and heat can affect your medication."
"What do I do if I have a problem?"	Give the client and family the names and numbers of health care providers the client can call for questions and in emergencies.

mood until 2 to 3 weeks after instituting an adequate dose of TCAs (it is a shorter time interval for SSRIs and serotonin and norepinephrine reuptake inhibitors [SNRIs]).

The principles guiding the use of MAOI and TCA medications are as follows:

- Drug treatment does not preclude psychotherapy, electroconvulsive therapy, or behavioral treatments if they are also indicated.
- Other antidepressant treatment should be given first unless contraindications are present, there are clinical indications for MAOIs, or there is a past history of unresponsiveness to other antidepressants.
- Dosage may vary and may be limited because of significant side effects.
- Clients with recurrent major depressive episodes with melancholia may require long-term maintenance treatment, although doses are usually lower than those needed in acute episodes.

Because clients who do not respond to other classes of antidepressants may respond to MAOIs, clients taking these medications are likely to have had negative experiences with antidepressant medication therapy. This history, in combination with the demands made of clients who take MAOIs such as dietary restrictions and medication limitations (discussed later in this chapter), requires careful attention by psychiatric–mental health nurses to the education needs of clients and their family members.

Teaching clients and families about antidepressant therapy is a challenge because the client may have symptoms of depression that interfere with learning. Special considerations for teaching, and evaluating your teaching efforts, are covered in Partnering With Clients and Families.

Side Effects of TCAs

Many of the common side effects of tricyclics are autonomic due to the anticholinergic characteristics of the medications discussed in Your Assessment Approach: Anticholinergic Side Effects on page 679. These side effects, discussed earlier in the section on antipsychotic medications, include dry mouth, blurred vision, constipation, palpitations, and urinary retention. Treat clients with glaucoma with caution. Some allergic skin reactions have been observed.

TCAs also cause changes in the normal electrical conduction of the heart and are cardiotoxic, which is particularly significant in treating clients with a history of cardiovascular disease, especially heart block. Sudden death has occurred during tricyclic treatment. TCAs are contraindicated in clients with mitral valve disease. Clients with known heart disease and most elderly clients require electrocardiograms (ECGs) before, and periodically during, the course of tricyclic therapy. Several CNS effects may occur, including tremor, twitching, paresthesias, ataxia, and convulsions.

Overdose Effects of TCAs

The consequences of overdosing are one aspect of TCA treatment that deserves attention. Significant overdoses may cause delirium, hyperthermia, convulsions, and even coma, shock, and respiratory failure. A lethal dose of an antidepressant such as amitriptyline (Elavil) is estimated at between 10 and 30 times the usual daily therapeutic dose. Drug intake deserves close attention, because many clients treated with these medications are severely suicidal. Serious overdosing is a medical emergency and may require resuscitative measures.

Side Effects of Monoamine Oxidase Inhibitors (MAOIs)

The main adverse effect with MAOIs is **hypertensive crisis**, where the blood pressure increases precipitously and can cause a cerebral vascular event or a cardiac arrhythmia. Hypertensive crisis is a significant danger when foods, fluids, or medications that contain tyramine are in the digestive tract together with an MAOI. Lower levels of side effects are sometimes called "cheese syndrome" because these side effects occur when an MAOI has been combined with any form of cheese. There is no firm formula to determine how much tyramine will cause an adverse event. Clients often test their capacity to tolerate tyramine by ingesting prohibited foods and fluids in small amounts as long as they are unable to detect side effects. (Prohibited foods and fluids are discussed later in this chapter.) The MAOI patch is largely not metabolized through the digestive system and thus is much less likely to require dietary restrictions.

More common side effects of MAOIs include lightheadedness, mild sedation or insomnia, muscle twitching, palpitations, and blurred vision. There are sexual side effects such as decreased libido, and typical anticholinergic side effects such as constipation and urinary retention can be a problem. Clients are usually taking MAOIs because no other antidepressant has worked to resolve symptoms or the client only responds to MAOIs. For these clients, management of side effects takes place on a long-term basis. Discuss with the client the side effects the client experiences and develop a plan to address the more durable and annoying ones.

Side Effects of Selective Serotonin Reuptake Inhibitors (SSRIs)

Although the side effects of SSRIs are less severe than those of other antidepressants, some may be intolerable for certain clients. The side effect profile for SSRIs is discussed in TABLE 31-3 ■ on page 688. Side effects of SSRIs are thought to be the result of an individual's sensitivity to higher levels of serotonin in the synapse as a consequence of SSRI treatment. Activation, a more energized state that includes decreased sleep and akathisia, is common. Take special care with clients who have histories of hypomania or mania, because SSRIs may precipitate a re-emergence or a relapse.

Because the level of serotonin in the synapse can be a physiological, as well as psychological, difficulty for a client, be sensitive to the possibility of serotonin syndrome. Similarly, when decreased levels of serotonin are experienced your client may have symptoms of this physiological state called serotonin discontinuation syndrome. The two Your Assessment Approach features on pages 688 and 689 describe the assessment, management, and prevention of serotonin syndrome and the SSRI discontinuation syndrome.

PARTNERING WITH CLIENTS AND FAMILIES

Teaching About Antidepressants

Proper client education enhances the effectiveness of medication therapy and can help make the difference between client adherence and nonadherence with the medication regimen. Client education begins when medication therapy begins and is repeated during the course of the client's hospitalization. Give instructions orally and in writing. Include family members or significant others if they will supervise home administration.

Initiating Antidepressant Therapy

- Make sure the client knows the name and dose of the medication(s) being taken. *(Rationale: This is basic information every client should know.)*
- Advise the client to arise slowly from a sitting or lying position, and to sit on the side of the bed before standing up. *(Rationale: This allows the body time to compensate for medications that have postural hypotension as a side effect.)*
- Encourage the use of ice chips, sugar-free gum, sugar-free hard candy, and increased fluids. *(Rationale: Alleviates dryness of mouth.)*
- Advise both client and family that it may take 2 to 4 weeks to see a therapeutic response to antidepressant therapy. *(Rationale: Prevents discouragement and impatience.)*
- Monitor for urinary retention or constipation, and take necessary actions. *(Rationale: These conditions may result from the anticholinergic effects of some antidepressants.)*
- Give medication early in the day if insomnia occurs as a side effect. *(Rationale: Some antidepressants have a stimulating effect.)*
- Give medication later in the evening if sedation occurs as a side effect. *(Rationale: Some antidepressants have sedating side effects.)*
- Monitor and record sleep patterns. *(Rationale: Normalization of sleep patterns should occur.)*
- Avoid giving TCAs or SSRIs and MAOIs concurrently. *(Rationale: To avoid hypertensive crisis, give 2 to 3 weeks apart.)*
- Observe the client for skin rashes, photosensitivity, weight gain, and signs of infection. *(Rationale: These are adverse side effects that you should evaluate.)*
- Advise the client that drowsiness, blurred vision, dry mouth, and jittery feelings will diminish after a few days on the medication. *(Rationale: Sedation and anticholinergic effects [except dry mouth] usually diminish over time. They will recur when dosage is raised, however.)*
- Monitor the client for suicide risk, particularly as depression begins to lift. *(Rationale: Profoundly depressed clients lack the energy to plan and implement suicide. As they begin to improve and energize but are still profoundly depressed, risk increases.)*
- Observe clients on high doses of TCAs closely for seizures. *(Rationale: High-dose tricyclics lower the seizure threshold.)*

Clients on SSRIs

- Depressive symptoms may resolve within 1 week. *(Rationale: SSRIs work more quickly than TCAs or MAOIs.)*
- Taking more than the prescribed dose will not resolve depression more quickly, nor is there a chance of toxic overdose effects. *(Rationale: More SSRI than prescribed will not hasten recovery and an excess of serotonin in the synapse is not dangerous. There may be physical discomfort associated with serotonin syndrome.)*
- There may be feelings of restlessness, headaches, GI upset, and vivid or disturbing dreams when first taking an SSRI. These are often temporary side effects. *(Rationale: The side effects may resolve within 3 weeks.)*
- There are no dietary restrictions with SSRIs. They cannot be taken simultaneously with MAOIs or with St. John's wort (which is a naturally occurring MAOI). *(Rationale: Co-administered SSRI and MAOI can cause CNS depression from ataxia and slurred speech to coma and death.)*

Clients on MAOIs

- Supervise the client's intake, and make sure no tyramine-rich agents are offered. *(Rationale: Tyramine may precipitate hypertensive crisis.)*
- Monitor the client closely for headaches and elevated blood pressure. Withhold medication, and report these signs to the prescribing professional immediately. *(Rationale: These may be early signs of hypertensive crisis.)*
- Keep phentolamine mesylate (Regitine) on hand for treating hypertensive crisis. *(Rationale: This is an alpha-adrenergic blocker and potent antihypertensive agent.)*
- Observe diabetic clients closely for hypoglycemia. *(Rationale: MAOIs promote hypoglycemia.)*

Prior to Discharge

- In collaboration with the client, work out a time schedule that fits the client's lifestyle. *(Rationale: This will increase the likelihood that the client will actually take the medication.)*
- Advise the client to take the medication as ordered and to avoid using alcohol or other central nervous system depressants during therapy. *(Rationale: Varying the dosage impairs the maintenance of therapeutic blood levels. Alcohol and other central nervous system depressants have a potentiating effect on antidepressants and may cause stupor or coma.)*
- Teach the client and family about possible adverse reactions and measures to initiate if they occur. *(Rationale: Ensures maximum comfort and safety.)*
- Caution the client not to operate dangerous equipment, drive a car, or engage in tasks requiring mental alertness if drowsiness persists. *(Rationale: Ensures safety.)*
- Teach the client not to discontinue the medication abruptly. *(Rationale: Antidepressant dosage should be gradually decreased to avoid withdrawal symptoms of nausea, dizziness, insomnia, and headache.)*
- For clients on MAOIs, provide a list of tyramine-containing substances and make sure the client and family understand the consequences of consuming tyramine. *(Rationale: Ensures client safety.)*
- Record accurately and completely what medication education the client and family have received. *(Rationale: Documenting client education provides legal protection for the nurse and institution in the event of an adverse reaction.)*

TABLE 31-3 ■ Side Effects of SSRIs Compared to Those of a Typical Tricyclic (Amitriptyline)

	Fluoxetine (Prozac)	Sertraline (Zoloft)	Paroxetine (Paxil)	Citalopram (Celexa)	Escitalopram (Lexapro)	Amitriptyline (Elavil)
Anticholinergic	0	1	1	1	0–1	4
Sedation	1–2	1–2	0–1	0–1	0–1	3
Activation	1–2	1–2	1–2	1–2	1–2	0
Hypotension	0	0	0	0–1	0	3
GI activation	1–2	1–2	1–2	1–2	1–2	0
Seizures	+	+	0	0	0	+

0 = low; 4 = high; + = present

An important consideration with clients taking SSRIs is the proximity of the administration of MAOIs. Fluoxetine (Prozac) and an MAOI together may cause serious and fatal interactions. The half-life of fluoxetine requires a 5-week gap between taking fluoxetine and taking an MAOI, and vice versa. Sertraline (Zoloft), paroxetine (Paxil), citalopram (Celexa), and escitalopram (Lexapro) have shorter half-lives, and there must be a 1- or 2-week gap (in both directions) between these medications and MAOIs.

Side Effects of Serotonin and Norepinephrine Reuptake Inhibitors (SNRIs)

Venlafaxine (Effexor) was the first in a class of medications called *phenethylamine antidepressants*. It has two

---

YOUR ASSESSMENT APPROACH   Serotonin Syndrome

Definition
- Mental, autonomic, and neuromuscular changes
- Mild in most people, and with supportive care recovery is complete within 24–72 hours, although it can cause death under certain circumstances (11%)
- Seen in people taking two or more medications that increase the levels of serotonin in the CNS, including SSRIs, TCAs, and MAOIs

Conditions of Diagnosis
- No antipsychotic medication used or increased in dose prior to onset of symptoms
- No other obvious causes of confusion or fever
- Recent addition or increased dose of an agent that raises serotonin levels

Symptoms
Three of the following must be present:

- Mental status changes (confusion, hypomania, anxiety, coma)
- Agitation
- Myoclonus
- Shivering
- Diarrhea
- Hyper-reflexia
- Ataxia/incoordination
- Diaphoresis
- Hyperpyrexia

Other Symptoms
Cardiovascular:
- Sinus tachycardia
- Hypertension
- Hypotension

Gastrointestinal:
- Nausea
- Abdominal pain
- Salivation

Motor Abnormalities:
- Muscle rigidity
- Restlessness
- Tremor
- Nystagmus
- Seizures

Other:
- Unreactive pupils
- Tachypnea

Management and Prevention of Serotonin Syndrome
- Use supportive measures to reduce hypertension, tachycardia, hyperthermia, and respiratory distress.
- Discontinue suspected agent.
- Discontinue OTCs that increase serotonin levels (dextromethorphan, pseudoephedrine, phenylpropanolamine).
- Benzodiazepines (lorazepam and diazepam) are used commonly to treat myoclonus and resultant hyperthermia.
- Severe cases not responding to benzodiazepines may respond to dantrolene (Dantrium) for relieving muscle rigidity and hyperthermia.
- Severe cases are treated with antiserotonergic agents (cyproheptadine [Periactin], methysergide [Sansert], propranolol [Inderal]).
- Reconsider using two or more serotonergic medications or consider switching to less serotonergic alternatives.

Note: Clonazepam is ineffective in treating serotonin syndrome.

YOUR ASSESSMENT APPROACH   SSRI Discontinuation Syndrome

- Withdrawal from an SSRI is characterized by symptoms including: dizziness, light-headedness, insomnia, fatigue, anxiety or agitation, nausea, headache, and sensory disturbances. Other possible symptoms include hypomania, worsening of mood, aggressiveness, and suicidality.

- Symptoms have occurred in less than 5% of clients taking long-acting agents, compared to 86% of clients treated with fluvoxamine for panic disorder.

- A possible cause of the syndrome could be a hyposerotonergic state because long-term use of SSRI therapy may down regulate (or desensitize) postsynaptic serotonin receptors. Abrupt discontinuation may restore or even enhance serotonin reuptake,

resulting in a depletion of synaptic serotonin. May take 2 to 3 weeks for these systems to readapt.

- Mild, transient symptoms such as jitteriness, sleep disturbance, and heart palpitations have been reported in newborns whose mothers received SSRIs during pregnancy.

- Short-acting SSRIs cause more numerous symptoms that appear earlier after discontinuation and typically last up to 3 weeks.

- Abrupt discontinuation or "drug holidays" should be avoided with short-acting SSRIs.

- These agents should be tapered if discontinued.

- If symptoms appear, the taper needs to be more gradual.

---

mechanisms of action: inhibiting the reuptake of serotonin and inhibiting the reuptake of norepinephrine. Medications that have this dual action are in a class known as SNRIs. Duloxetine (Cymbalta) has similar neurotransmission action and addresses the pain sensations amplified by depression, as well.

Anticholinergic-like side effects may occur with this category of medications. Sustained increases in blood pressure have also been reported with some clients taking venlafaxine. This last side effect seems to be dose related, so the nursing management of clients taking venlafaxine should include regular blood pressure monitoring. There is also a need for a time buffer with MAOIs: a 14-day gap after discontinuing an MAOI before starting venlafaxine, and at least a 7-day gap after discontinuing venlafaxine before starting an MAOI.

Medications that inhibit the reuptake of serotonin and norepinephrine, as SNRIs do, have an activation component that can cause anxiety. Anorexia may be a difficult side effect for underweight individuals. Other reported side effects include nausea, somnolence, dry mouth, dizziness, constipation, sweating, asthenia, absence of orgasm, delayed ejaculation, and anorexia.

The recommended starting dosage for venlafaxine is 75 mg/day, administered in divided doses and taken with food. The dose may be increased to 225 mg/day according to clinical needs, and even further increased to 375 mg/day. It is recommended that clients who have been taking venlafaxine for more than 1 week taper the dose when discontinuing the medication. Clients taking it for 6 weeks or more should time this taper over a 2-week period to minimize the risk of symptoms caused by discontinuing the medication.

Duloxetine dosing focuses on a total dose of 40 mg/day (20 mg twice daily) to 60 mg/day (given either once a day or as 30 mg twice daily). Duloxetine does not have to be taken on an empty or a full stomach; its bioavailability is not dependent on meals. There is no evidence that doses greater than 60 mg/day provide any additional antidepressant benefits. When discontinuing the medication, tapering the dose rather than abruptly stopping the medication is recommended to minimize discomfort. If intolerable symptoms occur after a decrease in the dose or when the medication is discontinued, then resuming the previously prescribed dose may be considered. Once the

client is stabilized, the prescriber may continue decreasing the duloxetine dose but at a more gradual rate.

Age-Related Considerations With Antidepressants

Overall, it is essential to carefully monitor any child, adolescent, or young adult who receives antidepressant therapy. The current concern is that antidepressants may contribute to an increased risk of suicidal behavior. Following an FDA Public Health Advisory in 2005, all antidepressants now have labeling that indicates that children, adolescents, and adults treated with antidepressants can experience greater suicidal ideation and behavior during the first few months of treatment. Clinically, suicidal thoughts are quite common in all age groups and particularly so with those individuals who have depression. What remains difficult is that suicidal thoughts have little relationship to suicidal behavior, in other words, while people may think about committing suicide it does not necessarily mean they will follow through (Gibbons & Mann, 2011).

An increase in suicidal ideation following weeks of treatment with antidepressants coincides with the clinical experience of most mental health professionals. Depressed individuals frequently become more activated by their medications and have considerably more energy while they are still actively depressed. Depressed thinking may include lethality. Therefore, closely monitor all clients who have expressed depressed, lethal thoughts and be aware of changes in behavior and comments indicating an intention to harm themselves. Competent and adequate use of antidepressants with clinical supervision reduces suicide. See Chapter 23∞ for a discussion of this phenomenon.

Client and Family Education

Because clients who do not respond to tricyclics may respond to MAOIs, they are likely to have had past negative experiences with antidepressant medication therapy. This, in combination with the demands of taking an MAOI, indicates the need for increased nursing involvement in educating clients and their family members.

MAOI antidepressants require an especially strong, concerted teaching effort from nurses. There are drawbacks to taking these medications that directly affect nursing intervention. For example, clients on MAOIs must avoid foods that contain even moderate amounts of tyramine; failure to do so will result in hypertensive crisis. Partnering With Clients and Families outlines the low-tyramine diet for clients taking MAOIs.

NURSING RESPONSIBILITIES WITH MOOD STABILIZERS

Detailed information on the category of psychiatric medications known as mood stabilizers is in Chapter 7∞. This section discusses the important clinical considerations for psychiatric–mental health nurses.

PARTNERING WITH CLIENTS AND FAMILIES

Teaching About a Low-Tyramine Diet

MAO inhibitors combined with certain foods and medications produce a significant increase in blood pressure, which can be a health hazard. In general, foods that can cause this reaction are those that have been *pickled, fermented, smoked, or aged*. The list below includes the main foods, fluids, and medications that clients should avoid while taking an MAOI and for the 2 weeks after the MAOI is discontinued. Keep in mind that fertilizers and preservatives can be tyramine based; therefore, the dietary restrictions should be updated regularly. This list may not include everything to be avoided (for example, the kind of fertilizer or preservative used may change over time) and may also include items that may be safe to consume at some later point in time.

Note: The monoamine oxidase inhibitor patch Emsam (selegiline) at its lowest strength can be used without the dietary restrictions that apply to all oral MAO inhibitors.

Foods and Beverages to Avoid Completely

Meats and fish	Pickled herring, dried fish, aged/dried/cured meats, unrefrigerated fermented fish, liver, caviar, fermented sausage (bologna, salami, pepperoni, summer sausage), hoisin sauce (fermented oyster sauce used in Asian dishes), any jerky, leftovers that may be partly fermented, meat extracts, commercial gravies, crackers made with cheese, miso (fermented soybean paste), soy sauce, teriyaki sauce, salad dressings with disallowed ingredients
Vegetables	English broad peas, Chinese pea pods, fava beans, banana peels, Italian or broad green beans, kim chee (fermented cabbage), lentils, lima beans, sauerkraut, spoiled or overly ripe fruits, peanuts, spinach
Dairy products	Yogurt, most cheeses (see Allowed Foods for exceptions). Tyramine content of some cheeses, per serving: English Stilton, 17.3 mg; mozzarella, 2.4 mg; grated Parmesan, 0.2 mg; cream cheese, 0
Beverages	Chianti, aged wines, imported beers, aged beers
Combination foods	Breads made with aged cheeses and meats, or yeast extracts; homemade or high-yeast breads; pizza; lasagna; soufflés; macaroni and cheese; quiche; liver pâté; Caesar salad; eggplant parmesan; all yeast products (such as brewer's yeast, bouillon or broth with yeast, and yeast extracts such as Marmite and other yeast spreads)

MSG	MSG is a flavor-enhancer used much more than in Asian dishes. Many prepared and processed foods use MSG (canned soups, taco and potato chips, packaged noodle meals, canned gravy, frozen prepared meals, salad dressings—especially the low-fat ones, and almost all the foods at convenience food restaurants include MSG). MSG is also labeled as hydrolyzed vegetable protein, Accent, Agino moto, natural meat tenderizer
Medications	Cold medications, nasal decongestants (tablets, drops, sprays, etc.), hay fever and allergy medications, weight reduction preparations, "pep" pills, antiappetite medications, asthma inhalant

Foods and Beverages to Take in Small Amounts

Dairy products	Processed American cheese
Fruits	Raisins, prunes, bananas, avocados, plums, canned figs
Caffeine sources	Coffee, chocolate, colas
Beverages	Domestic jug red wines; domestic beers, ales, and stouts; sherry *(Note: Alcohol is a depressant and should not be ingested by individuals in treatment for depression.)*

Allowed Foods

Beverages	White wines *(Note: Alcohol is a depressant and should not be ingested by individuals in treatment for depression.)*

Any baked goods raised with yeast, but not high yeast

Dairy products	Cottage cheese, cream cheese, milk, cream, ice cream

Additional Information

St. John's wort	Naturally occurring MAOI, less potent than pharmaceutical grade; is not regulated and may cause inconsistent access to the active ingredient; has the same dietary and medication restrictions as a pharmaceutical-grade MAOI

A variety of compounds are used as mood stabilizers. Mood stabilization, as well as activating and sedating side effects, must be addressed to ensure comfortable and consistent medication adherence. Because of the dangers of unmedicated bipolar disorder, an awareness of side effects and an effective response are important treatment and safety issues.

Lithium Carbonate

Lithium carbonate, used in the treatment and prevention of acute manic episodes since the 1960s, is used in preventing the recurrence of bipolar disorder as well. Lithium most likely alters neurotransmission in the central nervous system because it interferes with the ionic pump mechanism in brain cells. However, its exact mode of action is unknown. Its use is not recommended during pregnancy and breastfeeding or in clients with impaired renal function, congestive heart failure, sodium-restricted diets, organic brain disease, and impaired central nervous system functioning.

Administered orally, lithium's onset of action ranges from 1 to 3 weeks. The dosage is gradually increased until the recommended therapeutic blood level of 1.0 to 1.5 mEq/L is achieved. Once the desired effect is achieved, the dosage is adjusted downward to the maintenance blood level of 0.6 to 1.2 mEq/L. There are cultural considerations to the therapeutic blood level: persons of Asian descent may have toxic reactions at dosages as low as 0.6 mEq/L. Monitor therapeutic effect as well as side effects.

Include the following instructions in your teaching plan:

- The diet must include adequate salt and fluid intake, and the client should not take diuretics at any time.
- Regular testing of serum levels must be done, and the client should notify the prescriber of any illness, especially if vomiting and diarrhea occur.
- The client should also be aware of hydration levels and take care not to become dehydrated.
- The client should not vary the dosage and should continue to take the medicine even when feeling well because discontinuing lithium therapy often precipitates a manic episode.
- If symptoms of lithium toxicity occur—such as nausea, vomiting, diarrhea, polyuria, muscle weakness, fine hand tremors, headache, blurred vision, slurred speech, dizziness, sluggishness, abdominal cramping, and tinnitus—the client should immediately discontinue the medication and contact the prescriber.

Lithium has a significant number of side effects that can be troublesome and, in some cases, quite dangerous. Significant side effects are usually correlated with blood levels of lithium above 1.2 mEq/L. Common side effects include tremor, nausea, thirst, and polyuria. Thyroid goiter has also been seen as a side effect. See Your Intervention Strategies: Lithium Maintenance Toolbox for an elaboration of these details. It also includes teaching for clients and their families.

Severe lithium poisoning is a potential medical emergency. Early signs include vomiting and diarrhea, lethargy, and muscle twitching. These may progress to ataxia and

Care Plan: The Exercising Patient on Lithium

YOUR INTERVENTION STRATEGIES
Lithium Maintenance Toolbox

To keep a stable lithium level, nurses, clients, and family members should know the following:

1. Stabilize the dosing schedule (through sustained release formula or divided doses).
2. If a dose is missed, take within 2 hours. If more than 2 hours has elapsed, skip that one dose.
3. Ingest adequate dietary sodium.
4. Maintain hydration.
5. Replace fluids and electrolytes lost during exercise, exertion, or GI illness.
6. Monitor for signs of side effects and lithium toxicity.

Watch for these events to cause lithium level increases:

1. Hydration status change
2. Increases in other medications
3. Marijuana use
4. Carbamazepine
5. Lithium overdose
6. Decreased sodium intake
7. Diuretic treatments
8. Medical illness
9. Nonsteroidal anti-inflammatory drug therapy
10. Tetracycline use
11. Fluid and electrolyte loss through fever, sweating, diarrhea, vomiting, or dehydration

---

slurred speech. The client may become semiconscious or comatose; seizures may occur; and electrolyte imbalances may lead to cardiac arrest. This syndrome of severe toxicity ordinarily occurs only when the client has a blood lithium level of 2 to 3 mEq/L. The client may have overdosed or severely restricted food or salt intake (or taken diuretics) to induce this state.

Occasionally, very violent, agitated, or paranoid individuals with mania require antipsychotic medications as either a mood stabilizer (in the case of atypical antipsychotics) or as an adjunctive medication (for atypical and conventional antipsychotics). Antipsychotic medications used for delusions or agitation can be started simultaneously with the mood stabilizer, increased to whatever level is required to control the disintegrative behavior, then gradually reduced, and finally eliminated after therapeutic mood stabilizer levels have been effective for about 1 week.

NURSING RESPONSIBILITIES WITH ANXIOLYTICS

Detailed information on the category of psychiatric medications known as *anxiolytics*, or antianxiety medications, is in Chapter 7∞. This section discusses the important clinical considerations for psychiatric–mental health nurses.

Anxiolytic medications are used to treat a variety of problems, ranging from high levels of anxiety and panic to insomnia.

Side Effects

Common side effects include problems with daytime functioning, drowsiness, dizziness, and decreased coordination. These side effects can lead to an increase in accidents and falls, especially among older adults. Benzodiazepines induce hypnosis and sedation in addition to their muscle relaxant, anxiolytic, and anticonvulsant actions. Benzodiazepines are also known to induce respiratory depression, therefore always use caution with older adults, those with respiratory diseases, and those taking other medications that depress respiration, such as opiates. Regular use of benzodiazepines can lead to dependency on the benzodiazepine, rebound insomnia when the dose is reduced (a return of insomnia, sometimes greater than originally experienced), and withdrawal symptoms even if tapering is completed after long-term use (Kaiser, 2011).

Client and Family Education

Client teaching is an especially important element in the care of clients taking antianxiety medications. As you know from Chapters 8 and 18∞, anxiety is a generally uncomfortable experience. Self-medication often becomes the relief-seeking behavior used by many people with severe anxiety. Self-medication can be temporarily helpful in restoring a person's capacities and internal comfort. Some clients self-medicate by taking more anti-anxiety medication than is prescribed. Many of the anxiolytic drugs (especially benzodiazepines), however, carry a potential for dependence and tolerance. Therefore, nurses have a responsibility to help clients control anxiety in other safer and more effective ways.

Anxious clients often self-medicate when they have trouble sleeping. As with anxiolytics, insomnia preparations are generally intended for either occasional or short-term use. These medications are appropriate for clients newly admitted to a psychiatric inpatient unit or for clients in outpatient therapy who develop sleep disorders. As other medications (antidepressants, lithium, antipsychotics) begin to have a therapeutic effect, however, the need for sedative–hypnotic medication such as alprazolam (Xanax) or diazepam (Valium) should almost, if not completely, abate. Nurses working with clients in these situations need to help them regulate their sleep patterns.

NURSING RESPONSIBILITIES WITH MEDICATIONS FOR DEMENTIA

Detailed information on the categories of psychiatric medications used to treat dementias—both acetylcholinesterase inhibitors and glutamate pathway modifiers—are in Chapter 7∞. This section discusses the important clinical considerations for psychiatric–mental health nurses.

Dementia and other cognitive impairments are typically treated with acetylcholinesterase inhibitors such as donepezil (Aricept), galantamine (Reminyl), and rivastigmine (Exelon) and/or a glutamate pathway inhibitor such as N-methyl-d-aspartate (NMDA) receptor antagonist (memantine or Namenda). These medications perform actions that improve cognitive function.

The first of the acetylcholinesterase inhibitors was tacrine (Cognex). Problems with this medication included liver toxicity, which could be controlled, and several side effects such as GI disturbances and headache. From this beginning, subsequent compounds were developed. Donepezil, galantamine, and rivastigmine are more effective with dementia of the Alzheimer's type and have fewer and less problematic side effects. GI disturbances occur at a much lower level than with the original compound, and headaches are reported at only a slightly higher level than among clients taking a placebo. Acetylcholinesterase inhibitors are safe, effective, and well tolerated. They promise competent treatment for clients with dementia and other cognitive impairments. Alternative routes of administration, such as the rivastigmine's patch delivery system, offer choices for those with swallowing difficulties or issues about taking pills.

An entirely different route to treat dementia is to modify the glutamate pathway so the cells do not become overwhelmed and decay from overexcitation. Memantine, like other NMDA antagonists, causes behavioral activation associated with enhanced cerebral glucose utilization. Studies have shown that memantine can reverse the decreased metabolic activity associated with DAT, possibly accounting for its beneficial effects on cognition and global functioning. Chapter 14∞ discusses cognitive disorders.

NURSING RESPONSIBILITIES WITH HERBAL MEDICINES

Detailed information on herbal medicines can also be found in Chapters 7 and 33∞. Table 33-2∞ on page 732 identifies herbals and dietary supplements commonly used for psychiatric symptoms. This section discusses the important clinical considerations for psychiatric–mental health nurses.

Research involving complementary and alternative (CAM) medications assesses how safe and effective botanicals can be in treating psychiatric symptoms. It is vital to rigorously assess herbal side effects and drug–drug interactions because the CAM industry, unlike the pharmaceutical industry, is not regulated and monitored. Reports of contaminants and drug toxicity causing acute liver failure and general ineffectiveness for psychiatric symptoms abound (Nguyen & Vierling, 2011; Im, 2011).

People use CAM products for several different reasons—depression, anxiety, dementia, sleep disturbance, alcoholic encephalopathy, and peripheral neuropathy (refer to Table 33-2∞ on page 732). CAM substances used for depression—St. John's wort, tryptophan/5-hydroxytryptophan, S-adenosyl methionine, folate, and inositol—have been studied. However, no study was conclusively positive. A vital question that concerns the use of CAM substances by people who are depressed is: What happens when a CAM product such as St. John's wort, a naturally occurring MAOI, is used in combination with a prescriptive antidepressant? An earlier discussion in this chapter (see page 688) explores why combining SSRIs and MAOIs is contraindicated. Drug–CAM product interactions can and do occur. Inconclusive results and unequivocally negative results are regularly seen in the literature. If a depression does not respond to St. John's wort or other CAM within a brief and reasonable period of time, it is necessary to address the symptoms with a reliable and regulated medication. Although these results may make clinicians feel uncomfortable with and reluctant to recommend or advocate their use, CAM products may be an alternative for some.

CAM products do provide an opportunity for a client to feel empowered; however, it is important to note that symptoms of a moderate to severe level must be clinically monitored and effectively managed. Shortening the time interval until symptom relief is achieved while providing the client the neuroprotective nature of psychopharmacology (see Chapter 7∞) is the most responsible course of action. Selected CAM medications can have beneficial effects in some clients as an adjunctive treatment or as a low-potency treatment for those who are sensitive to pharmaceutical-grade compounds or cannot tolerate the lowest, weakest dosage form available. Keep your knowledge base up to date and refer to expert consultants (Fontaine, 2011; Kiefer, Pitluk, & Klunk, 2009).

Assessing Herbal Consumption

There are a variety of potentially adverse herb–drug interactions based on the pharmacologic properties of both herbal and prescription medications. Adverse herb–drug interactions seen clinically and in research are one of the three leading causes of acute liver failure (Nguyen & Vierling, 2011). This makes it vital that CAM–drug interactions become a topic of discussion for clients and caregivers.

Clients often combine prescription medications with complementary and alternative medications without telling their health care providers, and health care providers often fail to ask clients about CAM use. It is important to introduce a discussion of CAM use when assessing clients in order to avoid CAM–drug interactions. Table 33-3∞ on page 733 identifies commonly used natural medicines (including herbals) that should not be taken in combination with psychotropics. A nonjudgmental approach and an open dialogue about the use of CAM are more likely to yield relevant information. See Rx Communication on page 137 in Chapter 7∞ for examples of a conversation about this topic.

INCOMPATIBILITIES AND UNCOMMON MEDICATION COMBINATIONS

Nurses have many responsibilities to clients receiving neuroleptic drugs. To ensure the bioavailability and effectiveness of neuroleptic medications, it is important to understand the relationships between the medication and the liquid (or substance) with which it is administered, as well as the relationships between medications. Some medications are not compatible with all substances. For an overview of the compatibility of medications and typical liquids, see Table 31-4 ■.

In addition to liquid and drug compatibilities, you need to be aware of other problematic combinations—for example, the combination of grapefruit juice and several psychiatric medications, such as the anxiolytic medications triazolam (Halcion) and buspirone (BuSpar). When taken with grapefruit juice, triazolam is not metabolized efficiently and therefore remains at higher levels in the body, and buspirone blood levels can be raised to nine times the normal level. The explanation for this resides in the furanocoumarins in grapefruit juice and their ability to inhibit a liver enzyme (cytochrome $P_{450}3A4$ or CYP3A4) from metabolizing the medication out of the system (see Chapter 7∞). This action allows the medication and its metabolites to remain in the system longer than usual, where it accumulates, causing higher blood levels, enhanced effects of the medication, and greater side effects (Fagiolino, Vázquez, Eiraldi, Maldonado, & Scaramelli, 2011).

Ultimately, either of these mechanisms, cytochrome P_{450} activation or inhibition, can be accomplished through a variety of interactions among drugs, foods, liquids, or substances (e.g., nicotine). Maintaining a holistic view of your clients and their medications will alert you to drug–drug interactions as well as the dynamism of drug metabolism.

As drug combinations and innovative psychobiologic therapies become more commonplace in the practice of psychiatry, psychiatric–mental health nurses maintain vigilance for idiosyncratic responses among clients. Knowing the interactive effects of medications is an important feature of effective psychopharmacologic nursing. Planning and implementing care for this specialized client subpopulation are likely to be challenging, and your awareness of the underlying psychobiology allows early recognition of potential drug-related behaviors among clients who are on multiple-drug regimens (see Chapter 7∞).

Polypharmacy (using more than one medication to treat a set of symptoms) with second-generation antipsychotics (SGAs) is quite frequent among chronic clients who have severe and persistent mental illness. The practice of adding another medication as an adjunct to address persistent symptoms has become more frequent lately. When one SGA, such as risperidone, is used to treat psychotic symptoms, the client may still experience sleep difficulties. Adding another SGA such as quetiapine (Seroquel) at bedtime could further address the psychosis while providing sedation sufficient to allow quality sleep. Some research does not support the use of polypharmacy, but shortcomings have been noted in outcomes of clinical care where consistent avoidance of adjunctive pharmaceutical care is practiced (Barnes & Paton, 2011; Phillips, 2011).

ADHERENCE ISSUES

The current estimate of treatment adherence by recipients of psychiatric services, including adherence to prescribed medication regi mens, is that less than 28% take the medication that they should (Liu, Tepper, & Able, 2011). Responding to this treatment reality—almost three quarters do not adhere to their medication regimen—involves examining the reasons for nonadherence and generating creative nursing solutions to the problem. Your Assessment Approach lists possible factors that contribute to medication nonadherence.

Case Study: Medication Adherence

TABLE 31-4 ■ Overview of the Compatibility of Medications and Typical Liquids

	Chlor-promazine	Fluphen-azine	Haloperi-dol	Loxapine	Mesorida-zine	Thiorida-zine	Thiothix-ene	Trifluo-perazine	Lithium citrate
Liquid									
7-Up/Sprite	C	C		C		C		C	C
Apple juice/cider	X	X	C			X	X	X	X
Apricot juice	C	C				U	C	C	C
Coffee	U	X	X	C		X	X	U	C
Cola	U	X	C	C		X	X	C	C
Cranberry juice	X			C	C	C	C		C
Ginger ale		C				C			
Grapefruit juice	C	C	X	C	C	C	C	C	C
Grape juice	X		X		C	X		X	C
Lemonade						C			C
Mellow-Yellow		X				C		C	C
Milk	C	C	X			X	C	C	C
Orange juice	C	C	C	C	C	C	C	C	C
Orange soda	C	C				X		C	C
Pineapple juice		C		C		X	C	C	C
Prune juice	U	C				X	C	C	C
Saline	C	C	X			C		C	C
Soups/pudding	C	C	C				C	C	C
Tang	X			C					C
Tea	U	X	X			X	X	C	C
Tomato juice	C	C	C			X	C	C	C
V-8	C	C				X	X	C	C
Water	C	C	C		C	C	C	C	C
Medication									
Chlorpromazine						X			X
Haloperidol									X
Lithium citrate	X	C	U	C	C	X	C	X	
Thioridazine	X	X	X	X	X		X		X
Trifluoperazine									X

C = compatible; X = incompatible; U = unconfirmed, conflicting data; blank = no data available.

Source: Department of Pharmacy, Buffalo Psychiatric Center, Buffalo, NY, 2011.

YOUR ASSESSMENT APPROACH
Factors That Contribute to Medication Nonadherence

- Experiencing problems with prescribed psychotropic medications
- Severe level of symptomatology
- Cognitive impairments
- Negative effect of the medication on the client's adjustment
- Decreased motivation to collaborate in treatment
- Effect of the medication on the client's interpersonal relationships
- Paternalistic attitudes toward clients that interfere with partnering with clients in medication-based treatment planning decisions
- Substance use or abuse
- Lack of support from significant others
- Cultural attitudes and beliefs
- Insufficient or inadequate care planning

Many people who take prescribed psychotropic medications find it difficult to continue taking them over the long term. There are many factors that contribute to nonadherence to a medication regimen. Sometimes these medications can have uncomfortable or awkward side effects. Side effects are a major cause of nonadherence. Sometimes clients do not have a proper orientation about what to expect from these medications. The schedule of doses or the route of medication administration may be inconvenient or stressful for the client. Furthermore, the client's friends or relatives may not be entirely supportive of the client's continued adherence to the psychotropic regimen.

Because all these factors can impair medication adherence, it is important that treatment includes interventions designed to help overcome any or all of these difficulties to the extent possible. Make efforts to enhance adherence a standard feature of your psychiatric–mental health nursing care. Your Intervention Strategies suggests a number of avenues to explore when partnering with clients in this aspect of care.

YOUR INTERVENTION STRATEGIES   Adherence Enhancers

The following are ideas you can use to make it easier for clients to maintain their prescribed medication regimen:

- Discuss their health behaviors and perceptions with clients and their families.
- Use atypical antipsychotic medications—they have a lower side effect profile and can increase adherence because they are easier on the body.
- Try another medication with a different neurotransmitter action that may have a different or more tolerable side effect.
- Employ role-playing and assertiveness in practice sessions with clients that teach them how to report the range and severity of side effects, from dry mouth to priapism.
- Teach clients how to manage the side effects (and therefore continue taking the medication) by making side effects more tolerable (e.g., hard candy for dry mouth, rubber pillowcase liner for nighttime drooling [sialorrhea]).
- Arrange for reminders well before discharge from inpatient settings, especially with geriatric clients, to maximize both knowledge and adherence (knowledge can be the number-1 factor that determines whether a client adheres to his or her medication regimen).
- Simplify the medication regimen.
- Discuss with clients their expectations of the medication to determine whether those expectations are realistic.
- Use concrete educators that are known to enhance cognition—pamphlets, booklets, handbooks, workbooks, sheets, cards, videos, audiotapes, posters, magnets, logs, journals, computers, MP3 players, etc.
- Enhance the client's control over the treatment regimen by offering real choices.
- Teach the client how to self-administer medications as soon as possible in the inpatient setting.

- Involve the client in planning for problem solving as well as learning how to problem solve.
- Provide support from peers who will share how this medication could help with symptoms.
- Give depot medications weekly, biweekly, or monthly so that the client does not have to remember to take pills.
- Repeat relevant information on a number of occasions with patience, especially with clients who have schizophrenia and depression.
- Develop reminders to serve as cues to remembering. Wearing a rubber band on the wrist is a visual cue reminding the client "When I see this I need to take my pills" or "When I eat lunch I need to take my pills." Calendars, to-do lists, and alarm clocks or alarms on wristwatches or cell phones can also be helpful.
- Recommend the use of pillboxes, which come in many shapes, sizes, and organizational styles (marked for multiple daily doses, layers for time of day, timers with small alarm clock feature that opens compartment). If the medication cannot be taken out of its original container without affecting potency, placing a small button or candy in the pillbox will serve as a reminder.
- Keep all medications and information about them in one dry, cool place, not in the bathroom or by the sink or dishwasher in the kitchen.
- Refer the client to social services, where it can be determined whether financial assistance might be available.
- Arrange for the client to teach others (other clients or significant others) about their medications once they have learned sufficiently. Nothing speeds learning as much as teaching others.
- Encourage the client to be hopeful about his or her ability to manage symptoms.

These interventions can include supportive individual contacts with clients, family meetings, psychoeducation regarding specific medications and their effects, and communicating a basic interest in how the client is reacting to his or her course of medications. The goal in creating a collaborative environment of care is to incorporate better client-specific interventions than those contributing to nonadherence. Enlisting the cooperation and involvement of families in implementing interventions as appropriate also helps to promote adherence.

Pearson Nursing Student Resources

Find additional review materials at
nursing.pearsonhighered.com

Prepare for success with NCLEX®-style practice questions, interactive assignments and activities, web links, animations and videos, and more!

REFERENCES

Barnes, T. R. E., & Paton, C. (2011). Antipsychotic polypharmacy in schizophrenia: Benefits and risks. *CNS Drugs, 25*(5), 383–399.

Bhidayasiri, R., & Boonyawairoj, S. (2011). Spectrum of tardive syndromes: Clinical recognition and management. *Postgraduate Medical Journal, 87,* 132–141.

Bliss, D. Z., Savik, K., Jung, H.-J. G., Whitebird, R., & Lowry, A. (2011). Symptoms associated with dietary fiber supplementation over time in individuals with fecal incontinence. *Nursing Research, 60*(3S), S58–S67.

Connolly, K. R., & Thase, M. E. (2011). If at first you don't succeed: A review of the evidence for antidepressant augmentation, combination and switching strategies. *Drugs, 71*(1), 43–64.

Dabiesingh, D. S., Psevdos, G., & Sharp, V. L. (2011). Atazanavir-associated QT prolongation and torsades se points in a patient with liver cirrhosis: A rare but serious complication. *Infectious Disease in Clnical Practice, 19,* 226–228.

Fagiolino, P., Vázquez, M., Eiraldi, R., Maldonado, C., & Scaramelli, A. (2011). Influence of efflux transporters on drug metabolism: Theoretical approach for bioavailability and clearance prediction. *Clinical Pharmacokinetics, 50*(2), 75–80.

Fontaine, K. L. (2011). *Complementary and alternative therapies for nursing practice* (3rd ed.). Upper Saddle River, NJ: Pearson Education.

Fontenelle, L. F., Oostermeijer, S., Harrison, B. J., Pantelis, C., & Yücel, M. (2011). Obsessive–compulsive disorder, impulse control disorders and drug addiction: Common features and potential treatments. *Drugs, 71*(7), 827–840.

Galon, P. A., & Wineman, M. N. (2010). Coercion and procedural justice in psychiatric care: State of the science and implications for nursing. *Archives of Psychiatric Nursing, 24*(5), 307–316.

Gibbons, R. D., & Mann, J. J. (2011). Strategies for quantifying the relationship between medications and suicidal behavior: What has been learned? *Drug Safety, 34*(5), 375–395.

Hough, D. W., Natarajan, J., Vandebosch, A., Rossenu, S., Kraner, M., & Eerdekens, M. (2011). Evaluation of the effect of paliperidone extended release and quetiapine on corrected QT intervals: A randomized, double-blind, placebo-controlled study. *International Clinical Psychopharmacology, 26,* 25–34.

Im, E.-O. (2011). A situation-specific theory of Asian immigrant women's menopausal symptom experience in the United States. *Advances in Nursing Science, 33*(2), 143–157.

Kaiser, S. (2011). The importance of consultation in the treatment of chemical dependency. *Clinical Nurse Specialist,* May–June, 113–117.

Kiefer, D., Pitluk, J., & Klunk, K. (2009). An overview of CAM: Components and clinical uses. *Nutrition in Clinical Practice, 24*(5), 549–559.

Koreki, A., Tsunoda, K., Suzuki, T., Hirano, J., Watanabe, K., Kashima, H., & Uchida, H. (2011). Clinical and demographic characteristics associated with postural instability in patients with schizophrenia. *Journal of Clinical Psychopharmacology, 31,* 16–21.

Liu, X., Tepper, P. G., & Able, S. L. (2011). Adherence and persistence with duloxetine and hospital utilization in patients with major depressive disorder. *International Clinical Psychopharmacology, 26,* 173–180.

Masi, G., & Liboni, F. (2011). Management of schizophrenia in children and adolescents: Focus on pharmacotherapy. *Drugs, 71*(2), 179–208.

Nguyen, N. T. T., & Vierling, J. M. (2011). Acute liver failure. *Current Opinion in Organ Transplantation, 16,* 289–296.

Pae, C.-U., Forbes, A., & Patkar, A. A. (2011). Aripiprazole as adjunctive therapy for patients with major depressive disorder: Overview and implications of clinical trial data. *CNS Drugs, 25*(2), 109–127.

Phillips, R. M. (2011). The challenge of medication management in older adults. *Nursing Made Incredibly Easy!,* Jan/Feb, 24–31.

Seitz, D. P., & Gill, S. S. (2009). Neuroleptic malignant syndrome complicating antipsychotic treatment of delirium or agitation in medical and surgical patients: Case reports and a review of the literature. *Psychosomatics, 50*(1), 8–15.

Sulosaari, V., Suhonen, R., & Leino-Kilpi, H. (2011). An integrative review of the literature on registered nurses' medication competence. *Journal of Clinical Nursing, 20*(3–4), 464–478.

Thompson, J. W., & Johnson, A. C. (2011). Acute lithium intoxication: Properly directing an index of suspicion. *Southern Medical Journal, 104*(5), 371–372.

Veselinović, T., Schorn, H., Vernaleken, I. B., Schiffl, K., Klomp, M., & Gründer, G. (2011). Impact of different antidopinergic mechanisms on the dopaminergic control of prolactin secretion. *Journal of Clinical Psychopharmacology, 31,* 214–220.

Vigneault, P., Kaddar, N., Bourgault, S., Caillier, B., Pilote, S., Patoine, D., . . . Drolet, B. (2011). Prolongation of cardiac ventricular repolarization under paliperidone: How and how much? *Journal of Cardiovascular Pharmacology, 57,* 690–695.

Recovery and Psychiatric Rehabilitation Strategies

EILEEN TRIGOBOFF

LEARNING OUTCOMES

After completing this chapter, you will be able to:

1. Explain the central concepts of recovery and psychiatric rehabilitation to clients and their families.
2. Determine the adaptations in programming necessary to meet the needs of people with severe and persistent mental illness.
3. Design nursing care plans with recovery and rehabilitation goals for people with serious mental illness.
4. Analyze the effectiveness of a plan to promote recovery.
5. Modify a nursing care plan to promote and enhance rehabilitation.
6. Describe how your personal characteristics might influence your effectiveness in working with clients toward the goal of recovery.

CRITICAL THINKING CHALLENGE

Manny lives in a supervised residence for people who have major mental illnesses. His diagnosis, schizoaffective disorder with bipolar symptoms, means he has symptoms of schizophrenia as well as having mood instability. Although he takes his antipsychotic medication regularly (it is a long-acting injection administered by you on a monthly schedule), he self-administers his mood stabilizer medication. Lately Manny's mood has been unstable (manic symptoms) and he has become more delusional than usual (he believes he is married to a woman who lived down the street from him 40 years ago). He insists he is taking his oral medications. You discussed his treatment responses with other members of the treatment team during his recent clinic visit for his injection. During that appointment, Manny expressed "great joy" at now being perfect all because of you.

The team believes that Manny is either not consistently taking his oral mood stabilizers, that he has become unstable from the stress of a family friend's recent death, or both situations may be contributing to the exacerbation (worsening) of his symptoms. It has been suggested that Manny be rehospitalized.

1. How does readmission to a psychiatric hospital help a client's ultimate recovery?
2. What should Manny know about his treatment options at this point?
3. What behaviors are you likely to see if Manny's treatment plan is not altered?

For clients with mental health issues, rehabilitation and **recovery** means reaching a level of functioning which the client can maintain and with which the client is comfortable. Every environment—whether it is an inpatient setting, transitional housing, a community setting, the family home, or independent living—has the potential to further enhance a client's recovery. There are many methods that psychiatric–mental health nurses can use to promote the client's goals of rehabilitation and recovery. This chapter will focus on what it means to recover from mental illness and the proven strategies you can use to help clients achieve recovery.

Nurses accept the challenges of questioning, documenting, measuring, and determining—with evidence—the outcomes of their interventions, that is, the degree to which they succeed and fail. This pattern of determining effective strategies can be applied to helping a psychiatric–mental health client reach the goal of recovery. Your expertise in assessing and evaluating—learning what works best for a given set of circumstances—can be essential to an individual client's recovery.

READINESS FOR RECOVERY

Psychiatric–mental health clients working toward recovery may have discovered many ways to function effectively. However, the individual client needs to evaluate on an ongoing basis the usefulness of a particular coping strategy or interaction style, and develop an array of responses to problems. FIGURE 32-1 ■ illustrates the steps to take to learn about what works and what needs to be changed so clients can progress toward recovery.

Relapse is a return of significant symptoms that are problematic for the client in a number of areas of functioning. There are degrees of relapse from mild to total and severe, although frequently a severe level of relapse can be avoided if early symptoms are detected and addressed. This is discussed later in this chapter. Identifying stressors and triggers for relapse, developing coping skills, and recognizing each victory helps to make interactions effective and life meaningful. Examples follow of rehabilitation goals for clients range from basic functioning to quality-of-life issues.

- Washing their own clothes
- Shopping for their own food
- Maintaining healthy and appropriate nutrition
- Remaining active in the community—regardless of their living setting
- Seeking sufficient intellectual stimulation
- Enhancing their quality of life
- Continuing a relationship with mental health care providers
- Collaborating with caregivers to monitor psychotropic medications
- Participating in a plan to reduce or eliminate—when clinically safe to do so—psychotropic medications
- Expressing feelings assertively
- Coping with increases in symptoms and personal crises.

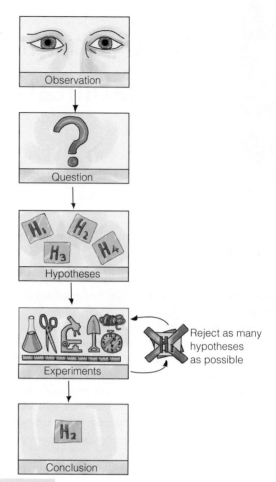

FIGURE 32-1 ■ Developing recovery skills that work for the individual client.

Clients are more likely to be able to strive for and achieve these goals when they acknowledge their own strengths and needs. As a nurse facilitating recovery you are involved in every aspect of a client's psychological growth and development (O'Baire-Kark & Kevay, 2011). The likelihood that a client will have symptom reduction to the point of recovery seems to be affected by the client's coping style (Staring, van der Gaag, & Mulder, 2011). In this 2011 study by Staring and associates, clients who integrated important features such as who they are, what their needs are, and what seems to help keep them stable and healthy, had significantly better odds for recovery. This study was conducted with people who have schizophrenia and was remarkable in that having insight and a therapeutic alliance did not contribute meaningfully to recovery. Recovery and remission seem to be more associated with putting the pieces together in a way that works for the individual, rather than insisting on a particular path or understanding how and why a problem exists (LeBel, 2011).

Once clients express a need for greater autonomy, planning for recovery can begin. All involved parties must be flexible to the changing circumstances of stress and illness, triggers and relapse, and barriers to overcoming them. Recovery is an individualized state defined by each client. It cannot be imposed from without; recovery must be achieved from within.

Prochaska Transtheoretical Model for Change

Clients continue to synthesize their experiences into a set of practices that is individually designed. The more experience a client has with his or her illness, the more information can be incorporated into a recovery plan. Someone who has been recently diagnosed might benefit from being in a group setting with healthier and more experienced clients. This experience encourages a sense of hope for the future and provides the client with an opportunity to see how others cope successfully. Over time, the client observes, refocuses, and readjusts to what works for him or her. Adjusting is part of the process of change. This section presents one model that can be used to guide clients through the process of change.

The Transtheoretical Model (TTM) of change formulated by Prochaska (Prochaska & DiClemente, 1986) suggests five stages of change through which people progress when behavioral change is desired. These stages are: precontemplation, contemplation, preparation, action, and maintenance. As the words imply, successful change involves thought and action before, during, and after change. The theoretical concept was examined within an addictions framework; however, more general applications are useful.

The five stages of TTM change are summarized in FIGURE 32-2 ■. The stages, processes, and principles that undergird the theory are described in TABLE 32-1 ■. While people tend to progress toward change, slipping back into familiar patterns

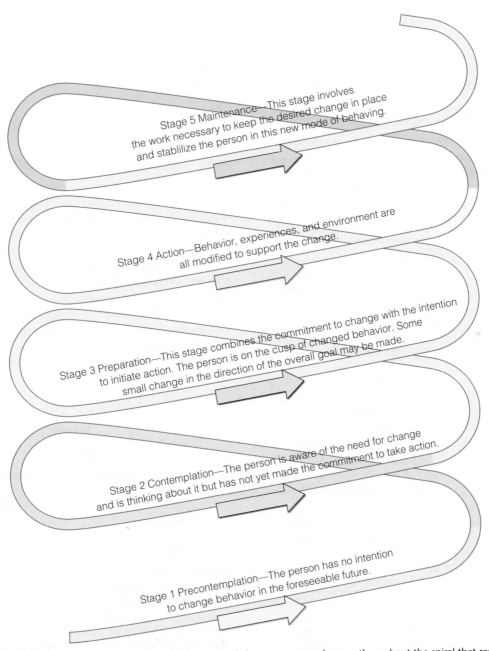

FIGURE 32-2 ■ Five stages of TTM. Movement through the stages of change waxes and wanes throughout the spiral that represents the progression of human behavior.

of previous behaviors is expected, especially during times of stress. When health-related behaviors are involved, this slipping back is called *relapse*. You may see clients who become frustrated, annoyed, and even demoralized at the amount of effort required for change, reverting to old, maladaptive behavior or thinking at various points in the change process.

Clinical Example

Michael is someone who has paranoid schizophrenia with frightening delusions. He was stabilized for several months. Michael became uncomfortable when he thought his neighbors were deliberately shining their headlights into his living room window in order to bother him. His symptoms steadily worsened and he stated at his clinic appointment, "Why do I have to revisit this hell? I was there already and got out. Now I'm back in hell again."

The transtheoretical model can help clients understand how to achieve healthier behaviors throughout their recovery period.

Those who have psychiatric illnesses in combination with substance abuse pose a particularly difficult clinical problem when it comes to making healthy change. Treatment programs and therapeutic approaches for this group are most effective when conceptualized along the lines of an organized change model such as TTM. This model has been applied successfully in the treatment of substance abuse as well as to co-occurring disorders such as substance abuse combined with mental illness (Finnell, 2009). A stage-based conceptual treatment approach such as this one highlights client responsibility and autonomy in decision-making and treatment outcomes.

Realistic and Attainable Expectations of Change

What kind of supports do clients need to begin the process of changing to recovery-focused behaviors? Expectations of change must be realistic and attainable, keeping in mind they may need to be flexible depending on crises and depleted resources (emotional and financial). The 10 main components of mental health recovery have been determined by an expert panel on mental health (see Box 32-1). Change is not immediate, instantaneous, or initially permanent. Every person trying to make a change in behavior must go through transitional stages before, during, and after the change is made. Use the TTM stages in your work with clients and ensure the resources necessary to achieve each one.

PSYCHIATRIC DISABILITY

The core feature of a severe and persistent disorder is not diagnosis or prognosis, but the experience of *psychiatric disability*. In 1980, the World Health Organization (WHO) developed and published a classification system (FIGURE 32-3 ■) for the phases of a long-term illness that also relates to mental illness or psychiatric disorders. Whether mild or severe, whether ongoing, recurring, or remitting, these disorders require services that go beyond the limits of an acute disease model. Severely and persistently mentally ill individuals have psychiatric disorders that disrupt major role functioning over time, involving some level of disability. FIGURE 32-4 ■ on page 702 shows the prevalence of serious mental illness in the United States.

TABLE 32-1 ■ The Transtheoretical Model (TTM) of Behavior Change

TTM explains the stages and processes of change. Knowing how change occurs throughout the stages, how decisional balance impacts the process of change, what an individual's vision of self-efficacy consists of, and how temptation is likely to be handled, make this perspective a useful one for promoting change.

Stage	Processes and Principles
1. Precontemplation	The client does not intend to change the health behavior in the near future, usually a 6-month period of time. The client avoids communication designed to help change occur.
2. Contemplation	The client does intend to change the health behavior in the next 6 months. There is awareness of the benefits of change, but the barriers to change are being attended to and ambivalence is potent.
3. Preparation	The client intends to make the change in the next month. A plan of action is developed with small, important steps taken toward change.
4. Action	The client overtly modifies risky behavior and makes the change. Considerable time and energy are necessary in order to resist reverting to previous risky behaviors.
5. Maintenance	The client works to prevent relapse. Temptation gradually recedes over 6 months to 5 years. This stage is meant to extend through the client's life.

FIGURE 32-3 ■ The WHO parallel sequence for long-term illness. The etiology of the disorder, known or unknown, gives rise to changes in structure or functioning, manifested as signs and symptoms and collectively known as *impairment*. If the impairment alters functional performance or behavior, it produces *disability*. When the impairment or disability places the person at a disadvantage within the community, a *handicap* occurs.

Box 32-1 National Consensus Statement on Mental Health Recovery: The 10 Fundamental Components of Recovery

The following are the fundamental components for recovery from a mental health problem:

- **Self-Direction.** Consumers lead, control, exercise choice over, and determine their own path of recovery by optimizing autonomy, independence, and control of resources to achieve a self-determined life. By definition, the recovery process must be self-directed by the individual, who defines his or her own life goals and designs a unique path toward those goals.
- **Individualized and Person Centered.** There are multiple pathways to recovery based on an individual's unique strengths and resiliencies as well as his or her needs, preferences, experiences (including past trauma), and cultural background in all of its diverse representations. Individuals also identify recovery as being an ongoing journey and an end result as well as an overall paradigm for achieving wellness and optimal mental health.
- **Empowerment.** Consumers have the authority to choose from a range of options and to participate in all decisions—including the allocation of resources—that will affect their lives, and are educated and supported in so doing. They have the ability to join with other consumers to collectively and effectively speak for themselves about their needs, wants, desires, and aspirations. Through empowerment, an individual gains control of his or her own destiny and influences the organizational and societal structures in his or her life.
- **Holistic.** Recovery encompasses an individual's whole life, including mind, body, spirit, and community. Recovery embraces all aspects of life, including housing, employment, education, mental health and healthcare treatment and services, complementary and naturalistic services, addictions treatment, spirituality, creativity, social networks, community participation, and family supports as determined by the person. Families, providers, organizations, systems, communities, and society play crucial roles in creating and maintaining meaningful opportunities for consumer access to these supports.
- **Nonlinear.** Recovery is not a step-by-step process; it is based on continual growth, occasional setbacks, and learning from experience. Recovery begins with an initial stage of awareness

in which a person recognizes that positive change is possible. This awareness enables the consumer to move on to fully engage in the work of recovery.

- **Strengths Based.** Recovery focuses on valuing and building on the multiple capacities, resiliencies, talents, coping abilities, and inherent worth of individuals. By building on these strengths, consumers leave stymied life roles behind and engage in new life roles (e.g., partner, caregiver, friend, student, employee). The process of recovery moves forward through interaction with others in supportive, trust-based relationships.
- **Peer Support.** Mutual support—including the sharing of experiential knowledge and skills and social learning—plays an invaluable role in recovery. Consumers encourage and engage other consumers in recovery and provide each other with a sense of belonging, supportive relationships, valued roles, and community.
- **Respect.** Community, systems, and societal acceptance and appreciation of consumers—including protecting their rights and eliminating discrimination and stigma—are crucial in achieving recovery. Self-acceptance and regaining belief in one's self are particularly vital. Respect ensures the inclusion and full participation of consumers in all aspects of their lives.
- **Responsibility.** Consumers have a personal responsibility for their own self-care and journeys of recovery. Taking steps toward their goals may require great courage. Consumers must strive to understand and give meaning to their experiences and identify coping strategies and healing processes to promote their own wellness.
- **Hope.** Recovery provides the essential and motivating message of a better future—that people can and do overcome the barriers and obstacles that confront them. Hope is internalized; but can be fostered by peers, families, friends, providers, and others. Hope is the catalyst of the recovery process.

Adapted from: The National Consensus Statement on Mental Health Recovery, U.S. Department of Health and Human Services, Substance Abuse and Mental Health Services Administration (SAMHSA), Center for Mental Health Services. National Mental Health Information Center: 1-800-789-2647, 1-866-889-2647 (TDD), http://www.samhsa.gov

---

People Who Are Seriously and Persistently Mentally Ill (SPMI)

The term **seriously and persistently mentally ill (SPMI)**, or serious mental illness (SMI), came into use because it acknowledges the extent and durability of the problem and avoids some of the more undesirable features of its predecessor term used to describe clients, the *chronically mentally ill*. There is no common course for SPMI. This is a clinically diverse population, with different diagnoses and varied patterns of illness, that needs access to caregivers who can provide a variety of strategies designed to enhance recovery.

Schizophrenia and similar disorders provide the prototype for SPMI; they are typically disabling on an intermittent or ongoing basis (see Chapter 16 ∞). However, even disorders on the schizophrenia spectrum vary considerably in

terms of symptom profile, pattern of relapse or acute exacerbations, and quality of long-term functioning. Bipolar disorders, recurrent depressions, and severe personality disorders can be just as disabling as some forms of schizophrenia.

The profile that emerges of people with SPMI is that of a highly vulnerable subgroup in our mental health care system, one of the groups least likely to access social resources to protect that vulnerability. This subgroup of our population accounts for the majority of persons being treated in hospital-based systems and in many community programs. They are at risk for developing secondary or concurrent psychiatric problems and for problems associated with socioeconomic status. They account for a significant percentage of homeless persons in our communities. These multiple, interacting problems require complex approaches to services.

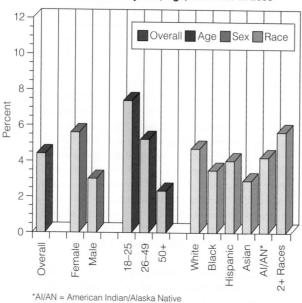

Prevalence of Serious Mental Illness Among U.S. Adults by Sex, Age, and Race in 2008

*AI/AN = American Indian/Alaska Native

FIGURE 32-4 ■ Prevalence of serious mental illness. Note the differences in each category of gender, age, and race.
Source: National Institute of Mental Health. Retrieved from http://www.nimh.nih.gov/statistics/SMI_AASR.shtml

Clinical Example

Xaviera is a 33-year-old woman with long standing mental health problems. Years of irregular adherence to treatment and intermittent episodes of substantial substance abuse have resulted in unacceptable behaviors. The unacceptable behaviors caused Xaviera to be evicted from her apartment. She is now homeless.

Yellen stopped taking his medication for bipolar disorder after he became homeless. Months later his symptom level began to interfere with every aspect of his functioning. Yellen began critiquing the outfits of people he passed on the street and then demanding consultation fees from them.

When Zephraim is able to collect enough money from passersby in center city where he panhandles, he abuses marijuana when he feels lonely or sad. After smoking marijuana he told the nurse at the clinic when he was receiving a depot injection of an antipsychotic medication, "I have the buffering of the best with the softness . . . of the world I want and deserve. Not the world. . . . you know, you . . . they . . . they've got nothing."

Natural Life History of a Disorder

Many disorders, especially chronic disorders, have a natural life history. The natural history of disorder refers to the course

of disorder over time in the absence of intervention. Chronic disorder may be viewed in a sequence of stages. Risk factors favoring the development of a disorder may be present early in life, preceding the appearance of symptoms by many years. We do not have a complete understanding of the natural history of many psychiatric disorders. Every disorder has its own life history, but in general, disorders have these four basic stages: susceptibility, presymptomatic disorder, clinical disorder, and disability. Their relationship to one other is illustrated in FIGURE 32-5 ■ .

Stage of Susceptibility

During this stage, the groundwork has been laid by the presence of risk factors that favor the occurrence of disorder. The individual is susceptible to the disorder, but the disorder has not yet developed. Identifying those at high risk for developing a disorder is a major mental health care challenge. For example, certain risk factors such as those in the clinical example, set the stage and place a client at increased risk for depression.

Clinical Example

Becky has three children under the age of 6, one of whom is autistic. Her husband felt that he could not cope with the chaos at home and left the family. Becky has not been employed since the first child was born and has few family of origin supports—her siblings live out of town, her father has COPD, and her mother died when Becky was 8 years old.

Stage of Presymptomatic Disorder

During this stage, there is no apparent disorder, but pathologic changes have started to occur. The disorder has begun but remains unrecognized because it may be asymptomatic. If signs of the disorder are present, they may be considered the ordinary discomforts of daily living. Mild depression serves as an example of this presymptomatic stage.

Stage of Clinical Disorder

This stage is characterized by recognizable signs and symptoms of disorder. For some disorders, people regularly come under nursing or medical care at some point over the course of an illness. These disorders are "high profile" because they cause such symptoms as peculiar behavior, failure to thrive, severe or chronic distress, or pain. Classification may be based on laboratory findings or on functional or therapeutic considerations. Cancer is usually classified by the location, extent, and type of tumor. The

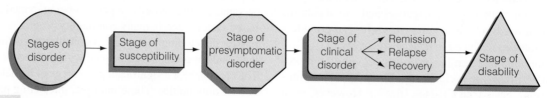

FIGURE 32-5 ■ Stages in the natural history of a disorder.

most current source of classification of psychiatric disorders is the American Psychiatric Association's *Diagnostic and Statistical Manual of Mental Disorders* (American Psychiatric Association, 2000). DSM criteria for psychiatric disorders rely on a descriptive diagnostic classification scheme. It is important to note that "clinical disorder" describes a disorder that has come under nursing or medical care and is then treated in a variety of ways that may alter the subsequent course of events. The disorders according to DSM criteria are thoroughly described in the chapters in Unit 4∞.

Stage of Disability

Some disorders run their course and resolve completely, either spontaneously or in response to therapy. However, some disorders leave residual impairment or disability of short or long duration. While there is a substantial amount of disability associated with acute disorders, the extended disability resulting from chronic disorders is of greater significance to society. The term SPMI is a descriptor of a stage of disability.

Community Support Programs for SPMI

Community support programs offer a range of treatment and rehabilitation services, with a case management component to assess needs, coordinate care, monitor outcomes, and assist the client to achieve recovery.

Case Management

Case management is the linchpin for community support programs. The case manager remains a consistent figure in the treatment plan. This avoids duplication and overlap of services. It also avoids shunting vulnerable clients between services because of fluctuations in their clinical status.

Case managers often find that they are fulfilling many roles for their clients that have not been satisfied by other clinical resources, including a sense of social support. High-risk groups such as clients with dual diagnoses, those who are homeless as well as mentally ill, and frequently hospitalized clients may receive more intensive and clinically sophisticated forms of case management to address their unique service requirements. The case management philosophy has generated enthusiasm in systems for psychiatric–mental health clients because it acknowledges the pervasive nature of their difficulties, their need for multiple services, the oscillating or unpredictable course of illness, and the ultimate triumph of clients managing their illness.

Support for Basic Needs

Community mental health programs generally emphasize the importance of self-support and gainful employment whenever possible. However, surveys of people who are severely mentally ill indicate generally low rates of competitive employment. Clinical example that follows gives two examples of situations in which employers are reluctant to hire.

Clinical Example

Rick has applied for a position as an architect. The employer does not want to hire Rick because he has been in the hospital for psychiatric problems. She is especially concerned that Rick would be distressed by the details of the engineering requirements for the skyscrapers that the firm designs and would be unable to draw up blueprints within the required time frame.

Emily applied for a job as a housekeeper in a condominium complex in a resort area. The building manager believes that because Emily has a history of mental illness she would have difficulty appropriately managing the complaints of irate vacationers and has denied her the position.

This situation reflects general economic conditions as well as work disability. In times of high unemployment, people with psychiatric disabilities may be pushed out of jobs that can be performed by competing groups in the labor force.

Certainly, many mentally ill individuals without "gainful" employment are meaningfully occupied in supported employment and/or volunteer work. However, low rates of competitive employment among members of this population underscore their dependence on income assistance programs such as Supplemental Security Income (SSI).

A community support system helps ensure the people who are severely mentally ill have both access to, and linkage with, appropriate services to secure income and obtain other entitlements (such as health benefits) and basic resources such as food, clothing, and transportation. This may be a more complex task than it appears because accessing financial resources may mean helping the client through difficult application procedures and even appeals. It may also involve providing money management services to help severely mentally ill individuals who cannot budget their monthly income independently.

Residential Services

Recent reports continue to document the lack of affordable and decent housing options for many who are severely mentally ill and their consequent concentration in what may be marginal or unsafe areas. Many people who are severely and persistently mentally ill live with families, but those who live alone frequently depend on residential hotels and boarding homes. It is difficult to generalize about the quality of these housing options because they vary a great deal. For example, some boarding arrangements encourage autonomy and provide a warm, stable environment for residents. Other arrangements, however, fall far below standards that should be applied to living environments for the chronically disabled, such as in the clinical example.

Clinical Example

Louis moved from one apartment to another in a different neighborhood. During his clinic appointment, he told the nurse that the new apartment had a bug problem. There were huge amounts of centipedes, spiders, and moths in every room. The building superintendent told Louis to "just handle it."

The question of housing satisfaction can also be highly subjective. Some people prefer the privacy of a hotel, despite what may be other negative features, such as location or limited living space. Other people prefer a more cozy, homelike environment. Programs with an active treatment component may be attractive to some people, but others appreciate a fairly calm and nondemanding environment despite its monotony. For this reason, a community support system focuses not only on accessing some form of acceptable housing but on evaluating the quality of that housing for the individual, working with the client to find "a good fit."

Medication Management

Medication regimens are the mainstay of treatment programs for the severely and persistently mentally ill. Research on the

WHY I PLAN TO BECOME A PSYCHIATRIC–MENTAL HEALTH NURSE

Madison's Story: I was 17 years old when I began working as a nurse's aide in a small long-term care facility. I was just starting college to become a nurse and wanted experience working in the field. There were not very many people being cared for in the facility because it was a private enterprise with the theme of making it as homelike as possible. I became close to all of the residents while learning to take care of them.

One woman, Louise, was extra special. She was only 50 years old but had such debilitating and deforming arthritis that she could not care for herself and was no longer able to work as a psychiatric-mental health nurse. She was bright and personable, and I admired her strength of character in dealing with a chronic illness. Her ability to see not just the content of a situation, but see the process of what was going on around her was so beyond what I could do that it seemed like magic to me. An interaction between her roommate and her roommate's granddaughter was an excellent example.

Louise's roommate, Ida, was a bitter and negative woman who rarely said anything neutral about her world or the people in it. A positive statement from Ida was unheard of. Ida's granddaughter came in to visit her grandmother and she was so excited to show off her boyfriend's gift—a pretty pearl ring in a gold band. Ida's only comment was, "Pearls mean sorrow." Ida's granddaughter was devastated and left in tears. Ida's response to her roommate was, "See, pearls do mean sorrow." Louise then reassured Ida that even though her granddaughter was becoming close to her boyfriend, no one could take Ida's place. Ida, Louise told her, would always be Grandmother and nothing could change that.

When I asked Louise later, in private, what was the connection between Ida being mean-spirited and Louise reassuring Ida, Louise's comment opened my eyes to the value of psychological sophistication. Louise said, "When people feel threatened about being hurt by someone, they will put the energy into hurting that person first. Ida wasn't being mean, she was being hurt." Being able to help someone cope with feelings with what I now know are psychiatric–mental health nursing interactions helped me choose the area for my nursing career.

efficacy of medication, particularly neuroleptic regimens for schizophrenia, demonstrates that these agents reduce rates of relapse and hospital readmission. However, they have not been problem free. Medication regimens demand adherence, tolerance of temporary side effects, and acceptance of the risk of long-term problems such as tardive dyskinesia. Secondary effects of medications can be uncomfortable and embarrassingly visible (e.g., tongue thrusting).

Medication services for the severely and persistently mentally ill should address the impact of medications on quality of life and should promote collaboration with clients to develop a regimen that is tolerable and beneficial. *Depot medication therapy,* usually consisting of an injection every 2 to 4 weeks, does not require the client to take medications several times a day and is a valuable strategy for some people. Current advances in psychopharmacology have produced new classes of medications that may prove less uncomfortable and socially limiting than standard treatments and may help people who have been resistant to medication, or nonadherent, in the past. The introduction of newer therapies makes the medication component of community care all the more important.

Clinical Example

Ms. Linnea is a 57-year-old widow who came into the medication clinic for her monthly injection, accompanied by her case manager. Ms. Linnea has had a diagnosis of schizophrenia, paranoid type, for many years but was maintained well with outpatient care and medications, requiring only brief crisis intervention and two short hospital stays by the time she was 50.

After her husband died, Ms. Linnea had a severe decompensation, experiencing frightening hallucinations and delusions, and threatened her neighbors. Police were called and she was hospitalized. Ms. Linnea was stabilized on depot medications and referred to a community-support program for assistance with both housing and rehabilitation. A case manager helped Ms. Linnea apply for SSI, arranged for a shared apartment, facilitated medication and clinic appointments, visited her weekly, and encouraged regular participation in a social rehabilitation program. Ms. Linnea has not required hospitalization in 6 years. Although she still "hears voices," she is able to monitor her symptoms and advises her son or her case manager when her symptoms increase.

Outpatient Treatment

Traditional outpatient psychotherapies that address *problems in living* may not meet the needs of all severely and persistently mentally ill persons because disabled people often require a broader range of support services to function well in the community. Many severely mentally ill individuals also require rehabilitation interventions that address their specific functional deficits and treatment goals, rather than insight-oriented therapies. Nevertheless, these clients need individual, family, and group treatments that are sensitive to their particular problems and needs. Because the principles of rehabilitation for people with SPMI are followed in community treatment centers, they are an ideal option for this population. See Chapter 13 ∞ for information about community treatment centers.

Crisis Stabilization

People with SPMI are at risk for acute exacerbations of their illness. This may be particularly true during times of stress or transition. But in some cases, acute exacerbations are entirely unpredictable and are more likely to be linked with fluctuations of the disease process than with environmental stressors. In any case, this population requires access to acute assessment and treatment services as part of a package of community support including 24-hour emergency and crisis units and outreach programs. Nursing expertise is extremely important in these emergency settings because of the need for skilled and comprehensive assessment of acute problems.

In addition to the need for crisis stabilization because of acute exacerbation of psychiatric illness, people with SPMI are also frequent victims of violent crime. Up to one third of people with severe mental illness are victims of violent crime and the rate of being victimized is, in some circumstances, double that of the general population. When alcohol and drug use is involved, the rate of victimization can be 140 times the rate of victimization of the general population (Maniglio, 2009). Crisis stabilization is often required in these situations, as well.

Mental Health in the News discusses an individual who had ups and downs and subsequent homelessness as a result of substance abuse. He achieved sobriety, but relapsed when stressors affected his stability.

General Health Care

People with SPMI are a medically underserved group in the community, with needs in the areas of primary health care, dental care, and vision care. Health needs are most pronounced in subgroups such as substance-abusing clients and the elderly mentally ill, who have concurrent physical disorders. However, many people who are severely mentally ill are, to some extent, at risk from lifestyle factors (problematic housing or nutrition) or from the consequences of psychiatric treatment (problematic medication side effects or medication interactions). Any person with a serious psychiatric diagnosis risks underdiagnosis of medical illness by both primary care and psychiatric providers.

In psychiatric services, clinicians may focus on mental disorders with inadequate attention to the total person. Only a small proportion of medical problems are diagnosed in physical assessments. Individuals most likely to be underdiagnosed are those who abuse substances, are elderly, or are female. Community support and case management interventions can help those with SPMI obtain services despite "falling between the cracks" in systems that are poorly organized to meet the needs of clients with multiple diagnoses.

Vocational Programs

When people with SPMI are surveyed about their preferences, they usually indicate a strong desire to work. Work not only provides income, it also helps create a sense of self-worth and social belonging. However, psychiatric disability limits access to employment by its impact on healthy functioning and because of the stigma attached to mental disorders. Vocational services address this problem by providing training and protected alternatives to the competitive workplace.

Vocational training may occur in specialized programs, or it may be integrated into other mental health modalities such as day treatment. It provides assessment of work capacities and preferences, technical preparation, and social skills training to prepare people for the workplace. However, not all people with psychiatric disabilities enter the competitive workplace. Many, by desire or by necessity, work within protected environments. Sheltered workshop programs have a long history of offering work in a low-stress, low-demand environment. Transitional vocational programs also provide a low-stress environment but emphasize the development of skills for movement to the competitive workplace. Therapeutic processes to address time use as well as occupational balance

MENTAL HEALTH IN THE NEWS

Ted Williams, The Golden Voice

It all began with a cardboard sign held by a disheveled homeless man standing on a wintry street. On the sign, the homeless man Ted Williams wrote that he had a golden voice and would gladly accept donations. A journalist asked Ted Williams to demonstrate his voice and Mr. Williams, on the spot, recorded an accomplished radio promo. During the interview with the journalist Mr. Williams detailed how he had been a radio voice-over artist until his fortunes changed as a result of substance abuse (narcotics and alcohol), and he became homeless. The video was posted on YouTube and immediately went viral.

Mr. Williams was subsequently interviewed on a number of television programs, discussed his life and his problems, and asserted he had been clean and sober for 2 years and wanted a chance to prove himself to be a capable voice-over artist. Subsequently, he received numerous job offers. He became the voice in advertisements for a food product, did network voice-over work, and hosted a television program. Reconciliations with many long-estranged family members accompanied the extensive media coverage.

Shortly thereafter, Mr. Williams began drinking again when it became difficult for him to manage the stress of the media attention. During a television interview with a psychologist, Mr. Williams agreed to enter a rehabilitation program. He was admitted but checked himself out 12 days later. Within 3 months, Mr. Williams returned to a rehabilitation facility and his job offers were withdrawn or put on hold indefinitely.

Ted Williams, the golden voice of radio, continues to pursue a successful course of recovery from substance abuse and a sober lifestyle. Along with many other similar clients, he has encountered some difficulties and setbacks. However, his continued motivation and efforts are necessary precursors to success.

Photo courtesy of Doral Chenoweth III/MCT/Newscom.

(balancing working with other life activities and needs) are helpful to those who have the challenge of a psychiatric disorder (Edgelow & Krupa, 2011). The clinical example describes several programs.

Clinical Example

House of Grace, a faith-sponsored organization, trains and prepares recently discharged female recipients of mental health services to enter the workforce. Donations of high end business clothing from business women help the women to "dress for success" in job interviews.

A sheltered workshop, located in a renovated and trendy downtown neighborhood that has become a haven for chic boutiques and antique stores, teaches recipients of mental health services how to refinish the antique furniture that young professionals and suburbanites purchase.

A transitional vocational program teaches welding to recipients of mental health services. Job coaches accompany the recipients to the job site to help them integrate into the new job.

Supported employment is an approach that provides training and support in one's place of employment. For example, a job coach might accompany a group of psychiatrically disabled workers to a place of employment where the coach learns the same job as the team, provides on-the-job training, and provides daily backup and support. This approach is based on the principle that people with a mental illness learn skills best in the environment in which they will be practiced. Supported employment models may become increasingly prominent because the Americans with Disabilities Act (ADA) guarantees people with psychiatric disabilities the right to reasonable accommodation in the workplace. To learn how the ADA applies to people with psychiatric disabilities, use the Online Student Resources for this book to access the policy guidelines of the Equal Employment Opportunity Commission at http://www.eeoc.gov

Day Programs

Day treatment and partial hospitalization programs provide continuity of care between the hospital and the outpatient sector in a less restrictive setting. These programs can also provide an alternative to hospital care for individuals who need complex treatment monitoring.

Day treatment programs offer groups and activities that provide for recreation and socialization and that help people function in the community. They may be used on a short-term basis for specific goals or on a long-term basis for relapse prevention. Day programs are increasingly incorporating a rehabilitation philosophy that maximizes opportunities for meaningful activities in environments that are as "normal" as possible, focusing on strengths rather than on pathology.

Family and Network Support

Family support interventions are directed at reducing stress in the client's interpersonal environment and minimizing the burden of care for family members. If clients have little contact with families, interventions may target the people in their networks who provide them with support: friends, landlords, service providers.

With this emphasis on support to the supporters, interventions include the following:

- Psychoeducational activities that increase knowledge about the disorder and reduce family stress
- Practical assistance with information about homemaking or legal services
- Respite services (short-term placements to relieve the family of the burden of care)

Such services have been widely recommended as a way to reduce the family's burden and enhance the quality of life of both client and family for the long term (Spijker et al., 2011).

When you work with families of the severely and persistently mentally ill, becoming attuned to their concerns promotes recovery. Families may express ambivalence about caregiving. For example, they may want to promote the client's autonomy yet feel discomfort or guilt about the type of living situation the client is able to maintain independently. Clear information and nonjudgmental attitudes from you and other providers can do much to alleviate a family's distress and assure them that there may not be a single ideal solution to their problems. Your Self-Awareness can help you clarify your attitudes about client autonomy.

Advocacy

Many of the difficulties severely mentally ill persons experience in the community reflect a poor understanding of psychiatric illness among the general population and inadequate resources for their needs. For example, access to housing is a function of resources and community acceptance. Attention to housing is futile if no residential resources exist; vocational programs require access to employers. For this reason, one component of community support for SPMI clients is advocacy, or activities that increase access to resources. Advocacy can occur on an individual basis; for example, a case manager might intervene with a landlord to help a client obtain housing. Advocacy activities also occur at the level of the community, such as in programs for community education or outreach to employers.

When you provide rehabilitation services to clients, you must have clear ideas of the client's rights as well as their responsibilities. Nurses often refer to these concepts in advocating for appropriate referrals and authorizations for treatment. A statement of rights helps focus our awareness on the most fundamental aspect of the nursing role, that of being a client advocate. When you carry out your role in this framework, you bring to the multidisciplinary team skills and knowledge that extend beyond biologic or pathologic aspects of care. You view the client through a holistic perspective. You piece together any fragmented pieces of the client's care to form a cohesive plan with the goal of recovery. This cannot be done in the isolation of an office or simply by telephone. It requires active, on-site presence, interviews, meetings, attendance at treatment planning conferences, and appropriate documentation. The extent of your involvement is detailed in the clinical example.

Clinical Example

Sheila wanted to work in a nearby hotel food service department. She was clear about her right to be hired without being discriminated against, but she was not clear about her responsibilities. Sheila's case management nurse discussed the following responsibilities with her: behaving appropriately even if she is experiencing symptoms, interacting civilly even if she is angry, and telling her supervisor when she is having difficulty and needs help or support.

Nurses working with clients toward rehabilitation and recovery may be caught in the middle of conflicting value systems. For example, clients with alcoholism or bulimia have been treated traditionally with intensive, extended inpatient treatment programs. Most health care insurance plans may authorize this treatment only in an outpatient setting. The nurse must respond to clients' needs for autonomy in making decisions regarding treatment as well as negotiate within the limitations of the health care insurance plan. You must use creativity and flexibility in negotiating among the conflicting needs of several parties. Clients and families who are accustomed to specific treatment models for illnesses with relapse potential often feel confused and misunderstood when new treatment approaches are suggested that appear economically motivated.

Families of SPMI clients have also assumed a much greater advocacy role than in the past. Family advocacy arose in response to problems accompanying the deinstitutionalization process that placed an enormous burden of care on families. It also developed in reaction to the stigmatization of parents by people who attributed serious mental disorders to child-rearing practices. The major family organization for people with severe and persistent mental disorders is the National Alliance on Mental Illness (NAMI). The national and local chapters of NAMI have grown tremendously over the past 30 years and have become a recognized force in mental health policy development. Chapter 29 ∞ discusses NAMI in greater detail.

PSYCHIATRIC REHABILITATION

Although the components of community support models provide the structure for services to people who are severely and persistently mentally ill, their effectiveness depends on the content of these component services. **Psychiatric rehabilitation**, an emphasis on the prevention or reduction of impairment or handicap as opposed to the treatment of disease, serves as a guide for the content of practice at many levels of care, and it includes an overall treatment philosophy as well as specific interventions and programs.

Psychiatric Rehabilitation Philosophy

Psychiatric rehabilitation has its roots in theory about physical disabilities and includes training and supportive interventions intended to increase functional status. Research in schizophrenia and related severe mental illness suggests that psychiatric rehabilitation facilitates recovery of social inclusion and functioning (Odes et al., 2011). Treatment addresses the disease process and its consequent symptoms. Rehabilitation approaches emphasize specific interventions to address targeted areas of functioning. Rehabilitation approaches are also strongly grounded in beliefs about empowerment of clients, emphasizing client feelings of control and worth.

Rehabilitation-oriented services begin with functional assessment and identification of highly individualized goals. A plan is developed to meet objectives by behavioral interventions that target specific functional deficits, or by environmental interventions that enable functioning with an existing deficit. From a rehabilitation perspective, it is important to extend support as long as possible. Support is not necessarily withdrawn because a client improves. For example, clients doing well in supported employment programs would not be expected to necessarily "graduate" to independent employment and thereby forfeit the support.

Rehabilitation philosophy is entirely consistent with self-care and symptom management interventions developed by psychiatric–mental health nurses. In fact, rehabilitation theory and conceptual models in nursing share a common focus on functional adaptation in supportive environments.

Psychosocial Rehabilitation Centers/Clubhouses

Although a rehabilitation philosophy can inform and enhance many treatment modalities, some specific rehabilitation programs make a unique contribution to service systems. One of the most important types of psychiatric rehabilitation programs is psychosocial rehabilitation. This particular model helps clients reintegrate within their communities and limit— or eliminate—revolving door admissions (Petersen, Lund, & Stein, 2011). Under a community support system structure, psychosocial rehabilitation modalities could be available at a day programming center. Psychosocial services emphasize a collaborative relationship between staff and clients, and provide experiences in a supportive but realistic milieu for the development of abilities for functioning in the real world, as in the clinical example.

Clinical Example

DeShawn has been attending a psychosocial rehabilitation center that functions as a clubhouse regularly for a number of weeks. Playing pool and cards and taking classes in hip-hop provide him with opportunities to socialize with his peers. He can bring up his concerns informally with the professional staff or in any one of a variety of planned group sessions.

Supported Employment

While all mental health programs have some emphasis on vocational rehabilitation, not all vocational programs conform to a psychiatric rehabilitation model. Supported employment models reflect a rehabilitation perspective because of their emphasis on adding support to the normal environment. This model delineates basic competencies that are necessary for employment and offers classes that prepare the client to set goals and choose a job focus. Once clients are placed, they are supported by job coaches who serve as role models, provide feedback, and act as liaisons to employers.

Clinical Example

Toddy was very good with numbers, organizing, and filing. His job coach found him a position in a shoe department of a large department store. His job was to take the shoes the customers tried on, return them to the proper box, and file the box according to its number in the shoe storage area. Alicia, the job coach, accompanied Toddy for the first several days in his new job. On his second day, there was a shoe sale and Toddy became distressed and agitated because customers left so many shoes lying about. The job coach helped Toddy calm down when he began yelling at the customers. Alicia ultimately had to find another placement for Toddy. This client's ability to manage stress turned out to be more important to his job success than his skill with numbers.

Social Skills Training

Social skills training methods are based on principles of social learning and use behavioral techniques such as role-playing, practicing, and reinforcement to promote the learning of instrumental role behavior as well as problem-solving abilities and interpersonal skills. Social skills training techniques may be incorporated into individual, group, and family treatment modalities (see Chapter 28∞ for examples), where they may add measurable benefits. Your Intervention Strategies suggests a useful analogy that you can use when encouraging clients to change their behavior.

HIGH-RISK SPMI CLIENTS

Subgroups of SPMI clients are at particularly high risk for poor outcomes and are also extraordinarily difficult to serve in conventional programs. These subgroups include the following:

- People who have substance-related problems
- People who are homeless
- People with frequent readmissions to acute care
- People who are frequently involved in the criminal justice system

The interrelationships among these problems are complex, making it difficult to separate them or to distinguish root problems from their consequences. For example, substance use may exacerbate symptoms and lead to rehospitalization. This in turn may disrupt stability of residence, increasing the possibility of arrest and reducing the likelihood of medication adherence. In other words, if individuals belong to one subgroup at risk, it is likely that they belong to several, thus increasing their overall vulnerability.

Concurrent Substance-Related Disorders

Psychiatric illness greatly increases the odds of having a substance-related disorder. Alcohol has typically been the drug of choice with people who are severely mentally ill, perhaps because it is relatively inexpensive and easily accessible. Psychostimulant use has also increased among this population, a phenomenon partially attributed to the emergence of crack cocaine and methamphetamine as major drugs of abuse. Concurrent substance-related disorders are probably the most consistent predictor of readmission to psychiatric hospitals.

Substance use contributes to a host of undesirable outcomes, which are thoroughly discussed in Chapter 15∞. It is highly correlated with homelessness and criminal justice system involvement (Maniglio, 2009). It is also a cause of concurrent medical morbidity, including exposure to HIV. Several of these risk-related behaviors are evident in the clinical example.

Clinical Example

On her last admission to the inpatient unit for treatment of a manic episode, Sadie had a persistent vaginal fungal infection that resisted treatment. HIV testing came back positive for the presence of HIV. Prior to this last admission, Sadie had not taken her lithium for 2 months. As Sadie's mania increased, so did her risk behavior. When elated, Sadie was game to try anything, from alcohol to crack cocaine to unprotected sex with men she met at several bars she frequented. Sadie felt invulnerable.

YOUR INTERVENTION STRATEGIES   Making Something Different Happen:
A Scenario You Can Use to Help Clients Change

Making a change involves specific steps. This is a scenario you can use with clients: A client is walking down a particular street and falls into a huge hole. This happens over and over again; the client walks down the same street and falls into the same hole. Imagine the hole is a stressor or an interaction with someone that doesn't go well.

Making something different happen in your life will not be an automatic or instantaneous event. Change is a process and requires progressive steps of mental action.

Think of the following five steps to making a change:

1. At some point, you realize you are unsatisfied with a particular behavior and you want it to change. "I keep doing this and I don't want to. I need to make a change." *The idea that change is needed is an important first step.*

2. Now you walk down the street with the huge hole in it and try to see the hole before you fall in it. *You may very well continue to perform the original, unsuccessful coping or interaction, but this step encourages you to recognize that you use it even though it does not work.*

3. Try to see the hole as soon as you walk down the street, then continue walking and fall in the hole. *The goal is to progress to anticipating earlier and earlier in the process your use of the unsuccessful coping or interaction.*

4. Walk down the street, see the hole as soon as you begin walking, and walk around the hole when you get to it. *This is an exciting step. You start coping or interacting, recognize your tendency to use the original unsuccessful coping or interaction, and use the healthier and more competent step instead.*

5. Walk down a street that does not have a huge hole in it. *From now on you will use the effective coping or competent interaction. You have successfully made a change in your life.*

Several hospital surveys indicate a high rate of seropositivity among adults who are severely mentally ill. Triple-diagnosis clients—such as those with HIV disorders, substance-related disorders, and psychiatric disorders—require a complex and demanding range of services. Clients need to be able to conceptualize change in a helpful and hopeful manner.

For a variety of reasons involving different funding streams and different treatment philosophies, substance abuse services and psychiatric care are often poorly integrated. In mental health care systems, the dually diagnosed client encounters little specific expertise related to drug or alcohol use. Severely mentally ill clients sometimes do poorly in substance abuse programs stressing confrontation or demanding sobriety as a precondition to treatment. Integrated programs for the dually diagnosed mentally ill include inpatient and day treatment programs as well as group interventions. Adjusting the psychotropic medications for these clients may help them deal with problems such as dysphoria and anxiety that lead to self-medication with drugs and alcohol.

FIGURE 32-6 ■ Estimates of the extent of homelessness among the mentally ill range from 25% to more than 50%. Whichever numbers are more accurate, it is clear that the mentally ill constitute a prominent subgroup among the homeless.
Photo courtesy of Wrangler/Shutterstock.

Homeless and Mentally Ill

Homelessness is at an all-time high among psychiatric clients (Paquin, 2011). The goal of providing acceptable and long-term housing remains elusive, particularly in urban centers. While the proportion of psychiatric clients in the community who are permanently homeless is thought to be relatively small, a large and heterogeneous group experiences spells of residential instability (see FIGURE 32-6 ■). Unfortunately, discharge from the hospital to no fixed address (a shelter or the street) is not uncommon (Williams & Stickley, 2011; Moore, Gerdtz, Hepworth, & Manias, 2011).

Clinical Example

Rob is a 29-year-old man who was referred to an intensive case management team after his third hospital admission within 1 year. Rob has a diagnosis of schizoaffective disorder, but it is unclear whether his diagnosis accounts for his frequent acute episodes or whether the episodes are precipitated by his use of stimulants and alcohol. Rob has no stable place of residence and has stayed in shelters over the past few years. He describes himself as too preoccupied with his survival needs to seek treatment between emergency episodes. He claims that alcohol helps him manage his anxiety and his "voices" when he is on the streets. The case management team will first address Rob's need for safe housing. The team will then work with Rob to help him acknowledge that alcohol and drugs can increase his discomfort, and to support his use of psychotropic medication. When Rob is stabilized, he will work with the team and consider other treatment goals.

Whether these periods of homelessness involve movement between transient accommodations or actual street dwelling, they impose very harsh living conditions on people who are highly vulnerable. Homelessness interferes with the ability to use services, including the use of psychotropic medications. It increases the risk of trauma, substance abuse, infectious disease exposure, and victimization. Homelessness also makes conventional services unworkable, because the undomiciled can rarely store medication and use regular outpatient services. Those who are homeless and mentally ill are likely to experience several barriers to beginning, maintaining, and completing treatment. Several practical matters—establishing a medication routine, having access to health care providers, having an actual address or telephone, and being supported by friends and family—are the usual barriers faced by homeless people. Living independently in the community is possible when there is a consistent set of circumstances, daily routines, privacy, and a secure base in which to feel capable (Pati, 2011). In many geographic locations, a dominant "treatment first" approach persists where individuals must meet a hierarchy of program requirements before becoming eligible for an apartment of their own. This persists as a barrier.

Services to the homeless include supported housing models with case management components, shelter-based rehabilitation and substance abuse services, and mobile outreach teams to identify cases and link them with services. Case management services are particularly important to maneuver through the labyrinth of services and entitlements. While shelters and emergency programs serve a critical short-term need, they also contribute to instability. It is preferable, by far, to develop permanent housing for people with psychiatric disabilities. The Homelessness Resource Center specifically focuses on the delivery of services to people who are homeless and have serious mental illnesses. Its website, http://www.nrchmi.samhsa.gov, can be accessed through the Online Student Resources for this book.

HIV

The homeless mentally ill who live in urban areas, particularly those who live in municipal shelters, are at particular risk for HIV and other communicable diseases. The high incidence of injection drug use in this population, along with exchanging sex for drugs or money, makes them extremely vulnerable. The specific cognitive barriers that result from mental illness and HIV infection add to the difficulty of obtaining prophylactic or early treatment.

An increasingly critical problem is the lack of decent, appropriate housing for the growing number of people with HIV disease. HIV disease is disproportionately prevalent among individuals already at the economic edge and those who are targets of discrimination in housing and medical care: people of color, homosexuals, injection drug users, and homeless and runaway youth. In many communities around the country, available housing and services fall short of the need for appropriate residential care for thousands of people who have been made homeless by HIV-related illnesses, or whose struggle to survive on the streets has been worsened by the disease. Fatigue, repeated hospitalizations, and recurring illnesses all require time off from work, resulting first in the loss of employment, then in the loss of housing. The lack of effective risk-reduction education programs among the homeless has led to predictable and dramatic increases in HIV seropositivity.

Although most people with an impaired immune system can live independently, they require a safe environment that helps them avoid exposure to infectious diseases, get adequate rest, meet their special nutritional needs, and have access to support services and home help when necessary.

Frequent Readmissions and Relapse

Virtually all severe and persistent disorders will involve some kind of relapse at some time; more than one or two admissions in 12 months exceed norms. Box 32-2 identifies why frequent admissions are unhealthy and problematic.

Client-based factors that contribute to recidivism include substance abuse, which may be the best predictor of readmission. Cycling through emergency and acute care has been attributed to a "chronic crisis" style among people in some diagnostic groups, particularly those with severe personality disorders. However, many younger clients with schizophrenia and bipolar disorder use alcohol and drugs to combat boredom and medication side effects, and to self-medicate or treat symptoms in what they consider a "normal" way.

On a systems level, readmission may reflect a failure to link the client with services that the client considers meaningful and accessible. The system as a whole may respond best to clients who "fit" into programs and benefit from treatment

---

Box 32-2 Why Frequent Readmissions Are Problematic

Recidivism, or frequent readmission, to acute psychiatric settings is a problem for several reasons, including:

1. It represents a considerable expense.
2. It is a signal of relapse, indicating severe difficulties for the individual.
3. It suggests a failure of the community system to link the client between acute episodes and to institute the type of treatment and monitoring that might manage symptomatic shifts without hospitalization.

---

alone. Those with more social needs or less acceptance of their illness may not consider ambulatory services relevant to their needs and may require assertive outreach to link with appropriate outpatient providers.

Frequent Criminal Justice System Involvement

Prevalence rates of major psychiatric disorders in the jails have increased gradually but continuously, at least in part because of deinstitutionalization policies. Society has a low tolerance for disordered behavior, and the lack of services for the severely and persistently mentally ill in the mental health care system leads to a funneling into the criminal justice system. According to the Bazelon Center for Mental Health Law (2011), mentally ill persons have a far greater chance of being arrested than those who are not mentally ill but have committed the same crime. Fact sheets offering specific information for advocates on combating the criminalization of people with mental illness can be found at http://www.bazelon.org and accessed through the Online Student Resources for this book.

Unemployment, homelessness, and substance abuse contribute to the profile of the severely mentally ill forensic client. Many forensic inpatient services are filled to capacity. Most mentally ill offenders end up in county jails rather than forensic mental hospitals; they rarely become connected with local mental health networks and are frequently counted among the homeless because they have no fixed address. Psychiatric–mental health nurses provide valuable case management and advocacy services for this specific population as well as for high-risk SPMI clients in general.

STEPS TO RECOVERY

Recovery is a process that has important components that are discussed in the next section. However, keep in mind that changes in an individual client's circumstances and preferences require ongoing needs assessment and adjustment of the plan for achieving recovery.

Assessing Needs

Nurses who work collaboratively with clients with the goal of recovery interact with all members of the health care team to create, with the client, a recovery plan. Trust, mutual support, and clear communication among team members are necessary. Meet with administrative personnel and employ tactful systems-entry strategies while laying the groundwork for the client's recovery program.

If the client is determined to need, and want, particular educational activities, your role as the nurse is to develop a plan in a collaborative manner to promote the successful acquisition of an educational experience. Similarly, stable living arrangements contribute significantly to the ability of a client to achieve recovery. Your involvement in client care includes prioritizing so that clients have the underpinnings that maximize the probability of success.

Planning for Rehabilitation and Recovery

In this phase of care, you can bring valuable information concerning benefits, limits, family resources, expectations, and

FIGURE 32-7 ■ Recovery for someone with SPMI is possible when people work together.
Photo courtesy of Yuri Arcurs/Shutterstock.

other pertinent data to the recovery planning table. Using the formal and informal support systems, the treatment team is able to set mutually agreed-upon goals with desired outcomes and can begin to plan action steps using client-driven timeframes or critical pathways as a guide. The team approach (see FIGURE 32-7 ■) promotes and maintains recovery.

Spirituality

An important component of coping with a chronic illness, and having successful experiences, is having an outlet for spirituality. This portion of the recovery plan honors the client's preferences and needs. Clients who find a system of meaning within which to function tend to have more satisfying outcomes (Onyango et al., 2011). Spirituality can enhance and support a client's recovery through strengthening psychosocial well-being.

There is no need to have formal religiosity in order to be a spiritual person, although many clients do prefer the structure of the rituals and religious practices. Being a member of a community seems to be the important feature. A spiritual person who has contact with other like-minded individuals, and feels accepted and appreciated, is unlikely to be alone in the world.

Voluntary Community Activities

As noted earlier in the chapter in occupational and vocational therapies, having a structure and purpose to ones daily activities provides healing and a sense of accomplishment (Arbesman & Logsdon, 2011). Voluntary activity is a way to be involved with others in a variety of settings that do not place premature demands on the client. Volunteering also offers a way for clients to master complex skills at their own pace while experiencing an activity level that can meet their individual needs.

Another benefit of volunteering comes from helping another cope with a problem similar to one's own. This is a feature of adult learning that reinforces learning. Most clients find that teaching others is an excellent way to incorporate meaningful information. This, along with contributing to

someone else's recovery, is a powerful message that the client has succeeded to a certain degree on the road to recovery and has something to offer the community.

Psychopharmacology and Recovery

Combining maintenance antipsychotic medication therapy with psychosocial approaches has been found to be more effective than pharmacotherapy alone in delaying or preventing relapse, and promoting recovery. Early intervention, when symptoms become less manageable or stressors increase, would be effective in preventing relapse in clients with mental disorder. This could be accomplished through close clinical or family monitoring for the client's particular *prodromal symptoms* (those symptoms that occur early in the relapse process for that client). Once identified, prompt clinical intervention with antipsychotic medication may reduce the overall frequency of the relapse event.

Programs for relapse prevention typically combine standard doses of maintenance antipsychotic medication with psychosocial treatment and result in lower relapse rates. Weekly group therapy for clients is an opportunity to monitor prodromal symptoms. Such clinical scrutiny may prevent or minimize relapse and rehospitalization. A multifamily group component is helpful to support and educate the families as well as provide peer contacts and here-and-now experiences.

Those clients who live more independently and experience relapses could benefit from a community treatment contact. Prevention is more effective when clients and their families understand the likely relapse triggers, as outlined in TABLE 32-2 ■.

Other aspects of relapse prevention have been implemented clinically with good results. Clients with a psychosis not responsive to pharmacotherapy may benefit from specific cognitive–behavioral therapies (see Chapter 30 ∞), while persons with persistent negative symptoms and limited social competence may find social skills training useful. Successful outcomes for clients and their families occur with psychological support, behavioral treatments, social and cognitive rehabilitation, assistance in social and scholastic activities, enhancement of social skills, and family support (Masi & Liboni, 2011). In addition, new programs of supported employment may enable some clients to maintain competitive employment. The impacts of regularly scheduled employment and improved social and job skills can be a helpful distracter from the onslaught of psychosis if it does not tax the client's coping abilities.

Implementing the Rehabilitation and Recovery Plan

The next phase of the recovery process is to ensure that the client obtains needed care. You and the client will take the opportunity to look at the whole picture of the client's needs and abilities and keep up to date on changes in the plan. Many times, a case manager will contribute time and resources needed to monitor the quantity and quality of care delivered.

Keep in mind during the implementation phase that your role involves conflict resolution. The skills needed to work

TABLE 32-2 ■ Relapse Triggers in Mental Disorder		
Physiological Stressors		
Infection	Pain	Rape
Acute illness	Fatigue	Surgery
Chronic illness	Side effects of medications	Injury
Dehydration Failure to take prescribed medications	Appetite changes	Insomnia
Personal Stressors		
Negative symptoms of schizophrenia	Financial difficulties Depression	Exacerbation/ relapse of illness
Spiritual distress	An increase in responsibility	Pet loss/illness/ aging
Recreational activity	Maturational/ developmental changes	Decreased access to resource choice
Interpersonal Stressors		
High expressed emotion	Loss of job or status within a job	Conflict, anger
Relationship changes (family, intimate relationships, friendships)	Altered contact with another or others	Perceived rejection/ abandonment
Community Stressors		
Difficulties making living arrangements	Disruption of living situation	Roommate/family stressors
	Transportation	Community disruption

with a client and manage relationships within a large mental health provision system include:

- Setting limits tactfully
- Arbitrating differences
- Maintaining the focus on successful outcomes for all

In order to contribute positively to an outcome of rehabilitation and recovery, you need patience, maturity, and experience. You may also be called upon to provide additional data or client/family education where a denial or extension of service is in question. As client advocate, you may identify gaps in care that require action in the community, in a treatment facility, or within the nursing system. Your recovery focus makes you the best consultant to nursing departments for improving quality because you view problems in the system from the client's perspective.

Evaluating the Rehabilitation and Recovery Plan

Evaluating progress toward the recovery goal consists of continuous monitoring of intervention responses and progress toward desired outcomes. This may include discussions to discover and ameliorate side effects of psychotropic medications (see Chapter 31∞), medication monitoring for dosage and adherence, as well as monitoring client response to other therapies such as counseling and activities. The evaluation is made together with the client, incorporating ancillary information when available. Perhaps the process is moving too slowly for the client, or the plan needs to be adjusted for more realistic shorter-term goals.

An important feature of any recovery plan is the active participation of the client. Flexibility and honest discussion help establish a workable document that is not static. Focus on proximal goals and make a point of acknowledging achievement at every stage. Every client has the right to expect recovery; every nurse has the responsibility to contribute faithfully and energetically to that goal.

Pearson Nursing Student Resources

Find additional review materials at
nursing.pearsonhighered.com

Prepare for success with NCLEX®-style practice questions, interactive assignments and activities, web links, animations and videos, and more!

REFERENCES

American Psychiatric Association. (2000). *Diagnostic and statistical manual of mental disorders* (4th ed., Text Revision). Washington DC: Author.

Arbesman, M., & Logsdon, D. W. (2011). Occupational therapy interventions for employment and education for adults with serious mental illness: A systematic review. *American Journal of Occupational Therapy, 65,* 238–246.

Bazelon Center for Mental Health Law. (2011). *Diversion from incarceration to reentry.* Retrieved from http://www.bazelon.org/Where-We-Stand/Access-to-Services/Diversion-from-Incarceration-and-Reentry-.aspx

Edgelow, M., & Krupa, T. (2011). Randomized controlled pilot study of an occupational time-use intervention for people with serious mental illness. *American Journal of Occupational Therapy, 65,* 267–276.

Finnell, D. S. (2009). How useful is the transtheoretical model (TTM) for individuals with psychotic disorders? *Alcoholism: Clinical & Experimental Research, Supplement 1,* 193A.

LeBel, J. L. (2011). Coercion is not mental health care. *Psychiatric Services, 62,* 453.

Maniglio, R. (2009). Severe mental illness and criminal victimization: A systematic review. *Acta Psychiatrica Scandinavia, 119*(3), 180–191.

Masi, G., & Liboni, F. (2011). Management of schizophrenia in children and adolescents: Focus on pharmacotherapy. *Drugs, 71*(2), 179–208.

Moore, G., Gerdtz, M. F., Hepworth, G., & Manias, E. (2011). Homelessness: Patterns of emergency department use and risk factors for re-presentation. *Emergency Medicine Journal, 28*, 422–427.

O'Baire-Kark, M., & Klevay, A. (2011). Another perspective on finger replantation surgery: Nursing support for the psychological levels of recovery. *Journal of Trauma Nursing, 18*(1), 34–42.

Odes, H., Katz, N., Noter, E., Shamir, Y., Weizman, A., & Valevski, A. (2011). Level of function at discharge as a predictor of readmission among inpatients with schizophrenia. *American Journal of Occupational Therapy, 65*, 314–319.

Onyango, G. R., Paratharayil, M., van den Berg, S., Reiffers, R., Snider, L., & Erikson, C. (2011). Spirituality and psychosocial work in emergencies: Four commentaries and a response. *Intervention, 9*(1), 61–73.

Paquin, S. O. (2011). Social justice advocacy in nursing: What is it? How do we get there? *Creative Nursing, 17*(2), 63–67.

Pati, A. (2011). Brighter prospects. *Nursing Standard, 25*(20), 20–21.

Petersen, I., Lund, C., & Stein, D. J. (2011). Optimizing mental health services in low-income and middle-income countries. *Current Opinion in Psychiatry, 24*, 318–323.

Prochaska, J. O., & DiClemente, C. C. (1986). Toward a comprehensive model of change. In W. Miller & N. Heather (Eds.), *Treating addictive behaviors* (pp. 3–27). New York, NY: Plenum Press.

Spijker, A., Wollersheim, H., Teerenstra, S., Graff, M., Adang, E., Verbey, F., & Vernooij-Dassen, M. (2011). Systematic care for caregivers of patients with dementia: A multicenter, cluster-randomized, controlled study. *American Journal of Geriatric Psychiatry, 19*, 521–531.

Staring, A.B. P., van der Gaag, M., & Mulder, C. L. (2011). Recovery style predicts remission at one-year follow-up in outpatients with schizophrenia spectrum disorders. *Journal of Nervous & Mental Disease, 199*(5), 295–300.

Substance Abuse and Mental Health Services Administration (SAMHSA). (2006). *National consensus statement.* Retrieved from http://store.samhsa .gov/product/National-Consensus-Statement-on-Mental-Health-Recovery/ SMA05-4129

Williams, S., & Stickley, T. (2011). Stories from the streets: People's experiences of homelessness. *Journal of Psychiatric & Mental Health Nursing, 18*(5), 432–439.

33

Complementary, Alternative, and Integrative Healing Practices

CAROL REN KNEISL

LEARNING OUTCOMES

After completing this chapter, you will be able to:

1. Explain the therapeutic uses for each of the complementary and alternative medicine (CAM) techniques discussed in this chapter.
2. Compare and contrast various CAM techniques, including their important characteristics and functions.
3. Integrate appropriate CAM techniques into a plan of care to promote, maintain, and restore emotional well-being for clients and their families.
4. Encourage clients and their family members to become educated consumers by educating them about the safety and effectiveness of CAM techniques, quackery and fraud, the qualifications of providers, and quality of service delivery.
5. Educate clients and their families in the effective use of CAM therapies.
6. Identify the natural medicines used for psychiatric symptoms and their effectiveness and safety.
7. Determine when a client should not use natural medicines in combination with prescribed psychopharmacologic medications.
8. Integrate CAM strategies into professional practice when appropriate.

CRITICAL THINKING CHALLENGE

You and three of your classmates are discussing your most recent clinical experiences. Jenny tells the story of a toddler she was caring for on the pediatric oncology unit. La Tonya and Shi-An share what it's like to work in the intensive care unit. You discuss the events of your day in the psychiatric emergency department. The four of you agree that stress is, and will continue to be, a part of your nursing life regardless of your area of clinical practice. The four of you also agree that living and working in a high-technology, stressful environment causes you to feel apprehensive and worried about your ability to live your life to its fullest potential.

1. Should you anticipate that stress will continue to be a part of your nursing life regardless of your area of clinical practice? Why, or why not?
2. How can this chapter help you and your classmates cope with the stresses in your nursing life?
3. Why should complementary and alternative healing practices be integrated into the care plan for a client when appropriate?

In many cultures around the world, health care and medical practices that are not currently an integral part of conventional Western medicine are used to relieve pain and cure illnesses. In Western culture, they are called *complementary and alternative medicine (CAM)*. **Complementary medicine** is used in conjunction with conventional medical practices. **Alternative medicine** is used in place of conventional medicine. **Integrative medicine** combines conventional medicine and CAM treatments for which there is quality evidence of safety and effectiveness. Integrative medicine is being used more often in hospitals, medical centers, and universities in North America as increasing numbers of contemporary Western health care providers incorporate the most appropriate, safe, and effective of ancient traditions and healing approaches into their practice. Programs in integrative medicine and CAM clinical centers are in existence in most academic centers throughout North America.

Nursing, with its tradition of holistic care—providing care for the whole person (mind, body, and spirit) in all its uniqueness—is especially well suited to deliver integrative therapy. Florence Nightingale herself encouraged holistic care by recognizing the importance of the environment, touch, light, aromatics, music, and quiet reflection to the healing process. Complementary and alternative approaches such as those described in this chapter will provide you with yet another way to promote clients' well-being. This chapter discusses complementary and alternative medicine as well as the research that documents, or fails to document, their usefulness.

REDISCOVERING CAM

Ancient traditions and healing practices such as those discussed in this chapter are being rediscovered by consumers and providers of health care in Western culture. Increasing numbers of consumers are seeking out CAM on their own, asking questions of their health care providers, and requesting that CAM be added to their plan of care. Health care providers are finding it easier to find articles on CAM in respected non-CAM medical and nursing journals. One woman's search to heal her spirit is presented in Mental Health in the Movies.

National Center for CAM

In 1992, the Office of Alternative Medicine was established at the National Institutes of Health (NIH) in response to increasing interest in CAM among the general population. This office has funded and studied a wide range of CAM therapies. Most early studies of CAM had serious methodologic problems, and their lack of scientific validity was justly criticized. The results of the office's scientifically designed and implemented studies led to greater acceptance by the medical community and increased credibility for CAM. As a result, the office was upgraded in 1998 to a fully recognized national center at the NIH and is now called the National Center for Complementary and Alternative Medicine (NCCAM). Much of the research in CAM today is funded by the NCCAM whose mission is to explore CAM practices using rigorous scientific methods to build an evidence base for the safety and effectiveness of these practices. However, as you will see later in this chapter, not all studies of CAM incorporate rigorous standards of scientific research. You can access the NCCAM database at http://www.nccam.nih.gov through a direct resource link on the Online Student Resources for this book.

Consumers of CAM

The National Health Interview Survey (NHIS) of over 30,000 adults and children, the latest findings by NCCAM and the National Center for Health Statistics, showed that almost 40% of American adults and 12% of children use some form of CAM treatment (Barnes, Bloom, & Nahin, 2008). In other national surveys, anywhere from 50% to 80% of respondents report using at least one CAM therapy at some point in their lifetime. Figure 33-1 ■ compares the 10 most common diseases or conditions for which CAM is used among adults and children. Figure 33-2 ■ identifies the 10 most common CAM therapies among adults and children.

Note that nonvitamin, nonmineral natural products are the most commonly used CAM treatments among adults and children. There are recent increases in the use of deep breathing, meditation, massage therapy, and yoga (discussed later in this chapter) among adults. Among children, chiropractic, deep breathing, and yoga are also frequently used. Chiropractic,

MENTAL HEALTH IN THE MOVIES
Eat, Pray, Love

Eat, Pray, Love is a portrayal of one woman's around-the-world journey to find herself after a painful divorce. Liz Gilbert (Julia Roberts) embarks to Italy, India, and Indonesia on a quest for self-discovery. The movie is based on the *New York Times* best seller memoir of the same name written by Elizabeth Gilbert.

Liz indulges herself in food and wine in Italy for 4 months and emulates the ascetic ways of yogis in hours of meditation at an ashram in India for 3 months during which she struggles to still her churning mind. Looking to balance the two—indulgence and asceticism—in Bali, Liz studies with a medicine man and reconnects with a healer. On this spiritual odyssey, she ponders the many paths to healing, falls in love, and finds a person to share her life. Elizabeth Gilbert remains in close contact with the many people she met along the way in her pilgrimage to find herself.

Critics of the movie say that it does not have the spiritual and emotional weight of the book that inspired it. Others say that the movie inspires one to ponder one's choices and forgive one's flaws—a mentally healthy thing to do.

Photo courtesy © Columbia Pictures/courtesy Everett Collection.

WebLink Application: Older Americans Not Disclosing CAM Use With Doctors

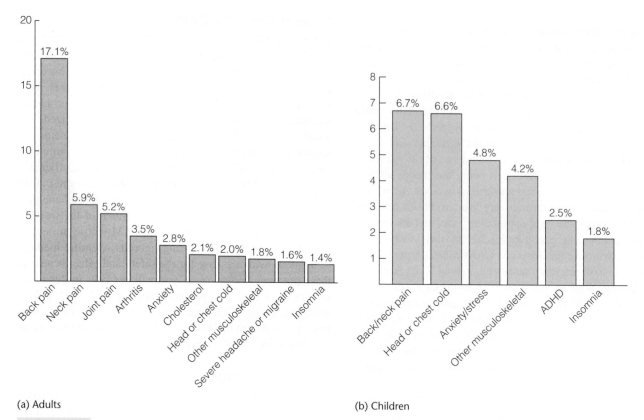

(a) Adults

(b) Children

FIGURE 33-1 ■ Ten most common diseases or conditions for which CAM therapies are used.
Source: National Center for Complementary and Alternative Medicine.

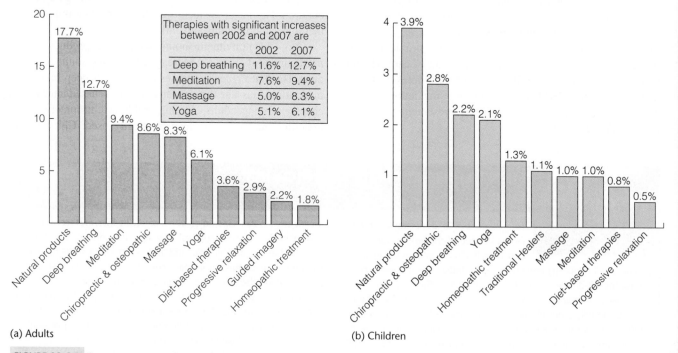

(a) Adults

(b) Children

FIGURE 33-2 ■ Ten most commonly used CAM therapies.
Source: National Center for Complementary and Alternative Medicine.

Box 33-1 Why People Seek CAM Therapies

- Wanting greater control over their lives
- Having a sense of responsibility for their own health care
- Wanting a more holistic orientation in health care so that body, mind, and spirit are addressed
- Finding that their health care provider does not have enough time or empathy for them
- Concern over the side effects of conventional therapies
- Concern over the financial cost of conventional medicine
- Finding the results of conventional treatments to be inadequate
- Identifying with a particular philosophy or practice because of cultural background

and some cautions associated with it, is also discussed later in this chapter. The report also tells us that among adults, CAM therapies are used more often by women, those with higher levels of education, and those with higher incomes.

Adults use CAM for a wide variety of conditions. The most common conditions are musculoskeletal—back, neck, and joint pain. The use of CAM to treat "chest and head colds" showed a decrease from statistics collected 5 years before the present NHIS. Other reports in the literature indicate that anxiety, depression, insomnia and other sleeping difficulties, gastrointestinal disorders, diabetes, HIV, allergies, and menopausal symptoms are also common reasons why adults use CAM. In addition to physical reasons, CAM is often used by parents to treat children with stress and attention deficit/hyperactivity disorder. The literature also reports that a majority of children with autism use some form of CAM treatment.

If you were to ask people why they use CAM therapies, they would likely give you the reasons listed in Box 33-1. It appears that undergirding the motivations of users of alternative medicine, at least in part, is their dissatisfaction with conventional medicine, and more specifically with the therapeutic relationship between the health care provider and the client. Many feel that their health care provider has too little time for them and not enough empathy. The health care consumer's message is clear—health care providers must place greater emphasis on the quality of their relationship with the client. There is no question that the move toward CAM reflects a consumer-driven health care enviro-nment.

Sociocultural Aspects

The use of CAM is related to cultural and health beliefs; thus, the reasons for using CAM are likely to vary among racial and ethnic groups. In an increasingly diverse society, understanding the rationales, motivations, and differences in and reasons for CAM use will enhance the cultural competence of health care professionals, shed light on cultural and social factors related to health behaviors, and help address the need for health care improvements among minority populations. Developing Cultural Competence discusses some of these rationales and motivations.

NURSING ROLE IN CAM

Nurses have several important roles in relationship to CAM approaches and integrative therapies. We are often in a position of being able to do the following:

- Identify whether a client is currently using CAM therapies
- Identify a client's need for CAM
- Identify when a CAM method is inappropriate for the client, or is contraindicated
- Suggest CAM therapies to treatment team members and to clients, their family members, or their friends
- Encourage clients to consider using a CAM therapy if appropriate

DEVELOPING CULTURAL COMPETENCE

Reasons for CAM Use in Various Cultures

Non-Hispanic white women are most likely to cite personal beliefs for CAM use while the cost of conventional medicine is the most prevalent reason among Mexican-American women. Media sources, family and friends, and physician referral seem to be most influential among non-Hispanic white women. Informal networks of family and friends were the most important social influences of CAM use among African-, Mexican-, and Chinese-American women.

Herbal medicines are used more often by Chinese Americans, and mind–body therapies by Asian Indians and Filipinos. Asian Americans, Hispanics, and non-Hispanic blacks are less likely than non-Hispanic whites to disclose the use of CAM methodologies to conventional health care providers. The use of herbal and natural supplements is also prevalent among Hispanics and lowest among African Americans. These findings from the literature suggest that it is particularly important to query these populations about CAM use.

CRITICAL THINKING QUESTIONS

1. Which actions on your part demonstrate your understanding that cultural forces are powerful determinants of health-related behaviors?
2. How could any prejudices or stereotypes that you have about mind-body therapies or herbal medicines affect your ability to provide holistic care?
3. How could any positive opinions that you have about mind-body therapies or herbal medicines negatively affect your ability to provide holistic care?

- Enlist the support of the treatment team, family members, and friends
- Help clients find providers

Also, we may be CAM practitioners ourselves. Nurses may be practitioners of CAM therapies in a variety of settings—hospital, outpatient clinic, home, community, private practice office, and so on. The most common CAM therapies that nurses provide are relaxation techniques (such as deep breathing, active progressive relaxation, visualization, and meditation), bodywork techniques (such as massage), and energy therapies (such as Healing Touch, Therapeutic Touch, and Reiki). These therapies are discussed in detail in this chapter. CAM therapies that require further training or equipment or are usually provided by others are discussed briefly.

We may be teachers of CAM therapies. Nurses play a significant role in helping clients and their families become aware of these methods and teaching them how to use them effectively. As health care educators, we have an important role in encouraging clients to be informed health consumers. And lastly, we can coordinate the integration of CAM services into a client's plan of care, as illustrated in the Evidence-Based Practice feature.

Helping Clients Become Informed Health Consumers

Integrative CAM approaches are creative and powerful tools under the following circumstances:

1. The approach used has been demonstrated to be safe and effective.

2. The method is appropriate for that particular client.
3. The client learns to use the method properly.

Consumers and professionals can access the Cochrane database system to help them evaluate safety and effectiveness. The Cochrane Collaboration has been in existence since 1993. It consists of 12 centers around the world and over 10,000 health expert volunteers from over 90 countries, who carefully review clinical trials in order to help people make well-informed decisions by preparing, maintaining, and promoting the accessibility of systematic reviews of the effects of interventions in all areas of health care. They have published hundreds of systematic reviews. There are some cautiously optimistic reviews of CAM methods for pelvic and back pain during pregnancy, low back pain, headaches, postoperative nausea and vomiting, chemotherapy-induced nausea and vomiting, and bedwetting. Some of these reviews are cited throughout this chapter. The appropriateness of individual CAM methods and guidelines for proper use are identified later in this chapter in the discussion of techniques.

Safety and Effectiveness

In general, the multi-billion dollar alternative therapy market fails to deliver the health benefits that it claims to offer. Many CAM therapies are not well regulated and researched. Some of the problems in determining the evidence base for CAM have to do with inconsistency across studies, variations in methodology, inadequate sample size, and problematic study design, making it difficult to judge the clinical significance

---

EVIDENCE-BASED PRACTICE

Helping Clients Become Informed CAM Consumers

Judy Krasinski is a psychiatric–mental health nurse and a member of the treatment team in the wellness center of a large urban medical center. Jammela, a new client, has recently been referred to the wellness center for evaluation of anxiety and depression, as well as an evaluation of the herbs and other natural medicines she is taking. Jammela has HIV and is on a HAART (highly active antiretroviral therapy) regimen to treat her symptoms. Judy was aware that some HIV clients use CAM as an alternative to their HAART regimen rather than to complement it. Using HAART inconsistently is problematic given its association with drug resistance.

Jammela has been on edge, worries about her future constantly, and has been moody and feeling blue. The results of the Beck Depression Inventory indicated that she is moderately depressed. Her depression has not improved despite treatment with paroxetine (Paxil) and then citalopram (Celexa). When Judy found that Jammela has also been taking St. John's wort and garlic supplements, she became even more concerned knowing that St. John's wort may potentiate the effects of antidepressants and garlic supplements have been found to inhibit the effectiveness of saquinavir,

one of the protease inhibitors in Jammela's medication protocol. Judy also learned that Jammela has not informed her prescribers of the herbs and other products she takes because she felt it was not important for them to have this information and, that in any case, they might not approve.

In addition to providing Jammela with information about the effects of St. John's wort on antidepressants and garlic supplements on protease inhibitors, Judy met with the other members of the team to discuss the possibility of CAM therapies other than herbs or dietary supplements to enhance Jammela's treatment for anxiety and depression. The team has suggested two programs based on the following research to augment her treatment: massage therapy and a mindfulness meditation program.

Action should be based on more than one study, but the following research would be helpful in this situation.

McDonald, K., & Slavin, S. (2010). My body, my life, my choice: Practices and meaning of complementary and alternative medicine among a sample of Australian people living with HIV/AIDS and their practitioners. *AIDS Care, 22*(10), 1229–1235.

CRITICAL THINKING QUESTIONS

1. Because Jammela is also anxious, what other herbal or dietary supplements should you assess for?
2. Why did the team recommend massage therapy?
3. How does mindfulness meditation help with anxiety?

of the results. Remember to be an inquiring consumer of research. The contents of many complementary and alternative medicine journals have only a limited number of randomized clinical trials. The proportion of positive articles is very high, thus suggesting bias. A limited number of studies reflect the best available evidence.

You can determine the safety and effectiveness of CAM methods and read any consumer advisories and news releases about the most recent research by accessing NCCAM's website at http://www.nccam.nih.gov. Another source is the current literature. The National Library of Medicine (NLM) and NCCAM have jointly developed a means of easy access to the literature on CAM from 1966 to the present. Over 12 million CAM journal citations can be found on NLM's PubMed at http://www.pubmed.gov, which can be accessed through a direct link on this text's Online Student Resources.

Encourage your clients to become informed health consumers. Help them to gather the following information about CAM:

- Advantages and disadvantages
- Risks
- Side effects and adverse effects
- Expected results
- Length of treatment
- Interaction with conventional Western medications

Clients can also gather information in informal ways, such as testimonials by others. However, while testimonials from others who are or have been clients may be helpful, they should never be the sole criterion in selecting a therapy. Informed health care consumers and health care practitioners will seek information on controlled scientific trials such as those summarized on the websites listed earlier. The clinical example discusses how one nurse was able to help the members of an advocacy and mutual-help organization become better informed health care consumers.

Clinical Example

Jesse is the father of an autistic son and the president of the local branch of an autism organization that works toward reducing stigma and promoting research and treatment for autism. Jesse was recently approached by a partnership of holistic practitioners who almost guaranteed that their services would help their autistic children. Jesse sought consultation from David, one of the other fathers, who was also a nurse. David was well aware of the statistics in Figures 33-1 and 33-2 on on page 716 and suggested caution. David volunteered to gather research information so that the board of the autism society could make an informed decision about whether or not to link with the partnership of holistic practitioners.

Remind clients that they can be led astray by television, newspapers—especially tabloid newspapers—and mass-market magazines. One popular television news program actually created a market for one of the most dubious alternative treatments—shark cartilage as a cancer treatment. The clinical example that follows illustrates some of the problems that can result from the promotion of dubious alternative treatments.

Clinical Example

A 9-year-old Canadian girl had undergone surgery to remove a malignant brain tumor. Her oncologist recommended radiation and chemotherapy as a follow-up treatment, which would have given her a 50/50 chance of survival. Her parents, impressed by the publicity surrounding shark cartilage, decided to forego conventional treatment in favor of alternative treatment. She died a few months later.

Clinical trials in the 1990s concluded that shark cartilage had no medicinal value. The question that continues to be debated in this and similar instances is: Did this alternative treatment negate any chance of her survival?

By helping clients become informed health consumers, you also help them to avoid fraudulently marketed products that are useless (such as electronic devices that claim to cure serious illnesses by sending electrical energy into the body), or products that have serious medication interaction risks (such as those that may cause a reduction in the therapeutic effect of oral contraceptives, a reduction in the therapeutic effect of medications used to treat HIV, or prevent transplant rejection). Interaction risks are discussed more fully later in this chapter. Tips on avoiding fraudulently marketed products and making a decision to use CAM are listed in Partnering With Clients and Families. A guide to fraud, quackery, and informed decision making is available on http://www.quackwatch.com, a website maintained by a physician. This data can be accessed through a link on the Online Student Resources for this text.

Practitioner Expertise

Encourage clients to examine the background, qualifications, and competence of a potential CAM practitioner. If there is licensure or certification for the particular CAM practice, is the practitioner licensed or certified? National organizations of CAM practitioners can provide referrals as well as information on legislation and state registration or licensing. Health regulatory bodies can provide information on state licensure or registration and any complaints lodged against specific practitioners. Nurses who practice CAM methods can be credentialed by any one of several specialty bodies and/or the American Holistic Nurses' Association, or licensed to practice specific CAM therapies in states where their use is governmentally regulated.

Clients should understand that just because a professional organization related to the CAM treatment exists, that, in and of itself, is not evidence that the treatments are safe or effective. Caution them about organizations—such as the American Academy of Medical Acupuncture, the General Chiropractic Council, and the Society of Homeopaths—that continue to promote their therapies for various inappropriate conditions, despite the lack of any evidence for the therapies' effectiveness in the case of acupuncture and homeopathy, or despite evidence demonstrating severe health risks such as in the case of chiropractic (Singh & Ernst, 2009).

CAM Safety

PARTNERING WITH CLIENTS AND FAMILIES

Educating Clients About CAM

Tips for Avoiding Fraudulent Health Claims

- Be suspicious of claims for a "miracle cure," an "exclusive product," or a "magical discovery."
- Check out claims on the Internet, in advertisements on television and radio, and in newspapers and magazines with reliable sources such as NCCAM.
- Understand that claiming to be "natural" doesn't necessarily mean that the product is safe.
- Be aware that impressive-sounding terminology may be a way to disguise a lack of good science.
- Be skeptical about claims that the government, research scientists, or the medical profession have conspired to suppress a product. Cures for serious disease are widely reported in the media. They are not hidden in obscure magazine ads, paid television advertisements, or website promotions.
- "Quick relief" or "quick cure" claims are unreliable, especially if the disease is serious.
- Beware of products that claim to treat a wide spectrum of unrelated illnesses.

Tips for Anyone Considering CAM as a Mode of Treatment

- First, consult and inform your health care provider to make sure that the treatment you have chosen does not interfere with any ongoing conventional treatment.
- Do not stop your conventional treatment unless your health care provider has given you this advice.
- Make sure there is evidence to support the benefit of the therapy you have chosen before you invest large sums of money. Alternative therapies can be expensive, especially if they involve long-term consultations.
- All therapies can involve the *placebo effect*. This sole reason does not justify its use if it involves risks to your health or constitutes a financial burden.
- Every treatment carries risks—conventional as well as alternative. Make sure that the benefits to you will outweigh the risks.

Encourage clients to also talk with other health care providers or former clients, who may be able to address the question of competence and the quality of the services provided by the practitioner. Clients should actually interview the CAM practitioner, asking about education, licensure, certification, treatment approach, and possible side effects or problems with the specific technique. This is an important step.

Quality and Costs of Service Delivery

Clients should visit the practitioner's office, clinic, or hospital to personally see the conditions under which treatment will be given. Are conditions safe and clean? Are regulated standards for medical care and safety adhered to?

Cost may also be an important consideration for clients. Although increasing numbers of insurers are covering costs of CAM services, not all do. Clients may have to pay directly for CAM services. Practitioners and health insurers should be able to tell clients which services are reimbursable.

Integrating CAM into a Treatment Plan

Integrating CAM into a treatment plan can take place only when clients discuss all CAM treatments and therapies with their primary physical or mental health care providers. Some CAM treatments affect physical or mental functioning, and certain products can interfere with or potentiate treatment with conventional medications.

Selecting Appropriate Clients

Most CAM techniques require that a client is motivated to participate in the interventions, is able to concentrate, and can follow directions, some of which may be quite complex.

Assess clients to see if they meet these criteria. Be sure to obtain informed consent before instituting CAM therapies.

Techniques that are lengthy and introspective or meditative should probably not be used with clients who are severely depressed, hallucinating, delusional, or have loss of contact with reality. Introspective techniques may lead to an increased loss of contact with reality, withdrawal, or increased rumination. Brief and externally focused techniques would be better for these clients. Clients who have multiple problems or are in extremely stressful situations may not have the time or energy to focus on or learn complex CAM techniques. Avoid adding another stressor to these clients' lives. Mental health problems that often respond well to CAM therapies are identified in Box 33-2.

Monitoring the Plan of Care

Clients using CAM therapies should first discuss the program with their health care provider. National population-based surveys and studies in primary care settings have documented inadequate communication about CAM between clients and their conventional health care providers. Although most clinicians recognize that their clients use CAM techniques, few consistently ask clients about their CAM use. Clients say that they do not inform their primary care practitioner of CAM use, most frequently because they were not asked.

The failure to assess for CAM use is problematic for several reasons. Be aware that some people, because of cultural background, may seek CAM therapies before they even access Western medicine. Because many of these techniques lower blood pressure, decrease heart rate, and reduce pain and anxiety, closely monitor clients' medications.

Box 33-2 Mental Health Problems and Related CAM Therapies

Alcohol Abuse

- Acupuncture
- Herbal therapy (kudzu)
- Meditation/medical meditation
- Yoga

Alzheimer's Dementia

- Herbal therapy (gingko)
- Dietary supplements (omega-3 fatty acids)
- Massage
- Medical meditation

Anxiety

- Acupressure
- Biofeedback
- Breathing and relaxation techniques
- Guided imagery
- Healing touch/therapeutic touch
- Self-hypnosis
- Massage
- Meditation/medical meditation

Attention Deficit/Hyperactivity Disorder

- Biofeedback

Depression

- Acupuncture
- Healing touch/therapeutic touch
- Herbal therapy (St. John's wort)
- Meditation/medical meditation
- Transcranial magnetic stimulation

Insomnia

- Breathing and relaxation techniques
- Herbal therapy (valerian/melatonin)
- Meditation

Obsessive–Compulsive Disorder

- Acupuncture
- Medical meditation

Stress

- Breathing and relaxation exercises
- Healing touch/therapeutic touch
- Massage
- Meditation/medical meditation

Monitoring is particularly important for psychiatric clients receiving psychotropic medications that may cause hypotension. Clients with cardiac problems may be at increased risk for cardiac arrhythmia because of vasovagal stimulation with certain techniques such as active progressive relaxation. The potential for medication–CAM interaction is considerable. Medication–CAM interactions are discussed later in this chapter, especially in the section on herbal therapy.

DEEP-BREATHING AND RELAXATION TECHNIQUES

Many clients can reduce the stress in their environmental, physiological, and cognitive lives. Doing so prevents involuntary fight-or-flight responses from taking over (see Chapter 8 ∞). Like clients in any other health care setting, psychiatric clients must endure time pressures, weather, noise, crowds, interpersonal demands, job performance demands, and various threats to security and self-esteem. And, perhaps more than clients in many of the other settings in which nurses practice, psychiatric clients experience cognitive stress because of how they interpret and label their experiences. For instance, a client might interpret the boss's facial expression as amused rather than pleased or as disgruntled rather than quizzical. This interpretation is likely to provoke anxiety. Dwelling on one's concerns and anxieties causes physical tension in the body, which in turn creates the subjective feeling of uneasiness and leads to more anxious thoughts.

Evidence for the effectiveness of relaxation techniques is mixed. They are useful for reducing stress and anxiety and possibly for insomnia and hypertension and they have been found to be helpful in controlling pain. Relaxation techniques may be a solution for people who are depressed and refuse antidepressants. In this instance, relaxation techniques can be a first-line treatment in a stepped-care approach to depression (Jorm, Morgan, & Hetrick, 2011). That is, those who do not respond within a set time could be offered more complex treatments for depression such as cognitive–behavioral therapy.

A major benefit is that in using them, clients are in charge of their own well-being and health. There are some techniques, identified later in this section, which may aggravate the conditions of clients with schizophrenia or severe depression. There are no serious risks with the use of relaxation techniques if used appropriately.

The deep-breathing and relaxation exercises that follow are based on the belief that mind and body are interrelated and that the condition of one will eventually affect the condition of the other. A relaxed body is incompatible with anxiety. If the body is relaxed, the mind will feel relaxed, as well.

Body Scanning to Assess Body Tension

The importance of body states and their relationship to stress have been emphasized by Eastern philosophies such as yoga and Zen. Because stress and body tension are simultaneous, one of the first steps in recognizing stress and anxiety is recognizing tension in the body. Body scanning helps you to become aware of where tension collects in your body and is an effective way to begin any of the relaxation techniques that follow. Use the step-by-step guide in Your Self-Awareness to help yourself become aware of the tension you carry in your body. You can use the same step-by-step guide to teach body scanning to your clients.

YOUR SELF-AWARENESS
Body Scanning to Assess Body Tension

In order to help others become aware of their own body tension, you must first become aware of where you carry tension in your own body. Use the following step-by-step guide to perform a self-assessment. You can follow these same guidelines when teaching clients and their families.

- Make sure that the spine is straight before beginning body scanning or any of the other exercises described in this chapter. Stand, sit, or lie on the floor, whichever is most comfortable, while maintaining good posture.
- Begin by closing your eyes and turning your attention to your own internal world, focusing on your body.
- Focus on your toes and move up slowly.
- As you do this, ask yourself: "Where am I tense?"
- Become aware of all of the muscles in your body and especially the parts of your body that feel tense or tight.
- Notice the location of the tenseness and talk to yourself about it, reminding yourself that muscular tension is self-induced. Perhaps you might say: "The muscles in the back of my neck feel tight. This means that I'm creating tension in my body. Tension causes me problems."

Enhancing Relaxation With Music

Many people find that listening to soothing music is relaxing. Music, on audiotape, compact disc (CD), videotape, or digital video disc (DVD), can help clients reduce anxiety and achieve relaxation and can also be a substitute for, or adjunct to, pain medication and tranquilizers. Oncology nurses and hospice nurses often use music as a nonpharmaceutical pain intervention. Recorded music may be used before or during surgery as in the clinical example, during dental work, chemotherapy, kidney dialysis, during recovery from spinal injury or burns, and to decrease anxiety in young children during treatment procedures.

Clinical Example

Benjamin is a cardiac surgeon. He plays soft jazz when he operates. Benjamin finds the music soothing and says that it helps him to keep his concentration fully on the client and the operative procedure. He also believes that the client, although anesthetized, and the other operating room staff also derive benefit from the music's soothing nature.

Music can be combined with body scanning and the breathing exercises discussed later in this chapter to help psychiatric clients reduce anxiety.

Music can also be effectively used in conjunction with guided imagery. You can teach clients to lower their blood pressure 10 to 20 points by using a combination of visual imagery and music. Music with 60 beats per minute can help those with cardiac arrhythmias achieve a better-regulated heart rate. Guided imagery (visualization) is discussed later in this chapter.

How does music achieve its relaxing effect? Soothing music produces endorphins in the brain, the same "feel-good" chemicals that running and meditation produce. These natural opiates, secreted by the hypothalamus, reduce the intensity with which pain is felt. Because people vary in their response to music, encourage clients to experiment with different kinds of music to discover which has positive effects and then to develop their own personal library. Tapes, CDs, and DVDs specifically for stress reduction are sold in bookstores and through catalogs. They are often available through local public libraries.

Recommend that clients pay attention to their breathing as they listen to music. Slow and deep breathing enhances the relaxing effect of music.

Breathing Exercises

Under most circumstances, people take breathing for granted as an automatic body function. They usually become aware of their pattern of breathing only when it has gone awry, such as when they are out of breath. Breathing properly can, by itself, reduce stress. Breathing calmly and deeply keeps the blood well oxygenated and purified. It helps remove waste materials from the blood and clears thinking. Poorly oxygenated blood may contribute to fatigue, mental confusion, anxiety, muscular tension, and feelings of depression.

As a nursing student, you may find deep breathing especially helpful when preparing for an anxiety-provoking experience such as taking a final examination, embarking upon a new clinical experience, or taking the RN licensure examination. Practicing a stress-management technique such as deep breathing on a regular basis helps to decrease test anxiety, nervousness, self-doubt, and concentration loss. Relaxation techniques may also reduce distraction and increase positive mood states. Be careful not to remove all traces of anxiety. As Chapter 8 ∞ reminds you, a mild level of anxiety is necessary for learning to take place.

The following exercises are designed to facilitate proper breathing.

Awareness of Breathing

Do you breathe properly, or does your breathing actually deprive you of oxygen? Take time to pay attention to your own breathing. Begin by placing one hand just below your rib cage and taking a deep breath. Notice what happens when you inhale. Does your hand move in? Does your hand move out? Does your hand move at all? If your hand moves out, you are breathing properly. But if your hand moves in or does not move at all, it is probably because you learned, as most of us have, to hold your stomach in and push your chest out while breathing. People who breathe this way do not fill the lungs to full capacity; they fill only the top third or top half.

Deep Breathing

During **deep breathing**, you move the diaphragm downward and fill the lower part of the lungs with air. The chest expands as the middle part fills with air, and the shoulders move upward as the upper part fills. To teach yourself or a client how to take deep, healthful breaths, follow the directions in Partnering With Clients and Families: Guidelines for Deep-Breathing Exercises. Remember also to use these same directions when you teach clients to deep breathe after surgery.

Deep breathing becomes easier with practice. It may become almost automatic. This is an exercise few resist—it is easy to do, it is inconspicuous, and it yields fast results.

10-to-1 Count

This exercise is also quick and simple. To teach yourself or a client how to perform the 10-to-1 exercise, follow the directions in Partnering With Clients and Families below. Some people use an abbreviated version and begin counting at the number 5; others require the full count of 10 to feel calm. If clients have problems with attention span, recommend that they begin with 5, rather than 10, deep breaths.

Clinical Example

Carolyn taught deep breathing to the clients on a long term psychiatric inpatient unit. First, she helped them to become aware of their breathing before she taught them to breathe properly. Next, she abbreviated the technique to 5 deep breaths because some clients found it difficult to maintain their attention for the 10 count. Carolyn also provided additional help to those clients who were able to perform the full 10 count. Once the clients mastered deep breathing, she intended to continue the program with alternate-nostril breathing for the clients who had tension and sinus headaches.

Alternate-Nostril Breathing

Although somewhat more difficult, alternate-nostril breathing, which stems from the practice of yoga, also helps reduce tension and sinus headaches. To teach yourself or a client how to perform alternate-nostril breathing, follow the directions in Partnering With Clients and Families below.

It may be easier to breathe through the right nostril at certain times of the day and through the left nostril at other times. The reason is that people breathe primarily through one nostril for approximately 4 hours and then breathe primarily through the other for the next 4 hours.

PARTNERING WITH CLIENTS AND FAMILIES

Guidelines for Deep-Breathing Exercises

Deep Breathing

- Sit, stand, or lie with your spine straight.
- Scan your body for tension.
- Place one hand on your chest and the other on your abdomen.
- Inhale slowly and deeply so that your abdomen pushes your hand up.
- Visualize your lungs slowly filling with air. Your chest should move only slightly as you inhale, but you should be aware of the movement of your abdomen.
- Exhale through your mouth, making a soft, whooshing sound by blowing gently. Keep your face, mouth, and jaw relaxed.
- Be aware of what it feels like and what you sound like when you breathe properly.
- Continue to take long, slow, deep breaths for at least 10 minutes at a time, once or twice a day.
- Increase the frequency if you wish, once you have mastered the technique.
- Scan your body again for tension, comparing the tension to what it was like before you began the deep-breathing exercise.

10-to-1 Count

- Sit, stand, or lie with your spine straight.
- Scan your body for tension.
- Incorporate the guidelines in the deep-breathing exercise described earlier.
- Inhale taking a deep breath, while saying the number "10" to yourself.
- Then exhale slowly, letting out all the air in your lungs.
- Inhale again, saying the number "9" to yourself.

- As you exhale, tell yourself: "I feel more relaxed than I did at number 10."
- With your next breath, say the number "8" to yourself.
- As you exhale, remind yourself: "I feel more relaxed than I did at number 9."
- Continue counting down and experience increasing calmness as you approach number 1.
- Scan your body again for tension, comparing the tension to what it was like before you began the deep-breathing exercise.

Alternate-Nostril Breathing

- Sit, stand, or lie with your spine straight.
- Scan your body for tension.
- Close off your right nostril by lightly pressing it with your right thumb.
- Then inhale through your left nostril as slowly and quietly as possible. (Do not exhale yet.)
- Remove your thumb from the right nostril and use your forefinger to close off the left nostril.
- Exhale slowly through your right nostril.
- Inhale through your right nostril as slowly and quietly as possible.
- Follow the procedure outlined earlier, closing your right nostril with your right thumb while exhaling through your left nostril.
- The basic cycle is 10 breaths; this can be increased up to 25 breaths.
- Scan your body again for tension, comparing the tension to what it was like before you began the deep-breathing exercise.

Progressive Relaxation

The technique of **progressive relaxation** is based on the premise that muscle tension is the body's physiological response to anxiety-provoking thoughts. Muscular tension increases the feeling of anxiety and reinforces it. Deep muscle relaxation, by contrast, decreases physiological tension and blocks anxiety.

Progressive relaxation decreases pulse and respiratory rates, blood pressure, and perspiration. In addition, it helps reduce anxiety. Clients with muscle spasms, lower-back pain, tension headaches, insomnia, anxiety, depression, fatigue, irritable bowel syndrome, hypertension, or mild phobias are among those who can achieve positive results using this technique. Some clients report feeling less alert after either active or passive progressive relaxation. When alertness is important, one of the other deep-breathing exercises is probably better.

It may take longer to master progressive relaxation than the deep-breathing techniques discussed earlier. With practice, however, one can learn to relax faster and more easily.

Active Progressive Relaxation

Active progressive relaxation helps people identify which muscles or muscle groups are chronically tense by distinguishing between sensations of tension (purposeful muscle tensing) and deep relaxation (a conscious relaxing of the muscles). You can teach yourself or your clients active progressive relaxation by implementing the procedure outlined in Partnering With Clients and Families: Guidelines for Active Progressive Relaxation. Be sure to attend to the cautions described there.

Passive Progressive Relaxation

In *passive progressive relaxation,* the muscles are not tensed. The goal is to relax the muscles without first tightening them. The sequence in which body parts are relaxed differs from that of the active progressive method. Begin with muscles easiest to relax (in the toes) and progress to muscles most difficult to relax (in the head). The sequence is as follows: feet, lower legs, knees and upper legs, hips and buttocks, lower back, lower arms and hands, chest and diaphragm, abdomen, pelvis and genitals, neck, forehead and upper face, mouth and jaw.

VISUALIZATION AND IMAGERY

Émile Coué, a French pharmacist, began to use the power of imagination with clients in the late 19th century. Carl Jung used it in his psychiatric practice during the early part of the 20th century. Nurses use it because it is time and cost effective and creates a healing partnership between nurse and client. Most recently, contemporary clinicians and individual clients have had remarkable success in the use of visualization to achieve control over serious physical illness and emotional discomfort and to improve quality of life.

Positive **visualization**, or **imagery**, uses the healing power of a person's own imagination and positive thinking to create powerful mental pictures or images to reduce stress or promote healing. Because of the vivid mental images that can be created, imagery has been considered by some to be a form of hypnosis (see the following section on hypnotherapy and self-hypnosis). Use visualization in conjunction with the body-scanning and deep-breathing exercises discussed earlier.

PARTNERING WITH CLIENTS AND FAMILIES

Guidelines for Active Progressive Relaxation

In active progressive relaxation, each muscle or muscle grouping is tensed for 5 to 7 seconds and then relaxed for 10 to 15 seconds. Repeat the cycle.

Four major muscle groups are covered in this order: (1) hands, forearms, and biceps; (2) head, face, throat, and shoulders; (3) chest, abdomen, and lower back; (4) thighs, buttocks, calves, and feet using this procedure:

- Practice progressive relaxation while lying down or seated in a chair with feet firmly on the floor.
- Begin active progressive relaxation by tightening the right fist (5 to 7 seconds) and paying attention to the tension. Allow the muscles of the right fist to relax (15 to 20 seconds), while noticing the pleasant difference.

- Do the same with the left fist—tensing, relaxing, and noticing the difference.
- Follow the same procedure for the forearms (tensing and relaxing as explained earlier), and then for the biceps, remembering to compare the difference in sensation between tensed and relaxed muscles.
- Progress through the next major muscle group—head, face, throat, and shoulders.
- Move to the third major muscle group—chest, abdomen, and lower back.
- End with the fourth major muscle group—thighs, buttocks, calves, and feet.
- Remember to return to muscle groups that are only partially relaxed to bring about deeper relaxation.

Caution: Counsel clients to observe some cautions while carrying out this technique. To avoid soft tissue and spinal injury, the client should not excessively tighten muscles of the neck and back. Tightening the muscles of the toes and feet too vigorously could also result in uncomfortable muscle cramps. Caution clients with cardiac arrhythmias against vasovagal stimulation by tensing muscles too tightly. Postoperative clients should probably avoid active progressive relaxation, a practice that could increase pain in the postoperative period. Teach these clients passive progressive relaxation instead.

Not everyone finds it easy to use the imagination in this way, and the technique may not work for everyone. Constructing a detailed, effective visualization requires time, patience, and practice. Some people find that **guided imagery**—using an outside resource such as an actual person who guides the imagery process or a voice on an audiotape or CD—helps to create a series of images. You can also implement the guidelines in Partnering With Clients and Families: Guidelines for Constructing a Visualization with soft background music to record your own guided imagery experience for relaxation, guidance, symptom control or pain relief, or to record a guided imagery for a client.

Nurses interested in gaining expertise in incorporating guided imagery into their practice might consider a certification program. Both the American Holistic Nurses Association and the Academy for Guided Imagery provide continuing education and certification programs. Such data can be accessed through a direct resource link on the Online Student Resources for this book. The website of the American Holistic Nurses Association also provides information on programs of study, standards of practice, and student memberships.

Visualization for Relaxation

Relaxing through visualization is enhanced by constructing in one's own mind a relaxing environment. Some people find the soothing sounds of the seashore calming; others prefer to imagine themselves floating above the world on a soft cloud or a magic carpet. Still others relax as they imagine themselves descending on a slow-moving escalator into a calmer and more relaxed state. If visualization seems difficult (and if a warm bath, hot tub, or swimming pool is relaxing), try constructing a visualization while in warm water, combining the physiological effects of the warm water with the products of the imagination.

Visualization for Guidance

Visualization can also be useful when seeking guidance, direction, or help with decision making. Upon reaching a special soothing place, visualize an "inner advisor" or "wise person." You can ask for an image to appear or use someone you know—a valued teacher, a historical figure (Florence Nightingale, Martin Luther King, Jr., Mother Theresa), a beloved grandparent (see Partnering With Clients and Families). Students often find this helpful during test taking.

Visualization for Symptom Control or Healing

Visualization techniques for symptom control or healing can be part of a well-rounded health program. For example, visualization can be used in conjunction with conventional medical treatment for people with cancer, people with pain, and to enhance tissue healing. Two suggestions for constructing visualizations for guidance and pain or symptom relief are given in Partnering With Clients and Families.

HYPNOTHERAPY AND SELF-HYPNOSIS

Hypnotherapy is the therapeutic use of suggestion during an altered state of consciousness to effect positive changes in a person's behavior and to treat a wide range of health conditions. Clinical trials show it is effective in reducing pain, anxiety, stress, hypertension, insomnia, and the symptoms of irritable bowel syndrome. It has also been used as an adjunct to anesthesia or in place of anesthesia, to treat tension and migraine headaches, to decrease dependence on tobacco, for weight control, in dentistry, and in trancelike states to access the deepest levels of the mind. However, it appears not to be effective for smoking cessation even though it is heavily promoted for this purpose (Singh & Ernst, 2009).

PARTNERING WITH CLIENTS AND FAMILIES

Guidelines for Constructing a Visualization

- Assume a position of comfort—either lying down or sitting up.
- Take five cleansing deep breaths. With each inhalation, imagine that you are taking in calmness and peacefulness. With each exhalation, imagine that you are releasing tension, discomfort, and worry.
- Allow your body to become increasingly relaxed with each deep breath.
- Use all your senses—seeing, hearing, touching, smelling, tasting—as you imagine yourself to be in an especially beautiful and wonderful place for you. What are the colors, shapes, and living things in your special place? What do you hear and smell? What objects and shapes do you feel? What do you usually taste in this place?
- If constructing a *visualization for guidance,* put your wise person into your special place. Use all your senses to imagine this

person. What color hair, eyes, and skin does your wise person have? What are the textures of that person's clothes? What smells do you associate with that person? What does it feel like to grasp that person's hand?
- If constructing a *visualization for pain or symptom relief,* the goal is to associate orange or red lights with the pain or symptom, and then to change the orange or red lights to blue lights that signify a change to pain-free or calm or symptom-free states. Another visualization involves attaching a symbolic visual image to the pain (a lump in the throat, a hammer pounding the head, a dog gnawing on a bone) and then imagining the symbol becoming weakened as the pain or symptom lessens.
- When you're ready, allow the images to fade. Take whatever time you need to bring yourself back to your outer world by slowly opening your eyes and stretching.

Although hypnotherapy has been practiced in many cultures for thousands of years, its use in health care became more common in the mid-20th century when the American Medical Association approved its use as a valid medical intervention. In hospitals today, it is not uncommon to find anesthesiologists, nurses, surgeons, psychologists, dentists, and social workers who use hypnosis in their therapeutic work. Nurses who wish to use hypnosis in their clinical practice must recognize that it is an advanced intervention that requires specialized training in hypnotherapy. It is also important to be aware of whether your state board of nursing identifies hypnosis as within the scope of practice of nurses.

Self-hypnosis has the potential to provide anxiety relief and reduce pain without undue cost. People practice **self-hypnosis**—hypnosis accomplished by oneself without the help of a second party as hypnotist—to achieve significant relaxation, to reduce anxiety, to manage low to moderate levels of chronic pain, to make positive suggestions for change (such as to lose weight, to overcome fear of the dark, or to overcome insomnia), and to increase learning and remembering. TABLE 33-1 ■ gives examples of some life problems and the hypnotic suggestions that can be used to overcome them.

Most people can achieve significant relaxation within 2 days with self-hypnosis. Self-hypnosis can be self-taught through books on the subject. Community adult education programs and holistic health centers often offer courses on self-hypnosis. Anyone with psychosis or severe mental problems should not use self-hypnosis.

MEDITATION

The increased use of meditation in North America owes much to Herbert Benson, a Harvard physician who identified and promoted the scientific benefits of meditation as a relaxation response almost 40 years ago (Benson & Klipper, 2000). **Meditation** helps one achieve inner peace and harmony by focusing uncritically on one thing at a time. Meditation has been associated with various religious and cultural practices and philosophies for thousands of years. It is seen as a way of becoming one with a higher power or the universe, finding enlightenment, and achieving such virtues as selflessness. However, the person who practices meditation need not associate it with religion or philosophy. It can be practiced as a means of reducing inner discord and increasing self-knowledge.

Effects of Meditation

The state of meditation is equivalent to a state of deep rest. The heart rate slows, the body uses less oxygen, and blood lactate—a waste product of metabolism—decreases sharply. Alpha brain waves, present during states of calm alertness, increase, as does the secretion of dopamine—the happiness neurotransmitter. There appear to be beneficial effects on cardiovascular functioning at rest and during acute stress situations. Meditation is also effective in decreasing mood disturbance and stress symptoms. The regular practice of meditation may even have neuroprotective effects and reduce the cognitive decline associated with aging.

TABLE 33-1 ■ Life Problems and Related Hypnotic Suggestions

Life Problem	Hypnotic Suggestion
Fear of coming into a dark house at night	I can come in tonight feeling relaxed and glad to be home.
Anxiety that prevents working or studying to meet deadlines	I can work steadily and calmly. My concentration is improving as I become more relaxed.
Insomnia	I will gradually become more and more drowsy. In just a few minutes, I will be able to fall asleep and will sleep peacefully all night.
Chronic fatigue	I can wake up feeling refreshed and relaxed.
Minor chronic headache or backache	As I become more relaxed, my headache (backache) lessens. In just a few minutes, it will go away. Soon, my head will be cool and relaxed. Gradually I will feel the muscles in my back loosen, and in an hour, they will be completely relaxed. Whenever these symptoms come back, I will simply turn my ring a quarter of a turn to the right and the pain will relax away.
Feelings of inferiority	The next time I see _____, I can feel secure in myself. I can feel relaxed and at ease because I am perfectly all right.
Anxiety about an upcoming evaluation or test	Whenever I feel nervous, I can say to myself…(insert your special key word or phrase here)…and relax.
Chronic anger or chronic guilt	I can turn off anger (guilt) because I am the one who turns it on. I will relax my body and breathe deeply.
Worry about interpersonal rejection	Whenever I lace my fingers together, I will feel confidence flowing through me.
Chronic tension or discomfort in a particular part of the body	I will think about my _____ every hour and let it relax.

YOUR INTERVENTION STRATEGIES
The Four Major Requirements for Successful Meditation

1. ***A quiet place.*** The environment for meditation should be one that minimizes distractions—a quiet place set aside as a haven from the urgencies of everyday life.
2. ***A comfortable position.*** A comfortable position that can be held for 20 minutes without stress facilitates meditation.
3. ***An object or thought to focus on.*** A repeated word (mantra), an object or symbol to look at or think about, or a specific thought or feeling helps keep distracting thoughts from entering the mind.
4. ***A passive attitude.*** A passive attitude requires understanding that thoughts and distractions will occur and can be cleared from the mind. If they occur, they should be noted and released without concern about their interference. It is counterproductive to worry about how well you are doing at meditating.

Clients who meditate have shown improvements in symptoms of depression and anxiety. Mindfulness-based (meditation) cognitive therapy is a cost-effective educational protocol (as an eight-session course) when delivered to participants in groups.

Steps in Meditating

Meditation exercises can be relatively easy to learn. Some people experience immediate relief and pleasure in only one session. To experience deeper effects, the person needs to practice meditation regularly for at least a month. There are four major requirements for successful meditation. They are discussed in Your Intervention Strategies.

Many people who meditate prefer to use a **mantra**, a syllable, word, or name that is repeatedly chanted aloud. Some teachers of meditation insist that each person have a special mantra with a specific meaning and vibration to achieve individual effects. Others recommend the use of any word or phrase the individual is drawn to, such as *love* or *calm*. Some popular mantras are *om* (I am), *so-ham* (I am he), *sa-ham* (I am she), *Shalom* (peace), and *The Lord is my shepherd*.

Avoid chanting too loudly or too vigorously. After about 5 minutes, shift to whispering the mantra as you relax more deeply. When it is not possible to chant aloud, you can chant silently.

Medical Meditation

More recently, scientific research has demonstrated that one of the newest and most cutting-edge advances in CAM is medical meditation. **Medical meditation** is meditation combined with adaptations of kundalini yoga (which is much more than simply a fitness-oriented practice). Medical meditation has specific physiological effects that can target such disorders as arthritis, anxiety disorder, diabetes, depression, hypertension, and many other physical and mental conditions (Khalsa & Stauth, 2001). Recent research demonstrates that medical meditation is a promising treatment for people with Alzheimer's disease and memory loss associated with aging (Newberg, Wintering, Khalsa, Roggenkamp, & Waldman, 2010).

Medical meditations unite the body, mind, and spirit by amplifying the energy system of the body that is, according to Hindu tradition, located in the seven major **chakras**. Chakras are concentrated areas of energy vertically aligned through the center of the body from the crown of the head to the pelvis (see FIGURE 33-3 ■). The chakras influence the physical body, the emotions, and the spirit. Each chakra corresponds to specific body structures and organs and has specific functions. The three lower chakras are primarily involved with basic elements of life such as survival, power, financial security, and procreation. The four higher chakras are involved with the higher, more advanced elements of life such as intellect, intuition, compassion, and spirituality.

Medical meditations are very specific. They involve special postures and movements, exact positioning of the hands and fingers, specific mantras, and specific breathing patterns in order to activate specific chakras.

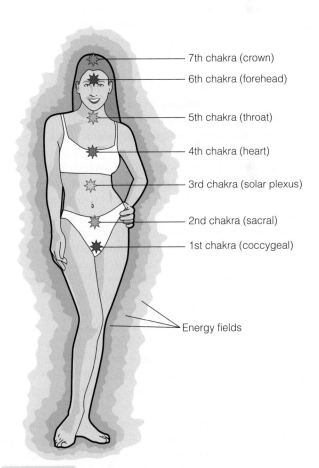

- 7th chakra (crown)
- 6th chakra (forehead)
- 5th chakra (throat)
- 4th chakra (heart)
- 3rd chakra (solar plexus)
- 2nd chakra (sacral)
- 1st chakra (coccygeal)
- Energy fields

FIGURE 33-3 ■ The seven major chakras, according to Hindu tradition, are concentrated areas of energy.

PRESSURE POINT THERAPIES

Several approaches use the application of pressure or stimulation to specific points on the body to promote healing, relieve pain, or promote wellness.

Acupuncture

Acupuncture originated in China more than 2,000 years ago and has grown in popularity in the United States over the past 20 years as more anesthesiologists, neurologists, nurses, specialists in physical medicine, and specialists in addictions are becoming trained and certified as practitioners by the National Certification Commission for Acupuncture and Oriental Medicine (http://www.nccaom.org). A national health interview survey of U.S. citizens found that 4.1% of the respondents reported lifetime use of acupuncture, and 1.1% (representing 2.13 million Americans) reported recent use (Burke, Upchurch, Dye, & Chyu, 2006). Musculoskeletal complaints were the most frequently reported condition, led by back pain (34%).

Acupuncture is based on the belief that the vital life energy of the body (*ch'i* or *qi*, pronounced "chee") circulates along 12 major and 8 secondary pathways, called *meridians* (note that scientists are unable to find evidence for the existence of meridians or ch'i). These pathways are linked to specific and organ systems. Hair-thin needles placed at acupuncture sites are used to stimulate the meridians and influence the flow of energy that affects internal organs.

According to the NIH consensus development statement on acupuncture (1997), stimulating acupuncture points causes biochemical changes in the central nervous system that either change the experience of pain or release other chemicals, such as hormones and neurotransmitters, which influence the body's self-regulating systems. The biochemical changes may stimulate the body's natural healing abilities and promote physical and emotional well-being. In 2003, the World Health Organization (WHO) published a misleading document on the effectiveness of acupuncture (Singh & Ernst, 2009). The document was based on several unreliable clinical trials and it endorsed acupuncture as a treatment for over 100 conditions. Systematic reviews by the Cochrane Collaboration indicate that acupuncture can reduce nausea and vomiting after surgery (Lee & Fan, 2011) and reduce the initial nausea associated with chemotherapy (Ezzo et al., 2011). There is some tentative evidence that acupuncture might be effective for some forms of pain relief as well; however, acupuncture fails to deliver any medical benefit in other situations (Singh & Ernst, 2009). There is no evidence that acupuncture is useful for the treatment of insomnia (Cheuk, Young, Chung, & Wong, 2011), depression (Smith, Hay, MacPherson, 2011), or schizophrenia (Rathbone & Xia, 2011).

Acupuncture, specifically auricular (ear) acupuncture, is widely used to ease withdrawal and treat addiction in alcoholics, drug addicts, and smokers in North America and in Europe (substance-related disorders are discussed in Chapter 15 ⚭). However, evidence from controlled studies regarding its effectiveness as a treatment for substance addiction has been inconclusive. The widespread acceptance of auricular acupuncture in the treatment of addictions remains controversial (Black, Carey, Webber, Neish, & Gilbert, 2011). Further research into the effectiveness of acupuncture as an ancillary therapy in addiction treatment is needed.

Acupressure

Acupressure is based on the same principles as acupuncture, but does not involve needles. Instead, finger pressure or implements are used to stimulate the meridians. Shiatsu massage, Jin Shin Jyutsu, and Jin Shin Do are forms of acupressure that stem from the Japanese tradition. **Reflexology** is the practice of acupressure on particular points of the feet, hands, and ears. There is no convincing evidence that reflexology can diagnose a health problem (the notion that resistance in one area of the foot is an indicator for a problem with a specific organ) or is effective for any condition. Reflexology offers the benefits of a relaxing foot massage. Several reflexology maps exist but do not agree among themselves how to apply the treatment. One such foot reflexology map is illustrated in FIGURE 33-4 ■.

1. Head and brain	11. Liver
2. Pituitary and pineal glands	12. Gallbladder
3. Throat and thyroid gland	13. Kidney
4. Sinus	14. Adrenal gland
5. Eyes and ears	15. Spleen
6. Shoulder	16. Pancreas
7. Heart	17. Small intestine
8. Lungs and thymus gland	18. Large intestine
9. Diaphragm and solar plexus	19. Bladder
10. Stomach	20. Sacrum and sciatic nerve

FIGURE 33-4 ■ Foot reflexology points.
Source: Fontaine, K. L. (2011). *Complementary and alternative healing therapies for nursing practice* (3rd ed.). Upper Saddle River, NJ: Prentice Hall, p. 216.

PARTNERING WITH CLIENTS AND FAMILIES

Self-Help Pressure Point and Finger Holding Techniques

Pressure Point Therapy to Ease Tension and Restore Energy

- Hold your left palm in front of you, fingers together.
- Using your right thumb, massage the fleshy spot between your thumb and index finger for a slow count of 15 (this spot is a key pressure point).
- Then switch hands, and repeat the process.

Finger Holds to Improve General Well-Being

Gently hold the appropriate finger on either hand while imagining negative emotions melting away and physical symptoms easing.

- **Thumb.** Corresponds to worrying, depression, and anxiety. Physical symptoms may be stomachaches, headaches, skin problems, and nervousness.

- **Index finger.** Corresponds to fear, mental confusion, and frustration. Physical symptoms are digestive problems and muscular problems such as backaches.
- **Middle finger.** Corresponds to anger, irritability, and indecisiveness. Physical symptoms are eye or vision problems, fatigue, and circulation problems.
- **Ring finger.** Corresponds to sadness, fear of rejection, grief, and negativity. Physical symptoms are digestive, breathing, or serious skin problems.
- **Little finger.** Corresponds to insecurity, effort, overdoing it, and nervousness. Physical symptoms are sore throat and bone or nerve problems.

Source: Fontaine, K. L. (2004). *Healing practices: Alternative therapies for nursing* (2nd ed.). Upper Saddle River, NJ: Prentice Hall, p. 214.

While these practices involve advanced training, you can incorporate noninvasive hand, foot, or ear massages into your clinical practice (Fontaine, 2011). Partnering With Clients and Families: Self-Help Pressure Point and Finger Holding Techniques discusses pressure points and finger holds that you can teach others as a self-help process.

TOUCH AND BIOFIELD THERAPIES

Touch therapies for healing, or the "laying on of hands" to help heal, are as old as history. However, the research on touch therapies is still in the early stages of development. Although the data are promising, to date they can only suggest that touch therapies may reduce anxiety, improve muscle relaxation, aid in promoting wound healing, and reduce pain. Most of what we call "laying-on-of-hands" modalities involves the transfer of energy (see the earlier discussion of chakras). For some modalities, it is somewhat of a misnomer to attach the word *touch*. In the nurse-developed biofield therapies discussed later in this section, the practitioner may not actually touch the client, or may only lightly touch.

Nurses around the globe use massage and biofield therapies to assist in easing pain and anxiety, promoting relaxation, accelerating wound healing, diminishing depression, and increasing the sense of well-being. Use caution in the use of any touch therapies with psychiatric clients. It is best not to touch psychiatric clients unless there is sound rationale. The principles and rationale for this caution are discussed in Chapters 4 and 10∞.

Massage

Massage is most probably helpful for people with pain and anxiety because it releases endorphins. Nurses have traditionally used massage to ease a client's discomfort and to develop a connection with the client. Increasing numbers of nurses, such as Melanie in the clinical example that follows,

focus on this CAM modality as licensed massage therapists in private practice and are affiliated with the American Massage Therapy Association (AMTA) (http://www.amtamassage.org, accessible through the Online Student Resources for this book).

Clinical Example

Melanie is a registered nurse who had had a private practice in massage therapy for 14 years. Melanie provides light touch Swedish massage, deeper sports massage, Reiki (discussed next), and finger acupressure, depending on the client's needs. Prior to beginning work with any client, Melanie uses her nursing assessment skills to determine whether the client is an appropriate candidate for massage and whether or not the client should be referred to a primary health care practitioner. Melanie incorporates aromatherapy in the massage oils she uses and provides a softly lighted environment with soothing background music.

A recent study found some evidence in favor of massage and touch interventions with dementia. As a complement to other therapies for dementia, massage can reduce anxiety, agitated behavior, and depression (Hansen, Jorgensen, & Ortenblad, 2011).

Another modality that uses the hands is **Reiki**, a gentle laying on of hands corresponding to the seven main chakras, discussed earlier on page 727. In Reiki, a popular form of spiritual healing, energy flows though the healer's hands. Clinical trial evidence to date fails to show its effectiveness for any condition. Currently, there is research underway to determine the effectiveness of Reiki for anxiety and depression.

Chiropractic

Chiropractic is the most frequently used alternative treatment—that is, it is often used in place of conventional medicine. It is

Therapeutic Touch

American Massage Therapy Association

based on the belief that symptoms can be relieved through the manipulation of misaligned spinal vertebrae. The chiropractor submits the vertebrae of the spine to a technique called *high-velocity, low-amplitude (HVLA) thrust,* a technique that pushes a joint beyond the point of resistance. The application of this force is called *spinal manipulation*; also called an *adjustment* by chiropractors. In its early development, chiropractic was based on the belief that all diseases stemmed from misaligned spinal vertebrae. Today, chiropractic takes a multicausational approach, although the chief modality for practice remains spinal manipulation.

Risks Associated With Chiropractic

Chiropractors can effectively treat some back problems, although chiropractic treatment for back problems is no more effective than conventional physical therapy, a much safer treatment (Walker, Frenchy, Grant, & Green, 2011; Rubinstein, van Middlekoop, Assendelft, de Boer, & van Tulder, 2011). According to the Cochrane Collection (Singh & Ernst, 2009), other claims are unsubstantiated and can carry a range of significant risks. Some of the most frequently cited risks in the literature have to do with applying heavy forces to adult necks (which can result in spinal compression fractures and dissection or rupture of the vertebral artery), manipulating the fragile bones of infants and young children, and exposing clients to excessive radiation.

Following are situations in which HVLA of the neck that causes dissection or rupture of the vertebral artery can result in death:

1. The formation of a blood clot because of damage to the vertebral artery can eventually become dislodged and travel into the brain where it blocks a distant part of the artery.
2. In vertebral artery dissection, blood can become trapped between the inner and outer layers of the artery causing swelling, and thus reducing the flow of blood to the brain.
3. Injury to the vertebral artery can cause it to go into spasm, thus reducing the flow of blood when the artery contracts.

Any one of these situations can lead to a stroke and/or permanent brain damage and death.

While some studies have shown the risk of traumatic rupture to the vertebral artery to be only 1.46 per million neck manipulations, experts suspect that the majority of incidents go unreported or unrecognized because vertebral dissection may not occur immediately and thus, may not be immediately connected to the chiropractic treatment. The incidence could actually be as high as 1 in 100,000 persons receiving neck manipulation (Singh & Ernst, 2009).

Nurse-Developed Biofield Therapies

There are two nurse-developed biofield therapies that have led to the development of the NANDA diagnosis, *disturbed energy field*—Healing Touch and Therapeutic Touch. To date, there has been limited research testing these interventions even though there is significant attention to these modalities in the nursing practice literature. Severe criticisms of biofield therapies have been leveled by several nurse researchers and theorists and by other scientists and researchers (see http://quackwatch.org on page 719) who note the lack of evidence-based research and the significant financial gain to be made from the sale of training materials for both HT and TT.

Therapeutic Touch (TT) was developed by Dolores Krieger (1979, 1993), a nursing professor, as a nursing activity. TT is defined as an intentionally directed process of energy exchange during which the TT practitioner uses the hands as a focus to facilitate the healing process. **Healing Touch (HT)** was developed by Janet Mentgen (2001), also a nurse. HT uses light touch or near-touch to activate the human energy system and direct it toward healing. Unlike TT which is practiced by nurses alone, HT is practiced by nurses and a broader variety of practitioners.

In these biofield therapies, the therapist's goal is to direct energy from a universal source, or transfer energy from one place to another within the body of the client.

Clinical Example

Dorothy is a teacher of medical-surgical nursing at a Midwestern university. She learned TT directly from Dolores Kreiger, her nursing professor when she was in graduate school. Dorothy provides TT to colleagues and students when requested to do so. Dorothy also provides TT for hospitalized clients upon their request or upon recommendation by their physician. Dorothy validates that she receives sensory cues during the assessment/scanning phase discussed below.

Much of the early research was flawed although increasingly more sophisticated studies are providing limited evidence-based support. For example, a study with a small sample size of 20 was designed to study the impact of TT on biobehavioral markers. In this study, the subjects had lower levels of pain, lower cortisol levels, and an increase in natural killer cells (Coakley & Duffy, 2010). A systematic review by the Cochrane Collaboration supported the use of both therapies for pain relief (So, Jiang, & Qin, 2011). However, clinical trial data for HT have not been evaluated using a systematic, evidence-based approach (Anderson & Taylor, 2011).

Both biofield therapies use the process of centering before beginning. *Centering* is a process of bringing the body, mind, and emotions to a quiet, focused state of consciousness in order to find an inner sense of equilibrium and connect with the inner core of wholeness and stillness. This phase serves to gather and focus the healer's energies on the client and exclude extraneous thoughts from the mind, a process akin to meditation. This state of centeredness is maintained throughout the process.

A second phase is *assessing/scanning*. Holding the hands 2 to 6 inches away from the client's body, the practitioner moves the hands from the head to the feet in a rhythmic and symmetric manner to determine the nature of the dynamic energy field. Sensory cues such as warmth, coolness, static, blockage, pulling, and tingling are described by some practitioners. These areas indicate a static condition, an imbalance, or congestion in the client's energy field that extends beyond the person's physical body.

The *intervention* phase is next. Interventions are based on interview and assessment data and the needs of the individual client. A commonly used intervention is called *clearing*, or unruf*fling*, to facilitate the flow of energy through the field. The practitioner uses sweeping hand movements, with the palms facing the client, moving from the midline to the outer edge of the body in a rhythmic and symmetric manner from the head to the feet. The intent is to balance, or rebalance, the bioenergetic field.

The bioenergy field is then reassessed and the practitioner uses professional, informed, and intuitive judgment to determine when to end the session. Feedback is elicited from the client and the session is evaluated. Evaluation guides the responses, intention, and interactions of the practitioner. Clients often report a sense of relaxation and relief from pain.

Nurse practitioners of TT in the United States can be contacted through http://www.therapeutic-touch.org. In Canada, there are TT groups in Ontario (http://www.therapeutictouch-netwk.com), British Columbia, Alberta, and the Canadian Atlantic Coast. Practitioners of HT can be contacted through http://www.healingtouchinternational.org and http://www.healingtouchprogram.com. These resources can be found on the Online Student Resources for this text.

HERBALS AND BOTANICALS

Natural herbs have been used as medicines across the ages and across all cultures. Their use has grown tremendously within the past 15 years and has become a billion-dollar market. Thousands of natural herbal products are used for symptom relief in a variety of conditions. Although only a few of these herbs are used for treatment of emotional symptoms or mental disorder, herbs are widely used by people with mental health problems (Rawen, Zimmerman, Schultz, & Wallace, 2011). TABLE 33-2 ■ lists the natural medicines that are likely to be effective and safe for clients with psychiatric-related symptoms.

Be careful of buzzwords such as "natural" and "traditional" and "organic" and "most often used to treat" in advertisements that avoid the use of the words "safe" or "effective." Also, be aware that there may be insufficient reliable information available to judge the effectiveness or safety of many herbs. Consumers who rely on portrayals in the media for information on herbals and botanicals are not being provided with information sufficient to make informed choices. There may be errors of omission in descriptions of clinical trial quality, interactions

with other medications, and underreporting of the risks of herbal remedies (Thakor, Leach, Gillham, & Esterman, 2011). Testing in clinical trials is relatively recent, and little long-term random testing has been conducted.

Misconceptions also abound. For example, one common misconception is that the herb goldenseal can be used to mask the results of laboratory tests for illicit drug use. Goldenseal has been found to be ineffective for this purpose. Other misconceptions are that Bach flower remedies (in spring water to which brandy is added), can cure emotional imbalances such as apathy, demandingness, despondency, anger, and self-blame. People who use these products are often unaware of their potential toxicities. Always encourage clients to discuss with their health care provider all natural remedies that they ingest.

Herbal medicines offer some interesting remedies, but they are outnumbered by the unproven, disproven, and dangerous herbals remedies on the market. Following are three potential dangers posed by herbal medicines:

1. Direct toxic reaction from the herbal medicine
2. Indirect reactions caused by interactions with other medications
3. Risk from ingesting contaminants and adulterants

The safety and effectiveness of herbs can be validated at the following websites:

1. U.S. Food and Drug Administration (FDA): http://www.fda.gov
2. National Center for Complementary and Alternative Medicine: http://www.nccam.nih.gov
3. University of Washington Medicinal Herb Garden: http://www.nnlm.gov/pnr/uwmhg/
4. NIH Office of Dietary Supplements: http://ods.od.nih.gov

Adverse effects from dietary supplements can be reported to the FDA's MedWatch program at http://www.fda.gov/medwatch. These data can also be found as resource links on the Online Student Resources for this book.

These products are widely used by clients who are also taking prescribed psychotropic medications (Rawen et al., 2011). Psychotropic medications and the herbs that affect them are listed in TABLE 33-3 ■. Some herbals and botanicals may potentiate the effects of psychotropic medications; others may block the effects. Others may increase the extent of adverse side effects.

BIOFEEDBACK

Visceral learning, known as **biofeedback**, is a technique for gaining conscious control over involuntary body functions such as blood pressure and heart rate, which are mediated by the autonomic nervous system. It has been shown, for example, that biofeedback is a promising alternative treatment for attention deficit/hyperactivity disorder, which is discussed in Chapter 26∞, and for migraine headaches, which can be

Herbal Safety and Effectiveness

TABLE 33-2 ■ Herbals, Botanicals, and Dietary Supplements Used for Psychiatric Symptoms

Psychiatric Symptom	Natural Medicine	Effectiveness and Safety[a]
Anxiety/restlessness	Kava[b]	■ Comparable to low-dose benzodiazepines for short-term treatment of anxiety ■ Possibly unsafe over the long term or in high doses (associated with liver failure)
Dementia	Ginkgo leaf extract	■ Likely effective; effect is similar to that of donezepil (Aricept) ■ Likely safe when used orally ■ Likely unsafe when used intravenously (IV) ■ Warrants large-scale trials
	SAMe (S-adenosylmethionine)[c]	■ Likely safe orally, IV, and intramuscularly (IM)
Depression	St. John's wort	■ Evidence is contradictory—possibly as effective as fluoxetine (Prozac) and sertraline (Zoloft), or perhaps no more effective than placebo ■ Likely safe when used orally and short term ■ Possibly unsafe in large doses (1,800 mg or more per day) ■ Interferes with prescription medications by metabolizing them and transporting them out of the body
	SAMe	■ Possibly as effective as oral tricyclic antidepressants
Encephalopathy (alcoholic) or peripheral neuropathy	Thiamine (vitamin B$_1$)	■ Likely safe when taken orally ■ Rare hypersensitivity when taken IM or IV
Sleep disturbance/insomnia	Melatonin/valerian	■ Possibly effective for jet lag and insomnia ■ Likely ineffective for work shift change adjustment ■ Possibly safe when used orally or parenterally
Dementia of the Alzheimer's type	Omega-3 fatty acids[d]	■ May possibly slow the cognitive and functional decline in Alzheimer's

[a]According to the sources listed, these natural medicines are thought likely to be effective and safe when used appropriately. It is important to validate safety and effectiveness with the most up-to-date sources.

[b]NCCAM has placed studies of kava on hold, pending further guidance from the Federal Food and Drug Administration (FDA). To view the FDA advisory, go to http://www.cfsan.fda.gov/

[c]Available studies are limited by small numbers of subjects, inconsistent diagnostic criteria, and short treatment periods.

[d]In May 2007, NIH announced the launching of a nationwide trial to test whether omega-3 fatty acids can affect the progression of, and lower the risk of, Alzheimer's disease.

Source: Adapted from Brenner, R., Azbel, V., Madhusoodanan, S., & Pawlowska, M. (2000). Comparison of an extract of hypericum (LI 160) and sertraline in the treatment of depression: A double-blind, randomized pilot study. *Clinical Therapies, 22*, 411–419; Freeman, M. P., Hibbeln, J. R., Wisner, K. L., Davis, J. M., Mischoulon, D., Peet, M.,...Stoll, A. L. (2006). Omega-3 fatty acids: Evidence basis for treatment and future research in psychiatry. *Journal of Clinical Psychiatry, 67*(12), 1954–1967; Jellin, J. M., Gregory, P. J., Batz, F., & Bonakdar, K. (2002). *Pharmacist's letter/prescriber's letter natural medicines comprehensive database* (4th ed.). Stockton, CA: Therapeutic Research Faculty; and Wettstein, A. (2000). Cholinesterase inhibitors and ginkgo extracts—are they comparable in the treatment of dementia? Comparison of published placebo-controlled efficacy studies of at least six months' duration. *PhytoMedicine, 6*, 393–401.

relieved by increasing blood flow to the hands. Biofeedback has also been found to be useful in treating tension headaches, insomnia, muscle or colon spasm, pain, hypertension, asthma, stuttering, bruxism (grinding of the teeth), and epilepsy. The psychological states achieved through biofeedback can be beneficial in decreasing anxiety and phobic reactions.

The technique is based on giving continuous feedback through the use of machines about the results of each attempt at control until the person is able to achieve control without the aid of a machine. In a typical session, a person might be given this feedback by equipment that amplifies body signals and translates them into a flashing light or a steady tone. Once people can "see" a heartbeat, for instance, and observe when it slows down or speeds up, they have the information they need to control their heart rate by slowing a flashing light or altering a tone. Inexpensive equipment for home use is available.

REPETITIVE TRANSCRANIAL MAGNETIC STIMULATION

In **repetitive transcranial magnetic stimulation (rTMS)**, an insulated coil of wire is placed on the client's head. Short pulses of an electrical current, sent through the insulated coil, generate a magnetic field that causes neurochemical changes in specifically targeted structures of the brain. In comparison to electroconvulsive therapy (ECT) that uses a direct electric current, rTMS uses an indirect electric current to stimulate neurons in the brain and disrupt neuronal firing. It is being examined as an alternative to ECT. Unlike ECT, with rTMS there is no seizure and no need for anesthesia. Preliminary results from active research indicate that there may even be less memory loss with this treatment than with ECT.

As a therapy, left prefrontal rTMS has recently been approved by the Food and Drug administration for the treatment of depression where it has the most promising

TABLE 33-3 ■ Commonly Used Natural Medicines That Should Not Be Taken in Combination With Psychotropic Medication[a]

Psychotropic Medication	Natural Medicine
Anticonvulsants	Sage
Carbamazepine (Tegretol)	Grapefruit juice, psyllium
Antidepressants	European mistletoe, SAMe, St. John's wort
Clomipramine (Anafranil)	Grapefruit juice
Monoamine oxidase inhibitors (MAOIs)	American ginseng, black tea, brewer's yeast, caffeine, cocoa, coffee, cola nut, ephedra, fenugreek, ginkgo leaf extract, green tea, guarana, panax ginseng, passionflower, phenylalanine, wine, yohimbe
Serotonin agonists	5-HTP
Serotonin antagonists	5-HTP
SSRIs	St. John's wort, SAMe
Fluoxetine (Prozac)	Melatonin
Fluvoxamine (Luvox)	Melatonin
Tricyclics	Belladonna, St. John's wort, SAMe, yohimbe
Antipsychotics	American ginseng, coffee, panax ginseng, Siberian ginseng (*Eleutherococcus*)
Central nervous system depressants	German chamomile, hawthorn, kava, melatonin, stinging nettle (above-ground parts), wine
Alcohol	Gamma hydroxybutyrate (GHB), kava, Siberian ginseng, valerian
Central nervous system stimulants	American ginseng, panax ginseng
Caffeine	Cocoa, black tea, ephedra, green tea, guarana, panax ginseng
Fenfluramine	St. John's wort
Clozapine (Clozaril)	Black tea, caffeine, cocoa, coffee, cola nut, green tea, guarana
Lithium	Black tea, caffeine, cocoa, coffee, green tea, guarana, psyllium
Phenothiazines	Evening primrose oil, yohimbe
Sedatives	Goldenseal, gotu kola, kava, passionflower, Siberian ginseng, valerian
Barbiturates	Ginger, goldenseal, kava, passionflower, Siberian ginseng, St. John's wort, valerian
Benzodiazepines	Kava, melatonin, valerian
Alprazolam (Xanax)	Kava
Buspirone (BuSpar)	Grapefruit juice
Midazolam (Versed)	
Triazolam (Halcion)	

[a]These combinations result in canceling out the therapeutic effect of the psychotropic medication, potentiating the effects above and beyond what is therapeutically intended, or causing untoward side effects. This table contains only those combinations that are likely to be clinically significant. It does not include all possible problematic combinations, nor does it include all incidents of case reports.

Source: Adapted from Blumenthal, M., Goldberg, A., & Brinkman, J. (2000). *Expanded commission E monographs.* Newton, MA: Integrative Medicine Communications; and Jellin, J. M., Gregory, P. J., Batz, F., & Bonakdar, K. (2002). *Pharmacist's letter/prescriber's letter natural medicines comprehensive database* (4th ed.). Stockton, CA: Therapeutic Research Faculty.

Case Study: Serotonin Syndrome

beneficial effects. A recent study of subjects with treatment-resistant depression found that mood improved and suicidal ideation was reduced in 67% of the subjects after 1 week of treatment (Hadley et al., 2011). Although rTMS has been used for treatment-resistant obsessive–compulsive disorder, there is insufficient data available to determine its usefulness with this condition (Rodriguez-Martin, Barbanoj, Perez, & Sacristan, 2011). Studies of rTMS as a treatment for schizophrenia and post-traumatic stress disorder (PTSD) are underway.

Treatment with rTMS is a noninvasive strategy. Clients are awake, alert, and require no sedation during treatment sessions. Treatment can be offered in office settings and, because there is no anesthesia or sedation, it can be conducted at any time and does not require the client to fast. Clients complete treatments and continue with daily activities without requiring recovery periods.

The side effects of rTMS are categorized into immediate and short term. These include seizures, cognitive impairment, cardiovascular side effects, auditory function changes, and headache. Long-term risks have not been identified. No neuronal damage has been observed in any of the animal long-term studies, and the seizures and cognitive deficits noted in shorter time frames have had no long-term sequelae.

EYE MOVEMENT DESENSITIZATION AND REPROCESSING

Eye movement desensitization reprocessing (EMDR) is a controversial intervention suggested for PTSD and dissociative identity disorder. Clients are asked to recall traumatic memories or a feared stimulus while making a series of rapid lateral eye movements. There is no definitive theoretical explanation of how EMDR might work other than the suggestion that it is the repetitive redirection of attention that induces a neurobiologic state, similar to that of rapid eye movement (REM) sleep, which assists in the integration of traumatic memories into the cortex of the brain. There is strong evidence for the effectiveness of EMDR to treat PTSD (Sharpless & Barber, 2011) especially by reducing the vividness of negative memories (van den Hout et al., 2011).

There is confusion in the literature about EMDR. For example, there is no empirically validated model that provides a convincing explanation of exactly how EMDR works, and there have been inaccurate and selective reporting of research, inadequately designed studies, and biased or inaccurate reviews. On the other hand, a randomized clinical trial that compared the short- and long-term benefits of medication (fluoxetine) with those of EMDR in subjects diagnosed with PTSD found that 75% of adult-onset subjects at 6-month follow-up were asymptomatic compared with none in the fluoxetine group (van der Kolk et al., 2007). For most childhood-onset trauma victims, neither medication nor EMDR produced complete symptom remission. This is clearly an area in which well-designed empirical studies are needed.

REFERENCES

Anderson, J. G., & Taylor, A. G. (2011). Effects of healing touch in clinical practice: A systematic review of randomized clinical trials. *Journal of Holistic Nursing, 29*(3), 221–228. doi: 10.1111/j.1742-1241.2008.01729.x

Barnes, P. M., Bloom, B., & Nahin, R. L. (2008). Complementary and alternative medicine use among adults and children: United States, 2007. *National Health Statistics Report, 10*(12), 1–23.

Benson, H., & Klipper, M. Z. (2000). *The relaxation response.* New York, NY: William Morrow.

Black, S., Carey, E., Webber, A., Neish, N., & Gilbert R. (2011). Determining the efficacy of auricular acupuncture for reducing anxiety in patients withdrawing from psychoactive drugs. *Journal of Substance Abuse Treatment, 41*(3), 279–287. doi: 10.1016/j.jsat.2011.04.001

Burke, A., Upchurch, D. M., Dye, C., & Chyu, L. (2006). Acupuncture use in the United States: Findings from the National Health Interview Survey. *Journal of Alternative and Complementary Medicine, 12*(7), 639–648.

Cheuk, D. K. L., Young, J., Chung, K., & Wong. V. (2011). Acupuncture for insomnia. *Cochrane Database of Systematic Reviews 2011*(5): Art. No.: CD005472. doi: 10.1002/14651858.CD005472.pub2

Coakley, A. B., & Duffy, M. E. (2010). The effect of therapeutic touch on post-operative patients. *Journal of Holistic Nursing, 28*(3), 193–200.

Ezzo, J., Richardson, M. S., Vickers, A., Allen, C., Dibble, S., Issell, B. F., ... Zhang, G. (2011). Acupuncture-point stimulation for chemotherapy-induced nausea or vomiting. *Cochrane Database of Systematic Reviews 2011*(5). Art. No.: CD002285. doi: 10.1002/14651858.CD002285.pub2

Fontaine, K. L. (2011). *Complementary and alternative therapies for nursing practice* (3rd ed.). Upper Saddle River, NJ: Prentice Hall.

Hadley, D., Anderson, B. S., Borckardt, J. J., Arena, A., Li, X., Nahas, Z., & George, M. S. (2011). Safety, tolerability, and effectiveness of high doses of adjunctive daily left prefrontal repetitive transcranial magnetic stimulation for treatment-resistant depression in a clinical setting. *Journal of Electroconculsive Therapy, 27*(1), 18– 25.

Hansen, N. J., Jorgensen, T., & Ortenblad, L. (2011). Massage and touch for dementia. *Cochrane Database of Systematic Reviews 2011*(5). Art. No.: CD004989. doi: 1002/14651858.CD004989.pub.2

Jorm, A. F., Morgan, A. J., & Hetrick, S. E. (2011). Relaxation for depression. *Cochrane Database of Systematic Reviews 2011*(5). Art. No.: CD007142. doi: 10.1002/14651858CD007142.pub.2

Khalsa, D. S., & Stauth, C. (2001). *Meditation as medicine: Activate the power of your natural healing force.* New York, NY: Simon & Schuster.

Krieger, D. (1979). *The therapeutic touch.* Upper Saddle River, NJ: Prentice Hall.

Krieger, D. (1993). *Accepting your power to heal.* Sante Fe, NM: Bear & Co.

Lee, A., & Fan, L. T. Y. (2011). Stimulation of the wrist acupuncture point P6 for preventing post-operative nausea and vomiting. *Cochrane Database of Systematic Reviews 2011*(5). Art. No.: CD003281. doi: 10.1002/14651858.CD003281.pub3

McDonald, K., & Slavin, S. (2010). My body, my life, my choice: Practices and meanings of complementary and alternative medicine among a sample of Australian people living with HIV/AIDS and their practitioners. *AIDS Care, 22*(10), 1229–1235.

Mentgen, J. (2001). Healing touch. *Nursing Clinics of North America, 36*(1), 143–157.

National Institutes of Health Consensus Panel. (1997). *Acupuncture: National Institutes of Health consensus development statement.* Bethesda, MD: National Institutes of Health.

Newberg, A. B., Wintering, N., Khalsa, D. S., Roggenkamp, H., & Waldman, M. R. (2010). Meditation effects on cognitive function and cerebral blood flow in subjects with memory loss: A preliminary study. *Journal of Alzheimer's Disease, 20*(2), 517–526.

Rathbone, J., & Xia, J. (2011). Acupuncture for schizophrenia. *Cochrane Database of Systematic Reviews 2011*(5). Art. No.: CD005475. doi: 10.1002/146511858.CD005475

Rawen, S. E., Zimmerman, M. B., Schultz, S. K., & Wallace, R. B. (2011). 12-month herbal medicine use from the national comorbidity survey replication (NCS-R). *Annals of Clinical Psychiatry, 23*(2), 83–94.

Rodriguez-Martin, J. L., Barbanoj, J. M., Perez, V., & Sacristan, M. (2011). *Cochrane Database of Systematic Reviews 2011*(5). Art. No.: CD003387. doi: 10.1002/14651858.CD003387

Rubinstein, S. A., van Middlekoop, M., Assendelft, W. J. J., de Boer, M. R., & van Tulder, M. W. (2011). Spinal manipulation therapy for chronic low-back pain. *Cochrane Database of Systematic Reviews 2011*(2). Art. No.: CD008112. doi: 10.1002/14651858.CD008112.pub2

Sharpless, B. A., & Barber, J. P. (2011). A clinician's guide to PTSD treatments for returning veterans. *Professional Psychological Research and Practice, 42*(1), 8–15.

Singh, S. S., & Ernst, E. (2009). *Trick or treatment*. New York, NY: WW Norton.

Smith, C. A., Hay, P. P. J., & MacPherson, H. (2011). Acupuncture for depression. *Cochrane Database of Systematic Reviews 2011*(1). Art. No.: CD004046. doi: 10.1002/14651858.CD004096.pub.3

So, P. S., Jiang, Y., & Qin, Y. C. (2011). Touch therapies (healing touch, therapeutic touch and Reiki) for the treatment of pain relief for adults. *Cochrane Database of Systematic Reviews 2011*(5). Art. No.: CD006535. doi: 1002/14651858.CD006535.pub.2

Thakor, V., Leach, M. J., Gillham, D., & Esterman, A. (2011). The quality of information on websites selling St. John's wort. *Complementary Therapeutic Medicine, 19*(3), 155–160.

van den Hout, M. A., Engelhard, I. M., Rijkeboer, M. M., Koekebokker, J., Hornsveld, H., Leer, A, ... Akse, N. (2011). EMDR: Eye movements superior to beeps in taxing working memory and reducing vividness of recollections. *Behavioral Research and Therapy, 49*(2), 92–98.

van der Kolk, B. A., Spinazzola, J., Blaustein, M. E., Hopper, J. W., Hopper, E. K., Korn, D. L., & Simpson, W. B. (2007). A randomized clinical trial of eye movement desensitization and reprocessing (EMDR), fluoxetine, and pill placebo in the treatment of posttraumatic stress disorder: Treatment effects and long-term maintenance. *Journal of Clinical Psychiatry, 68*(1), 37–46.

Walker, B. F., Frenchy, S. D., Grant, W., & Green, S. (2011). Combine chiropractic interventions for low back pain. *Cochrane Database of Systematic Reviews 2011*(5). Art. No.: CD005427. doi: 10.1002/14651858.CD005247.pub2

34

Crisis Intervention

EILEEN TRIGOBOFF
CAROL REN KNEISL

LEARNING OUTCOMES

After completing this chapter, you will be able to:

1. Describe the types of maturational and situational crises a person can experience.
2. Differentiate between a crisis that is a turning point in a person's life and making an important life decision.
3. Analyze the sequence of a crisis and determine its significance for the nursing care of a client in crisis.
4. Incorporate an understanding of the origins of a crisis, risk factors, and balancing factors during the assessment phase of crisis management.
5. Synthesize crisis intervention modalities into a plan of care for a person in crisis.
6. Incorporate the ABCs of crisis counseling in a plan of care for a client in crisis.
7. Develop a psychoeducational plan for clients and families who are disaster victims.
8. Analyze personal feelings and attitudes that may affect professional practice when caring for clients in crisis.

CRITICAL THINKING CHALLENGE

Katrinka V., a 43-year-old nurse, is a survivor of domestic violence. She and John, her husband of 15 years, have two children. Last night after a long period of drinking, John threatened Katrinka and the children with a gun. Katrinka managed to get herself and the children out of the house and into her car, where they spent the night. In the morning, Katrinka, distraught, highly anxious, and in crisis, arrived at the psychiatric emergency department. She said, "I can't think of what to do. I've got to get to my job and the kids have to go to school. It's not safe for any of us at either place. What should I do?"

1. How do you understand her current situation?
2. What critical areas do you need to assess?
3. Which interventions would be helpful?

On September 11, 2001, in the most devastating terrorist act waged against the United States to that point in time, hijackers crashed two airliners into New York City's World Trade Center, toppling its twin 110-story towers.

The deadly calamity was witnessed on television screens across the world as a third plane slammed into the Pentagon, and a fourth crashed outside Pittsburgh. The death toll, numbering almost 3,000, also included firefighters, police officers, and medical personnel killed while attempting to rescue victims. The impact on New York City was horrific. Many people lost their jobs because businesses were demolished and tourists stayed away. Even the usual winter holiday festivities for which New York City is famous were conducted with an air of great sadness. The impact on the rest of the country—survivors, citizens, and visitors alike—and around the world was tremendous, as these clinical examples illustrate.

Clinical Example

Nguyen, a visitor from Malaysia, was walking across the Brooklyn Bridge, admiring the view of lower Manhattan, when he saw the plane hit the first tower. He stood on the bridge in horror, watching the fireball as people jumped from the buildings. Although he has long since returned to Malaysia, he has nightmares in which he relives the experience over and over.

Two teenagers were at home in Arizona watching TV while getting ready for school when they saw the news. First they experienced sadness, then disbelief, confusion, anger, and, finally, fear. One said, "Now I know that terrorism isn't just something you see on the evening news that happens on the other side of the world. My life has been changed forever."

Tadeusz works at an airport outside Warsaw, Poland. People were gathered around him, chatting about the disaster, crying, and praying. Tadeusz left work sick that day. He told his supervisor that he felt nauseated and weak in the knees at the thought that airplanes at his airport could be targeted and that life was so fragile.

The research literature suggests that more people need treatment for mental health difficulties than for physical symptoms following an injury-causing agent or event. The mental health risks include not only post-traumatic stress disorder (PTSD), but also acute stress disorder, depression, complicated bereavement reactions, substance use disorders, fear, anxiety, somatization, anger control, and arrest or regression of childhood developmental progression (DelGaizo, Elhai, & Weaver, 2011; Claassen, Kashner, Kashner, Xuan, & Larkin, 2011). Communities exposed to a crisis, even communities distant from the threat or the disaster, face an acute "mental health surge" that can overwhelm available community mental health resources. Recent developments in health care preparedness have addressed some of these needs; however, further investigation and investment are required (Raphael & Ma, 2011).

Do you remember how you felt on Tuesday, September 11, 2001? Did you feel helpless? Did you know what to do or say to others? Did you believe you were in danger? Did you call anyone? Did you talk about the event with others? Did you want it all to go away? If you answered "yes" to any of these questions, you know what a crisis feels like. Chances are that you, your family, and your community were in crisis, along with many other individuals, families, and communities.

A **crisis** is an acute, time-limited state of disequilibrium resulting from situational, developmental, or societal sources of stress. An individual can be said to be in crisis when that person is in a situation in which usual problem-solving or adaptive methods are inadequate to resolve a problem or conflict, causing a state of disequilibrium. People involved in these incidents may be unable to effectively manage stressful events or environmental changes. They may be unable to function and may feel paralyzed and powerless. FIGURE 34-1 ■ illustrates the progression of a crisis to either successful or unsuccessful resolution.

It is likely that the terrorist attack (and other large-scale crisis events) will continue to have effects such as PTSD far into the future (Raphael & Ma, 2011). Years after the event, mothers and adolescents—who were children when 9/11 occurred—had symptoms of depression and post-traumatic stress disorder (Gershoff, Aber, Ware, & Kotler, 2010). Those who study what happens to the survivors of catastrophes—natural or manmade—find similar disruptions of psychosocial health of great concern (Berger, 2011). Adolescents who experienced or witnessed violence had different coping mechanisms regardless of gender (Reid-Quiñones, Kliewer, Shields, Goodman, Ray et al., 2010). Aggressive and avoidant responses by victims as well as witnesses indicate that more attention should be given to how youth cope with violence. Other examples of situations that have caused a crisis on a more limited scale are discussed in the following clinical example.

Clinical Example

An ex-employee comes into an office building and shoots 15 people; a tragic school bus accident claims five 6-year-old children and their teacher; two teenagers from the same high school commit suicide the same week; a 66-year-old man retires and feels useless and considers suicide; a 23-year-old woman finds out that she has a fatal illness; a premature baby is born; a 12-year-old child is kidnapped while walking home from school.

FIGURE 34-1 ■ Rescue workers cover up bodies near a bomb-damaged train in Madrid, Spain. The explosion killed more than 170 rush-hour commuters and wounded more than 500 in 2004.
Photo courtesy of AP Wide World Photos, Paul White.

Nurses are intimately connected with crises. We often interact with people who are faced with new, frightening, and troublesome situations. Because of who we are, where we work, and our accessibility to individuals and families, we are in a position to offer supportive and therapeutic interventions that can change people's lives. You can help if you understand how to effectively intervene, that is, if you understand how to implement crisis intervention skills. **Crisis intervention** is a conceptual framework for intervention that calls for short-term, action-oriented assistance focused on problem solving, with a goal of restoring the individual's equilibrium. Effective crisis intervention will call for all the skills that a well-prepared nurse can muster (Yin, He, Arbon, & Zhu, 2011).

Crisis intervention is not the specialty of any one professional group. People who intervene in crises come from the fields of nursing, medicine, psychology, social work, and theology. Police officers, teachers, school guidance counselors, rescue workers, and bartenders, among others, are often on-the-spot crisis interveners. Obviously, crisis intervention can be the business of many different people. The Association of Traumatic Stress Specialists provides training programs and board certification for qualified interveners. The association represents those who serve victims of crime, veterans (such as Justin whose story is told on page 267), refugees, survivors of natural disasters and terrorist attacks, holocaust survivors, persons with line-of-duty–related injuries, individuals coping with a death, victims of school and workplace violence, victims of political persecution, and others who have experienced traumatic stress. The association can be accessed through the Online Student Resources for this book.

CRISIS AS A TURNING POINT

The word *crisis* stems from the Greek *krinein,* "to decide." In Chinese, two characters are used to write the word; one is the character for danger and the other the character for opportunity. The interaction between *danger* and *opportunity* will become clearer as you read this chapter.

Crisis situations are turning points or junctures in a person's life that result in a new equilibrium. The new equilibrium may be close to that of the precrisis state, or it may be a more positive or more negative state. If the new equilibrium is more positive, the person experiences personal growth, increased competence, a better social network, newfound problem-solving abilities, or an improved self-image. If the new equilibrium is more negative, the individual may lose skills, regress to an earlier developmental stage, develop socially unacceptable behaviors, or develop a mental disorder. Unsuccessful negotiation of a crisis leaves the person feeling anxious, threatened, and ineffective. Individuals may also respond to a crisis event with disturbed personal coping or with frankly psychotic behavior. This process is illustrated in FIGURE 34-2. ■

Because a state of disequilibrium is so uncomfortable, a crisis is self-limiting. That is, even without intervention, a crisis will resolve itself with either a favorable or unfavorable conclusion. Studies indicate those who do not seek or are not involved in some form of mental health treatment tend to be more vulnerable to mental health issues such as depression and post-traumatic stress disorder. The Centers for Disease Control and Prevention (CDC) has information on coping with stress after a traumatic event. This is why crisis intervention is sometimes called *primary prevention for PTSD* (refer to Chapter 18 ∞ for details about PTSD). Evidence-Based Practice discusses the characteristics of those at risk for mental health problems following an attack.

Common Characteristics of Crises

To understand the concept of crisis fully and to appreciate the interaction of risk factors, we must differentiate among levels of distress to illustrate what a crisis is not. Stress is not crisis. Everyone feels stress at various times, in a variety of forms

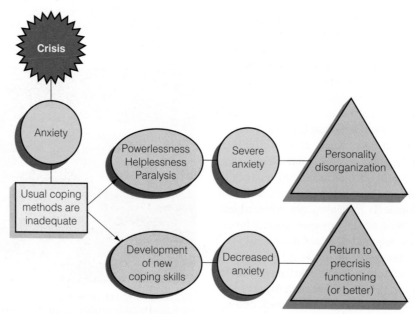

FIGURE 34-2 ■ The progression of a crisis to either successful or unsuccessful resolution depends on what people do when they discover that their usual coping mechanisms are ineffective.

EVIDENCE-BASED PRACTICE

Tangible Support for a Client in Crisis

Crises occur when someone is personally attacked, has a dire set of circumstances, or has their worldview disrupted. Nurses practice with people in these situations in a variety of settings. One of the main goals is to minimize the risk of psychological disorder, or a worsening of a disorder, for people experiencing the crisis. The set of common symptoms to assess and address would be depressive symptoms.

Mrs. Suny, a middle-age Indian-American woman, has been admitted for a crisis evaluation and brief stay at the behavioral unit in the general hospital in which you work. It has been several weeks since a terrorist attack has been averted due to police action. In reviewing her records, you note that she has had multiple hospitalizations for crisis-type episodes, severe anxiety, and depression during this recent time period.

She is tearful and anxious, as well as depressed, and connects most of her anxiety to the fact that she lives in a housing project where considerable discrimination has been experienced by people of Indian ethnicity. This has increased in recent weeks after the news stories of the planned attack. Her greatest fear is for her own safety and the safety of her family. She is articulate and without ideas of suicide or homicide. She is not psychotic.

You know by your review of the literature that the risk of depression ranges between 20% and 30% in direct victims and between 4% and 10% in the general population in the first few months after terrorist attacks. Characteristics that tend to increase risk of depression after a terrorist attack are female gender, having experienced more stressful situations before or after the attack, peritraumatic reactions during the attack, loss of psychosocial resources, and low social support.

You are working the full week, and Mrs. Suny will be your client for the next 5 days. On the third day, she tells you that right after the news reports of the thwarted terrorist plan, she was held captive for 6 hours and brutally beaten and raped by a man who lived in her building. He proclaimed how he would, "not let people like her see him scared," and that he would show her who had power in this world. Mrs. Suny shared with you her fear that she is "going crazy." You implement the following interventions:

- Explain to Mrs. Suny that many of her problems could be related to the attack.
- Explore with her the coping styles that emerged from this event.
- Encourage her to make connections between the event and her current situation.
- Provide tangible support by helping her select an outpatient therapist who is competent to treat trauma victims and arrange for her to meet the therapist while she is still in the hospital.

Your interventions are based on your review of the literature and other relevant studies, as well as the following research that indicates that many individuals who seek psychiatric help have been traumatized and the trauma has not been recognized or adequately treated.

Salguero, J. M., Fernandez-Berrocal, P., Iruarrizaga, I., Cano-Vindel, A., & Galea, S. (2011). Major depressive disorder following terrorist attacks: A systematic review of prevalence, course, and correlates. *BMC Psychiatry, 11*(1), 96. doi: 10.1186/1471-244X-11-96

CRITICAL THINKING QUESTIONS

1. In what ways can racist and sexist stereotypes influence rape blame attribution—that is, how do the victim, family and friends, and even health care providers attribute blame?
2. How is it possible that all of Mrs. Suny's symptoms can be explained by a diagnosis of PTSD?

(see the discussion in Chapter 8 ∞). Stress is pressure and tension. Stressful situations may demand our attention and may be exhausting, but they are not crises. An emergency is a situation that often demands an immediate response to ensure the survival of an individual. Although neither stress nor an emergency are themselves a crisis, stress or an emergency can ultimately precipitate a crisis. A crisis is not a mental disorder. A crisis can happen to someone who has never had a mental disorder or to someone who is currently experiencing a mental disorder. Common characteristics of crises are discussed in Box 34-1.

Resilience, Risk Factors, and Balancing Factors

Why do some people effectively manage disequilibrium while others go into crisis? This capacity is called *resilience*. Resilience is the ability not only to survive and bounce back from difficult and traumatic experiences, but also to continue to grow and develop emotionally and psychologically. The notion of resilience encompasses the biologic and psychological characteristics intrinsic to an individual, such as personality style and quality of interpersonal relationships,

that confer protection against the development of psychopathology (Bhui & Dinos, 2011). Resilience probably explains why not all people who are stressed and socially isolated

---

Box 34-1 Common Characteristics of Crises

- Many situational crises are experienced as sudden. The person is usually not aware of a warning signal, whether or not others could "see it coming." The individual or family may feel they have had little or no preparation for the event or trauma.
- The crisis may be experienced as ultimately life threatening, whether this perception is realistic or not.
- Communication with significant others is often reduced or cut off.
- There may be perceived or real displacement from familiar surroundings or significant loved ones.
- All crises have an aspect of loss, whether actual or perceived. The losses can include an object, a person, a hope, a dream, or any significant factor for that individual.

Box 34-2   Risk Factors for Crisis

- Intensity of exposure to the situation
- Pre-existing psychiatric symptoms and diagnosis
- Prior history of traumatic exposure
- Family history of psychiatric problems, anxiety, and/or antisocial behavior
- Early separation from parents
- Childhood abuse
- Poverty
- Cultural expectations that prohibit asking others for help
- Degree of threat to life (being on a plane that crashes versus watching a plane crash from a distance)

---

experience mental health problems (Cacioppo, Reis, & Zautra, 2011). Researchers and clinicians alike have been surprised by the prevalence of the capacity for resilience, and clinicians are beginning to focus on uncovering and energizing pathways to resilience in their clients. The concept of resilience in relation to mental health is discussed in Box 1-1∞ on page 4.

There are several risk factors, in addition to the nature of the trauma or the experience itself, that place individuals at high risk for crisis. These factors are identified in Box 34-2.

In addition to these risk factors, the presence or absence of certain other events or situations are important to the successful resolution of disequilibrium. For example, how do individuals perceive and understand the event/crisis in their lives? Are they being punished? Is this happening only to them and never to anyone else? How will the event affect their future? Do they see the situation realistically, or is it distorted? Situational supports are also important. Are there people in their lives who can help them solve the problem? Meaningful relationships with others give support and assistance during the crisis. Individuals with inadequate support are likely to experience a decrease in self-esteem. In turn, lowered self-esteem may make an event appear more threatening. An individual's coping mechanisms may add or detract from the successful resolution of disequilibrium caused by crisis. All people use mechanisms to cope with anxiety and tension. Because the individual has used these coping mechanisms with success in the past, they become part of the coping repertoire. These tension-relieving mechanisms can be obvious or subtle (see the discussion in Chapter 8∞). If an individual has a realistic perception of the traumatic event or crisis, adequate situational support, and adequate coping mechanisms the problems will be resolved and equilibrium will be regained, making it unlikely that a crisis will result. If, however, one or more of these important factors are absent, the problem is likely to be unresolved, disequilibrium is likely to continue, and a state of crisis will result.

BIOPSYCHOSOCIAL THEORIES OF CRISIS

The recognition of crisis has a long history. As long ago as 400 B.C.E., physicians understood that a crisis was a hazardous life event. It was not until the 20th century, however, that strategies for helping people to cope with crisis were developed. Theories of crisis and crisis intervention resulted from early research studies that are now classics, as well as more recent events in the field of mental health. Some of these are described in the following section.

- Lindemann's (1944) landmark study of the survivors of the tragic Coconut Grove nightclub fire in Boston identified symptoms common to individuals experiencing acute grief. Lindemann determined that if grieving was delayed or absent, the crisis resulted in negative outcomes.
- The observations of, and treatment by, military psychiatrists of World War II battle-weary and emotionally upset soldiers at the front lines allowed the soldiers to return to duty rather than having to be sent to inpatient psychiatric facilities.
- Tyhurst's (1957) studies of the stages individuals go through when experiencing transition states such as migration, retirement, and civilian disasters led to the identification of three phases—a period of impact, a period of recoil, and a posttraumatic period of recovery.
- Federal funding was made available in 1961 for community-based mental health programs such as suicide prevention and crisis services, including crisis telephone counseling services, known popularly as *hotlines*.
- Caplan's (1964) work in preventive psychiatry and anticipatory guidance in the early days of the Peace Corps expanded on Lindemann's work. Caplan studied developmental crises and accidental crises. He determined that successfully navigating the stages of a crisis required using new coping skills.
- The publication by the American Psychiatric Association of the *Diagnostic and Statistical Manual of Mental Disorders* in 1980 provided, for the first time, a system to measure the severity of psychosocial stressors and to reflect that severity with the psychiatric diagnosis via Axis IV (see Chapter 11∞).
- More contemporary methods of crisis intervention include Roberts' seven-stage crisis intervention model for frontline crisis workers (Roberts, 2005).
- Six precipitants of a crisis for those with intellectual disabilities have been identified as: a change in residence, serious interactional problem, difficulty with an authority (police, etc.), unemployment for more than 1 month, recent trauma/abuse, or a drug or alcohol problem (Lunsky & Elserafi, 2011).

The etiology, psychobiology, epidemiology, comorbidity, and treatment of crisis and its sequelae are complicated. Mental Health in the News highlights one such complicated crisis. Some theories that attempt to explain what happens in a crisis and how to intervene in a crisis are described next.

Tyhurst's Stages of Disaster

Tyhurst (1957) identified three overlapping stages in response to a disaster. They are as follows:

1. Impact
2. Recoil
3. Posttrauma

MENTAL HEALTH IN THE NEWS

Anna Nicole Smith

Anna Nicole Smith, famous for transforming herself from an exotic dancer to the wife of an elderly billionaire, has had a life full of crises. She was 17 years old when she had a son, Daniel, who she had to raise on her own. She was a Playboy playmate and popular celebrity.

When her husband died, she had a 12-year public court battle fighting for the right to her inheritance. Her newsworthy performances included admitting to addictions and eating disorders and having a reality show about her life. Through it all, her son Daniel had been labeled a sensitive grounding force. They were in the Bahamas when Anna Nicole gave birth to her daughter, Dannielynn Hope. Dannielynn came into the world with many questions about who her father might be. Several men claimed fatherhood, and there was one theory that Anna Nicole used her deceased husband's sperm to impregnate herself.

While Daniel was visiting Anna Nicole, he died of an apparent heart attack in Anna Nicole's hospital room of what was determined to be an accidental drug-related death (high blood levels of methadone and two antidepressant medications).

Following her son's death, Anna Nicole was reportedly devastated and had difficulty coping with that fresh assault on her much-publicized fragile state. Five months later, Anna Nicole was found unresponsive in her hotel room and died of an apparent accidental overdose of chloral hydrate (a sedative/hypnotic) and at least eight other prescription medications including methadone, lorazepam (Ativan), and diazepam (Valium).

Even though Anna Nicole Smith has died, the chaos and controversy that marked her life continue as several lawsuits are still pending regarding the estate, assets, and outstanding debts. Dannielynn's father, Anna Nicole's former boyfriend Larry Birkhead, is raising his daughter.

Photo courtesy of Kathy Hutchins Photography/Newscom.

These stages are as relevant today as they were then, and they help mental health care workers understand the experiences of the victims of hurricanes, floods, fires, terrorist attacks, and other disasters as well as the people who experienced the disaster by watching it at home on their television sets.

Impact

The first stage, *impact,* is stimulated by the catastrophe. Victims recognize what is happening to them and are concerned mainly with the present. During this acute phase, the victim's major concern may be staying alive. According to Tyhurst, about 75% of victims experience shock and confusion. Although they appear dazed, they also exhibit the physical signs of fear. Another group of people, up to 25%, remain coherent. They logically and rationally assess the situation and develop and implement a plan for dealing with the immediate problems brought on by the catastrophe. A third group, also up to 25%, may panic or become immobilized with fear. They may behave hysterically, or they may be overlooked because they sit and silently stare into space as the man and the woman in the Critical Thinking Challenge on page 139 page 139.

Recoil

In *recoil,* the second stage, the initial stress of the disaster has passed, and victims may no longer find their lives in immediate danger, although injuries and other discomforts come to their awareness. Emergency shelter, food, and clothing become available. The victims' behavior is usually dependent—they want to be taken care of. Weeping is common as survivors begin to realize all that has happened to them.

Posttrauma

The full impact of the losses the victims have experienced comes in the third, or *posttrauma,* period. Grief is a predominant response to the losses in their lives. Disturbed and psychotic responses may occur.

Caplan's Stages of a Crisis Reaction

Caplan (1964) studied various developmental crisis reactions to premature births, infancy, childhood, and adolescence, as well as accidental crises such as illness and death. Caplan built upon Tyhurst's work with disaster victims. According to him, the four stages of a crisis reaction are as follows:

1. *Phase 1:* The individual experiences an initial increase in tension because of the emotionally hazardous crisis-precipitating event.
2. *Phase 2:* When the individual is unable to resolve the crisis quickly, tension and disruption of daily living increase.
3. *Phase 3:* If the individual attempts but fails to resolve the crisis by the usual problem-solving techniques, tension increases to such a level that the individual may become depressed.
4. *Phase 4:* At the final stage, the person may partly resolve the crisis by using new coping skills. Mental disruption or disorder may occur if the person does not develop new coping skills to manage the crisis.

Roberts' Model of Crisis Intervention

Roberts' seven-stage model of crisis intervention (2005) has been used to help people in acute psychological crisis and acute situational crisis, persons in high-risk populations such as suicidal juvenile offenders (Roberts & Bender, 2006), and persons diagnosed with acute stress disorder. The seven stages are as follows:

1. Plan and conduct a thorough assessment (including lethality assessment [refer to Chapter 23 Chapter 23], assessment of dangerousness to self or others, and assessment of immediate psychosocial needs).
2. Make interpersonal contact, establish rapport, and rapidly establish the relationship (conveying genuine regard and respect for the client, acceptance,

WHY I BECAME A PSYCHIATRIC–MENTAL HEALTH NURSE

Sandra Niemann, RN, PhD

Although I didn't plan to become a psychiatric nurse when I entered nursing school, a clinical rotation at a state mental hospital during my last semester changed that. That semester I cared for a client with chronic schizophrenia. Although in retrospect I realize I understood very little about her world, her aloneness and daily struggle touched me. And her obvious pleasure in my visits solidified something I'd recently learned but didn't yet believe—that a relationship is often the most powerful treatment of all.

This same realization brought me back to a doctoral program in nursing many years later, this time to do research in infant mental health. I had recently adopted my daughter from Taiwan, where she spent her first 7 months in an orphanage. I could see the imprint of these early months on her development, but there was very little research to tell me what lay ahead or the best practices for mitigating early deprivation. I would like to contribute to this field by conducting research that helps clarify what those best practices are.

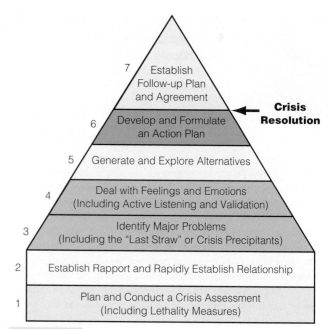

FIGURE 34-3 ■ Roberts' seven-stage model of crisis intervention. *Source:* From Roberts, A. R. (2005). Bridging the past and present to the future of crisis intervention and crisis management. In A. R. Roberts (Ed.), *Crisis intervention handbook: Assessment, treatment, & research* (3rd ed.) (Figure 1-1, p. 20). New York, NY: Oxford University Press. Used by permission of Oxford University Press, Inc.

reassurance, and a nonjudgmental attitude; refer to Chapter 4∞).

3. Examine the dimensions of the problem in order to define it (including the "last straw" of the precipitating event).

4. Encourage an exploration of feelings and emotions through active listening (refer to Chapter 10∞).

5. Explore and assess past coping attempts and generate and explore alternatives and previously untried coping methods or solutions.

6. Restore cognitive functioning through the implementation of an action plan based on cognitive mastery (refer to Chapter 30∞).

7. Follow up with the client and leave the door open for future contact, especially around the time of the anniversary of the event (exactly 1 month or 1 year after the victimization).

FIGURE 34-3 ■ illustrates Roberts' seven-step model. This model is integrated throughout the Nursing Process section later in this chapter.

TYPES OF CRISES

In the contemporary view, the origin of a crisis is as important as the type of crisis. Roberts (2005) points out that if we know how the crisis began, we have a better opportunity to intervene effectively. Two general categories of crisis origins are situational and maturational.

Situational Crisis

A **situational crisis** can originate from three sources: material or environmental (fire, natural disaster, manmade biohazards, terrorist attacks); personal or physical (heart attack, diagnosis of fatal illness, bodily disfigurement); and interpersonal or social (death of a loved one or divorce). Often, these life-threatening events motivate people to take significant action in their close relationships that alter their life course.

Because the event leading to the situational crisis is usually unanticipated, one generally cannot do anything directly to prevent it. In a more indirect sense, an individual can attempt to keep healthy and focus on the most effective methods of interacting with others. However, the complexity of the experience influences the ability of the individual to resolve the trauma. For instance, a person coping with one traumatic incident is more likely to resolve the experience than someone faced with multiple traumas or factors (Melamed & Castro, 2011). An example of a situational crisis (in which the origin of the crisis is the husband's diagnosis of terminal cancer) follows.

Clinical Example

Jessie, age 52, is a social worker at a local mental health clinic who is feeling increasingly less able to function since she learned that her husband has a terminal, inoperable form of cancer. Many arrangements need to be made, including finding adequate medical treatment and doing appropriate evaluations of her husband.

Jessie has been unable to work for 2 to 3 days and now tells a psychiatric–mental health nurse that she can no longer function—she has been unable to make any of the required phone calls, despite knowing she is the person who must coordinate everything. Jessie speaks of feeling overwhelmed, shakes her head, and says, "Can you believe it? I do this all the time for others, but I can't do it now. Isn't that a joke?"

Maturational Crisis

A **maturational crisis** involves life cycle changes or normal transitions of human development. These are the traditional stages of human development that include infancy, childhood, puberty, adolescence, adulthood, middle age, and old age. During each stage, the individual is subject to unique stressors. Each stage of development is characterized by developmental tasks the individual must accomplish in order to progress to the next level. A failure at any one level compromises the next stage of development.

Maturational crises also include such changes as marriage, retirement, and the transition from student to worker. Crises associated with these states arise when the individual enters a new area of development or functioning and cannot adatpt to functioning at that level. If the person experiences additional trauma or change, the risk for experiencing a crisis increases. Whenever people experience more than two life changes or traumatic events, their coping capacity may be strained, and the potential for crisis becomes greater.

An example of a maturational crisis, in which the origin of the crisis is a decision to divorce complicated by multiple stressors, follows.

Clinical Example

Bernie is a 62-year-old man who has been hospitalized several times for paranoid schizophrenia over the past 40 years. Bernie's wife Alice moved out of their apartment and told Bernie that she has decided to seek a divorce. After Alice moved out, the apartment caught fire and burned. Bernie moved to a boardinghouse and became depressed and stopped taking his medication. He began to have auditory hallucinations. Bernie has come to the crisis center accompanied by the police, who found him on the street crying, sobbing, and mumbling incoherently.

NURSING SELF-AWARENESS

It is important that you develop increased awareness of yourself and are able to handle your feelings so that you can intervene in a crisis situation. It will help you to reflect upon your answers to the questions posed in Your Self-Awareness.

To remain effective in crisis work, and to continue to grow personally and professionally, you should practice the following important behaviors:

- Respect and believe in a person's capacity to grow and change.
- Be aware of the impact on yourself of repeatedly listening to horrible stories.
- Formulate your own outlets for stress, frustration, and anger.
- Deal with your own fears about violence and your own vulnerability to stress and conflict.
- Develop realistic expectations about what you can do for others.
- Respect each person's own unique timetable for crisis resolution.
- Collaborate with other crisis interveners and community groups.

YOUR SELF-AWARENESS
Am I Ready for Crisis Work?

Thoughtfully consider and reflect on your answers to the following questions:

- Do I believe that people who are in crisis are helpless?
- Can I contain my own anxiety when I am working with someone who is severely anxious?
- How do I feel when I'm not in control in certain situations?
- How do I react to people who are frightened?
- How do I react to people who are angry?
- How do I react to people who threaten me?
- Do I have ideas that will hinder my ability to help others? For example, do I believe any of the following: Women who are raped are asking for it; men should be strong and not show emotions; children should be seen and not heard?

You will become more skilled as you incorporate each of these behaviors into your professional repertoire.

Some additional activities that you can undertake to take care of yourself and lessen the personal impacts of disaster and crises involve self-nurturance. Focus on what you did right every day, monitor your own reactions, keep a journal in which you write your personal thoughts and feelings, and practice the self-care tips in Your Self-Awareness, "Self-Care Tips for Emergency and Disaster Response Workers." People in crisis will expect you to help them regain control of themselves, not to control them. Being self-assured and composed will help your clients to regain control.

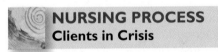

NURSING PROCESS
Clients in Crisis

Crisis intervention as a therapeutic strategy is strongly humanistic. People are viewed as capable of personal growth and as having the ability to influence and control their own lives. According to these concepts, the task of the intervener is to help the individual in crisis understand the combination of events that led to the crisis and guide the individual, prior to a maladaptive response, toward a resolution that will meet the person's unique needs and foster future growth and strength. Especially during the acute phase, the goal of crisis intervention is to restore the person to the pretrauma level of functioning as quickly as possible.

In addition to the interventions discussed in this section, other strategies that are employed with clients in crisis can be found in other chapters. They are cognitive–behavioral therapy interventions (Chapter 30∞), pharmacologic interventions (Chapters 7 and 31∞), and stress management techniques (Chapter 33∞). Providing psychoeducation for survivors of trauma helps them to better understand their own stress responses. Learning coping strategies provides a sense of control over these responses.

YOUR SELF-AWARENESS
Self-Care Tips for Emergency and Disaster Response Workers

Normal Reactions to a Disaster Event

- No one who responds to a mass casualty event is untouched by it.
- Profound sadness, grief, and anger are normal reactions to an abnormal event.
- You may not want to leave the scene until the work is finished.
- You will likely try to override stress and fatigue with dedication and commitment.
- You may deny the need for rest and recovery time.

Signs That You May Need Stress Management Assistance

- Difficulty communicating thoughts
- Difficulty remembering instructions
- Difficulty maintaining balance
- Uncharacteristic argumentativeness
- Difficulty making decisions
- Limited attention span
- Unnecessary risk taking
- Tremors/headaches/nausea
- Tunnel vision/muffled hearing
- Colds or flulike symptoms
- Disorientation or confusion
- Difficulty concentrating
- Loss of objectivity
- Greater tendency toward feeling easily frustrated
- Inability to engage in problem solving
- Inability to let down when off duty
- Refusal to follow orders
- Refusal to leave the scene

- Increased use of drugs/alcohol
- Unusual clumsiness

Ways to Help Manage Your Stress

- Limit on-duty work hours to no more than 12 hours per day.
- Make work rotations from high-stress to lower-stress functions.
- Make work rotations from the scene to routine assignments as feasible.
- Use counseling assistance programs available through your agency.
- Drink plenty of water and eat healthy snacks like fresh fruit or dried fruit, nuts, trail mix, whole grain breads, and other energy foods at the scene.
- Keep yourself hydrated with water, mineral water, decaffeinated coffee or tea, juice, and electrolyte supplements.
- If you are able to, take calcium supplements, which can counteract high levels of lactic acid produced by tension, and vitamin C, which may help you to maintain alertness.
- Take frequent, brief breaks from the scene as feasible.
- Talk about your emotions to process what you have seen and done.
- Stay in touch with your family and friends.
- Participate in memorials, rituals, and use of symbols as a way to express feelings.
- Pair up with another responder so that you may monitor one another's stress.

Source: Adapted from USDHHS Substance Abuse and Mental Health Services Administration. (2011). *Self-care tips for emergency and disaster response workers.* Retrieved from http://www.samhsa.gov

---

It is equally important that, in this era of heightened security brought on by terrorist concerns, nurses also are educated and prepared to respond to crisis and disasters. Disaster preparedness plans are created by individual health care facilities, and most nurses undergo a program of continuing education training in their agency. However, it would be an effective primary prevention strategy to prepare nursing students for just such contingencies. For example, psychological crisis intervention has been identified as a core nursing skill for disaster response training (Yin et al., 2011).

Assessment

Assessment takes place on three levels: individual, family, and sociocultural.

Individual Assessment

Assessment of the individual is the first phase of crisis intervention. The nurse or helper must focus on assessing the following elements that relate to the person and the problem. Collect data about the following:

- The client's resilience
- The client's coping style
- The precipitating event

- The situational supports
- The client's perception of the crisis
- Any guilt a disaster survivor may feel about having survived or about actions taken in order to survive
- The client's ability to handle the problem

Rx Communication shows an example of assessing a client's coping style.

Assessment is an essential step of crisis intervention and the basis for later decisions about how and when to intervene, and whom to call (the first step of Roberts' model). Another feature of an individual assessment in the face of a crisis is how the client is managing spiritually. See Caring for the Spirit as a tool to help clients use their faith to heal. Intellectual capabilities would also contribute to decisions about needed interventions (Lunsky & Elserafi, 2011).

Also assess and evaluate the client's suicide potential. (See Chapter 23∞ for lethality assessment.) During this time, a client may need to be hospitalized to ensure safety, and a referral to a therapist or an emergency department in a general hospital or a psychiatric emergency room may be necessary. Part of the overall assessment is to determine what is necessary to return this client to a state of equilibrium; this may be different from what is necessary to solve the problem.

COMMUNICATION

Client in Crisis

CLIENT: "How will I ever be able to get my son back from the foster home that child services put him in? I never seem to do anything right with him."

NURSE RESPONSE 1: "Jim, if you could rank yourself as a Dad on a scale of 1 to 10, with 10 meaning always doing everything 'right' and 1 meaning never doing anything 'right,' where would you rank yourself?" *RATIONALE:* Using a scaling question will open the door to discussing with Jim the skills and competencies that are within his control and need to be worked on.	**NURSE RESPONSE 2:** "Let's talk about what you have been doing with Jimmy that is 'right.'" *RATIONALE:* This intervention has two goals: eliciting a behavioral description of the interaction between father and son and helping the client identify his parenting strengths.

Family Assessment

Family assessment is important when an individual has been traumatized, because trauma reverberates through an entire family as well as when a crisis involves all or several members within a family (de Jong & Schout, 2011). Meet with as many family members as possible to assess family resilience, family resources, coping skills, and interpersonal styles. Crises often accompany role changes in families or increased stresses in families that do not have the resources to meet the challenge.

Some common family crises are the death of a family member, the terminal illness of a family member, single parenting, divorce, drug/alcohol dependence, family violence, infidelity, remarriage, mental illness, incest, and "empty nest syndrome."

Sociocultural Assessment

A critically important source of the meaning of an individual's response to stress or trauma is the broader sociocultural context in which the person lives. A client's culture influences the sources of distress a client experiences, as well as the client's symptomatology, interpretation of symptoms, and methods of coping.

How one is raised influences how one experiences distress, whether one seeks help, and whether one allows oneself to be disabled by a mental health problem. For example, in some cultures, anxiety is considered a problem of individual

strength or moral code, as opposed to a mental health problem. In some cultures, it may be more acceptable to have a physical problem than an emotional problem.

Cultural competence requires knowledge about other cultures and sensitivity to the culture of your clients in order to select the interventions that will likely be most helpful. Cultural sensitivity involves much more than simply identifying a family's ethnic origins or health practices. Think about developing a cultural family genogram as an aid to assessing culturally diverse families. The cultural family genogram is discussed in Chapter 29 ∞ as it applies to family-based interventions. It is just as relevant a tool for working with culturally diverse families in crisis.

To be effective in sociocultural assessment, you must also become aware of the influences and beliefs from your own experiences. If you are not familiar with a client's culture, ask respectful questions to help the client fully express his or her distress. For example, "I want to understand how all of this might affect you. Tell me more about how you feel about this situation. Tell me how your neighbors (your friends/your family) might feel about it."

Disaster Assessment

Nurses as citizens are often at the scene of natural disasters or may be called on to help. Nurses can be particularly helpful during the initial stage of a disaster because, in addition

---

CARING FOR THE SPIRIT

Crisis as a Test of Faith

It may be that a psychiatric crisis has also brought forth a spiritual crisis. The client may, for the first time, be faced with looking at the three spiritual questions of life.

1. "What have I placed on life's altar? Of what value is my life? Why was I born, anyway? I have nothing to give." These are the words of someone who is depressed or actively suicidal.
2. "What do I hold to be sacred?" What things are important to the client, what things have meaning?
3. "How do I know what's true?" The client with anxiety or psychosis has great difficulty sorting out what's

real and what's not real, determining what's true and what's not true. Life as we know it has many dichotomies. The unanswerable becomes even more of a challenge when a psychiatric crisis emerges.

Recall what happened to your relationships with friends and family when you were in a personal crisis. Did the relationships change? Our cognitive sphere, our affective sphere, and our relational sphere are all affected. We lose our centering of purpose, of sacredness, of reality. We lose our spirit and become disconnected. Do you think your clients' relationships change when they are in a crisis?

MENTAL HEALTH IN THE MOVIES
Disaster Movies

The themes of disaster movies tend to challenge us to think about our abilities to cope in a crisis. The film can take the form of a special vacation trip we can all relate to being spoiled by volcanoes, asteroids, or dinosaurs. Or a futuristic view of the world can spark our imaginations and then introduce the element of intrusions by alien beings or dark mega-deities from the nth dimension. There will be different venues presented; however, the overarching question seems to be, "What would you do if faced with …"

The main themes of disaster movies can be categorized by our responses to the story. Generally, these themes, and our possible responses, are as follows:

Escapism—The movie takes you away from your everyday difficulties and can prompt you to say to yourself, "At least my current problems are not as bad as that."

Reinforcing our current skill level—Throughout the film, you could say to yourself, "I can manage that situation better than the people in the movie are doing."

Shock and awe—Being surprised or not having any idea what is coming can give you an adrenalin surge while you are sitting comfortably at the movies.

Challenging our coping—This movie theme can give us pause, where we consider, "What could be done to deal with this set of circumstances?"

Despite the seemingly superficial manner with which disaster movies treat our psychological underpinnings, they do awaken our sensibilities to the human condition. Whether it is appreciating how people have the strength of character to perform under horrible conditions or to be able to imagine yourself managing and coping, disaster movies can serve a purpose beyond pure entertainment.

Photo courtesy of Everett Collection Inc.

to having the ability to provide care to the injured, they have the skills needed to perform physical assessments and assess psychological distress. The Red Cross trains health care professionals as responders in disasters. Their Web site can be accessed via a direct link on the Online Student Resources for this book and provides information on the different training programs available.

Mental Health in the Movies discusses the ways in which disaster movies increase our awareness of our skills and stimulates thinking about how we would behave in certain circumstances.

Nursing Diagnosis: NANDA

People in crisis may have a variety of problems and symptoms. They may appear overwhelmed, calm, or agitated. They may speak clearly or they may ramble. Some appear rational, others psychotic. An individual's personal response and perception of the event will guide you toward determining the nursing diagnoses. The most common nursing diagnoses for people in crisis are as follows:

- Ineffective Coping
- Interrupted Family Processes
- Risk for Self-Directed Violence
- Anxiety
- Acute Confusion
- Spiritual Distress
- Sleep Deprivation
- Risk for Post-Trauma Syndrome
- Complicated Grieving
- Impaired Social Interaction

Outcome Identification: NOC

Determine outcome criteria for clients in crisis in collaboration with the client to avoid irrelevant goals and unworkable solutions. Consider the following as possible outcome criteria for a client in crisis:

- The client will be able to identify effective, as well as ineffective, coping patterns.
- The client will be able to employ effective coping strategies.
- The client will ask for help when necessary.
- The client will use available social support.
- The client will report an increase in psychological comfort and a decrease in negative feelings.

Planning and Implementation: NIC

Effective planning for crisis intervention must be as follows:

- Based on careful assessment and an understanding of human dependence needs
- Developed in active collaboration with the person in crisis and the significant people in that person's life
- Focused on immediate, concrete, contributing problems
- Appropriate to the person's level of thinking, feeling, and behaving
- Consistent with the person's lifestyle and culture
- Time limited, concrete, and realistic
- Mutually negotiated and renegotiated
- Organized to provide for follow-up

Many of these principles form the basis for therapeutic communication strategies.

Effective intervention is based on the ability to implement the second step of Roberts' model—make interpersonal contact, establish rapport, and rapidly establish the relationship (conveying genuine regard and respect for the client, acceptance, reassurance, and a nonjudgmental attitude). One-to-one interventions to make interpersonal contact, establish

CARING FOR THE SPIRIT

Helping Clients to Recuperate from Crisis

It is important for people who have experienced a crisis or trauma to stay grounded. Suggest the following exercises to someone who is feeling confused, upset, in disbelief, or hopeless.

1. Sit on a chair, feel your feet on the ground, press on your thighs, feel your behind on the seat and your back supported by the chair. Look around you and pick six objects that have red or blue in them. This should allow you to feel in the present, more grounded, and in your body. Notice how your breath gets deeper and calmer. You may want to go outdoors and find a peaceful place to sit on the grass. As you do, feel how your body is held and supported by the ground.

2. Gently pat the different parts of your body with your hand, with a loose wrist. Your body may feel more tingling, more alive, sharp, and you may feel more connected to your feelings.

3. Tense your muscles, each group at a time. Hold your shoulders with your arms across your chest, tighten your grip, and pat your arms up and down. Do the same with your legs, tighten them and hold them from the outside, patting through their length. Tighten your back, tighten your front, then gently release the tension. This may help you to feel more balanced.

4. If you believe in prayer or in a greater power, pray for the rest of the souls of the dead, for the healing of the wounded, and for the consolation of the grieving. Pray for peace, understanding, wisdom, and for the forces of good to prevail. Do not give up faith in the ultimate goodness of being and keep your trust in humanity.

Take comfort in knowing that we humans are extremely resilient and have been able to recuperate from the most horrendous tragedies.

Source: Adapted from USDHHS Substance Abuse and Mental Health Services Administration. *After a disaster: Self-care tips for dealing with stress.* Retrieved from http://www.samhsa.gov

---

rapport, and establish the relationship are important to an individual in crisis. However, nurses who work with people in crisis often need to use many nontraditional interventions, which can be as important as any verbal interventions. Working successfully with people in crisis is based on having a flexible, open view of what may be therapeutic with different individuals. You must have a full repertoire of skills and interventions that can be individualized to help all types of clients in crisis, including the ability to assist with spiritual needs. Caring for the Spirit offers suggestions that help a person in crisis integrate body, mind, and spirit.

Several different types of crisis intervention are discussed next.

Crisis Counseling

Crisis counseling is a type of brief, solution-focused therapy. Unlike therapies that focus on bringing about major personality change, crisis counseling focuses on strengths and solving immediate problems. Focusing on strengths is a resilience-oriented approach (Honig, 2010).

Crisis counseling usually lasts for five or six sessions and involves individuals, groups, or families. The following techniques are used:

- Listening actively and with concern (Your Intervention Strategies discusses communication strategies specific to working with a person in crisis.)
- Exploring the dimension of the problem, including the "last straw," in order to define it (Roberts' third step)
- Encouraging the open expression of feelings (Roberts' fourth step)
- Helping the client gradually accept reality

- Assessing past coping attempts and helping the client explore new ways of coping with problems (Roberts' fifth step)
- Linking the client to a social network
- Engaging in decision counseling or problem solving with the client, thus restoring cognitive mastery (Roberts' sixth step)
- Reinforcing newly learned coping devices
- Following up on the case after resolution of the crisis and leaving the door open for future contact, especially around the time of the anniversary of the event (Roberts' seventh step)

Telephone Counseling

Suicide prevention and crisis intervention centers rely heavily on telephone counseling by volunteers who have professional consultation available to them. Also known as *hotlines* and often available around the clock, they allow callers to remain anonymous and test what it feels like to ask for assistance. No appointment, travel time, or money is necessary, and help is immediately available. The volunteers usually work within a protocol that indicates what information they need from the client to assess the crisis. Their goal is to plan steps to provide immediate relief and then long-term follow-up, if necessary.

The calls made to a hotline usually fall into one of four categories: crisis calls, ventilation calls (getting a problem "off one's chest"), combinations of ventilation and information calls, or information-only calls. Calls that request information and ventilation are handled by supportive listening and giving information. Crisis calls need special techniques. Workers in crisis intervention centers generally follow a step-by-step agency protocol. For more information on suicide prevention hotlines, refer to Chapter 23 ∞.

YOUR INTERVENTION STRATEGIES Communication Strategies in Crisis Work

- **Use silence**—this gives the person time to reflect and become more aware of feelings. Silence can prompt elaboration. Simply being with the person is supportive.
- **Use nonverbal communication**—maintaining eye contact, head nodding, caring facial expressions, and occasional "uh-huhs" lets the person know that you are in tune.
- **Paraphrase**—understanding, empathy, and interest are conveyed by repeating portions of what the person said. Paraphrasing also checks for accuracy, clarifies misunderstandings, and lets people know they have been heard. You could say, "So, you are saying that…" or "I have heard you say that…."
- **Reflect feelings**—this helps the person identify and articulate emotions. You could say, "You sound angry, scared, etc. Does that fit for you?"
- **Allow the expression of emotions**—this is an important part of healing. Venting often helps the person work through feelings in order to better engage in constructive problem solving.

Some Things to Say

- "These are normal reactions to an abnormal situation."
- "It is understandable that you feel this way."
- "It wasn't your fault; you did the best you could."
- "I am sorry that this happened."
- "Things will get better, and you will feel better, although they may never be the same again."
- "You had a special relationship with your pet/car/house/child."
- "It is a good idea for you to talk about how you feel."
- "I care about how you feel."
- "You have the right to have these feelings."

Source: Adapted from USDHHS Substance Abuse and Mental Health Services Administration. *Disaster counseling.* Retrieved from http://www.samhsa.gov

---

Assisting With Environmental Changes

Working with an individual or a family in crisis may require taking steps to provide shelter. It may be necessary to find shelter for a homeless person, to obtain shelter in a safe house for an abused woman and her children, or to arrange for in-home health care.

Anticipatory Guidance

Anticipatory guidance is providing assistance in anticipation of the potential for crisis, thus averting it. These are some examples of anticipatory guidance: discussing methods of contraception with adolescents or young adults, preparing a child and the family for a tonsillectomy, arranging for a volunteer from the Reach for Recovery Program to visit a woman who has had a mastectomy, and preparing a list of helpful phone numbers for the newly discharged schizophrenic client.

Helping Develop Social Supports

Immediate and tangible social support is crucial for clients in crisis. Many people who are at risk for major depressive episodes following a crisis perceive their social supports to be very low (Salguerro et al., 2011). Many people in crisis have limited social supports and are not always sure about how to access supports or develop them. You can help a client develop tangible social supports by: introducing a woman whose husband is an alcoholic to Al-Anon groups in her community, referring a family with a terminally ill member to a local hospice, giving a rape victim the telephone number of the rape crisis hotline, or informing the newly discharged client with bipolar disorder and his family of the National Alliance on Mental Illness (NAMI) local group or national Web site (http://www.nami.org).

Critical Incident Stress Management

Critical incident stress management (CISM) is a comprehensive, integrative, and multifaceted approach to crisis intervention that spans the time sequence of a crisis. It is based on the notion that no single intervention alone is effective in crisis work. CISM consists of multiple components that can be applied to individuals, families, small groups, large groups, communities, and organizations. It can be best understood as a strategic delivery platform for primary, secondary, and tertiary prevention programs in the wake of large and small critical incidents (crises) rather than simply a crisis intervention treatment (Strand, Felices, & Williams, 2010; Yin et al., 2011). TABLE 34-1 ■ describes the elements of CISM described by Everly and Mitchell (2008) and their intents.

The term CISM replaces the term *critical incident stress debriefing (CISD)* to describe this approach. CISD was originally formulated in the 1980s by Mitchell and Everly (1996) in response to an air disaster in Washington, DC. The original approach, known as critical incident stress debriefing, was intended to include four major elements—on-scene crisis intervention; postincident small group discussion (known as *defusing*); a more formalized several-phase group discussion, which included debriefing; and follow-up support services. In practice, however, only one element, the group discussion, often to the exclusion of the others, became the focus of disaster mental health intervention. Its ease of use and the perception that it prevented PTSD led to its popularity. Although the small group meeting has both psychological and psychoeducation elements, described later in this section, it should not by itself be considered psychotherapy. According to the criticisms voiced by its developers, Everly and Mitchell (2008), and evidence in recent research (Strand, Felices, & Williams, 2010; Wei, Szumilas, & Kutcher, 2010), CISM is not a singular standalone crisis intervention or an effective way to prevent PTSD. Its

TABLE 34-1 ■ Components of Critical Incident Stress Management (CISM)

Component	Intent
1. Pre-event planning and preparation	To provide anticipatory guidance and foster resilience
2. Assessment	To determine the need for intervention for those directly and indirectly exposed
3. Strategic planning	To improve the crisis response
4. Individual crisis intervention	To provide psychological first aid to individuals
5. Large group crisis intervention	To provide large group psychological first aid
6. Small group crisis intervention	To provide small group psychological first aid and powerful event group support
7. Family crisis intervention	To provide psychological first aid to families
8. Organizational and community intervention	To deliver services to organizations and communities and to improve preparedness
9. Pastoral crisis intervention	To provide faith-based support
10. Follow-up and referral	To ensure continuity of care for those directly and indirectly exposed

most effective use appears to be in mitigating (decreasing, but not preventing) PTSD in soldiers and emergency services personnel. CISM is a more contemporary and broader approach and includes debriefing as one of its several components.

The debriefing process remains a valuable crisis intervention. The debriefing process offers an opportunity for individuals affected by a traumatic event to share their thoughts and feelings in a safe and controlled environment. Box 34-3 discusses the phases of the small group debriefing process in detail.

The typical settings in which debriefing as a component of CISM is used are: with staff on an inpatient unit after a suicide, with inmates after a murder in a jail, with military medical teams, with crisis line volunteers, with schoolchildren and school personnel after a multiple shooting in a school, with law enforcement personnel, as well as with rescue and health care workers after natural disasters or terrorist attacks (Everly & Mitchell, 2008; Strand, Felices, & Williams, 2010; Honig, 2010).

Disaster Assistance

The type of help needed by victims of a disaster changes as the disaster unfolds. Initially, people need information about evacuation plans, rescue efforts, and the location of food, shelter, and medical care. The media can provide this information, especially when there is time to plan and anticipate need (as with floods or hurricanes).

After acute needs are met at the disaster scene, in makeshift hospitals, or in emergency rooms, morgues, and shelters,

more far-reaching interventions are necessary. People need housing, jobs, and help in reconstructing their emotional lives. Two federal agencies assist with meeting the needs of both survivors and responders. The Federal Emergency Management Agency (FEMA) has a crisis counseling assistance and training program that provides mental health services to all individuals affected by a disaster (http://www.fema.gov). The Substance Abuse and Mental Health Services Administration (SAMHSA) of the Department of Health and Human Services also meets the mental health needs of survivors and responders (http://www.mentalhealth.samhsa.gov). Such data can be accessed on the Online Student Resources for this book.

Following are the psychological needs of victims both during and after a disaster:

- Talking about the experience and expressing their feelings of fear, panic, loss, and grief
- Becoming fully aware and accepting of what has happened to them
- Resuming concrete activities and reconstructing their lives with the social, physical, and emotional resources available

To guide victims and their families through the crisis, crisis workers employ the following skills:

- Listen with concern and sympathy, and ease the way for them to tell their tragic story, weep, and express feelings of anger, loss, frustration, and despair.
- Help them accept in small doses the tragic reality of what has happened. This means staying with them during the initial stages of shock and denial. It also may mean accompanying them back to the scene of the tragedy and being available for support when they are faced with the full impact of their loss.
- Help them make contact with relatives, friends, and other resources required for beginning the process of social and physical reconstruction. This could mean making telephone calls to locate relatives, accompanying someone to apply for financial aid, or giving information about social and mental health care agencies for follow-up services.

People who are panicked should receive prompt attention to minimize the potential for contagious panic that sometimes occurs in large groups. One strategy to help a panic-stricken person is to give the person a small, structured task that focuses energies constructively. Remember, however, that assigning tasks beyond the person's capabilities will add to the person's anxiety and feeling of helplessness. When in a disaster situation, remember to also incorporate concepts and intervention strategies related to death and loss such as those described in Chapter 17∞.

The effects of a disaster are felt long after the disaster is over. Provide anticipatory guidance that includes self-care tips to victims and their families so that they can manage their postdisaster experiences. Self-care tips are in Partnering With Clients and Families on page 751.

Box 34-3 The Small Group Debriefing Process

Introduction Phase (Setting the Tone for the Subsequent Phases)

- Explain the purpose of the meeting.
- Explain and give an overview of the process.
- Motivate the participants.
- Assure the participants that information will be confidential.
- Explain the guidelines.
- Identify the team members.
- Answer questions or concerns.

Fact Phase (Imparting Power to the Participants Through Giving Information)

- Assist the participants to discuss the facts of the incident.
- Ask the participants to tell who they are.
- Ask the participants to tell how they were involved in the incident.
- Ask the participants to tell what happened from their perspective.

Thought Phase (Transitioning Between Impersonal Outside Facts and That Which Is Internal, Close, and Personal)

- Ask each participant to discuss his or her first thoughts or most prominent thoughts about the traumatic event.
- Expect to hear emotional comments.

Reaction Phase (Ventilating With a Potential for Emotional Abreaction)

- Most of the discussing is done by the participants.
- Discussion is freewheeling.
- Ask participants what the worst thing was about the situation, what they would choose to erase, and what aspect of the situation causes the most pain.

Symptom Phase (Normalizing and Attacking the Myth of Unique Weakness or Vulnerability)

- Move the group toward more cognitively oriented material.
- Ask participants to describe any cognitive, physical, emotional, or behavioral experiences they encountered at the scene of the incident.
- Ask about any symptoms that followed subsequently.

Teaching Phase (Moving Further Away From the Emotional Content of the Reaction Phase)

- Acknowledge symptoms described in the symptom phase.
- Reaffirm that symptoms are normal, typical, or predictable after what they've been through.
- Forewarn the group about possible symptoms they might experience in the future.
- Involve the participants in stress management activities.

Re-Entry Phase (Identifying Homogenizing Themes That May Be Used to Facilitate Closure and Provide a Psychological Uplift)

Participant Roles

- Introduce any new material they wish to discuss.
- Review old material already discussed.
- Ask any questions.
- Discuss whatever would help them to bring closure to the debriefing.

Debriefing Team Roles

- Answer any questions.
- Inform and reassure.
- Provide appropriate handouts and other written material.
- Provide referral sources for assessment, therapy, and so on.
- Summarize the debriefing experience with words of respect, encouragement, appreciation, support, and direction.

Evaluation

Nurses in acute care or short-term settings may not see the long-term effects of their interventions. Typically, nurses in these settings need to evaluate the crisis, set up the plan, and begin implementing it.

In long-term settings, you can evaluate the client or family response to the intervention by determining whether clients have resumed their precrisis level of functioning or show evidence of increased functioning (growth). A nurse in either a long-term or short-term setting may also have an opportunity to evaluate whether a similar problem might lead to another crisis for the client.

It is difficult to evaluate the effectiveness of disaster intervention because of the large numbers of people involved and the disruptive nature of a disaster. Evaluation can take place at many different levels. Nurses can evaluate their work with individual clients; mental health care agencies can monitor statistics on groups of clients; government agencies can assess the numbers of unemployed and homeless; public health departments can measure the extent of disease and disability.

The most important aspect of evaluation is to review how the interventions were implemented and the effectiveness of the relief work. Disaster preparedness is needed to effectively intervene when the unthinkable—a disaster—occurs. Many hospitals and clinics have ongoing drills to prepare for the possibility of a disaster. It is important that you understand your role and the tasks and functions for which you are responsible.

CASE MANAGEMENT

Case management services for crisis may include any one or several activities. Arranging for crisis intervention or forensic intervention services may be necessary. In disaster situations, triaging—e.g., rapid medical and psychological evaluation—and hospitalization, if necessary, may be a case management activity. The case manager in all crisis situations will mobilize necessary mental health resources and monitor outcomes for clients. Referral for vocational training, family crisis

PARTNERING WITH CLIENTS AND FAMILIES

Self-Care Tips After a Disaster

Things to Remember When Trying to Understand Disaster Events

- No one who sees a disaster is untouched by it.
- It is normal to feel anxious about your and your family's safety.
- Profound sadness, grief, and anger are normal reactions to an abnormal event.
- Acknowledging your feelings helps you to recover.
- Focusing on your strengths and abilities will help you to heal.
- Accepting help from community programs and resources is healthy.
- Everyone has different needs and different ways of coping.
- It is common to want to strike back at people who have caused great pain. However, nothing good is accomplished by hateful language or actions.

Signs That Adults Need Stress Management Assistance

- Difficulty communicating thoughts
- Difficulty sleeping
- Difficulty maintaining balance
- Easily frustrated
- Increased use of drugs/alcohol
- Limited attention span
- Poor work performance
- Headaches/stomach problems
- Tunnel vision/muffled hearing
- Colds or flulike symptoms
- Disorientation or confusion
- Difficulty concentrating
- Reluctance to leave home
- Depression, sadness
- Feelings of hopelessness
- Mood swings
- Crying easily

- Overwhelming guilt and self-doubt
- Fear of crowds, strangers, or being alone

Ways to Ease the Stress

- Talk with someone about your feelings—anger, sorrow, and other emotions—even though it may be difficult.
- Encourage others, as well as yourself, not to tell your stories in a repetitive way—this ultimately deepens the trauma. Instead, support and hear one another, but with breaks and interruptions of the story from beginning to end.
- Remember not to hold yourself directly responsible for the disastrous event or be frustrated because you feel that you cannot help directly in the rescue work.
- Take steps to promote your own physical and emotional healing by staying active in your daily life patterns or by adjusting them (i.e., healthy eating, rest, exercise, relaxation, meditation). This healthy outlook will help you and your family.
- Maintain a normal household and daily routine, limiting demanding responsibilities for yourself and your family.
- Spend time with family and friends.
- Participate in memorials, rituals, and use of symbols as a way to express feelings.
- Use existing support groups of family, friends, and house of worship.
- Establish a family emergency plan—this can be very comforting.
- Seek outside professional assistance if these self-help strategies are not helping you or you find that you are using drugs/alcohol in order to cope.

Source: Adapted from USDHHS Substance Abuse and Mental Health Services Administration. *After a disaster: Self-care tips for dealing with stress.* Retrieved from http://www.samhsa.gov.org

intervention services, or grief counseling may be called for. Case managers for clients with prolonged postdisaster distress may refer clients for cognitive–behavioral therapy, implemented no sooner than 60 days postdisaster (Kar, 2011). This can function as an intermediate step between traditional crisis counseling and longer-term mental health treatments.

COMMUNITY-BASED CARE

Most communities have a wealth of community-based services, such as hotlines (see Chapter 23∞) or crisis centers appropriate for persons in crisis. After disasters, local communities and various government agencies band together to provide additional services to meet the expected surge in the need for mental health services.

Mobile crisis units (MCUs) are community-based programs that are designed to deliver crisis services to any location in the community. MCUs are staffed by teams that may include psychiatrists, psychiatric–mental health nurses, substance abuse counselors, psychologists, psychiatric social

workers, child welfare workers, or other trained professionals. The specific functions of MCUs vary by community. Following are the typical advantages that MCUs provide:

- Intervening in crisis situations without delay
- Providing increased community access to services
- Assessing clients in their own community environment
- Avoiding unnecessary hospitalizations
- Facilitating hospitalization or detoxification when needed
- Avoiding unnecessary arrests
- Consulting to law enforcement
- Working together with the person's family and network (Sjlie, Karlsson, & Kim, 2010).

HOME CARE

Home visits are made when telephone counseling does not suffice or when the crisis workers need to obtain additional information by direct observation or to reach a client who is unobtainable by telephone. Home visits are appropriate when crisis workers need to initiate contact rather than waiting for clients to come to them—for example, when a telephone caller is assessed to be highly suicidal or when a concerned family member, neighbor, physician, or clergyman informs the agency of clients in potential crisis. Home crisis visits are also an effective intervention for persons with serious mental illnesses who are having a mental health crisis (Bookle & Webber, 2011), helping to keep them functioning in the community.

Often, clients in crisis are too disorganized or distraught to seek help by themselves. The police may arrange for a home crisis visit to avoid imprisoning or hospitalizing a client. Problems for which home crisis visits are usually instituted are spousal abuse, child abuse, psychiatric emergencies (such as drug overdose, suicide attempt or other life-threatening self-abuse, stalking, assault, rape, and homicide), and medical emergencies.

In many agencies, the crisis team often consists of a man and a woman who are highly skilled and experienced in crisis intervention. The male–female team is generally perceived as less threatening than two men, two women, or a single person. Their goal is to defuse the situation with as little disruption and violence as possible and to engage the client in longer-term treatment. They may also be members of mobile crisis units (discussed in the previous section).

There are others who intervene in community crises, as well. The public health nurse is in an excellent position to identify, assess, and intervene with clients experiencing a life crisis. Public health nurses often have access to community resources as well as informal communication lines, and they usually maintain contact with families and clients for longer periods of time than nurses in other settings. They are often recognized by the community as knowledgeable experts who are available for immediate assistance, as in the following clinical example.

Clinical Example

Emily, age 78, and her sister Frances, age 84, lived in a run-down part of town. Frances became seriously ill with pneumonia and became progressively weaker. Emily's anxiety about Frances's health grew when her sister refused to see a doctor. Emily feared that her sister would die or need to go to a nursing home. Emily felt paralyzed and didn't know what to do. When the visiting nurse came by to visit Emily's neighbor, Emily asked the nurse to see Frances. Together, they were able to persuade Frances to get medical care so that she could stay home.

VICARIOUS TRAUMATIZATION

Disasters and traumatic experiences shake the foundations of our beliefs about how other people behave toward one another, and can shatter our assumption that the world is a safe place. In evaluating the aftereffects of a disaster, remember that there may be an impact on those who are not direct victims.

Clinical Example

Matilda worked as a short-order cook in a restaurant in Wichita, Kansas. On Monday morning, Matilda decided to call in sick, although she was well. Matilda's fiancé, a waiter at the same restaurant, was killed along with several others when a propane gas talk in the restaurant's storage area exploded. Matilda now has vivid nightmares. She alternates between feeling sad and angry. She refuses to attend church anymore, asking God, over and over, why He spared her and not the others at the restaurant.

Janelle frantically pressed the redial button on her cell phone, trying to reach her mother, who lived in an area of southern California plagued by wildfires. After 3 hours of frantic but unsuccessful activity, Janelle, exhausted, sat down on a curb and sobbed. When her cell phone finally rang, it was Janelle's mother calling from a fire station that had evacuated residents threatened by the wildfires. She was dirty and scared, but okay. Despite this good news, Janelle couldn't stop crying. Months later, she still feels anxious.

A disaster can affect the mental health of various groups—a condition known as **vicarious traumatization**. Also known as *secondary trauma response*, vicarious traumatization is a condition in which psychological aftereffects are experienced by those who are not direct victims of the traumatic event. The groups most commonly at increased risk are identified in the following list. Those individuals who are most affected are listed first.

1. Next-of-kin
2. Injured survivors and their close ones
3. Uninjured survivors
4. Onlookers (the helpless helpers, who are at particularly high risk)
5. Rescuers
6. Body handlers
7. Health personnel (many mass-injury situations may demand difficult prioritizing)
8. People responsible for the disaster
9. Coworkers in workplace disasters
10. Evacuees

The World Trade Center attack has focused a great deal of attention on the responses of survivors and their families in the posttrauma period. The impact of the event has resonated deeply with those who survived. The overall prevalence of PTSD among over 3,200 civilian survivors was 15%, with almost 96% reporting at least one ongoing PTSD symptom (DiGrande, Neria, Brackbill, Pulliam, & Galea, 2011). Those at greatest risk for PTSD had direct exposure to the terrorist attacks by being on a high floor in the towers, initiating evacuation late, being caught in the dust cloud that resulted from the tower collapses, personally witnessing horror, and sustaining an injury.

Nurses and other crisis workers are routinely exposed to victim suffering and to the aftereffects of crisis, trauma, and inhumane acts (see FIGURE 34-4 ■). They are at risk for becoming what has been called "wounded healers." Awareness of the psychological risk can prevent the loss of necessary personnel (Walden, 2010). This clinical example illustrates how vicarious traumatization can affect rescue workers.

Clinical Example

Brian is a police officer from Buffalo, New York, who volunteered to assist the New York City Police Department in the days immediately after the terrorist attack at the World Trade Center. He was on a team looking for people who might still be alive in the rubble. Although Brian considered himself "tough" and had a macho image among his fellow officers, he burst into tears and had to be led away from the site to meet with a mental health counselor. Brian acts tougher than ever, but still occasionally bursts into tears and has difficulty controlling his emotions.

Sheila was a mental health nurse at a hospital in Gulfport, Mississippi, located only a few blocks from the Gulf of Mexico. She was also a volunteer who assisted survivors of Hurricane Katrina and first responders (firefighters, police officers, paramedics) and counseled them for several weeks. Sheila became preoccupied with the stories of her clients. Her insomnia and angry outbursts at home prompted Sheila to seek counseling for herself.

FIGURE 34-4 ■ Exhausted nurses and other crisis workers.
Photo courtesy of AP Wide World Photos, Jeff Beiermann.

Expect to be vulnerable to this condition if you work with clients in the highly disorganized crisis period; with those who are victims of sexual assault, violence, or disaster; or with those, such as sexual offenders, who traumatize others. Vicarious traumatization can also affect your own physical health by inducing gastrointestinal problems (such as gastritis or peptic ulcer), hypertension, and fatigue. In the home or the workplace, you could experience the following:

- An increase in the number of sick days
- Indecision or difficulty with problem solving
- Isolation or withdrawal
- Behavioral outbursts

Should this happen, seek additional support, supervision, and referral for professional assistance.

The opposite of vicarious traumatization, *vicarious resilience*, is an emerging topic for study. Vicarious resilience is a new concept put forth by Hernandez, Gangsei, and Engstrom (2007) that addresses the question of how psychotherapists who work with survivors of political violence or kidnapping are affected by their clients' stories of resilience. Their study illustrates, yet again, that therapists are affected by their clients' stories (this time positively) and that stories of resilience and constructive coping with adversity can contribute to sustaining and empowering trauma therapists.

Pearson Nursing Student Resources

Find additional review materials at
nursing.pearsonhighered.com
Prepare for success with NCLEX®-style practice questions, interactive assignments and activities, web links, animations and videos, and more!

REFERENCES

Berger, J. T. (2011). Imagining the unthinkable: Illuminating the present. *Journal of Clinical Ethics, 22*(1), 17–19.

Bhui, K., & Dinos, S. (2011). Preventive psychiatry: A paradigm to improve population mental health and well-being. *British Journal of Psychiatry, 198*, 417–419.

Bookle, M., & Webber, M. (2011). Ethnicity and access to an inner city home treatment service: A case-control study. *Health & Social Care in the Community, 19*(3), 280–288.

Cacioppo, J. T., Reis, H. T., & Zautra, A. J. (2011). Social resilience: The value of social fitness with an application to the military. *American Psychologist, 66*(1), 43–51.

Caplan, G. (1964). *Principles of preventive psychiatry.* New York, NY: Basic Books.

Centers for Disease Control and Prevention, National Center for Injury Prevention and Control, Division of Violence Prevention. Coping with stress after a traumatic event. Retrieved from http://www.cdc.gov/violenceprevention/pdf/Coping_with_Stress-a.pdf

Claassen, C., Kashner, T. M., Kashner, T. K., Xuan, L., & Larkin, G. L. (2011). Psychiatric emergency "surge capacity" following acts of terrorism and mass violence with high media impact: What is required? *General Hospital Psychiatry, 33*(3), 287–293. doi: 35400018984980.0110

de Jong, G., & Schout, G. (2011). Family group conferences in public mental health care: An exploration of opportunities. *International Journal of Mental Health Nursing, 20*(1), 63–74.

DelGaizo, A. L., Elhai, J. D., & Weaver, T. L. (2011). Posttraumatic stress disorder, poor physical health and substance use behaviors in a national trauma-exposed sample. *Psychiatry Research, 188*(3), 390–395. doi: 10.1016/j.psychres.2011.03.016

DiGrande, L., Neria, Y., Brackbill, R. M., Pulliam, P., & Galea, S. (2011). Long-term posttraumatic stress symptoms among 3,271 civilian survivors of the September 11, 2001 terrorist attacks on the World Trade Center. *American Journal of Epidemiology, 173*(3), 271–281.

Everly, G. S., & Mitchell, J. T. (2008). *Integrative crisis intervention and disaster mental health*. Ellicott City, MD: Chevron Publishing Corporation.

Gershoff, E. T., Aber, J. L., Ware, A., & Kotler, J. A. (2010). Exposure to 9/11 among youth and their mothers in New York City: Enduring associations with mental health and sociopolitical attitudes. *Child Development, 81*(4), 1142–1160.

Hernandez, P., Gangsei, D., & Engstrom, D. (2007). Vicarious resilience: A new concept in work with those who survive trauma. *Family Process, 46*(2), 229–241.

Honig, A. L. (2010). War then and now: From surviving to thriving. *International Journal of Emergency Mental Health, 12*(3), 207–212.

Kar, N. (2011). Cognitive behavioral therapy for the treatment of posttraumatic stress disorder: A review. *Neuropsychiatric Diseases and Treatment, 7*, 167–181.

Lindemann, E. (1944). Symptomatology and management of acute grief. *American Journal of Psychiatry, 101*, 141–148.

Lunsky, Y., & Elserafi, J. (2011). Life events and emergency department visits in response to crisis in individuals with intellectual disabilities. *Journal of Intellectual Disability, 55*(7), 714–718. doi: 10.1111/j.1365-2788.2011.01417.x

Melamed, B. G., & Castro, C. (2011). Observations and insights about strengthening our soldiers (SOS). *Journal of Clinical Psychology in Medical Settings, 18*(2), 210–223. doi: 10.1007/s10880-011-9253-4

Mitchell, J. T., & Everly, G. S., Jr. (1996). *Critical incident stress debriefing: An operations manual*. Ellicott City, MD: Chevron Publishing.

Raphael, B., & Ma, H. (2011). Mass catastrophe and disaster psychiatry. *Molecular Psychiatry, 16*(3), 247–251.

Reid-Quiñones, K., Kliewer, W., Shields, B. J., Goodman, K., Ray, M. H., & Wheat, E. (2010). Cognitive, affective, and behavioral responses to witnessed versus experienced violence. *American Journal of Orthopsychiatry, 814*(1), 51–60.

Roberts, A. R. (Ed.). (2005). *Crisis intervention handbook: Assessment, treatment, and research* (3rd ed.). New York, NY: Oxford University Press.

Roberts, A. R., & Bender, K. (2006). Juvenile offender suicide: Prevalence, risk factors, assessment, and crisis intervention protocols. *International Journal of Emergency Mental Health, 8*(4), 255–265.

Salguero, J. M., Fernandez-Berrocal, P., Iruarrizaga, I., Cano-Vindel, A., & Galea, S. (2011). Major depressive disorder following terrorist attacks: A systematic review of prevalence, course, and correlates. *BMC Psychiatry, 11*(1), 96. doi: 10.1186/1471-244X-11-96

Sjlie, H., Karlsson, B., & Kim, H. S. (2010). Crisis resolution and home treatment: Structure, process, and outcome—a literature review. *Journal of Psychiatric and Mental Health Nursing, 17*(10), 881–892.

Strand, R., Felices, K., & Williams, K. (2010). Critical incident stress management (CISM) in support of special agents and other first responders to the Fort Hood shooting: Summary and recommendations. *International Journal of Mental Health, 12*(3), 151–160.

Tyhurst, J. S. (1957). The role of transition states—including disasters—in mental illness. In *Symposium on preventive and social psychiatry* (pp. 1–23). Washington, DC: Walter Reed Army Institute of Research.

Walden, P. (2010). Wounded healers: Nurses and depression. *Nursing Made Incredibly Easy!, 8*(6), 6–7.

Wei, Y., Szumilas, M., & Kutcher, S. (2010). Effectiveness on mental health of psychological debriefing for crisis intervention in schools. *Educational Psychology Review, 22*(3), 339–347.

Yin, H., He, H., Arbon, P., & Zhu J. (2011). A survey of the practice of nurses' skills in Wenchuan earthquake disaster sites: Implications for disaster training. *Journal of Advanced Nursing, 67*(10), 2231–2238. doi: 10.1111/j.1365-2648.2011.05699.x

Anger Management and Intervention in Psychiatric–Mental Health Settings

35

SUE C. DELAUNE

LEARNING OUTCOMES

After completing this chapter, you will be able to:

1. Describe theoretical perspectives that are useful in understanding anger and violent behavior.
2. Assess for the presence of behavioral and verbal cues that indicate escalation of anger.
3. Identify risk factors that contribute to violent behavior.
4. Incorporate nursing measures to de-escalate potentially violent behavior within the context of the principle of least restrictiveness.
5. Develop nursing care plans that balance the issue of safety maintenance with the need to ensure the individual freedom of the violent client.
6. Implement a variety of nonpharmacologic nursing strategies for intervening with violent clients.
7. Describe common staff responses to anger and violence.
8. Analyze personal feelings and attitudes that may affect professional practice when caring for clients exhibiting anger and/or violent behavior.

CRITICAL THINKING CHALLENGE

Harold, an 80-year-old retired jeweler, was admitted to the inpatient unit after hitting a personal care aide at the extended care facility where he has resided for 10 years. On admission, he is mute, does not eat, wanders in and out of other clients' rooms, and is easily frustrated. Sometimes he strikes out at the nursing staff when they attempt to assist him with routine self-care activities. The staff has requested a case conference to develop a new approach to his care.

1. How do you rate Harold's potential for violence?
2. What primary need should Harold's treatment team address?
3. What are some specific measures staff members could implement to increase safety for Harold, other clients, and care providers?

AN OPEN LETTER TO THE STUDENT

Does the title of this chapter make your heart beat a little faster or cause you to become somewhat fearful? If your philosophy is "Don't tell me about danger," then certain sections of this chapter may cause you some discomfort. However, if you understand that our imaginations can be the fertile ground in which worry and anxiety grow, then you also understand that you have a choice. You can choose to worry about something, or you can take precautions and take action to find solutions. Taking precautions is constructive; remaining in a state of fear or worry is destructive.

The truth is that most psychiatric–mental health nurses live their professional lives without being victims of violence by mental health clients. The distorted and sensationalist views in the media—striking visuals and excited news anchors—combine to add to our fears of the people who happen to be our clients in the mental health settings in which we practice.

Whether you realize it or not, you use your ability to predict behavior in everyday life. You often know when a car will edge over into your lane without signaling. We often refer to that as our "intuition." The root of the word intuition means to guard or protect. Don't dismiss it. It is a cognitive process that tells us it is time to call on our better judgment skills. The great scientist Albert Einstein once said that when you follow your intuition the solutions come to you and you don't know why or how. Many great discoveries have followed on the heels of a hunch, an intuition. You need to know how to harness your intuition by developing your assessment skills.

In this chapter we will show you how your assessment skills will help you to anticipate and avoid violence and how specific nursing strategies can be used to de-escalate anger and aggressive behavior if it occurs. Our goal is to help you to become safer and more comfortable, and reduce your fear, while acknowledging that a certain element of danger does exist in mental health settings.

Gavin de Becker, an expert on violent behavior who has successfully proposed new laws to help manage violence, identifies three ways in which we can use our fears to improve our lives:

1. *When you feel fear, listen.*
2. *When you don't feel fear, don't manufacture it.*
3. *If you find yourself creating worry, explore and discover why (de Becker, 1997).*

We intend that this chapter will help you to avoid unwarranted fear and harness and respect your ability to recognize, prevent, and de-escalate anger and aggressive behavior.

Carol Ren Kneisl and Eileen Trigoboff

Anger is a universal emotional response to a threat or feeling of powerlessness and a common automatic response to anxiety (see Chapter 8∞ for the relationship between anger and anxiety). When they experience fear, many people become angry, as evidenced by the adage, "I don't get sad, I get mad." When dealing with a client, it is important that you determine if fear is an underlying factor so that the fear can be discussed and, hopefully, decreased. Everyone is entitled to their feelings of anger. However, no one has the right to express anger in an aggressive manner.

Aggression, behavior that violates the rights of other individuals, results in harm to others. **Violence** (a term used interchangeably with *aggression*) refers to behavior that is harmful to others. Violence can be expressed verbally (e.g., screaming, threatening, abusive remarks) and nonverbally (e.g., physical assault). Violent behavior can occur on a continuum, ranging from threatened assault, to physical abuse, to acts of terrorism. Anger (the emotion) usually precedes aggression; therefore, it is important for you to assess the client's degree of anger. Individuals who have healthy outlets for angry emotions rarely escalate to aggressive, violent behavior.

Society in general, and nursing in particular, increasingly recognizes that violence is a significant health problem. Violence is also an ever-increasing problem in health care environments. According to the Bureau of Labor Statistics, U.S. Department of Labor (2010) health care and social assistance occupations experienced the highest rate of occupational injuries (3 out of 10 categories) than the other occupations surveyed. Literature supports the fact that nurses are frequently exposed to workplace violence (Campbell et al., 2011; Gillespie, Gates, Miller, & Howard, 2010; Magnavita & Heponiemi, 2011).

Health care providers in every setting—not just psychiatric treatment facilities—are potential targets of violent behavior. For example, emergency departments are especially prone to increased incidents of workplace violence (Taylor & Rew, 2011). Nurses in every practice area encounter clients and family members who may be potentially violent. Perpetrator risk factors in health care settings include drug or alcohol abuse, mental illness, inability to deal with crises, and possession of weapons (Gillespie et al., 2010). Following are other factors that have contributed to the increasing violence in health care facilities:

- Downsizing of staff
- Change in skill level of staff members, who now include greater numbers of paraprofessionals
- Increased client acuity levels
- Absence of workplace violence prevention programs

One other factor that contributes to aggression toward nurses is the mistaken belief that violence is part of the job (Allen, de Nesnera, Cummings, & Darling, 2011). These factors, and the fact that nurses are the most frequent victims of assault in health care facilities, magnify the need for psychiatric–mental health nurses to learn to accurately assess and intervene with clients in order to maintain safety.

This chapter provides theoretic perspectives for understanding anger and aggressive (or violent) behavior. It also describes successful preventive measures such as exploring potential causative factors, recognizing warning signs of escalating anger, nursing interventions, and client and staff education. Evidence-Based Practice illustrates the steps that can be taken to avoid the escalation of aggressive behavior.

EVIDENCE-BASED PRACTICE

De-Escalating Strategies for Aggression

Marty, a 42-year-old client on an inpatient unit, is becoming more aggressive toward staff and other clients. He paces in the hall and mutters to himself. When approached by the nursing staff, he shouts and curses at them. You know that these behaviors are indicative that Marty's aggressive behavior is escalating.

In an attempt to avoid using seclusion and restraints, the nursing staff decides to use the following interventions aimed at de-escalating Marty's behavior:

- Identify the intensity of Marty's behavior.
- Make a personal connection with Marty by having a one–to–one interaction.
- Determine the meaning of Marty's behavior (i.e., understand what he needs).

Additional approaches that may be useful in helping Marty calm down are deep breathing, distraction, and the therapeutic use of music, dance, and movement therapy. The treatment team decides to use observation and role-modeling of expected behavior. Also, after Marty's behavior has stabilized, teaching him anger management techniques may be very useful.

These intervention approaches are based on the following research:

De Benedictis, L., Dumais, A., Sieu, N., Mailhot, M. P., Letourneau, G., Tran, M. A., . . . Lesage, A. D. (2011). Staff perceptions and organizational factors as predictors of seclusion and restraint on psychiatric wards. *Psychiatric Services, 62*(5), 484–401.

Lanza, M. L., & Witkower, A. (2010). Concentric Interactive Group Model: A unique experience for patients and staff. *Perspectives of Psychiatric Care, 46*(4), 294–300.

LaRue, C., Dumais, A., Drapeau, A., Menard, G., & Goulet, M. H. (2010). Nursing practices recorded in reports of episodes of seclusion. *Issues in Mental Health Nursing, 31*(12), 785–792.

CRITICAL THINKING QUESTIONS

1. What is the basis for the belief that anger management can be taught successfully?
2. What is the rationale for adding deep breathing and distraction?
3. Why would music, dance, and movement therapy be helpful?

The strategies in Evidence-Based Practice are more fully discussed in the Nursing Process section later in this chapter.

NURSING SELF-AWARENESS

Not every nurse can work with angry, aggressive, or violent mentally ill clients. Because such work can be frightening and upsetting, it is important to take the time for self-reflection and to examine your reactions to others. This is particularly important when working with violent clients, because your own stress and anxiety can greatly interfere with your ability to attend to subtle cues and to initiate sensitive interventions in a timely manner.

Self-awareness is a process that helps you to avoid personalizing client comments and behaviors. Whenever we "take it personally," as Brenda did in the clinical example that follows, objectivity is lost and therapeutic effectiveness decreases.

Clinical Example

Brenda, a nursing student, was immediately drawn to Maria, a client who vigorously paced the outdoor recreation area. On her part, Maria seemed taken with Brenda and they spent a comfortable morning together on Brenda's first day on the inpatient unit. Brenda's classmates were envious of the easy relationship she seemed to have with Maria. When Brenda returned to the unit one week later, Maria would have nothing to do with Brenda, shouting at her to "go away." Brenda felt confused and hurt. She could not understand what went wrong. Finding out that Maria was diagnosed with bipolar disorder, and that her behavior reflected the rapid mood swing cycle she was in, did not help Maria feel any better.

As you can see in the clinical example, intellectual knowledge is not always enough. Often, our responses to client aggressiveness reflect the beliefs that we incorporated as children. For example, as young children, some of us learned that anger was something to be feared and avoided at all costs. Some of us have learned to take responsibility for the anger of others. Others of us may have learned that the aggressive expression of anger is powerful. These beliefs adopted in childhood often govern our behavior as adults. Self-reflection helps us to determine how our own beliefs influence our responses to clients. Your Self-Awareness lists some areas that are important for you to consider when you work with angry or potentially violent clients.

YOUR SELF-AWARENESS
Factors That Influence Your Response to Violence

When working with violent clients, be sure to monitor yourself for the following:

- Ability to use anger constructively and to not take clients' anger personally
- Capacity for clear verbal communication
- Ability to listen actively with a nonjudgmental attitude
- Capacity to both establish and maintain empathic linkages with clients and to disengage when appropriate
- Willingness to understand your fears and anxieties about violence
- Belief that violent clients are amenable to treatment

BIOPSYCHOSOCIAL THEORIES

The ongoing debate in psychiatry of "nature versus nurture" (what we are born with versus what we learn) extends into the study of the causes of violence. The expression of aggressive behavior is affected by a complex interaction of biologic and psychosocial factors. Therefore, there is no simple answer for the etiology of violent behavior, and no single theoretic framework can sufficiently explain or predict violence.

Even though there are no specific diagnostic classifications for anger and violence, there are some mental disorders in which aggressiveness is more likely to occur. Box 35-1 lists some of the mental disorders in which aggressive behavior is prominent; note that the list is not inclusive. It is also important to note that the diagnosis alone does not make the client violence prone. Rather, clients who have these disorders are likely to experience impairments in impulse control, sensory–perceptual functioning, cognitive functioning, and social skills. Individuals who have poor coping skills and feelings of helplessness and powerlessness are at high risk of exhibiting violent behavior. There is wide diversity among individuals and the situations in which they live. It is, therefore, more valuable to consider violence from a variety of perspectives.

Biologic Factors

Current research is exploring the biologic basis of aggression. While it is likely that violence may be influenced by many biologic variables—genetic factors, hormonal factors, neurotransmitters, and neurophysiological factors—the exact relationship remains uncertain.

Physiological changes within the brain may result in violent behavior. Trauma and other disturbances that produce anoxia (e.g., cardiorespiratory arrest) are likely culprits in the development of aggression in some individuals. For example, some people who experience brain tumors or cerebral vascular accidents (strokes) demonstrate violent behavior. Metabolic disorders such as severe hypoglycemia, encephalitis, and dementia may also lead to violence.

In order to understand the underpinnings of violence, it is important for nurses to understand the following structures of the brain and their effects on emotion and behavior:

  ■ The amygdala, located in the lateral temporal lobe, directs emotional responses, including the aggressive expression of anger.

Box 35-1 Mental Disorders in Which Aggressiveness Often Occurs

  ■ Antisocial personality disorder
  ■ Borderline personality disorder
  ■ Conduct disorder
  ■ Delusional disorder
  ■ Dementia of the Alzheimer's type
  ■ Intermittent explosive disorder
  ■ Mania
  ■ Schizophrenia
  ■ Substance-related disorders

  ■ The hippocampus regulates the recall of recent experiences and new information. Impairment in this area interferes with learning from past experiences, as is often demonstrated by individuals with impulsive behavior.
  ■ The hypothalamus, which serves as a relay between the cerebral cortex and the lower autonomic centers and the spinal cord somatic centers, is the route through which the mind influences bodily function.
  ■ Temporal lobe dysfunction (which occurs with seizures) may cause people to become aggressive. It is not unusual for some individuals to become violent in the postictal phase of a seizure.
  ■ The limbic system (a functional grouping rather than an anatomic one; includes nuclei, tracts, and structures along the border between the cerebrum and the diencephalon) mediates primitive emotions and basic drives, such as appetite, sexual urges, and aggression. Dysfunction of the limbic system may result in an increase or decrease in aggressive behavior.

Chapter 6∞ discusses these issues in detail.

Numerous research studies substantiate that neurotransmitters, hormones, enzymes, and signaling molecules influence aggression (Booij et al., 2010; Parsey, 2010; Rosell et al., 2010; Takahashi, Quadros, de Almeida, & Miczek, 2011). TABLE 35-1 ■ provides an overview of the effects of selected neurotransmitters on aggression.

Genetic Theories

No one gene or variant thereof has yet been identified as the causative factor of aggressive behavior. However, one study (Beaver, Sak, Vaske, & Nilsson, 2010) indicates that it may be possible to measure the risk of antisocial behaviors, such as aggression, by examining gene x environmental alterations. Another study (Roaldset, Bakken, & Biorkly, 2011) suggests that violent behavior may be associated with low cholesterol levels due to a specific gene mutation. Additional research related to the complexity of the genetic contribution to aggressive behavior is needed (Jasinska & Freimer, 2009). Study of the relationship between heredity and violence is continuing at a rapid pace and is focusing on specific molecular genetic markers for aggressiveness.

Psychosocial Theories

Psychoanalytic, psychological, and sociocultural theories contribute to our understanding of the complex behavior of aggression. Freud (1989) theorized that aggression is one of the two innate drives, the other being the pleasure principle. This viewpoint states that it is instinctive for humans to express anger in aggressive ways. When aggression is directed inward, depression results.

Aggression may be viewed as a direct result of unmet needs and wants. Whenever an individual's basic needs are unmet, the resulting threat to his or her existence may cause the person to respond in an aggressive manner. The frustration that arises from unmet needs may escalate to aggressiveness.

TABLE 35-1 ■ Role of Neurotransmitters in Aggression

Transmitter	Function	Description
Acetylcholine	Exerts excitatory effect Facilitates transmission of nerve impulses across myoneural junction	A deficiency (such as that occurring in dementia of the Alzheimer's type) may increase aggressive behavior by lowering the threshold for confusion and impairing memory
Dopamine	Regulates emotional responses and movement	Increased levels heighten sexual activity, aggressive behavior, and vigilance
Gamma-aminobutyric acid (GABA)	Exerts inhibitory response on brain activity	Exerts regulatory effect on violence
Norepinephrine	Exerts excitatory response Is inactivated by monoamine oxidase (MAO)	May increase vigilance and aggression
Serotonin (5-HT)	Influences the processing of information Modulates sleep, sensory responses, and mood	Variations in 5-HT levels lead to misperception of stimuli, which may result in aggressive behavior

There are numerous psychosocial variables that influence the development and expression of violent behavior. Current research is examining the effects of child abuse, emotional rejection in childhood, and parenting styles as precursors to the development of violence (Fassino, Amianto, Gastaldo, & Leombruni, 2009; Ferguson, San Miguel, & Hartley, 2009; Mrug & Windle, 2010). Dysfunctional family dynamics and negative factors in the childhood home may contribute to violence. Many violent individuals have had childhood experiences of abuse (Thornberry, Freeman-Gallant, & Lovegrove, 2009).

It is critical to be culturally sensitive when interacting with clients, especially those demonstrating the potential for violence. Because the expression of aggressive behavior is significantly influenced by culture, there is a potential for discrimination (especially for sexism and racism) unless you are culturally sensitive when assessing the onset of violence.

Behavioral Theories

Is aggressive behavior learned by witnessing violence? There is ongoing debate about the impact on children of viewing violence as portrayed in television, movies, music, and video games. Currently, there is vigorous debate about the long-term effects of exposure to violent behavior through the media (Ferguson et al., 2009). Children who witness domestic violence are at risk for developing "intergenerational linkages in antisocial behavior" with numerous subsequent problems, such as depression, anxiety, and violence directed at peers (Thornberry et al., 2009, p. 82). Adolescents who are victimized at home have higher rates of delinquency (Mrug & Windle, 2010).

Humanistic Theories

Being valued as a person and judged to be worthy affects one's self-esteem, a basic need (Maslow, 1970). Valuing oneself as a significant person with something to contribute is part of self-esteem. When individuals feel they are inadequate, they begin to feel hopeless—for themselves and the future. If a person feels undervalued, unneeded, or insignificant, self-esteem becomes threatened. One response to such an existential threat may be aggressiveness. Acting out in an aggressive manner may be an individual's attempt to communicate self-importance.

NURSING PROCESS
Clients Who Are Angry, Aggressive, or Violent

In order to maintain safety and self-esteem of clients, you must intervene effectively with clients who express anger. Remember that every person has the right to feel every emotion they are experiencing. However, no one has the right to be aggressive (demonstrate violent behavior) toward others. Using the nursing process as the framework for delivery of care to angry or aggressive/violent clients results in continuity of care, which improves the quality of care.

Assessment

Assessing clients for their violence potential is an ongoing process and occurs across the continuum of care (in both inpatient and community-based settings). The determination of who in a given setting poses a risk for violence, and the perception that someone is more likely to be violent, is known as **dangerousness**. An assessment that someone is dangerous determines fundamental decisions about the need for hospitalization, special supervision, emergency psychopharmacologic intervention, and community placement options. Identifying whether a state of dangerousness exists is the result of an assessment and is essential for guiding treatment decisions.

An increased risk for violence among acutely disturbed clients is associated with the following variables:

- History of violence
- Severity of psychopathology
- Higher levels of hostility–suspiciousness, thinking disturbance, and agitation–excitement (as measured on the Brief Psychiatric Rating Scale [BPRS])
- Length of time in the hospital
- Early age of onset of psychiatric symptoms
- Frequency of admission to psychiatric hospitals

In the following clinical example, Theodore meets most of these criteria.

Clinical Example

Theodore, a 40-year-old single man, was brought to the psychiatric emergency department by the police in response to a call from his mother. He had been pounding on the door of his mother's home, screaming obscenities and wielding a knife. She was terrified. The staff recognized Theodore immediately—he had been hospitalized there more than 20 times over the past several years. He was diagnosed with paranoid schizophrenia at age 18. Early in his illness, he responded well to the supportive hospital environment and medications but did not follow up with day treatment, residential care, or medication when released from the inpatient setting.

It is important to begin your assessment by taking a comprehensive violence history on admission. The goal of history taking is to find patterns or trends in behaviors in order to identify the conditions under which an individual is likely to act aggressively. Your Assessment Approach lists factors for which to be alert when eliciting a violence history.

Clients and significant others are important sources of information. Interview questions about the violent client's history should be open and direct, as if you were questioning a suicidal individual. Ask, "How much have you thought about violence?" "Tell me what you do when you feel angry." "What is the most violent thing you have done?" Do not, however,

YOUR ASSESSMENT APPROACH
Risk Factors for Violence

Look for the presence of these factors when assessing clients for potential aggressive behavior:

- Availability of and/or possession of weapons
- Cognitive impairment
- Cruelty to animals
- Fire setting
- History of childhood abuse
- History of drug/alcohol abuse
- History of medication nonadherence
- History of violence directed toward others
- History of witnessing family violence
- Impulsivity
- Psychotic symptoms (e.g., hallucinations, paranoid delusions)
- Suicidal behavior

rely on client responses as the sole basis for your assessment. Also review the client's history, as stated by significant others and in the clients' medical record.

Managing and reducing the risk of violence is based on careful assessment of client behaviors. In addition to interviewing, observation is a most useful tool for gathering data about client aggressiveness. Your Assessment Approach lists behavioral and verbal clues that indicate violence. Determining the potential for violence helps one to anticipate and prevent aggressive outbursts. Some agencies have a structured violence assessment tool that can be helpful in identifying the likelihood of violence.

Substance abuse increases the potential for aggressive behavior. Determine whether the client is under the influence of drugs including CNS depressants (e.g., alcohol, benzodiazepines), stimulants (e.g., cocaine, amphetamines), hallucinogens (e.g., PCP, LSD), and narcotics (e.g., morphine, oxycodone).

A thorough assessment also collects data about the client's sleep pattern (discussed later in this chapter), nutritional status, and history of medical problems such as temporal

YOUR ASSESSMENT APPROACH
Determining the Risk of Violence

To help determine the risk of violence, you might use the following questions and statements with the client:

- How do you know when you are getting angry at others? At yourself?
- On a scale of 1 to 10, with 1 meaning not angry to 10 meaning extremely angry, how would you rate your anger right now?
- Describe one instance in which you have had a problem with anger.
- What types of things trigger anger in you?
- Tell me what you usually do when you feel angry.
- What do you do to help decrease your feelings of anger?

To help determine the risk of violence, you might observe the client for the following behaviors:

- Clenched jaws and fists
- Dilated pupils
- Intense staring
- Flushing of the face and neck
- Frowning, glaring, or smirking
- Pacing
- Increased vigilance

To help determine the risk of violence, you might listen to the client for the following verbal clues:

- Threatening harm
- A loud, demanding tone of voice
- Abrupt silence
- Sarcastic remarks
- Pressured speech
- Illogical responses
- Yelling, screaming
- Statements of fear
- Statements of suspicion

lobe epilepsy. Also note the client's ability to solve problems and cope with stressors. It is important to note how the client expresses anger. Does verbalization decrease the intensity of anger, or is the client showing signs of escalating violence? Once these questions have been answered, you can then establish appropriate nursing diagnoses.

Nursing Diagnosis (NANDA)

Clients who are violent usually have numerous problems, including poor impulse control, low self-esteem, and dysfunctional interpersonal relationships. Following are the relevant nursing diagnoses for clients exhibiting violence:

- Risk for Other-Directed Violence
- Risk for Self-Directed Violence
- Anxiety
- Ineffective Coping
- Chronic Low Self-Esteem
- Situational Low Self-Esteem

Outcome Identification: NOC

Clients who demonstrate violent behaviors challenge the entire treatment team. It is imperative that team members agree on the expected client outcomes. Following are some outcomes that apply to clients with aggressive behavior:

- Identifies precipitating events prior to losing control
- Refrains from self-injury and from injuring others
- Identifies alternative methods for expressing anger
- Refrains from impulsive behavior

Even though we have provided a list of suggested outcomes, remember that each client, violent or not, is an individual with unique needs.

Planning and Implementation: NIC

The major goal for all clients is maintenance of safety; this is especially true for those who are at risk for violence. Protecting the client and others from harm is the primary goal for all health care providers in every setting, not only psychiatric settings. What Every Nurse Should Know suggests strategies for use in crisis situations.

You must balance the issue of safety maintenance with the need for ensuring the aggressive client's individual freedom. Providing treatment in the least restrictive environment, while maintaining safety, is of paramount importance. Chapter 12∞ discusses the legal and ethical ramifications of the least restrictive environment concept.

Working successfully with clients who demonstrate violence, or the potential for violence, calls for teamwork, critical thinking, and creativity on the part of the entire treatment team. FIGURE 35-1 ■ provides a model for analyzing the risks versus the benefits of several different interventions for a violent client. You may employ a variety of methods, including developing a therapeutic relationship, milieu management, limit setting, pharmacologic agents, behavioral interventions, restrictive measures, and client education. Refer to Your Intervention Strategies: Guidelines for Working With the Angry Client on page 763 for specific approaches.

WHAT EVERY NURSE SHOULD KNOW

Assessing Anger and Preventing Violence

Imagine that you are a nurse working in an emergency department:

- Remember that there is a difference between anger (a subjective feeling) and aggression (a harmful behavior).
- When clients enter your emergency department, it is important to assess their level of anger—just as you assess every client's vital signs and pain level.
- Knowing how angry your client is will help determine your next action.
- Approach each client with a calm, reassuring manner. This will help the client feel less threatened and more secure.
- Involve clients in their own care as much as possible. This will increase their sense of control, which helps decrease anger.
- When a client's aggression is escalating, you must protect the safety of that client, other clients, yourself, and other staff.
- Call for help immediately if your interventions have not de-escalated the client's aggressive behavior.

Therapeutic Relationship

Establishing rapport with the client helps reduce suspiciousness on the client's part by building trust. When clients feel that they are in a supportive, trusting relationship, there is less need to respond aggressively. Safety maintenance is a key element of a therapeutic relationship. Safety refers not only to physical but also to psychological factors; the environment must be one in which the client feels safe to express feelings and risk learning new behaviors. However, being suspicious and fearful of people simply because they are psychiatric clients will interfere greatly with your ability to establish a therapeutic relationship. Suspiciousness and fear prevented the nursing student in the clinical example from establishing rapport with clients.

Clinical Example

Luanne was very nervous about beginning her psychiatric nursing clinical experience. She was pale and looked stunned when she first entered the inpatient unit. For the first few days of her clinical experience, Luanne made sure that she placed herself in the midst of her fellow classmates, avoiding any individual contact with the clients on the unit. She startled whenever clients spoke to her. It took several days before Luanne was able to discuss her irrational fear of violence with her instructor. Once she was able to do so, Luanne became more comfortable in the clinical setting and was able to demonstrate her ability to put her knowledge and skills into practice.

Jason is a voluntary client hospitalized on an open unit who punched another client, fracturing his jaw. You assess Jason after he hit his peer and find him very calm. You determine that he needs 1:1 supervision with staff until you can decide on a course of action. You review his record and discover that he has been in prison for assault and battery. While hospitalized he has not engaged in any violence before today. You call the doctor, the nursing supervisor, the social worker and security; you also call in extra staff to maintain safety.

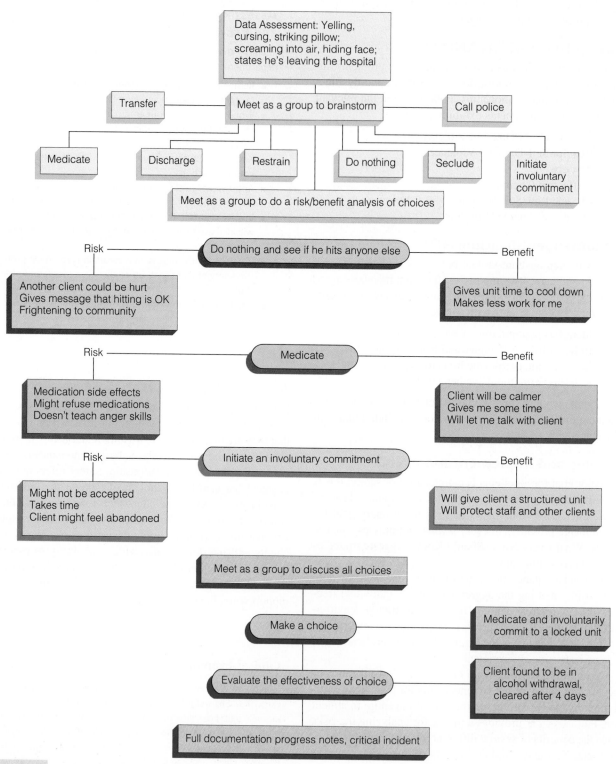

FIGURE 35-1 ▓ Risk/benefit analysis as a means of making decisions about the treatment of a violent client.

YOUR INTERVENTION STRATEGIES   Guidelines for Working With the Angry Client

Nursing Intervention	Rationale
■ Use a calm, unhurried approach.	■ Calmness promotes security.
■ Do not touch client indiscriminately.	■ Touch may be misinterpreted as aggressive or sexual.
■ Respect personal space.	■ Space provides insulation/protection.
■ Use active listening skills.	■ Attention and direct eye contact promote trust.
■ Remain aware of your feelings.	■ This helps to avoid countertransference reactions.
■ Use statements to provide feedback and identify sources of anger: "I notice your fists are clenched—what's happening?"	■ Feedback on feelings increases client awareness.
■ Assure client that staff will not allow the client to hurt self or others.	■ This conveys the presence of external controls.
■ Observe for escalation of anger (increased activity, verbal and nonverbal acting out).	■ Early awareness prevents crisis.
■ Institute precautions against suicide, homicide, assault, or escape, as indicated.	■ This ensures safety of client and others.
■ Discuss alternate means of releasing tension and physical energy.	■ This increases self-esteem through adaptive outlets.
■ Provide physical outlets to reduce tension, such as exercise, gardening, clay work, music, art (avoid competitive or contact sports).	■ Exercise releases anxiety/tension.
■ Protect other clients from verbal/physical abuse.	■ This ensures safety of all clients.
■ Clearly communicate and enforce agency regulations concerning acting-out behavior.	■ People behave according to expectations.
■ Postpone discussion of consequences of acting out until client is in control.	■ This avoids triggering aggressive behavior.
■ Role-model appropriate assertions of angry feelings: "I dislike it when—"	■ New behaviors can be learned by watching others.
■ Communicate desire to help client maintain/regain control.	■ Offering self helps to establish trust.
■ Hold client responsible for behavior; remind client of the ability to make choices.	■ This promotes internal control.
■ Use contracts for behavioral control, including seeking out staff people when feelings emerge.	■ This reinforces personal responsibility.
■ Teach assertiveness skills, relaxation, imagery, thought stopping, thought control.	■ This defuses anxiety and reinforces the ability for self-control.

A therapeutic nurse–client relationship also involves the nurse's demonstration of compassion and caring, which is actualized through presence, or therapeutic use of self. Be aware of the need to help clients learn to enhance self-esteem. Avoid labeling aggressive behavior as "attention seeking" without doing a complete assessment to determine the precipitating events that led to the aggressive outburst.

Active listening is essential when working with violent clients or those who are at risk for becoming violent. Listen for the expression of unmet needs (such as control and dependency) and for the expression of the ability to regain/maintain control. Active listening, or mindful listening, is a communication technique discussed in Chapter 10∞. When interacting with violent clients, it is important that you constantly assess the potential for aggressive behavior.

Milieu Management

Some mental health care environments can be dehumanizing and depersonalizing. When clients feel devalued,

aggressiveness usually escalates. Environmental elements contributing to violence in mental health settings include space and location, architectural design, staffing patterns, and activity levels.

Space and Location Space and location factors include territoriality, privacy, and overcrowding. The concept of territoriality involves defending physical objects or the space a client has identified or "staked out" as personal space. For example, a client often "claims" a special chair on the unit, and a new client comes along and sits in it. The resulting conflicts over special territory also raise the issue of privacy. Overcrowding is also related to the issue of privacy. Clients who are suspicious or have been abused as children often have difficulty tolerating people near them or touching them.

Architectural Design Architectural designs that create blind spots and opportunities for nonobservation can also increase the risk of violence. Mirrors have been used effectively to cope with particular architectural design problems in psychiatric units. Assess the environment for structures that lend themselves to frustration or blind spots. Sometimes the simple installation of one additional client telephone or a minor structural alteration on a unit can significantly reduce the number of violent incidents.

How an inpatient unit and its staff choose to handle potentially dangerous items such as glass, belts, and matches is complex and is related not only to institutional policy and unit philosophy but also to individual clinical judgment. On many units, staff members monitor these items, by using sign-up procedures or by locking them up and distributing them at the discretion of a member of the staff or a member of the client government in milieus that provide for client government.

Staffing Patterns The relationship between staffing patterns and violence is not well understood. Optimal staffing, often cited as a prerequisite for achieving treatment objectives, is being rigorously studied by the American Nurses Association and other professional groups. Whether a given health care facility has sufficient staff to manage potentially violent clients depends on the amount of care required by the total client population at that time.

Activity Level Activity level refers to the client's degree of participation in therapeutic activities. Peak times for violent incidents tend to be mealtimes and periods of concentrated treatment programming. In both situations, there is a high concentration of clients, and performance and participation are demanded.

Peak activity levels can be modified through adjustments such as scheduling, coordinating, and temporary withdrawal to allow the agitated client some interpersonal space. Scheduling staff breaks and mealtimes during client meals can create a situation of temporary understaffing on the unit. Staggering mealtimes for clients and staff is a simple mechanism that may prevent violent behavior. Coordinating client activities with the nursing staff schedule is an important consideration.

Staff who attempt to cajole or coerce clients into participation often create a situation in which the client feels trapped, and striking out becomes the only defense. Sometimes the most valuable intervention with any client—but particularly with one who is agitated, angry, or frightened—is temporary withdrawal. This allows the client quiet time free from the anxiety of interpersonal demands. Making frequent, brief, individualized contact with the client is more reassuring and does more to de-escalate a situation than forcing the client to attend a community meeting or other activity where the client's behavior is likely to be the focal point of discussion. Individualizing the milieu activities of clients may be as important to advancing their treatment and preventing violence as the proper medication regimen.

Limit Setting

Setting limits on inappropriate behavior is necessary when the client becomes increasingly agitated and aggressive. But remember to use limit setting as a therapeutic intervention, not as a punitive tool. The intent of limit setting is not to control the client but rather to provide consistent expectations and

YOUR INTERVENTION STRATEGIES
Limit Setting

Nursing Intervention	Rationale
▪ State limits in specific and direct language.	▪ This decreases the possibility of misunderstanding.
▪ Use a calm, unhurried approach.	▪ This promotes a sense of security.
▪ Offer time-out periods/one–to–one sessions in a quiet area.	▪ This diminishes sensory stimuli.
▪ Explain the limits and consequences during initial interactions (i.e., tell the client what is expected and the related outcomes).	▪ This promotes the tendency to behave according to expectations.
▪ Assure client that the staff will not allow client to hurt self and/or others.	▪ This promotes a sense of safety and conveys external controls.
▪ Expect all staff to consistently reinforce limits.	▪ This promotes behavior shaping.
▪ Accept the client while rejecting the inappropriate behavior.	▪ This protects self-esteem and reinforces behavioral limits.
▪ Reward the desirable behavior(s).	▪ This promotes continued demonstration of expected behavior(s).
▪ Continuously evaluate the need for limits; discontinue external limits as soon as the client is able to self-regulate.	▪ This empowers the client to exercise self-control.

guidelines for self-control. Setting limits must be viewed as a temporary process to protect the client and others. Limits are implemented only until the client demonstrates, either verbally or behaviorally, the ability to establish and maintain self-control. The rationales and recommendations for setting limits are explained in Your Intervention Strategies.

Pharmacologic Interventions

Many pharmacologic agents, such as haloperidol (Haldol) and olanzapine (Zyprexa), are currently used to reduce aggression. Medications with an extended half-life, i.e., risperidone (Risperdal Consta) and fluphenazine decanoate (Prolixin-D), are administered as injections to clients in the community. These medications are also used with inpatients with histories of medication nonadherence. Trazodone (Desyrel) is also used to minimize aggressiveness. Selective serotonin reuptake inhibitors (SSRIs) are being used to control impulsive violent behavior because of the association between serotonergic dysfunction and aggressive behavior (Butler et al., 2010).

In addition to these medications, several others are used specifically to minimize violent behavior in older clients.

Atypical antipsychotics are effective in decreasing aggression, as are the SSRIs. The SSRIs may be safer, especially for older clients, due to decreased cardiotoxicity (Mohundro, Pope, Shaw, & Hitchcock, 2010). Anticholinesterase inhibitors—for example donepezil (Aricept), rivastigmine (Exelon), and galantamine (Reminyl)—have also been effective in modifying aggressive impulses in the elderly. These and other medications used with older clients are discussed in Chapters 14 and 27∞.

The second-generation antipsychotic agents such as clozapine (Clozaril) and risperidone (Risperdal) reduce the symptoms of agitation and aggression while producing fewer extrapyramidal side effects than conventional antipsychotics. An anticonvulsant agent, valproic acid (Depakene), potentiates GABA-induced inhibition and thus leads to decreased aggressiveness in many individuals (Sadock & Sadock, 2010). SSRIs, such as fluoxetine (Prozac) and paroxetine (Paxil), are often effective in decreasing aggressive behaviors in some clients. TABLE 35-2 ■ lists pharmacologic agents commonly used in reducing aggression. Refer to Chapters 7 and 31∞ for a thorough discussion of these medications.

Although medication is the most widely used treatment for the control of violent behavior in institutional settings, it is important to recognize that pharmacologic agents alone are not the answer to violence. Psychotropic medications must be used with greater caution in older clients, as discussed in Chapter 27∞. Nonpharmacologic interventions (and their rationales) for elders are discussed in What Every Nurse Should Know.

Educating Clients

Education is an important intervention for clients who have a history of violence or who are at risk of becoming violent. Client teaching focuses on empowering the client by providing

WHAT EVERY NURSE SHOULD KNOW

Avoiding Violence by Elders Through Nonpharmacologic Interventions

Imagine that you are caring for an elderly client:

- Be aware of your own biases about older adults. *Negative biases influence your attitude and approach and may engender anger.*
- Do not expect all elders to be kindly and docile. *It is a myth that all elders are docile; their personalities and behavior may be exaggerated with increasing age. An angry young adult may become an even angrier older adult.*
- Assess mental status, including orientation level. *Confusion and disorientation can be frightening and may lead to impulsive or aggressively self-protective behavior.*
- Avoid touching confused elders. *Your touch may be frightening or misinterpreted as an attack. Touch should always be used judiciously after assessing that it is appropriate.*
- Use a calm approach to decrease the client's anxiety level. *Just as anxiety can be interpersonally communicated, so can calmness and a sense of peace.*
- Establish rapport to lessen the older adult's sense of alienation. *Establishing rapport builds trust and helps the elder to feel connected to another.*
- Include the elder in decision making that affects his or her interests. *Including the elder avoids dehumanization and provides the elder with a sense of control.*

tools for increasing self-responsibility. Following are some specific topics for teaching aggressive clients:

- Anger management
- Social skills training (discussed in Chapter 28∞)
- Problem solving
- Communication skills (discussed in Chapter 10∞)
- Relaxation skills (discussed in Chapter 33∞)
- Assertiveness training (see Partnering With Clients and Families: Teaching About Assertiveness)

An outline for a five-session anger management class that includes these topics is listed in Partnering With Clients and Families: Teaching About Anger Management. The classes can be modified as needed.

De-Escalating Aggressive Behavior

Avoiding client injury that can occur with the use of seclusion and restraints requires an attempt to use alternative methods to calm clients whose anger is escalating. It is imperative that you fully attend to the client in order to determine where the client's behavior falls on the continuum of aggression. You also need to be able to understand the meaning underlying the client's behavior in order to intervene appropriately. Some strategies for reducing escalation and averting a crisis are given in Your Intervention Strategies on page 767. The techniques listed are directed at de-escalating anger and aggressive behavior. Use them before the client loses self-control.

TABLE 35-2 ■ Psychopharmacologic Agents Commonly Used to Reduce Aggression		
Classification	**Generic Name**	**Trade Name**
Anticonvulsant	carbamazepine lamotrigine valproic acid	Tegretol Lamictal Depakene
Anxiolytic	buspirone	BuSpar
Benzodiazepine	clonazepam lorazepam	Klonopin Ativan
Beta blocker	propranolol	Inderal
Mood stabilizer	lithium	Eskalith, Lithane, Lithobid
Neuroleptic	clozapine fluphenazine haloperidol risperidone	Clozaril Prolixin Haldol Risperdal
Selective serotonin reuptake inhibitor (SSRI)	fluoxetine paroxetine	Prozac Paxil

PARTNERING WITH CLIENTS AND FAMILIES

Teaching About Assertiveness

Discuss the following elements of assertive behavior with clients and their families in order to encourage self-confidence and self-control.

1. Identify your usual patterns of behavior. Are you passive, aggressive, or assertive in dealing with others?
2. Deliberately work on changing your pattern of thinking. Assertive people do not respond automatically; they take time to look at a situation and plan their response. Avoid being pressured into a quick decision. Instead, say "I need some time to think about that."
3. Choose not to be responsible for the feelings of others when you know your actions were reasonable. In other words, avoid feeling guilty about being assertive.
4. Stand firm without precipitating an argument. Use the broken-record technique—calmly repeat an assertive statement over and over ("I really don't like violent movies") until the other person hears you.
5. Recognize that it is unrealistic to expect others to read your mind. Instead, use assertive statements of feeling such as: "Something is bothering me. I feel as if my movie preferences don't matter to you."
6. Choose to remain in control of yourself. Focus on remaining relaxed and calm. Breathe deeply, consciously relax your muscles, make eye contact, and speak in an even tone of voice.
7. Use "I" statements, such as: "I am feeling on the spot. I want to have a nice evening with you, but I also want to see a movie I can enjoy." By making it clear that you are expressing your own feelings and opinions, you help the other person to be nondefensive and able to listen to what you are saying.
8. Be patient, give yourself a chance, and don't expect too much too soon. Change comes about slowly with repeated practice.
9. Begin with small steps. A few successes will give you confidence. Go slowly and build a solid foundation.
10. Remember to give yourself due credit for successfully asserting yourself. Ask for qualified help—a teacher, a counselor, an assertive person—when you need it.

Restrictive Measures: Verbal Interventions

Consider all interventions within the context of the principle of least restrictiveness. This principle requires staff to use less restrictive measures of control before resorting to more restrictive interventions. Staff members must document their efforts to intervene with a client using verbal strategies before they intervene physically.

Forming a therapeutic relationship with the potentially violent client is often the first step to containing the violent behavior. It is important to convey control in the situation by using clear, calm statements and a confident physical stance rather than through remarks or cues that can be interpreted as challenging. A confrontational, aggressive, or threatening manner or a tendency to overidentify with the client's experience can make the staff member a target of violence and can actually precipitate it.

Some violent behavior occurs impulsively and without warning. Most episodes, however, involve an escalation of behavior and are therefore more appropriate for verbal intervention. Establishing quick rapport and an alliance with the potentially violent client is essential. Examples of nonconfrontational verbal interventions and positional strategies for working with potentially violent clients are provided in Your Intervention Strategies on page 767. The overall goal is to protect the client's already damaged self-esteem as much as possible in order to decrease the potential for violent behavior. Clinical judgment and the situation itself must dictate the appropriateness of their use. Sometimes verbal interventions

PARTNERING WITH CLIENTS AND FAMILIES

Teaching Anger Management

Session 1: What Is Anger?

- Signs and symptoms
- Causes: just or unjust anger
- Responses: thoughts, feelings, and actions

Session 2: Managing Anger Through Relaxation

- Importance and advantages
- The relaxation response
- Demonstration and practice

Session 3: Managing Anger Through Communication

- Importance and advantages
- Communication process
- Assertive communication
- Demonstration, role-play, practice

Session 4: Problem Solving

- Importance and advantages
- Process of problem solving
- Demonstration and practice

Session 5: Closure: Putting It All Together

- Review of processes
- Exercise: responding to a situation
- Self-evaluation

YOUR INTERVENTION STRATEGIES
De-Escalation Strategies for Angry or Aggressive Clients

- Diversion
- Exercise
- Change of surroundings
- Release from schedule or "demands"
- Relaxation
- Music
- Quiet periods
- Being read to or talked to by staff
- A quiet walk
- Reciting phrases or counting
- Thought stopping (a cognitive–behavioral technique in which the client examines angry thoughts and feelings that drive action; see Chapter 30∞)

are insufficient to contain the situation, particularly when the violent behavior occurs impulsively. In these instances, additional interventions—including medications, behavioral techniques, and seclusion and restraint—can be used with or instead of the verbal strategies.

Restrictive Measures: Seclusion and Restraint

Several intervention approaches can reduce the use of restraints. Some of these approaches include improved staff–client ratios, behavioral strategies, antipsychotic medications, and crisis response teams. Various behavioral strategies established around the principle of progressive isolation are often attempted before initiating seclusion and restraint. The therapeutic intent is to reduce disruptive stimulation and provide the client with a contained, well-defined space for reassurance and protection. Depending on unit construction, the client can be encouraged to seek quiet refuge at the back of the unit, in a specially designed serenity room or in a private room. Isolation can progress from the back of the unit to the client's room to open seclusion or a quiet room as indicated. These strategies are typically used in conjunction with medications to avoid the more restrictive procedures of seclusion and restraint. The ethics of seclusion and restraint are discussed in Chapter 12∞.

When efforts to contain the client's behavior using verbal techniques or administering medications and behavioral techniques do not prevent the violent behavior, or if an assault occurs without warning, staff members must intervene to seclude or mechanically restrain the client in order to protect the client and others. **Seclusion** consists of confining a person to a room or area where the person is physically prevented from leaving. If seclusion is not effective in helping the individual regain behavioral control, then restraints may be instituted. A **restraint** is any device attached to a person's body that cannot be easily removed by the person; the device restricts the individual's freedom of movement. As indicated earlier in this chapter, restraint is a measure of last resort that is used with caution.

YOUR INTERVENTION STRATEGIES   Verbal Interventions and Positional Strategies

Technique	Rationale
Approach the client from the side. Do not stand face-to-face with a potentially violent person.	This decreases the tendency of the violent person to project and externalize the assault.
Leave plenty of space between yourself and the client.	This reduces anxiety and the opportunity for assault.
Speak slowly, directly, in a normal tone of voice, using simple statements such as "Mr. Jones, put the chair down," or "Mrs. Clark, let's sit down and talk about what's bothering you." Encourage the client to sit down. If the client is pacing and cannot sit down, pace with the client.	This reduces anxiety, communicates control, increases the client's self-esteem, and models negotiation.
Center your statements on the issues concerning the client. For example, if the client states, "The nurse said I'm too sick to leave the hospital," a response such as, "You're upset at this big disappointment" will likely be more effective than "I can see how you must be upset by that."	Deflects attention away from the staff member who has become the target for the violent behavior.
When responding to the client's anger at not being allowed to leave, try saying, "I'm interested in understanding how terrible that is for you, Mr. Lewis."	This avoids challenging the client and expresses interest in the client's perspective.
Express clear expectations of control. For example, "I expect you can control yourself." Resist touching clients when they are upset and posing an immediate danger.	This communicates clarity and emphasizes the client's ability to control own behavior. It also communicates respect for the client and maintains a comfortable distance, thereby reducing the client's sense of threat.
Acknowledge nonviolent behavior. When the client sits down to talk, try saying, "Thank you for sitting with me. I can listen better this way."	This focuses on the client's strength and maintains the client's self-esteem.

Client Rights In the past several years, there has been a concerted effort by federal and state agencies, professional associations, and health care facilities to reduce the use of seclusion and restraint. Client safety is the primary reason for the trend toward eliminating seclusion and restraint in health care settings. According to Mental Health America (2011), formerly the National Mental Health Association, the use of restraints results in physical and psychological harm. Asphyxiation and cardiac arrest are the causes of most deaths associated with restraints used in psychiatric and geriatric settings.

Proposed federal legislation requires improved staff training in crisis de-escalation techniques and advocates for improved access to medication and community-based treatment for individuals with severe mental illness. The Children's Health Act of 2000 enacted by the 104th Congress requires any public or health care facility that receives federal funding to protect and promote the rights of each resident with regard to restraints or involuntary seclusion. This act also mandates that restraints and seclusion may be imposed only to ensure physical safety and only on the written order of a physician or other licensed practitioner. Another significant part of this legislation is implementing regulations for appropriate staffing levels and training.

The movement toward a restraint-free environment of care is the exemplification of least restrictive measures. *Seclusion and restraint are to be used only in the case of behavioral emergency.* The following clinical example, which continues the story of Theodore, first described on page 760, illustrates a situation in which seclusion may be therapeutic.

Clinical Example

Upon Theodore's admission to the psychiatric emergency department, he is disheveled, unable to cooperate with the staff, and is screaming and flailing. He is tormented with delusions and hallucinations that frighten him and lead him to strike out at others in the belief that they are trying to hurt him. He has a history of assaults against his mother and the nursing staff. The staff assesses Theodore's risk for imminent violence to be high and administer haloperidol IM and place him in a seclusion room where they hope he will rest and feel safer.

The American Psychiatric Nurses Association (APNA) has developed a position statement on the use of seclusion and restraint. Box 35-2 provides an overview of these principles (APNA, 2007). Be sure to familiarize yourself with the policies of your agency and your state mental health statutes.

Facilities using seclusion and restraint require staff attendance at assault training programs. These programs teach policies and procedures for dealing with assaultive clients, including assessment, prevention of escalating aggressiveness, and legal and clinical documentation requirements, as well as appropriate physical contact for use with violent clients. *At no time should students or other untrained personnel intervene using these techniques because they involve actual physical contact with clients, thereby increasing the risk of personal injury.*

Box 35-2   Summary of the American Psychiatric Nurses Association Position Statement on the Use of Seclusion and Restraint

- Emphasizes prevention and reduction of the use of seclusion and restraint
- Calls for their use only in behavioral emergencies that pose an immediate risk of harm to a client or others
- Calls on psychiatric–mental health nurses to provide leadership in establishing a treatment environment that is client focused and noncoercive
- Urges working within a collaborative relationship with the client and family
- Focuses on the need for an individualized treatment plan that promotes the client's self-management

Source: American Psychiatric Nurses Association. (2007). *Position statement on the use of seclusion and restraint.* Retrieved from http://www.apna.org

---

Care of the Client in Seclusion and Restraint Psychiatric–mental health nurses have a major responsibility in the decision to isolate and restrain as well as in caring for the client while in seclusion and restraints. Once the decision has been made to seclude and restrain a potentially violent client, a leader is chosen from among the available staff. The leader is responsible for designating roles to be performed by the remaining staff and for directing the steps in the seclusion and restraint procedure. Choice of the leader is important and can be based on various factors, one of which is familiarity with the client. Remember that the goal is to gain maximum cooperation from the client and minimize violence.

After a leader is chosen, a sufficient number of personnel must be gathered. This support staff should convey confidence and calm, reflecting a detached, professional approach to a familiar procedure. Avoid intimidating language and physical stances, because these behaviors may provoke the client's potential for violence. It is often sufficient to have the support staff gather around the leader the first time the client is approached. This show of force may be enough, and the client may comply without further intervention.

One staff member is assigned responsibility for managing the unit environment and other clients. This person is responsible for supporting and calming the other clients, who may become anxious during the procedure. In addition, the area near the seclusion room must be cleared of clients or physical obstructions to minimize the potential for injury.

Once the unit environment is safe, the team approaches the violent client. The leader offers a clear, brief statement of the purpose and rationale for seclusion or restraint. For example, the client is told that his or her behavior is out of control and that time in seclusion is required to help him or her regain control. The other team members position themselves around the client for easy access to the client's limbs. The leader then asks the client to walk into the seclusion room accompanied by staff. At this point, further discussion or negotiation should be avoided because it frequently aggravates the situation.

The behavioral options given to the client must be kept simple, clear, and minimal. Specific procedures for placing a client in restraints should follow governmental regulations, professional association standards, and agency policies.

Once a client is placed in seclusion or restraint, nursing observations of the client's behavior are required every 15 minutes. These checks include a description of the client's behavior, as well as routine care activities, including meals, circulation checks, and toileting. These observations should be conducted by nursing staff entering the seclusion room and participating in a verbal exchange with the client. Document the content of these dialogues, paying particular attention to a reduction in the client's symptoms, responsiveness to limits, capacity to discuss options, and increased capacity to tolerate frustration. Documentation of these behavioral checks and routine physical care activities is required.

Release From Seclusion and Restraint The client may be released from seclusion and restraint when his or her behavior is under control and the client no longer poses a danger to self or others. The decision to release a client from seclusion or remove restraints is based on an assessment of data gathered while the client is in seclusion. The ability of the client to control his or her behavior has been observed many times during the course of seclusion or restraint and is the basis for the decision to release.

Professional Education

Education about the reduction of violence in the workplace, especially the de-escalation of violence, should be ongoing. The focus of the staff must be on the prevention, rather than the management, of aggressive behavior. The educational programs are designed to help you do the following:

- Understand the ways in which you increase your own vulnerability to assault.
- Develop a provocation profile based on recognizing your own personal triggers for aggression (refer back to Your Self-Awareness on page 757) to increase your sensitivity and awareness.
- Role-play conversations with violent clients.
- Practice teamwork for physical restraint procedures.
- Promote a safe, nonblaming environment to discuss your experiences of working with violent clients.
- Develop sensitivity to the effects your own experiences of violence have in your daily work.

Resistance to restraint reduction may exist despite the strong stances taken by professional organizations, regulating agencies, and mental health facility administrators. Staff educational programs must identify barriers to restraint reduction such as concern for personal safety, lack of practice using alternate de-escalation skills, and fear of disrupting the therapeutic milieu.

Collegial Support

Nurses and other staff members who have been assaulted by clients need the support of their coworkers in a safe, supportive environment. An initial approach is to encourage those who have been attacked to discuss their feelings and experiences. Critical incident stress management (CISM) is often used to help staff members come to terms with violent assaults. CISM is an interaction facilitated by mental health clinicians to allow personnel to talk about their thoughts, feelings, and reactions to a stressful event. The most serious psychological harm to clinical nurses is post-traumatic stress disorder (Pai & Lee, 2011). CISM has been found to be beneficial for alleviating PTSD symptoms in health care providers and emergency first responders. Refer to Chapter 34∞ for a complete explanation of CISM.

Evaluation

There are many elements to consider in evaluating the effectiveness of strategies for violence management. Individual characteristics, biologic factors, conditions in the social environment, and the interpersonal styles of both clients and staff contribute to violent behavior. Despite our theoretic understanding of violent behavior and efforts to implement management strategies to decrease the likelihood of its occurrence, we are not yet able to predict with absolute certainty when someone will act in a violent manner. We can, however,

WHY I BECAME A PSYCHIATRIC–MENTAL HEALTH NURSE

Diane Hess, RN, BSN

In nursing school, I discovered that I enjoyed my psychiatric–mental health nursing rotation best. After graduation, I worked in several medical–surgical units where I found that the emotional needs of clients were mostly unmet. This was especially true when I worked on an oncology unit. Then, I took a job on a subacute psychiatric unit and knew that I'd found my niche.

Partnering with clients to design a plan of care to address emotional problems was very gratifying and sometimes frustrating, but nevertheless, this unit was a place where I could use my skills to change behavior. Discovering more successful coping skills, and helping clients to implement them, was exciting. My next adventure in psychiatric–mental health nursing was working with a person who was schizophrenic and had been hospitalized for many years. Her new psychiatrist wanted a nurse to help her transition from the hospital to her new home. The daunting task of helping her to adjust in the community and finding a house and suitable staff fell to me.

Dealing with her visual hallucinations while we were out eating in a restaurant was not something that I had experience with. But, I learned. The most wonderful event for my client was the discovery of the second-generation psychotropic medications that decreased the most disabling of her hallucinations. Seventeen years later, having experienced birthdays, holidays, deaths, and hurricanes together, the rest of the staff and I have been blessed with the insight that living within this very symptomatic schizophrenic person is an intelligent, funny, warm, and loving woman.

use the information presented earlier in this chapter to help predict based on the following:

- Identifying persons with mental disorders in which aggressiveness often occurs (see Box 35-1 on page 758)
- Assessing a client's risk factors for violence (see Your Assessment Approach on page 760)
- Assessing clients for indicators of impending violence (see Your Assessment Approach on page 760)
- Determining a client's violence history

The fact remains: Violence occurs in health care settings, and psychiatric–mental health nurses are at risk for assault from psychiatric clients. Another fact: Through accurate assessment and prompt intervention, the incidence of violence can be decreased.

Consider specific criteria when evaluating violent clients. Determine whether the client is able to do the following:

- Refrain from verbal outbursts.
- Refrain from striking others.
- Refrain from violating others' personal space.
- Identify factors that precipitate violent behaviors.
- Identify feelings of anger or frustration.
- Vent negative feelings appropriately.
- Identify alternative ways to cope with problems.

CASE MANAGEMENT

The concept of least restrictive environment is used to guide the planning of nursing care for all clients. However, when aggressive behavior begins to intensify, the safety of everyone involved—client, staff, and others in the community—overrides the client's right to freedom. Therefore, the case manager's role is often very challenging when coordinating care for the aggressive client in community settings. When referring clients with a history of violence to care providers, the case manager functions as an educator and an advocate. It is also important that the case manager assesses the client's adherence to the medication regimen and follow-up appointments as prescribed.

COMMUNITY-BASED CARE

Milieu management is not limited to inpatient treatment settings. When working in outpatient areas, such as clinics and offices, be aware of the relationship between the physical environment and the potential for violence. For example, a safe office arrangement calls for the furniture to be arranged in such a way that you can exit without being trapped. Having easy access to an emergency call system is also essential in maintaining the safety of both staff and clients.

HOME CARE

In order to assist aggressive clients to function in the home, it may be helpful to teach family members, friends, and significant others specific techniques for defusing violence. Refer to the de-escalating strategies in Your Intervention Strategies on page 767. You can teach these same strategies to family members, friends, and significant others, as well as the indicators for impending violence identified in Your Assessment Approach on page 760. Prior to discharge to home, encourage the client to use anger management and relaxation skills as needed. Also, review the section on home care in Chapter 13.

Pearson Nursing Student Resources
Find additional review materials at
nursing.pearsonhighered.com
Prepare for success with NCLEX®-style practice questions, interactive assignments and activities, web links, animations and videos, and more!

REFERENCES

Allen, D. E., de Nesnera, A., Cummings, K., & Darling, F. E. (2011). Transforming the culture of caring. *Journal of Psychosocial Nursing & Mental Health Services, 49*(1), 45–49.

American Psychiatric Nurses Association. (2007). *Position statement on the use of seclusion and restraint.* Retrieved from http://www.apna.org

Beaver, K. M., Sak, A. Vaske, J., & Nilsson, J. (2010). Genetic risk, parent-child relations, and antisocial phenotypes in a sample of African-American males. *Psychiatry Research, 175*(1–2), 160–164.

Booij, L., Trembley, R. E., Leyton, M., Seguin, F. R., Vitaro, F., Gravel, P., . . . Benkelfat, C. (2010). Brain serotonin synthesis in adult males characterized by physical aggression during childhood: A 21-year longitudinal study. *PLoS One, 5*(6), e11255.

Bureau of Labor Statistics, U.S. Department of Labor. (2010). 2009 survey of occupational injuries and illnesses: Summary estimate charts package. Retrieved from http://www.bls.gov/iif/oshwc/osh/os/osch0042.pdf

Butler, T., Schofield, P., Greenburg, D., Allnutt, S. H., Indig, D., Carr, V., . . . Ellis, A. (2010). Reducing impulsivity in repeat violent offenders: An open label trial of a selective serotonin reuptake inhibitor. *Australian and New Zealand Journal of Psychiatry, 44*(12), 1137–1143.

Campbell, J. C., Messing, J. T., Kub, J., Agnew, J., Fitzgerald, S., Fowler, B., . . . Bolyard, R. (2011). Workplace violence: Prevalence and risk factors in the safe at work study. *Journal of Occupational & Environmental Medicine, 53*(1), 82–89.

de Becker, G. (1997). *The gift of fear: Survival signals that protect us from violence.* Boston: Little, Brown and Company.

De Benedictis, L., Dumais, A., Sieu, N., Mailhot, M. P., Letourneau, G., Tran, M. A., . . . Lesage, A. D. (2011). Staff perceptions and organizational factors as predictors of seclusion and restraint on psychiatric wards. *Psychiatric Services, 62*(5), 484–401.

Fassino, S., Amianto, F., Gastaldo, L., & Leombruni, P. (2009). Anger and functioning amongst inpatients with schizophrenia or schizoaffective disorder living in a therapeutic community. *Psychiatry and Clinical Neurosciences, 63*(2), 186–194.

Ferguson, C. J., San Miguel, C., & Hartley, R. D. (2009). A multivariate analysis of youth violence and aggression: The influence of family, peers, depression, and media violence. *Journal of Pediatrics, 155*(6), 904–908.

Freud, S. (1989). *Civilization and its discontents* (J. Strachey, Ed.). New York, NY: Norton. (Original work published 1930.)

Gillespie, G. L., Gates, D. M., Miller, M., & Howard, P. K. (2010). Workplace violence in healthcare settings: Risk factors and protective strategies. *Rehabilitation Nursing, 35*(5), 177–184.

Jasinska, A., & Freimer, N. B. (2009). The complex genetic basis of simple behavior. *Journal of Biology, 8*(8), 71.

Lanza, M. L., & Witkower, A. (2010). Concentric Interactive Group Model: A unique experience for patients and staff. *Perspectives of Psychiatric Care, 46*(4), 294–300.

LaRue, C., Dumais, A., Drapeau, A., Menard, G., & Goulet, M. H. (2010). Nursing practices recorded in reports of episodes of seclusion. *Issues in Mental Health Nursing, 31*(12), 785–792.

Magnavita, N., & Heponiemi, T. (2011). Workplace violence against nursing students and nurses: An Italian experience. *Journal of Nursing Scholarship, 43*(2), 203–210.

Maslow, A. (1970). *Motivation and personality* (2nd ed.). New York, NY: Harper & Row.

Mental Health America. (2011). *Position Statement 24: Seclusion and restraints.* Retrieved from http://www.mentalhealthamerica.net

Mohundro, B. L., Pope, K., Shaw, V., & Hitchcock, K. (2010). Clinical inquiries. Which drugs are best when aggressive Alzheimer's patients need medication? *Journal of Family Practice, 59*(10), 595–604.

Mrug, S., & Windle, M. (2010). Prospective effects of violence exposure across multiple contexts on early adolescents' internalizing and externalizing problems. *Journal of Child Psychology & Psychiatry, 51*(8), 953–961.

Pai, H. C., & Lee, S. (2011). Risk factors for workplace violence in clinical registered nurses in Taiwan. *Journal of Clinical Nursing, 20*(9), 1405–1412.

Parsey, R. V. (2010). Serotonin receptor imaging: Clinically useful? *Journal of Nuclear Medicine, 51*(1), 1295–1298.

Roaldset, J. O., Bakken, A. M., & Biorkly, S. (2011). A prospective study of lipids and serotonin as risk markers of violence and self-harm in acute psychiatric patients. *Psychiatric Research, 186*(2–3), 293–299.

Rosell, D. R., Thompson, J. L., Silfstein, M., Xu, X., Frankie, W. G., New, A. S., . . . Siever, L. J. (2010). Increased serotonin 2A receptor availability in the orbitofrontal cortex of physically aggressive personality disordered males. *Biological Psychiatry, 67*(12), 1154–1162.

Sadock, B. J., & Sadock, V. A. (2010). *Kaplan & Sadock's pocket handbook of clinical psychiatry* (5th ed.). Philadelphia, PA: Lippincott Williams & Wilkins.

Takahashi, A., Quadros, I. M., de Almeida, R. M., & Miczek, K. A. (2011). Brain serotonin receptors and transporters: Initiation vs. termination of escalated aggression. *Psychopharmacology, 13*(2–3), 183–212.

Taylor, J. L., & Rew, L. (2010). A systematic review of the literature: Workplace violence in the emergency department. *Journal of Clinical Nursing, 20*(7–8), 1072–1085.

Thornberry, T. P., Freeman-Gallant, A., & Lovegrove, P. J. (2009). Intergenerational linkages in antisocial behavior. *Criminal Behaviour and Mental Health, 19*(2), 80–93.

APPENDIX A

DSM-IV-TR CLASSIFICATION

NOS = Not Otherwise Specified

An *x* appearing in a diagnostic code indicates that a specific code number is required.

An ellipsis (. . .) is used in the names of certain disorders to indicate that the name of a specific mental disorder or general medical condition should be inserted when recording the name (e.g., 293.0 Delirium Due to Hypothyroidism).

If criteria are currently met, one of the following severity specifiers may be noted after the diagnosis:

Mild

Moderate

Severe

If criteria are no longer met, one of the following specifiers may be noted:

In Partial Remission

In Full Remission

Prior History

DISORDERS USUALLY FIRST DIAGNOSED IN INFANCY, CHILDHOOD, OR ADOLESCENCE

Mental Retardation

Note: *These are coded on Axis II.*
317 Mild Mental Retardation
318.0 Moderate Mental Retardation
318.1 Severe Mental Retardation
318.2 Profound Mental Retardation
319 Mental Retardation, Severity Unspecified

Learning Disorders

315.00 Reading Disorder
315.1 Mathematics Disorder
315.2 Disorder of Written Expression
315.9 Learning Disorder NOS

Motor Skills Disorder

315.4 Developmental Coordination Disorder

Communication Disorders

315.31 Expressive Language Disorder
315.32 Mixed Receptive–Expressive Language Disorder
315.39 Phonological Disorder
307.0 Stuttering
307.9 Communication Disorder NOS

Pervasive Developmental Disorders

299.00 Autistic Disorder
299.80 Rett's Disorder
299.10 Childhood Disintegrative Disorder
299.80 Asperger's Disorder
299.80 Pervasive Developmental Disorder NOS

Attention Deficit and Disruptive Behavior Disorders

314.xx Attention Deficit/Hyperactivity Disorder
   .01 Combined Type
   .00 Predominantly Inattentive Type
   .01 Predominantly Hyperactive–Impulsive Type
314.9 Attention Deficit/Hyperactivity Disorder NOS
312.xx Conduct Disorder
   .81 Childhood-Onset Type
   .82 Adolescent-Onset Type
   .89 Unspecified Onset
313.81 Oppositional Defiant Disorder
312.9 Disruptive Behavior Disorder NOS

Feeding and Eating Disorders of Infancy or Early Childhood

307.52 Pica
307.53 Rumination Disorder
307.59 Feeding Disorder of Infancy or Early Childhood

Tic Disorders

307.23 Tourette's Disorder
307.22 Chronic Motor or Vocal Tic Disorder
307.21 Transient Tic Disorder
   Specify if: Single Episode/Recurrent
307.20 Tic Disorder NOS

Elimination Disorders

_____.__ Encopresis
787.6 With Constipation and Overflow Incontinence
307.7 Without Constipation and Overflow Incontinence
307.6 Enuresis (Not Due to a General Medical Condition)
   Specify type: Nocturnal Only/Diurnal Only/Nocturnal and Diurnal

Other Disorders of Infancy, Childhood, or Adolescence

309.21 Separation Anxiety Disorder
   Specify if: Early Onset
313.23 Selective Mutism

Reprinted with permission from the *Diagnostic and Statistical Manual of Mental Disorders,* Fourth Edition, Text Revision. (Copyright 2000). American Psychiatric Association.

313.89 Reactive Attachment Disorder of Infancy or Early Childhood
Specify type: Inhibited Type/Disinhibited Type
307.3 Stereotypic Movement Disorder
Specify if: With Self-Injurious Behavior
313.9 Disorder of Infancy, Childhood, or Adolescence NOS

DELIRIUM, DEMENTIA, AND AMNESTIC AND OTHER COGNITIVE DISORDERS

Delirium

293.0 Delirium Due to... *[Indicate the General Medical Condition]*
____.___ Substance Intoxication Delirium *(refer to Substance-Related Disorders for substance-specific codes)*
____.____ Substance Withdrawal Delirium *(refer to Substance-Related Disorders for substance-specific codes)*
____.____ Delirium Due to Multiple Etiologies *(code each of the specific etiologies)*
780.09 Delirium NOS

Dementia

294.xx Dementia of the Alzheimer's Type, With Early Onset *(also code 331.0 Alzheimer's disease on Axis III)*
.10 Without Behavioral Disturbance
.11 With Behavioral Disturbance
294.xx Dementia of the Alzheimer's Type, With Late Onset *(also code 331.0 Alzheimer's disease on Axis III)*
.10 Without Behavioral Disturbance
.11 With Behavioral Disturbance
290.xx Vascular Dementia
.40 Uncomplicated
.41 With Delirium
.42 With Delusions
.43 With Depressed Mood
Specify if: With Behavioral Disturbance
Code presence or absence of a behavioral disturbance in the fifth digit for Dementia Due to a General Medical Condition:
0 = Without Behavioral Disturbance
1 = With Behavioral Disturbance
294.1x Dementia Due to HIV Disease *(also code 042 HIV on Axis III)*
294.1x Dementia Due to Head Trauma *(also code 042 HIV on Axis III)*
294.1x Dementia Due to Head Trauma *(also code 854.00 head injury on Axis III)*
294.1x Dementia Due to Parkinson's Disease *(also code 332.0 Parkinson's disease on Axis III)*
294.1x Dementia Due to Huntington's Disease *(also code 333.4 Huntington's disease on Axis III)*
294.1x Dementia Due to Pick's Disease *(also code 331.1 Pick's disease on Axis III)*
294.1x Dementia Due to Creutzfeldt–Jakob Disease *(also code 046.1 Creutzfeldt–Jakob disease on Axis III)*
ICD-9-CM code valid after October 1, 2000.
294.1x Dementia Due to . . . *[Indicate the General Medical Condition not listed above] (also code the general medical condition on Axis III)*

____.___ Substance-Induced Persisting Dementia *(refer to Substance-Related Disorders for substance-specific codes)*
____.___ Dementia Due to Multiple Etiologies *(code each of the specific etiologies)*
294.8 Dementia NOS

Amnestic Disorders

294.0 Amnestic Disorder Due to... *[Indicate the General Medical Condition]*
Specify if: Transient/Chronic
____.___ Substance-Induced Persisting Amnestic Disorder *(refer to Substance-Related Disorders for substance-specific codes)*
294.8 Amnestic Disorder NOS

Other Cognitive Disorders

294.9 Cognitive Disorder NOS

MENTAL DISORDERS DUE TO A GENERAL MEDICAL CONDITION NOT ELSEWHERE CLASSIFIED

293.89 Catatonic Disorder Due to... *[Indicate the General Medical Condition]*
310.1 Personality Change Due to... *[Indicate the General Medical Condition]*
Specify type: Labile Type/Disinhibited Type/Aggressive Type/Apathetic Type/Paranoid Type/Other Type/Combined Type/Unspecified Type
293.9 Mental Disorder NOS Due to... *[Indicate the General Medical Condition]*

SUBSTANCE-RELATED DISORDERS

The following specifiers apply to Substance Dependence as noted:
[a]With Physiological Dependence/Without Physiological Dependence
[b]Early Full Remission/Early Partial Remission/Sustained Full Remission/Sustained Partial Remission
[c]In a Controlled Environment
[d]On Agonist Therapy
The following specifiers apply to Substance-Induced Disorders as noted:
[I]With Onset During Intoxication/[W]With Onset During Withdrawal

Alcohol-Related Disorders

ALCOHOL USE DISORDERS
303.90 Alcohol Dependence[a,b,c]
305.00 Alcohol Abuse
ALCOHOL-INDUCED DISORDERS
303.00 Alcohol Intoxication
291.81 Alcohol Withdrawal
Specify if: With Perceptual Disturbances
291.0 Alcohol Intoxication Delirium
291.0 Alcohol Withdrawal Delirium
291.2 Alcohol-Induced Persisting Dementia
291.1 Alcohol-Induced Persisting Amnestic Disorder

291.x Alcohol-Induced Psychotic Disorder
   .5 With Delusions[I,W]
   .3 With Hallucinations[I,W]
291.89 Alcohol-Induced Mood Disorder[I,W]
291.89 Alcohol-Induced Anxiety Disorder[I,W]
291.89 Alcohol-Induced Sexual Dysfunction[I]
291.89 Alcohol-Induced Sleep Disorder[I,W]
291.9 Alcohol-Related Disorder NOS

Amphetamine (or Amphetamine-Like)–Related Disorders

AMPHETAMINE USE DISORDERS

304.40 Amphetamine Dependence[a,b,c]
305.70 Amphetamine Abuse

AMPHETAMINE-INDUCED DISORDERS

292.89 Amphetamine Intoxication
   Specify if: With Perceptual Disturbances
292.0 Amphetamine Withdrawal
292.81 Amphetamine Intoxication Delirium
292.xx Amphetamine-Induced Psychotic Disorder
   .11 With Delusions[I]
   .12 With Hallucinations[I]
292.84 Amphetamine-Induced Mood Disorder[I,W]
292.89 Amphetamine-Induced Anxiety Disorder[I]
292.89 Amphetamine-Induced Sexual Dysfunction[I]
292.89 Amphetamine-Induced Sleep Disorder[I,W]
292.9 Amphetamine-Related Disorder NOS

Caffeine-Related Disorders

CAFFEINE-INDUCED DISORDERS

305.90 Caffeine Intoxication
292.89 Caffeine-Induced Anxiety Disorder[I]
292.89 Caffeine-Induced Sleep Disorder[I]
292.9 Caffeine-Related Disorder NOS

Cannabis-Related Disorders

CANNABIS USE DISORDERS

304.30 Cannabis Dependence[a,b,c]
305.20 Cannabis Abuse

CANNABIS-INDUCED DISORDERS

292.89 Cannabis Intoxication
   Specify if: With Perceptual Disturbance
292.81 Cannabis Intoxication Delirium
292.xx Cannabis-Induced Psychotic Disorder
   .11 With Delusions[I]
   .12 With Hallucinations[I]
292.89 Cannabis-Induced Anxiety Disorder[I]
292.9 Cannabis-Related Disorder NOS

Cocaine-Related Disorders

COCAINE USE DISORDERS

304.20 Cocaine Dependence[a,b,c]
305.60 Cocaine Abuse

COCAINE-INDUCED DISORDERS

292.89 Cocaine Intoxication
   Specify if: With Perceptual Disturbances

292.0 Cocaine Withdrawal
292.81 Cocaine Intoxication Delirium
292.xx Cocaine-Induced Psychotic Disorder
   .11 With Delusions[I]
   .12 With Hallucinations[I]
292.84 Cocaine-Induced Mood Disorder[I,W]
292.89 Cocaine-Induced Anxiety Disorder[I,W]
292.89 Cocaine-Induced Sexual Dysfunction[I]
292.89 Cocaine-Induced Sleep Disorder[I,W]
292.9 Cocaine-Related Disorder NOS

Hallucinogen-Related Disorders

HALLUCINOGEN USE DISORDERS

304.50 Hallucinogen Dependence[b,c]
305.30 Hallucinogen Abuse

HALLUCINOGEN-INDUCED DISORDERS

292.89 Hallucinogen Intoxication
292.89 Hallucinogen Persisting Perception Disorder (Flashbacks)
292.81 Hallucinogen Intoxication Delirium
292.xx Hallucinogen-Induced Psychotic Disorder
   .11 With Delusions[I]
   .12 With Hallucinations[I]
292.84 Hallucinogen-Induced Mood Disorder[I]
292.89 Hallucinogen-Induced Anxiety Disorder[I]
292.9 Hallucinogen-Related Disorder NOS

Inhalant-Related Disorders

INHALANT USE DISORDERS

304.60 Inhalant Dependence[b,c]
305.90 Inhalant Abuse

INHALANT-INDUCED DISORDERS

292.89 Inhalant Intoxication
292.81 Inhalant Intoxication Delirium
292.82 Inhalant-Induced Persisting Dementia
292.xx Inhalant-Induced Psychotic Disorder
   .11 With Delusions[I]
   .12 With Hallucinations[I]
292.84 Inhalant-Induced Mood Disorder[I]
292.89 Inhalant-Induced Anxiety Disorder[I]
292.9 Inhalant-Related Disorder NOS

Nicotine-Related Disorders

NICOTINE USE DISORDER

305.1 Nicotine Dependence[a,b]

NICOTINE-INDUCED DISORDER

292.0 Nicotine Withdrawal
292.9 Nicotine-Related Disorder NOS

Opioid-Related Disorders

OPIOID USE DISORDERS

304.00 Opioid Dependence[a,b,c,d]
305.50 Opioid Abuse

OPIOID-INDUCED DISORDERS

292.89 Opioid Intoxication
   Specify if: With Perceptual Disturbances

292.0 Opioid Withdrawal
292.81 Opioid Intoxication Delirium
292.xx Opioid-Induced Psychotic Disorder
   .11 With Delusions[I]
   .12 With Hallucinations[I]
292.84 Opioid-Induced Mood Disorder[I]
292.89 Opioid-Induced Sexual Dysfunction[I]
292.89 Opioid-Induced Sleep Disorder[I,W]
292.9 Opioid-Related Disorder NOS

Phencyclidine (or Phencyclidine-Like)–Related Disorders

PHENCYCLIDINE USE DISORDERS

304.60 Phencyclidine Dependence[b,c]
305.90 Phencyclidine Abuse

PHENCYCLIDINE-INDUCED DISORDERS

292.89 Phencyclidine Intoxication
   Specify if: With Perceptual Disturbances
292.81 Phencyclidine Intoxication Delirium
292.xx Phencyclidine-Induced Psychotic Disorder
   .11 With Delusions[I]
   .12 With Hallucinations[I]
292.84 Phencyclidine-Induced Mood Disorder[I]
292.89 Phencyclidine-Induced Anxiety Disorder[I]
292.9 Phencyclidine-Related Disorder NOS

Sedative-, Hypnotic-, or Anxiolytic-Related Disorders

SEDATIVE, HYPNOTIC, OR ANXIOLYTIC USE DISORDERS

304.10 Sedative, Hypnotic, or Anxiolytic Dependence[a,b,c]
305.40 Sedative, Hypnotic, or Anxiolytic Abuse

SEDATIVE-, HYPNOTIC-, OR ANXIOLYTIC-INDUCED DISORDERS

292.89 Sedative, Hypnotic, or Anxiolytic Intoxication
292.0 Sedative, Hypnotic, or Anxiolytic Withdrawal
   Specify if: With Perceptual Disturbances
292.81 Sedative, Hypnotic, or Anxiolytic Intoxication Delirium
292.81 Sedative, Hypnotic, or Anxiolytic Withdrawal Delirium
292.82 Sedative, Hypnotic, or Anxiolytic-Induced Persisting Dementia
292.83 Sedative-, Hypnotic-, or Anxiolytic-Induced Persisting Amnestic Disorder
292.xx Sedative-, Hypnotic-, or Anxiolytic-Induced Psychotic Disorder
   .11 With Delusions[I,W]
   .12 With Hallucinations[I,W]
292.84 Sedative-, Hypnotic-, or Anxiolytic-Induced Mood Disorder[I,W]
292.89 Sedative-, Hypnotic-, or Anxiolytic-Induced Anxiety Disorder[W]
292.89 Sedative-, Hypnotic-, or Anxiolytic-Induced Sexual Dysfunction[I]
292.89 Sedative-, Hypnotic-, or Anxiolytic-Induced Sleep Disorder[I,W]
292.9 Sedative-, Hypnotic-, or Anxiolytic-Related Disorder NOS

Polysubstance-Related Disorder

304.80 Polysubstance Dependence[a,b,c,d]

Other (or Unknown) Substance-Related Disorders

OTHER (OR UNKNOWN) SUBSTANCE USE DISORDERS

304.90 Other (or Unknown) Substance Dependence[a,b,c,d]
305.90 Other (or Unknown) Substance Abuse

OTHER (OR UNKNOWN) SUBSTANCE-INDUCED DISORDERS

292.89 Other (or Unknown) Substance Intoxication
   Specify if: With Perceptual Disturbances
292.0 Other (or Unknown) Substance Withdrawal
   Specify if: With Perceptual Disturbances
292.81 Other (or Unknown) Substance-Induced Delirium
292.82 Other (or Unknown) Substance-Induced Persisting Dementia
292.83 Other (or Unknown) Substance-Induced Persisting Amnestic Disorder
292.xx Other (or Unknown) Substance-Induced Psychotic Disorder
   .11 With Delusions[I,W]
   .12 With Hallucinations[I,W]
292.84 Other (or Unknown) Substance-Induced Mood Disorder[I,W]
292.89 Other (or Unknown) Substance-Induced Anxiety Disorder[I,W]
292.89 Other (or Unknown) Substance-Induced Sexual Dysfunction[I]
292.89 Other (or Unknown) Substance-Induced Sleep Disorder[I,W]
292.9 Other (or Unknown) Substance-Related Disorder NOS

Polysubstance-Related Disorder

304.80 Polysubstance Dependence[a,b,c,d]

Other (or Unknown) Substance-Related Disorders

OTHER (OR UNKNOWN) SUBSTANCE USE DISORDERS

304.90 Other (or Unknown) Substance Dependence[a,b,c,d]
305.90 Other (or Unknown) Substance Abuse

OTHER (OR UNKNOWN) SUBSTANCE-INDUCED DISORDERS

292.89 Other (or Unknown) Substance Intoxication
   Specify if: With Perceptual Disturbances
292.0 Other (or Unknown) Substance Withdrawal
   Specify if: With Perceptual Disturbances
292.81 Other (or Unknown) Substance-Induced Delirium
292.82 Other (or Unknown) Substance-Induced Persisting Dementia
292.83 Other (or Unknown) Substance-Induced Persisting Amnestic Disorder
292.xx Other (or Unknown) Substance-Induced Psychotic Disorder
   .11 With Delusions[I,W]
   .12 With Hallucinations[I,W]
292.84 Other (or Unknown) Substance-Induced Mood Disorder[I,W]
292.89 Other (or Unknown) Substance-Induced Anxiety Disorder[I,W]

292.89 Other (or Unknown) Substance-Induced Sexual Dysfunction[I]

292.89 Other (or Unknown) Substance-Induced Sleep Disorder[I,W]

292.9 Other (or Unknown) Substance-Related Disorder NOS

SCHIZOPHRENIA AND OTHER PSYCHOTIC DISORDERS

295.xx Schizophrenia

The following Classification of Longitudinal Course applies to all subtypes of Schizophrenia:

Episodic With Interepisode Residual Symptoms (*Specify if:* With Prominent Negative Symptoms)/Episodic With No Interepisode Residual Symptoms

Continuous (*Specify if:* With Prominent Negative Symptoms)

Single Episode in Partial Remission (*Specify if:* With Prominent Negative Symptoms)/Single Episode in Full Remission

Other or Unspecified Pattern

.30 Paranoid Type
.10 Disorganized Type
.20 Catatonic Type
.90 Undifferentiated Type
.60 Residual Type

295.40 Schizophreniform Disorder

Specify if: Without Good Prognostic Features/With Good Prognostic Features

295.70 Schizoaffective Disorder

Specify type: Bipolar Type/Depressive Type

297.1 Delusional Disorder

Specify type: Erotomanic Type/Grandiose Type/Jealous Type/Persecutory Type/Somatic Type/Mixed Type/Unspecified Type

298.8 Brief Psychotic Disorder

Specify if: With Marked Stressor(s)/Without Marked Stressor(s)/With Postpartum Onset

297.3 Shared Psychotic Disorder

293.xx Psychotic Disorder Due to... *[Indicate the General Medical Condition]*

.81 With Delusions
.82 With Hallucinations

____.____ Substance-Induced Psychotic Disorder *(refer to Substance-Related Disorders for substance-specific codes)*

Specify if: With Onset During Intoxication/With Onset During Withdrawal

298.9 Psychotic Disorder NOS

MOOD DISORDERS

Code current state of Major Depressive Disorder or Bipolar I Disorder in fifth digit:

1 = Mild
2 = Moderate
3 = Severe Without Psychotic Features
4 = Severe With Psychotic Features

Specify: Mood-Congruent Psychotic Features/Mood-Incongruent Psychotic Features

5 = In Partial Remission

6 = In Full Remission
0 = Unspecified

The following specifiers apply (for current or most recent episode) to Mood Disorders as noted:
[a]Severity/Psychotic/Remission Specifiers/[b]Chronic/[c]With Catatonic Features/[d]With Melancholic Features/[e]With Atypical Features/[f]With Postpartum Onset

The following specifiers apply to Mood Disorders as noted:
[g]With or Without Full Interepisode Recovery/[h]With Seasonal Pattern/[i]With Rapid Cycling

Depressive Disorders

296.xx Major Depressive Disorder
.2x Single Episode[a,b,c,d,e,f]
.3x Recurrent[a,b,c,d,e,f,g,h]

300.4 Dysthymic Disorder
Specify if: Early Onset/Late Onset
Specify if: With Atypical Features

311 Depressive Disorder NOS

Bipolar Disorders

296.xx Bipolar I Disorder
.0x Single Manic Episode[a,c,f]
Specify if: Mixed
.40 Most Recent Episode Hypomanic[g,h,i]
.4x Most Recent Episode Manic[a,c,f,g,h,i]
.6x Most Recent Episode Mixed[a,c,f,g,h,i]
.5x Most Recent Episode Depressed[a,b,c,d,e,f,g,h,i]
.7 Most Recent Episode Unspecified[g,h,i]

296.89 Bipolar II Disorder[a,b,c,d,e,f,g,h,i]
Specify (current or most recent episode): Hypomanic/Depressed

301.13 Cyclothymic Disorder

296.80 Bipolar Disorder NOS

293.83 Mood Disorder Due to... *[Indicate the General Medical Condition]*
Specify type: With Depressive Features/With Major Depressive-Like Episode/With Manic Features/With Mixed Features

____.____ Substance-Induced Mood Disorder *(refer to Substance-Related Disorders for substance-specific codes)*
Specify type: With Depressive Features/With Manic Features/With Mixed Features
Specify if: With Onset During Intoxication/With Onset During Withdrawal

296.90 Mood Disorder NOS

Anxiety Disorders

300.01 Panic Disorder Without Agoraphobia

300.21 Panic Disorder With Agoraphobia

300.22 Agoraphobia Without History of Panic Disorder

300.29 Specific Phobia
Specify type: Animal Type/Natural Environment Type/Blood-Injection-Injury Type/Situational Type/Other Type

300.23 Social Phobia
Specify if: Generalized

300.3 Obsessive–Compulsive Disorder
Specify if: With Poor Insight

309.81 Post-Traumatic Stress Disorder
Specify if: Acute/Chronic
Specify if: With Delayed Onset
308.3 Acute Stress Disorder
300.02 Generalized Anxiety Disorder
293.84 Anxiety Disorder Due to . . . *[Indicate the General Medical Condition]*
Specify if: With Generalized Anxiety/With Panic Attacks/ With Obsessive–Compulsive Symptoms
____.____ Substance-Induced Anxiety Disorder *(refer to Substance-Related Disorders for substance-specific codes)*
Specify if: With Generalized Anxiety/With Panic Attacks/ With Obsessive–Compulsive Symptoms/With Phobic Symptoms
Specify if: With Onset During Intoxication/With Onset During Withdrawal
300.00 Anxiety Disorder NOS

SOMATOFORM DISORDERS

300.81 Somatization Disorder
300.82 Undifferentiated Somatoform Disorder
300.11 Conversion Disorder
Specify type: With Motor Symptom or Deficit/ With Sensory Symptom or Deficit/With Seizures or Convulsions/With Mixed Presentation
307.xx Pain Disorder
.80 Associated With Psychological Factors
.89 Associated With Both Psychological Factors and a General Medical Condition
Specify if: Acute/Chronic
300.7 Hypochondriasis
Specify if: With Poor Insight
300.7 Body Dysmorphic Disorder
300.82 Somatoform Disorder NOS

Factitious Disorders

300.xx Factitious Disorder
.16 With Predominantly Psychological Signs and Symptoms
.19 With Predominantly Physical Signs and Symptoms
.19 With Combined Psychological and Physical Signs and Symptoms
300.19 Factitious Disorder NOS

Dissociative Disorders

300.12 Dissociative Amnesia
300.13 Dissociative Fugue
300.14 Dissociative Identity Disorder
300.6 Depersonalization Disorder
300.15 Dissociative Disorder NOS

Sexual and Gender Identity Disorders

SEXUAL DYSFUNCTIONS

The following specifiers apply to all primary Sexual Dysfunctions:
Lifelong Type/Acquired Type

Generalized Type/Situational Type
Due to Psychological Factors/Due to Combined Factors

SEXUAL DESIRE DISORDERS

302.71 Hypoactive Sexual Desire Disorder
302.79 Sexual Aversion Disorder

SEXUAL AROUSAL DISORDERS

302.72 Female Sexual Arousal Disorder
302.72 Male Erectile Disorder

ORGASMIC DISORDERS

302.73 Female Orgasmic Disorder
302.74 Male Orgasmic Disorder
302.75 Premature Ejaculation

SEXUAL PAIN DISORDERS

302.76 Dyspareunia (Not Due to a General Medical Condition)
306.51 Vaginismus (Not Due to a General Medical Condition)

SEXUAL DYSFUNCTION DUE TO A GENERAL MEDICAL CONDITION

625.8 Female Hypoactive Sexual Desire Disorder Due to . . . *[Indicate the General Medical Condition]*
608.89 Male Hypoactive Sexual Desire Disorder Due to . . . *[Indicate the General Medical Condition]*
607.84 Male Erectile Disorder Due to . . . *[Indicate the General Medical Condition]*
625.0 Female Dyspareunia Due to . . . *[Indicate the General Medical Condition]*
608.89 Male Dyspareunia Due to . . . *[Indicate the General Medical Condition]*
625.8 Other Female Sexual Dysfunction Due to . . . *[Indicate the General Medical Condition]*
608.89 Other Male Sexual Dysfunction Due to . . . *[Indicate the General Medical Condition]*
____.____ Substance-Induced Sexual Dysfunction *(refer to Substance-Related Disorders for substance-specific codes)*
Specify if: With Impaired Desire/With Impaired Arousal/With Impaired Orgasm/With Sexual Pain
Specify if: With Onset During Intoxication
302.70 Sexual Dysfunction NOS

PARAPHILIAS

302.4 Exhibitionism
302.81 Fetishism
302.89 Frotteurism
302.2 Pedophilia
Specify if: Sexually Attracted to Males/Sexually Attracted to Females/Sexually Attracted to Both
Specify if: Limited to Incest
Specify type: Exclusive Type/Nonexclusive Type
302.83 Sexual Masochism
302.84 Sexual Sadism
302.3 Transvestic Fetishism
Specify if: With Gender Dysphoria
302.82 Voyeurism
302.9 Paraphilia NOS

GENDER IDENTITY DISORDERS

302.xx Gender Identity Disorder
.6 in Children
.85 in Adolescents or Adults

Specify if: Sexually Attracted to Males/Sexually Attracted to Females/Sexually Attracted to Both/Sexually Attracted to Neither

302.6 Gender Identity Disorder NOS

302.9 Sexual Disorder NOS

EATING DISORDERS

307.1 Anorexia Nervosa
  Specify type: Restricting Type; Binge-Eating/Purging Type
307.51 Bulimia Nervosa
  Specify type: Purging Type/Nonpurging Type
307.50 Eating Disorder NOS

SLEEP DISORDERS

Primary Sleep Disorders

DYSSOMNIAS

307.42 Primary Insomnia
307.44 Primary Hypersomnia
  Specify if: Recurrent
347 Narcolepsy
780.59 Breathing-Related Sleep Disorder
307.45 Circadian Rhythm Sleep Disorder
  Specify type: Delayed Sleep Phase Type/Jet Lag Type/ Shift Work Type/Unspecified Type
307.47 Dyssomnia NOS

PARASOMNIAS

307.47 Nightmare Disorder
307.46 Sleep Terror Disorder
307.46 Sleepwalking Disorder
307.47 Parasomnia NOS

Sleep Disorders Related to Another Mental Disorder

307.42 Insomnia Related to . . . *[Indicate the Axis I or Axis II Disorder]*
307.44 Hypersomnia Related to . . . *[Indicate the Axis I or Axis II Disorder]*

Other Sleep Disorders

780.xx Sleep Disorder Due to . . . *[Indicate the General Medical Condition]*
  .52 Insomnia Type
  .54 Hypersomnia Type
  .59 Parasomnia Type
  .59 Mixed Type
_____._____ Substance-Induced Sleep Disorder *(refer to Substance-Related Disorders for substance-specific codes)*
  Specify type: Insomnia Type/Hypersomnia Type/ Parasomnia Type/Mixed Type
  Specify if: With Onset During Intoxication/With Onset During Withdrawal

IMPULSE-CONTROL DISORDERS NOT ELSEWHERE CLASSIFIED

312.34 Intermittent Explosive Disorder
312.32 Kleptomania

312.33 Pyromania
312.31 Pathological Gambling
312.39 Trichotillomania
312.30 Impulse-Control Disorder NOS

ADJUSTMENT DISORDERS

309.xx Adjustment Disorder
  .0 With Depressed Mood
  .24 With Anxiety
  .28 With Mixed Anxiety and Depressed Mood
  .3 With Disturbance of Conduct
  .4 With Mixed Disturbance of Emotions and Conduct
  .9 Unspecified
  Specify if: Acute/Chronic

PERSONALITY DISORDERS

Note: *These are coded on Axis II.*
301.0 Paranoid Personality Disorder
301.20 Schizoid Personality Disorder
301.22 Schizotypal Personality Disorder
301.7 Antisocial Personality Disorder
301.83 Borderline Personality Disorder
301.50 Histrionic Personality Disorder
301.81 Narcissistic Personality Disorder
301.82 Avoidant Personality Disorder
301.6 Dependent Personality Disorder
301.4 Obsessive–Compulsive Personality Disorder
301.9 Personality Disorder NOS

OTHER CONDITIONS THAT MAY BE A FOCUS OF CLINICAL ATTENTION

Psychological Factors Affecting Medical Condition

316 . . . *[Specified Psychological Factor] Affecting . . . [Indicate the General Medical Condition]*
Choose name based on nature of factors:
Mental Disorder Affecting Medical Condition
Psychological Symptoms Affecting Medical Condition
Personality Traits or Coping Style Affecting Medical Condition
Maladaptive Health Behaviors Affecting Medical Condition
Stress-Related Physiological Response Affecting Medical Condition
Other or Unspecified Psychological Factors Affecting Medical Condition

Medication-Induced Movement Disorders

332.1 Neuroleptic-Induced Parkinsonism
333.92 Neuroleptic Malignant Syndrome
333.7 Neuroleptic-Induced Acute Dystonia
333.99 Neuroleptic-Induced Acute Akathisia
333.82 Neuroleptic-Induced Tardive Dyskinesia
333.1 Medication-Induced Postural Tremor
333.90 Medication-Induced Movement Disorder NOS

Other Medication-Induced Disorder

995.2 Adverse Effects of Medication NOS

Relational Problems

V61.9 Relational Problem Related to a Mental Disorder or General Medical Condition

V61.20 Parent–Child Relational Problem

V61.10 Partner Relational Problem

V61.8 Sibling Relational Problem

V62.81 Relational Problem NOS

Problems Related to Abuse or Neglect

V61.21 Physical Abuse of Child
(*code 995.54 if focus of attention is on victim*)

V61.21 Sexual Abuse of Child
(*code 995.53 if focus of attention is on victim*)

V61.21 Neglect of Child
(*code 995.52 if focus of attention is on victim*)

_____._____ Physical Abuse of Adult

V61.12 (if by partner)

V62.83 (if by person other than partner) (*code 995.81 if focus of attention is on victim*)

_____._____ Sexual Abuse of Adult

V61.12 (if by partner)

V62.83 (if by person other than partner) (*code 995.83 if focus of attention is on victim*)

Additional Conditions That May Be a Focus of Clinical Attention

V15.81 Noncompliance With Treatment

V65.2 Malingering

V71.01 Adult Antisocial Behavior

V71.02 Child or Adolescent Antisocial Behavior

V62.89 Borderline Intellectual Functioning

Note: *This is coded on Axis II.*

780.9 Age-Related Cognitive Decline

V62.82 Bereavement

V62.3 Academic Problem

V62.2 Occupational Problem

313.82 Identity Problem

V62.89 Religious or Spiritual Problem

V62.4 Acculturation Problem

V62.89 Phase of Life Problem

ADDITIONAL CODES

300.9 Unspecified Mental Disorder (nonpsychotic)

V71.09 No Diagnosis or Condition on Axis I

799.9 Diagnosis or Condition Deferred on Axis I

V71.09 No Diagnosis on Axis II

799.9 Diagnosis Deferred on Axis II

MULTIAXIAL SYSTEM

Axis I Clinical Disorders

Other Conditions That May Be a Focus of Clinical Attention

Axis II Personality Disorders

Mental Retardation

Axis III General Medical Conditions

Axis IV Psychosocial and Environmental Problems

Axis V Global Assessment of Functioning

MULTIAXIAL ASSESSMENT

A multiaxial system involves an assessment on several axes, each of which refers to a different domain of information that may help the clinician plan treatment and predict outcome. There are five axes included in the DSM-IV multiaxial classification:

Axis I	Clinical Disorders
	Other Conditions That May Be a Focus of Clinical Attention
Axis II	Personality Disorders
	Mental Retardation
Axis III	General Medical Conditions
Axis IV	Psychosocial and Environmental Problems
Axis V	Global Assessment of Functioning

The use of the multiaxial system facilitates comprehensive and systematic evaluation with attention to the various mental disorders and general medical conditions, psychosocial and environmental problems, and level of functioning that might be overlooked if the focus were on assessing a single presenting problem. A multiaxial system provides a convenient format for organizing and communicating clinical information, for capturing the complexity of clinical situations, and for describing the heterogeneity of individuals presenting with the same diagnosis. In addition, the multiaxial system promotes the application of the biopsychosocial model in clinical, educational, and research settings.

The rest of this section provides a description of each of the DSM-IV axes. In some settings or situations, clinicians may prefer not to use the multiaxial system. For this reason, guidelines for reporting the results of a DSM-IV assessment without applying the formal multiaxial system are provided at the end of this section.

AXIS I: CLINICAL DISORDERS—OTHER CONDITIONS THAT MAY BE A FOCUS OF CLINICAL ATTENTION

Axis I is for reporting all the various disorders or conditions in the Classification except for the Personality Disorders and Mental Retardation (which are reported on Axis II). The major groups of disorders to be reported on Axis I are listed in the Axis I box. Also reported on Axis I are Other Conditions That May Be a Focus of Clinical Attention.

When an individual has more than one Axis I disorder, all of these should be reported. If more than one Axis I disorder is present, the principal diagnosis or the reason for the visit should be indicated by listing it first. When an individual has both an Axis I and an Axis II disorder, the principal diagnosis or the reason for visit will be assumed to be on Axis I unless the Axis II diagnosis is followed by the qualifying phrase "(Principal Diagnosis)" or "(Reason for Visit)." If no Axis I disorder is present, this should be coded as V71.09. If an Axis I diagnosis is deferred, pending the gathering of additional information, this should be coded as 799.9.

AXIS I	Clinical Disorders

Other Conditions That May Be a Focus Of Clinical Attention

Disorders Usually First Diagnosed in Infancy, Childhood, or Adolescence (*excluding Mental Retardation, which is diagnosed on Axis II*)

Delirium, Dementia, and Amnestic and Other Cognitive Disorders

Mental Disorders Due to a General Medical Condition

Substance-Related Disorders

Schizophrenia and Other Psychotic Disorders

Mood Disorders

Anxiety Disorders

Somatoform Disorders

Factitious Disorders

Dissociative Disorders

Sexual and Gender Identity Disorders

Eating Disorders

Sleep Disorders

Impulse-Control Disorders Not Elsewhere Classified

Adjustment Disorders

Other Conditions That May Be a Focus of Clinical Attention

AXIS II	Personality Disorders

Mental Retardation

Paranoid Personality Disorder	Narcissistic Personality Disorder
Schizoid Personality Disorder	Avoidant Personality Disorder
Schizotypal Personality Disorder	Dependent Personality Disorder
Antisocial Personality Disorder	Obsessive–Compulsive Personality Disorder
Borderline Personality Disorder	Personality Disorder Not Otherwise Specified
Histrionic Personality Disorder	Mental Retardation

AXIS II: PERSONALITY DISORDERS AND MENTAL RETARDATION

Axis II is for reporting Personality Disorders and Mental Retardation. It may also be used for noting prominent maladaptive personality features and defense mechanisms. The listing of Personality Disorders and Mental Retardation on a separate axis ensures that consideration will be given to the possible presence of Personality Disorders and Mental Retardation that might otherwise be overlooked when attention is directed to the usually more florid Axis I disorders. The coding of Personality Disorders on Axis II should not be taken to imply that their pathogenesis or range of appropriate treatment is fundamentally different from that for the disorders coded on Axis I. The disorders to be reported on Axis II are listed in the Axis II box.

In the common situation in which an individual has more than one Axis II diagnosis, all should be reported. When an individual has both an Axis I and an Axis II diagnosis and the Axis II diagnosis is the principal diagnosis or the reason for visit, this should be indicated by adding the qualifying phrase "(Principal Diagnosis)" or "(Reason for Visit)" after the Axis II diagnosis. If no Axis II disorder is present, this should be coded as V71.09. If an Axis II diagnosis is deferred, pending the gathering of additional information, this should be coded as 799.9.

Axis II may also be used to indicate prominent maladaptive personality features that do not meet the threshold for a Personality Disorder (in such instances, no code number should be used). The habitual use of maladaptive defense mechanisms may also be indicated on Axis II.

AXIS III: GENERAL MEDICAL CONDITIONS

Axis III is for reporting current general medical conditions that are potentially relevant to the understanding or management of the individual's mental disorder. These conditions are classified outside the "Mental Disorders" chapter of ICD-9-CM (and outside Chapter V of ICD-10). A listing of the broad categories of general medical conditions is given in the box on page 781.

As discussed in the "Introduction," the multiaxial distinction among Axis I, Axis II, and Axis III disorders does not imply that there are fundamental differences in their conceptualization, that mental disorders are unrelated to physical or biologic factors or processes, or that general medical conditions are unrelated to behavioral or psychosocial factors or processes. The purpose of distinguishing general medical conditions is to encourage thoroughness in evaluation and to enhance communication among health care providers.

General medical conditions can be related to mental disorders in a variety of ways. In some cases it is clear that the general medical condition is directly etiologic to the development or worsening of mental symptoms and that the mechanism for this effect is physiological. When a mental disorder is judged to be a direct physiological consequence of the general medical condition, a Mental Disorder Due to a General Medical Condition should be diagnosed on Axis I and the general medical condition should be recorded on both Axis I and Axis III. For example, when hypothyroidism is a direct cause of depressive symptoms, the designation on Axis I is 293.83 Mood Disorder Due to Hypothyroidism, With Depressive Features, and the hypothyroidism is listed again and coded on Axis III as 244.9.

In those instances in which the etiologic relationship between the general medical condition and the mental symptoms is insufficiently clear to warrant an Axis I diagnosis of Mental Disorder Due to a General Medical Condition, the appropriate mental disorder (e.g., Major Depressive Disorder) should be listed and coded on Axis I; the general medical condition should be coded only on Axis III.

There are other situations in which general medical conditions are recorded on Axis III because of their importance

AXIS III	**General Medical Conditions (With ICD-9-CM Codes)**

Infectious and Parasitic Diseases (001–139)

Neoplasms (140–239)

Endocrine, Nutritional, and Metabolic Diseases and Immunity Disorders (240–279)

Diseases of the Blood and Blood-Forming Organs (280–289)

Diseases of the Nervous System and Sense Organs (320–389)

Diseases of the Circulatory System (390–459)

Diseases of the Respiratory System (460–519)

Diseases of the Digestive System (520–579)

Diseases of the Genitourinary System (580–629)

Complications of Pregnancy, Childbirth, and the Puerperium (630–676)

Diseases of the Skin and Subcutaneous Tissue (680–709)

Diseases of the Musculoskeletal System and Connective Tissue (710–739)

Congenital Anomalies (740–759)

Certain Conditions Originating in the Perinatal Period (760–779)

Symptoms, Signs, and Ill-Defined Conditions (780–799)

Injury and Poisoning (800–999)

to the overall understanding or treatment of the individual with the mental disorder. An Axis I disorder may be a psychological reaction to an Axis III general medical condition (e.g., the development of 309.0 Adjustment Disorder With Depressed Mood as a reaction to the diagnosis of carcinoma of the breast). Some general medical conditions may not be directly related to the mental disorder but nonetheless have important prognostic or treatment implications (e.g., when the diagnosis on Axis I is 296.30 Major Depressive Disorder, Recurrent, and on Axis III is 427.9 Arrhythmia, the choice of pharmacotherapy is influenced by the general medical condition; or when a person with diabetes mellitus is admitted to the hospital for an exacerbation of Schizophrenia and insulin management must be monitored).

When an individual has more than one clinically relevant Axis III diagnosis, all should be reported. If no Axis III disorder is present, this should be indicated by the notation "Axis III: None." If an Axis III diagnosis is deferred, pending the gathering of additional information, this should be indicated by the notation "Axis III: Deferred."

AXIS IV: PSYCHOSOCIAL AND ENVIRONMENTAL PROBLEMS

Axis IV is for reporting psychosocial and environmental problems that may affect the diagnosis, treatment, and prognosis of mental disorders (Axes I and II). A psychosocial or environmental problem may be a negative life event, an environmental difficulty or deficiency, a familial or other interpersonal stress, an inadequacy of social support or personal resources, or other problem relating to the context in which a person's difficulties have developed. So-called positive stressors, such as job promotion, should be listed only if they constitute or lead to a problem, as when a person has difficulty adapting to the new situation. In addition to playing a role in the initiation or exacerbation of a mental disorder, psychosocial problems may also develop as a consequence of a person's psychopathology or may constitute problems that should be considered in the overall management plan.

When an individual has multiple psychosocial or environmental problems, the clinician may note as many as are judged to be relevant. In general, the clinician should note only those psychosocial and environmental problems that have been present during the year preceding the current evaluation. However, the clinician may choose to note psychosocial and environmental problems occurring prior to the previous year if these clearly contribute to the mental disorder or have become a focus of treatment—for example, previous combat experiences leading to Post-Traumatic Stress Disorder.

In practice, most psychosocial and environmental problems will be indicated on Axis IV. However, when a psychosocial or environmental problem is the primary focus of clinical attention, it should also be recorded on Axis I, with a code derived from the section "Other Conditions That May Be a Focus of Clinical Attention."

For convenience, the problems are grouped together in the following categories:

- **Problems with primary support group**—e.g., death of a family member; health problems in family; disruption of family by separation, divorce, or estrangement; removal from the home; remarriage of parent; sexual or physical abuse; parental overprotection; neglect of child; inadequate discipline; discord with siblings; birth of a sibling
- **Problems related to the social environment**—e.g., death or loss of friend; inadequate social support; living alone; difficulty with acculturation; discrimination; adjustment of life-cycle transition (such as retirement)
- **Educational problems**—e.g., illiteracy; academic problems; discord with teachers or classmates; inadequate school environment
- **Occupational problems**—e.g., unemployment; threat of job loss; stressful work schedule; difficult work conditions; job dissatisfaction; job change; discord with boss or coworkers
- **Housing problems**—e.g., homelessness; inadequate housing; unsafe neighborhood; discord with neighbors or landlord
- **Economic problems**—e.g., extreme poverty; inadequate finances; insufficient welfare support
- **Problems with access to health care services**—e.g., inadequate health care services; transportation to health care facilities unavailable; inadequate health insurance
- **Problems related to interaction with the legal system/ crime**—e.g., arrest; incarceration; litigation; victim of crime
- **Other psychosocial and environmental problems**— e.g., exposure to disasters, war, other hostilities; discord with nonfamily caregivers such as counselor, social worker, or physician; unavailability of social service agencies

AXIS IV	Psychosocial and Environmental Problems

Problems with Primary Support Group
Problems Related to the Social Environment
Educational Problems
Occupational Problems
Housing Problems
Economic Problems
Problems with Access to Health Care Services
Problems Related to Interaction with the Legal System/Crime
Other Psychosocial and Environmental Problems

When using the Multiaxial Evaluation Report Form, the clinician should identify the relevant categories of psychosocial and environmental problems and indicate the specific factors involved. If a recording form with a checklist of problem categories is not used, the clinician may simply list the specific problems on Axis IV.

AXIS V: GLOBAL ASSESSMENT OF FUNCTIONING

Axis V is for reporting the clinician's judgment of the individual's overall level of functioning. This information is useful in planning treatment and measuring its impact, and in predicting outcome.

The reporting of overall functioning on Axis V can be done using the Global Assessment of Functioning (GAF) Scale. The GAF Scale may be particularly useful in tracking the clinical progress of individuals in global terms, using a single measure. The GAF Scale is to be rated with respect only to psychological, social, and occupational functioning. The instructions specify, "Do not include impairment in functioning due to physical (or environmental) limitations."

The GAF scale is divided into 10 ranges of functioning. Making a GAF rating involves picking a single value that best reflects the individual's overall level of functioning. The description of each 10-point range in the GAF scale has two components: The first part covers symptom severity, and the second part covers functioning. The GAF rating is within a particular decile if **either** the symptom severity **or** the level of functioning falls within the range. For example, the first part of the range 41–50 describes "serious symptoms (e.g., suicidal ideation, severe obsessional rituals, frequent shoplifting)" and the second part includes "any serious impairment in social, occupational, or school functioning (e.g., no friends, unable to keep a job)." It should be noted that in situations where the individual's symptom severity and level of functioning are discordant, the final GAF rating always reflects the worse of the two. For example, the GAF rating for an individual who is a significant danger to self but is otherwise functioning well would be below 20. Similarly, the GAF rating for an individual with minimal psychological symptomatology but significant impairment in functioning (e.g., an individual whose excessive preoccupation with substance use has resulted in loss of job and friends but no other psychopathology) would be 40 or lower.

In most instances, ratings on the GAF Scale should be for the current period (i.e., the level of functioning at the time of the evaluation) because ratings of current functioning will generally reflect the need for treatment or care. In order to account for day-to-day variability in functioning, the GAF rating for the "current period" is sometimes operationalized as the lowest level of functioning for the past week. In some settings, it may be useful to note the GAF Scale rating both at time of admission and at time of discharge. The GAF Scale may also be rated for other time periods (e.g., the highest level of functioning for at least a few months during the past year). The GAF Scale is reported on Axis V as follows: "GAF =," followed by the GAF rating from 0 to 100, followed by the time period reflected by the rating in parentheses—for example, "(current)," "(highest level in past year)," "(at discharge)."

In order to ensure that no elements of the GAF Scale are overlooked when a GAF rating is being made, the following method for determining a GAF rating may be applied:

STEP 1: Starting at the top level, evaluate each range by asking "is either the individual's symptom severity OR level of functioning worse than what is indicated in the range description?"

STEP 2: Keep moving down the scale until the range that best matches the individual's symptom severity OR the level of functioning is reached, **whichever is worse.**

STEP 3: Look at the next lower range as a double-check against having stopped prematurely. This range should be too severe on **both** symptom severity **and** level of functioning. If it is, the appropriate range has been reached (continue with step 4). If not, go back to step 2 and continue moving down the scale.

STEP 4: To determine the specific GAF rating within the selected 10-point range, consider whether the individual is functioning at the higher or lower end of the 10-point range. For example, consider an individual who hears voices that do not influence his behavior (e.g., someone with long-standing Schizophrenia who accepts his hallucinations as part of his illness). If the voices occur relatively infrequently (once a week or less), a rating of 39 or 40 might be most appropriate. In contrast, if the individual hears voices almost continuously, a rating of 31 or 32 would be more appropriate.

In some settings, it may be useful to assess social and occupational disability and to track progress in rehabilitation independent of the severity of the psychological symptoms.

GLOBAL ASSESSMENT OF FUNCTIONING (GAF) SCALE

Consider psychological, social, and occupational functioning on a hypothetical continuum of mental health illness. Do not include impairment in functioning due to physical (or environmental) limitations.

Global Assessment of Functioning (GAF) Scale

Code (Note: Use intermediate codes when appropriate, e.g., 45, 68, 72.)

100/91	Superior functioning in a wide range of activities, life's problems never seem to get out of hand, is sought out by others because of his or her many positive qualities. No symptoms.
90/81	Absent or minimal symptoms (e.g., mild anxiety before an exam), good functioning in all areas, interested and involved in a wide range of activities, socially effective, generally satisfied with life, no more than everyday problems or concerns (e.g., an occasional argument with family members).
80/71	If symptoms are present, they are transient and expectable reactions to psychosocial stressors (e.g., difficulty concentrating after family argument), no more than slight impairment in social, occupational, or school functioning (e.g., temporarily falling behind in schoolwork).
70/61	Some mild symptoms (e.g., depressed mood and mild insomnia) OR some difficulty in social, occupational, or school functioning (e.g., occasional truancy, or theft within the household), but generally functioning pretty well, has some meaningful interpersonal relationships.
60/51	Moderate symptoms (e.g., flat affect and circumstantial speech, occasional panic attacks) OR moderate difficulty in social, occupational, or school functioning (e.g., few friends, conflicts with peers or coworkers).
50/41	Serious symptoms (e.g., suicidal ideation; severe obsessional rituals, frequent shoplifting) OR any serious impairment in social, occupational, or school functioning (e.g., no friends, unable to keep a job).
40/31	Some impairment in reality testing or communication (e.g., speech is at times illogical, obscure, or irrelevant) OR major impairment in several areas, such as work or school, family relations, judgment, thinking, or mood (e.g., depressed man avoids friends, neglects family, and is unable to work; child frequently beats up younger children, is defiant at home, and is failing at school).
30/21	Behavior is considerably influenced by delusions or hallucinations OR serious impairment in communication or judgment (e.g., sometimes incoherent, acts grossly inappropriately, suicidal preoccupation) OR inability to function in almost all areas (e.g., stays in bed all day; no job, home, or friends).
20/11	Some danger of hurting self or others (e.g., suicide attempts without clear expectation of death; frequently violent; manic excitement) OR occasionally fails to maintain minimal personal hygiene (e.g., smears feces) OR gross impairment in communication (e.g., largely incoherent or mute).
10/1	Persistent danger of severely hurting self or others (e.g., recurrent violence) OR persistent inability to maintain minimal personal hygiene OR serious suicidal act with clear expectation of death.
0	Inadequate information.

The rating of overall psychological functioning on a scale of 0–100 was operationalized by Luborsky in the Health-Sickness Rating Scale (Luborsky, L. [1962]. "Clinicians' judgments of mental health." *Archives of General Psychiatry, 7,* 407–417). Endicott and colleagues developed a revision of the Health-Sickness Rating Scale called the Global Assessment Scale (GAS) (Endicott, J., Spitzer, R. L., Fleiss, J. L., & Cohen, J. [1976]. "The Global Assessment Scale: A procedure for measuring overall severity of psychiatric disturbance." *Archives of General Psychiatry, 33,* 766–771). A modified version of the GAS was included in DSM-ILL-R as the Global Assessment of Functioning (GAF) Scale.

INDEX

Page numbers followed by *f* indicate figures and those followed by *t* indicate tables, boxes, or special features.